Textbook of Psychiatry

Textbook of Psychiatry

Nilesh B. Shah
Professor and HOD
Department of Psychiatry
LTMMC & GH
Sion
Mumbai 400022

Avinash Desousa
Research Associate and Consultant Psychiatrist
Department of Psychiatry
LTMMC & GH
Sion
Mumbai 400022

Sagar Karia
Assistant Professor
Department of Psychiatry
LTMMC & GH
Sion
Mumbai 400022

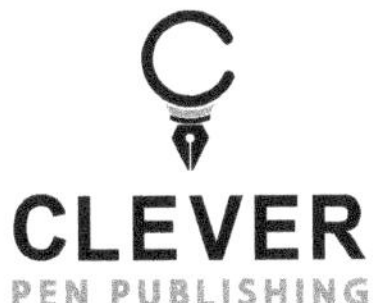

First Edition: 2023

Published by:

Clever Pen Publishing
D-2 Neelkanth Business Park Co-op. Premises Society Ltd.
Nathani Road
Vidyavihar (West)
Mumbai 400086
Mob.: 09867214519

Email: cleverpen9@gmail.com

ISBN 978-93-92215-38-4

Printed & Bound in India

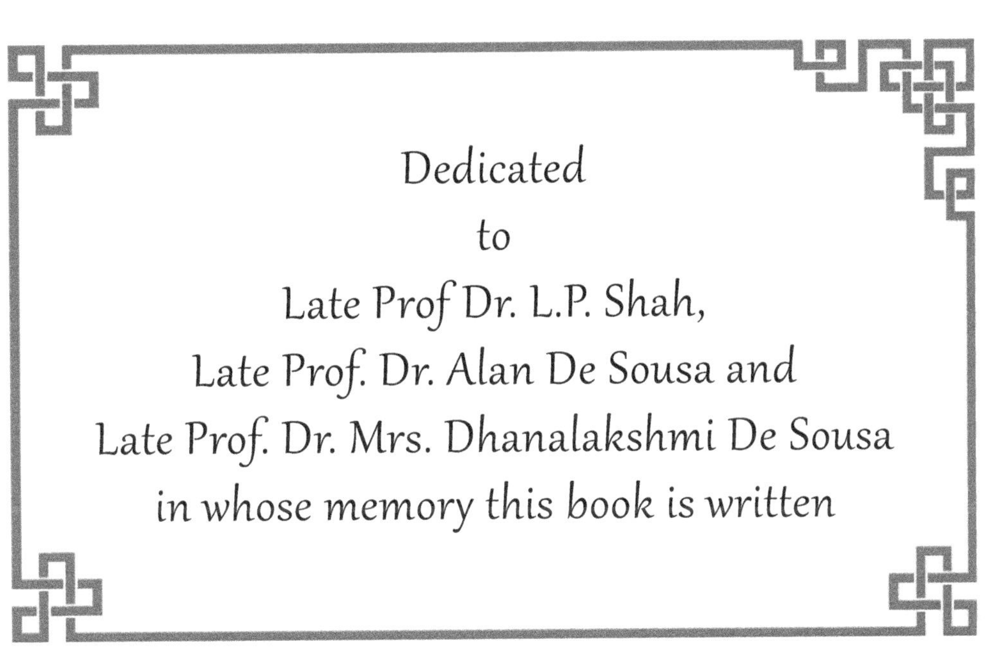

Dedicated
to
Late Prof Dr. L.P. Shah,
Late Prof. Dr. Alan De Sousa and
Late Prof. Dr. Mrs. Dhanalakshmi De Sousa
in whose memory this book is written

PREFACE

Psychiatry is an expanding specialty in medicine. With the advent of recent advances in Psychiatry, we have come out with this textbook that is a basic book on psychiatry written keeping in mind the needs of medical undergraduate students, nursing students, occupational and physiotherapy students as well as students of social work and psychology. The book is also intended for general practitioners that aim to get grip on the subject of Psychiatry. The book has been written keeping in mind the needs of readers that may have little or no idea about Psychiatry as subject.

We hope that readers welcome this contribution by us with enthusiasm and happiness.

Nilesh B. Shah
Avinash De Sousa
Sagar Karia

ACKNOWLEDGMENTS

Thankful to all the authors that contributed chapters to the textbook and to all students that have inspired us to write this book

I am grateful to my publisher, **Mr. Rajesh Bhalani** and **Mrs. Harsha Shah** from **Clever Pen Publishing** along with the DTP typesetter for making persistent efforts to complete the book in time.

Nilesh B. Shah
Avinash Desousa
Sagar Karia

CO-AUTHORS AND EDITORS

Akanksha Sharma
Assistant Professor
Department of Psychiatry
Dr Ram Manohar Lohia Institute of Medical Sciences and Hospital
Lucknow

Akshay Chordia
Director and Consultant
Anandwan Wellness Centre
Nalasopara

Alka A. Subramanyam
Associate Professor
Department of Psychiatry
TNMC & BYL Nair Ch. Hospital
Mumbai

Ami Pawar
Assistant Professor
Department of Psychiatry
H.B.T. Medical College &
Dr. R.N. Cooper Hospital,
Mumbai

Amit Singh
Assistant Professor
Department of Psychiatry
King George Medical University
Lucknow

Amulya Koneru
Junior Consultant Psychiatrist
Asha Hospital
Hyderabad

Anil Dokhale
Senior Resident Doctor
Department of Psychiatry
Lokmanya Tilak Municipal Medical College & General Hospital,
Mumbai

Anup Subhash Bharati
Professor
Department of Psychiatry
MVPs Dr Vasantrao Pawar Medical College and Hospital
Nashik

Aparna Ramakrishnan
Assistant Professor
Department of Psychiatry
D.Y. Patil Medical College and Hospital
Navi Mumbai

Astik Mane
Assistant Professor
Department of Psychiatry
H.B.T. Medical College &
Dr. R.N. Cooper Hospital
Mumbai

Atul Ambekar
Professor
National Drug Dependence Treatment Centre
All India Institute of Medical Sciences
New Delhi

Avinash De Sousa
Consultant Psychiatrist & Founder
Desousa Foundation
Research Associate
Department of Psychiatry
Lokmanya Tilak Municipal Medical College & General Hospital
Mumbai

Bindoo S. Jadhav
Professor and Head
Department of Psychiatry
K.J. Somaiya Medical College, Hospital and Research Centre
Mumbai

Chetan Vispute
Assistant Professor
Department of Psychiatry
D.Y. Patil Medical College & Hospital
Navi Mumbai

Chethana Kishore
Department of Psychiatry
NIMHANS
Bangalore

Cicilia Chettiar
Assistant Professor and Head
Department of Psychology
Maniben Nanavati Women's College
Mumbai

Damodharan Dinakaran
Assistant Professor
Department of Psychiatry
NIMHANS
Bangalore

Delnaz Palsetia
Ex-Assistant Professor
Department of Psychiatry
Lokmanya Tilak Municipal Medical
College & General Hospital
Mumbai

Devakshi Dua
Former Senior Resident
Department of Psychiatry
PGIMER
Chandigarh

Dhanshree Waghmare
Psycholgist – Re-New-You &
Discover Yourself
PGT Psychology and Sociology
The Millennium School Surat

Dhruv Parmar
Consultant Psychiatrist, Sexologist &
De-addiction Specialist
Neurospychiatric Care Hospital
Valsad
Gujarat

Dinesh Saroj
Developmental Behavioral Pediatrician
Fellowship in Learning Disability &
Neurodevelopmental Pediatrics
Sion Hospital
Mumbai

Disha Parikh
Consultant Psychiatrist
The Beautiful Mind
Specialty Psychiatry Clinic
Pune

Elvin Lukose
Assistant Professor
Department of Psychiatry
Seth G.S. Medical College &
K.E.M. Hospital
Parel
Mumbai

Fiona Mhapatrao
Professor and Head
Department of Psychiatry
D.Y. Patil Medical College
Navi Mumbai

G. Prasad Rao
Director
Schizophrenia & Psychopharmacology
Asha Hospital
Hyderabad

Ganesan Venkatasubramanian
Professor
Department of Psychiatry
NIMHANS
Bangalore

Harshal Sathe
Assistant Professor
Department of Psychiatry
MGIMS Sevagram
Wardha

Havovi Hyderabadwalla
Co-Founder – Mind Mandala
Clinical Psychologist
Forensic Psychologist
Private Practice
Mumbai

Heena Merchant Pandit
Associate Professor
Department of Psychiatry
Lokmanya Tilak Municipal Medical
College & General Hospital
Mumbai

Henal R. Shah
Professor
Department of Psychiatry
TNMC and BYL Nair Ch. Hospital
Mumbai

Heta N. Shah
Counseling Psychologist
Private Practice
Mumbai

Hrishikesh Nachane
Specialty Doctor,
CAMHS Secure Services
St Andrew's Healthcare
Northampton
UK

Jagadisha Thirthalli
Professor
Department of Psychiatry
NIMHANS
Bangalore

Jahnavi Kedare
Associate Professor
Department of Psychiatry
TNMC and BYL Nair Ch. Hospital
Mumbai

Janardhanan C. Narayanaswamy
Professor
Department of Psychiatry
NIMHANS
Bangalore

Janki Mehta
Co-Founder – Mind Mandala
Counseling Psychologist
Private Practice
Mumbai

Jitender Jakhar
Consultant Psychiatrist
Department of Mental Health and
Behavioral Science
Fortis Hospital
New Delhi

Kalpana Pawar
Ex – Assistant Professor
Department of Psychiatry
TNMC and BYL Nair Ch. Hospital
Mumbai

Karishma Rupani
Assistant Professor
Department of Psychiatry
Seth GS Medical College & K.E.M.
Hospital
Mumbai

Kirti Yeshwant Tandel
Consultant Psychiatrist
VIBHAS Hospital &
Manasparsh Clinic
Virar

Krishnapriya Murlimanohar
Senior Resident Doctor
Department of Psychiatry
HBT Medical College &
RN Cooper Hospital
Mumbai

Maithili Umate
Associate Professor
Department of Psychiatry
Grant Govt. Medical College
Mumbai

Manasa Ram
Consultant Psychiatrist & Head
Indlas Child Guidance Clinics
Vizag

Manjiri Desphpande Shenoy
Consultant Psychiatrist & Head
Indla Child Guidance Clinics
Mumbai

Mansi Somaiya
Assistant Professor
Department of Psychiatry
TNMC and BYL Nair Ch. Hospital
Mumbai

Nahid Dave
Consultant Psychiatrist
Mindfulness Trainer
Private Practice
Navi Mumbai

Navoneela Bardhan
Assistant Professor
Department of Psychiatry
K.J. Somaiya Medical College, Hospital and Research Centre
Mumbai

Neena Sawant
Professor and Unit Head
Department of Psychiatry
Seth GS Medical College and K.E.M. Hospital
Mumbai

Nilesh Shah
Professor and Head
Department of Psychiatry
Lokmanya Tilak Municipal Medical College and General Hospital
Mumbai

Nitin B. Raut
Specialist (Psychiatry)
Lady Hardinge Medical College
New Delhi

Omkar Nayak
Senior Resident Doctor
Department of Psychiatry
Lokmanya Tilak Municipal Medical College & General Hospital
Mumbai

Parag Shah
Professor and Head
Department of Psychiatry
SMIMER
Surat

Parmod Kumar
Consultant Psychiatrist
Dr. Parmod's Clinic
Chandigarh

Pavitra KS
Professor and Head
Department of Psychiatry
BMCH
Chitradurga

Poornima Khadanga
Assistant Professor
Department of Psychiatry
Grant Govt Medical College
Mumbai

Poornima Rao
Registrar
North Western Mental Health Service
Melbourne
Victoria, Australia

Pragya Lodha
Clinical Psychologist & Research Associate
Desousa Foundation
Mumbai

Pranav U. Pohane
Consultant Psychiatrist
ESIS Hospital &
New Era Hospital
Nagpur

Prashant Chaudhari
Consultant Psychiatrist
Bandra Care Clinic &
Shivaji Park Care Clinic
Mumbai

Preeti Sinha
Department of Psychiatry
NIMHANS
Bangalore

Prerna Khar
Consultant Psychiatrist
Mind Temple Clinic &
Rotary Service Centre
Mumbai

Priyanka Anup Bharati
Director
Sarathya Rehabilitation Centre
Nashik

Radhika MS
Post Doctoral Fellow
Child Psychiatry
VIMHANS
Vijaywada

Ravi Gupta
Addl. Professor
Department of Psychiatry
AIIMS
Rishikesh

Riteeka Deshpande
Fellow Psychiatry
Top End Mental Health Service
NT, Australia

Rizwana Qureshi
Addl. Professor
National Drug Dependence Treatment
Centre, AIIMS
New Delhi

Ruksheda Syeda
Consultant Psychiatrist
Trellis Family Centre
Mumbai

Rupali Shivalkar
Consultant Psychiatrist & Head
St. Stephen's Hospital
Delhi

Sagar Karia
Assistant Professor
Department of Psychiatry
Lokmanya Tilak Municipal Medical
College & General Hospital
Mumbai

Sandeep Grover
Professor
Department of Psychiatry
PGIMERS
Chandigarh

Sarika Dakshikar
Associate Professor
Department of Psychiatry
Grant Govt Medical College
Mumbai

Satish Suhas
Assistant Professor
Department of Psychiatry
NIMHANS
Bangalore

Sayalee Daberao
Senior Resident Doctor
Department of Psychiatry
Lokmanya Tilak Municipal Medical
College & General Hospital
Mumbai

Shalini S. Naik
Assistant Professor
Department of Psychiatry
PGIMERS
Chandigarh

Sheela Dang
Counseling Psychologist
Private Practice
Mumbai

Shipra Singh
Assistant Professor
Department of Psychiatry
Pandit BD Sharma University of Health Sciences
Rohtak

Shivani Chande
Research Associate
Desousa Foundation
Mumbai

Shubham Kamal
Visiting Research Scientist
Department of Psychiatry
Yale School of Medicine
New Haven, Connecticut
USA

Shubrata Kalmane
Professor
Department of Psychiatry
Subbaiah Institute of Medical Sciences
Shimoga

Shyam Sundar Arumugham
Associate Professor
Department of Psychiatry
NIMHANS
Bangalore

Sriramya Vemulakonda
Research Officer – Psychiatry
Asha Hospital
Hyderabad

Sushant Sarang
Associate Professor
Department of Occupational Therapy
Seth GS Medical College &
KEM Hospital
Mumbai

Suyog Jaiswal
Associate Professor
Department of Psychiatry
AIIMS
Nagpur

Swati Chaudhary
Assistant Professor
Department of Psychiatry
AIIMS
Jodhpur

Swati Shelke
Assistant Professor
Department of Psychiatry
TNMC and BYL Nair Ch. Hospital
Mumbai

Tejal Doshi
Department of Psychiatry
Lokmanya Tilak Municipal Medical
College and Hospital
Mumbai

Tejesvi Dave
Clinical Psychologist
Department of Psychiatry
Lokmanya Tilak Municipal Medical
College & Hospital
Mumbai

Varun Mehta
Associate Professor
Department of Psychiatry
Central Institute of Psychiatry
Ranchi

Veena Kumar
Assistant Professor and Head
Department of Psychology
KC College & HSNC University
Mumbai

Vijay Krishnan
Assistant Professor
Department of Psychiatry
AIIMS
Rishikesh

Vinyas Nisarga
Assistant Professor
Department of Psychiatry
KJ Somaiya Medical College, Hospital
and Research Centre
Mumbai

Vishal Indla
Director
Indlas VIMHANS and Indlas Child
Guidance Centres
Vijaywada

Yusuf Matcheswalla
Honorary Professor
Department of Psychiatry
Grant Govt Medical College &
GT Hospital
Mumbai

CONTENTS

Ch No.	Title	Author	Pg. No.
1.	Growth of Psychiatry as a Medical Specialty	*Krishnapriya Murlimanohar* *Prashant Chaudhari*	1
2.	Normality and Mental Health	*Pragya Lodha* *Avinash De Sousa*	7
3.	History Taking in Psychiatry	*Delnaz Palsetia* *Avinash De Sousa*	11
4.	Common Signs and Symptoms in Psychiatry	*Krishnapriya Murlimanohar* *Prashant Chaudhari*	15
5.	Basics of Mental Status Examination	*Elvin Lukose* *Heena Merchant Pandit*	21
6.	Communication, Empathy and Rapport Building	*Pragya Lodha* *Nilesh Shah*	33
7.	Essential Investigations in Patients having Psychiatric Disorders	*Elvin Lukose* *Heena Merchant Pandit*	38
8.	Basics of EEG for Undergraduates	*Suyog Jaiswal* *Pranav U. Pohane*	48
9.	Biopsychosocial Model of Mental Illness	*Pragya Lodha* *Avinash De Sousa*	55
10.	Transference and Countertransference	*Shivani Chande* *Avinash De Sousa*	59
11.	Neuroanatomy Review	*Jitender Jakhar* *Satish Suhas* *Shailini S. Naik*	70
12.	Basics of Neurotransmitters	*Ami Pawar* *Astik Mane*	82
13.	Schizophrenia and Related Psychotic Disorders	*Damodharan Dinakaran* *Ganesan Venkatasubramanian*	101
14.	Depression	*Neena Sawant*	113
15.	Bipolar Disorder	*Pragya Lodha* *Avinash De Sousa*	121
16.	Anxiety Disorders	*Jahnavi Kedare* *Hrishikesh Nachane*	127

Ch No.	Title	Author	Pg. No.
17.	Obsessive Compulsive and Related Disorders	*Karishma Rupani* *Avinash De Sousa*	143
18.	Stress and Trauma Related Disorders	*Mansi Somaiya* *Alka A. Subramanyam* *Henal R. Shah*	154
19.	Substance Use Disorders	*Atul Ambekar* *Amit Singh* *Rizwana Qureshi*	169
20.	Basics in Psychosomatic Medicine	*Elvin Lukose* *Heena Merchant Pandit*	187
21.	Personality Disorders	*Chetan Vispute*	200
22.	Psychocutaneous Disorders	*Sayalee Daberao* *Avinash De Sousa*	209
23.	Eating Disorders	*Reetika Dikshit* *Avinash De Sousa*	215
24.	Factitious Disorder	*Nahid Dave*	223
25.	Sexual Disorders	*Parag Shah*	228
26.	Gender Identity Disorder	*Sagar Karia* *Tejesvi Dave*	244
27.	Paraphilias	*Sagar Karia* *Tejesvi Dave*	252
28.	Psychiatric Aspects in LGBTQ+ Populations	*Pragya Lodha* *Avinash De Sousa*	256
29.	Sleep Disorders – an overview	*Vijay Krishnan* *Ravi Gupta*	262
30.	Overview of Child Psychiatric Disorders	*Vishal Indla* *Radhika M.S.* *Manjiri Deshpande* *V. Manasa Ram*	276
31.	Autism Spectrum Disorders	*Manjiri Deshpande Shenoy* *V. Manasa Ram* *Vishal Indla*	297
32.	Intellectual Disability	*Kalpana Pawar* *Henal Shah*	306
33.	Learning Disability	*Sheela Dang* *Avinash De Sousa*	324

Ch No.	Title	Author	Pg. No.
34.	Role of Parents and Teachers in Prevention of Child Abuse	*Yusuf Matcheswalla* *Avinash De Sousa*	332
35.	Child Sexual Abuse	*Tejal Doshi* *Avinash De Sousa*	342
36.	Fussy Infants and Temper Tantrums	*Dinesh Saroj*	377
37.	Organic Mental Disorders	*G. Prasad Rao* *Amulya Koneru* *Sriramya Vemulakonda*	385
38.	Delirium	*Sandeep Grover*	397
39.	Dementia	*Sandeep Grover* *Swati Chaudhari*	407
40.	Geriatric Psychiatry	*Alka A. Subramanyam* *Nitin. B. Raut* *Shipra Singh*	425
41.	Suicide, Deliberate Self Harm (DSH) & Non-Suicidal Self Injury (NSSI)	*Alka A. Subramanyam* *Shipra Singh*	446
42.	Psychiatric Emergencies	*Harshal Sathe*	459
43.	Psychopharmacology	*Akshay Chordia*	471
44.	Electroconvulsive Therapy and Brain Stimulation Therapies for Psychiatric Conditions	*Shalini Naik* *Preeti Sinha* *Jagadisha Thirthalli*	491
45.	Surgeries for Psychiatric Conditions: a brief overview	*Chetana Kishore* *Janardhanan* *C. Narayanaswamy* *Shyam Sundar Arumugham*	508
46.	Rehabilitation in Psychiatry	*Kirti Yeshwant Tandel*	514
47.	National Mental Health Programme	*Delnaz Palsetia* *Sagar Karia*	530
48.	Ethics in Psychiatry	*Anup Subhash Bharati*	536
49.	Overview of Forensic Psychiatry	*Prerna Khar* *Disha Parikh*	539
50.	Criminal Responsibility and Mental Illness	*Sagar Karia*	556
51.	Family Psychoeducation in Psychiatry	*Anil Dokhale* *Omkar Nayak* *Sushma Sonavane*	559

Ch No.	Title	Author	Pg. No.
52.	Overview of Psychotherapy and the Psychotherapeutic Process	*Janki Mehta* *Avinash De Sousa*	563
53.	Psychology - Basics	*Pragya Lodha* *Avinash De Sousa*	573
54.	Cognitive Behaviour Therapy (CBT) & Rational Emotive Behaviour Therapy (REBT)	*Heta N. Shah*	576
55.	Family Therapy – an overview of key constructs	*Avinash De Sousa* *Nilesh Shah*	578
56.	Behaviour Therapy	*Sushma Sonavane* *Avinash De Sousa*	593
57.	Psychiatric Aspects of TB and HIV	*Maithili Umate* *Varun Mehta*	599
58.	Psychiatric Aspects of Epilepsy	*Sarika Dakshikar* *Poornima Rao* *Poornima Khadanga*	608
59.	Neuropsychiatric Aspects of Headache and Migraine	*Bindoo S. Jadhav* *Navoneela Bardhan*	618
60.	Role of Psychiatric Social Worker in Mental Health	*Priyanka Anup Bharati*	633
61.	Rape – Psychiatric Aspects	*Havovi Hyderabadwalla* *Avinash De Sousa*	636
62.	Occupational Therapy in Psychiatry – an overview	*Sushant Sarang*	642
63.	Psychiatric Disorders in Pregnancy and related to Menstruation and Menopause	*Ruksheda Syeda* *Rupali Shivalkar*	657
64.	Consultation Liaison Psychiatry	*Sandeep Grover* *Devakshi Dua*	666
65.	Disaster Psychiatry	*Fiona Mhapatrao* *Aparna Ramakrishnan*	672
66.	Transcultural Psychiatry	*Pavitra KS* *Shubrata Kalmane*	689
67.	Newer Psychiatric Disorders	*Prerna Khar* *Vinyas Nisarga* *Swati Shelke*	701

Ch No.	Title	Author	Pg. No.
68.	Mental Health	*Pragya Lodha* *Avinash De Sousa*	713
69.	Stress – its nature and management	*Nahid Dave*	726
70.	Psychology of Learning and Memory	*Veena Kumar*	733
71.	Psychology of Motivation	*Dhruv Parmar* *Avinash De Sousa*	747
72.	Psychology of Emotions	*Dhanashree Waghmare* *Avinash De Sousa*	754
73.	Psychology of Adolescence	*Shivani Chande* *Avinash De Sousa*	760
74.	Parenting - Basics	*Avinash De Sousa* *Sushma Sonavane*	767
75.	Theories of Psychosexual Development	*Avinash De Sousa* *Sushma Sonavane*	774
76.	Anger Management	*Avinash De Sousa* *Pragya Lodha*	781
77.	Parenting – Past, Present and Future	*Cicilia Chettiar*	786
78.	Enuresis	*Sagar Karia* *Avinash De Sousa*	795
79.	Gaming Disorder	*Parmod Kumar* *Shubham Kamal*	805
Index			814

Growth of Psychiatry as a Medical Specialty

1

Krishnapriya Murlimanohar • Prashant Chaudhari

The history of psychiatry as a medical specialty has to be distinguished from the history of psychiatric medical knowledge which began in ancient Greece with the birth of medicine as a science. For more than 2000 years, only physicians observed and treated mental illnesses, and institutions were created in which the patients which were then referred to as 'lunatics' and the 'insane' were received.[1]

History of Psychiatry as a medical profession parallels history of growth of medicine in terms of moving ahead from faith healing to evidence based scientific inquiry. In his book on epilepsy, *On the Sacred Disease,* Hippocrates (460 to 377 BC) attacked the prevailing belief that those afflicted with epilepsy were possessed by gods or goddesses.

Despite this initial view, throughout most of human history, epilepsy constituted demonic possession or the accumulation of bad humours, and attempts at exorcism involved trephination, cautery of the back of the skull, diuretics, emetics, bloodletting, purging, sweating, and even intercourse to release sperm. In the 18th century, the first so-called scientific treatise on epilepsy since ancient times attributed seizures to masturbation. By happenstance, bromides, which were introduced to diminish libido and masturbation, proved to be the first successful antiepileptic medication. With the development of effective antiepileptic drugs and the introduction of EEG, physicians have come full circle to Hippocrates' belief that epilepsy is rooted in organic brain disease. Similarly the difference between organic brain disease vs Psychiatric disease is null and void now that we understand the brain as the seat of behavioral diseases and need to look inward to understand the pathogenesis than only outward. And if the brain is the principal organ of psychiatry, then an understanding of brain science is the starting point for a comprehensive knowledge of the field.

Although as early as in 1667, Thomas Willis, one of the fathers of neuroscience, described in detail the anatomy of the brain and nervous system. He developed theories relating to neurological explanations for psychiatric illnesses, it was not until middle of the eighteenth century that 'some degree of specialization occurred [in England] among respectable physicians' when the monopoly of Bethlem was broken and new mental asylums, such as St Luke's were opened. But the narrative still remained the same as 2 millennia before to institutionalize the mentally ill.[2]

The deinstitutionalization of the mentally ill represents an important set of changes in the provision of mental health services which began with the advent of psychopharmacological agents such as Chlorpromazine and for the first time in history community integration of severely mentally ill was possible in 1960s.[3]

From then in 1999 — fluoxetine became the third best-selling prescription drug in America.

This drug was approved for release in 1987, and its impact on the treatment of depression was extraordinary. Today, fluoxetine is used for the treatment of major depressive disorder and OCD worldwide.

Electroconvulsive therapy (ECT), which is among the oldest and most controversial treatments in the field of psychiatry is more than 80 year old now. It is one of the few lifesaving modalities in Psychiatry considering dramatic improvements in suicidality, resistant Psychosis and affective ailments, catatonia and peripartum mental illnesses. The effectiveness of these modalities having been tested against placebo in various studies in last century attests to the fact that Psychiatry is not just about talking someone out of the illness, but these are actual mental and behavioral diseases which require systematic identification, classification and categorization for targeted interventions.[4]

The question of the identity of psychiatry as a medical profession has been the subject of much discussion in this first decade of the new century. The question that advances in neurosciences such as electroencephalography, functional MRI, PET scans and others are trying to answer. It has been found that advancement in neurobiology takes the centre stage at the background of ongoing discussion about position of Psychiatry as a medical speciality. Psychiatry seems to be well on its way to achieving this integration and successfully facing the challenges from inside and outside as an integral part of medicine in the 21st century provided Psychiatrists actively face these challenges head on.[5]

In our quest to assume the status as a medical speciality, we also have come up with classification of diverse symptoms into syndromic clusters in DSM and ICD which was probably pounced on too hard for administrative reasons than clinical ones to the point that these categorization merely serves as guidelines to stroll through the unknown tributaries of the brain. Some also believe that this lead to death of phenomenological inquiry in the field of Psychiatry.[6] Whilst the detailed phenomenological inquiry taking Bio-Psycho-Social variations into account is what sets a psychiatrist apart across medical specialities.

It is also important to acknowledge that before the DSM, the field was disjointed. The publication of the first American diagnostic manual, the precursor of the DSM, mirrored society's interest in organized record keeping and prevention rather than treatment of mental illness. DSM thus represents the current status of the field-not only with regard to science but also reflecting the place of global Psychiatry in medicine today.[7]

The broad range of affective, cognitive, and behavioral characteristics of humans arises as a consequence of specific patterns of activation in networks of neurons that are distributed across the central nervous system (CNS). These patterns of activation are mediated by the connections among specific brain structures. This network model has been used to further research in Psychiatry.[8]

A novel approach in evolution since 1990 is Cognitive neuropsychiatry which represents a systematic and theoretically driven approach to explain clinical psychopathologies in terms of deficits to normal cognitive mechanisms.[9]

The term epigenetics is used to describe "changes in gene expression that lead to predictable, stable, and possibly heritable alterations in cell function that are not due to changes in DNA sequence." This definition is particularly relevant in psychiatry where environmental factors, such as stress or substance abuse, alter the expression of genes in postmitotic neurons that are not heritable, but contribute to psychiatric pathologies such as major depression, anxiety, and addiction. Epigenetic factors are found to have been playing major role in psychopathology and hence psychopharmacology have joined hands with pharmacogenomics to trace this path.[10]

Over the past few decades, electrophysiology has contributed substantially to the understanding of normal brain functions as well as brain function deviations in psychopathological conditions. EEG methodology is exquisitely applied in perusal of current theories on the pathogenesis of psychiatric illness, no longer conceptualized as the result of a dysfunction of one or more brain regions, but as a consequence of the failure to integrate neural activity through networks engaged across multiple brain regions. Advances in electrophysiological measurement of brain function has been aided by technological advances at levels of bio-amplification, electrode sensors, and computational algorithms for signal processing and quantification.[11]

In the early 21st century, neuroscience has captured the public imagination like never before. One of the reasons was Neurocentrism. It basically presumes to explain everything in the language of neurotransmitters passing between neurons measured with functional imaging techniques.[12]

These new approaches along with the advent of dynamic imaging techniques have furthered the position of Psychiatry in being a medical subspeciality. Nonetheless, psychiatrists have a clinical, scientific, and humanistic imperative to advance their understanding of the neurobiology of psychiatric disorders and to see that this knowledge informs the clinical practice of psychiatry.[13]

The position of Psychiatry as evidence based medicine has been fairly established in last century. Now the question arises to implement the said evidence in practice. To make evidence-based practice feasible in real-life clinical practice, a number of problems need to be solved at each stage of the process.[14]

Psychiatry faces these problems on multiple levels such as Biological, Social and Psychological. Hence the implementation of Bio-Psycho-Social model in diagnostic formulation becomes imperative moving forward. There is still lot of work needed to counter the arguments of arbitrary definitions of illnesses and finding the neurobiological nidus for illnesses. A Psychiatrist has to fight this battle every day in the clinics while educating patients about what's happening to them.

Psychiatry is no longer perceived as a 'different' discipline and has successfully embraced the medical model without abandoning its biopsychosocial principles. As a matter of fact Major advances in the evolutionary explanation of behavior and emotions from the second half of the 20th century have yet to be fully applied in psychiatry.[15]

The twentieth century has witnessed significant improvements in general health in most countries.

Although a number of key public health threats have been eradicated or brought under control under the leadership of WHO, priority was given to communicable diseases in view of their inherent potential to spreading. At the present time, a focus on non-communicable diseases and mental health would now appear as the next natural step in public health priorities.[16]

Increasing awareness about mental health and government support has led to improvement in perception of general public as these ailments as something to be treated and taken seriously. New mental health care law aims to give rights of mental health in hands of public with its share of criticisms.[17]

It remains the fact though that science has conceptualized the building blocks of nuclear fission more readily than the building blocks of mental health. In these years the implicit assumption that mental health is absence of mental illness is challenged and there is increasing efforts to define normality in mental health.[18]

Culture influences the process of diagnosis in many ways: the experience and expression of symptoms, signs, and behaviors that are criteria for diagnosis; the configuration of symptoms into culturally distinctive syndromes; the stigma attached to specific symptoms and syndromes that may prevent their clinical reporting and influence the subsequent course of illness; and the conduct of the clinical encounter through which diagnosis is made. This has been addressed with cultural formulation in DSM.

Psychiatric diseases, do not follow simple Mendelian inheritance patterns but rather are examples of etiologically complex traits. Etiological complexity may be due to many factors, including incomplete penetrance (expression of the phenotype in only some of the individuals carrying the disease-related genotype), the presence of phenocopies (forms of the disease that are not caused by genetic factors), locust erogeneity (different genes associated with the same disease in different families or populations), or polygenic inheritance (risk for disease increases only if susceptibility variants at multiple genes act in concert). Mapping a complex disorder involves several component steps, including definition of the phenotype to be studied, epidemiological studies to determine the evidence for genetic transmission of that phenotype, choice of an informative study population, and determination of the appropriate experimental and statistical approaches.[19]

Interactions between the immune system and the central nervous system play a critical role in the maintenance of bodily homeostasis and the development of diseases, including psychiatric disease. The relative role of cytokines and their signalling pathways in the various psychiatric diseases is an area of active investigation, as is the role of infectious and autoimmune diseases in the pathophysiology of psychiatric disorders. Taken together, these findings highlight the importance of interdisciplinary efforts involving the neurosciences and immunology for gaining new insights into the etiology of psychiatric disorders. It has been known for years that psychosocial factors can mitigate or worsen the effects of stress, not only on immune functioning but also on the long-term outcomes of medical conditions in which the immune system is known to play a role. Therefore, behavioral interventions aimed at maximizing protective psychosocial factors might be predicted to have a beneficial effect, not only in terms of mitigating the effect of stress on immune functioning but perhaps also on diminishing emotional disturbances that arise in the context of immune system dysregulation.[19]

Endocrine disorders are frequently associated with secondary psychiatric symptoms, such as depressed mood and disturbances in thought. In addition, certain psychiatric syndromes are associated with distinct patterns of endocrine dysfunction. The term *psychoneuroendocrinology* encompasses the inextricable structural and functional relationships between hormonal systems and the CNS and behaviors that modulate and are derived from both. Classically, *hormones* have been defined as the products of endocrine glands transported by the blood to exert their action at sites distant from their release. Advances in neuroscience have shown, however, that in the CNS the brain not only serves as a target site for regulatory control of hormonal release but also has secretory functions of its own and serves as an end-organ for some hormonal actions. These complex interrelationships make classic distinctions between the origin, structure, and function of neurons and those of endocrine cells dependent on physiological context. Multiple interactions between the endocrine and immune systems have pointed to a parallel regulatory complexity.[19]

With all the changes taking place in Modern practice of Psychiatry, and seeing the evolution of Psychiatrists into Physicians it reaffirms the place of Psychiatry as a branch of medicine and an all-encompassing term may be Psycho-Socio-Neuro-Immuno-Endocrinology.

BIBLIOGRAPHY

1. Pichot P. The history of psychiatry as a medical specialty. New Oxford Textbook of Psychiatry. 2012 Feb;17–27.
2. Yohanna D. Deinstitutionalization of people with mental illness: Causes and consequences. Virtual Mentor. 2013;15(10):886–91.
3. Gronfein W. Psychotropic Drugs and the Origins of Deinstitutionalization. Social Problems. 1985 Jun;32(5):437–54.
4. Gazdag G, Ungvari GS. Electroconvulsive therapy: 80 years old and still going strong. World Journal of Psychiatry [Internet]. 2019 Jan 4 [cited 2022 Jan 23];9(1):1. Available from: /pmc/articles/PMC6323557/
5. Gaebel W, Zielasek J, Cleveland HR. Psychiatry as a medical specialty: challenges and opportunities. World Psychiatry [Internet]. 2010 [cited 2022 Jan 22];9(1):36. Available from: /pmc/articles/PMC2816931/
6. Andreasen NC. DSM and the death of phenomenology in america: an example of unintended consequences. Schizophrenia bulletin [Internet]. 2007 Jan [cited 2022 Jan 22];33(1):108–12. Available from: https://pubmed.ncbi.nlm.nih.gov/17158191/
7. Fischer BA. A review of American psychiatry through its diagnoses: the history and development of the Diagnostic and Statistical Manual of Mental Disorders. The Journal of nervous and mental disease [Internet]. 2012 Dec [cited 2022 Jan 22];200(12):1022–30. Available from: https://pubmed.ncbi.nlm.nih.gov/23197117/
8. Shah NJ, Arrubla J, Rajkumar R, Farrher E, Mauler J, Kops ER, et al. Multimodal Fingerprints of Resting State Networks as assessed by Simultaneous Trimodal MR-PET-EEG Imaging. Scientific Reports [Internet]. 2017 Dec 1 [cited 2022 Jan 23];7(1). Available from: https://pressrelease.brainproducts.com/mr-pet-eeg/
9. Halligan PW, David AS. Cognitive neuropsychiatry: towards a scientific psychopathology. Nature reviews Neuroscience [Internet]. 2001 [cited 2022 Jan 22];2(3):209–15. Available from: https://pubmed.ncbi.nlm.nih.gov/11256082/
10. Mahgoub M, Monteggia LM. Epigenetics and Psychiatry. Neurotherapeutics [Internet]. 2013 Oct [cited 2022 Jan 23];10(4):734. Available from: /pmc/articles/PMC3805856/
11. Newson JJ, Thiagarajan TC. EEG Frequency Bands in Psychiatric Disorders: A Review of Resting State Studies. Frontiers in Human Neuroscience. 2019 Jan 9;12:521.
12. Neurocentrism: Implications for psychotherapy practice and research. - PsycNET [Internet]. [cited 2022 Jan 23]. Available from: https://psycnet.apa.org/record/2015-56839-003
13. Fusar-Poli P, Broome MR. Conceptual issues in psychiatric neuroimaging. Current opinion in psychiatry [Internet]. 2006 Nov [cited 2022 Jan 22];19(6):608–12. Available from: https://pubmed.ncbi.nlm.nih.gov/17012940/
14. Geddes JR. From science to practice. New Oxford Textbook of Psychiatry. 2012 Feb;122–30.
15. Integrating psychiatry with other medical

specialties | MDedge Psychiatry [Internet]. [cited 2022 Jan 23]. Available from: https://www.mdedge.com/psychiatry/article/64023/practice-management/integrating-psychiatry-other-medical-specialties

16. Moore BA, Barnett JE. Oxford Clinical Psychology Military Psychologists ' Desk Reference. Case Studies in Clinical Psychological Science: Bridging the Gap from Science to Practice [Internet]. 2015 [cited 2022 Jan 23];(August):1–7. Available from: http://books.google.com/books?hl=en&lr=&id=aT1Z84G5S0sC&pgis=1
17. Mishra A, Galhotra A. Mental Healthcare Act 2017: Need to Wait and Watch. International Journal of Applied and Basic Medical Research [Internet]. 2018 [cited 2022 Jan 23];8(2):67. Available from: /pmc/articles/PMC5932926/
18. Normality and Mental Health: analysis of a multivalent relationship [Internet]. [cited 2022 Jan 23]. Available from: http://www.scielo.org.co/scielo.php?script=sci_arttext&pid=S2011-30802015000100004
19. Sadock BJ, Sadock VA, Ruiz P. Kaplan & Sadock's comprehensive textbook of psychiatry. [cited 2022 Jan 23]; Available from: https://www.wolterskluwer.com/en/solutions/ovid/kaplan--sadocks-comprehensive-textbook-of-psychiatry-761.

Normality and Mental Health 2

Pragya Lodha • Avinash De Sousa

World Health Organization (WHO) defines mental health as "a state of welfare in which the individual realizes his own abilities, can cope with the normal stresses of life, can work productively and fruitfully, and is able to make a contribution to his community "(WHO, 2007). Health is holistically understood as a combination of physical and mental well-being. Thus, there is no health without mental health. Mental health can be conceptualized as above normal and a mental state that is objectively desirable, as in Sigmund Freud's definition of mental health which is the capacity to work and to love. Second, from the viewpoint of healthy adult development, mental health can be conceptualized as maturity. Third, mental health can be conceptualized in terms of positive psychology—as epitomized by the presence of multiple human strengths. Fourth, mental health can be conceptualized as emotional intelligence and successful object relations. Fifth, mental health can be conceptualized as subjective well-being—a mental state that is subjectively experienced as happy, contented, and desired. Sixth, mental health can be conceptualized as resilience, as the capacity for successful adaptation and homeostasis.

Model A: Mental Health as Above Normal

This first perspective differs from the traditional medical approach to health and illness. No manifest psychopathology equals mental health. In this medical model, if one were to put all individuals on a continuum, normality would encompass the major portion of adults, and abnormality would be the small reminder. This definition of health correlates with the traditional role model of the doctor who attempts to free his patient from grossly observable signs of illness. In other words, in this context health refers to a reasonable, rather than an optimal, state of functioning. Yet, as already pointed out, mental health is not normal; it is above average. Some believe that true mental health is the exception, not the rule. Moreover, until recently some believed that mental health was imaginary.

Model B: Mental Health as Maturity

Unlike other organs of the body that are designed to stay the same, the brain is designed to be plastic. Therefore, just as optimal brain development requires almost a lifetime, so does the assessment of positive mental health. A 10-year-old's lungs and kidneys are more likely to reflect optimal function than are those of a 60-year-old, but that is not true of a 10-year-old's central nervous system. To some extent, then, adult mental health reflects a continuing process of maturational unfolding. Statistically, physically healthy 70-year-olds are mentally healthier than they were at age 30 years. However, if prospective studies of adult development reveal that the immature brain functions less well than the mature brain, does that mean that adolescents are mentally healthier than toddlers? Are the middle-aged mentally healthier than adolescents? The answer is both yes and no, but the question illustrates that in order to understand mental health we must first understand what we mean by maturity. To confirm the hypothesis that maturity and positive mental health are almost synonymous, it is necessary to study the behavior and emotional states of persons over a lifetime. Although such longitudinal studies have come to fruition only recently, all of them illustrate the association of maturity with increasing mental health. After age 50 years, of course, the association between mental health and maturity is contingent on a healthy central nervous system. The ravages of illnesses like brain trauma, major depression, arteriosclerosis, Alzheimer's, and alcoholism must all be avoided.

The association of mental health to maturity is probably mediated not only by progressive brain myelination into the sixth decade but also by the evolution of emotional and social intelligence through experience. Erik Erikson conceptualized that such development produced a "widening social radius." In such a view, life after age 50 years was no longer to be a staircase leading downward, but a path leading outward. In Erikson's model the adult social radius expanded over time through the mastery of certain tasks such as "Identity versus Identity Diffusion," "Intimacy versus Isolation," "Generativity versus Stagnation," and "Integrity versus Despair."

Model C: Mental Health as Positive or "Spiritual" Emotions

This model defines both mental and spiritual health as the amalgam of the positive emotions that bind us to other human beings. Love, hope, joy, forgiveness, compassion, faith, awe, and gratitude comprise the important positive and "moral" emotions included in this model. Of great importance, these selected positive emotions all involve human connection. None of the emotions listed is just about the self. These positive emotions appear to be a common denominator of all major faiths. Omitted from the list are five other positive emotions—excitement, interest, contentment (happiness), humour, and a sense of mastery, for a person can feel these latter five emotions alone on a desert island. Negative emotions originating in the hypothalamus such as fear and anger are elaborated in the human amygdala (larger in humans than in other mammals). Of tremendous importance to individual survival, the negative emotions are all about "me." In contrast, positive emotions, apparently generated in the limbic system and unique to mammals, have the potential to free the self from the self.

The effect of positive emotion on the autonomic (visceral) nervous system has much in common with the relaxation response to meditation. In contrast to the metabolic and cardiac arousal that the fright-or-flight response of negative emotion induces in our sympathetic autonomic nervous system, positive emotion via our parasympathetic nervous system reduces basal metabolism, blood pressure, heart rate, respiratory rate, and muscle tension.

Model D: Mental Health as Socioemotional Intelligence

High socioemotional intelligence reflects above-average mental health in the same way that a high intelligence quotient (IQ) reflects above-average intellectual aptitude. Such emotional intelligence lies at the heart of positive mental health. In the Nicomachean Ethics, Aristotle defined socioemotional intelligence as follows: "Anyone can become angry—that is easy. But to be angry with the right person, to the right degree, at the right time, for the right purpose, and in the right way—that is not easy." All emotions exist to assist basic survival. Although the exact number of primary emotions is arguable, seven emotions are currently distinguished according to characteristic facial expressions connoting anger, fear, excitement, interest, surprise, disgust and sadness. The capacity to identify these different emotions in ourselves and in others plays an important role in mental health. The benefits of being able to read feelings from nonverbal cues have been demonstrated in almost a score of countries. These benefits included being better emotionally adjusted, more popular, and more responsive to others.

Emotions are critical to mammalian communication. Because such communications are not always consciously recognized, the more skillful individuals are in identifying their emotions, the more skilled the individual will be in communicating with others and in empathically recognizing their emotions. Put differently, the more one is skilled in empathy, the more one will be valued by others, and thus the greater will be social supports, self-esteem, and intimate relationships.

Social and emotional intelligence can be defined by the following criteria:

- Accurate conscious perception and monitoring of one's emotions.
- Modification of emotions so that their expression is appropriate. This involves the capacity to self-soothe personal anxiety and to shake off hopelessness and gloom.
- Accurate recognition of and response to emotions in others.
- Skill in negotiating close relationships with others.
- Capacity for focusing emotions (motivation) toward a desired goal. This involves delayed gratification and adaptively displacing and channelling impulse.

Model E: Mental Health as Subjective Well-Being

Positive mental health does not just involve being a joy to others; one must also experience subjective well-being. Long before humankind considered definitions of mental health, they pondered criteria for subjective happiness. Subjective wellbeing is not just the absence of misery, but the presence of positive contentment. Subjective happiness can have maladaptive as well as adaptive facets. The search for happiness can appear selfish, narcissistic, superficial, and banal. Pleasures can come easily and be soon gone. Happiness is often based on illusion or on dissociative states. Illusory happiness is seen in the character structure associated with bipolar and dissociative disorders. Maladaptive happiness can bring temporary bliss but has no sticking power. Subjective well-being makes available personal resources that can be directed toward innovation and creativity in thought and action.

Model F: Mental Health as Resilience

Adversity is a fact of life. Resilience is that ineffable quality that allows some people to be knocked down by life and come back at least as strong as before. Rather than letting difficulties or failure overcome them and drain their resolve, they find a way to rise. There are three broad classes of coping mechanisms that humans use to overcome stressful situations. First, there is the way in which an individual elicits help from appropriate others: Namely consciously seeking social support. Second, there are conscious cognitive strategies that individuals intentionally use to master stress. Third, there are adaptive involuntary coping mechanisms (often called "defense mechanisms") that distort our perception of internal and external reality in order to reduce subjective distress, anxiety, and depression.

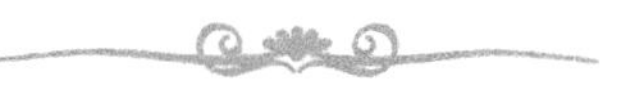

History Taking in Psychiatry 3

Delnaz Palsetia • Avinash De Sousa

INTRODUCTION

Effective communication is fundamental for a good history taking by establishing an adequate rapport with the patient which leads to making a more accurate diagnosis, establishing a management plan and improved adherence by patient to it.

Important points to note while conducting a psychiatric interview:

- The interview need not be conducted in a particular order. Flexibility can be exercised.
- It is better to interview the patient first to avoid creating any bias based on informant's account of the patient's condition.
- It is useful to record Patient and informant history separately, if found to be discordant.
- Empathy is essential while taking history as this puts the patient at ease.
- Non verbal communication is as important as verbal communication.
- Patient's responses should be recorded verbatim rather than using medical jargon.
- Preferably use open-ended and non-directive questions
- Active listening helps to improve rapport and makes the patient feel that he/she is being heard.
- Confidentiality is necessary except in certain situations like suicidal/homicidal risk and child abuse.
- Safety measures to be taken when interviewing agitated and aggressive patients.
- Lack of insight and disturbance of thought, perception and judgment can interfere while communicating with patients during a psychiatric interview.

A) **Personal Data**: Name, Age, Sex, Marital status, Education, Occupation, Income, Address, Religion, and Socioeconomic background

B) **Informant**: The reliability of the information provided by the informants should be assessed based on:

1. Relationship with patient,
2. Whether they stay with the patient or not,
3. Intellectual and observational ability,
4. Degree of concern regarding the patient.

C) **Reason for referral**: The immediate reason which made the patient seek treatment or to be brought to hospital.

D) **Presenting complaints and duration**:

It is important to use patient's own words and to note the duration of each presenting complaint. Some of the additional points which should be noted include:

1. Onset of present illness/symptom.
2. Duration of present illness/symptom.

3. Course of symptoms/illness.
4. Predisposing factors.
5. Precipitating factors (include life stressors).
6. Perpetuating and/or relieving factors.

E) **History of presenting complaints:** When the patient was last well or asymptomatic should be mentioned. The symptoms of the illness should be recorded chronologically with clarity. A life chart helps to describe course of illness, severity, frequency, relationship to stressors, and response to treatment.

1. How the symptoms began, and how the symptoms changed with time (e.g. Began suddenly, Increased gradually, whether episodic in nature)
2. Changes in biological functions (e.g. Sleep, appetite, weight)
3. How symptoms affect patient's socio-occupational functioning
4. Association between symptoms and any stressors or life events
5. Presence of suicidal ideation, ideas of self-harm and ideas of harm to others with details about any possible intent and/or plans
6. Any other relevant information

F) **Past psychiatric and medical history**: Patient's understanding of their illness may be different from the formal diagnosis. Corroborative evidence such as previous notes are often helpful. Note if illness is episodic or was the patient continuously unwell.

A past history of any serious medical or neurological illness, surgical procedure, accident or hospitalisation should be obtained.

G) **Treatment history:** Patient's beliefs about their medication can give useful insight into what they believe is wrong with them. Any treatment received in present and/or previous episode(s) should be asked along with history of treatment adherence, response to treatment received, any adverse effects or any drug allergies. Also, ask about previous hospitalizations.

H) **Family history**

The family history usually includes the 'family of origin' (i.e. the patient's parents, siblings, grandparents, uncles, etc.). The 'family of procreation' (i.e. the patient's spouse, children and grandchildren) is conventionally recorded under the heading of personal history. Family history includes

1. Family structure: A pedigree chart can be used to record all the relevant information.
2. Age and occupations of parents
3. General information about siblings
4. Note whether family is a nuclear, extended or joint family and who is the nominal and functional leader of the family.
5. Any consanguineous relationships
6. The age and cause of death (if any) of family members
7. Family history of similar or other psychiatric illnesses, major medical illnesses, alcohol or drug dependence and suicide and suicidal attempts should be recorded.
8. The patient's relationship with his parents and siblings
9. Knowledge, attitudes and perception of family members towards the patient's illness should be noted.

10. The communication patterns in the family
11. Cultural and religious values, and social support system and socioeconomic status

I) Personal history

Relevant information should be asked depending on age of the patient. In a younger patient, more attention to details can be given regarding earlier personal history. In older patients, it is difficult to get a detailed account of the early childhood history

1. Birth and Developmental History: Breastfeeding, weaning and any history suggestive of maternal deprivation should be noted. Important developmental milestone should be asked. History of neurotic traits such as stuttering, stammering, tics, enuresis, encopresis, night terrors, thumb sucking, nail biting, head banging, body rocking, phobias, somnambulism, temper tantrums, and food fads.
2. Schooling: Age of beginning formal education, academic achievements and relationships with peers and teachers, any school phobia, truancy, learning difficulties and reasons for giving up schooling should be noted.
3. Friendships: Relationships with peers. Assessment of play history is more important in the younger patients.
4. Puberty: Age at menarche, and reaction to menarche, the age at appearance of secondary sexual characteristics in both females and males and any anxiety related to changes in puberty should be asked.
5. Menstrual and Obstetric History: The regularity, the length of each cycle, the last menstrual period, any abnormalities, the number of children born, and termination of pregnancy, if any to be noted.
6. Employment History: Age at which began working, jobs held in chronological order, whether jobs changed frequently and reasons for the same, relationships with authorities, peers and subordinates and approximate income.
7. Marital History: The duration of marriage or relationships, arranged marriage with or without consent or by choice with or without parental consent, number of marriages, divorces or separations, marital role.
8. Psychosexual History: sexual activity and sexual practices, contraceptive measures used, sexual satisfaction and psychosexual dysfunction to be mentioned.
9. History of substance use: Alcohol and drugs like alcohol, nicotine, cannabis and other drugs of use can often lead to several psychiatric symptoms, duration, amount and frequency of use, social, legal or financial problems secondary to substance use.

J) Premorbid personality

This information is recorded to get an idea about what sort of a person the patient was before he fell ill. It is not necessary to ask all of the questions at all times especially if patient is acutely distressed. Some of the history can be gathered from old notes, and from speaking to an informant. Temperament to be mentioned if the age is less than 16 years.

1. Interpersonal relationship with family members, friends and colleagues
2. Hobbies; interests;
3. Predominant mood

4. Attitude to self and others
5. Attitude to work and responsibility
6. Religious beliefs and moral attitudes

After the history, General and Systemic examination is done. Mental Status Examination is done. And then Differential diagnosis/ Diagnosis is given.

BIBLIOGRAPHY

1. Ahuja N. Psychiatric History and Examination (from A Short Textbook of Psychiatry, Chapter 2, 7th Ed) Jaypee Brothers Medical Publishers (P) Ltd, New Delhi.
2. Dr. Hughes S. History Taking and Risk Assessment, Chapter 2, University of Bristol.
3. Phelan M.; Blair G. Medical history-taking in psychiatry, Cambridge University Press.

Common Signs and Symptoms in Psychiatry

4

Krishnapriya Murlimanohar • Prashant Chaudhari

Prevalence rates for psychiatric disorders vary from 9.5 to 370/1000 population in India in epidemiological studies. Almost 20% of the adult population in the community is affected with some or the other psychiatric disorder. There is a shift in conundrum in mental health from psychotic disorders to common mental disorders and from mental hospitals to primary health centres. Increase in mental health problems such as suicidal attempts, aggression and violence, use of substances, marital discord emphasize on the necessity to prioritize and make substantial changes in the strategies to promote adequate mental health care.[1]

Knowing signs and symptoms of psychopathology is the first step in learning psychiatry and further few pages will cover common signs and symptoms of the speciality, the language of psychiatry.

Signs are objective evidence of disease perceptible to the examining practitioner.

Symptoms are subjective evidence of disease perceived by the patient.[2]

Neurosis: Psychiatric illnesses in which judgment, insight, personality, reality content are intact.

Psychosis: Psychiatric illnesses in which judgment decreases, insight is absent, personality deteriorates and there is loss of reality content.

Thinking: Normal thinking is a goal directed flow of ideas, symbols and associations initiated by a problem or a task, characterized by rational connections between successive ideas or thoughts, and leading towards a reality oriented conclusion.

Thought form disorders: It is how the person's thoughts are expressed in their speech.

Thought stream disorders: It refers to the constant movement and appearance of thoughts in the conscious mind.

Thought possession disorders: It includes thought insertion, thought withdrawal, thought broadcast.

Thought content disorders: It describes what the patient is thinking and includes the presence or absence of delusional or obsessional thinking and suicidal or homicidal ideas.

Loosening of associations: Thought process characterized by a series of ideas without apparent logical connections.

Neologisms: These are idiosyncratically formed new words whose derivation cannot be understood easily.

Verbigeration/word salad: Senseless repetition of same words or phrases over and over again.

Tangentiality: Sudden and oblique digression in to unnecessary details that completely distract from the central theme; however, the patient never returns to the original theme after digression (unlike in circumstantiality).

Flight of ideas: Rapid speech with sudden shifts in ideas, without losing logical connection.

Clang association: Jumping from one rhyming word to another.

Prolixity of speech: Lively embellishment of speech.

Thought block: It is defined as any experience where a person suddenly finds themselves unable to think, speak, or move in response to events that are happening around them.

Circumstantiality: Digression in to unnecessary details that distract from the central theme; however, the patient returns to the original theme after digression (unlike in tangentiality).

Poverty of speech: Decreased speech production.

Poverty of content of speech: The speech production is adequate, but the content conveys little information.

Pressure of speech: Rapid production of speech output, with a subjective feeling of racing thoughts.

Perplexity: Puzzled bewilderment.

Perseveration: Persistent repetition of words or themes beyond the point of relevance.

Thought insertion: Subject experiences thoughts imposed by some external force on his passive mind.

Thought withdrawal: Thoughts cease and subject experiences them as removed by external force.

Thought diffusion or Broadcasting: Subject experiences that his thoughts are escaping the confines of his self and are being experienced by others around.

Delusional ideas: False belief or thought.

Overvalued idea: A solitary, abnormal belief that is neither delusional nor obsessional in nature, but which is preoccupying to the extent of dominating the sufferer's life.

Delusion: A false, unshakable belief which is not amenable to reasoning, and is not in keeping with the patient's socio-cultural and educational background.

Delusional perception: Normal perception has a private and illogical meaning.

Grandiosity: Excessive and exaggerated feeling of one's importance.

Mood: The pervasive feeling tone which is sustained (lasts for some length of time) and colors the total experience of the person. Mood is assessed by seeing its congruency to affect, reactivity, lability, whether restricted/blunted/flat and its appropriateness to the surroundings.

Affect: The outward expression of the immediate (cross-sectional) experience of emotion at a given time.

Blunted affect: Severe reduction in the intensity of affect.

Labile affect: Rapid and abrupt changes in affect, unrelated to external stimuli.

Emotional incontinence: Complete loss of control over affect (represents an extreme form of emotional lability).

Incoherence: Thought process that is disconnected, disorganised, or incomprehensible.

Euthymia: Normal range of mood, with absence of depressed or elevated mood.

Ecstasy: Very severe elevation of mood (seen in delirious or stuporous mania); Intense sense of rapture or blissfulness (stage IV).

Exaltation: Severe elevation of mood (seen in severe mania; Stage III); Intense elation with delusions of grandeur.

Elation: Moderate elevation of mood (seen in mania; Stage II); Feeling of confidence and enjoyment along with increased psychomotor activity.

Euphoria: Mild elevation of mood (seen in hypomania); Increased sense of psychological well-being and happiness, not in keeping with on-going events (stage I).

Dysthymia: It is a continuous long-term (chronic) form of depression. One may lose interest in normal daily activities, feel hopeless, lack productivity, and have low self-esteem and an overall feeling of inadequacy.

Depression: It is a common and serious medical illness that negatively affects how you feel, the way you think and how you act. It causes feelings of sadness and/or a loss of interest in activities you once enjoyed.

Anhedonia: Loss of interest in previously pleasurable activities.

Alexithymia: Inability to verbally describe one's emotional feelings.

Anergia: Lack of energy for day-to-day activities.

Anxiety: An unpleasurable emotional state, associated with psycho-physiological changes in response to an intrapsychic conflict.

Dysphoric mood: It includes depression with anxiety and irritability.

Panic: An acute, intense, overwhelming episode of anxiety, often associated with feelings of impending doom.

Phobia: An irrational fear of an object, situation or activity.

La bella indifference: Mood indifferent to presentation. Can be seen in conversion disorder.

Illusion: A misinterpretation of stimuli arising from external objects.

Hallucination: A perception that occurs in the absence of a stimulus.

Thought echo: Voices speaking out thoughts aloud; also called as echo de la pense. **First person auditory hallucination.**

Second person auditory hallucinations: Patients hear a voice, or voices, talking directly to them. It can be persecutory, highly critical, complimentary or issue commands to the patient (**command hallucination**).

Third person auditory hallucinations: Patients hear a voice or voices speaking about them, referring to them in the third person. This may take the form of two or more voices arguing or discussing the patient among themselves; or one or more voices giving a **running commentary** on the patient's thoughts or actions.

Extra-campine hallucinations: Hallucinations beyond the sensory fields. Example – Hearing of voices inaudible to others from outer space.

Reflex hallucinations: A stimuli is required for the hallucination. Stimuli and hallucination occur in different modalities. Example – **synaesthesia.**

Functional hallucinations: Here hallucinations are triggered by a stimulus in the same modality, and co-occur with it.

Pseudo-hallucination: It is an involuntary sensory experience vivid enough to be regarded as a hallucination, but which is recognised by the person experiencing it as being subjective and unreal.

Formication: A false sense of insects crawling on one's skin.

Somatic passivity: Bodily sensations, especially sensory symptoms, are experienced as imposed on body by some external force.

Depersonalization: An alteration in the perception of self, so that the feeling of one's reality is (as if) temporarily changed or lost.

Derealization: An alteration in the perception of external world, so that the feeling of the reality of external world is (as if) temporarily changed or lost.

Fugue: Physical and psychological flight (wandering) from one's usual place.

Attention: It is the ability to actively process specific information in the environment while tuning out other details.

Concentration: It refers to the mental effort you direct toward whatever you're working on or learning at the moment. It's sometimes confused with attention span, but **attention span** refers to the length of time you can concentrate on something.

Distractibility: Inability to concentrate or focus attention.

Orientation: Awareness of the self and of outer reality; that is, the ability to identify one's self and to know the time, the place, and the person one is talking to.

Disorientation: A disturbance in orientation in time, place and/or person.

Memory: The ability to retain information or a representation of past experience, based on the mental processes of learning or encoding, retention across some interval of time, and retrieval or reactivation of the memory.

Working memory/Recent memory: It is the small amount of information that can be held in mind and used in the execution of cognitive tasks.

Remote memory: Remote memory typically refers to memory for the distant past, measured on the order of years or even decades. It encompasses episodic (autobiographical), personal semantic, and general semantic memory involving historical people and events.

Confabulation: A false memory that the patient believes to be true.

Judgment: An ability to assess a situation correctly and act appropriately within that situation. It is assessed by looking for test judgment, personal judgment and social judgment.

Abstract thinking: Abstract thinking is the ability to assume a mental set voluntarily, shift voluntarily from one aspect of a situation to another, keep in mind simultaneously the various aspects of a situation, grasp the essentials of a 'whole' (e.g. situation or concept), and to break a 'whole' into its parts.

Concrete thinking: Cannot think beyond the literal meaning. Seen in schizophrenia.

Intelligence: The ability to think logically, act rationally, and deal effectively with the environment.

Insight: The ability to understand one's own behavior and emotions. In the context of psychiatric disorders, it implies the degree of awareness and understanding that the patient has regarding his/her illness. It is also known as epiphany.

Ambitendency: Due to ambivalence, tentative actions are made, but no goal directed action occurs.

Ambivalence: Inability to decide for or against, due to co-existence of two opposing impulses for the same thing at the same time in the same person.

Catatonia: Abnormality of movement and behavior arising from a disturbed mental state (typically schizophrenia). It may involve repetitive or purposeless overactivity, or catalepsy, resistance to passive movement, and negativism.

Stupor: A clinical syndrome of akinesis and mutism, with relative preservation of conscious awareness. No psychomotor activity; not actively relating to environment.

Catalepsy: The person maintains body posture in to which it is placed. Passive induction of a posture held against gravity.

Waxy flexibility: Slight, even resistance to positioning by examiner; Parts of body can be placed in positions that will be maintained for long periods of time, even if very uncomfortable; flexible like wax. The process is called as waxy flexibility, while the end result is called as catalepsy.

Mutism: Complete absence of speech. No, or very little, verbal response to instructions or external stimuli.

Negativism: An apparently motiveless resistance to all commands and attempts to be moved, or doing just the opposite.

Posturing: Spontaneous assumption and active maintenance of an inappropriate and often bizarre posture usually against gravity for long periods of time.

Mannerisms: Odd, repetitive and goal-directed movements. Circumstantial caricature of normal actions.

Stereotype: Odd, repetitive, abnormally frequent and non-goal directed movement (can also be verbal).

Agitation: Presence of anxiety with severe motor restlessness (In cases of catatonia, not influenced by external stimuli).

Grimacing: Contorted facial movement.

Rigidity (Catatonic): Maintenance of a rigid posture against efforts to be moved.

Echolalia: Repetition, echo or mimicking of phrases or words heard.

Echopraxia: Repetition, echo or mimicking of actions observed.

Cataplexy: Abrupt loss of muscle tone without impairment of consciousness. Often seen in Narcolepsy.

Biopsychosocial model: Given by George Engel. States that social factors, past history, communications skills, biological predisposition, family involvement, psychological factors all contribute to mental illness.

Tic: Involuntary, sudden, rapid, recurrent, nonrhythmic and stereotyped movement (can also be verbal)

Coprolalia: Vocal tics characterized by shouting of obscene words.

Deja entendu: A false sense of familiarity when hearing something new.

Deja vu: A false sense of familiarity with unfamiliar circumstances or scenes.

Jamais entendu: A sense of unfamiliarity when hearing something familiar.

Jamais vu: A sense of unfamiliarity with familiar circumstances or scenes.

Folie å deux: Delusions shared between two closely connected persons. Also known are folie å trios, folie å quatre, and folie å famille.

Somnolence: Inability to maintain a state of alertness without constant stimulation.

Suicide: A human act of self-intentioned and self-inflicted cessation (death).

Trance: A sleep like state of reduced consciousness and suggestibility.[3]

Signs and symptoms are window to the psychopathology. It has been found with the advents in neuroimaging that at times these peculiar clinical features may also point towards neurobiological nidus of a given psychiatric disease.

BIBLIOGRAPHY

1. Math SB, Srinivasaraju R. Indian Psychiatric epidemiological studies: Learning from the past. Indian Journal of Psychiatry [Internet]. 2010 [cited 2022 Jan 23];52(Suppl1):S95. Available from:/pmc/articles/PMC3146182/
2. Sign or Symptom (Concept Id: C3540840) - MedGen - NCBI [Internet]. [cited 2022 Jan 23]. Available from: https://www.ncbi.nlm.nih.gov/medgen/761917
3. Sadock BJ, Sadock VA, Ruiz P. Kaplan & Sadock's comprehensive textbook of psychiatry. [cited 2022 Jan 23]; Available from: https://www.wolterskluwer.com/en/solutions/ovid/kaplan--sadocks-comprehensive-textbook-of-psychiatry-761

Basics of Mental Status Examination

5

Elvin Lukose • Heena Merchant Pandit

INTRODUCTION

Mental Status Examination (MSE) is a structured method of assessment of psychiatric symptoms in a patient. It is a psychiatrist's equivalent of a physical examination. It is designed to determine symptoms under parameters that are observable, reliable and stable over a period of time thus helping the clinician to maintain a consistent record of findings. MSE provides an insight into the patient's pathological thought processes and allows evaluation of every observable aspect of behavior from their attire to their judgment of the context of his surroundings. In case of an uncooperative patient or in situations where history is inadequate or filled with discrepancies, MSE provides enough information to allow prompt management. MSE done consecutively on multiple visits enables us in understanding the course of illness. MSE thus is not only a diagnostic aid but also a tool to measure changes and response to therapy over a period of time during the course of treatment.

MSE begins from the moment a patient enters the examination room till the completion of interview. Observation of how a patient responds to the hospital staff or caregiver; the mannerisms in walking or talking and the information conveyed by the patient lead to an effective MSE.

FOR THE CLINICIAN

Not every patient is forthcoming with information about one's experience of symptoms and some hostile patients may even attempt to deflect the conversation and hinder the MSE. Due to the defensive nature of patients in general, following techniques by the clinician may help in obtaining a good MSE.

Use of 'open ended' questions

The interview may begin with the clinician asking open ended questions like *"What has been troubling you since a few days?"* or *"How have you been feeling lately?"* which can facilitate responses by building rapport. Active listening without interruption allow the clinician to assess any formal thought disorder or underlying delusional ideas of the patient.

Use of 'summary statements' and clarification

Summarizing the patient's responses from time to time during the interview may provide the patient, a sense of validation and reinforce his willingness to provide more details about his/her mental status.

Non-Judgmental stance

Patients with formal thought disorders or bizarre psychotic experiences may feel defensive and hence withhold information out of fear of invalidation or embarrassment. Keeping a non judgmental stance by the clinician with validating statements like *"I can understand how you feel when those voices are mocking you"* can circumvent the defensiveness and allow better appraisal of the mental status of the patient.

Use of 'close-ended' questions

Close ended questions like *"Are those voices coming from an outside source or is it your inner self talk?"* or *"Do you feel someone might be doing this to you?"* can help in clarifying certain points and resolve any ambiguities in symptomatology. It also helps in ruling out other disorders and thus, arrive at a particular diagnosis.

MSE has to be conducted in a patient friendly setting with optimal privacy and minimal coercion. Security personnel may be required on standby in case of hostile or aggressive patients for the safety of both the patient and the clinician.

GENERAL ATTITUDE AND APPEARANCE

The general attitude and appearance provide the first clue to a patient's mental status and require observation of the following aspects of the patient's presentation and behavior.

- *Level of consciousness* (conscious, stuporous, drowsy etc.)
- *Level of co-operation* (willingness to be examined and questioned; indicates interest in the interview).
- *Level of Self care* (overall manner of dressing whether kempt or ill kempt, appropriateness to the context and surroundings; dishevelled, minimally clothed or dressed in a flamboyant fashion).
- *Interaction with the interviewer and the accompanying family members or relatives during the course of the interview* (hostile, argumentative, indifferent, agreeable or over-familiar etc.).
- *Eye contact*- initiation and maintenance (avoidance gaze, fleeting or downcast gaze etc.).

Table 5.1: The outline of the mental status examination

Mental Status Examination
GENERAL ATTITUDE AND APPEARANCE
PSYCHOMOTOR ACTIVITY
SPEECH
• Spontaneity
• Rate
• Rhythm
• Volume
• Word Output
MOOD
THOUGHT
• Form
• Stream
• Content
• Possession of thought
PERCEPTION
ORIENTATION
ATTENTION AND CONCENTRATION
MEMORY
• Immediate
• Recent
• Remote
INTELLIGENCE
• General knowledge
• Comprehension
• Arithmetic
• Abstraction
JUDGMENT
• Personal
• Social
• Test
INSIGHT

PSYCHOMOTOR ACTIVITY

It is the motor activity associated with the emotional experience of the patient including overall amplitude of bodily movements (accelerated or retarded), character (overactive/hyperactive, restless, rocking motion, manneristic expressions, stereotype etc.) and any involuntary or abnormal movements (tremors, dystonias, chorea, posturing, waxy flexibility etc.).

SPEECH

Speech is assessed by its *Rate*, *Rhythm*, *Volume*, *Word output* and *Spontaneity*. Additional information such as *response latency* or *reaction time* (time taken to respond to a question), *coherence* (intelligibility) and *relevance* can also be taken note of. *Pressure of Speech*, which is the inability to stop talking even after providing a sufficient answer despite repetitive indication from the interviewer to do so when present, can also be mentioned.

MOOD

Assessment of mood includes both the subjective experience (mood) reported and the objective evaluation of the expressed mood (affect).

Mood is defined as the subjective emotional experience of a patient which influences his/her perception of external phenomena and events in the world. It is longitudinal and described in patient's own words (sad, happy, angry etc.). Patient needs to be asked how he/she has been feeling since a few days and how it has affected his/her daily activities and interpersonal relationships in order to get a better understanding of the pervasive nature of the abnormal emotional experience.

Affect is the objective evaluation of a patient's emotional state of mind. It is clinically gauged partly by the facial expressions and partly by the body language and the emotional intonation of speech.

Affect can be described by its *Character/quality* (tearful, happy, fearful, anxious etc.), *Mood-congruency* (whether it's in keeping with the mood described), *Range* (overall amplitude and depth of different emotions expressed throughout the interview), *Reactivity* (the degree to which the affect shows a change in response to stimuli corresponding to different emotions), *Appropriateness* (whether it's in or out of keeping with the context of surrounding or the thought expressed) and *Lability* (rapid fluctuations in the expression). Abnormal neurological affects include emotional incontinence or emotional lability observed in lesions affecting the frontopontine pathways responsible for voluntary control and regulation of emotional expressions. It is also seen in pseudobulbar palsy where it is known as *Pseudobulbar Affect* (PBA).

THOUGHT

Thought processes need to be examined for the following aspects:

- *Form*
- *Stream*
- *Content*
- *Possession of Thought*

Form of Thought

Normal thought is said to be constant, organised and continuous. Formal thought disorder is a manifestation of error in conceptual and abstract thinking leading to lack of association between conveyed ideas resulting in changing and unclear concepts. This leads to a thought process that lacks constancy; is disorganised and discontinuous. These were hypothesised to arise from morbid processes occurring in the patient and form one of the core features that suggest a psychopathology. The morbid processes include loss of adequate connection between successive thoughts; clusters of more or less related thoughts; thoughts inclusive of irrelevant material; imprecise approximations of the thought intended to be expressed; use of words or concepts having a private meaning etc..

The various formal thought disorders are as follows:

Loosening of associations is the lack of connection between different elements of the same thought or successive thoughts. The entire speech sample of the patient may sound irrelevant and not convey anything meaningful. The type in which a thought slips into another unrelated thought is known as *Derailment* or *Knight's move*.

Tangentiality is the tendency of the patient to start his/her answer initially in the premise relevant to the question but gradually deviating from it in a way that he/she does not return to the original point of the conversation.

Clang Association is the use of words or phrases associated with each other by way of a rhyming quality to the syllables involved. For example *"Bitter batter splattered on my platter."*

Neologism is a word constructed by the patient de novo or by distorting an existing word. They could be ordinary words used in an unconventional way to express a particular thought or concept that holds a private meaning to the patient. Neologisms represent an attempt by the afflicted patient (as in Schizophrenia) to make sense of the ongoing experiences which maybe too bizarre to be understood or expressed using conventional words. For example Patient may use the term *'food vessel'* consistently to refer to his stomach.

Verbigeration is the meaningless repetition of words irrelevant to the topic at hand.

Word Salad is severe form of disorganization of thought leading to breakdown of grammar, syntax and overall meaning. Historically, word salad was found more prevalent in Schizophrenia and hence, was termed as Schizophasia.

Stream of Thought

The stream of thought is the train of thought or the manner in which each thought succeeds another thought without losing sense of what is being communicated. Disorders of stream of thought are as follows:

Flight of Ideas consists of rapid succession of ideas which bear chance association to each other accompanied by a high speech rate such that the patient does not return to the point by the end of the conversation. It is characteristically seen in Mania. *Prolixity* is a variant of this thought disorder in which there is an ordered manner in the succession of ideas and wherein the patient eventually returns to the point of conversation. It is not accompanied by high rate of speech and is more commonly seen in Hypomania.

Circumstantiality is the tendency of the patient to include unnecessary but relevant details while conveying a thought with the patient ultimately reaching to the point of conversation. It may clinically appear as if the patient is 'beating around the bush'. For example, on asking the patient how he reached the hospital, he may reply with a speech sample like this-

"I woke up and I looked out of the window and saw that it's a nice and sunny day---
I went to the station but the line was too long and I was getting bored---
I took a taxi from the station and he charged me big money---
I was arguing with him about it---
I saw the sign and reached the hospital".

Perseveration is the persistence of a response beyond its point of relevance. In perseveration, the patient's response is relevant to the first question and irrelevant thereafter whereas in the case of verbigeration, the responses are irrelevant right from the start for example, in the following conversation-

Doctor- *"Where do you live?"*

Patient- *"Delhi"*

Doctor- *"What is your age?"*

Patient- *"Delhi"*.

Thought Block is an arrest in the train of thought of the patient which manifests itself as a brief pause which may be followed by a new thought. A patient with thought block is lucid during the pause and may have an accompanying delusion that his thoughts are being extracted by an external agency or force.

It is important to keep a verbatim account of the patient's speech sample and mention in the MSE.

Content

Examination of thought content may give rise to following findings:

Delusion is a false, firm, fixed unshakeable belief not in keeping with a patient's educational or socio-cultural background which persists despite the evidence to the contrary. The following are different types of delusions-

Delusion of Persecution is the false belief that the patient or his/her loved ones are being harmed. Delusion of persecution could take form as a delusion of reference where the patient believes he/she is being talked about or is being watched. The patient may believe the news on the television or the newspaper or a song on the radio is referring to him/her and contains encrypted messages intended to influence or harm him/her in some way. Patients with such delusional content tend to be hostile, hyper vigilant, guarded or aggressive.

Delusion of Grandiosity is the false belief that the patient is or is associated with a powerful or supernatural figure (grandiose identity) or possesses some special power, talent or a huge amount of wealth (grandiose ability). Such a delusional content maybe accompanied by an elevated expansive mood as seen in Mania. Behavior may reveal an air of authority or over-familiarity with speech consisting of pseudo-philosophical comments, chants, jokes or songs sung inappropriately during the interview.

Delusion of Love is the false belief that some person is in love with the patient even in the absence of any form of liaison between them that could indicate so. Any refusal to acknowledge the relationship or defensiveness on the part of the person will be perceived by the patient as an attempt to hide their relationship from the scrutiny and criticism of the society. Such behavior is called *paradoxical conduct* characteristic of this disorder. *Erotomania* or *De Clerambault's syndrome* is the variant more commonly seen in females where the person they allege to be in love with them is usually a male who is older; of a higher social status and a well known public figure. Delusion of love mixed with persecutory ideas or delusion is known as *Old Maid's Insanity*.

Delusion of Infidelity is the false belief that the patient's spouse or romantic partner is engaged in an illicit relationship with someone else. Such a delusion may result in aggressive behavior towards his/her spouse partner and at times, even involve violence or homicide.

Delusional Misidentification is based on the concept of 'double'. In *Capgras' delusion*, the patient perceives that his/her loved one or someone closely related to them has been replaced by an impostor bearing the same face. In *Fregoli's delusion*, the patient falsely perceives an unfamiliar person as a familiar one. The false belief that one person can transform into a second person with a different physical or psychological identity is called *Syndrome of Intermetamorphosis.* In *Syndrome of Subjective Doubles*, a patient may believe in the existence of his/her 'duplicates' bearing physical similarities but with or without unique psychological identities.

Delusion of Guilt is the false belief that the patient has committed some sin and has brought wrath upon himself or his family. The guilt feelings are out of proportion to the 'sin' alleged to have been committed and the content is usually self-deprecatory or reproachful in its tone. Such patients may have accompanying psychomotor retardation and suicidal ideations as in depressive disorders.

Nihilistic Delusion is the false belief that one is dead or his/her organs; his mind; his loved ones and the whole world are dead. *Cotard Syndrome* is a variant of nihilistic delusion wherein a patient believes his/her organs are rotting away.

Delusional Parasitosis or *Ekbom's Syndrome* is a false belief wherein the patient believes his/her body has been infested with insects or microscopic organisms. They may be accompanied by tactile hallucinations of something crawling or moving inside the body or on the surface of the skin.

Negative Ideas of Hopelessness, Worthlessness or Helplessness are critical thoughts about one's future; sense of self-worth and potential of getting help from the given environment respectively. Classically known as *Beck's triad*, it is seen as a core thought process in depressive disorders. Suicidal ideas whether present or absent need to be elicited and mentioned in the content compulsorily. A patient may not have suicidal ideas but have wishes to be killed involuntarily by way of an accident, life-threatening illness or some procedure which may be documented as *passive death wishes.*

Possession of Thought

Disorders of possession of thought cause the patient to experience a loss of control or loss of sense of agency of one's own thinking process.

Obsessions and Compulsions

Obsessions are thoughts, images or impulses that are irrational, recurrent and intrusive to a patient's consciousness that are difficult to dismiss causing significant anxiety and associated distress. Common obsessive thoughts include obsession of contamination or symmetry. Compulsions are either mental or observable behaviors that are repetitive and are intended to reduce the anxiety caused by obsessions. Common compulsive behaviors include compulsive hand washing and checking.

Thought Alienation

Thought Alienation occurs when the patient experiences his thoughts as being under the control of an external agency and at times perceive them to be occurring against his/her will. In *thought withdraw*al, the patient finds himself losing his train of thought and believes his/her thoughts are being extracted out of his/her mind by an external agency or influence. It frequently accompanies thought block. In *thought insertion*, the patient believes the ongoing thoughts as not being his/hers and instead, are being 'put into' in his/her her mind by an external agency. In *thought broadcast*, the patient feels his/her thoughts are being revealed to others through some external medium. The patient may also say that others can know or are aware of his/her thoughts. Thought alienation is one of Schneiderian first rank symptoms for Schizophrenia.

PERCEPTION

Perception is the subjective interpretation by a patient of his/her experience of one or more stimuli in the environment.

Hallucination

Hallucination is defined as the perception of a stimulus in the absence of the corresponding stimulus in the external environment. They are false perceptions and occur simultaneously alongside real perception. Hallucinations can be classified based on modality affected- Auditory, Visual, Tactile, Gustatory and Olfactory. They can be even described by nature of its experience such as the following special varieties:

Autoscopy (Phantom Mirror Image) - The visual perception of an image of oneself in external space. Negative Autoscopy is described as the perception of the absence of one's mirror image.

Hypnogogic and Hypnopompic Hallucination- These are hallucinations experienced during the transition into sleep (Hypnogogic) or from sleep to wakefulness (Hypnopompic).

The different aspects of hallucinatory experience should be documented such as follows:

- *Type of hallucination* (auditory, visual, tactile etc.)
- *Whether occurring in first person, second person or third person* (for auditory hallucinations)
- *Content of hallucination* (derogatory, threatening, accusatory, commanding etc.)

Auditory hallucinations of first person consist of hearing one's own thoughts audibly and is known as *thought echo*. Second person auditory hallucinations consist of voices talking to the patient. When these voices appear to comment on the patient's daily activities, it is known as *thought commentary*. Third person auditory hallucinations consist of voices talking amongst themselves. Hallucinations that command a patient to perform an act are called *command* or *imperative hallucinations*.

COGNITIVE FUNCTIONS

Following domains need to be assessed for gauging the status of cognitive functions:

- *Orientation*
- *Attention/Concentration*
- *Memory*
- *Intelligence*
- *Judgment*

Orientation

Orientation is the awareness and the capacity of a patient to accurately gauge time, space and person in his/her current setting. It is dependent on availability of multiple cues in the environment and the intellectual capacity of the patient to derive and deduce meaningful conclusions about his environment. Assessment of orientation requires patient to be evaluated in the presence of adequate light in an environment that includes persons familiar to the patient.

Disorientation occurs with respect to *time*, *place* and *person* and is affected in that order.

Evaluation for *orientation to time* includes questions enquiring about *the time of the day*, *period of the day* (morning, noon, evening and night); *the time passed since last meal*; *day of the week*; *current month* and the *current year*. Looking at calendars, clocks or watches should be avoided to prevent anchoring of responses by the patient. In case of illiterate patients or in those with lower intellectual capacity, questions about the current season or the time elapsed since the last festival or occasion can be asked.

Evaluation for *orientation to place* includes questions enquiring about *the current setting of examination (is it a hospital, railway station or police station? etc.)*; *the particular floor of the building* and *name of the town/city or even State.*

Evaluation for *orientation to person* includes identification of the caretaker or family member beside the patient; the attending doctor or personnel; identity of self (full name and relationship to family members) and other family members or relatives (names and relatedness).

Attention/Concentration

Attention is the act of focusing of consciousness on a particular stimulus. Concentration is sustained attention over a period of time.

It is clinically assessed under two broad categories:

Active Attention

Active attention is the level of attention deliberately paid to a given task. It is described as whether *arousable* and whether it is *sustained* or *ill-sustained*. It can be gauged clinically by observing the relevance of responses of the patient to the questions and the extent to which the patient maintains the thread of the conversation without interruption.

Passive Attention

Passive attention is the ability to switch attention to a novel stimulus or a significant change in any stimulus in the background of the environment. For example, passive attention is said to be intact when during the interview, a patient directs his/her attention to the source of a loud noise in the room or to the flickering of a light source. Passive attention is said to be decreased if no such response is noted and is said to be increased if the patient is distracted by insignificant or any irrelevant stimuli in the environment.

Various tests that can aid an objective assessment of Attention and Concentration are–

- *Serial Subtraction*
- *Naming days of the week or months of the year forwards and backwards*
- *Digit Span test*

Serial Subtraction

The patient is asked to subtract 7 from 100 and then further subtract 7 from the answer without any hints or prompts. The time taken to complete the task should also be noted. Up to 5 such serial subtractions (100-7=93, 93-7=86, 86-7=79, 79-7=72, 72-7=65) have to be performed without the interviewer correcting or reinforcing any response. One point can be deducted for every wrong answer and the total score out of 5 should be mentioned. Whether an answer is right or wrong is judged on whether the patient is correctly applying the rule of 'subtracting 7 from the current number' correctly for consecutive responses.

Depending on the intellectual capacity or lucidity of the patient, easier combinations like serially subtracting 5 from 50 or 3 from 20 can be tried.

Naming Days of the Week or Months of the Year

This test can be done provided the patient has knowledge of the same. Avoid exposure to a calendar or any such cues near the patient.

Digit Span Test

Digit Span test includes providing combination of numbers that need to be repeated by the patient in the same order as instructed. The patient may be given a mock combination of 2-3 numbers with some facilitation to check if he/she has understood the instruction. The combinations are to be recalled both *forwards* and *backwards* using separate sets of digits for both.

Memory

Memory is a cognitive process by which information is encoded, stored and retrieved for later recall.

Memory has been broadly divided into three types for assessment namely *Immediate*, *Recent* and *Remote*.

Immediate Memory can be tested by using the Digit span test or provision of combination of 5 unrelated names. Combinations can include name of an object, animal, place, abstract idea and color (for example, Hammer-Giraffe-Nagpur-Sadness-Yellow). Any relation between the names in as in rhyme, association or same initial letters etc. can cause the patient to form a mnemonic and hence give an erroneous evaluation of immediate memory. Once provided to the patient, he/she has to repeat the combination in the same order once *(Registration)* and repeat a second time after an interval of 5 minutes *(Recall)* during which the rest of the interview can be continued to avoid mental rehearsal by the patient.

Recent Memory can be tested by asking the patients about the activities of the day at different time intervals; the different interactions with people; the details of travelling and the various meals etc. The provided information has to be corroborated and validated by the informant or the hospital staff depending on circumstances.

Patient can also be given 3-4 lines of an unfamiliar address to repeat once and again after 5 minutes during which the patient has to be distracted by continuing the rest of the interview. The answers need to be noted down verbatim and cross checked for any discrepancy or distortion.

Remote Memory can be assessed by questions about date of birth; year of passing Matriculation or an equivalent examination/graduation; year of obtaining employment or change of jobs; year of marriage and time since marriage and details about children like their age, order of birth and names.

Preferably those questions have to be asked the answers of which can be validated and cross checked from a relative or spouse.

In case of illiterate patients, questions about the previous season or details about the important events of a last few months can be asked.

Intelligence

Intelligence is the aggregate or global capacity of an individual to act purposefully; to think rationally and to deal effectively with his/her environment. Three areas of intelligence that are important from clinical point of view are abstract, practical and social intelligence.

Assessment of Intelligence involves areas of *General knowledge*, *Comprehension*, *Arithmetic* and *Abstraction*.

General Knowledge can be gauged by asking the general questions like name of State's Chief Minister/Country's President or Prime Minister; names of states or important cities/capitals (around 5 names may be sufficient); important dates of national or socio-cultural importance; information about ongoing events in sports, politics or current affairs.

Questions pertaining to the occupation and socio-cultural background can be asked to patients with limited educational background. For example, festivals and associated attire; significance of certain traditions; crops growing in different seasons; how to use tools relevant to the patient; current prices of vegetables etc.

Comprehension

Comprehension implies the ability to understand a question or a command and make sense of incoming information in order to formulate an appropriate response. Clinically, comprehension can be gauged by the appropriateness of answers to different questions during the interview. Additional testing can include questions about the nature of his/her occupation and steps of routine household procedures like washing or making tea. Hypothetical questions like *"What will you do if there is a small fire at your home?"* or *"What all will you pack for a trip to a hill station/ beach?"* relevant to the patient's educational and socio-cultural background can also be provided.

In children, comprehension can be assessed by asking them the meaning of the first few lines of a memorised poem or a simple passage can be given or read out to the child as per his/her educational level and asked what it means.

Arithmetic

Arithmetic computational skill can be assessed by asking basic calculations using each operator (addition, subtraction, division, multiplication, square etc.) appropriate to the patient's educational background (for example, *"What is 8 plus 9?")* and arithmetic reasoning can be tested using word problems involving complex series of calculations (for example, *"If one pencil costs 8 rupees and you buy 6 of them, then how much change should you receive from the shopkeeper if you pay 200 rupees?")*.

Abstraction

Abstract reasoning is the ability of the patient to shift back and forth between general concepts and specific examples. It is clinically assessed by questions about similarities, differences and interpretation of proverbs.

Differences

In differences, the patient is asked to mention the various aspects in which two given examples are dissimilar or don't share the same properties. e.g. *Aeroplane and Bird (artificial-natural, requires pilot-flies on its own etc.)*.

Similarities

In similarities, the patient is asked to mention the different aspects in which two given examples are similar or alike. For example *Table and Chair (both are wooden; types of furniture; brown in color etc.)*

Interpretation of Proverbs

The patient is asked about the famous proverbs he/she has adequate knowledge of. Other than that, the patient could be provided with universally popular quotes. For example, phrases like *"a stitch in time saves nine"* and *"as you sow so shall you reap"*.

All the examples used and the responses (whether correct or incorrect) obtained should be documented verbatim in the final MSE.

Care needs to be taken that the chosen proverbs are familiar and relevant to the patient's socio-cultural background and popular in the language known best by the patient.

Judgment

Judgment is defined as the ability to think rationally and behave appropriately as per the implicit rules of a given situation and context. Judgment is assessed in the following areas; *Personal*, *Social* and *Test*

Personal Judgment

Personal Judgment is assessed by clinical observation and from details in the history regarding patient's level and nature of self care; impulsivity; behavior that can potentially harm self or others; substance use despite ongoing physical complications or from the patient's explanations about his/her symptoms or interpersonal conflicts; his/her compliance to treatment etc. Questions can be directed towards current or future plans that patient may convey.

Social Judgment

Social Judgment is assessed by clinical observation and from details in the history regarding patient's attitude toward family members, caretakers, authoritative figures (police, security, superiors etc.) and the interviewer. Patients who appear too over-familiar or hostile with the interviewer or the hospital staff and those who appear to be smiling to themselves or expressing bizarre mannerisms are said to have impaired social judgment.

Test Judgment

Test Judgment is assessed by posing a question that involves clear choices and clear outcomes with minimal ambiguity. For example *"What would you do if your house is on fire?"* (Answers include putting out the fire by water or calling the fire brigade) or *"What would you do if you find a stamped envelope carrying 2000 rupees on the road with a name and an address on it?"* (Answers include submitting it to the post office or informing the addressee). Even when the patient gives appropriate answers, one must check for his/her reasoning which maybe erroneous to some extent. For example, *"I will submit that letter to the post office because I don't want the Secret Society to know that I stole something"*. Such reasoning will suggest impaired test judgment.

INSIGHT

Insight is a patient's awareness of his/her own illness. It is the capacity of the patient to recognise that his/her symptoms are suggestive of a psychiatric condition and that it warrants treatment. Insight can be elicited either directly through questioning or observation of the patient's behavioral responses to his/her ongoing symptoms and willingness for treatment.

Direct questioning can be done using the Socratic Method whereby the patient is asked about the nature of his/her symptoms; sources to which they are attributed; consideration of other plausible alternative explanations and the degree to which his/her reasoning is consistent or inconsistent with his/her prior belief systems and those of the consensus. Insight is not a fixed or stable cognition hence can vary with treatment, remission or exacerbation. Hence, insight can be graded from time to time as:

***GRADE I*:** Denies he/she has any psychiatric symptoms.

***GRADE II*:** Admits some of his/her psychiatric symptoms. *("Yes, I do hear someone talking to me from nowhere")*.

***GRADE III*:** Attributes his/her psychiatric symptoms to an external cause or agency. (*"I am experiencing these problems because I haven't had food properly"*).

***GRADE IV*:** Ambivalent whether his/her symptoms are due to an internal cause or an external cause. (*"I am really not sure why this is happening to me, maybe I am losing my mind"*).

***GRADE V*:** Admits his/her symptoms are due to a psychiatric illness (*Intellectual Insight*). (*"No one else is experiencing these things like I am; this is probably some mental condition")*.

***GRADE VI*:** Admits he/she has a psychiatric illness and wants treatment for the same (*Emotional Insight* or *True Insight*). (*"I will take whatever treatment I may need to make these voices go away"*).

In cases where questions cannot be asked or adequate answers are not provided by the patient, insight can be graded as *No Insight*, *Partial Insight* or *Good Insight*.

OTHER APPROACHES

The Folstein Mini-Mental State Examination (MMSE) tests orientation, immediate and short-term memory, concentration, arithmetic ability, language and praxis, calculated over a total score of 30. The Cognitive Capacity Screening Examination (CCSE) tests orientation, serial subtraction, memory, and similarities. It is less sensitive in cases of delirium or dementia in the elderly. The Neurobehavioral Cognitive Status Examination (NCSE) is favorable for medically ill patients and it focuses on consciousness, orientation, attention, language, construction, memory, calculations, and reasoning and is more sensitive in detecting impairment. Kirby's method involves evaluation of observable parameters like eye contact; pupillary reflexes; vitals, overall psychomotor activity; involvement with the environment etc. It is designed for assessment of mental status examination in cases of unconscious, uncooperative and catatonic patients.

A good MSE is a key tool for psychiatrists. Astute observational skills through informal assessment and formal exams help the clinician orient himself to subtle aberrations in affect, speech, and behavior over the course of meetings. Gradual development of expertise in detecting subtleties is a critical component of becoming a skilled psychiatric clinician.

BIBLIOGRAPHY

1. Fish FJ, Casey PR, Kelly B. *Fish's clinical psychopathology: signs and symptoms in psychiatry*. RCPsych Publications; 2007.
2. Oyebode, Femi. Sims' *symptoms in the mind: an introduction to descriptive psychopathology*. Fifth Edition. Elsevier Health Sciences; 2015
3. Sadock BJ, Sadock VA. *Kaplan and Sadock's synopsis of psychiatry: Behavioral sciences/clinical psychiatry*. Eleventh Edition. Lippincott Williams & Wilkins; 2016.
4. Tasman, A. E., Kay, J. E., Lieberman, J. A., First, M. B., & Maj, M. E. *Psychiatry*, Vols. 1-2. Wiley Blackwell, 2015
5. Weschler D. *The Measurement of Adult Intelligence*. Baltimore, MD. Willaims & Wilkins, 1944.

Communication, Empathy and Rapport Building

6

Pragya Lodha • Nilesh Shah

Communication is one of the foundational requirements for any relationship and likewise for the doctor-patient relationship as well. Studies have shown that good communication skill in a doctor improve patient's compliance and overall satisfaction. There are certain basic principles of practicing good communication. Patient listening, empathy, and paying attention to the paraverbal and non-verbal components of the communication are the important ones that are frequently neglected. Proper information about the nature, course and prognosis of the disease is important. Besides, patients and attendants should always be explained about the necessity and yield of expensive investigations and risks/benefits involved in invasive procedures. One should be extremely cautious while managing difficult encounters and breaking bad news. Formal training of the doctors in improving communication skills is necessary and has proven to improve overall outcome. The need for good communication skills has been an increasing need among the doctor fraternity in our country.

Communication is not only verbal in nature but also includes non-verbal communication. It is verbal and non-verbal communication together that enhance the communication process between two individuals. Verbal communication is the spoken (and or written) words whereas non-verbal communication entails body language, eye contact, gestures, tone and pitch of language. Effective communication can be established by engaging in active listening.

Components of Active Listening

Pay Attention

One goal of active listening is to set a comfortable tone that gives your patient an opportunity to think and speak. Allow "wait time" before responding. Don't cut patients off, finish their sentences, or start formulating your answer before they've finished. Pay attention to your body language as well as your frame of mind. Be focused on the moment, and operate from a place of respect.

Being Non-Judgmental

Active listening requires an open mind. As a listener and a doctor, be open to new ideas, new perspectives, and new possibilities apart from the factual information that you are aware of. Even when good listeners have strong views, they suspend judgment, hold any criticisms, and avoid arguing or selling their point right away.

Reflect

Don't assume that you understand your patient correctly — or that they know you've heard them. Mirror your patient's information and emotions by periodically paraphrasing key points. Reflecting is a way to indicate that you and your counterpart are on the same page.

Clarify

Don't be shy to ask questions about any issue that is ambiguous or unclear. If you have doubt or confusion about what your patient has said, say something like, "Let me see if I'm clear. Are you talking about ...?" or "Wait a minute. I didn't follow you."

Summarize

Restating key themes as the conversation proceeds confirms and solidifies your grasp of the other person's point of view. It also helps both parties to be clear on mutual responsibilities and follow-up. Briefly summarize what you have understood as you listened, and ask the other person to do the same. Giving a brief restatement of core themes raised by the patient might sound like: "Let me summarize to check my understanding.....Did I get that right?" Restating key themes helps both parties to be clear on mutual responsibilities and follow-up.

Share

Active listening is first about understanding the other person, then about being understood. As you gain a clearer understanding of the other person's perspective, you can begin to introduce your ideas, feelings and suggestions. You might talk about a similar experience you had or share an idea that was triggered by a comment made previously in the conversation.

Ask Open Ended Questions

Open-ended, clarifying, and probing questions are important tools that encourage the patient to do the work of self-reflection and problem solving, rather than justifying or defending a position, or trying to guess the "right answer." Open ended questions allow the person to think beyond yes and no answers.

Paraphrase

Sometimes patients go on talking about their distress, it is best not to interrupt them, allow them to complete and pay attention while they speak. Once they are done, it is good to summarize and sometimes paraphrase what they said so patients feel that you are on the same page as them. Paraphrasing is saying the same what patients say but in different words while maintain the essence of what they said.

Listening not only involves understanding the verbal component but also eliciting patient's attitudes, needs and motives behind the words. The goal of listening is, also, to delve into the physical, social and emotional impact of these problems on the patient's quality of life so as to provide holistic care and satisfaction.

Benefits of Good Communication

The practice of good communication skills in the medical profession is integral for the following:

- Development of meaningful and trustworthy relationship between the doctors and patients
- It is beneficial to both the doctors and patients
- The diagnostic capability of the doctor is greatly enhanced because of better understanding of patient's problems
- It is also useful in managing difficult clinical encounters and thus decreases the frustration of both the doctor and the patient or attendant in situations of emotional outbursts
- It has also been shown to decrease work stress and increase job satisfaction for doctors
- Patients feel more understood and heard out which can enhance their prognostic ability

The Role and Need for Empathy

Empathy is defined as, "the ability to understand and share the feelings of another." It is the capacity to put one's self in another's shoes and feel what that person is going through and share their emotions and feelings. It is the recognition and validation of a patient's fear, anxiety, pain and worry. It is the ability to understand patients' feelings and facilitate a more accurate diagnoses and more caring treatment. Empathy extends far beyond a patient's medical history, signs and symptoms. It is more than a clinical diagnosis and treatment. Empathy encompasses a connection and an understanding that includes the mind, body and soul. Expressing empathy is highly effective and powerful, which builds patient trust, calms anxiety and improves health outcomes. Research has shown empathy and compassion to be associated with better adherence to medications, decreased malpractice cases, fewer mistakes, and increased patient satisfaction. Expressing empathy, one patient at a time, advances humanism in healthcare. Nevertheless, it goes without saying that physicians cannot fully experience the suffering of each patient.

Physicians can engage in empathy by ensuring:

- To keep in check personal prejudices and stereotypes
- Make eye contact with the patient
- Paying attention to non-verbal cues of the patients and of self as well
- Listen to the patient attentively, engage in active listening

Rapport Building in Patient Care

Establishing rapport is central to any health professional-patient encounter. O'Toole defines rapport as the development of a therapeutic relationship based on mutual understanding (respect, empathy and trust). Developing a positive relationship with a patient enables the health practitioner to elicit pertinent information and make informed clinical decisions about their treatment and ongoing care. However, rapport is more than that. It promotes communication, collaboration, and a shared understanding of the patient's perspective.

The most important reason for health professionals to establish rapport with patients is the positive impact this has on patient outcomes. A positive trusting relationship between a health care practitioner and patient facilitates the garnering of information vital to the establishment of a diagnosis and correct treatment options. In addition, a patient in a collaborative relationship with a health care practitioner they trust and respect is more likely to adhere to their treatment. Key studies in this area have confirmed the link between the establishment of this positive relationship and patient outcomes. Furthermore, patients who have experienced positive rapport with their health practitioners report better levels of satisfaction with their treatment and are less likely to make a complaint or file malpractice suits. With communication and the skill of

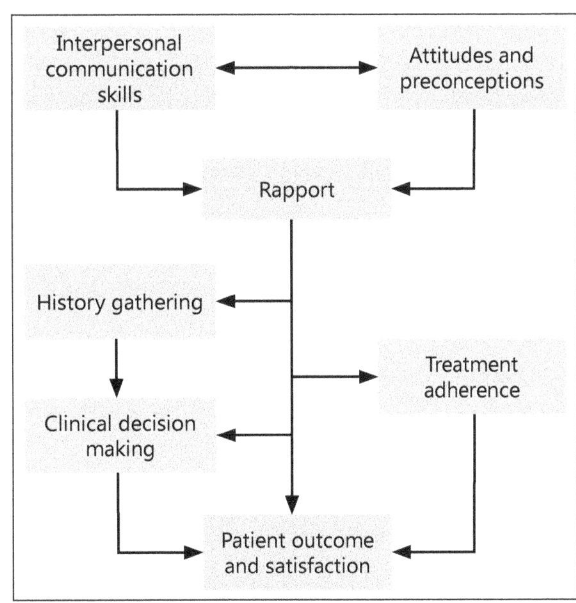

Figure 6.1: Relationship between rapport and patient outcomes.

building patient rapport integral to patient care and outcomes it is vital that the teaching of these skills be included in undergraduate health care professional education.

Steps to Build a Rapport with Your Patient

1. Many a times patients do not walk in your cabin with a lot of comfort, they may be distressed for various reasons. Make sure one of the first things you do is to make them comfortable, which could start with a simple introduction of yourself or you asking about them.
2. Small talks on how was their day or how did they manage to reach to your clinic are some ways to reduce distress.
3. Most of us are experts at listening to a patient's lung and bowel sounds, as well as their answers to our questions about symptoms. But we don't always listen in a way that builds our understanding of where our patients are coming from or what's truly on their minds. At some point, just leave everything and sit to listen.
4. When you validate what your patient says, you're telling them that you hear and understand their concerns, but you're not telling them what you think they should do about it. By validating your patient's feelings, you open the door to learning more about their feelings and experience, and this can improve care.
5. Be open and honest about what you have to tell your patient including what your limitations are as a professional. Being defensive doesn't help.
6. Attend to the inconveniences of your patient and let your staff do the same.
7. Keep the patient well informed about procedures and reasons for if you have to excuse yourself for getting medications or attend to an emergency.
8. Medical experiences can be frightening and disorienting, so patients find it reassuring to be kept informed of what care is being given and planned for them.
9. Answer the questions of your patients if they want to know either out of curiosity or anxiety. Addressing their concerns make patients feel better.

Communication Skills and Handling Difficult Patients

With effective communication skills, doctors can ensure to be confident while handling difficult patients. Anywhere between 15%-20% of encounters between doctor-patient are labelled as difficult. Difficult patient relationships involve imbalance between the expectations, perceptions and the conduct of the doctor and the patient. Difficult encounters may occur when a doctor deals with a patient having several medical complexities, at times, a patient may present with misleading information from internet and pose challenging situation leading to professional burnout of the physician. Furthermore, lack of adequate knowledge or time or even negative bias towards the patient's ailment may attribute to difficult encounter. Besides, poor communication skills and psychosocial attitudes along with lesser job satisfaction among the doctors may also contribute to such difficult encounters. Being honest and transparent about the information asked by patients, revealing balanced details requested by the patient, asking open ended questions, addressing the patient's emotional concerns and sometimes mutually planning the treatment agenda with patients are some helpful components of effective communication that can help a doctor handle difficult patient encounters.

The Role of Communication in Breaking Bad News

Though it may be a daily affair of doctors to see patients lose their lives, it is an equally important skill to be able to convey the bad news to the caregivers / family of the patient. Disclosing bad news is a complex communication art that not only involves verbal component of actual news breaking but also includes empathetic response of the doctor to tackle the reaction. Poor communication skills of an inexperienced clinician can ruin the goal of providing support to the patient and eliciting patient's collaboration for future treatment. Studies have demonstrated that many doctors lack competence as well as confidence in their ability to divulge bad news and there is necessity to provide didactic training.

7 Essential Investigations in Patients having Psychiatric Disorders

Elvin Lukose • Heena Merchant Pandit

Medical investigation and testing in psychiatric patients have received credible interest in the last half a century given the increasing prevalence of deaths secondary to non-psychiatric illnesses resulting either from the use of psychotropic medications or from co-existing morbidities exacerbated as a result of the psychiatric illness and its treatment. Risk factors associated to medical co-morbidity include tobacco use, alcohol, poor dietary habits and obesity. Comorbid illnesses arising from the use of psychotropic medications include obesity, metabolic syndrome and hormonal disturbances. Testing can also help in ruling out organic disorders mimicking psychiatric syndromes and therefore, utilize time in adequate and appropriate treatments. These can have a cumulative effect on the overall health related quality of life and the mortality rate in the psychiatric population. Hence, identifying modifiable medical risk factors and illnesses early on during treatment can act as an intervention aimed at primary prevention. A holistic management will thus enable in improving the quality of life and in prolongation of survival.

Essential investigations in psychiatric care will be studied under as follows:

- *Clinical Biochemistry*
- *Vitamin Assays*
- *Toxicology Studies*
- *Electro-Encephalography*
- *Polysomnography*
- *Electro-cardiogram*
- *Hormonal Studies*

CLINICAL BIOCHEMISTRY

Serum electrolyte levels are done in the routine initial evaluation of a psychiatric patient. Levels of serum electrolytes often are abnormal in patients in confusional states like delirium and substance related intoxication or withdrawal. Abnormalities are also commonly seen in response to the administration of psychotropic medications

Blood Electrolytes

Sodium: Low Sodium levels are seen in psychogenic polydypsia and more commonly seen secondary to SSRIs, mood stabilizers like Carbamazepine and first generation anti-psychotics, the probable etiology of hyponatremia due to first two causes being SIADH i.e. Syndrome of inappropriate secretion of Anti-Diuretic Syndrome. Symptoms of hyponatremia may range from irritability to frank delirium.

Chloride: Low serum chloride levels occur in eating disorders: in patients who purge by self-induced vomiting who present with hypochloremic alkalosis.

Bicarbonate: Serum bicarbonate levels may be elevated in patients who purge or who abuse laxatives in purgative type of eating disorders. Bicarbonate levels are commonly low in patients who hyperventilate in response to anxiety.

Potassium: Low Potassium levels may be present in Anorexia Nervosa and Bulimia Nervosa patients who purge or abuse laxatives. Non-potassium sparing diuretic abuse by these patients also may produce hypokalemia. Characteristic ECG changes in hypokalemia include U waves, flattened T waves and ST-segment depression..

Calcium: Low serum calcium levels are associated with depression, delirium and irritability. Elevated levels are associated with depression, psychosis and weakness. Laxative abuse, common in eating disorder patients, can be associated with hypocalcemia.

Magnesium: Magnesium levels may be low in patients with alcohol dependence. Low magnesium levels are associated with agitation, confusion and delirium. If untreated, convulsions and coma may follow.

Phosphorus: Low levels of serum phosphorus are seen in eating disorders with purging behavior. Phosphorus levels may also be low in hyperventilation syndrome. Hyperparathyroidism independently or secondary to Lithium may produce low serum phosphorus levels.

Copper: Serum copper levels are low in Wilson's disease. Laboratory assessment for Wilson's disease includes the measurement of serum ceruloplasmin (low) and urine copper, measured in a 24-hour specimen (elevated).

Liver Function Tests

The drugs used in psychiatry and neurology are the second most important group of drugs implicated in liver injury after anti-infectious drugs. Serum ammonia levels are often elevated in patients with hepatic encephalopathy. High levels are associated with the delirium of hepatic encephalopathy. Serum ammonia levels also may be elevated in patients undergoing treatment with valproate.

Table 7.1: Classifies the types of drug induced liver injury and the causative agents.

Acute Liver Injury	*Hepatocellular type* Bupropion Fluoxetine Nefazodone Paroxetine Sertraline Risperidone Sodium Valproate Agomelatine *Cholestatic type* Chlorpromazine Phenothiazines TCAs (Imipramine, Amitryptiline) *Mixed type* Amitryptiline Carbamazepine Phenytoin
Chronic Liver injury	*Steatosis* Sodium Valproate (micro-vesicular) Clozapine Olanzapine
Others	Naltrexone Disulfiram Divalproate Sodium (Divalproex) Diazepam Chlordiazepoxide

LFT should thus be considered in high risk population (history of alcohol dependence, liver disease, multiple organ disease etc.) before initiation of the above mentioned drugs.

Renal Function Tests

Tests of renal function include BUN, Creatinine and Creatinine Clearance. Most of psychotropics are considered to be safe in renal disorders. However, drugs that may require additional attention during treatment on account of their action on kidney function and possible exacerbation of any underlying renal disease are as follows:

- Lithium
- Acamprosate
- Topiramate
- Pregabalin
- Gabapentin
- Disulfiram
- Diazepam
- Chlordiazepoxide

BUN and 24 hour- creatinine clearance are sensitive indicators of drug related kidney injury, hence initial and later semi-annual monitoring may be required during treatment with the above mentioned drugs.

Apart from routine investigations, urinary level of porphobilinogen is valuable in diagnosis of Acute intermittent porphyria which presents with psychiatric symptoms of agitation and paranoia during acute attacks

TOXICOLOGY STUDIES

Toxicological studies in psychiatric population include therapeutic drug monitoring and screening tests for drugs of abuse. Commonly screened drugs include alcohol, barbiturates, benzodiazepines, cocaine metabolites, opiates, phencyclidine and tetrahydro-cannabinol.

Different specimens that can be tested for substances of abuse are–

- *Urine*
- *Blood*
- *Saliva*
- *Sweat patch*
- *Hair*
- *Fingernails*

Analytical methods of detection are *Enzyme Immuno-assays(EIAs)* and *Chromatography* techniques that include Gas Liquid- Mass Spectrometry (GL-MS) and Thin layer Chromatography (TLC)

Blood alcohol level (BAL) may be useful in patients with acute alcohol intoxication and levels commonly lie in between 100 and 300 mg/dL. The degree of alcohol intoxication can also be assessed using the concentration of alcohol using a breath analyzer.

Findings in Alcoholic Liver Disease

Alcoholic liver disease includes Fatty Liver, Alcoholic hepatitis and Liver Cirrhosis. Hepatic Encephalopathy is a late stage complication with fatal outcomes. Alcoholic liver disease is characterized by elevations in AST and ALT, typically in a ratio of AST to ALT of 2:1 or greater. The γ-glutamyl transpeptidase (GGT) level may be elevated. Following findings and investigations can help in diagnosis and starting appropriate interventions for pharmacotherapy and prevention.

Table 7.2

Fatty Liver	Elevated AST, ALT, Bilirubin
Alcoholic Hepatitis	Elevated AST, ALT & bilirubin, prolonged prothrombin time
Liver Cirrhosis	Elevated AST (more specific), Bilirubin, prolonged PT, low serum albumin low, diagnostic liver biopsy, altered cirrhotic echotexture on USG, portal Doppler for porto-systemic shunts
Hepatic Encephalopathy	Deranged LFTs, elevated serum ammonia, prolonged PT, abnormal EEG (triphasic complexes)

Useful findings in Alcohol use related complications

Alcohol dependence may provide a very diverse hematological profile owing to the direct damage by alcohol, changes secondary to nutritional deficiencies and disorders affecting organs involve in blood circulation like liver and spleen.

Table 7.3

Anemia	Macrocytosis, stomatocytes (hemolysis), siderocytes, low ferritin
Folate Deficiency	Macro-ovalocytes with hypersegmented neutrophils, MCV > 110 fL, low serum folate, elevated homocysteinemia.
Liver disease	Target cells, Spur cells (advanced cirrhosis)
Hypophosphatemia (especially during withdrawal)	Microspherocytosis, hypochromasia, serum phosphate level < 0.5 mg/dL
Hypersplenism	Macrocytosis (mild), anisocytosis, spherocytosis

VITAMIN ASSAYS

Vitamin B9 (Folate) and Vitamin B12 (Cyanacobalamin)

Folate and B12 deficiencies are most commonly seen in patients with alcohol dependence. Folate and B12 deficiencies are associated with dementia, delirium, paranoid ideation, fatigue, and personality disturbances.

Low folate levels may be also found in patients who use OCPs or other forms of estrogen, who drink alcohol, or who are on anti-epileptic treatment with Phenytoin.

Folate and B12 deficiencies are also responsible for majority of reversible dementias hence Vitamin B12 and folate are included in routine work up for Dementia.

THERAPEUTIC DRUG MONITORING

Lithium

Lithium is a mood stabilizer with anti-suicidal properties. On account of its narrow therapeutic index, blood levels of lithium must be monitored to achieve therapeutic dosing and avoid toxicity. Effective serum concentrations for mania are 1.0 to 1.5 mEq/L with the recommended range for maintenance treatment being 0.4 to 0.8 mEq/L. Symptoms of toxicity may begin to manifest with serum levels greater than 1.2 mEq/L. Clinical toxicity, especially in elderly persons, has been documented within the therapeutic range of 0.5 to 1.5 mEq/L. Regular therapeutic drug monitoring of Lithium levels should be obtained every 2 to 6 months. Weekly levels may be required in cases where there are signs of toxicity, during dosage adjustments, and in persons suspected to be noncompliant to treatment. When obtaining blood for lithium levels, patients should be at steady-state lithium dosing (usually after 5 days of constant dosing) and the blood sample must be drawn 12 hours after a given dose. Artefacts and false laboratory values may result from the collection of blood in tubes with lithium-heparin anticoagulant. Effective serum concentration for mania is in the range of 1.0 to 1.5 mEq/L. The recommended range for maintenance treatment is 0.4 to 0.8 mEq/L. Side effects have to be managed based on clinical presentation of signs and symptoms even when the Lithium levels are within the therapeutic range.

Clozapine

TDM of Clozapine levels is determined by its trough levels before administration of the morning dose of medication. Statistical data correlating serum levels with onset of response and side effects recommend a level of 100 mg/mL as the minimum therapeutic threshold. At least 350 mg/mL is considered to be requisite to achieve therapeutic response in patients with refractory schizophrenia. There is a 4% risk of seizures in users taking doses greater than 600 mg/day with a linear increase in the likelihood of seizures and other side effects with levels greater than 1,200 mg/mL. Clozapine also causes leucopenia and agranulocytosis in 1% of user population. Hence, WBC monitoring weekly for first 6 months of treatment can help in early diagnosis and prevention of fatal outcomes. A leukocyte count of less than 3000-3500 cells/mm^3 on CBC conducted prior to treatment is a contraindication to starting Clozapine.

Carbamazepine

The anticonvulsant blood concentration range for carbamazepine is 4 to 12 μg/ml. Most side effects are seen at levels above 9 μg/ml. There is no consistent data on therapeutic levels in mood disorders although a level between 4-7 μg/ml corresponding to a dose of approximately 600 mg/day is recommended. Carbamazepine is seen to cause clinically insignificant suppression of the WBC count commonly occurs during carbamazepine treatment however potential serious hematologic effects of carbamazepine include pancytopenia, agranulocytosis, and aplastic anemia occurring in about 1 in 125,000 patients necessitating pretreatment hematological work up. Routine liver and renal function tests can help in diagnosis of Carbamazepine induced hepatitis and hyponatremia respectively. Carbamazepine treatment should be discontinued if total WBC count is below 3,000/mm^3, erythrocytes below 4.0×10^6/mm^3, neutrophils below 1,500/mm^3, hematocrit less than 32 percent, hemoglobin less than 11 g/100 mL, platelet count below 100,000/mm3, reticulocyte count below 0.3 percent, and if a serum iron concentration is below 150 mg/100 mL.

Valproate

Antimanic response is generally associated with levels greater than 50 μg/mL, in a range of 50 to 150 μg/mL. Routine liver function tests are indicated due to incidence of hepatic damage on treatment. Valproate and divalproex may cause a sustained elevation in liver transaminase levels upto three times the upper limit of normal posing a high risk for serious hepatotoxicity. Hematological abnormalities include leucopenia and thrombocytopenia. Treatment with valproate may cause hyperammonemia with resultant cognitive impairment and in extreme cases, hyperammonemia-induced encephalopathy. Suspected cases with altered mental status or lethargy may thus, require monitoring of serum levels of ammonia for diagnosis. Thrombocytopenia and platelet dysfunction occur most commonly at high dosages and result in the prolongation of bleeding times. A pretreatment urine pregnancy test is usually obtained in women of childbearing years for early detection of birth defects known to occur from folate deficiency as a consequence of valproate treatment.

ELECTRO-ENCEPHALOGRAPHY

Many neurological syndromes like dementia, epilepsy and movement disorders have significant psychiatric overlap and EEG can serve to distinguish or rule out an organic diagnosis. EEG is also used during electroconvulsive therapy (ECT) to monitor seizure activity, and as a component of polysomnography in the evaluation of sleep disorders. A standard array consists of 21 electrodes. Placement of the electrodes is based on the 10/20 International System of Electrode Placement.

Table 7.4: Common EEG Abnormalities

Diffuse slowing	Most common however non specific for encephalopathies
Focal slowing	Local parenchymal disorder Local epileptic focus (space occupying lesions, hematomas etc.)
Triphasic waves	Hepatic Encephalopathy Toxic and metabolic encephalopathies
Spike and wave discharges	Epileptic disorders
Periodic lateralizing epileptiform discharges	Focal destructive brain lesions (eg. HSV Encephalitis)
Periodic sharp waves (PSWs)	Creutzfeldt- Jakob Disease
Beta fast activity	Alcohol withdrawal Benzodiazepine and Barbiturate use
Increased voltage of alpha activity	Cocaine Marijuana Nicotine
Increased voltage of theta activity	Alcohol use Caffeine withdrawal Opioid overdose

Psychiatrists utilize EEG to rule out non-psychiatric disease in cases where behavioral abnormalities in seizure disorders or delirium can present as psychiatric syndromes. In the presence of suspected strokes, tumors, subdural hematomas, or dementia, the yield is usually higher with neuro-imaging. In addition, the EEG is commonly obtained when there is an abnormal CT or MRI.

POLYSOMNOGRAPHY

Polysomnography is an array of multiple parametric observations utilized in sleep studies for sleep and sleep related disorders. Electro-encephalogram, electromyogram (ocular muscle movements, submental activity, leg muscles), electrocardiogram, nasal–oral airflow, respiratory effort, oxyhemoglobin saturation, heart rhythm, and leg movements during sleep are measured.

Indications for polysomnography include:

- Diagnosis of sleep-related breathing disorders
- Positive airway pressure titration and assessment of treatment efficacy (CPAP)
- Sleep Related Behavior Disorders (Somnambulism, REM Sleep Behavioral Disorder)

ELECTROCARDIOGRAM

The ECG is commonly used in psychiatry for:

- Differential diagnoses in Anxiety disorders
- Pre-anesthetic assessment for Electro-Convulsive Therapy (ECT)
- Assessment of side effects of psychotropic medications

Following disorders can be assessed using an ECG for organic differential diagnosis of anxiety symptoms:

- *Myocardial Infarction*
- *Paroxysmal Atrial Tachycardia*
- *Mitral Valve Prolapse*
- *Hypertension (hypertrophic changes)*
- *Pulmonary Embolism*

Most of the psychotropics affect heart rate and cause slowing in conduction pathways with development of ectopic beats; arrhythmias and prolongation of QTc interval >440 ms.

Table 7.5

QTc prolongation	Anti-psychotics: IV Anti-psychotic, Pimozide, Sertindole, Haloperidol, Quetiapine, Ziprasidone, Asenapine, Olanzapine, Thioridazine Anti-Depressants: TCAs, Citalopram, Trazodone
Atrial/Ventricular ectopic beats	Reboxetine
Ventricular tachycardia	Duloxetine
Asystole	Venlafaxine
Prolongation of the PR, QT and QRS intervals ***ST-segment*** ***T-wave abnormalities***	Tricyclic Antidepressants Lithium
Bundle Branch Blocks ***Brugada Syndrome***	Tricyclic Antidepressants Lithium

Hence, ECG is advisable before starting the above mentioned medications. Echocardiogram (2D- Echo) may also be necessary to rule out any cardiac insufficiency or anatomical pathology like Mitral Valve Prolapse before procuring fitness for ECT. Holter monitoring could be useful for the evaluation of dizziness, palpitations and syncope.

HORMONAL STUDIES

Many endocrine disorders like hypothyroidism and Cushing's disease have been known to show psychiatric symptoms. The confounding nature and presence of comorbid hormonal disturbance in primary psychiatric disorders have created further interest in the endocrine disorders. Modern use of second generation/atypical antipsychotics has ushered in a diverse metabolic profile of side effects compared to the first generation anti-psychotics. Due to their long term nature, hormonal studies are vital in the management of psychiatric illnesses for appropriate choice of anti-psychotics and mitigation of side effects.

Prolactin

Prolactin is synthesised from the anterior lobe of the pituitary gland. The secretion of prolactin is under direct inhibitory regulation by dopaminergic neurons located in the tuberoinfundibular section of the hypothalamus. Blockade of these neurons by psychotropics therefore result in elevated prolactin levels.

Pathological causes of hyperprolactinemia include pituitary adenomas, infiltrative tumors of the pituitary gland and hypothalamic disease. More relevant to psychiatry are the pharmacological causes that include anti-psychotics (Amisulpride, Risperidone, Phenothiazines), SSRIs (Esitalopram, Paroxetine, Sertraline), TCAs (Imipramine, Clomipramine, Dosulepin), Synthetic opioids (Methadone) and some MAO inhibitors (Clorgyline).

If the prolactin level is less than 2,000 mIU/L (~95 ng/mL), elevations are most likely secondary to psychotropic medication; if the level is greater than 2,500 mIU/L (~118 mg/mL), in the absence of breast-feeding or pregnancy, a pituitary tumor may be suspected and neuro-imaging advised.

Prolactin levels may peak 10-20 minutes following a seizure returning to baseline after 6 hours. For this reason, a two fold increase in baseline levels of prolactin after possible seizure activity may assist in differentiating a seizure from a pseudoseizure.

Thyroid hormone

Hypothyroidism can cause depressive symptoms while hyper-thyroidism can cause mania, anxiety and irritability. Indications of thyroid function tests in psychiatry include ruling out primary hypothyroidism. Subclinical hypothyroidism can often complicate and create treatment resistance in the pharmacological treatment of depression and cause rapid cycling in bipolar mood disorder. In elderly population, thyroid abnormalities are reversible causes of dementia. Mood stabilizers like Lithium and Carbamazepine can cause secondary hypothyroidism and cognitive impairment. Hence, TFTs should be periodically conducted in patients on Lithium and Carbamazepine.

Human Chorionic Gonadotropin

Urine Human chorionic gonadotropin (hCG) test is a routine test for pregnancy. Due to evidence of teratogenicity, pregnancy tests are considered before initiating certain psychotropic medications, such as lithium, carbamazepine, and valproate, which are associated with congenital anomalies especially in those in the reproductive age group.

Steroids

Both Hypo-adrenalism and Cushing's syndrome can cause psychiatric symptoms like psychosis, depression, fatigue, delirium and cognitive slowing. Low plasma levels of cortisol are found in Addison's disease whereas elevated levels of cortisol are seen in Cushing's syndrome.

Anabolic steroid abuse is associated with irritability, aggression, depression, and psychosis. Athletes and bodybuilders and patients with Body dysmorphic disorder (with muscle dysmorphia) are common abusers of anabolic steroids. Urine specimens can be used to screen for anabolic steroid and its metabolites. Generally, androgens other than testosterone can be detected by gas chromatography and mass spectroscopy.

Anti-Diuretic Hormone

Polydipsia in psychiatry can be either due to psychogenic factors or secondary to psychotropic use. Levels of ADH may thus help in ruling out iatrogenic from primary pathology of ADH secretion.

Lithium has been shown to decrease the sensitivity of renal tubules to AVP and hence cause Lithium induced Diabetes Insipidus (nephrogenic type). Syndrome of inappropriate secretion of ADH (SIADH) may develop in response to head injury to the base of the brain or from psychotropic use (including phenothiazines, butyrophenones, Carbamazepine, Oxcarbazepine and SSRIs).

ADDITIONAL NOTES

Anti-Depressants

Routine laboratory studies like CBC, serum electrolytes, and liver function tests should be considered before initiation of antidepressants. Because TCAs (tricyclic antidepressants) affect cardiac conduction, electrocardiogram (ECG) maybe required to assess for the presence of abnormalities in cardiac rhythm and prolonged PR, QRS and QTc (torsades de pointes) complexes before initiation. Treatment with MAOIs is occasionally associated with hepatotoxicity. For this reason, liver function tests usually are obtained at the initiation of treatment and periodically after.

Electroconvulsive Therapy

Electroconvulsive therapy (ECT) is non-invasive form of brain stimulation indicated routinely in cases with suicidal behavior, aggression and treatment resistance. Typical laboratory tests obtained for the pre-anesthetic check up prior to the administration of ECT include CBC, serum electrolytes, liver function tests, ECG and Chest X-ray.

Neuroleptic Malignant Syndrome

Neuroleptic malignant syndrome (NMS) is potentially fatal, consequence of neuroleptic administration in 0.01 to 0.02 percent of patients treated with antipsychotics. The syndrome consists of autonomic instability, hyperpyrexia, severe extrapyramidal symptoms like tremors and rigidity and in some cases, delirium. Rhabdomyolysis from the sustained muscle contraction results in elevated levels of creatine kinase (CK). In NMS, CK levels greater than 1000 international units/L, however, are more specific and the degree of CK elevation correlates with disease severity and prognosis. Myoglobinuria can occur due to acute kidney injury or acute renal failure. Elevated liver enzymes will reveal incipient liver failure. A typical laboratory workup for NMS includes a CBC, serum electrolytes, BUN, Cr, CPK (both total and MB). Additionally, urine myoglobin can be done to assess for any renal damage. Pronounced elevations in the white blood cell (WBC) count may occur in NMS typically in the range from 10,000 to 40,000 per mm^3. A low serum iron concentration (mean 5.71 μmol/L; normal 11 to 32 μmol/L) is commonly seen in NMS patients and is a sensitive but not specific marker for NMS among acutely ill psychiatric patients.

NEURO-IMAGING

Computed tomography and Magnetic Resonance Imaging are routinely performed in cases with neuro-psychiatric overlap symptoms. Additionally, tests like PET, SPECT, Magnetic Resonance Spectroscopy, functional MRI and Diffusion Tensor Imaging are only indicatedin special cases.

Neuro-imaging is commonly advised in psychiatric cases to rule out:

- Head Injury
- Epileptic foci
- Cerebro-vascular accidents
- Space-occupying lesions
- Encephalitides
- Dementia
- Demyelinating disorders

Computed Tomography

CT Scans take a series of X-ray pictures from all vantage points, 360 degrees around a patient's head. The computer uses matrix algebra calculations to assign a specific density to each point within the head; the end result of which is a set of two-dimensional images. Iodine based contrast agents allow for better appreciation of space-occupying lesions and areas of inflammation by the extent of radiation absorbed by the iodine. The value of CT scan over MRI remains in its ability to detect hemorrhage, hematomas and bone fractures in emergency cases.

Magnetic Resonance Imaging

MRI is currently the choice of neuro-imaging in non-emergency cases. MRI is based on the principle of nuclear magnetic resonance (NMR) of hydrogen atoms. The rate of realignment of the hydrogen axis is determined by a combination of both the nature of the molecule of which it is a part and the degree to which it is surrounded by water. Hydrogen nuclei within different tissue contents align and re-align at different rates and hence, soft tissues appear well delineated in MRI as compared to CT scans. **MRI protocol for epilepsy** is a group of MRI sequences put together to improve sensitivity and specificity in identifying possible structural abnormalities that underlie seizure disorders (e.g. mesial temporal sclerosis) using 3 tesla MRI (3T MRI).

Common types of findings assessed in neuro-psychiatric disorders include:

- ✓ Ischemic/Infarct zones (water-shed infarcts)
- ✓ White Matter Hyper-intensities (peri-ventricular and deep white matter)
- ✓ Ventricular dilatations
- ✓ Atrophy of cortex or deep nuclei (caudate nucleus, globus pallidus)

Special additional variations include Perfusion Weighted Imaging (PWI) and Diffusion Weighted Imaging (DWI) usually performed in patients with strokes to delineate salvageable brain tissue and decide on thrombolysis.

BIBLIOGRAPHY

1. Bottomley, S. (2019). Nutritional Syndromes with Anemia: Alcohol. In R. Means Jr (Ed.), *Nutritional Anemia: Scientific Principles, Clinical Practice, and Public Health* (pp. 175-188). Cambridge: Cambridge University Press. doi:10.1017/9781139023993.015
2. Lal, Rakesh. "Substance use disorder–manual for physicians." *New Delhi: National Drug Dependence Treatment Centre, All India Institute of Medical Sciences* (2005).
3. Berman, Brian D. "Neuroleptic malignant syndrome: a review for neurohospitalists." *The Neurohospitalist* 1.1 (2011): 41-47.
4. Walters, James, and Ian Jones. "Clinical questions and uncertainty—prolactin measurement in patients with schizophrenia and bipolar disorder." *Journal of Psychopharmacology* 22.2_suppl (2008): 82-89.
5. David, Daniel, et al. *Lishman's Organic Psychiatry: A Textbook of Neuropsychiatry*. John Wiley & Sons, 2012.
6. Ellingrod, Vicki L. "How to modify psychotropic therapy for patients who have liver dysfunction." *Current Psychiatry* 13.12 (2014).

8 Basics of EEG for Undergraduates

Suyog Jaiswal • Pranav U. Pohane

KEY POINTS

- There has been a shift to common genetic and mechanistic factors across psychiatric disorders; electroencephalography (EEG) measures are well suited to be used as putative biomarkers within this approach.
- In order to be more effective biomarkers of neural circuit activity, EEG research must successfully contend with controversies within the field regarding:
  1. The use of different EEG measurements (event-related potentials, quantitative EEG and time frequency measures)
  2. Analysis of cortical sources rather than scalp signals.
- Advances in signal processing software are making it increasingly feasible for researchers to successfully address both controversies within their own research.
- Future directions using advanced signal processing and statistical methods will result in identification of better, more effective biomarkers and a reconceptualization of a diagnostic or treatment target to a map of translational domains that will define a richer landscape within which individual and group differences can be quantified.

HISTORY & OVERVIEW OF EEG

Brain has always been an organ of fascination for the clinicians and scientists across the globe, especially because though the knowledge that brain acts as a central command system for the body was commonplace, but not much was known about the complex functions of brains such as emotional regulations and cognition. Owing to lack of sophisticated non-invasive techniques to study the functions of brain, the human brain had remained a mystery to early brain researchers. One method to study the brain function is to study the electric discharges generated by the brain and this is done through scalp electrodes and it's termed as electroencephalogram (EEG). First EEG was recorded by Richard Caton from exposed brain cortices of animals. This proved the existence of brain derived electric potential. Subsequently brain researcher works by various scientists like Vaisili Danilevsky, Adolph Beck & Napolean Cybulski established the facts that the electrical activity of brain responds to photic stimulation, local injury. The electric stimulus to the cortex was used to induce brain-wave seizure discharges, thus prestaging the use of EEG in epilepsy. For fifty years since the first EEG recording in animal, the human EEG elusive, till the German professor of psychiatry Hans Berger in 1924 successfully recorded the first human EEG. In subsequent years he published several papers to bring the EEG in position of acceptance and clinical usefulness. He is also the one who coined the term *electroencephalogram*.

Over next two decades the EEG was extensively studied in various psychiatric and neurological conditions. In 1934 Fred Gibbs discovered the classic three per second spike and wave complex of petit mal seizure. Subsequently he and his team discovered the diffuse spike and wave EEG patterns associated with grand mal and myoclonic seizure. The complex partial seizure was described as psychomotor seizure with EEG manifestations during the ictal psychomotor disturbance. Similarly, there was also a rejuvenation of interest in uncovering the brain secrets of psychiatric disorders through EEG investigations and the quest to find answers had one more tool to wield. The various investigation revealed that almost all psychiatric disorders are associated with increased minor abnormalities in EEG when compared to healthy individuals. These EEG changes were however neither consistent nor specific to single or a spectrum of known psychiatric disorders. With the emergence of latest technology & sophistication in EEG recording the quest for finding specific EEG marker for psychiatric disorders is progressing again. Today EEG forms one of the basic and fairly popular investigations for various neuropsychiatric disorders due to its non-invasive nature and load of information it delivers in a cheaper way. The high degree of skill required in recording and interpreting along with dynamic nature of brain electrical activity are still few of the drawbacks of modern EEG.

BASIC SCIENCE OF EEG

The EEG is in its most simplistic sense is a voltmeter which measures the potential difference between two electrodes of a channel (and there are multiple channels). The potential difference is measured in μV, which generally ranges from 30 to 80 μV. Depending on the sensitivity & calibration of the machine, the readings above and below the range can be recorded. The beginning of EEG started with recordings in single channel i.e. recording the potential difference between only two electrode sites on scalp. It soon evolved to multichannel and simultaneous recordings. EEG machines capable of recording up to 256 channels are available in market, but for most clinical purposes one with 32 channels suffices. Higher channel may be required in research settings. EEG is recorded through multiple electrodes placed on scalp and it records whatever electrical impulses accessible to it at the site which may or may not be exclusively originating from the brain cortex. It has multiple interferences from adjacent sites. These interferences are termed as artefacts and nullified digitally as well as manually to obtain good EEG record. The EEG record does not originate from a single neuron or group of neurons closer to the recording site of scalp. It is primarily generated by the summation field potential of excitatory and inhibitory postsynaptic potentials (EPSPs/IPSPs) of cerebral cortical pyramidal neurons. Interactions between thalamic and cortical networks also play a role in generation of rhythmical EEG activity. But because the way the dominant brain waves are generated EEG is recorded represents more of the electrical activities of the cortical areas than the subcortical processes. EEG electrodes record a pool of around 2.5 lacs neurons synchronously to generate a signal at the scalp. Synchronization occurs among neighboring neurons to produce a local field potential. High-frequency waves are likely to be originated from smaller neuronal assemblies, whereas low-frequency oscillations span larger neuronal populations.

EEG RECORDING

EEG recording is generally done in outpatient settings within a controlled environment. Lately 'plug and play' portable EEG machines are available which are a single unit which can be attached to any computer and specific electrode caps to record the EEG.

Electrode Placement

The EEG electrodes are made of high conducting metals and are placed on the scalp after preparation of scalp. The hairs need to be washed and free of oil or grease to facilitate conduction and minimize the impedance. It is a common practice to rub local area slightly with cleansing material to remove superficial epidermis. The electrodes are placed at specific points for EEG recording and conducting gel is used for improving the conduction and stabilizing the electrodes. The 10-20 International System of Electrode Placements is commonly followed in India. From readily identifiable bony landmarks (nasion, inion, and preauricular point), specific measurements are made and then 10% and 20% of a specified distance is used as the interelectrode interval. This enables replication consistently over time, between technicians, and among different laboratories. Each electrode placed is designated an upper-case letter denoting the brain area beneath the electrode and a number. Odd numbers are for left hemisphere and even numbers for right hemisphere. The subscript z is used for denoting the midline electrodes.

Montage

The voltage measurement always requires a reference point to define the potential difference. For EEG readings, the voltages or potentials on the scalp are measured with respect to another point, usually on the scalp or at least on the body. For analogue EEGs the two points are selected and physically connected to the amplifier at the time of the recording and are non-changeable thereafter. For the digital EEGs the signals are recorded with a common reference point and then are converted to digital signals. Digital recordings not only allow combinations of different electrodes but also digital filtering post recording. Significant spatial information is lost by recording with handful of electrodes. This loss is compensated for by recording the signals in orderly arrangement of different electrode derivations, known as montages. Montages allow the localization of EEG data.

In *referential* montages, each electrode is displayed with respect to a common electrode which is relatively inactive. Commonly used reference electrodes are auricular (A1, A2), vertex (Cz), common non cephalic electrode and an average of all scalp electrodes. However, no single reference electrode can be used for all the activities of interest. The reference point needs to be chosen and changed as per the required activity. Another commonly used montage is bipolar montage. Bipolar montages link sequential pairs of electrodes to form chains in the longitudinal (sagittal), transverse (coronal), or circular (axial) directions. In these montages, each electrode is recorded in two adjacent channels. Bipolar montages are ideal for highlighting activity that changes rapidly in space, that is, has a fairly localized field.

Optimal EEG recording combines both referential and bipolar montages. It is recommended that a standard record should include a longitudinal bipolar montage, a transverse bipolar montage, and a referential montage for a comprehensive recording and localization of activities recorded.

Activation Procedures

EEG is a dynamic record and the abnormal electrical discharges are paroxysmal. To increase the chances of recording the EEG abnormalities certain activating procedures are employed. There are various techniques which are used as activation procedures, some of the common ones are *hyperventilation* (patient is asked to over breath deep with mouth open, eyes closed in reclining position for 1-4 minutes), *photic stimulation* (high intensity strobe lights are flashed in a frequency ranging from 1 to 50 Hz), *sleep deprivation* (of 24 hours) & *sleep*.

Artefacts

Artefacts are the unwanted electrical waves arising outside the brain which are picked up on EEG recording. The artefacts may be physiological or non-physiological in origin. Non-physiological artefacts are result of the ambient electrical noise (50 Hz), monitoring equipment, electronics and malfunctioning of electrode due to various reasons. Whereas artefacts of physiological origin include head/neck movements, eye movements/blinking, pulse rate/ECG, muscles and sweat. The artefacts are removed using frequency filters (low & high) to a great extent. Though it may not be possible for new learners to identify all the artefacts in a given EEG recording but an expert reader of EEG can identify most artefacts from pathological EEG oscillations.

WAVEFORMS OF EEG (INCLUDING NORMAL EEG)

Electrical activity from brain consists primarily of rhythms and these rhythms are classified based on its frequency.

- Delta: 3.5 Hz or below.
- Theta: 4-7.5 Hz
- Alpha:8-13 Hz.
- Beta: > 13 Hz.

These different rhythms are found at different ages of the patient and also under different

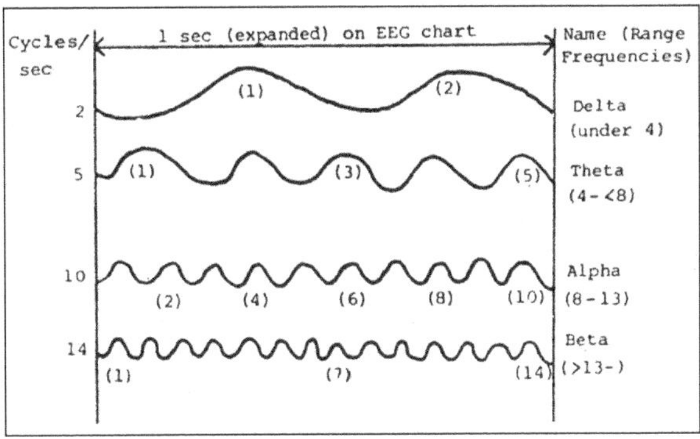

Fig. 8.1

conditions. Usually, there is one dominant frequency, one which is the most prominent in the record which is called as "background rhythm".

- Background rhythm in wake:

  In infants: 4 to 5 Hz (Delta and Theta waves)

  In children: 5 to 8 Hz (Theta)

  In adults: 8 to 10 Hz (Alpha)
- Background rhythm in sleep:

  In light sleep: 5 to 6 Hz (Theta)

  In deep sleep: 2 to 3 Hz (Delta)

Abnormal Patterns

These are mainly divided into two types

1. Slow waves: These are rhythms, appearing especially during wakefulness, that are slower than in the normal. Abnormal slow waves appear when the brain cells are damaged regardless of the etiology of the damage.
2. Spikes (Sharp waves): The spike is the suddenly appearing electrical explosion that looks on the paper record like a spike or large nail. The sharp wave is the same as spike, except for a difference in the duration of the event. Spikes are shorter in duration, usually under 70 milliseconds, while sharp waves range from 70 to 200

milliseconds. These two related patterns usually signify an epileptogenic region of the brain and are found in the patients with seizures.

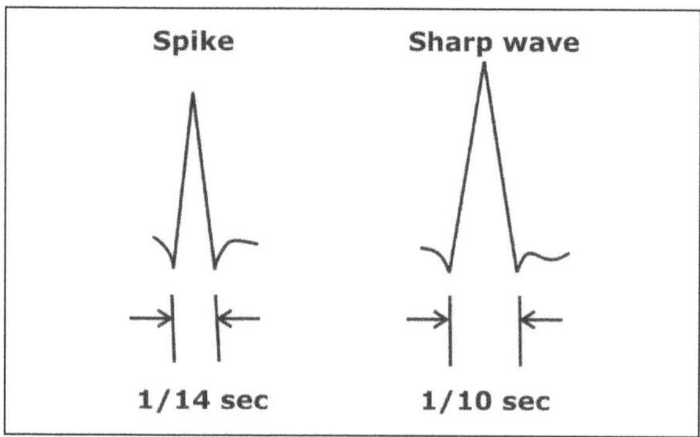

Fig. 8.2

EEG FINDINGS IN ORGANIC PATHOPHYSIOLOGY

Seizures

The interictal background EEG is usually normal in patients with epilepsy. Abnormal interictal EEG waveforms may include non-epileptiform abnormalities and interictal epileptiform discharges (IEDs). The typical EEG findings of an active seizure are spikes or spike-wave discharges. These can be generalized, hemispheric or focal, depending on the origin of the electrical activity. Generalized tonic-clonic or "grand mal" seizures, are often the most dramatic of the generalized seizures with a motor tonic and clonic component. The EEG demonstrates a "recruiting rhythm" that is composed of repetitive alpha frequencies in the maximal anterior head regions. EEG findings shows generalized bursts of sharp and slow waves throughout the EEG. Absence or "petit mal" seizure have a typical 3-Hz spike-and-wave pattern on EEG. When bursts of 3-Hz spike-and-waves are generalized, regular, symmetrical, synchronous, and maximal in the anterior head regions and are longer than 3 sec, the EEG strongly suggests the diagnosis of absence seizures. The focal seizure tends to begin with localized or regional rhythmic activities that slow in frequency as they build in amplitude. As they evolve they propagate to adjacent brain regions. The net result of this is to create an appearance on EEG like a crescendo mark in music. Spike foci, usually in anterior temporal in origin and associated with complex partial seizures are of specific interest to the psychiatrist. Focal clonic seizures often arise from the central region. Tonic seizures may have an origin from nearly any region in the brain, but commonly the frontal lobe.

Space Occupying Lesion

Structural lesions tend to induce focal slowing of rhythms. The irritation caused by the lesion to the surrounding brain area may give rise to the spike along with focal slowing of the rhythm. Cerebral abscess is highly localized lesion which identifies with abnormal slowing of rhythm and spike due to high degree of irritation it induces to the surrounding tissues. Deeper subcortical lesion is less likely it is to generate changes on scalp EEG. The superficial tumors generate more irregular delta waves along with suppression of background rhythms whereas deep tumors have more rhythmical theta waves. Midline tumor are likely to be associated with bilaterally synchronous slow waves maximal frontal or occipital. The cortical tumors are detected 90% of the times on routine EEG investigation, therefore it is advisable to repeat the EEG after reasonable time in cases where minor focal slowing is observed to study the increase in magnitude of activity suggesting growth of tumor.

Vascular Events of Brain

Cerebrovascular accident or transient ischemic attacks present with slowing of activity in the region, whereas hemorrhage is often represented as sharp waves or spike in addition to slow waves. Focal slowing is the sequalae of head trauma at the site of trauma or countercoup site. It may be transient in nature, but if focal spikes appear, it may be regarded as onset of post traumatic seizure disorder. Subdural hematoma identified as slow waves, usually appearing after depression of normal rhythms.

Metabolic and Endocrine Disorders

Since these affect brain in a generalized manner what we see in brain is generally diffuse slowing of background rhythm in wakeful state but no focal changes. The degree of abnormality is correlated with the severity of the disorder and its effect on brain. In cases of hepatic (renal) coma Triphasic waves are seen in the EEG. Subacute sclerosing panencephalitis (SSPE) has a pathognomonic pattern on EEG and consists of short bursts of irregular, bilateral sharp and slow wave complexes, appearing periodically, usually every 5 to 6 sec.

EEG IN PSYCHIATRIC DISORDERS

None of the psychiatric disorders have any specific EEG changes help the diagnosis, therefore it is not an investigation advised very frequently by the psychiatrists. However, it holds a unique position in psychiatry and is requested from time to time. When evaluating the complex and episodic behavioral syndromes, EEG comes as a helpful tool to rule out the complex partial seizure especially temporal lobe epilepsy. EEG is also useful to monitor the seizure activity during the electroconvulsive therapy (ECT) sessions. The EEG changes associated with various psychiatric diagnoses are non-specific and are not of diagnostic value (**Table 8.1**).

Table 8.1: EEG abnormalities associated with Psychiatric disorders

Attention deficit hyperkinetic disorder (ADHD)	EEG abnormalities can be seen in 60 percent cases with ADHD which are Spikes or sharp wave discharges.
Alcohol use disorders	Prominent slowing with in active dependence. In delirium tremens excessive fast activities are seen
Antisocial personality disorder	Increased non-specific abnormalities in the EEG in those with aggressive behavior.
Borderline personality disorder	Spikes can be seen in the 25 percent patients with the Borderline personality disorder.
Schizophrenia	EEG studies indicate that many schizophrenia patients have abnormal records, increased sensitivity to activation procedures, decreased alpha activity, increased theta and delta activity. Evoked Potentials: Large number of abnormalities in evoked potential have been described. Abnormalities in the P300 wave have been reported which smaller in schizophrenia patients than comparison groups. It is large positive evoked-potential wave that occurs about 300 milliseconds after a sensory stimulus is detected.

Table 8.2: EEG changes with psychotropics and substances of abuse

Benzodiazepines	Increased Beta activities
Alcohol	Decreased Alpha and increased Theta activities.
Barbiturates	Increased Beta activities.
Cocaine, Cannabis	Increased Alpha activities
Lithium	Slow and paroxysmal activities
Antipsychotics	Non-specific changes

STANDARD VS QUANTITATIVE EEG

Traditionally EEG is used to see the abnormality in the recorded waveform via visual inspection, going through the whole record looking for the pathological oscillation complexes. Older analogue EEG records needed to be stored on papers with no scope of looking at the data from a different perspective (montages, filtering etc.) than the one which was used to record. Then as the technology evolved the digital EEGs are commonplace which allow the digital conversion and storage of EEG data. This data can be looked into by multiple ways for visual inspections as well as digital quantification and analysis of the electrical activities of brain termed as Q-EEG.

Spectral analysis i.e. analysis of EEG frequencies, is the most commonly used quantification analysis. It allows the measurement of power of frequency bands as well as specific frequencies in the EEG. The findings of Q-EEG are promising, especially when psychiatric disorders are investigated. It is now known that synchronization of neural groups associated with different sensory inputs is the basic binding process of brain, leading to a complete percept. Q-EEG findings suggest that slower waves are associated with cognitive processes of the brain. Delta waves are related to internal concentration, theta with working memory, slow alpha with attention & fast alpha is involved in memory functions.

Coherence is a quantitative tool to measure the shared electrical activity among different scalp sites and evaluation of functional interaction of those. This gives a spatial idea of interactions between the brain areas. These quantitative analyses of EEGs have rejuvenated the study of EEG in psychiatric disorders and looks a promising field for biomarker research in psychiatry.

FUTURE RESEARCH

Currently, many applications of EEG research within child psychopathology are being proposed and interpreted within the context of endophenotypes and biomarkers for disease and treatment response. Biomarkers are defined as, "a characteristic that is objectively measured and evaluated as an indication of normal biological processes, pathogenic processes, or pharmacologic responses to a therapeutic intervention. In the past 10 to 15 years, our understanding of psychopathology (in both child and adult forms) has evolved from a focus on unique factors (genetic, environmental, neurobiological, and cognitive) underlying specific psychiatric disorders to one aimed at examining shared factors across different forms of psychopathology. This paradigmatic shift started in large part due to advances made by the Human Genome Project and subsequent focus on identifying genetic factors underlying complex traits.

BIBLIOGRAPHY

1. Marcuse LV, Fields MC, Yoo JJ. Rowan's Primer of EEG E-Book. Elsevier Health Sciences; 2015 Sep 22.
2. Ebersole JS, Husain AM, Nordli DR. Current practice of clinical electroencephalography. Lippincott Williams & Wilkins; 2014 Apr 10.
3. Tatum IV WO, editor. Handbook of EEG interpretation. Demos Medical Publishing; 2014 Mar 19.
4. Misulis KE. Atlas of EEG, seizure semiology, and management. Oxford University Press; 2013.
5. Feyissa AM, Tatum WO. Adult EEG. In Handbook of clinical neurology 2019 Jan 1 (Vol. 160, pp. 103-124). Elsevier.

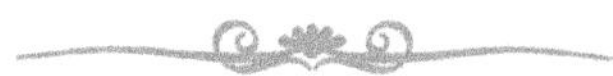

Biopsychosocial Model of Mental Illness

9

Pragya Lodha • Avinash De Sousa

INTRODUCTION

Tracing the footprints to understand mental health, it comes to light that history regards various models to understand the etiology of mental disorders. Some of the various models comprise- supernatural model, psychoanalytical model, behavioral and cognitive model, sociological model, developmental model, recovery model, wellness model, biological model, psychological model, bio-psycho-social model (BPS model), biomedical model and the most recent neuropsychiatric model of mental health and illnesses.

Psychiatry began with a biomedical approach and later adopted the psychoanalytic approach by 1950s and 1960s. It was around the same time when George Engel proposed the biopsychosocial model (BPS model, 1977), in an attempt to explain a more comprehensive alternative to the biomedical model (which he critiqued) for understanding mental illnesses. He formulated this model at a time when science was evolving from an exclusively analytic and reductionistic endeavour to become more contextual and cross-disciplinary.

BIOPSYCHOSOCIAL MODEL OF MENTAL ILLNESSES

G. Engel's BPS model addresses a challenge against the reductionist biomedical model, in a quest to empower the patients and humanize the treatment for mental illnesses. The biopsychosocial model attempts to explain the vulnerability and development of psychopathology from multiple views. Mental illnesses are not an end-product of a single factor causation and the biopsychosocial model thus fits to explain the various combination of factors. There is no one straightforward etiological explanation for illnesses and till 2018, we are struggling to make our understanding as comprehensive as we can in order to better treat mental illnesses. Thus, the need for understanding all factors that influence an individual are important while understanding the phenomena of mental illnesses. This further builds a stronger scaffolding while looking at the treatment of mental illnesses. The seven components of the biopsychosocial model that make it a relevant paradigm to address mental illnesses more holistically comprise- (1) self-awareness; (2) active cultivation of trust; (3) empathic curiosity; (4) self-calibration as a way to reduce bias; (5) educating the emotions to assist with diagnosis and forming therapeutic relationships; (6) using informed intuition; and (7) communicating clinical evidence to foster dialogue. The model says that each dynamic- biological, psychological and sociological- reciprocally influence other dynamics in the model and also affect mental health- and the dynamics change over time.

The BPS model proposes a multidimensional perspective, stating, that clinicians must address illnesses from biological (genetic, brain structure and function), psychological (personal, emotional, family) and sociological (environment, culture and society) standpoints. What the model posits is how the factors come to influence health only in interaction and not as stand-alone elements.

Further, it is a humanistic approach, where George Engel and John Romano (1977) mention that the patient's subjective experiences are crucial to treatment along with an establishment of provider-patient relationship (PPR) and patient-centred interviewing. What is further crucial to note is the successful establishment of the General Adaptation Syndrome (Hans Selye, 1936) that explains how psychological stressors may also have injurious consequences on health and that the response system to stress is not merely biologically dysregulated but is also equally affected by stressful life events and harmful behaviors.

The BPS model furthers to explain the relevance of the model in psychiatry, stating that humans are biopsychosocial beings, affected not solely by the molecular biology but also by their psychological processes and social factors in the environment. The model looks at human beings beyond their molecular construction and assigns them an identity beyond biology. Though a biological underpinning of human development and mental illnesses is inevitable, the biopsychosocial model encompasses the same in a larger context with other important variables that ascribe to being human-emotions, personality, cognition, environment, family and social stimuli. Psychosocial factors co-determine patient's vulnerability along with the severity and course of mental illnesses. Environmental factors play a role to increase the probability of the clinical expression of a mental disorder, along with determining the time of onset of an illness's manifestation. Environmental factors can also protect a vulnerable person from the illness. For example, for someone who has a one parent with depression but the parent has received treatment for depression, they stay in a joint family where there is ample social support, strong familial relationships, decent socio-economic status and an engaging lifestyle with less stressors, the risk for developing depression reduces (however, there may be several other risk factors that may also lead to a greater vulnerability which may be encountered in the course of life).

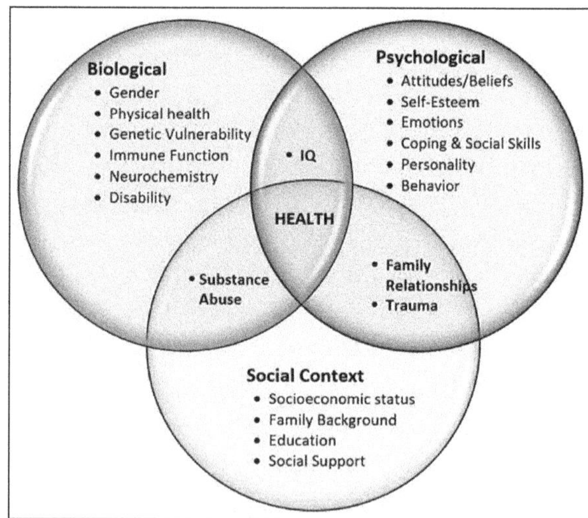

Fig. 8.1

One reason why the biopsychosocial perspective is so useful is because it explains how some people who are seemingly "healthy" can get mental illnesses and why some are more prone to mental illness than others. Those who are mentally healthy most likely exercise, have positive energy and strong social bonds does not exempt them from mental illness. The biopsychosocial perspective gives evidence that although someone can be mentally healthy at some point in their life, they can still experience mental illness if their biopsychosocial balance is disturbed.

It is a well-documented fact that stressful experiences modify immunological response and influence treatment compliance. Non-adherence to pharmacotherapy as well as to the psychosocial interventions, may deteriorate recovery of psychosocial functioning, relapse of the disorder and increase the burden of treatment cost. Psychoeducation of mental illnesses from a biopsychosocial standpoint plays an important role in patient wellness and overall preventive care. Simply put, the BPS model explains how interactions between people's genetic makeup (biology), mental health and personality (psychology), and sociocultural environment (social world) contribute to their experience of health or illness.

From a treatment point of view, psychotherapy along with psychopharmacotherapy has best results, as document in research and clinically, for the simple reason that where drug therapy takes care of the necessary biological intervention, psychotherapy incorporates the psycho-social aspects from patient responsibility and family support to optimal utilisation of environmental support for well-being.

BIOPSYCHOSOCIAL FRAMEWORK

The biopsychosocial model is understood to have a philosophical as well as clinical connotation. Philosophically, it considers the multiple levels of understanding suffering, disease and illnesses- from a molecular level to a societal level. Clinically, it pays heed to the subjective experiences of the patients in order to accurate a diagnosis, health outcome and care. In its holism, awareness of levels in nature, and inclusiveness of diverse perspectives, the BPS model argues that social and behavioral factors play an obvious and major role in human health overall (e.g., poor eating habits, nicotine dependence, alcoholism, risk-taking behavior, stress, anxiety, depression among many others), and a sole reductionistic physicalism does not aid understanding of such phenomena.

The BPS model is the fundamental framework for understanding health and illness. In the realm of psychology, it is argued that the biopsychosocial framework provides the central pathway to unify the field of professional psychology which is a combined approach of psychiatric and psychotherapeutic practice. On a diurnal basis, the practice of psychiatry heavily benefits from a biopsychosocial perspective where the management of mental illness can happen at biopsychosocial level, leading to a better prognostic possibility. There are nuances in mental illnesses that are not as well managed at the biomedical level but are better taken care of at the psychological or sociological level.

Engel's argument to develop the biopsychosocial model was to overcome the challenges of dualism (mind-body being separate), reductionism (all behaviors and illnesses determined by molecular biology) and detached observer (pure objectivity and missing dimension of physician and patient humanity). The BPS model serves to be a beneficial understanding when psychiatric treatment is coupled with psychotherapeutic approach. This approach not only helps in better management of mental illnesses but is profusely conducive towards the well-being of the patients. There is documented validation for the relevance of the biopsychosocial model in psychiatric practice. Where at one hand, the medical model may provide with clarity of evidence and target specific management and treatment of illnesses, it fails to provide etiological exactness as well as a holistic understanding of manifested illnesses. There are various aspects of several illnesses that may not have a medical explanation but are better explained due to psychological and social phenomena (situational anxiety and depression, conversion, phobia and several other adjustment related problems).

CONCLUSION

Despite its usefulness, there are issues with the biopsychosocial model, including the degree of influence that each factor has, the degree of interaction between factors, and variation across individuals and life spans. Though the biopsychosocial model, like all other and biomedical model has its limitation, it stands a wider chance to be developed as a further holistic model of understanding mental illnesses in the combined matrix of biology, psychology and sociology with the added advents of revolutionised biomedicine and neuropsychiatry. In adding to the strengths, the BPS model aids in the development of preventive skills in an individual and also helps predict the susceptibility of a mental illness in an individual. Biopsychosocial approach can continue to remain relevant as far as the ongoing approaches to biology can be integrated and the model may be modified to suit the needs of the time. Nevertheless, in comparison to a solely biomedical approach, the biopsychosocial model of mental health/ illnesses stands a better chance of clinical explanation and relevance in psychiatry. Though there is no clear-cut explanation of how the bio-psycho-social variables exactly interact, the model has the potential to remain the axiom of progressive unification of psychiatry, moving towards better understanding and management of mental health.

BIBLIOGRAPHY

1. Babalola E, Noel P, White R. The biopsychosocial approach and global mental health: Synergies and opportunities. Indian Journal of Social Psychiatry. 2017 Oct 1;33(4):291.
2. Engel GL. The need for a new medical model: a challenge for biomedicine. Science. 1977 Apr 8;196(4286):129-36.
3. Kandel ER, Squire LR. Neuroscience: Breaking down scientific barriers to the study of brain and mind. Science. 2000 Nov 10;290(5494):1113-20.
4. Papadimitriou G. The" Biopsychosocial Model": 40 years of application in Psychiatry. Psychiatrike= Psychiatriki. 2017;28(2):107-10.
5. Saxena S, Funk M, Chisholm D. World health assembly adopts comprehensive mental health action plan 2013–2020. The Lancet. 2013 Jun 8;381(9882):1970-1.

Transference and Countertransference

10

Shivani Chande • Avinash De Sousa

TRANSFERENCE

The Therapeutic Relationship

More than the techniques or the theoretical approach that a therapist takes, what influences the outcome of the therapeutic process is the relationship between the client and the therapist. The ability of the therapist and client to work together efficiently and effectively largely depends upon the relationship that they develop. It is very important for both parties to have mutual trust and respect for each other. There are few cases wherein the therapist and client dislike each other or have incompatible personalities (Welfel & Patterson, 2005). However, it is important for the therapist and client to work together to understand, explore the phenomenon of transference and countertransference that are caused by feelings, thoughts, and emotions that they express to each other.

What is Transference?

Transference is the client's projections of past or present feelings, attitudes or desires onto the therapist (Brammer et al., 1993).

The notion of transference in a therapeutic relationship is clearly embedded in the psychoanalytical theory and many view it as only occurring in psychoanalysis or analytically based therapy. However, Gelso and Carter (1985), among others view transference and countertransference as universal and occurring in almost all counselling or therapeutic relationships. They also suggested that the transference phenomenon occurs across theoretical approaches and it occurs regardless of the treatment duration (short term or long term). Transference may develop from the first moment the client interacts with the therapist, or maybe even before that, as the client anticipates meeting the therapist and may have certain expectations.

However, it is true that transference develops differently across different situations. How it develops, its extent, and its effects on the therapeutic process depends upon a number of factors. These factors include the therapist's view about its importance (or lack of it) in the therapeutic process, the particular client and their individual characteristics, the particular therapist, and the setting.

Furthermore, according to Gelso and Carter (1985), all therapists have something known as a transference pull, which is an image generated through the use of their personality and a particular theoretical viewpoint. The way a therapist looks, gestures, speaks, or sits may trigger a client's reaction. However ambiguous they try to be, therapists can never be total blank screens, which then influences the kind and intensity of the transference reactions.

Transference can be of two types. Either direct or indirect. (Cavanagh, & Levitov, 2002). An example of a direct transference is when the client thinks of the therapist as his sister. Indirect transference is trickier to recognize. It is unearthed by how the client behaves or says to the therapist during therapy, actions or statements that may not directly be related to the therapist. For example.

According to Watkin (1983), most transference behaviors fit into one of five patterns: The client may perceive the therapist as ideal, seer, nurturer, frustrator or nonentity

Theoretical Views of Transference

Freud viewed transference as repressed or unsatisfied wishes and experiences from the patient's past, generally originating from childhood, which gets transferred onto the therapist, revealing where their neurosis originated from. For example, they may see the therapist as a strict or overbearing mother, or at other times a romantic partner. If transference is handled appropriately and correctly, it allows for patients to re-experience and work through past childhood conflicts with the help of the therapist's interpretation, in the safety of the therapist's clinic or consulting room.

The term "Transference" was first used by Freud in the year 1905 in his reports regarding his work with patients. He noted the changes in his patient's attachment to him and their experience of strong positive or negative feelings. Freud gave the term Transference to these feelings, which he considered to be a result of a 'false connection'. He observed transference to be 'new editions' of old impulse and phantasies aroused during psychoanalysis, in which a person from the patient's past is replaced with the therapist.

According to Freud (1912), Transference cannot be created by a therapeutic situation, it is merely revealed by it. Most Psychoanalysts agree with this statement and suggest that a therapeutic relationship only brings to light for example, a patient's idealising tendencies or how he or she reacts to authority.

According to the classical Freudian view, the analyst or therapist understands that transference is a repetition of the past which is in line with Freud's idea of 'repetition compulsion' This reflected his view that repressed past experiences cannot be communicated or expressed verbally, instead, he stated, they are acted out, i.e. they are transferred into repeated actions performed compulsively.

Freud wrote "The patient does not say that he remembers that he used to be defiant and critical towards his parents' authority, instead he behaves in that way to the doctor. . . He does not remember having been intensely ashamed of certain sexual activities and afraid of their being found out, but he makes it clear that he is ashamed of the treatment on which he is now embarked and tries to keep it secret from everybody. This is his way of remembering" (Freud, 1914).

Hence, Transference was explained to be a form of resistance to memory, wherein it is represented as a bypassing of memory and creating instead a re-enactment of desires and conflict to the analyst or therapist.

Originally Freud viewed the therapist as a mirror onto which the patient's projections were seen. However, nowadays, we also view the patient to be projecting into the therapist. This is an important change in our understanding whereby not only is the patient's behavior based upon a distorted perception of the therapist, but also, they may act on the therapist's mind by projecting into the therapist, so that the therapist themselves may be affected.

Unlike Freud, according to whom, transference was a misreading of the present, in terms of the past, many contemporary theorists view transference as a process in which current feelings and emotions are externalised into their relationship with their therapist. Contemporary psychoanalytic practice is governed by the interpretation of transference occurring in the 'here and now'.

Classical Adlerian psychotherapy holds a different view of transference as compared to that of traditional psychoanalysis. It does not view transference or countertransference as important pillars or cornerstones of therapeutic treatment. According to the Adlerian perspective, Transference is the tendency of the client to transfer inappropriate feelings (negative or positive), originally experienced toward their parent, sibling or any other significant individual from their childhood, towards the therapist. In Adler's view, the client's transference is a device to protect and justify the pursuit of a hidden, fictional, hypothetical goal. The therapist's role is to diplomatically bring to attention the transfer of perception and feelings as a long-standing habit that needs to be worked upon and corrected. This perspective considers transference to be a resistance to the cooperation that is important between a client and therapist. The client generally tries to place the therapist into a familiar relationship where they can imagine winning an eventual secret victory.

Carl Jung wrote a book entitled "*The Psychology of the Transference*" (1969) where he uses alchemical symbolism to explain the transference phenomena. He describes how within the transference dyad, both participants experience an assortment of emotional constellations and opposites, from love to hatred, and the key to success and psychological growth is the ability to tolerate the tension of the opposites without deserting the process. According to Jung, the tension is itself the force that allows one to transform and to grow.

According to Carl Rogers, Clients would always experience certain positive and negative emotions during therapy sessions. A proportion of those feelings would be based upon past experiences but it is not important to pay any special attention to those feelings (Nye, 2000). The transference process occurs in every human relationship (Jacobs, 2010). Rather, they are so much a part of everyday interactions that we do not need any sort of elaborate manipulations to bring them out (Lomas, 1973). Roger's view is that there is no need for the therapist to make transference interpretations because if he uses genuineness, acceptance and empathy, the meanings of these positive and negative feelings will automatically become clear to the client.

The Quality of Transference:

The client can develop a range of transferences. It can be either positive or negative. Cavanagh (1982) considers both to be forms of resistance. However, both types can benefit therapy in different ways. Positive transference leads the client to view the therapist as kind, concerned, or otherwise helpful. Negative transference might cause the client to direct angry or painful feelings toward the therapist, but the therapist may still be able to use these feelings to help the client achieve greater understanding about themselves.

It is important to remember that whatever is transferred is an object relationship attached to a particular affect. This means that in formulating the transference at any given moment, the therapist must keep in mind how the client experiences themselves in relation to an affectively laden representation of the other person (e.g. the client as an abandoned victim of a neglectful therapist).

The Positive Transference

In many cases, transferences smoothen the therapeutic process. For example, a positive transference helps the therapeutic work as the client's attachment to the therapist allows for a greater ease of communication and engagement. However, an idealising transference can build roadblocks to treatment. The client who wishes to recreate an all gratifying relationship with the therapist may find it to give up on this kind of relationship and would be inhibited in understanding the range of feelings that they have towards the therapist. Such an idealising transference may appear to be associated with dramatic changes in the client. This would be viewed as a transference cure, wherein the client bypasses a working through loss, disappointments and frustrations. Such a sudden jump to a cure is not usually accompanied by long lasting change. If the transference contains painful or fearful impulses (either loving or aggressive), it may cause some kind of resistance. Often, the client may persist in a particular transference towards the therapist as a method of avoiding less tolerable feelings; for example, a client who strives to be agreeable all the time as a defence against certain paranoid notions or anxieties about the therapist's intentions (Joseph, 2000). It is necessary to interpret these feelings so as to liberate the client to open up to the therapist about what they need in any given moment and to show the client that the therapist can bear to be experienced as the object of not only their love but also of their hate.

The Erotic and Sexualised Transference

More research has been done on transference and resistance arising from aggressive impulses than those arising from loving or sexual feelings of the client towards the therapist. However erotic transference is a kind of transference that arises considerable anxiety in the therapist. Freud viewed loved as not only problematic in life but also in therapy (Freud, 1915). He broke down the boundary between real love and transference love, arguing that the distinction between both was a matter of degree rather than kind. Freud stated that when erotic feelings start emerging in a therapeutic relationship, they represent an attempt to disrupt the therapeutic work by recruiting the therapist into being the client's lover. The intimacy of a therapeutic relationship can be an arousing experience, especially if the client is generally isolated or has difficulty maintaining a relationship or sharing themselves with others. When such a client finds a receptive therapist, who listens to them and gives them a feeling being taken care of, this can give rise to a desire for the intimacy to go beyond the consulting room. Loving or erotic feelings in transference are ubiquitous and are very common. Development of erotic feelings in a therapeutic relationship can become problematic, and when it does, it is referred to as eroticised transference. Eroticised transference is more tenacious and is resistant to interpretations as the client becomes persistent on the gratification of their erotic feelings and fantasies. Such erotic transference can emerge, for example, while working with a client who has previously been sexually abused or where their relationships in childhood were sexualised, even if actual abuse did not occur.

The development of erotic feelings in a therapeutic relationship is problematic for both the client as well as the therapist: As therapy offers a chance for the re-working of parent-child dependency issues, its erotic components will carry the illegitimate quality characteristic of incestuous feelings (Rosenberg, 1999). Erotic feelings may hence be experienced as illicit and may have to be repressed. However, they generally continue to exert their impact on the relationship: In the therapeutic relationship, both members fear the development or activation of erotic feelings, and this causes the erotic dimensions of transference and countertransference to be one of the fundamental problems of analytic treatment (Kernberg, 2000: 87'7). In psychoanalysis, effective exploration of sexual thoughts, behavior, phantasies - conscious and unconscious-and dreams is often stalled by resistances that affect both client and the therapist. This prevents an understanding of the connotation of these feelings and leaves the therapeutic situation at risk of a standstill or of acting out.

Around five to seventeen percent of mental health professionals admit to having sexual intimacies with their patients (Pope et al., 1995). The confusion arises in therapists because the passion and intensity of the feelings and emotions that the client may develop towards the therapist is often convincing. Instead of being content for doing a good enough job, the therapist may begin to feel like a long sought-after parent, friend or lover. The therapist may confuse being the object of realistic love with the powerful seductive experience of being the object of the client's idealisation, dependence and passion. These reactions, if unexplored, may seriously compromise the therapeutic relationship and its effectiveness. The lure of turning into the perfect partner who will help cure the client of his problems can lead a therapist down a slippery slope of enactment. To avoid such enactments, a therapist needs to be vigilant to the difference between the positive pleasure that therapists can derive in doing competent work and the "illusory gains of fantasy gratification" (Novick and Novick, 2000) that turn into an occupational hazard. Viewing from a clinical perspective, the critical question is how intervention should be carried out when erotic feelings arise. In a general sense, therapists should be receptive to any feelings that the client experiences towards them, including sexual ones. Given that feelings such as these are also often frequently associated with fear or shame, therapists help the client if they can approach this exploration without anxiety or judgment on their part. Working with erotic feelings in therapy elicits anxiety, regardless of how experienced a therapist is. A very helpful discussion of issues like these can be found in a paper by Rosenberg (1999). Here are a few aspects of working with erotic feelings:

- Notice the emergence of erotic feelings in the client or in oneself and take them to supervision.
- Explore whether the erotic feelings have an infantile quality. This would suggest that they probably reflect the development, in the relationship, of attachment needs suffused with incestuous fantasies, for example, a client who had been brought up in an orphanage developed a very strong attachment towards the therapist. Six months into the therapy, he hesitantly declared that he loved her and that he often entertained conscious fantasies of the two of them living together. As the therapist and client explored these feelings, it became clearer to them both that he was giving expression to a wish for closeness to an attachment figure that he had never experienced in his life because of being placed in an orphanage. This wish was mixed with more erotic feelings related

to a fantasy of being held in the therapist's arms and soothed to sleep. This client's longing for closeness with the therapist had an erotic dimension, but these wishes and feelings originated from a more childlike part of him.

- Explore whether the client is sexualising the therapeutic relationship. In contrast to the client described above, a client who sexualises the therapeutic relationship is using sexual fantasies and feelings to attack the therapy and the therapist. An example of such a client would be one who would often come to the session reporting the previous night's sexual exploits with young girls. He would give the therapist detailed descriptions of what he did to the young girls and the therapist regularly found herself both repelled and intimidated by these revelations. It felt as if he was relating to the therapist as one of the powerless young girls in relation to whom he felt powerful. This kind of sexualisation is very hostile in nature.
- Think about whether the type of relationship that the client strives to establish is a defence against erotic feelings. For example, the client's search for a more dependent, childlike relationship with a therapist may be a defence against the activation of such erotic feelings: the client may defensively fall back into wishing to be seen as a child in relation to the therapist and deny erotic feelings that threaten to overwhelm him and cause anxiety.
- Explore how the erotic feelings are being used in the transference. The erotic transference can be used in a variety of different dynamic ways, for example, as a cover-up for hostility or in an effort to seek reassurance from the therapist. Whatever its use, it signifies an attempt to lure the therapist away from their therapeutic role and this represents a form of resistance. Working through an erotic transference has important significance: If the client can tolerate sexual feelings while deeply accepting that they will not be gratified in the therapeutic situation, then sublimation, working through and mourning may consolidate an intense relationship in the transference while helping both client and therapist to begin their process of separation (Kemberg, 2000).

The Negative Transference

A positive transference is quite common in the early stages of therapy as the client is mobilised by his desire to get better and usually hopes that the therapist will be of help to him. Nevertheless, as with any relationship, the therapeutic one will also need to undergo the test of the client's mistrust or his hostility. These feelings are not always expressed at the beginning. Some clients may find it very threatening to own up to and/or express such feelings in themselves. Consequently, they may be displaced onto other relationships in client's life so as to shield the therapeutic relationship. The client will, for example, report conflicts or arguments with a boss or partner safely keeping their anger "out there in the real world" rather than in the relationship with the therapist. Generally, negative feelings are more readily voiced when the client trusts that the therapist can tolerate their expression of emotions without retaliating or trying to minimise their significance. The development of such feelings in the therapeutic relationship is referred to as negative transference. There are differences between the various schools as to how to work with the emergence, in therapy, of negative feelings and attitudes towards the therapist. Emphasis on the negative transference and its initial early interpretation are characteristic of the Kleinian technique. Anna Freud and her followers argued, on the contrary, that interpretation of the negative transference should be avoided early on, before the establishment of a solid therapeutic alliance. These days, more attention is paid to the negative transference across different schools and its interpretation early on in the therapeutic relationship. Interpretation of the negative transference is a risky intervention since it brings into focus the client's hostile feelings and emotions towards the therapist. Once exposed, such negative feelings may leave the client fearing the therapist's retaliation. This could lead to the generation of anxiety which could lead a client to break off treatment and at the very least, demands of the client, a capacity to bear his own aggression and paranoid anxieties. In light of these considerations, it is thus often suggested and preferable to explore negative transference in the context of an established therapeutic alliance in which the client has felt supported and has had experience of work with a helpful therapist. However, there are certain clinical situations in which the interpretation of the negative transference, even if it is a relatively new therapeutic relationship - may be essential so as to help the client to remain in therapy by giving him the experience of being with a therapist who can understand and think about more aggressive feelings without retaliating. In other words, although the negative transference will often be visible in the first session itself, whether the therapist explores it will depend on our assessment of how helpful it will be at that stage of therapy. the interpretation of the negative transference in the initial sessions is justified where the client's ambivalence about being in therapy is prominent and could undermine the viability of the therapy, or where the client's aggression is so apparent that not interpreting it could be experienced by the client as the inability to manage such feelings. This in itself could be the reason, the client breaks off treatment as he would not have had the experience of the therapist being able to understand, and think about the meaning of, his hostility. Managing the client's negative feelings towards the therapist with equanimity is important, but under their pressure the therapist may be tempted to seduce the client away from their distrust or anger. This is another instance when supervision is vital as it supports the therapist to stay with such uncomfortable feelings.

Interpreting the Transference

If a therapist catches on to the fact that transference has taken place and is affecting the working of the therapeutic relationship, they may foster, deepen and work through the transference misperceptions with interpretations. For example, a therapist might, at an appropriate time in the treatment, interpret to a client who often shows rebelliousness and an oppositional style during the sessions, that her behavior may be shaped in response to a controlling and authoritarian mother. This kind of behavior might have been necessary as a young girl in the face of such a mother, however it is less appropriate for a mature adult in response to a therapist who is neither looking to dominate nor control.

There are some general considerations to keep in mind when constructing a transference interpretation:

- The therapist must ask themselves what is the purpose of the interpretation? How does this relate to the aims of treatment?
- The therapist should explore if there is a fit between the thematic content of the interpretation and the overall formulation of the client's difficulties and the goals of

treatment. This is especially essential in short term therapy where it is important that the interpretations are related to the focal area/conflict that has been agreed upon with the client.

- Consider what evidence there is available for the interpretation. Like any other type of interpretation, a transference interpretation is only but a working hypothesis.
- Before sharing and explaining the interpretation to the client, consider its timing: is the client ready to hear it? How would it be experienced by him? Is the therapist feeling a pressure to speak and give back a projection to the client? If so, it would be better to hold back from verbalising what may be going on until the therapist have a clearer understanding of this.
- Especially with clients who are not well versed in therapeutic treatment, structuring the interpretation by starting with what the client has said or done (or not said or done) that suggests that he may be feeling in a particular way about the therapist.
- Keeping the interpretation relatively simple is, without too many sub clauses is important.
- When offering it, the interpretation needs to include clear references to the here-and-now. Especially in short term therapy, it is essential to link more systematically the here-and-now experience to parallel relationship patterns in the client's life.
- Where appropriate, it would be important to acknowledge that the stimulus for the client's transference perception and reaction may partially come from something the therapist may have said or done (or not said or done).
- Too great an emphasis on transference may be associated with a negative outcome and weakening of the therapeutic alliance when the client's immediate need is to process and verify actual historical events (e.g. with clients who have undergone trauma).

As a therapist listens to their clients' narratives, they must listen out for the following:

- Who does what to whom? This involves understanding perceived intentions (benign and/or malign) towards the self and of the self towards other people.
- Who feels what towards whom? This involves identifying the main feelings and emotions present in the narrative.
- How do we feel as we listen? This involves identifying countertransference (e.g. does the therapist feel swamped, seduced or excited by the story?)

Once a skeleton pattern of actions and affects has been formulated, the therapist can proceed to think about whether these have any relevance to the here-and now scenario. They rely on their capacity to sustain an internal process of supervision (Casement, 1985) and try to identify the ways in which they may have also contributed to the client's experience. Thus, the aim is to identify the trigger for the activation of a particular transference - the trigger may be either internal (e.g. a conscious or unconscious phantasy) or external, that is, an actual event.

COUNTERTRANSFERENCE

What is counter transference?

Countertransference occurs when a therapist transfers emotions to a client in therapy, it is many a times, a reaction to transference, a phenomenon in which the client in treatment redirects feelings for others onto the therapist. It refers to the therapist's projected emotional reaction to or behavior towards the client (Fauth & Hayes, 2006; Hanses, Rossberg, & Cramer, 1994).

Sigmund Freud originally described the concepts of transference and countertransference. He explained countertransference as a largely unconscious process in which the therapist's emotions and feelings are influenced by the client during therapy, and the therapist reacts with countertransference. Carl Jung had documented his own struggles with the process of countertransference. He characterizes it as a problematic phenomenon that can restrict psychological treatment when left unchecked.

It is essential for therapists to overcome the tendency to participate in unconscious countertransference by developing healthy boundaries and remaining mindful of the threat posed by countertransference, both to the therapeutic alliance and a therapist's work with people seeking treatment.

Contemporary psychologists typically distinguish between helpful and unhelpful countertransference. Many therapists openly share their own thoughts and feelings with their clients and may use countertransference, consciously, to understand differences between their own experiences and the experiences of the client.

Not all countertransference is unhelpful or problematic. For example, a therapist may meet with a client who has extreme difficulty making conversation. The therapist may begin, unknowingly, to lead the conversation and provide additional prompts to the client in order to encourage discussion. A therapist who acknowledges this can then point to the countertransference to help the client better understand the effect that difficulty making conversation can have on others. A therapist who has experienced the same issues as the client may also be able to empathize with that person at a deeper level, whether the therapist decides to engage in self-disclosure and share those personal stories or not.

Unhelpful countertransference, or even harmful countertransference, takes place when the therapist transfers to the client, feelings that are misplaced or when a therapist uses the client to meet personal psychological needs. For example, a therapist may give the "advice" of leaving her husband to a client who is undergoing similar relationship problems as her. Another example of problematic countertransference, when a client triggers a therapist's issues with the therapist's own child. The client, for example, might be rebellious towards the therapist and may transfer defiance felt toward a parent onto the therapist. If the therapist reacts to the client as one would behave towards one's own child, by becoming increasingly dominant or controlling, for example, without recognizing the presence countertransference, this could severely impact the therapeutic relationship in a negative way and perpetuate unhealthy patterns in the life of the client.

A therapist might also feel ill-equipped to deal with a client who expresses beliefs, values and personal preferences that are different from the therapist's own, such as sexist, racist or homophobic views, however, a therapist can still help a client who has differing opinions by attempting to explore where any harmful or potentially damaging beliefs stem from and discussing that history with the client.

Watkins (1985) classified counter transference into four forms:

- Overprotective

- Benign
- Rejecting
- Hostile

The first two forms are examples of identification. In these forms of countertransference, the therapist overidentifies with the client and is unable to remain emotionally distant from them. The last two, that is rejecting and hostile forms of countertransference are example of misidentification or disidentification. Here the therapist becomes distant and emotionally removed from the client. Disidentification may cause the therapist to behave in manner which is aloof, nonempathetic, cold, antagonistic, or even hostile. This highlights the importance both of awareness of one's motivation (for example, a therapist was aware that a 59-year-old male client's manipulative manner triggered anxieties in her because she reminded her of how her father sometimes controlled how she should feel and think when a child) and also of behaving ethically.

Recognizing and Dealing with Countertransference

Signs of countertransference in therapy can include a variety of behaviors, including excessive self-disclosure on the part of the therapist or an unhealthy interest in irrelevant details from the life of the client. A therapist who acts on their feelings toward the client or their situation, or engages in behavior not appropriate to the treatment process, may not be fruitfully managing countertransference. They may not be working on or even recognize the presence of countertransference. Therapists can make an effort to be particularly mindful about recognizing and understanding their own fears and feelings when working with a client who has experienced a personal trauma or stress the therapist has also experienced recently or even in the past.

During the course of therapy, a therapist may come to develop an attraction towards the client. While an attraction to the client in itself is not an unnatural occurrence, the therapist must be able to recognize these feelings and endeavour to deal with them in an appropriate manner to prevent the development of an inappropriate attachment or relationship with a client.

Guidelines for Working with Countertransference

- A therapist must get accustomed to noting their own emotional responses to the client's verbal and non-verbal behavior.
- A therapist must not dismiss seemingly unconnected associations that may come to mind as they listen to their client (e.g. a song or a character from a movie or book).
- Therapist must question if the feelings they are experiencing (or that they think they should be experiencing but are not) accountable for in terms of issues in their own life at the time?
- Even if a therapist thinks that the feelings are personally relevant to them, they may still be also responding to the client's projection. It may simply be that the therapist is especially sensitive to that particular projection at the time. The therapist must be careful to monitor what belongs to them so as to create enough mental space to reflect on what their emotional reaction may also be telling them about their client.
- A therapist should try to stay with the feeling(s) evoked in them. Note what it made them feel like doing or what it makes them feel about themselves (e.g. powerful, attractive, incompetent). If they feel under pressure to say something, it may be a further indication that projective identification is operative.

- Generally, the process of internal reflection eases the psychological tension as one gains essential emotional distance and hence perspective. When the therapist has reached this stage internally, they are probably ready to begin to formulate a possible interpretation and to judge the patient's receptivity to it.

BIBLIOGRAPHY

1. Gladding, S. T. (2018). *Counseling: A comprehensive profession*. Pearson.
2. Welfel, E. R., & Patterson, L. E. (2009). *The counseling process: A multitheoretical integrative approach*. Brooks/Cole.
3. Gelso, C. J., & Carter, J. A. (1985). The Relationship in Counseling and Psychotherapy. *The Counseling Psychologist, 13*(2), 155-243. doi:10.1177/0011000085132001
4. Pickman, A. J. (1995). *Complete guide to outplacement counseling*. Lawrence Erlbaum Associates.
5. Watkins, C. E. (1983). Transference Phenomena in the Counseling Situation. *The Personnel and Guidance Journal, 62*(4), 206-210. doi:10.1111/j.2164-4918.1983.tb00187.x
6. Cavanagh, M. E., & Levitov, J. E. (2002). *The counseling experience: A theoretical and practical approach*. Waveland Press.
7. Transference and Countertransference. (2008). *Introduction to the Practice of Psychoanalytic Psychotherapy,* 230-273. doi: 10.1002/9780470713426.ch7
8. Jacoby, M. (1984). The analytic encounter: Transference and the human relationship. Toronto: Inner City Books.
9. Jacobs, M. (2010). Psychodynamic counselling in action (4th edn). London: Sage.
10. Lomas, P. (1973). True and false experience. London: Penguin.
11. Malan, D.H. (2004). Individual psychotherapy and the science of psychodynamics. London: Arnold.
12. Rogers, C. R. (2003). *Client-centred therapy*. Constable & Robinson.
13. Ladson, D., & Welton, R. (2007, April). Recognizing and managing erotic and eroticized transferences. Retrieved from https://www.ncbi.nlm.nih.gov/pmc/articles/PMC2921238/
14. What passes between client and therapist? (n.d.). Retrieved from https://thepsychologist.bps.org.uk/volume-28/july-2015/what-passes-between-client-and-therapist
15. Jung, C. G. (1969). *The psychology of transference*. Princeton University Press.
16. Fauth, J., & Hayes, J. A. (2006). Counselors' Stress Appraisals as Predictors of Countertransference Behavior With Male Clients. *Journal of Counseling & Development, 84*(4), 430-439. doi:10.1002/j.1556-6678.2006.tb00427.x
17. Hansen, J. C., Rossberg, R. H., & Cramer, S. H. (1994). *Counseling: Theory and process*. Allyn and Bacon.

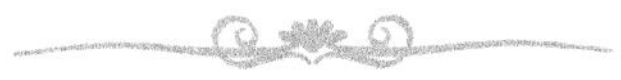

11 Neuroanatomy Review

Jitender Jakhar • Satish Suhas • Shailini S. Naik

INTRODUCTION

This chapter will provide an insight into the current neurobiological understanding of psychiatric disorders, transforming intellectual curiosity from behavioral science to their biological underpinnings. To understand the fundamental aspect of pathophysiology, we need to revise the functions of various chemical neurotransmitters in the brain and receptors involved, intraneural signaling pathways, different neuroanatomical organizations of the brain network, and various structures involved in the biology of neuropsychiatric disorder. Psychiatry has progressed from the days of attributing causation to paranormal influences to a more neuroscience approach that is based on the following fundamental assumptions.

1. All psychological phenomena across perception, thinking, emotions, behavior, and experiences are intricately associated with neural processes.
2. All psychological disorders can be explained by alterations in healthy neural operations irrespective of the cause that triggers these experiences. For example, although a failure in an exam can precipitate depression, it is associated with neurobiological correlations that lead to clinical signs and symptoms.
3. Interaction between Nature and Nurture: Genes and the environment share a complex relationship with the neural processes that can be adaptive or pathoplastic. The environment, including perinatal asphyxia, adverse childhood experiences, parenting practices, social experiences, life events, stressors, support systems, can cross-talk with genetic expression [For example though, epigenetics] to mediate health and disease.

The next important thing to understand is that neurobiology does not mean one process or a circuit. It involves a complex interaction of genes, neural circuits, neurotransmission, molecular biology. This chapter will focus on the neurobiological correlates of individual psychiatry disorders and assumes that the readers are primed with basic knowledge of neuroanatomy, neurochemistry, and neurophysiology.

NEUROANATOMY

The neuroanatomy of psychiatric disorders is currently understood based on brain regions' interconnectivity, also termed "neural circuitry." While a few specific findings are found for each neuropsychiatric disorder, there are common findings across different neuropsychiatric disorders. Most of the neuroanatomical associations in each disorder are drawn from the convergence of classical animal lesion studies, rigorous observation of psychiatric symptoms in patients with neurological disorders, and the application of modern brain imaging methodologies in both psychiatric patients and healthy controls.

The two important structures strongly implicated in most psychiatric disorders are the prefrontal and limbic structures. The frontal lobe deals with intelligence, inhibition of undesirable behavior, language. The frontal lobe's structural and functional disturbance is implicated in psychiatric disorders such as schizophrenia, depression, obsessive-compulsive disorder, unprovoked aggression and dementia. The limbic system includes structures viz., ventromedial temporal lobe (hippocampus), thalamus, nucleus accumbens, and amygdala. It is a seat for the processing of emotion, religious experience, recovered memory, and its damage is known to cause auras, paroxysmal limbic disorders, schizophrenia, depression, and drug addiction.

Prefrontal Cortex

It comprises three parts, as elucidated in **Table 11.1**. It is implicated in executive functions, including short-term memory, planning, decision making. Additionally, aspects of personality expression, social behavior modulation, and aspects of language regulation are also attributed to prefrontal cortex.

Limbic System [Formerly Rhinencephalon]

It is a set of brain regions situated on both sides of the thalamus, immediately beneath the medial temporal lobe. Its gray matter includes cortical gyri and subcortical nuclei.

- Cortical gyri
  - Cingulate gyrus: It receives inputs from the thalamus and neocortex and projects to the entorhinal cortex via the cingulum.
  - Hippocampus: Part of the ventromedial temporal lobe and it is vulnerable to long-term stress
- Subcortical nuclei
  - Amygdala
  - Mammillary bodies
  - Anterior nucleus of the thalamus

Table 11.1: Prefrontal cortical structures

Neuroanatomical structure	Function	Clinical manifestations	Psychiatric disorders
Dorsolateral prefrontal cortex [DLPFC]	Attention, planning and verbal working memory, ability to initiate, plan ahead and carry out goal-directed behavior	Difficulty in sustaining attention, problems in planning and executing tasks	Cognitive symptoms of schizophrenia, Depression, Addictive disorders
Orbitofrontal cortex or Ventromedial prefrontal cortex [OFC/vmPFC]	Regulation of mood and social behaviors. Inhibit interfering external or internal influences	Heightened emotional responsivity, euphoria, poor decision-making in social circumstances, impulsivity	Obsessive-compulsive disorder, frontotemporal dementia, Witzelsucht
Medial prefrontal or Anterior cingulate cortex [mPFC/ACC]	Drive, motivation, reward appraisal	Lack of initiative and motivation, significant apathy or blunting of affect	Negative symptoms of schizophrenia, Depression, Obsessive-compulsive disorder, Addictive disorders

Table 11.2: Important structures of the Limbic system

Structure	Function	Clinical manifestations
Hippocampus	Spatial memory, declarative/ explicit memory, formation of new memories, and retrieval of past memories	Transient global amnesia, anterograde amnesia > retrograde amnesia. Hippocampal atrophy is seen in Alzheimer's dementia, schizophrenia, severe depression, post-traumatic stress disorder
Cingulate gyrus	Reward center (a sense of satisfaction after the fulfilment of basic instincts), emotion formation and processing, and memory	Negative symptoms of schizophrenia, Depression, Obsessive-compulsive disorder, Addictive disorders
Mammillary bodies	Episodic and spatial memory	Damage of mammillary bodies due to thiamine deficiency found in Wernicke-Korsakoff syndrome Mammillary body atrophy seen in Alzheimer's dementia and schizophrenia
Amygdala	Memory formation and storage associated with emotional events, autobiographical memory, fear conditioning, facial emotion recognition, and processing	Hyperactivity: Mood disorder, obsessive and compulsive disorder, post-traumatic stress disorder, generalized anxiety disorder, social anxiety disorder, and schizophrenia. Hypoactivity [Kluver-Bucy syndrome]: hypoemotionality/docility, loss of fear and anger, hypersexuality, and hyperorality (inappropriate objects are placed in the mouth)
Fornix	Consolidation of short-term memory to long-term memory	Acute amnestic syndrome

A bundle of projection fibers (axons) connects the hippocampus with the mammillary body, called the fornix, and constitutes the "efferent system" of the hippocampus. Various functions and clinical manifestations of limbic structures are mentioned in **Table 11.2**.

Papez Circuit

It is a neural loop beginning from hippocampal formation to the mammillary body (via fornix) in the hypothalamus to the anterior nucleus of the thalamus (AN) to cingulate gyrus and back to the hippocampal formation (**Fig. 11.1**). It is the functional connectivity within the limbic system involved in processing emotion and controlling emotional expression.

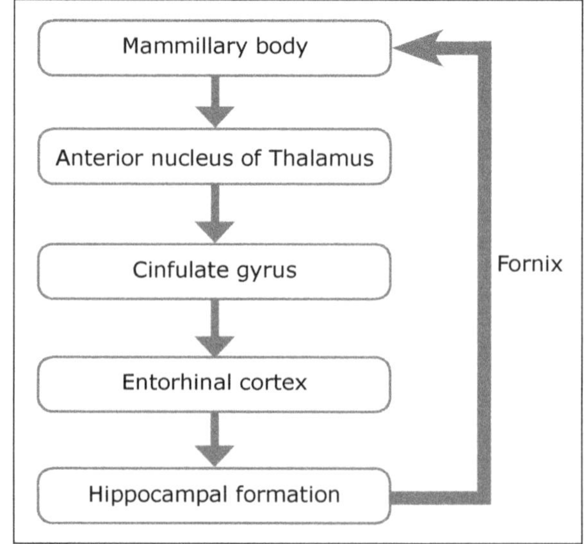

Fig. 11.1: Papez circuit.

NEUROTRANSMITTER

Neurotransmitters are molecules released after membrane stimulation and either excite or inhibit the adjacent neuron by acting on the postsynaptic receptor. Excitatory transmission (e.g., Glutamate) promote depolarization, and inhibitory (e.g., GABA) promotes hyperpolarization of the target neuron. Neurotransmitter receptors are mainly located on the postsynaptic neuron, sometimes on the presynaptic neuron, divided into two types; Ligand-gated ion channel, which is intrinsic to the receptor, and the other metabotropic, which activates guanosine triphosphate (GTP) binding protein. The receptor acts through ion channel, typically depolarize via sodium or calcium, and hyperpolarize by chloride channel, while metabotropic receptor acts through second messenger pathway that produces a series of complex effect via modulating the gene expression on the target cell, exerting slow or fast synaptic effects. GABAa, 5-HT3, Glycine, and Nicotinic receptors are ligand-gated pentameric receptors comprising five subunits and exert fast response in synaptic signaling. NMDA receptor, AMPA, and kainate receptor are the main ligand gated excitatory ion channels for glutamate. G protein-coupled receptor exerts slow changes and acts by the generation of second messengers cCAMP and Di-acylglycerase (DAG), which leads to activation of specific protein kinases and cascading the release of gene transcription factor and hence contributing to synaptic plasticity. Increasing evidence from the neuropharmacological study highlighted that psychotropic medication therapeutic response results from many changes in intracellular structure and long intake induce a neuroadaptive response by underpinning remodeling of target neural pathway and circuit and hence altering gene expression and protein synthesis. Blocking the normal functioning of the neurotransmitters hampers the propagation of the action potential in a designated neural path. For the last few decades, biogenic amine has dominated the role of neurotransmitters in the neuroscience of psychiatric disorders; however, since the last two decades, significant evidence has been generated about the potential involvement of aminoacid-neurotransmitter in the pathophysiology of the broad range of psychiatric disorders. Over 100 unique neuropeptides have been identified in the brain, and a subset of them are relevant in psychiatry. Classification of Neurotransmitter based on specific class is shown in **Table 11.3**.

Neurotransmitters can directly or indirectly influence human behavior by regulating neuronal

Table 11.3: Classification of Neurotransmitter

Class	Neurotransmitter
Biogenic amine NT	Catecholamines (dopamine, norepinephrine, and epinephrine)
	Serotonin (5- hydroxytryptamine, 5HT)
	Histamine
	Acetylcholine
Amino Acid NT	Glutamate
	Gamma-Aminobutyric acid (GABA)
	Glycine
Neuropep-tide NT	Thyrotropin-releasing hormone (TRH), Corticotrophin- releasing factor (CRF), Oxytocin, Arginine Vasopressin (AVP), Adrenocorticotropin hormone (ACTH), Neuropeptide Y, Neurotensin, etc.
Gas NT	Nitric Oxide (NO)
	Carbon Monoxide (CO)
Other NT	Endocannabinoids: Anandamide, 2- arachidonoyl- glycerol (2-AG)
	Neurotrophic factors: Neurotrophins (for example, BDNF, NGF), Insulin-like growth factor (IGF), Vascular endothelial growth factor (VEGF)

function through specific receptor-ligand interaction. Subtle changes in this receptor neurotransmitter function, either qualitative or quantitative, can significantly exert profound alteration in social behaviors. This behavioral manifestation results from dysregulated neuronal communication between neurons due to an imbalance in the neurotransmitter messenger system. The neurotransmitters of principal interest in psychiatry are biogenic amines serotonin, norepinephrine, and dopamine, extensively studied in affective disorder and schizophrenia. Also, the brain's decreased synthesis or expression of various other neurotransmitters implicated as the causative agent for neurobehavioral changes includes GABA, Glutamate, histamine, Glycine, and acetylcholine. The essential role of some important neurotransmitters is discussed here.

Acetylcholine:

Acetylcholine (Ach) is the most abundant neurotransmitter found in the brain, autonomic ganglia, spinal cord, and nerve ending in muscle. It is synthesized in the presynaptic nerve terminal from choline and acetyl-CoA by the enzyme choline acetyltransferase. Central dysfunction in Ach release can produce memory deficit and alteration in consciousness, and hence it has a prime role in memory, learning, and arousal in human beings. Neurons containing Ach as a principal neurotransmitter in the brain can send short projections and act as interneurons or send long projections to different brain regions. Cholinergic long projection from basal forebrain to cortex serves memory and attention, whereas ascending projection from cell bodies of pons and midbrain regulates sleep-wake cycles, arousal, and rapid eye movements. Progressive neurofibrillary degeneration of cholinergic projection from the basal forebrain is seen in Alzheimer's dementia, and subsequent gradual changes occur in the nicotinic or muscarinic receptor in a different area of the cerebral cortex perturbates the synaptic physiology and long-term potentiation.

Serotonin

Serotonin or 5-hydroxytryptamine (5-HT) is one of the most important monoamine neurotransmitters and constitutes approximately 1% of all CNS neurons. Serotonin, norepinephrine, and epinephrine are synthesized in various steps from the same amino acid Tryptophan. The majority (80%) of periphery serotonin is produced in the gastrointestinal system and platelets. Centrally, serotonergic projection begins from midline raphe nuclei of the brainstem, and through the rostral and caudal pathway, innervate the majority of brain regions. Serotonin plays a vital role in mood, slow-wave sleep, appetite regulation, and aid in the release of hormones such as ACTH and prolactin, and that's why most antidepressant medications help by increasing serotonergic transmission in the human brain. Subtypes of serotonergic receptors identified in humans are $5HT_{1A-1F}$, $5HT_{2A-2C}$, $5HT_3$, $5HT_4$, $5HT_{5A-5C}$, $5HT_6$, and $5HT_7$.5HT1 and 5HT5 are inhibitory and act by reducing cAMP level, whereas other receptors are excitatory and act by increasing cAMP level. All serotonin receptors are G-protein coupled receptors, except 5-HT3, which is ion channel-dependent. Out of these, 5HT1 and 5HT2 receptors are predominately studied in the mechanism of antidepressant medication, specific antipsychotic medication, and ECT. Selective serotonin reuptake inhibitor medication increases the synaptic concentration of serotonin by blocking presynaptic serotonin transporter (SERT) in both the soma and dendritic area of neurons. Indeed, serotonergic dysfunction has been proposed in most psychiatric disorders ranging from depression, anxiety, impulse control disorder, aggression to autism, schizophrenia, and suicidal behaviors.

Several studies reported a reduced 5-hydroxy indole acetic acid (5-HIAA) level in cerebrospinal fluid linked to suicidal behaviors. Also, genetic polymorphism in the serotonin transporter gene is linked to depression and obsessive-compulsive disorder and indicates a poor prognosis to treatment. Recently 5-HT receptors are extensively studied in the area of psychosis also, and the latest antipsychotics are exploring the potential of 5HT3 receptors in therapeutic effects.

Noradrenaline

Norepinephrine or noradrenaline (NA) neurons project mainly from the locus ceruleus in the pons of the brain stem to different regions in the brain and modulate complex behavioral regulation. Dorsal fiber projects to the neocortex, cerebellum, limbic cortex, and hippocampus. Other ventral bundles project mainly to the limbic system and hypothalamus. NA release is both tonic and phasic and profoundly influences arousal and vigilance in humans. It maintains a low concentration during the sleep phase and reaches peak secretion during any stress-inducing or alarming situation. NA functional significance is understood in classical fear-flight response during emergency reaction or "alarm reaction in stress," as hypothesized by Selye. The non-locus ceruleus noradrenergic projections from another region in the brain are connected directly to the hypophysis-adrenocortical and center of the sympathetic system. Beta-blocker is clinically helpful for this autonomic surge and are used to allay symptoms during a panic attack, performance anxiety, or fear-provoking situations. Recent studies also implicated the role of norepinephrine in ADHD pathophysiology, and medication that blocks noradrenaline transporter(NAT), e.g., Stimulant methylphenidate, has shown beneficial results. The hyperarousal symptoms of Post-traumatic stress disorder in war veterans /survivors are linked with tonically elevated CSF concentration of NA, and medication such as clonidine, prazosin, or beta-blocker helps in these hyperarousal symptoms. Clinical studies support the link between arousal symptoms and Noradrenergic dysfunction. Excessive surge increases the arousal level and amplifies body reaction to stressful stimuli in the form of irritability, exaggeration of fear, insomnia, anxiety, and emotional instability (Hyperarousal symptoms). In contrast, the decreased activity could result in insensitivity to stress, amotivation, and decreased emotional reactivity (Hypo arousal symptoms).

Dopamine (DA)

DA is synthesized from amino acid tyrosine and critically plays a role in learning, emotion, creativity, motor activity, reward, and motivation. Within the Central nervous system, principal dopamine neurons originate from cell bodies in the midbrain and hypothalamus. Also called the molecule of reward, it is responsible for the motivation and reward system in the human brain. There are five different dopamine receptors in humans: D1, D2, D3, D4 & D5. D1 receptors are most abundant, and D1 and D5 are stimulatory and activate adenylyl cyclase and second messenger system, while D2, D3, and D4 receptors are inhibitory and deactivate the adenylyl cyclase system. Dopaminergic neurons originating from the ventral tegmental area to the nucleus accumbens regulate the reward pathway and incentive motivation. Patients with substance use disorder have a critical urge and craving, which is due to a transient and steep dopamine surge in this pathway, leading to abuse and addiction. Predominately D3 receptors have a role in sensitization, and repetitive target lead to the addictive behavioral syndrome. Dopamine also regulates fine coordination of body movements through the extrapyramidal pathway, which projects dopaminergic fibers from the substantia nigra of the midbrain to the basal ganglia. Most Antipsychotic drugs produce extrapyramidal side effects due to the involvement of this pathway. Delay and Deniker, in 1952 first time reported the use of chlorpromazine in psychosis, which acts by blocking the D-2 receptor and afterwards, many antipsychotic evolved over time targeting dopamingeric receptor.

Gamma-aminobutyric Acid Deficit (GABA)

There is growing evidence towards the role of the Gamma-aminobutyric acid deficit (GABA) in a patient with psychiatry disorder. GABA, the most abundant inhibitory neurotransmitter in the central nervous system, has a critical role in modulating cortical reactivity and neuroplasticity. GABAergic neurons comprise 25–30% of the neurons in the motor cortex, and their connection horizontally can extend up to a distance of 6 mm or more which are known to modulate and fine-tune excitatory neurotransmission of various other neuronal systems in the brain, including the cholinergic and monoaminergic projections to the forebrain. This balance of inhibitory and excitatory postsynaptic potentials synchronizes the activity of pyramidal cells. When this GABAergic interneuron terminates on pyramidal cells, then inhibitory postsynaptic potentials are generated. This neurophysiological mechanism of GABA inhibitory interneuron attenuating the activity of another pyramidal neuron in the cortex is known as cortical inhibition. It is known that depression, anxiety disorders, autism spectrum disorder, and schizophrenia are associated with low GABAergic states. These disorders also improve with pharmacologic drugs that increase the activity of this GABAergic neurotransmission. GABA shows its actions by interacting with two different subtypes of receptor a)GABAA receptors (GABAARs)-ionotropic and b)GABAB receptor (GABABRs)-metabotropic.GABAARs are predominately responsible for anxiety and mood disorders due to considerable evidence suggesting altered GABAAR signaling in both. Benzodiazepines act as an allosteric modulator of a major subset of GABAARs, demonstrating potent anxiolytic activity and playing key control elements of anxiety state. GABABRs, coded by GABAB (1) and GABAB (2) gene, are members of the G-protein coupled receptor family, and their role in the causation of affective disorder have been recently implicated in mice which demonstrated alerted anxiety and depression-related behavior after subjecting to pharmacological and genetic manipulations of these receptors. In 2010, one review suggested compelling evidence of both GABA A and GABAB inhibitory deficit in the pathophysiology of MDD and anxiety disorder.

BIOLOGICAL CORRELATES OF SPECIFIC COMMON PSYCHIATRIC DISORDERS

Biological factors play a key role in the pathophysiology of neuropsychiatric disorders, including major depression, bipolar disorder, anxiety, panic disorder, OCD, and schizophrenia. Brain and behavior are immensely muddled complicated, and our knowledge about them is still sparse in contrast to what we still have to learn. With more propelling research, a more refined hypothesis will generate, and learning will continue to grow. In this section, we will summarize the available existing evidence in the neurobiology of common mental disorders.

Neurobiology of Psychosis and Schizophrenia

To understand the neurobiology of schizophrenia, we need to deconstruct it into different symptom domains to understand the neurobiology better. The following symptoms domains characterize schizophrenia and related psychosis spectrum disorders

1. Positive psychotic symptoms: Positive psychotic symptoms include abnormal experiences that are *not* usually present in the general population. They include
   - Disorders of experience: These include delusions [false, firm, fixed beliefs that persist despite evidence to the contrary and are not culturally shared], hallucinations [perception without stimulus].
   - Disorganization symptoms: These include disorganized thinking [thinking that does not have logical continuity, coherency, or constancy] and disorganized behavior [self-contradictory, inconsistent behavior including silly, unpredictable, or inappropriate].
2. Negative psychotic symptoms: Negative psychotic symptoms include the absence of healthy experiences that should be present in healthy individuals. These include alogia, asociality, avolition, apathy, anhedonia, decreased emotional expressivity.
3. Other symptoms: In addition to these symptoms, poor self-care, cognitive symptoms, the decline in healthy social and occupational functioning is almost always present. There may be other symptom clusters such as catatonic symptoms, mood symptoms, aggression, or suicidal behavior that may be additionally present.

Table 11.4 maps these symptom domains to neurobiological areas.

Table 11.4: Simplistic localization of symptom domains of schizophrenia to specific neuro-anatomical areas

Symptom domain	Neuro-anatomical correlates
Positive psychotic symptoms*	Mesolimbic dopamine pathway [hyperdopaminergia]
Negative psychotic symptoms*	Meso-cortical [hypodopaminergia] and abnormal reward processing at nucleus acumbens
Cognitive symptoms	Dysfunctional information processing at Dorsolateral prefrontal cortex
Aggression	Disordered impulse control at Orbitofrontal cortex + amygdala dysfunction leading to disordered threat control override
Affective symptoms	Ventromedial prefrontal cortex dysfunction

* Implies symptom domains that are more specific to psychosis

Genetics of Schizophrenia

Schizophrenia is heritable and associated with several candidate genes. It has been proven beyond doubt that the model that explains the role of genetics in schizophrenia is the stress-diathesis model [Genetic predisposition + environmental stress (second hit) leading to decompensation and schizophrenia]. This association has been proven through twin studies, adoption studies, family studies, linkage analysis, and genome-wide association studies. The risk for schizophrenia with identical twin affected is 46%, both parents affected is 40%, one sibling, the parent or fraternal twin affected is 12-15%, one grandparent is 6%, and with no relatives is 0.5-1%. The major genetic loci implicated are summarized in **Table 11.5**. 22q deletion, also known as the velocardiofacial syndrome, is associated with a 30% risk of schizophrenia.

Neurotransmitter Pathways in Schizophrenia

Dopamine was one of the first neurotransmitters whose role was explored in psychosis. The primary dopamine, glutamate neurotransmitter

Table 11.5: Genetics of Schizophrenia

Implicated genes/ loci	Chromosome locus	Mechanism on
DTNBP1	6p	Synaptic glutamate release
NRG1	8p	Multiple pathways
COMT	22q	Cerebral monoamines
DISC 1	1q	Synaptogenesis and neurodevelopment
mGLU3	7q	NMDA receptor
PRODH	22q	Synaptic transmission
DAOA	13q	NMDA modulation

DTNBP – Dystrobrevin binding protein aka Dysbindin; NRG – Neuregulin;
COMT – Catechol-O-Methyl Transferase;
DISC – Disrupted in schizophrenia;
mGLU3 – metabotropic Glutamate receptor 3;
PRODH – proline dehydrogenase;
DAOA – A-amino acid oxidase activator.

pathways and their role in psychosis are summarized in Table 6. Dopamine is probably the final common pathway through which psychosis is mediated. Among the four primary dopamine circuits involved in schizophrenia is the hyperdopaminergia at the mesolimbic and hypodopaminergia at the mesocortical circuits. Glutamate regulates dopaminergic function, and its dysfunction can explain all the major symptom domains of psychosis. The pathways through which glutamate causes psychosis are elucidated in **Table 11.6**. Aberrant salience [implies a tendency for irrelevant stimuli to be attributed motivational importance that could lead to abnormal thinking and behavior] plays an essential role in expressing psychotic symptoms secondary to the neurotransmitter abnormality. Table 6 summarizes the important role of Dopamine and Glutamate pathways in schizophrenia.

Neuroimaging Correlates

Persons with schizophrenia exhibit larger ventricles, reduction in the gray matter especially involving the prefrontal cortex. Additionally, decreased volumes of subcortical structures such as the amygdala, hippocampus, parahippocampus, and thalamus. Decreased volumes of the superior temporal gyrus have been seen in persons with prominent delusions, hallucinations, and thought disorganization.

Table 11.6: Dopamine and Glutamate pathways and their role in psychosis

Neurotransmitter / Neural Pathway	Projection	Dysfunction	Symptoms explained
Mesolimbic Dopamine pathway	Ventral tegmental area to nucleus acumbens in ventral striatum [part of the limbic system]	Hyperactivity	Delusions and Hallucinations
Mesocortical Dopamine pathway	Ventral tegmental area to the prefrontal cortex	Hypoactivity	Negative symptoms
NMDA [Type pf Glutamate receptor]	Reduced receptor or functioning of the GABAergic interneurons leading to disinhibition of glutamatergic projections on the midbrain dopamine neurons	Hypofunction on GABAergic interneurons + Downstream Increased Glutamate release leading to increased dopamine activity of dopaminergic neurons	Positive, Negative, and Cognitive

Mood Disorders

The neurobiology of depression can be discussed in the following domains

Genetic

Mood disorders are heritable. Polymorphisms of the 5HT2C and 5HT transporter protein are associated with mood disorders.

Neuroendocrine Model

The hypothalamic-pituitary-adrenal axis [HPA axis] has been extensively studied in stress-mood disorder etiology. Various components of the HPA axis can lead to mood disorders that are summarized below:

- Cortisol hypersecretion – One in two patients with depression have direct or indirect evidence of excess cortisol [excess serum cortisol, hypertrophied adrenal glands]
- Non-suppression with Dexamethasone challenge test – Corticosteroid administration is expected to reduce the release of Corticotrophin release hormone and downstream pituitary release of the adreno-cortico-trophic hormone. In this test, despite exogenous administration of a dexamethasone challenge, up to half of the patients with severe depression cannot suppress endogenous cortisol levels.

Neurochemical Theories

Depression and mania are explained by the role of monoamine transmitters. Serotonin, noradrenaline, and dopamine have all been implicated. A functional decrease of these NTs in a synaptic cleft or increased has been implicated with depression and mania. This is proved by studies demonstrating reduced plasma levels of Tryptophan [5HT precursor], reduced 5HTIAA CSF levels in depression.

Sleep Correlates

Depression is associated with sleep disturbances. Disturbed sleep figures as one of the minor diagnostic criteria for depression. Delayed initiation of sleep and early morning awakening is associated with depression and is associated with decreased REM latency and increased REM sleep [with the possibility of increased dreams]

Neuroimaging Correlates

In the elderly, depression is associated with subcortical white matter hyperintensities secondary to vascular insults. Functional neuroimaging data reflect a decrease in subcortical anterior neural structures such as the prefrontal cortex and cingulate cortex. Non-specific ventricular enlargement and sulci widening can also be seen.

Neuroanatomical Correlates

Different neural structures can be associated with different symptom domains in depression, and they are summarized in **Table 11.7**. These factors, in combination, lead to disordered neuroplasticity and depression.

Table 11.7: Neural correlates of Depression symptom domains

Structures	Domain
Neocortex and hippocampus [decreased neurotropic support, e.g., BDNF]	Cognitive domain – depressed cognitions [worthlessness, hopelessness, helplessness], guilt, memory impairments, and suicidal ideation
Nucleus acumbens [part of the ventral striatum] and amygdala	Trigger of emotional memories, reduced motivation, anhedonia [lack of interest in previously pleasurable activities]
Hypothalamus	Neurovegetative symptoms – disturbed sleep, appetite, libido, energy

Obsessive-compulsive Disorders

Obsessive-compulsive disorders (OCD) are characterized by

- Obsessions - a psychic phenomenon that is intrusive, unwanted [ego-dystonic], repetitive, not easily controlled, can involve domains of thought including forms of image, or memory [including perceptual memory – visual and auditory are most common], and they may be associated with
- Compulsions – repetitive motor or mental acts that serve to decrease distress associated with obsessions.
- Obsessions and compulsions are almost always associated with psychological distress, anxiety.

Genetics

To date, although OCD is deemed as a heritable polygenic disorder, inconsistent genetic variations in candidate genes such as SLC1A1, DLGAP1, and PTPRD, have been reported with OCD. However, genetic underpinnings of OCD are mainly unknown.

Neurobiological Model

To understand the neurobiology of OCD, it is essential to understand the frontal circuits and their connection with the basal ganglia. Frontal subcortical circuits usually have two pathways – a direct loop and an indirect loop.

- Direct pathway – Disinhibits the thalamus and activates the circuitry in a positive feedback loop for a complex sequence of pre-planned activity
- Indirect pathway – Inhibits the thalamus and provides a negative feedback loop to the activity

Complex motor commands are carried out with coordinated activity between the direct and the indirect pathway. In OCD, there is a bias towards some internal or external stimuli involving themes of danger, sex, violence, order. Due to the increased tone of the direct pathway, persons with OCD have a low threshold for socio-territorial concerns, leading to them performing compulsions. This is associated with impaired response inhibition and difficulty in shifting to more adaptive behaviors. Imaging studies have demonstrated this imbalance through the hyperactive orbito-fronto-thalamic circuit, especially the hyperactivity of the OFC, cingulate, and the head of caudate.

Anxiety Disorder

Anxiety disorders are a broad rubric encompassing phobic and neurotic disorders. They are associated with autonomic arousal, avoidance of the object/ situation mediating anxiety, psychological and physical features of anxiety. Anxiety disorders are associated with dysregulation of serotonergic systems, increased adrenergic activity [noradrenergic activity originating in locus ceruleus mediate arousal and anxiety], hypersensitivity to presynaptic alpha-2 receptors, reduced GABA activity.

Symptoms such as panic involve the dysfunction in the fear network [i.e., the triad of the amygdala, hypothalamus, and brain stem.] Panic disorder is associated with genomic duplication on chromosome 15. Locus ceruleus, limbic system, and prefrontal cortex are implicated in panic disorder. Locus ceruleus activity affects the hypothalamic-pituitary-adrenal axis functioning. The amygdala plays a pivotal role in mediating emotionally charged conditioned fear response. Specific phobias are associated with hyperactivity of the paralimbic brain structures, thalamus, and visual association areas that trigger a conditioned fear response. PTSD is atypical because it may be associated with reduced cortisol and increased glucocorticoid receptor sensitivity with a blunted HPA response to stress. In PTSD, the ventromedial prefrontal cortex is dysfunctional and fails to extinguish the responses to innocuous stimuli that evoke memories and recollection from the traumatic experience.

Substance use and Addiction

To understand the neurobiology of addiction, it is essential to understand the different phases of the addiction cycle in a recurring fashion. The altered neurocircuitry functioning is due to disruption of the dopamine and glutamate systems and the stress-control systems of the brain, which are influenced by corticotropin-releasing factors and dynorphin. The behaviors during the three stages of addiction evolve as a person transitions from drug experimentation [due to novelty seeking, peer group influences, low harm avoidance, impulsivity] to addiction as a function of the progressive neuroadaptations that occur in the brain

- Binge and intoxication stage – All known drugs lead to activation of the reward pathway leading to dopamine-induced 'high.' This is then subjected to behavioral conditioning with associated stimulus leading to the expectation of a reward and induces craving. The neural structures involved in this process include the ventral striatum [nucleus acumbens], globus pallidus, and thalamus
- Withdrawal and negative affect stage – When the substance is withheld, it leads to withdrawal [psychological and physical]. These withdrawal experiences lead to pathological changes in the amygdala and forebrain, negative emotions, and increase sensitivity to stress. This activates the 'anti-reward' system and resulting dysphoria [Thus, the patient, in addition to a current craving for the substance, seeks out the drug to be relieved from the withdrawal effects]. This is mediated through the amygdala, basal nucleus of stria terminalis, and ventral striatum
- The preoccupation and anticipation stage involves the prefrontal cortex, where the person can make healthy decisions and execute decisions. Both glutamate and dopamine are implicated in this dysfunction leading to repeated failure by individuals to stop taking drugs. Over some time, compulsivity of drug use becomes the norm unless appropriately treated. The neural structures involved in this process include the orbitofrontal cortex, anterior cingulate cortex, and hippocampus.

CONCLUSION

These neurobiological processes explained are simplistic and meant to prime the readers to primary neural correlates of psychiatric disorders. Understanding these mechanisms has led to significant advancements in the field of psychiatry diagnosis and treatment.

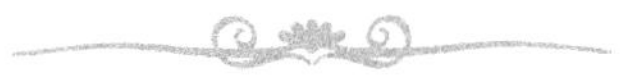

12 Basics of Neurotransmitters

Ami Pawar • Astik Mane

INTRODUCTION

The story of how chemicals communicate in our brain forms the basis of understanding many core psychiatric illnesses. It is also the foundation on which modern psychopharmacology is based.

A *neuron* is the basic cell of chemical communication in the brain. The human brain is made up of billions of neurons which are linked to each other through specialized connections known as *synapses*. Neurons communicate with one another and with their target tissues by releasing specific chemical substances into synapses known as *neurotransmitters*. The process is called chemical *neurotransmission* and happens within chemical synapses. These neurotransmitters not only affect the way we think, feel and behave but also have an effect on motor coordination and other physiological functions such as heart rate, blood pressure etc. Psychiatric medications act by altering the levels of neurotransmitters in the synapse or by altering neurotransmission itself.

In this chapter, the basic mechanism of neurotransmission is highlighted in brief, followed by properties, classification and details of individual neurotransmitters.

MECHANISM OF NEUROTRANSMISSION

Neurotransmitters (NTs) are chemicals which help to transmit information from one cell to another. They are synthesized in the ribosomes of the presynaptic neurons and stored in vesicles present in the cytoplasm of the presynaptic neuron. A nerve impulse basically means a propagated action potential which is nothing but the rapid sequential change in the membrane potential of the neuron. When the presynaptic neuron is depolarized by this propagated action potential, it causes the calcium channels located in the presynaptic neuron to open. The influx of calcium in the presynaptic neuron leads to the fusion of synaptic vesicles with the presynaptic membrane. This leads to release of the neurotransmitter from the presynaptic neuron. The neurotransmitter released binds to its specific receptor which could be located on the presynaptic membrane or post synaptically. Depending on the type of neurotransmitter and the specific receptor it binds to, the post synaptic neuron is either excited or inhibited. Neurotransmitters which lead to excitation are more likely to cause the post synaptic neuron to generate an action potential and those that lead to inhibition prevent the post synaptic neuron from generating an action potential.

However, we can't always sort neurotransmitters clearly as either excitatory or inhibitory. It is important to note that there isn't just one type of receptor for each neurotransmitter and the same neurotransmitter can bind to and activate multiple different receptor proteins.

Receptor proteins that are activated by neurotransmitters can be divided into two broad types, *ionotropic* and *metabotropic* receptors:

Ionotropic receptors (ligand or ion channel receptors) are membrane spanning ion channel proteins which open directly in response to ligand binding. They have specific NT binding sites on them. When a neurotransmitter binds, they change shape and cause the channel to open. They may be excitatory or inhibitory depending on the ions that pass through them. They produce quick physiological responses and the NT is cleared off quickly from the synapse by enzymes or by reuptake into nearby cells.

Metabotropic receptors on the other hand are G-protein coupled receptors. NT binding triggers an intracellular signaling pathway which may directly or indirectly open or close channels or have some entirely different effect. Neurotransmission through these receptors frequently involves a second messenger pathway. Due to the multiple steps involved, neurotransmission through these receptors is slower than with ion channel receptors.

A special type of receptors which are normally located on the presynaptic neuron are *auto receptors*. When stimulated these auto-receptors *inhibit* the release of neurotransmitter from that neuron. The basic structure of a synapse and mechanism of neurotransmission are as shown in **Figs. 12.1 and 12.2**.

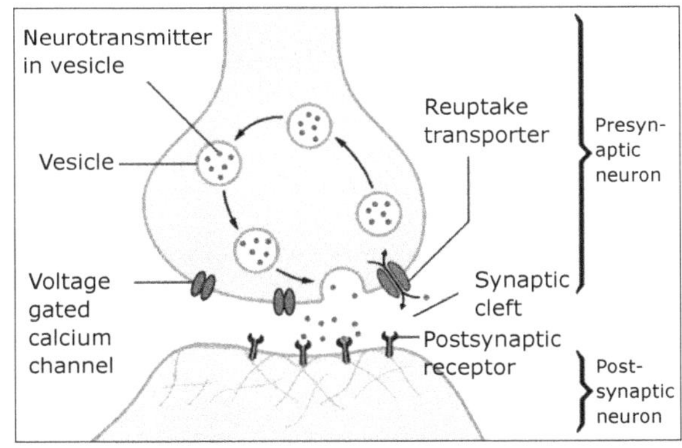

Fig. 12.1: Neurotransmission in a synapse.

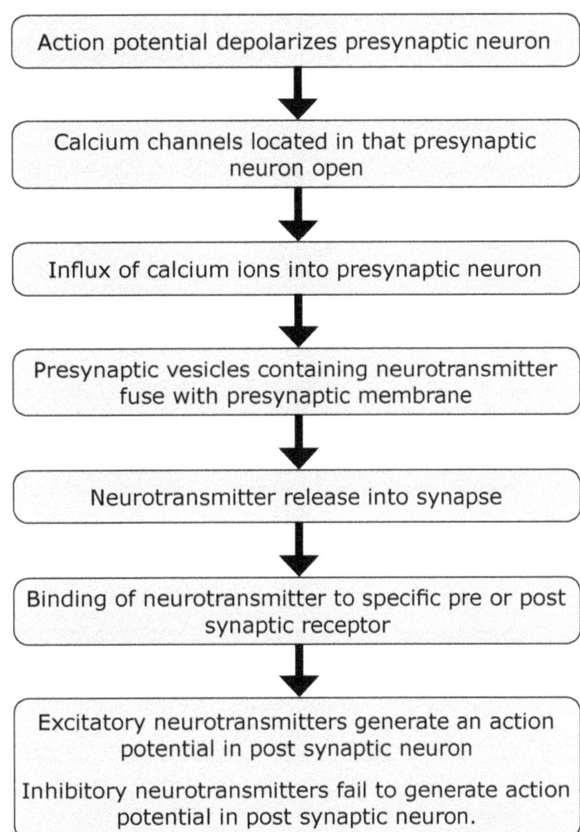

Fig. 12.2: Mechanism of neurotransmission.

CRITERIA TO DEFINE NEUROTRANSMITTERS

Having understood the mechanism of neurotransmission, we now look at what it is that makes a molecule in the neuron a neurotransmitter. The following criteria have been used over the years to confirm that a molecule acts as a neurotransmitter at a given chemical synapse:

1. The molecule should be present in the presynaptic neuron.
2. The molecule must be released in response to presynaptic depolarization, and the release must be Ca^{2+}-dependent.
3. Specific receptors for the substance must be present on the postsynaptic cell.

PROPERTIES OF NEUROTRANSMITTERS

SYNTHESIS
- Neurotransmitters are synthesized in the presynaptic neurons.

STORAGE
- Neurotransmitters are stored in vesicles which are located in the presynaptic neurons.

RELEASE
- Neurotransmitters are released in the synaptic cleft in response to change in the presynaptic electrical activity which requires calcium influx into the presynaptic terminal.

RECEPTOR
- Neurotransmitters have specific receptors on the post synaptic "target" cell (e.g. neuron, muscle cell or gland cell)

ACTION
- Neurotransmitters exert their biological action on binding to the specific post synaptic receptors.

REMOVAL
- Neurotransmitters are rapidly removed from the synaptic cleft by the process of reuptake into the neuron, or by degradation in the cleft itself.

Fig. 12.3: Properties of neurotransmitters.

Accordingly, all neurotransmitters have certain common properties pertaining to their synthesis, storage, release, receptor action and removal. These properties are highlighted in **Fig. 12.3**.

CLASSIFICATION OF NEUROTRANSMITTERS

Broadly speaking, there are two main ways to classify neurotransmitters. Firstly, we can classify them based on their function (i.e. inherent effect in the nervous system) as either excitatory or inhibitory. Another way to classify neurotransmitters is based on their chemical structure (**Fig. 12.4**). As discussed earlier, since all neurotransmitters cannot clearly be compartmentalised into inhibitory and excitatory, and overlap may occur, individual neurotransmitters are further discussed based on their structural classification.

CLASSIFICATION OF NEUROTRANSMITTERS		
BASED ON FUNCTION	INHIBITORY	GABA, GLYCINE, SEROTONIN, DOPAMINE
	EXCITATORY	GLUTAMATE, NOR-EPINEPHRINE, EPINEPHRINE, DOPAMINE
BASED ON STRUCTURE	MONOAMINE	SEROTONIN, DOPAMINE, NOREPINEPHRINE, HISTAMINE & ACETYLCHOLINE
	AMINO ACID	GABA, GLUTAMIC ACID
	NEUROPEP-TIDES	HORMONES, SUBTANCE P, SUBSTANCE K etc.
	NOVEL NT	NITRIC OXIDE, CARBON MONOXIDE, CANNABINOIDS,, EICOSANOIDS & NEUROSTEROIDS

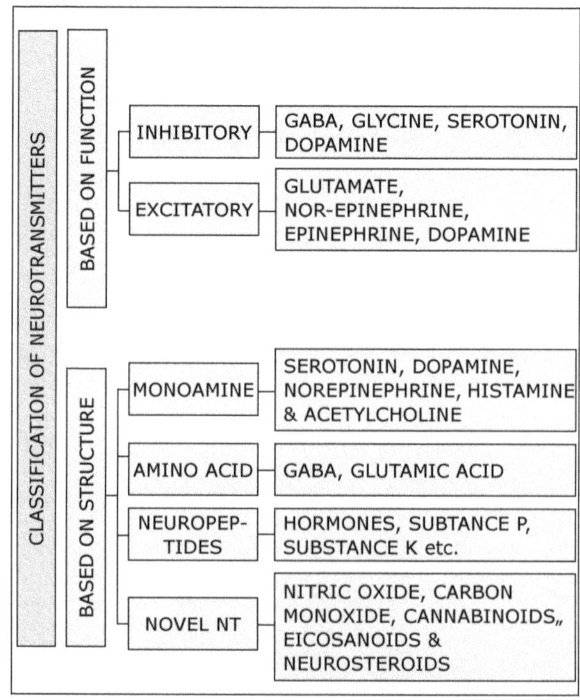

Fig. 12.4: Classification of neurotransmitters.

MONOAMINE NEUROTRANSMITTERS

SEROTONIN

a) Type

Serotonin or 5-Hydroxytryptamine (5HT) is a monoamine which can act as both an excitatory and inhibitory neurotransmitter.

b) Anatomy

Serotonergic neurons are present in the brainstem raphe nuclei which give projections to a wide region in the brain. The ascending fibers project to the prefrontal cortex, striatum and thalamus while the descending fibers project down the brainstem and spinal cord (**Image 12.1**).

c) Life cycle

i) Synthesis: Serotonin is synthesized by hydroxylation of the amino acid tryptophan to 5- hydroxytryptophan (5 HTP). The 5HTP undergoes decarboxylation to form serotonin (5-Hydroxytryptamine, i.e. 5-HT.

ii) Storage and release: 5-HT is taken up into the vesicles with the help of Vesicular Monoamine Transporter (VMAT). When the cell is depolarized, the vesicles fuse with the presynaptic axon terminal and serotonin is released.

iii) Reuptake/Breakdown: The 5-HT further acts on the postsynaptic or the presynaptic receptors. In the synaptic space, it can be either degraded or taken back by the pre-synaptic neuron. Monoamine Oxidase Type A (MAO-A) oxidises serotonin which is the first step in degradation. Further oxidation leads to formation of 5-Hydroxyindoleacetic Acid (5-HIAA) (**Fig. 12.5**).

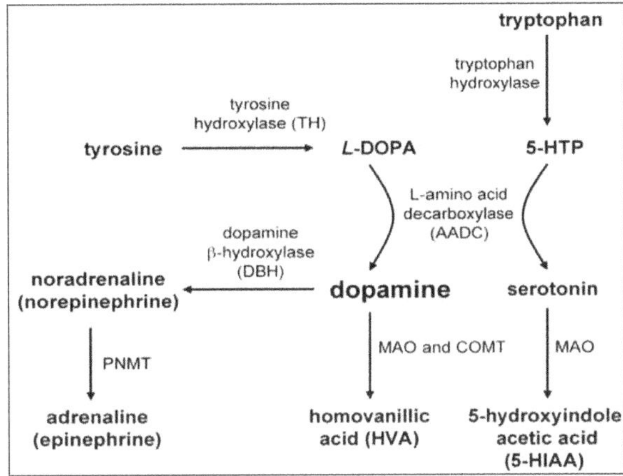

Fig. 12.5: Synthesis and breakdown of monoamine neurotransmitters.

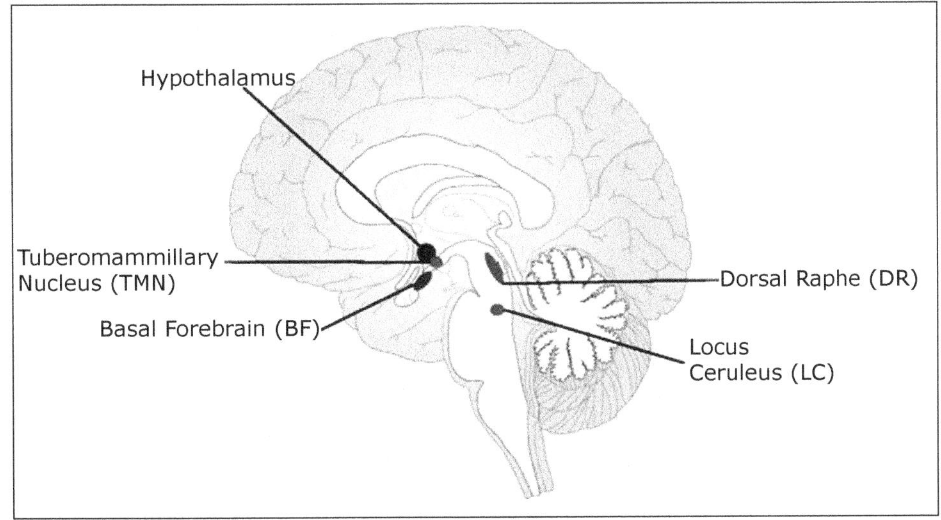

Image 12.1: Monoamine nuclei in the brain.

d) Receptors & their function:

Serotonergic receptors can be either ligand gated (ionotropic) or G- protein coupled (metabotropic) receptors. There are 7 subtypes of serotonergic receptors: 5HT1-5HT7. Their location and function are explained in brief in **Table 12.1**.

e) Psychiatric correlates

i) *Depression:* The monoamine hypothesis of depression postulates that depression is associated with low serotonin levels in the brain. Selective serotonin reuptake inhibitors (SSRIs) are effective in the treatment of depression, which indicates that serotonin is a neurotransmitter related to depression. Most classes of antidepressant drugs exert their effect by modulating serotonin levels in the brain. Examples of SSRIs include: Escitalopram, Citalopram, Fluoxetine, Sertraline, Fluvoxamine and Paroxetine. Other antidepressant drugs which modulate serotonin are SNRI (serotonin norepinephrine reuptake inhibitors) e.g. Venlafaxine, Tricyclic antidepressants e.g. Amitriptyline, and Noradrenergic and Specific Serotonergic Antidepressant (NaSSA) e.g. Mirtazapine.

ii) *Obsessive compulsive disorder:* SSRIs such as fluvoxamine, fluoxetine and sertraline are amongst the first line medications in the treatment of recurrent intrusive thoughts and acts which form a part of OCD. This highlights the possibility of serotonergic imbalance in these patients.

iii) *Anxiety disorders:* Serotonergic antidepressant drugs serve as first line medications in the treatment of panic disorder, agoraphobia and generalized

Table 12.1: Serotonin receptors

Receptor type	Location	Function
5-HT1 (5-HT1A, 5-HT1B, 5-HT1D, 5-14T1E and 5-HT1F)	Cerebral cortex, striatum, hippocampus, amygdala, septum, entorhinal cortex, hypothalamus, raphe nuclei	5-HT1A -Serotonergic auto receptor. Stimulation decreases serotonin release
5-HT2 (5-HT2A, 5-HT2B and 5-HT2C)	Globus pallidus, cerebral cortex, hypothalamus, septum, substantia nigra, spinal cord	5-HT2A -Stimulation decreases dopamine release in striatum 5-HT2C- Regulates dopamine and norepinephrine release. Agonists at this receptor may be used for treatment of obesity
5-HT3	Hippocampus, entorhinal cortex, amygdala, nucleus accumbens, solitary tract nerve, trigeminal nerve, motor nucleus of the dorsal vagal nerve, area postrema, spinal cord	Peripheral 5HT3 receptors are responsible for bowel regulation. Central 5HT3 receptors mediated vomiting and nausea
5-HT4	Hippocampus, striatum, olfactory tubercle, substantia nigra	Stimulation causes GI motility
5-HT5 (5-HT5A, 5-HT5B)	Olfactory bulb, hebenula	Unknown
5-11T6	CNS: caudate, putamen, hippocampus	Modulation of CNS Ach release
5-HT7	Cerebral cortex, septum, thalamus, hypothalamus, amygdala, superior colliculus	Regulates serotonin release. Antagonist have antidepressant action. Smooth muscle relaxation

anxiety disorder highlighting the role of serotonin in their etiopathogenesis.

iv) *Eating Disorders:* SSRIs and TCAs are the first line medications useful in the treatment of eating disorders such as anorexia and bulimia nervosa.

v) *Schizophrenia:* The role of serotonin is pathophysiology of schizophrenia is based on the observation that atypical antipsychotics such as olanzapine, quetiapine etc. act as serotonergic dopaminergic antagonists and are effective in reducing both positive and negative symptoms of schizophrenia.

vi) *Sleep regulation and sexual drive:* Serotonin in an important neurotransmitter in the regulation of sleep. L-tryptophan is a precursor for serotonin, decreased levels of L-tryptophan cause a decrease in REM sleep. Serotonin has also been observed to have an inhibitory effect on sexual function: i.e. it decreases sexual desire and delays ejaculation.

DOPAMINE

a) Type

Dopamine is a monoamine neurotransmitter and can act as both excitatory and inhibitory.

b) Anatomy

There are four dopaminergic pathways which are of clinical importance in psychiatry. They are the *mesocortical pathway, mesolimbic pathway, nigrostriatal pathway* and *tubero-Infundibular pathway.* Dopaminergic neurons which project from the Ventral Tegmental Area in the midbrain to the cortex form the *mesocortical* pathway, and those going to limbic system form the *mesolimbic pathway*. Dopaminergic neurons projecting from the substantia nigra pars compacta in the brainstem to the striatum of basal ganglia form the *nigrostriatal pathway.* Dopaminergic neurons projecting from the hypothalamus to the pituitary gland form the *tubero-infundibular pathway* (**Image 12.2**).

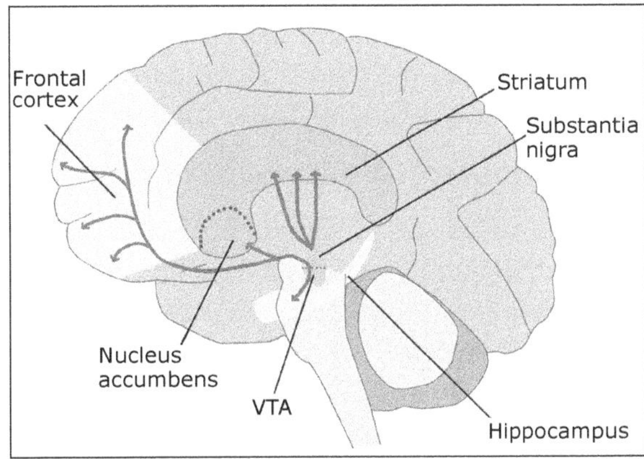

Image 12.2: Dopamine pathways.

c) Life cycle

i) *Synthesis:* Dopamine is synthesized from the amino acid tyrosine. Tyrosine hydroxylase is the rate limiting enzyme in biosynthesis and converts the tyrosine to DOPA which is then acted upon by the decarboxylase enzyme to form dopamine.

ii) *Storage and release*: Dopamine is taken up into the vesicles with the help of Vesicular Monoamine Transporter (VMAT). When depolarised, the vesicles fuse with the presynaptic axon terminal and dopamine is released. Dopamine then proceeds to act on the postsynaptic or the presynaptic receptors.

iii) *Reuptake/Breakdown*: Once in the synapse, dopamine can either be degraded by an enzyme or taken back by the presynaptic neuron. Monoamine Oxidase (MAO) and Catechol-O-Methyltransferase (COMT) are the enzymes responsible for the degradation of dopamine to form homovanillic acid (HVA). Whereas MAO-A is more specific for serotonin and norepinephrine, MAO-B is more specific for dopamine (**Fig. 12.5**).

d) **Dopamine Receptors:**

All the dopamine receptors are metabotropic G- protein coupled receptors. There are five subtypes of dopamine receptors D1, D2, D3, D4 and D5. Their location and functions are explained in brief in **Table 12.2**.

e) **Neuropsychiatric correlates**

i) *Schizophrenia:* The Dopamine hypothesis of schizophrenia was based on the fact that dopamine antagonists reduce the symptoms of the disorder. It was found that increased dopamine was related to positive symptoms of schizophrenia such as delusions and hallucinations. Antipsychotic medications such as haloperidol and olanzapine act as dopamine receptor antagonists and help in controlling the symptoms of schizophrenia.

ii) *Parkinson's disease:* A loss of dopaminergic neurons in the substantia nigra is the core pathology in Parkinson's disease which leads to dopamine deficit state associated with cogwheel rigidity, tremors and slow movements along with mask-like facies. Pro-dopaminergic drugs like levodopa and inhibitors of degrading enzymes COMT and MAO are also useful in management of this condition.

iii) *Extrapyramidal symptoms*: The nigro-striatal pathway (Substantia Nigra Pars Compacta to Striatum) has dopaminergic neurons. When dopamine receptor antagonists are given in disorders like schizophrenia, the striatal dopaminergic receptors are also blocked. This pathway is involved in regulation of smooth movements. Blocking them can cause symptoms like rigidity, bradykinesia and tremors.

iv) *Depression:* It has been observed that reduced dopaminergic activity is present in depression and increased in mania. Therefore, drugs like Bupropion which are norepinephrine dopamine reuptake inhibitors (NDRIs), increase Dopamine levels and are effective in the treatment of depression.

v) *Substance use disorders:* Dopamine is an important neurotransmitter in the reward

Table 12.2: Dopamine receptors

Receptors	Location	Function
D1	Striatum, nucleus accumbens, olfactory bulb, amygdala hippocampus, substantia nigra hypothalamus, frontal cortex	Locomotion, learning and memory, attention, impulse control, sleep, regulation of renal function
D2	Striatum, VTA, olfactory bulb, cerebral cortex	Locomotion, learning and memory, attention, sleep, reproductive behavior. D2 receptor antagonism reduces positive symptoms of schizophrenia
D3	Striatum, cortex	Locomotion, cognition, attention, impulse control, sleep, regulation of food intake
D4	Frontal cortex, amygdala, hypothalamus, nucleus accumbens	Cognition, impulse control, attention, sleep, reproductive behavior
D5	Cortex, substantia nigra, hypothalamus	Cognition, attention, decision making, motor learning, renin secretion

pathway. Dopaminergic neurons from the Ventral Tegmental Area to the Nucleus Accumbens (NA) form the final part of the reward circuit. Increased dopamine level in the NA is associated with a feeling of pleasure which motivates drug seeking behavior.

vi) *Attention Deficit Hyperactivity Disorder (ADHD)*: In ADHD dysfunction is observed in both dopamine and norepinephrine neurotransmission in the prefrontal cortex. Impaired dopamine levels are associated with increased distractibility seen in ADHD.

NOREPINEPHRINE

a) Type

Norepinephrine is a catecholamine neurotransmitter and is excitatory in nature.

b) Anatomy

CNS: The locus ceruleus of the brainstem is the main nucleus from which brain norepinephrinergic pathways emerge. Noradrenergic neurons project bilaterally (send signals to both sides of the brain) from the locus ceruleus along distinct pathways to many locations, including the cerebral cortex, limbic system, and the spinal cord, forming a neurotransmitter system. Effects of norepinephrine release are alertness and arousal, and influences on the reward system (**Image 12.1**).

PNS: Norepinephrine is also released from postganglionic neurons of the sympathetic nervous system, to transmit the fight-or-flight response in each tissue respectively. The adrenal medulla can also release norepinephrine into the blood as a physiological response to a stressful event.

c) Life cycle

i) Synthesis: Norepinephrine is synthesized in a series of steps from the amino acid tyrosine, the same amino acid from which dopamine is synthesized. Tyrosine undergoes hydroxylation into dihydroxyphenylalanine (DOPA) catalysed by tyrosine hydroxylase. This is followed by decarboxylation into the neurotransmitter dopamine catalysed by DOPA decarboxylase. Last is the final β-oxidation into norepinephrine by dopamine beta hydroxylase. Hence, it is from dopamine that norepinephrine gets synthesized.

ii) Storage and release: Between decarboxylation and final oxidation, dopamine is transported into the vesicles in the neuron, and converted into norepinephrine by dopamine hydroxylase and stored till further release. Many substances modulate the release, some inhibiting it and some stimulating it. For instance, there are inhibitory α2 adrenergic receptors presynaptically, which act as autoreceptors and give negative feedback on the release of norepinephrine.

iii) Reuptake/Breakdown: Monoamine Oxidase -A (MAO-A) is more specific for serotonin and norepinephrine degradation. Monoamine oxidase breaks down the norepinephrine in the synaptic cleft hence terminating its action. Norepinephrine action can also be terminated by reuptake by its transporter NET (Norepinephrine transporter) back into the neuron (**Fig. 12.5**).

d) Receptors & their function

There are two main families of adrenergic receptors: alpha and beta. Alpha receptors have two subtypes α1 and α2, of which α2 are present on both presynaptic and postsynaptic neurons which are further divided as shown below. Beta receptors have three subtypes, namely β1, β2 and β3. Details of these receptors are as shown in **Table 12.3**.

Table 12.3: Norepinephrine receptors

Receptor type	Location	Function
α1 has 3 subtypes: α1A, α1B and α1D α2 has 3 subtypes: α2A, α2B and α2C	Periphery > CNS	α1 receptors are involved in smooth muscle contraction α2 antagonists enhance mood by increasing norepinephrine
β are divided to β1, β2 and β 3	Periphery > CNS	β2 agonists help in smooth muscle relaxation e.g. bronchodilation

e) Psychiatric correlates

i) *Depressive disorders:* Norepinephrine projections go from the locus ceruleus to the limbic system, a part of the brain involved in regulating emotions. Deficits in norepinephrine levels in the brain are associated with depression which gets treated on administering antidepressants with norepinephrine reuptake properties such as SNRIs, NDRIs and NRIs.

ii) *Anxiety disorders:* Enhanced central noradrenergic activity is associated with the activation of fear and anxiety circuits. Paradoxically SNRIs which increase norepinephrine levels are employed with considerable success in the treatment of anxiety disorders, though one needs to be watchful for the transient increase in anxiety symptoms at the outset of treatment.

iii) *Schizophrenia:* In schizophrenia patients can have impairment in cognition, motivation and executive functions. Anhedonia (inability to experience pleasure in normally pleasurable acts) is another feature of schizophrenia and may be attributed to norepinephrine dysfunction.

iv) *Sleep-wake cycle:* Norepinephrine also regulates sleep. Locus ceruleus, when stimulated reduces the REM sleep, causing wakefulness.

v) *Attention Deficit Hyperactivity Disorder (ADHD)*: Sustained and selective attention is regulated by norepinephrine. Dysfunction in norepinephrine levels cause inattention. Norepinephrine reuptake inhibitors like atomoxetine are useful in the treatment of ADHD.

iv) *Opioid withdrawal*: Opioid withdrawal is associated with autonomic instability and an increase in noradrenergic activity. α2 receptor agonists like Clonidine reduce the release of norepinephrine and are useful in the management of opioid withdrawal.

HISTAMINE

a) Type

Histamine acts as an excitatory neurotransmitter. Activation of H1 histaminergic receptors causes increase in excitatory neuronal responses.

b) Anatomy

Histamine is located both peripherally and centrally in the body. Only a small portion is located centrally in the brain. Histaminergic cell bodies are found in the posterior hypothalamus in an area called the tuberomammilary nucleus. In addition, the monoaminergic and cholinergic nuclei also have a dense histaminergic innervation. From these locations, histaminergic fibers project diffusely through the brain and spinal cord (**Image 12.1**).

c) **Life cycle**

i) *Synthesis*: Histamine is synthesized by decarboxylation of amino acid histidine in the brain by the L- histidine decarboxylase enzyme (**Fig. 12.6**).

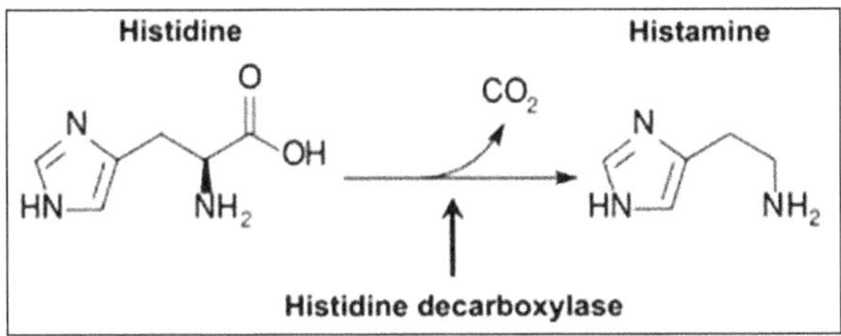

Fig. 12.6: Histamine synthesis.

ii) *Storage and release:* Peripheral histamine is stored in mast cells and released on cellular interaction with allergens. Enterochromaffin- like cells of the stomach also have stores of histamine. Central (non-mast cell) histamine found in the brain serves as a neurotransmitter and also acts like a hormone, in that it exerts its action at a site distant from its site of release.

iii) *Reuptake/Breakdown*: Histamine is metabolized by histamine *N*-methyltransferase in the synapses in the brain and produces methylhistamine which undergoes oxidative deamination by MAO-B enzyme. Diamine oxidase is another enzyme responsible for histamine degradation.

d) **Receptors & their function**

Histamine exerts its effects by binding to G-protein coupled histamine receptors. These histamine receptors are of four types: H1, H2, H3 and H4. Their respective location and function is explained in brief in the **Table 12.4**.

Table 12.4: Histamine receptors

Receptor type	Location	Function
H1	CNS> Periphery	Affects sleep wake cycle Regulates appetite Causes bronchoconstriction, vasodilatation & itch perception in periphery
H2	CNS> Periphery	Stimulates gastric acid production in the stomach Modulates gastrointestinal function Causes vasodilatation in the periphery
H3	CNS> Periphery	Auto-receptor and hetero-receptor function wherein stimulation decreases release of histamine, serotonin, norepinephrine and acetylcholine. Modulates pain perception, gastic acid secretion and food intake.
H4	Periphery> CNS	Cognition, impulse control, attention, sleep, reproductive behavior
D5	Cortex, substantia nigra, hypothalamus	Role in mast cell chemotaxis

e) **Psychiatric correlates**

i) H1 Antagonist drugs are useful as anti-allergic and anti-inflammatory agents. These medications can also cause weight gain and sedation. Various antidepressant and antipsychotic medications with H1 antagonism lead to sedation and help in the treatment of insomnia associated with these disorders. The same properties can also account for daytime drowsiness and weight gain as a side effect of these drugs.

ii) H2 Antagonist agents are used in treatment of GI reflux, peptic ulcers and GI bleeding.

iii) H3 Antagonists increase histamine release and have been promoted as wakefulness promoting agents in treatment of Narcolepsy. They also have a proposed role in treatment of obesity and dementia.

iv) H4 Antagonists have a possible role as anti-inflammatory agents.

ACETYLCHOLINE

a) Type

Acetylcholine can exert an excitatory or inhibitory effect depending upon the type of receptor present on the post synaptic (target) cell. For example, acetylcholine is excitatory at the neuromuscular junction in skeletal muscle. In this case, acetylcholine binding to its post synaptic ion channel receptor makes the target cell more likely to fire an action potential. This causes the skeletal muscle to contract. In contrast, it is inhibitory in the heart, where it decreases the heart rate. In this case, acetylcholine binds to a G- protein coupled receptor which triggers a downstream response leading to decreased muscle contraction.

b) Anatomy

Acetylcholine is found as a neurotransmitter in the peripheral and central nervous system. In the periphery, it is released at the neuromuscular junction as well as in the autonomic nervous system in the preganglionic sympathetic and parasympathetic neurons. It is the neurotransmitter at all the parasympathetic innervated organs. Within the brain (i.e. centrally), cholinergic transmission occurs locally in interneurons or to distant areas through projection neurons. Local cholinergic transmission occurs in interneurons in the striatum of the basal ganglia. There are two main regions in the basal forebrain region from which cholinergic neurons project: the *nucleus basalis of Meynert* and the *meso-pontine complex* in the area of the midbrain and pons. Cholinergic fibers project from these areas in the brain upwards towards cortex and other cerebral structures, and downwards to other brainstem areas and cranial nerve nuclei (**Image 12.1**).

c) Life cycle

i) *Synthesis:* Acetylcholine is synthesized through a single step reaction mediated by enzyme Choline Acetyl Transferase *(ChaT)*. Choline transported from the blood to the brain is taken up into cholinergic neurons where an acetyl group is transferred from acetyl coenzyme A. Acetyl coenzyme A is made from glucose present in the mitochondria of the neuron (**Fig. 12.7**).

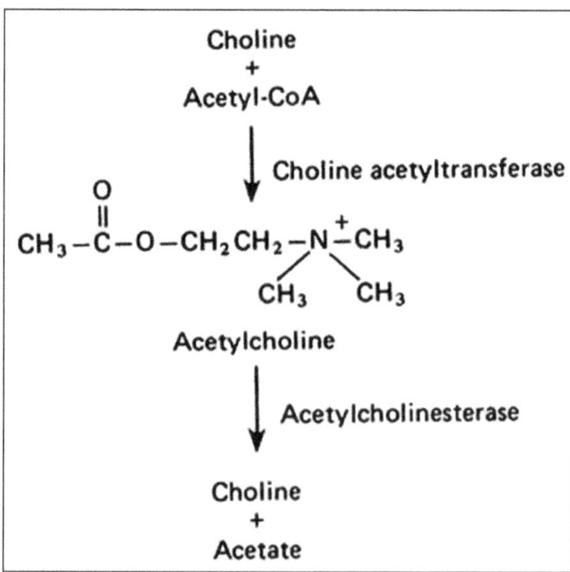

Fig. 12.7: Acetylcholine synthesis and breakdown.

ii) *Storage and release:* The acetylcholine synthesized is taken up for storage in synaptic vesicles with the help of a *vesicular acetylcholine transporter.* When a nerve impulse arrives at the terminal, acetylcholine is released from these vesicles. This release occurs at preganglionic and post ganglionic parasympathetic neuronal synapses as well as at the neuromuscular junction.

iii) *Reuptake/Breakdown*: After its release, the action of acetylcholine can be terminated by the action of two enzymes: *acetylcholinesterase (AChE)* and *butyrylcholinesterase (BuChE)* respectively. Acetylcholinesterase is found intracellularly as well as extracellularly whereas butyrylcholinesterase is found in glial cells, liver and plasma. AChE is the main enzyme for inactivating acetylcholine at the cholinergic synapses. BuChE breaks down the acetylcholine which reaches the glia. Through the effect of either enzyme, acetylcholine gets rapidly broken down by *hydrolysis* to choline and acetate. The choline from the synapse gets transported back by reuptake into presynaptic vesicles via the *choline transporter*. In the presynaptic neuron, this choline is recycled into acetylcholine and packaged into vesicles as already discussed.

d) Receptors & their function

There are two major subtypes of acetylcholine receptors: *muscarinic* and *nicotinic* types. Details on their location and function are given in **Table 12.5**.

Muscarinic receptors are metabotropic G- protein linked receptors and are both pre- and post- synaptic. Binding of acetylcholine to these receptors triggers a signaling pathway and often involves second messenger system in the cell which eventually can open or close ion channels, and lead to excitatory or inhibitory effects.

Table 12.5: Acetylcholine receptors

Acetycholine receptor	**Location**	**Function**
MUSCARINIC RECEPTORS		
M1	Cerebral cortex, hippocampus, autonomic ganglia (post synaptic) Gastric glands	Key role in memory and cognition Salivation
M2	Brain and heart (presynaptic autoreceptor)	Cardiac inhibition
M3	Smooth muscles of eye, viscera, blood vessels. Lower levels in cortex and hippocampus	Regulates GI movements, lacrimation, blood vessel contraction
M4	Basal ganglia, cortex, hippocampus	Regulates potassium and calcium channels
M5	Substantia nigra	Regulate dopamine release
NICOTINIC RECEPTORS (CNS)		
Alpha 7 nicotinic receptors	Prefrontal cortex (post synaptic) Cholinergic, dopaminergic and glutamatergic neurons (presynaptic)	Mediates cognitive function Facilitates release of acetylcholine, dopamine and glutamate respectively
Alpha-4 beta-2 nicotinic receptors	Nucleus accumbens of the basal ganglia (post synaptic)	Regulates dopamine release, contributes to reinforcing and addicting properties (tobacco)

Due to the multiple steps involved, signaling through these receptors is slower than signaling through ion channel receptors. They are found in the myocardium, certain smooth muscles, and in the CNS.

Nicotinic receptors are ligand activated ion channel receptors. They have specific binding sites for the neurotransmitter acetylcholine. They are post synaptic, membrane spanning, rapid onset, excitatory receptors which open directly in response to ligand (acetylcholine) binding. They are located at neuromuscular junctions, autonomic ganglia, and to a small extent in the CNS. Two of the most important CNS nicotinic cholinergic receptors are those with alpha 7 subunits and those with alpha 4 beta 2 subunits.

e) Neuropsychiatric correlates

i) Alzheimer's dementia: A significant degeneration of cholinergic neurons in the nucleus basalis of Meynert and a resultant decrease in cholinergic innervation is seen in patients with Alzheimer's disease, leading to the memory and cognitive changes seen in this condition. Accordingly, cholinesterase inhibitors like Donepezil, Rivastigmine, Tacrine and Galantamine which act by increasing acetylcholine levels have been useful in the treatment of Dementia.

ii) Tobacco dependence: The alpha-4 beta-2 subtype of nicotinic cholinergic receptors regulates the release of dopamine in the reward pathway. The nicotine in tobacco binds to the alpha-4 beta-2 nicotinic receptor, causing it to open, which in turn leads to release of dopamine. The dopamine thus released is responsible for the reinforcing and addictive properties of the substance. The nicotinic partial agonist Varenicline, which is used in smoking cessation acts through these receptors. It binds to the alpha 4 beta 2 receptor, allowing it to open less frequently, hence controlling the amount of dopamine released, accounting for its anti- addictive properties.

iii) Parkinson's disease: Parkinson's disease is characterized by loss of nigrostriatal dopaminergic neurons. Dopamine neurotransmission in the striatum is regulated by cholinergic interneurons. Studies have shown that nicotine and/or nicotinic agonists may prove beneficial in the management of Parkinson's disease.

iv) Extrapyramidal side effects of antipsychotics: Extrapyramidal symptoms like tremors, rigidity and slowness of movements which are common side effects of antipsychotic medications are known to improve on treatment with anticholinergic drugs such as trihexyphenidyl, promethazine etc. Antipsychotic medications decrease dopamine levels in the nigrostriatal pathway leading to a relative excess of nigrostriatal acetylcholine and the associated side effects of tremors, rigidity, slow movements and masking of face. Adding an anticholinergic medication helps relieve these side effects.

v) Schizophrenia: The gene coding for the alpha-7 nicotinic acetylcholine receptor subtype has been implicated as one of the susceptibility genes for development of schizophrenia.

vi) Myasthenia gravis: It is an autoimmune disease of the neuromuscular junction where the acetylcholine receptors are destroyed by the patient's own antibodies. Drugs such as physostigmine and neostigmine inhibit the hydrolysis and breakdown of acetylcholine and are useful in the diagnosis and treatment of myasthenia gravis.

vii) *Sleep:* Cholinergic neurons continue to fire during REM sleep and can play a role in REM sleep induction.

viii) *Delirium:* Lower levels of acetylcholine are associated with impaired cognition and a confused state with fluctuating orientation. Anticholinergic drugs should hence be used with caution in patients with impaired cognition/brain damage etc.

AMINO ACID NEUROTRANSMITTERS

GABA

a) Type

GABA (Gamma Amino Butyric Acid) is the main inhibitory neurotransmitter in the brain. It regulates the activity of many other neurons by reducing their activity.

b) Anatomy

GABA is found in maximum concentrations in the midbrain and diencephalon as an inhibitory neurotransmitter. It is also found in lower concentrations in the cerebral hemispheres, pons and medulla. It coexists with glycine and other biogenic amine and peptide neurotransmitters.

c) Life cycle

i) *Synthesis*: GABA is synthesized from the amino acid glutamate by the action of the enzyme glutamic acid decarboxylase (GAD) as shown in **Fig. 12.8**.

ii) *Storage and release:* Once synthesized in the presynaptic neurons, GABA is transported into synaptic vesicles by vesicular inhibitory amino acid transporters for storage. It is stored there till release into the synapse during inhibitory neurotransmission.

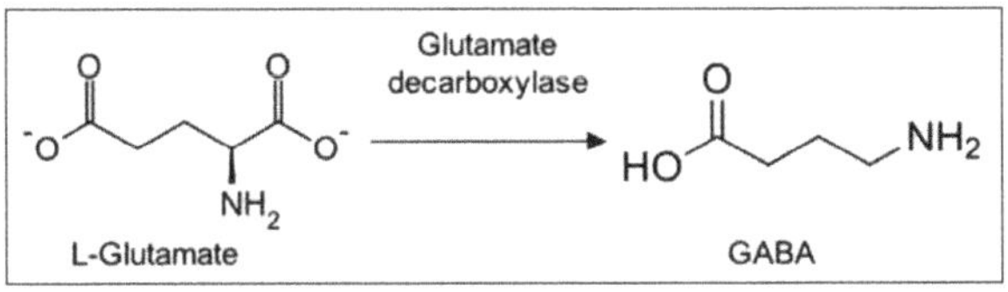

L-Glutamate —Glutamate decarboxylase→ GABA

Fig. 12.8: GABA synthesis.

iii) *Reuptake/Breakdown*: The action of GABA is terminated by reuptake through a GABA reuptake pump known as *GABA transporter* (GAT). Its action can also be terminated by the enzyme *GABA transaminase* which converts GABA into an inactive substance.

d) Receptors & their function

GABA neurotransmission is regulated through three types of post synaptic GABA receptors: $GABA_A$, $GABA_B$ and $GABA_C$. Of these receptors $GABA_A$ and $GABA_C$ are ligand gated ion channel receptors and are part of a complex inhibitory chloride channel. The $GABA_A$ receptor channel complex is a hetero-pentamer made of five subunits clustered together with a chloride channel in the centre. $GABA_A$ receptors have binding sites for benzodiazepines as well as GABA on them. The physiological role of $GABA_C$ receptors is poorly defined. $GABA_B$ receptors are G- protein coupled receptors and may be coupled with potassium or calcium channels. Details of the GABA receptors are shown (**Table 12.6**).

e) Psychiatric correlates

i) *Anxiety disorders:* Low levels of GABA are associated with increased anxiety. The amygdala which is the part of the brain that mediates fear responses is overactive in states of anxiety. Benzodiazepines exert their anxiolytic effects by acting on the post synaptic GABAergic receptors and enhancing their inhibitory output, reducing the symptoms of anxiety, fear and worrying.

ii) *Schizophrenia* has been associated with GABAergic deficit in the cerebral cortex. GABAergic neurons have a regulatory effect on the glutamatergic neurons in the pyramidal cells of the cortex, i.e.

Table 12.6: GABA receptors

Gaba receptor type	Location	Function
$GABA_A$	Widespread in the brain. For example found in interneurons of the cerebral cortex, cerebellum, amygdala, basal ganglia. (post-synaptic location)	Critical for inhibitory neurotransmission. Specific subunits are involved in mediating sleep and anxiety. Targets of anxiolytic benzodiazepines. Binding site for inhaled anesthetics, alcohol, neuro-steroids and barbiturates.
$GABA_B$	Widespread (pre-synaptic inhibition by decreasing calcium entry and post-synaptic inhibition by increasing potassium permeability)	Involved in regulating pain, mood, memory and other CNS functions.
$GABA_C$	Retina of eye	Role in retinal signal processing.

they decrease the glutamate output. In schizophrenia, a decrease in GABA inhibition leads to disinhibition of the glutamatergic output. This disinhibition leads to the excessive dopamine release associated with schizophrenia and also accounts for the cognitive and negative symptoms of schizophrenia.

iii) *Alcohol use and delirium tremens:* Acute alcohol intoxication leads to an increase in GABAergic activity and accounts for the anxiolytic effect alcohol can have in this state. When alcohol is taken over prolonged periods in a dependence pattern, the sustained increase in GABA causes the $GABA_A$ receptors to get downregulated. Sudden discontinuation of alcohol leads to a GABA deficit and a hyperexcitable state associated with delirium known as delirium tremens. Benzodiazepines regularize the GABAergic activity and are useful in the management of acute alcohol withdrawal and associated delirium.

iv) *Epilepsy:* Anticonvulsant medications such as Topiramate, Gabapentin, Tiagabine act via various mechanisms which potentiate GABAergic activity and exert their anti-seizure effect.

GLUTAMIC ACID

a) Type

Glutamate or glutamic acid is actually an amino acid which acts as the key excitatory neurotransmitter of the central nervous system. It can increase the excitability of nearly all the CNS neurons. It is often called the "master switch". It is also important as an amino acid and is used as a building block for protein synthesis.

b) Anatomy

Glutamate is the excitatory neurotransmitter for nearly 80 percent of brain synapses. The major primary sensory input pathways in the retina of the eye, cochlea of the ear, spinal cord or the trigeminal nerve are glutamatergic. In addition, certain specific glutamatergic pathways have important psychiatric implications. For example, the glutamatergic pathway going from cortex to brainstem regulates monoamine neurotransmitter release. Excitatory glutamatergic neurons project from the cortex to brainstem neurotransmitter centres such as: raphe nucleus for serotonin, locus ceruleus for norepinephrine, and substantia nigra for dopamine, stimulating neurotransmitter release from these respective areas. Excitatory glutamatergic pathways also run from the cortex to other cortical areas, cortex to striatum and cortex to thalamus respectively. The projections which relay sensory information in turn from the thalamus to various parts of the cortex are also glutamatergic. An important circuit involved in formation of new memories involves a series of glutamatergic synapses in the temporal lobe involving the hippocampus. Hence glutamate has an important role to play in regulating many other brain pathways and influences neurotransmitter release.

c) Life cycle

i) *Synthesis*: Glutamate for use as a neurotransmitter is synthesized from glutamine by the action of glutaminase enzyme. The glial cells have the enzyme glutamine synthetase which converts the glutamate back to glutamine (**Fig. 12.9**).

ii) *Storage and release:* Once synthesized, glutamate is taken up for storage in synaptic vesicles by vesicular glutamate transporter. It is stored there till release into the synapse during excitatory neurotransmission.

iii) *Reuptake/Breakdown*: After release of glutamate in the synapse, it is taken up by the glial cells through the Excitatory Amino Acid Transporter. No enzymatic breakdown of glutamate occurs in the synapse. The enzyme *glutamine synthetase* in the glial cells converts the glutamate taken back to glutamine. Glutamine is released by the process of *reverse transport* from the glial cells and taken up by the presynaptic glutamate neurons where the glutaminase enzyme converts it to glutamate for neurotransmission as discussed.

d) Receptors & their function

Glutamate receptors can be of two main types: metabotropic and ionotropic receptors. Metabotropic glutamate receptors are linked to G-proteins and can be found pre- and post-synaptically. The ionotropic receptors are ligand gated ion channels and are post synaptic in location. These receptors are open cation permeable channels which mediate sodium (Na+), potassium (K+) or calcium (Ca2+) ion flow after glutamatergic agents bind to them. These ionotropic glutamate receptors are further classified into three subtypes based on the agonists that bind to them as: N-methyl-D-aspartate (NMDA) receptors, alpha-amino-3-hydroxy-5-methyl-4-isoxazole-propionic acid (AMPA) receptors and Kainate (KA) receptors.

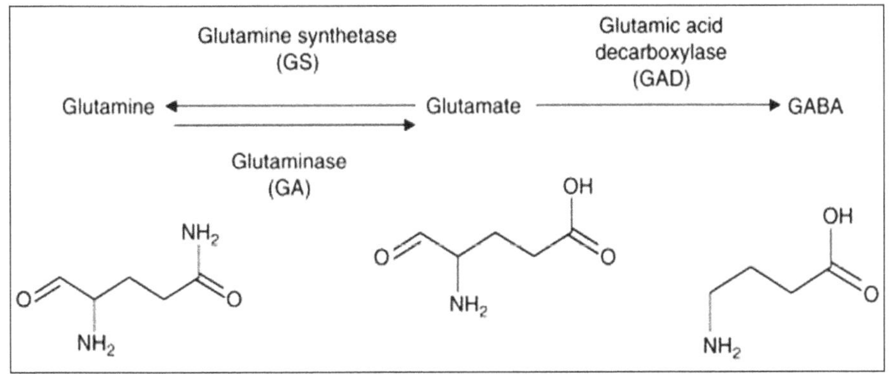

Fig. 12.9: Glutamate synthesis.

The NMDA receptors are unique in that post synaptic glutamate neurotransmission requires the presence of co-transmitters, namely *glycine* or *D-serine*. Glutamate neurotransmission can only occur through these receptors when three things occur at the same time: *glutamate binds* to its site on the NMDA receptor and the *co-transmitter glycine or D-serine binds* to the co-transmitter binding site, leading to *depolarization* and removal of the magnesium plug, finally allowing for the calcium entry and post synaptic glutamatergic effects. Glutamate receptors and their role is as shown in **Table 12.7**.

e) **Psychiatric correlates**

i) *Anxiety disorders:* Stress is an important risk factor in the genesis of anxiety disorders. Animal studies have shown that stress precipitates glutamate release in limbic regions that may in part act to stimulate the hypothalamus-pituitary-adrenal axis and contribute to glucocorticoid-induced neurotoxicity. Drugs which act through NMDA receptors are being studied for their role as anxiolytic agents.

e.g. the NMDA antagonist memantine is being studied for its role in treatment of anxiety.

ii) *Schizophrenia:* Glutamatergic dysfunction has been shown to play a major role in development of schizophrenia. Psychotic symptoms are known to occur with *decreased* glutamatergic function at the NMDA receptors and an *increased* glutamatergic function at AMPA and Kainate receptors.

The *NMDA hypofunction hypothesis* of schizophrenia explains a link between

Table 12.7: Glutamate receptors

Type of glutamate receptor		Location	Function
METABOTROPIC (G- protein coupled receptors)	Eight subtypes: mG1u1-8 divided into groups I, II and III.	Presynaptic are autoreceptors	Stimulation blocks glutamate release and protects against glutamate excitotoxicity.
		Post-synaptic	Stimulation facilitates glutamate release and strengthens excitatory transmission via ionotropic receptors.
IONOTROPIC (ligand gated ion channel receptors)	NMDA (N-methyl-D-aspartate)	Post- synaptic, some presynaptic and glial. Have a wide distribution	Show slow kinetics. Role in memory formation through synaptic plasticity and long term potentiation. Excitotoxicity
	AMPA	Post-synaptic and glial. Have a wide distribution	Mediate fast, excitatory post synaptic neurotransmission mediated by glutamate by allowing Na+ entry and neuron depolarization.
	Kainate (KA)	Pre- and Post- synaptic. Have a limited distribution	Mediate fast, excitatory post synaptic neurotransmission mediated by glutamate by allowing Na+ entry and neuron depolarization.

hypo functioning NMDA receptors and GABAergic neuropathology in the cortex which in turn influences the dopamine output in these patients. A decrease in the glutamate due to hypo functioning glutamate receptors decreases the GABA output. The decrease in inhibitory GABA output disinhibits the glutamatergic neurons which in turn are linked to dopaminergic neurons. The result is an increase in dopamine release. These findings can explain the symptoms of psychoses seen in patients with schizophrenia. Studies show that newer drugs acting at the glycine site on the NMDA receptor may be useful in the treatment of some symptoms in schizophrenia.

iii) *Mood disorders:* Glutamate dysfunction has been implicated in the genesis of depressive symptoms. Ketamine, an NMDA antagonist, when given at low doses does not cause psychoses. It has been shown to have rapid, substantial and persistent reduction in depressive symptoms including suicidal thoughts when given for the treatment of depression.

iv) *Memory and dementia:* NMDA receptors and AMPA receptors are involved in long term potentiation which is essential to the formation of long-term memory. The pathophysiology of Alzheimer's dementia involves aggregates of beta amyloid being deposited in the brain. The beta amyloid aggregates remove the magnesium block in NMDA receptors and increase the extracellular glutamate which causes excitotoxic damage to neurons. Hence, Memantine which is an NMDA antagonist is useful in the management of mild to moderate Alzheimer's disease since it decreases the rate of neuronal degeneration.

v) *Alcohol dependence:* Acute alcohol intoxication not only increases the GABA transmission as mentioned before, it also decreases the glutamate NMDA receptor function. Accordingly, prolonged use of alcohol in a dependence pattern causes glutamate deficit state which leads to upregulation of the NMDA receptors. Suddenly stopping alcohol in these patients causes the hyperexcitable state of delirium. In this state the NMDA receptors are supersensitive. When coupled with thiamine deficiency, this leads to the excitotoxic neuron degeneration of Wernicke -Korsakoff's syndrome. Acamprosate which is used in the management of alcohol withdrawal is an anti-craving agent which acts by inhibiting the hyperexcitable NMDA receptors.

NEUROPEPTIDES AND NOVEL NEUROTRANSMITTERS

Neuropeptides are signaling molecules present in the CNS and may act as neurotransmitters, neuromodulators or neurohormones. They regulate a variety of behavioral and physiological processes such as hunger, sleep, sex, temperature control, movement, learning and memory. They also exert an influence on the body's response to stress and pain, emotion, social understanding and behavior. They are released in the synaptic cleft along with other neurotransmitters and can modulate the effect of neurotransmitters. The main difference between neuropeptides and neurotransmitters is that neuropeptides are slow-acting and produce a prolonged action whereas neurotransmitters are fast-acting and produce a short-term response. A brief comparison between neurotransmitters and neuropeptides is shown in **Table 12.8**.

Novel neurotransmitters and neurosteroids: Recent studies have shown the role of certain gases such as nitric oxide, carbon monoxide; endocannabinoids and neuro-steroids in

Table 12.8: Neuropeptides versus neurotransmitters

Receptors	Location	Function
D1	Striatum, nucleus accumbens, olfactory bulb, amygdala hippocampus, substantia nigra hypothalamus, frontal cortex	Locomotion, learning and memory, attention, impulse control, sleep, regulation of renal function
D2	Striatum, VTA, olfactory bulb, cerebral cortex	Locomotion, learning and memory, attention, sleep, reproductive behavior. D2 receptor antagonism reduces positive symptoms of schizophrenia
D3	Striatum, cortex	Locomotion, cognition, attention, impulse control, sleep, regulation of food intake
D4	Frontal cortex, amygdala, hypothalamus, nucleus accumbens	Cognition, impulse control, attention, sleep, reproductive behavior
D5	Cortex, substantia nigra, hypothalamus	Cognition, attention, decision making, motor learning, renin secretion

psychiatric disorders. They are novel in that their mechanism of action is not exactly like the classic neurotransmitters. They are like neurotransmitters in that they physiologically influence the electro-chemical state of adjacent cells. Where the novel neurotransmitters have been postulated to have a role in psychoses and schizophrenia, neurosteroids may play a distinct role in depression and anxiety disorders. Knowledge about these novel neurotransmitters may pave the way for newer psychiatric medications in the near future.

BIBLIOGRAPHY

1. Sadock, Benjamin J., Virginia A Sadock, and Pedro Ruiz. *Kaplan & Sadock's Synopsis of Psychiatry: Behavioral Sciences/clinical Psychiatry*. 11th edition/Philadelphia: Wolters Kluwer, 2015.
2. Stahl, S. M. (2008). *Stahl's essential psychopharmacology: Neuroscientific basis and practical applications*. Cambridge: Cambridge University Press.
3. https://pdfs.semanticscholar.org/106c/bf8ac-6cc219ed64bcceaeb002d5d5bc7d4ee.pdf?_ga=2.168543521.1009651782.1573382563-2110234351.1573382563
4. https://www.khanacademy.org/science/biology/human-biology/neuron-nervous-system/a/neurotransmitters-their-receptors
5. https://www.caam.rice.edu/~cox/wrap/norepinephrine.pdf
6. Glutamate and psychiatric disorders APT (2002), vol. 8, p. 193.

Schizophrenia and Related Psychotic Disorders

13

Damodharan Dinakaran • Ganesan Venkatasubramanian

Schizophrenia is a heterogeneous disorder with substantial impairment in thinking (delusions), speech (formal thought disorders), perception (hallucinations), judgment and behavior (disorganised/catatonia). Loss of touch with the reality, lack of insight about the illness and noticeable deterioration in everyday functioning are typical of schizophrenia. Eugene Bleuler coined the term *"Schizophrenia"* (Schiz – to split, Phren – the mind) which was previously known as *"Dementia Praecox"* termed by Emil Kraeplin. Kraeplin had conceptualised this mental condition as an unremitting illness with its onset in the early adulthood and has a chronic, deteriorating course finally leading the individual to develop Dementia. However, the current understanding is clear that only a proportion of schizophrenia patients have such a deteriorating course. Bleuler conceptualised Schizophrenia as putative fundamental disturbances of 4 'A's *(affect, associations, ambivalence and autism)*

1. Autism (preoccupation with self & diminished social interactions)
2. Ambivalence (apparent inability to make decisions)
3. Loosening of Association (lack of association within the thought process)
4. Affective flattening (markedly reduced expression of emotion)

Classification Systems (See Table 13.1)

The International classification of diseases version 10 (ICD -10) produced by World Health Organization (WHO) in 1992 had classified Schizophrenia into various subtypes (paranoid, hebephrenic, catatonic, undifferentiated, residual etc.). However, the recent version ICD -11 has moved away from categorising the illness due to the lack of longitudinal stability and predictive validity of such subtypes. This is consistent with the classification of schizophrenia provided by the Diagnostic and Statistical Manual of Mental disorders recent version 5 (DSM-5) developed by the American Psychiatric Association (APA) in 2013. The key difference between these classificatory systems is the duration criteria employed for diagnosing schizophrenia. DSM-5 criteria mandates the duration of illness to be six months with at least one month of active florid symptoms while ICD-11 provides duration criteria as 1 month.

Epidemiology

Schizophrenia is a globally prevalent psychotic disorder with gross prevalence of 1 in 100 adult general population (1%) and mean annual incidence of 0.2-0.4 per 1000 population. Illness usually has an illness onset specifically during late adolescence to adulthood. It is clear that the sexual predilection is nil and both sexes are affected almost equally. However, men tend to have relatively increased risk, earlier age at onset and poor prognosis compared to women. Women tend to have a delayed onset during late adulthood, post partum or post-menopausal period and generally the

Table: 13.1 Schizophrenia Diagnostic guidelines

International Classification of Diseases (ICD-11)

Schizophrenia:

Diagnostic guidelines: Essential features

1. **At least two** of the following symptoms *must* be present (by the individual's report or through observation by the clinician or other informants) most of the time for a period of **one month or more**. At least one of the qualifying symptoms should be from item a) through d) in the list below:
   a) Persistent delusions – false beliefs (e.g., Persecutory, referential, grandiose etc.,)
   b) Persistent hallucinations – false perceptions (auditory, visual, olfactory etc.,).
   c) Disorganized thinking (formal thought disorder) (e.g., tangentiality, loose associations, neologisms etc., When severe, the person's speech may be so incoherent or incomprehensible)
   d) Experiences of influence, passivity or control (e.g., the phenomenon that one's thoughts, impulses, actions are not originated by self but being placed in/withdrawn from one's mind by others/agency, or that one's thoughts are being broadcast to others).
   e) Negative symptoms – (apathy, alogia or paucity of speech, avolition, asociality and anhedonia) Note: It must be clear that the symptoms are primary (idiopathic) and not secondary to affective disorder or use of a substance or medication.
   f) Grossly disorganized behavior (e.g., behavior that appears bizarre or purposeless, unpredictable or inappropriate emotional responses that interfere with the organization of behavior.)
   g) Psychomotor disturbances (e.g. catatonia)
2. The symptoms or behaviors are not a secondary presentation of another medical condition (e.g., a brain tumor/epilepsy) and are not due to the effect of a substance or medication on the central nervous system (e.g., corticosteroids), including withdrawal effects (e.g., alcohol).

Diagnostic and Statistical Manual of Mental Disorders (DSM-5)

Schizophrenia:

Diagnostic guidelines

A. **Two or more** for **at least a one-month (actively present)** period of time, and at least one of them must be 1, 2, or 3:
   1. Delusions – false beliefs
   2. Hallucinations – false perceptions
   3. Disorganized speech – formal thought disorder
   4. Grossly disorganized behavior or catatonia
   5. Negative symptoms (apathy, alogia, asociality etc.,)

B. Impairment in one of the major areas of daily functioning for a significant period of time since the onset of the psychotic disturbances (e.g. work, self care, interpersonal relationships etc.,)

C. Some features of the illness must last for a **continuous period of at least six months**. This period

(Continued)

Table: 13.1 Schizophrenia Diagnostic guidelines (Continued)

	must include at least one month of active symptoms (or less if treated) that meet criterion A (active phase symptoms) and may include periods of residual symptoms. During residual periods, only negative symptoms may be present.
D.	Schizoaffective disorder and bipolar or depressive disorder with psychotic features have been ruled out: (differential diagnoses) 1. No major depressive or manic episodes occurred concurrently with active phase period 2. If mood episodes (depressive or manic) have occurred during active phase period, they have been present only for a minority of the total duration of the active and residual phases of the disorder.
E.	The disturbance is not secondary to or caused by the effects of a substance (alcohol) or another medical condition (brain tumor/epilepsy etc.,)
F.	If there is a history of autism spectrum disorder or a communication disorder (childhood onset), the diagnosis of schizophrenia is only made if prominent delusions or hallucinations, along with other symptoms, are present for at least one month

prognosis is better. Relative high prevalence in urban upbringing and higher socio-economic status environment had been reported but the evidence is not definitive.

Pathogenesis

Despite decades of research on possible putative mechanisms and the etiology of schizophrenia is yet to be categorically elicited and is noted to be in the early budding phase. Nonetheless, the general agreement by renowned international expert committees is that there is interaction between putative environmental factors and psychosis susceptibility genes that leads to the ultimate expression of Schizophrenia phenotype.

1. Neurodevelopmental Hypothesis:

   This hypothesis suggests that the developing brain is vulnerable to sustain insults right from conception, womb (prenatal period) through late adolescence. The cumulative insults are believed to be detrimental to the developmental trajectory of specific neurotransmitters, synapses, neural circuits in specific brain region. These insults result in pathophysiologic and morphologic alterations in the brain and ultimately behavioral manifestations. Environmental factors that are conceptualized to be the risk factors include prenatal infection, maternal malnutrition, paternal age, neonatal hypoxia, infections, childhood abuse, cannabis use, epilepsy etc.

2. Genetic Factors:

   The Psychiatric Genetics Consortium (PGC) had recently reported the findings of Genome Wide Association Studies (GWAS) which included data from 36000+ patients and 110000+ healthy controls. They had identified 108 independent genomic risk loci. The promising genes include dopamine receptor related (DRD2), Glutamatergic neurotransmission (GRIN2A, GRIA1), Neuronal calcium signaling (CACNA1C, CACNA2), Synaptic functioning (CNTN4, PAK6), Brain derive neurotropic factor (BDNF), Neuregulin (NRG) and also Major Histocompatibility Complex (MHC) locus in chromosome 6. Interestingly, deletion at chromosome 22.q.11 that results in Velo-cardio-facial Syndrome (DiGeorge syndrome) substantially increases the risk to develop schizophrenia.

3. Stress Diathesis Model:

   Consensus agreement is that neither of the above mentioned models independently leads to the psychotic manifestation but it is the interaction between such environmental insults with the genetic mutation. In a susceptible population with genetic predisposition (e.g. mutations in the Major Histocompatibility Complex (MHC – HLA complex), environmental insults (e.g. Prenatal infection) interact to produce a cascade of events making the developing brain vulnerable to manifest psychosis.

4. Neurotransmitters Model:

   Abnormalities in various neurotransmitters have been postulated to be implicated in the manifestations of psychosis like Dopamine, Glutamic acid, Gamma Amino Butyric Acid (GABA), Nicotine, Acetyl Choline, serotonin etc.

a) Dopamine: Hypothesis of dopamine's involvement evolved after the serendipitous discovery of antipsychotic medicine chlorpromazine's effect on calming individuals with psychosis. Antipsychotics exert their effects by blocking dopamine D2 receptor in the brain. Excess of dopamine in meso-limbic pathway has been postulated to be the mechanism of developing psychosis. Many drugs (cannabis, stimulants like amphetamine, cocaine etc.,) that are implicated in predisposing individuals to develop psychosis predominantly act by increasing the availability of dopamine in the meso-limbic pathway ultimately culminating in the behavioral manifestations of psychosis

b) Glutamate - GABA: Recent evidence suggests the involvement of abnormal glutamate neurotransmission and deficient GABA interneurons in the brain that results in excitation – inhibition imbalance leading to psychotic manifestations. Hypofunctioning glutamate receptor (N-methyl D-aspartate receptor - NMDAR) leads to poor neuroplasticity and ultimately poor learning and cognition in psychotic patients. Sudden alcohol withdrawal in an individual with chronic alcohol use leads to hallucinations (auditory, visual and tactile) with or without delirium. Glutamate – GABA imbalance has been the postulated mechanism underlying such psychotic presentation.

c) Nicotine – Acetyl choline: Both the transmitters are implicated to be involved in regulating the motivation, attention, memory and cognition in psychotic patients. *"Self Medication"* hypothesis suggests psychotic patients have decreased attention and concentration and to overcome such difficulties they tend to use nicotine (smoking). Nicotine use has been noted to be more prevalent in schizophrenia patients than in general public. Nicotinic receptors in brain (nACHR) are novel targets for newer drug development to treat cognitive dysfunction in psychotic patients.

d) Serotonin: Drugs like Lysergic acid Diethylamide (LSD), psilocybin, mescaline etc. cause mental effects primarily acting through serotonin 5-HT2A serotonin receptors. Second generation (SGA) or newer antipsychotics or atypical antipsychotics exert their action predominantly by blocking serotonin receptors (5-HT2A) along with dopamine receptor (D2) blocking.

5. Autoimmune and other inflammatory conditions:

   Psychotic symptoms could occur in association with certain autoimmune conditions that has nervous system manifestations like systemic lupus erythematosus (SLE). Cross reactivity of auto-antibodies towards GluNR1 sub unit of NMDA receptors are postulated to be the mechanism. Immune encephalitis secondary to certain paraneoplastic syndromes, ovarian teratomas, post- viral encephalitis (Herpes virus) produces similar psychotic symptoms as in schizophrenia.

6. Neuropathology:

   Earlier computed tomography (CT) Brain studies reported abnormal lateral ventricular enlargement in schizophrenia patients as compared to healthy controls. Recent Magnetic Resonance Imaging (MRI) Brain studies had published significant brain gray mater volume reductions in specific foci like dorsolateral prefrontal cortex (DLPFC), hippocampus, middle temporal and parietal regions. Specialized brain potentials recorded through Electro-Encephalography (EEG) called "Event Related Potentials (ERP)" that are elicited secondary to auditory, visual, motor or cognitive events are found to be abnormal in psychotic patients. They primarily exhibit reduced attention and concentration, abnormal attention salience, poor cortical inhibition and poor integration between different brain regions.

Clinical Features

Clinically schizophrenia symptoms/signs can be broadly classified to following domains namely positive symptoms (exaggerated), negative symptoms (diminished), cognitive deficits, motor symptoms and affective symptoms.

Positive symptoms: These are mainly *delusions* and *hallucinations*. Delusion (latin meaning; delude – to deceive) is a false, firm, fixed beliefs (thoughts) that are out of keeping with the person's social, educational living background that arise from a morbid internal process. Delusional beliefs are usually held with extraordinary conviction and subjective self certainty and are usually impervious to counter-arguments and available evidence. Persecutory, referential, grandiose and control delusions are common in schizophrenia. Historically, Kurt Schneider had grouped 11 signs and symptoms and called them *"First Rank Symptoms (FRS)"*of schizophrenia. He conceptualised them to occur predominately and be pathognomonic of schizophrenia. However these symptoms do occur in other psychotic and mood disorders and hence their status is deemphasised in recent classificatory systems (ICD-11 & DSM-5). See **Table: 13.2** for types of delusional themes and Schneider's first rank symptoms. Hallucinations are simply perceptions without any stimulus. Based on the sensory modality they are further divided into auditory, visual, olfactory, gustatory, tactile and kinesthetic hallucinations. Auditory hallucinations occur most commonly in schizophrenia followed by visual hallucinations. Presence of visual or olfactory hallucinations in a psychotic patient should raise the suspicion about the possible organic etiology like temporal lobe seizures, encephalitis or substance intoxication/withdrawal.

Negative symptoms: Amotivation (diminished drive), Avolition (reduced actions), Asociality (diminished social interactions), Apathy (decreased emotional response), Alogia (decreased speech output) and Anhedonia (reduced interest/desire). These symptoms can be primary (idiopathic) or secondary to factors such as positive symptoms, depression, anxiety, side effects of medications, chronic institutionalization etc. In primary form, the cluster of negative symptoms is also known

Table 13.2: Delusional themes & Schneiderian First Rank Symptoms (FRS)

Delusional themes: Based on the content of the belief, delusions are classified as follows	
Persecutory delusions	Belief that people/group/agency is behind an individual with malicious intent to harm him/her or acting to bring bad reputation
Referential delusions	Insignificant events or remarks in an individual's environment are believed to be referred to him/her
Grandiose delusions	Belief that an individual possess extraordinary powers or him/her is of a greater identity (e.g. I am God/I am the president of USA)
Infidelity delusions (Othello syndrome)	Belief that his/her spouse is in an affair with some other individual. More common in the context of alcohol use
Control delusions	delusion that one's thought/impulses/mood/actions are under the control of an external person/agency
Delusion of Love (erotomania/ De-Clerambault's)	Belief that a particular individual is in love with the affected person. Usually the particular individual is from a superior social status is believed to be in love with affected person
Cotard syndrome	Belief that one does not exist or has died. Also belief that body organs are removed/not functioning
Delusional Parasitosis	Belief that one is infested with insects, worms, mites, bacteria etc.
Capgras syndrome	Belief that a close aide/relative is being replaced by an impostor
Fregoli syndrome	Belief that different people are in fact the same person keeps changing the appearances/disguise
Folie a deux (Shared delusion)	Same delusional belief shared by more affected individuals related by family/ living arrangement
Schneiderian First Rank Symptoms (FRS)	
Delusional Perception	A primary delusion. A normal perception is given a delusional significance in a self referential way.
Thought Echo	One's own thoughts are audible like an echo (to self and others)
3rd person auditory hallucinations (3 PAH)	Voices that discusses about the affected patient in third person (e.g. "He" is a bad person. "He" did many mistakes. "She" has a knife)
Running commentary	Voices giving running commentary about the individual's actions (e.g. He is going to the kitchen, starting to wash vessels, cooking)
Thought insertion	Thoughts are believed to be not arising from self but inserted against will into one's mind
Thought withdrawal	Thoughts are believed to be withdrawn against will from one's mind
Thought Broadcast	Belief that thoughts are broadcasted out of one's mind and others may have access to those thoughts
Made Impulse	An impulse to carry out the current action is not felt as one's own
Made Act	One's acts are completely controlled by external agency
Made Feelings	One's feelings that do not seem to his/her own
Somatic Passivity	Bodily sensations produced by external agency

as deficit schizophrenia or deficit syndrome. Secondary negative symptoms usually respond when underlying cause is appropriately treated but treatment of primary negative symptoms is usually challenging and often characterized as poor prognostic factor.

Cognitive symptoms: Impaired functioning of dorsolateral prefrontal cortex has been implicated in cognitive deficits in schizophrenia. Attention, processing speed, vigilance, working memory, verbal/visual memory and social cognition domains are found to be impaired in schizophrenia patients. These are impaired also in patient's first degree relatives, individuals with high risk to develop psychosis and early in the development of psychosis. Hence cognitive deficits are conceptualised as trait related deficits and endophenotypes. Cognitive deficits are already worse at the onset of the illness before treatment initiation and worsen further at each exacerbation of the illness. Social cognitive deficits mean patients exhibit theory of mind deficits. Difficulties arise in inferring the intentions in social situations that is central to cognitive distortions developing delusions and eventually social withdrawal.

Motor Symptoms: Marked psychomotor agitation or retardation is common in Schizophrenia. Motor symptoms are expressed in a wide range from mild restlessness to catatonia. *Karl Leonhard* had explained a variety of cycloid psychoses called motility psychosis in which striking changes in psychomotor activity is noted from akinetic to hyperkinetic range (akinetic-resembles catatonic stupor, hyperkinetic – resembles excitement). Catatonia concept was formulated and coined by *Karl Ludwig Kahlbaum*. Catatonia syndrome is described in **Table 13.3**: includes mutism, stupor, posturing, negativism, retardation, echolalia, echopraxia, mannerisms, stereotype, waxy flexibility, automatic obedience and

Table 13.3: Catatonia – signs and symptoms

Sign/Symptom	Description
Mutism	Verbal unresponsiveness, diminished speech output
Stupor	Motor unresponsiveness, hypoactivity, reduced arousal levels
Posturing	Actively assuming and maintaining postures for long periods
Catalepsy	Posture passively initiated by examiner held against gravity
Negativism	Senseless opposition/resistance to examiner's attempts to move
Gegenhalten	Patient resists with the strength equal and opposite to examiner's action
Mannerism	Odd, purposeful, exaggerated caricature movements
Stereotype	Non-goal directed, repetitive motor movements
Verbigeration	Repetitive speech like a scratched record (verbal stereotype)
Waxy flexibility	There is an initial resistance offered by the patient and gradually later allows the movement, like bending a candle
Echolalia	Spontaneously repeats examiner's speech
Echopraxia	Spontaneously repeats examiner's motor actions
Ambitendency	Patient appears "stuck"/indecisive when contradicting verbal and non-verbal commands are given. e.g.- Examiner says "Don't shake my hand" but offers hand shake
Automatic obedience	Despite instruction to the contrary, patient allows his/her hand to be moved by the examiner's slight pressure and maintains that posture for a prolonged period
Autonomic instability	Fluctuations in pulse, temperature, blood pressure, respiratory rate, sweating etc.

autonomic instability. DSM-5 conceptualised catatonia to be a separate syndrome that could manifest in organic illnesses, substance intoxication/withdrawal, primary psychotic disorder and mood disorders. Presence of 3 or more symptoms/signs is taken to denote the presence of catatonia.

Affective symptoms: Depressive symptoms are common during the prodromal phase of the illness. Depression also predominate the clinical picture during the convalescence from the illness. During recovery, development of insight about the illness along with guilt and stigma might predispose the individual to attempt suicide or self harm. Anxiety is also noted to be co-morbid during the prodrome phase, illness and convalescence phases of the illness. Especially social anxiety co-morbidity is quite high in patients with schizophrenia. When syndromal mood symptoms occur along with active florid psychotic symptoms a diagnosis of Schizoaffective disorder is considered.

Course and Outcome

WHO had reported 5 common courses of Schizophrenia as described in Figure 13.1. As suggested in the figure only a proportion of patients have poor chronic course. Early intervention and treatment leads to recovery in almost 30-40% of individuals. Co-morbidity in the form of substance use predominate the course. As much as 80% patients have co-morbid nicotine use disorder and varying proportions have other substance dependence. Family history, poor pre-morbid level of functioning, early age at onset, longer duration of untreated psychosis, substance use, marked non-adherence to treatment and lack of social support are reported to be poor prognostic indicators.

Course	Visual representation
One episode with complete recovery	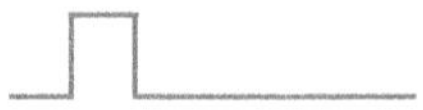
One episode with incomplete recovery (persisting symptoms)	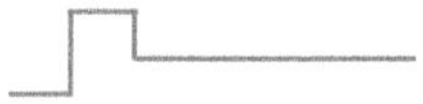
Many episodes with complete recovery in-between episodes	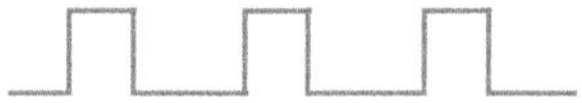
Many episodes with incomplete recovery in-between episodes	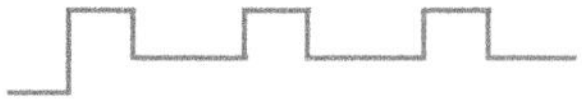
Continuous prolonged course	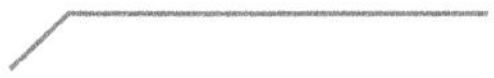

Fig. 13.1: WHO Schizophrenia course.

Treatment

Pharmacological

Antipsychotics are the mainstay of treatment. Chlorpromazine was the first antipsychotic discovered by *Delay and Deniker* in 1952 serendipitously by the calming effect it produced on psychotic patients. Haloperidol was the first synthetic antipsychotic produced in laboratory by 1958. They are broadly classified as first generation or second generation based on the receptor blocking profiles. First generation antipsychotics (e.g. Chlorpromazine, Haloperidol etc.) are also known as typical antipsychotics and exert their action by blocking Dopamine D2 receptors. Second generation drugs (e.g. Clozapine, olanzapine etc.) on the other hand exert their action by blocking serotonergic 5-HT2 receptors in addition to dopamine blockade. Approximately 40-60% patients respond to first antipsychotic drug. When a patient fails to respond to two or more antipsychotics given in adequate dosage for adequate time (at least 6 weeks), the illness is said to be treatment resistant. Clozapine is the first line choice in treatment resistant schizophrenia.

First generation antipsychotics have more extra-pyramidal side effects like dystonia, tremors, bradykinesia, rigidity, akathisia and chronic use might lead to tardive syndromes (tardive dyskinesia, tardive dystonia etc.). Second generation agents are notorious in producing metabolic side effects like weight gain, obesity, deranged lipids, deranged sugar control that might in turn predispose the individual to develop cardio-vascular disorders. See **Table 13.4** for commonly prescribed antipsychotics, their dosage range and notable side effects.

Table 13.4: Commonly prescribed Antipsychotic Drugs

Drug	Dosage range	Common side effects
First generation drugs		
Chlorpromazine	Oral 400-1000 mg/day	Sedation, extra-pyramidal, constipation, postural hypotension, skin photosensitivity
Haloperidol	Oral 5-20 mg/day Inj. 5-10 mg i.mor i.v for sedation Depot Inj.100 mg i.m once a month	Extra-pyramidal, postural hypotension, sedation, hyperprolactinemia, cardiac rhythm disturbances especially in i.v route
Flupenthixol	Oral - 3-12 mg/day Depot Inj. 20-40 mg i.m once a week/ fortnightly	Extra-pyramidal, postural hypotension, sedation, hyperprolactinemia
Trifluoperazine	Oral 5-20 mg/day	Extra-pyramidal, postural hypotension, sedation, hyperprolactinemia
Fluphenazine	Depot Inj. 25-50 mg i.m once a week/ fortnightly	Extra-pyramidal, postural hypotension, sedation, hyperprolactinemia
Second generation drugs		
Olanzapine	Oral 5-20 mg/day Inj. 10 mg i.m for sedation Depot Inj. 210-405 mg i.m once fortnightly or monthly	Sedation, increased appetite, weight gain, deranged glucose and lipids. Post injection confusion to be monitored after depot injection
Risperidone	Oral 2-8 mg/day Depot Inj. 50 mg once fortnightly or monthly	Extrapyramidal side effects, hyperprolactinemia, postural hypotension. Weight gain
Quetiapine	Oral 200-800 mg/day	Sedation, postural hypotension, weight gain
Amisulpride	Oral 200-1200 mg/day	Hyperprolactinemia, sedation
Lurasidone	Oral 40-160 mg/day	Akathisia, nausea, cardiac rhythm abnormalities
Ziprasidone	Oral 40-160 mg/day	Akathisia, nausea, cardiac rhythm abnormalities
Aripiprazole	Oral 5-45 mg/day Depot Inj. 400 mg i.m Once a month	Akathisia, extrapyramidal side effects
Paliperidone	Oral 3-12 mg/day Depot Inj. 100-150 mg i.m Once a month	Akathisia, extrapyramidal side effects, hyperprolactinemia,
Clozapine	Oral 150-400 mg/day	Common: Sedation, tachycardia, hypersalivation, postural hypotension, constipation Serious: Seizures, myocarditis, agranulocytosis

Benzodiazepines (clonazepam, lorazepam etc.) are used commonly along with antipsychotics during acute agitation, sleep disturbances and co-morbid anxiety or panic symptoms. Anticholinergic agents (trihexyphenidyl, promethazine, Benztropine, Glycopyrollate etc.) are used to ameliorate the extra-pyramidal side effects like dystonia, tremors, rigidity and slowness. Antidepressants (fluoxetine, escitalopram etc.) are used for co-morbid anxiety, depressive symptoms and for secondary negative symptoms.

Brain Stimulation Techniques

Electro-Convulsive Therapy (ECT)

Electro-convulsive therapy is a treatment modality that involves the application of electric current under light anesthesia to induce seizures in brain. Mechanism of action of ECT is postulated due to the secondary changes that happen in brain following seizures involving increased epileptic threshold, secretion of neurotropic factors and eventually neurogenesis. ECT is advised in schizophrenia usually in catatonia phases, risk of suicide, unmanageable aggression and as an augmenting agent to clozapine in resistant patients. ECT as a treatment modality is highly efficacious but the effects are usually short lasting (up to 3 months). However for selected patients, maintenance ECT is considered at variable intervals.

Non-Invasive Brain Stimulation Techniques

Recently repetitive Transcranial Magnetic Stimulation (rTMS) that involves induction of current in the cortex through magnets and electric stimulation (Transcranial Direct Current Stimulation – tDCS) that involves induction of current in the cortex through battery are utilised for specific indications in schizophrenia. These are safe, non-invasive brain stimulation techniques which do not involve anesthesia. Evidence of efficacy is emerging and has a potential application to ameliorate cognitive deficits, negative symptoms, affective symptoms and hallucinations in schizophrenia. Though both modalities are considered safe, rTMS tend to induce action potential thereby has a risk of inducing seizures. However tDCS is considered safe in patients with co-morbid seizures.

Psychosocial Management

Apart from pharmacological agents and brain stimulation modalities, various psychological and social therapy modules are available for focussed needs. Cognitive therapy is useful in retraining the individual while motivation enhancement therapy helps quitting substance use. Family therapy is employed when the understanding of patient's illness is poor among family members leading to criticality and poor social support. Adherence monitoring helps to improve overall compliance of the patient with the formulated treatment plan. Physical exercises and yoga therapy are utilised to improve cognitive deficits and manage weight gain secondary to antipsychotic treatment.

Other Psychotic Disorders

Schizotypal Disorder

Also known as the Schizotypal personality disorder is an under-recognised clinical entity classified along with Psychotic disorders. Classical onset is ill-defined and the presentation is usually traced back to the childhood. It is characterized by referential beliefs, quasi psychotic thinking, abnormal perceptual experiences, oddities in thoughts/ speech, self centered ideas, inappropriate affect and peculiar eccentric behavior with few friends. Common co-morbid conditions include other personality disorders (paranoid, schizoid) and anxiety disorders like social phobia, obsessive compulsive disorder etc., Antipsychotics play a primary or adjunct role based on the dominant clinical presentation. Antidepressants and benzodiazepines are used to relieve manifestations of anxiety. Individual therapy is usually provided when obsessive compulsive symptoms are prominent.

Delusional Disorder

Diagnosis of delusional disorder is considered when a person has one or more delusions present for 3 or more months leading to distress and dysfunction in the affected domains. Hallucinations are usually absent and if present are fleeting. General functioning in the unaffected domains are generally adequate. E.g. A person having delusion of infidelity might have dysfunction only in spouse relationship domain whereas other areas of social-occupational functioning would be adequate. It usually has an onset in the middle age. Persecutory type of delusions is the most common type. Treatment is usually difficult with marked lack of insight. A good doctor – patient relationship is the key for treatment. Antipsychotic drugs are the first line. Prognosis is good with proper treatment and monitored adherence.

Schizoaffective Disorder

Schizoaffective disorder is considered when both psychotic syndrome (hallucinations, delusions) and affective syndrome (mania, depression or mixed episode) occurs simultaneously or within a few days of each other. ICD defines an episode as "Schizoaffective, manic or depressive" cross-sectional while DSM defines it after taking into consideration the longitudinal course of the illness. DSM mandates the presence of psychotic phenomena (delusions/ hallucinations) even after affective syndrome has subsided to characterize the schizoaffective episode. Diagnostically schizoaffective disorder assumes an intermediary position between schizophrenia and bipolar mood disorder. Men and women are equally affected. Treatment is usually Antipsychotics and mood stabilizers (Lithium, Valproate, carbamazepine, Lamotrigine etc.). Antidepressants are used during depressive episodes.

Acute Psychotic Disorders

When the onset of the psychotic illness happens within two weeks, it is referred to as acute in onset. Usually the onset is precipitated by mental or physical stress. The presentation is generally polymorphic in nature with a mixture of psychotic, anxiety and mood symptoms. The illness has a good prognosis and remits mostly within a month. If the illness persists more than a month, based on the presentation can be categorised to schizophrenia or delusional disorder. The longitudinal stability of the diagnosis is questionable since more than $2/3^{rd}$ of the patients eventually develop mood disorders. Treatment during acute phase is usually with antipsychotics and benzodiazepines.

Shared Psychotic Disorders

Shared psychotic disorders also known as induced psychotic disorders or *"Folie –au-deux"* are reported when a normal individual shares delusions from an affected patient. Usually the recipient of the delusion is disadvantaged socially or economically or dependent on the affected person or the inductor. Case reports and series are available describing shared delusions between individuals and among all members from the same family. Separating the recipient from the inductor usually leads to resolution of symptoms in the recipient. However persistent symptoms are treated with antipsychotic drugs.

Secondary Psychotic Disorders

As discussed in etio-pathogenesis, psychosis could manifest secondary to various other conditions and hence referred to as secondary psychotic disorders.

Medical conditions related: Psychosis might appear secondary to chronic epilepsy as post-ictal and inter-ictal psychosis. As a complication with autoimmune disorders especially systemic lupus erythematosus, NMDA- receptor autoantibody encephalitis secondary to paraneoplastic syndrome etc.

Medications related: Psychosis may happen secondary to various medicines used to treat tuberculosis (Isoniazid, rifampicin), Cushing's syndrome (steroids), stimulants used to treat Attention – Deficit Hyperactive Disorder – ADHD (methylphenidate, amphetamine, modafinil), dopamine agonists used for Parkinson's disease (levodopa, amantidine etc.)

Substance related: stimulant drug abuse involving drugs like amphetamine, cocaine etc. leads to development of paranoid psychosis. Party drugs like Methylene Dioxy Methamphetamine MDMA (Ecstasy), Lysergic acid diethylamide (LSD, Acid), Phencyclidine (Angel dust) are all implicated as precipitants of psychosis. Cannabis (Marijuana, Ganja or Weed) use has been strongly associated in triggering the onset of psychotic breakdown and perpetuating the syndrome. Chronic alcohol use is associated with development of psychosis especially during relative alcohol withdrawal period. Delusion of infidelity is more common in individuals with chronic alcohol use. Nicotine use do not directly influence psychotic breakdown but it is strongly associated as a co-morbid feature with psychosis. Smoking induces Cytochrome P450 enzymes thereby reducing the bio-availability and efficacy of antipsychotic drugs. Patients with psychosis reportedly smoke more and inhale deeply thereby predisposing them to various respiratory system morbidities.

Treatment of secondary psychoses usually involves treating the underlying causative illness or removing the offending agent wherever feasible. Antipsychotics, if used are only for a brief period. Education about the underlying illness, harms caused by the substance/medication used, ways to prevent relapse and promote well-being needs to be discussed with the affected individual for better quality of life.

Acknowledgement

GV acknowledges the support of the SwarnaJayanti Fellowship by the Department of Science and Technology, Government of India (DST/SJF/LSA-02/2014–15).

BIBLIOGRAPHY

1. ICD-11:https://gcp.network/en/private/icd-11-guidelines/categories/schizophrenia-and-other-primary-psychotic-disorders
2. DSM-5: Diagnostic and statistical manual of mental disorders : DSM-5: Fifth edition. Arlington, VA : American Psychiatric Publishing, [2013] ©2013;
3. SIMS: Symptoms in the mind: Oyebode F. Sims' Symptoms in the Mind: Textbook of Descriptive Psychopathology E-Book: Elsevier Health Sciences; 2018
4. Schizophrenia: Weinberger DR, Harrison P. Schizophrenia: Wiley; 2011.
5. Taylor DM, Barnes TRE, Young AH. The Maudsley Prescribing Guidelines in Psychiatry: Wiley; 2018.
6. Cowen P, Harrison P, Burns T. Shorter Oxford Textbook of Psychiatry: OUP Oxford; 2012.
7. Sadock BJ, Sadock VA, Ruiz P. Kaplan and Sadock's Comprehensive Textbook of Psychiatry: Wolters Kluwer Health; 2017.

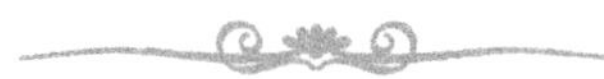

14 Depression

Neena Sawant

INTRODUCTION

Depression is one of the most commonly occurring psychiatric illnesses with prevalence from 5 to 17%. It also happens to be one of the leading causes of death due to suicide worldwide. Depression also accounts for health related disability as it causes economic burden and reduced productivity. Hence the early diagnosis and treatment of depression is very important to reduce the burden of illness.

Depression is classified under mood disorders. Mood is defined as a pervasive sustained emotion that influences a person's behavior and colors his perception of being in the world. Currently patients having depressive episodes are considered to have major depressive disorder or unipolar depression. But there is a current debate on whether depression is a part of the bipolar spectrum as many patients on detailed questioning do reveal history of manic or hypo manic symptoms which went undiagnosed.

However we will learn about depression in this chapter.

HISTORY

It was Hippocrates who used the terms mania and melancholia to describe mental disturbances. Melancholia comes from the Greek word melan [black] and chole [bile] which was used to explain human behavior not in relation to Gods and the dark viscous liquid excreted by the bile was considered to be responsible for the dark state of mind.

EPIDEMIOLOGY

The lifetime prevalence of depressive disorders in India is about 15%.The mean age of onset is between 30-35 years, though it is also seen in children and geriatric population. Depressive disorders are twice more common in females as compared to males. Marriage is a protective factor for men whereas married women with children are found to have high rates of depression. Racial, ethnic and socioeconomic differences have not been correlated with depression though it is found to occur more in rural areas.

ETIOLOGY

A variety of factors contribute to the causation of depression.

Biological factors

Recently apart from the monoamine neurotransmitter system which has been the major cause for depression, other neurotransmitters are also being implicated. Among the biogenic amines there is enough evidence to cite the role of norepinephrine and serotonin in the pathogenesis of depression. Norephinephrine is reduced in depression and there is a correlation between the down regulation or decreased sensitivity of ß adrenergic receptors and clinical antidepressant responses of antidepressants drugs with noradrenergic effects.

Serotonin is the most common biogenic amine associated with depression and the efficacy of serotonin specific reuptake inhibitors (SSRIs). There is reduced serotonin in depression and in those with suicidal behaviors the level of serotonin in the CSF is also low.

Dopamine is the other biogenic amine associated with depression and mania with reduced dopaminergic activity found in depression and increased activity is seen in mania.

The other neurotransmitters in depression include glutamate, glycine, GABA, and acetylcholine. Glutamate and glycine bind to sites on NMDA receptors causing neurocognitive effects. Reduced GABA levels are seen in depression and chronic stress can deplete GABA levels. Cholinergic agonists can exacerbate depressive symptoms.

Hormonal Factors

Hypercortisolemia is seen in depression and there is elevated HPA activity due to the underlying stress. Elevated TSH levels are seen in 5 to 10% of the depressed population.

Sleep Patterns

Depression is associated with increase in nocturnal arousal due to reduced REM sleep latency, increased REM density with a total reduction in sleep time.

Immunological Disturbances

There are several immunological abnormalities seen in depression resulting in impaired immunity due to reduction in neuromodulators and interleukins.

Genetic Factors

Family, adoption and twin studies have documented the role of genetic factors in the causation of depressive disorders. Family studies indicated that if one parent has mood disorder the risk increases between 10 and 25% for the child. Also if more family members are affected then the risk also greatly increases for the child. There is also evidence regarding gene –environment interaction in the development of major depression.

Psychosocial Factors

There is enough data to implicate those life events and environmental stresses are strongly associated with depression like losing a parent before 11 years of age, loss of spouse, unemployment etc. Negative life events may precede a depressive episode and it is important to understand the meaning attached by the patient to the event as though it could be perceived as a mild stressor by outsiders, the event could be perceived as devastating to the patient.

Psychodynamic Factors

Sigmund Freud and Karl Abraham theorized that the faulty infant-mother relationship in the first 10-18 months of life, real or imagined object loss, and ambivalent feelings towards the lost object with the anger directed towards self is responsible for depression. John Bowlby felt that the damaged early attachment and traumatic separation in childhood predispose to depression as adult losses then revive the childhood trauma.

Cognitive Theory

As per Aaron Beck depression occurs due to

cognitive distortions and postulated a cognitive triad where there is (1) a negative self percept, (2) environment is viewed as hostile, (3) future looks bleak due to expectations of failure and suffering. The feelings of hopelessness, helplessness and worthlessness are to be challenged in the cognitive therapy.

DIAGNOSIS

The DSM5 Diagnostic criteria for Major Depressive Disorder are listed in **Table 14.1**.

Table 14.1: DSM5 Diagnostic Criteria for Major Depressive Disorder

A. 5 or more of the 9 symptoms should be there in the same 2 week period with either (1) or (2) being present
1. Pervasive depressed mood or anhedonia; children/adolescents can have irritable mood
2. Loss of interest or pleasure in most of the daily activities
3. Loss of appetite with weight loss not due to dieting or increase in appetite
4. Insomnia or Hypersomnia
5. Psychomotor agitation or retardation as observed by others
6. Loss of energy or fatigue
7. Feelings of worthlessness or inappropriate guilt
8. Impaired concentration or indecisiveness
9. Recurrent thoughts of death, suicidal ideation or a suicide attempt
B. Symptoms cause significant distress or impairment in socio-occupational functioning
C. Episode is not attributable to effects of a substance or medical disorder
D. Episode is not explained by any psychotic disorder
E. There is no previous history of mania or hypomania

ICD 10 Diagnostic Criteria for Depressive episode are listed in **Table 14.2**.

Table 14.2: ICD 10 Diagnostic Criteria for Depressive episode

Requires 4 or more (of 10) symptoms present for at least 2 weeks	
Symptoms must include ≥ 2 of: **Depressed mood** **Anhedonia** **Energy loss**	
Key symptoms include:	
1.	Depressed mood
2.	Loss of interest and enjoyment
3.	Reduced energy leading to: Increased fatigability Diminished activity
4.	Reduced concentration and attention
5.	Reduced self-esteem and self confidence
6.	Ideas of guilt and unworthiness
7.	Bleak and pessimistic views of the future
8.	Ideas or acts of: Self-harm Suicide
9.	Disturbed sleep
10.	Diminished appetite

CLINICAL FEATURES

Patients with depressive disorders primarily present with mood symptoms. Mood is defined as a pervasive and sustained emotion or feeling tone that colors a person's perception of the world and influences his/her behavior. Mood symptoms should be present for most of the day for at least a minimum of 2 weeks to qualify for a disorder.

Depressed mood: Patients express the mood as being sad, empty, feel hopeless or at times irritable most of the day. They could be observed to be tearful and cry easily during conversations. Children and adolescents may express more of irritability rather than sadness.

Loss of Interest: Depressed patients often find a lack of initiative to do things that were previously enjoyed by them e.g. watching TV, going out, routine daily household chores etc. They may express reduced pleasure or anhedonia.

Suicidal Ideations

About 60-70% of the patients do give suicidal ideations which could be active thoughts with contemplation and planning or just passive thoughts where they feel life is not worth living and it is better to die. About 10-15% of the depressed patients do commit suicide. Suicide is the major cause of death worldwide.

Physiological/Vegetative Disturbances

Most patients have sleep related problems which would include early awakening seen in about 80% of the patients, delayed initiation, multiple awakenings with inability to fall back asleep, parasomnias or at times hypersomnia. Similarly majority complain of reduced appetite with weight loss which is not attributed to dieting or other causes. Weight loss may often be significant in some people. There is associated bowel disturbance with constipation being a major problem. Patients with atypical depression may show increased appetite with hypersomnia. There may also be associated gastrointestinal symptoms of bloating, nausea, flatulence etc. due to underlying anxiety. Females may also have menstrual irregularities. Decreased libido as well as sexual problems often go unrecognized as symptoms of depression and may lead to wrong referrals to a sex therapist or marital counselor.

Psychomotor Disturbances

Most patients usually complain of agitation observed as restlessness, pacing, nervousness and apprehension due to underlying anxiety. There could also be psychomotor retardation where the person feels slowed down, not having the usual pace and energy to do routine work. Associated feelings of tiredness, fatigue and anergia accompany the retardation.

Cognitive Disturbances

The thought process of a depressed person has predominant negative themes which ruminate due to which there is slowing of the thought process too. Feelings of hopelessness, helplessness and worthlessness predominate due to which the person has lowered self esteem, self loathing with a lot of guilt which is a vicious cycle often resulting in the person having suicidal thoughts/ideations which can lead to a suicidal attempt. There is often lack of concentration in other areas of functioning and the person only focuses on the negative themes. This results in a lot of cognitive distortions which often intensifies the depressive episode.

Psychotic Features

Severe depressive episodes maybe accompanied with mood congruent psychotic features (in harmony with the mood disorder) like delusions of sin, nihilism, illness, guilt etc. or mood incongruent psychotic features (not in harmony with the mood disorder) like delusions of persecution, reference. Patients with mood incongruent psychotic features could have schizoaffective disorder or schizophrenia.

Somatic Complaints

In India many depressed patients first express somatic symptoms instead of mood symptoms. Initially this was called as masked depression. The most common symptoms include body aches, pains in various locations, giddiness, dizziness etc. Most of these symptoms do not have any underlying pathology and are often treated by physicians as pain syndromes with minimum improvement.

Anxiety

Anxiety is a common symptom of depression seen in about 90% of all depressed patients. Patients complain of agitation, restlessness, ruminations and worries.

Diurnal variation may be seen in 50% of the patients where the patients report feeling worse in the morning or on waking up with a reduction in symptoms in the evening as the day progresses.

Case Vignette 1

A 40 year old middle aged man was admitted with history of suicidal attempt by hanging. He expressed feelings of hopelessness, helplessness as he was under debt of Rs 3 lakhs and had creditors asking him to repay at the earliest. His business for which he had taken the loan had failed and he had no financial support from his family. His wife was a homemaker and he had 2 school going children. His stressors were ongoing for nearly 2 years but were precipitated by a threat from one of the creditors 15 days prior to his attempt. He gave sadness of mood, crying spells and increased withdrawn behavior. At times he felt as if he could hear his creditors threatening to do something to him. Patient started feeling scared and would be vigilant at all times. He refused to go out of the house thinking that something would happen to him on the streets. His family tried to explain to him but to no avail. He also was having total loss of sleep the last few days when one night due to extreme feelings of hopelessness he tried to hang himself.

Bereavement

Depressive symptoms may occur during grief and bereavement but are a part of the grief process. However if the intensity of the symptoms lasts beyond 3 months with the person having morbid preoccupation of the deceased person or guilt feelings that they were responsible for the death then it may ensue in suicidal behaviors and requires treatment.

Case Vignette 2

A 65 year old widow, who lost her husband 2 months ago was brought by her daughter with severe body ache, dizziness and loss of balance while walking and pulling sensation in both legs at bedtime. As per her daughter, patient used to be persistently worried about her 2 sons who were alcohol dependent and not working. Her husband had died 2 months ago due to alcohol induced hepatitis. She expressed a bleak future, hopelessness and had active suicidal ideations. She was a vegetable seller but had stopped working since 1 month, as she felt dizzy. She said that her entire life was a misery as her husband used to abuse and beat her under influence of alcohol, felt her sons were becoming like their father and she expressed decreased desire to do anything and just wanted to die. Her condition deteriorated after her husband's death and she could not handle her activities till her married daughter brought her for treatment. She had diabetes and was taking her medicines irregularly. However her investigations and MRI brain were normal. Patient improved on medications and was taken up for counseling. She restarted her job as a vegetable vendor and is doing well. Her daughter accompanies her for a regular psychiatric follow up, though both her sons denied treatment for alcohol dependence.

DIFFERENTIAL DIAGNOSIS

There are several mental and physical conditions which could have depressive symptoms and have to be ruled out (**Table 14.3**).

Table 14.3: Mental and physical disorders with depressive symptoms

Mental Disorders with Depressive Symptoms
1. Adjustment disorder with depressed mood
2. Anxiety Disorders: Generalized anxiety disorder, Panic Disorder, Mixed anxiety-depressive disorder, Obsessive compulsive disorder, posttraumatic stress disorder
3. Schizophrenia
4. Mood disorders: Dysthymia, Bipolar mood disorders,Cyclothymia
5. Substance induced mood disorders: Alcohol
6. Somatoform disorders : Somatization, Hypochondriasis, Pain disorders
7. Eating Disorders: Anorexia Nervosa, Bulimia Nervosa
Physical Disorders with Depressive Symptoms
1. Neurological: Head injury, CVA, Parkinson's disease, Dementia, Cerebral tumors, Meningitis, Migraine, Multiple sclerosis
2. Endocrine disorders: Hypothyroidism, Hyperthyroidism, Cushing's disease, Diabetes mellitus, Hyperparathyroidism
3. Infections: AIDS, Kochs, Hepatitis, Syphilis, Viral fevers, Pneumonia
4. Nutritional deficiency: Anemia, Pellagra, Folate
5. Autoimmune disorders: SLE, Rhematoid arthritis
6. Medications : Steroids, NSAIDs, antihypertensives, antipsychotics, antibacterials, antineoplastics, sedatives, hypnotics, antiparkinsonian drugs

COURSE AND PROGNOSIS

The first depressive episode usually occurs before 40 years of age in about 50% of the patients. An untreated depressive episode remits by self within 6 months. Stoppage of antidepressants within 3 months of treatment usually leads to a relapse. As the disorder progresses the frequency and duration of the episodes increases. 50% patients admitted for first episode usually recover, 25% experience recurrence in the first 6 months after hospitalization and about 30-50% in the following 2 years.

Mild episodes, short hospital stay, good psychosocial support, absence of psychotic symptoms are good prognostic factors. Comorbid medical and mental disorders, substance use, personality factors, unstable family dynamics are poor prognostic factors.

TREATMENT

Most cases of mild depressive episodes present to general practitioners and may resolve spontaneously along with de-stressing techniques, empathic listening and reassurance. Treatment is usually initiated after detailed history, mental status examination, ruling out medical conditions and routine investigations. Moderate and severe depressive episodes can be treated on outpatient basis unless patients are suicidal and need to be hospitalized. A combination of both pharmacotherapy and psychotherapy works for most patients.

Pharmacotherapy

A patient of depressive disorder can be treated with antidepressant medications which usually help in symptom reduction and symptom remission. Patients generally do start feeling better and recover within 4 weeks if the dose

Table 14.4: List of antidepressant medications

No.	Class	Medications
1	**Selective serotonin reuptake inhibitors (SSRIs)**	• Citalopram • Escitalopram • Fluoxetine • Fluvoxamine • Paroxetine • Sertraline
2	**Serotonin-norepinephrine reuptake inhibitors (SNRIs)**	• Desvenlafaxine • Duloxetine • Levomilnacipran • Milnacipran • Venlafaxine
3	**Serotonin modulator and stimulators (SMSs)**	• Vilazodone • Vortioxetine
4	**Serotonin antagonist and reuptake inhibitors (SARIs)**	• Nefazodone – withdrawn/discontinued in most countries • Trazodone
5	**Norepinephrine reuptake inhibitors (NRIs)**	• Atomoxetine - approved to treat ADHD • Reboxetine • Teniloxazine • Viloxazine
6	**Norepinephrine-dopamine reuptake inhibitors (NDRIs)**	• Bupropion
7	**Tricyclic antidepressants (TCAs)**	• Amitriptyline • Amoxapine • Clomipramine • Desipramine • Dosulepin • Doxepin • Imipramine • Melitracen • Nortriptyline • Opipramol • Trimipramine
8	**Tetracyclic antidepressants (TeCAs)** Mianserin, mirtazapine, are also sometimes described as **noradrenergic and specific serotonergic antidepressants (NaSSAs)**	• Mianserin • Mirtazapine • Maprotiline
9	**Monoamine oxidase inhibitors (MAOIs) approved to treat depression**	• Isocarboxazid • Phenelzine • Selegiline • Tranylcypromine

of the medications is adequate. Hence it is important that the patient does a regular follow up for monitoring of side effects and improvement in his symptom profile. Though most drugs exert their therapeutic effects within 3 to 4 weeks, some newer agents may show their actions earlier.

The most common mistake is giving a low dose of medication with frequent changing of the molecule. Antidepressant medications should be maintained for at least 6-9 months or the length of the previous episode, whichever is greater. Sometimes prophylactic treatment with antidepressants also helps in reducing the frequency and intensity of the symptoms during the recurrences.

Management of depression begins with choosing an appropriate antidepressant, ensuring treatment adherence, monitoring treatment outcomes and psycho education regarding early signs of relapse or recurrence in the maintenance phase help in achieving remission.

The commonly used antidepressant medications are listed in **Table 14.4**.

PSYCHOTHERAPY

Cognitive Therapy

This therapy was developed by Aaron Beck which helps to identify the cognitive distortions present in the patients so as to help them identify these automatic negative thoughts and develop alternative flexible ways of thinking and thus improve the patients thinking and behavior. Therapists in the early phase of therapy (1 to 6 sessions) establish a therapeutic relationship, educate patients about cognitive model of treatment, identify target symptoms, set short term goals and establish relationship between depressive feelings and automatic negative thoughts. The middle phase of therapy (sessions 7 to 12) use a systematized approach to addressing the automatic negative thoughts. The latter phase of therapy(session 13 to termination)prepare patient for termination of therapy, identify risk factors for relapse and implement a life plan that will support a balanced way of thinking about self, life and the world.

Behavior Therapy

Depression is associated with reduced goal directed behaviors with a decrease in positive reinforcement. In this therapy the goal is to make the patients understand and monitor their mood and activities with the help of an activity planner, homework assignments etc. Behavioral strategies to reduce anxiety like relaxation techniques, breathing exercises, desensitization etc. are taught to patients. Social skills training, assertiveness training and a step wise approach to problem solving also help the patients to cope with the impact of interpersonal stressors.

Interpersonal Therapy

Interpersonal therapy works on the principle that addressing the interpersonal problems in the patient's life, whether contributing or facilitating the depressive symptoms would help in symptom resolution. In about 12 to 16 sessions, the therapist works on themes like unresolved grief, role transitions, role disputes, loneliness, social isolation etc. to help the patient understand, clarify, resolve and cope with the interpersonal issues.

Family Therapy

Family therapy is usually done when it is seen that the patient's mood disorder creates an impact on the family functioning, marriage stability and is responsible for a relapse.

Repetitive Transcranial Magnetic Stimulation (rTMS)

rTMS is now showing emerging as an upcoming treatment for patients of depression who have failed to achieve satisfactory improvement on medication. It involves giving short pulses of magnetic energy to stimulate the nerve cells in the brain. It is noninvasive and does not require sedation or anesthesia.

BIBLIOGRAPHY

1. Sadock BJ, Sadock VA, Ruiz P. Synopsis of Psychiatry, 11th ed. Delhi: Wolters Kluwer Pvt Ltd, 2015: 347-380.
2. World Health Organization. The ICD 10 Classification of Mental and behavioral Disorders: Clinical descriptions and diagnostic guidelines. Oxford: Oxford University Press, 1992.
3. Prescribers Guide: Stahl's essential Psychopharmacology, 5th ed. Cambridge, 2014.

Bipolar Disorder 15

Pragya Lodha • Avinash De Sousa

INTRODUCTION

Bipolar Disorder was earlier known as manic depressive illness or manic depression. Bipolar disorder is one of the severe mental illnesses characterized by unusual shifts in mood, energy, activity levels, concentration, and the ability to carry out day-to-day tasks. Bipolar disorder is a mood disorder that involves the patient experiencing depressive moods and euphoric moods. Bipolar Disorder can be broadly classified as Bipolar Disorder Type I and Bipolar Disorder Type II along with another condition that is less frequently observed called as Cyclothymia. All these three conditions involve clear changes in mood, energy, and activity levels. These moods range from periods of extremely "up," elated, irritable, or energized behavior (known as manic episodes) to very "down," sad, indifferent, or helpless periods (known as depressive episodes). Less severe manic periods are known as hypomanic episodes.

Bipolar Disorder Type I is defined by manic episodes that last at least 7 days, or by manic symptoms that are so severe that the person needs immediate hospital care. Usually, depressive episodes occur as well, typically lasting at least 2 weeks. What is a marker of type I is that the depressive episode occurs always after the manic episode the manic episode is usually never hypomanic. Bipolar Disorder Type II is characterized by a pattern of depressive episodes and hypomanic episodes, but not the full-blown manic episodes that are typical of Bipolar I Disorder. Cyclothymia, also known as cyclothymic disorder is a milder form where there are experiences of low and high mood swings however these mood swings never meet the criteria of major depressive episode or full-blown mania. The patient experiences low mood, hypomania and mania but without meeting the actual criteria for any.

Another phenomenon that is tied to bipolar disorder is known as rapid cycling. Rapid cycling is a term used when a person with bipolar disorder experiences four or more mood swings (episodes) within a twelve-month period. An episode may consist of depression, mania, hypomania, or a condition known as a mixed state in which depression and mania are co-occurring. Sometimes a person might experience symptoms of bipolar disorder that do not match the three categories listed above, which is referred to as "other specified and unspecified bipolar and related disorders."

EPIDEMIOLOGY & ETIOLOGY

The annual incidence of bipolar illness is considered generally to be less than 1 percent, but it is difficult to estimate because milder forms of bipolar disorder are often missed. The prevalence of bipolar disorder is equal in men as in women. However, manic episodes are more common in men whereas depressive episodes are more commonly seen in women. The age of onset of bipolar disorder is during late adolescence or young adulthood with a mean age of 30 years. However, the illness can manifest at any age. Among children, it is referred to as pediatric bipolar disorder. It is rare for the onset of this illness to start after the age of 50-55 years.

Some research suggests that people with certain genes are more likely to develop bipolar disorder. Many genes are involved, and no one gene can cause the disorder. Genetically, family, adoption and twin studies have long documented the heritability of bipolar disorder. Bipolar disorder runs in families and family history pays a strong role in the onset of the disorder. A family history of schizophrenia, psychosis or major development disorder also increases the risk for bipolar disorder. Biologically, disturbances in neurotransmitter levels, neural circuits and neuroregulatory mechanisms have been implicated.

SYMPTOMS

One may look for the following signs in order to identify a depressive episode in bipolar disorder:

- Low mood and feelings of sadness
- Loss of interest in doing day to day tasks that were earlier pleasurable
- Being unable to enjoy things that were enjoyable earlier
- Feelings of restlessness and being agitated
- Low self-confidence
- Feelings of hopelessness
- Feelings of helplessness
- More than usual irritability
- Suicidal ideas or thinking.
- Finding it hard to make simple decisions about day to day activities
- Difficulty in starting and maintaining doing a task
- Difficulty in concentrating on tasks
- Increased or decreased sleeping
- Increased or decreased eating
- Fatigue and easy tiredness
- Lack of interest in maintaining sexual relationships
- Crying spells
- Lack of interest to socialize

One may look for the following signs in order to identify a manic episode in bipolar disorder:

- Feeling overly happy or “high” for long periods of time
- May also feel irritable, agitated or may also become very sensitive on certain issues
- Having a decreased need for sleep
- Talking in a very fast manner, often with racing thoughts where the person feels that his/her thoughts go faster than the ability to talk about them
- Moving from one idea to another while talking
- Loss of inhibition in general behavior
- Feeling extremely restless or impulsive at sudden spurs of moments
- Easily distracted
- Behaviors may sometimes be bizarre and unexplainable
- Feeling overconfidence in their abilities
- Making grandiose and unrealistic plans Thinking that they can do too many things at once

- Engaging in risky behaviors such as involving in impulsive (and may be multiple) sexual encounters, gambling with money that is required for more important needs, or spending without much thought and judgment.
- There may be signs that individual is hearing, seeing and/or talking to individuals who only he/she can see. These are psychotic symptoms which are seen in schizophrenia as well.
- Person may attempt impulsive suicide in the state of mania

Between episodes: Some people with bipolar disorder may go back to normal, while many of them continue to experience low levels of depressive symptoms and mild problems even when they appear, to other people, to be 'back to normal'.

Sometimes people experience both manic and depressive symptoms in the same episode. This kind of episode is called an episode with mixed features. People experiencing an episode with mixed features may feel very sad, empty, or hopeless, while, at the same, time feeling extremely energized.

DSM 5 CRITERIA FOR BIPOLAR DISORDER

To be diagnosed with bipolar disorder, a person must have experienced at least one episode of mania or hypomania.

To be considered mania, the elevated, expansive, or irritable mood must last for at least one week and be present most of the day, nearly every day. To be considered hypomania, the mood must last at least four consecutive days and be present most of the day, almost every day.

During this period, three or more of the following symptoms must be present and represent a significant change from usual behavior:

Table 15.1: Difference in signs and symptoms between a manic and depressive episode

People having a manic episode may:	People having a depressive episode may:
Feel very "up," "high," elated, or irritable or touchy	Feel very sad, "down," empty, worried, or hopeless
Feel "jumpy" or "wired"	Feel slowed down or restless
Have a decreased need for sleep	Have trouble falling asleep, wake up too early, or sleep too much
Have a loss of appetite	Experience increased appetite and weight gain
Talk very fast about a lot of different things	Talk very slowly, feel like they have nothing to say, forget a lot
Feel like their thoughts are racing	Have trouble concentrating or making decisions
Think they can do a lot of things at once	Feel unable to do even simple things
Do risky things that show poor judgment, such as eat and drink excessively, spend or give away a lot of money, or have reckless sex	Have little interest in almost all activities, a decreased or absent sex drive, or an inability to experience pleasure ("anhedonia")
Feel like they are unusually important, talented, or powerful	Feel hopeless or worthless, think about death or suicide

1. Inflated self-esteem or grandiosity
2. Decreased need for sleep
3. Increased talkativeness
4. Racing thoughts
5. Distracted easily
6. Increase in goal-directed activity or psychomotor agitation
7. Engaging in activities that hold the potential for painful consequences, e.g., unrestrained buying sprees

The depressive side of bipolar disorder is characterized by a major depressive episode resulting in depressed mood or loss of interest or pleasure in life. The DSM-5 states that a person must experience five or more of the following symptoms in two weeks to be diagnosed with a major depressive episode:

1. Depressed mood most of the day, nearly every day
2. Loss of interest or pleasure in all, or almost all, activities
3. Significant weight loss or decrease or increase in appetite
4. Engaging in purposeless movements, such as pacing the room
5. Fatigue or loss of energy
6. Feelings of worthlessness or guilt
7. Diminished ability to think or concentrate, or indecisiveness
8. Recurrent thoughts of death, recurrent suicidal ideation without a specific plan, or a suicide attempt

COMORBIDITY

Bipolar disorder may not always exist as the primary illness. Often, it is found to be comorbid with substance use in men. Whereas, among women, anxiety and eating disorders. However, in general, anxiety and substance use are seen to be commonly seen comorbid conditions with bipolar disorder. Another comorbidity that is seen clinically are psychotic features. Sometimes, psychotic features may overlap with those of a full-blown mania and must be differentiated and identified with a detailed case history.

TREATMENT

The first step to treatment for bipolar disorder is a detailed case history that helps the clinician to clearly identify the diagnosis and plan for a treatment accordingly. An effective treatment plan usually includes a combination of medication and psychotherapy. Bipolar disorder is a lifelong illness. Episodes of mania and depression typically come back over time. Between episodes, that is, in remission, many people with bipolar disorder are free of disabling symptoms, but some people may have lingering symptoms which may not be severe. Long-term, continuous treatment can help people manage these symptoms and improve quality of life.

Medications generally used to treat bipolar disorder include mood stabilizers and second-generation ("atypical") antipsychotics. Treatment plans may also include medications that target sleep or anxiety. Health care providers often prescribe antidepressant medication to treat depressive episodes in bipolar disorder, combining the antidepressant with a mood stabilizer to prevent triggering a manic episode. Medication for bipolar disorder, like any other mental disorder must be taken consistently, as prescribed, even when one is feeling better.

1) Mood Stabilizers: These are invariably prescribed to ensure moods stay stable and within a manageable range.

2) Anti-Psychotics: may also be prescribed depending on the symptoms exhibited by an individual

3) Antidepressants: these are to be administered with great caution to BD patients because they can precipitate mania.

4) Tranquilisers

The Role of Medication

- Medications are very important as they control the mood swings present in these patients.
- In episodes of mania, there are anger outbursts which can be controlled with regular dosage of medicines.
- There are sleep disturbances and patients need to get enough sleep for early recovery and medicines help in maintaining this.
- Some patients may be suicidal and/or homicidal which needs to be managed properly and can be done medically.
- In a depressive phase, to elevate mood, to regain interest in earlier activities medicines definitely help along with therapeutic help and social support from the family.
- Also, proper and timely use of mood stabilizers helps to prevent further recurrence of these episodes. More the mood episodes, more difficult it becomes to control them as severity and recurrence rates of episodes increases.

People Taking Medication Should

- Understand the risks and benefits of the medication from your doctor.
- Tell the doctor about any prescription drugs, over-the-counter medications, or supplements they are already taking.
- Report any concerns about side effects to the doctor right away. They may need to change the dose or try a different medication.

What Else Can Help in the Patient's Recovery?

1. **Psychotherapy**: Regular therapy sessions with a Psychologist can be very beneficial. In the depressive phase especially, CBT (Cognitive Behavioral Therapy) is of particular benefit. It helps the patient identify and correct faulty thought patterns.
2. **Exercise**: Regular exercise, say even a half hour walk everyday helps in multiple ways. Exercise improves physical and mental well-being.
3. There are other holistic approaches that can be adopted in consultation with the treating Doctor, such as Yoga, Art Therapy, Mindfulness meditation, picking up a hobby, etc.
4. **Peer Support Groups** are great communities for patients as well as their caregivers to engage in. They encourage adherence and are a rich pool of knowledge and shared experiences.
5. If applicable, getting them to earn a living increases their self-esteem and makes them feel more responsible.

Ways to Enhance Home Environment for Better Management Of BD

➔ Changing your home environment to suit the needs of a BD patient is not as difficult as it may seem. Start by making simple changes to your home design such as choosing a softer, warmer color scheme for your walls and furniture. These colors are less harsh and can be calming for BD patients.

- Lighting also plays a key role — keep bright lights only where it is needed (example, in a study room) and keep soft and soothing lights in other areas, especially areas where one can rest (living room, bedroom).
- Ensure valuables and hazardous materials, particularly those that can be used for suicide or self-harm, are put away.
- It is possible for patients to become irritable and violent during an episode of mania (or sometimes depression as well), and they may attempt to harm themselves or others with things around. Buy furniture that is too heavy to lift, or if possible, bolster it to the floor/wall. Don't have too many fragile objects around.
- It may be helpful for you to have a designated area where the patient can go to calm down if they are very angry or anxious. This is particularly useful for children with BD. Fill this room with objects that can be calming such as puzzles and books. Ensure you keep potential hazards away from here.
- Aside from redesigning your home, it is important to have everyone living in the home aware of BD and any crisis plans that have been put into place. Encourage everyone to be patient with and understanding, and to practice self-care. It's perfectly okay to need space and time away just for yourself.
- If you are a working parent, have your partner or another family member who the patient is familiar with, stay at home with the patient. This can be useful even if the patient is an adult. In case the patient has children, make a plan so that the children have a safe place to go if the situation at home becomes too stressful for them. This may take time depending on the patient's episode so ensure the children are left with someone they like and trust.
- Dividing the caregiving responsibilities helps better care as the burden gets shared.

BIBLIOGRAPHY

1. Cutler JL. Kaplan and Sadock's synopsis of psychiatry.
2. Belmaker RH. Bipolar disorder. New England Journal of Medicine. 2004 Jul 29;351(5):476-86.
3. Grunze H. Bipolar disorder. In Neurobiology of brain disorders 2015 Jan 1 (pp. 655-673). Academic Press.
4. Geddes JR, Miklowitz DJ. Treatment of bipolar disorder. The lancet. 2013 May 11;381(9878):1672-82.
5. Basco MR, Rush AJ. Cognitive-behavioral therapy for bipolar disorder. Guilford Press; 2005 May 20.

Anxiety Disorders 16

Jahnavi Kedare • Hrishikesh Nachane

Anxiety is a thin stream of fear trickling through the mind.
If encouraged, it cuts a channel into which all other thoughts are drained.

— ***Arthur Somers Roche***

INTRODUCTION

Before we begin understanding the phenomenon of anxiety disorders, take a look at these statements you might have come across in your day to day life:

How will I be able to travel alone to US? I have never travelled alone before this!

How will the exam be? Will I get a good score?

Tomorrow I have to make a presentation in the office? Will I be able to do it? All my superiors will be there!

Do you think these statements constitute as anxiety?

These are some of the situations which make us feel apprehensive and make us uneasy. This vague sense of apprehension is known as 'anxiety' and is experienced by all of us at some point in time. It is normal to feel anxious once in a while. Anxiety is an unpleasant feeling which makes us nervous and is very common in our day to day life. It is a warning signal. It alerts us about an impending danger and helps us in facing it.

Anxiety gives rise to a variety of physiological and psychological symptoms

Worry Being upset Nervousness
Inability to concentrate Confusion
Inability to recall- forgetfulness

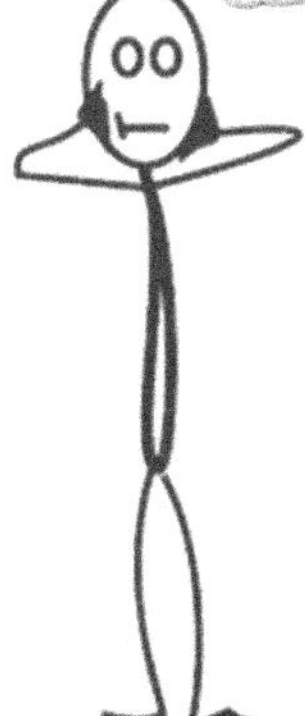

Palpitations
Light headedness
Perspiration
Hyperhidrosis
Breathlessness
Shortness of breath
Tremulousness
Syncope
Dizziness
Stomach upset
Restlessness e.g. pacing, fidgety
Urinary frequency, hesitancy, urgency
Constricting sensation in chest

ANXIETY V/S FEAR

Anxiety warns of an impending danger, but it is an internal threat which is vague and conflictual in nature i.e. related to conflicts in mind. Fear is also a warning signal towards a threat. However, the threat is an external, known, definitive and nonconflictual object or situation. e.g. fear of a tiger, a speeding car approaching a person. Fear arises suddenly and anxiety is an insidious feeling. Fear typically gives rise to a 'Flight or Fight' response in response to a dangerous situation leading to running away or freezing in a fearful situation and helps a person in facing the situation.

ADAPTIVE FUNCTION OF ANXIETY

Anxiety helps in adapting to various situations successfully. It helps the individual in preparing for and facing impending danger. The treat perceived may be of bodily harm, of pain, illness, of unknown situations. The threat may be of frustration, of failure Vs success, of being alone(loneliness), of separation from loved ones and a threat to unity of self. Anxiety prompts a person to take necessary actions to ward off the dangers. E.g. A person travelling alone for the first time gathers enough information and seeks advice from experienced people; a student makes a schedule of his study and prepares well for the exam and a person making a presentation in front of superiors practises enough number of times to feel confident. Activation of sympathetic and parasympathetic nervous system takes place in this process.

An event or a situation may be perceived as stressful when the person is unable to cope with it. Such a stressful event gives rise to anxiety. When a person cannot handle stress, anxiety becomes severe, lasts for a long time and causes disturbances in the individual's day to day functioning. Then the anxiety becomes ***'pathological anxiety'.***

EPIDEMIOLOGY

Anxiety disorders are one of the commonest psychiatric disorders in the population. One person in four suffers from at least one anxiety disorder. 17.7% of the population suffers from anxiety disorders. Anxiety disorders are seen more frequently in women than in men, occurring in a ratio of approximately 2:1.

ETIOLOGY

I] Biological factors

1) Neurotransmitters

   An excess of norepinephrine due to a poor regulation of secretion of norepinephrine in locus ceruleus has been shown to be present in anxiety disorders.Serotonin is another important neurotransmitter involved in causing anxiety disorders. Any stress causes an increase in the turnover of 5-Hydroxytryptamine (5HT) in various parts of the brain. A hypothesis of serotonin as a causative factor for anxiety also stems from the fact that serotonergic drugs like Specific serotonin reuptake inhibitors (SSRIs) are effective in treating anxiety disorders.GABA (Gamma amino butyric acid) also seems to play some role in causing anxiety. GABAergic drugs like benzodiazepines are quite effective in relieving anxiety and on the other hand benzodiazepine antagonists like Flumazenil cause severe panic attacks.

2) Hypothalamic –Pituitary-Adrenal Axis:

   Stress leads to an increase in the synthesis and release of cortisol. Hypothalamic levels of Corticotropin Releasing Hormone (CRH) are increased in stress.

This causes activation of HPA axis and thus increases the release of cortisol and dehydroepiandrosterone (DHEA). This leads to anxiety.

3) Neuroimaging studies:

Neuroimaging studies have shown various findings. There are cerebral asymmetries with the right side of the brain showing some abnormalities, but not the left side. CT scans and MRIs have shown increased ventricular size. fMRI and PET studies have demonstrated abnormal findings in frontal cortex, occipital and temporal areas and parahippocampal gyrus in panic disorder. In OCD there are abnormalities in caudate nucleus and in PTSD amygdal is implicated.

4) Neuroanatomical findings:

Limbic system- Septohippocampal pathway of the limbic system and cingulated gyrus are responsible in anxiety disorders.

Cerebral cortex- As the frontal cortex is connected to parahippocampal region, cingulated gyrus and hypothalamus it may be involved in causation of anxiety. Temporal cortex is also implicated in anxiety disorders.

5) Genetic factors: Genetic factors are important in anxiety disorders and hereditary predisposition makes a person more vulnerable to develop anxiety disorder.

II] Psychological factors

1) Psychoanalytical theories:

Freud described anxiety as a 'signal' of presence of danger in the unconscious mind. Anxiety is said to arise from conflicts between sexual or aggressive impulses and the superego and external reality.

2) Behavioral theories:

This theory describes anxiety as a conditional response to a specific environmental stimulus.

3) Existential theories:

A person who perceives his existence as being in a purposeless universe develops anxiety. He thinks there is a void in existence and that it is meaningless.

CLASSIFICATION OF ANXIETY DISORDERS

Over the years, the classification of anxiety disorders has undergone considerable change. Initially classified under the umbrella of 'Neurosis', recent data based on genetic, behavioral, pharmacological, biochemical, and psychophysiological investigation of these so called neurotic disorders, their placement has varied over the years in the various classification systems. The term neurosis was coined by William Cullen in 1769 to refer to "disorders of sense and motion". Cullen used the term to describe various nervous disorders and symptoms that he could not be explained physiologically. He observed that physical features were almost inevitably present. The term 'neurosis' has undergone several changes over the early and middle 20th century, owing to the likes of Sigmund Freud and Carl Jung. It is still used in psychology and philosophy. They include what we now classify as anxiety disorders, depression, obsessive-compulsive disorders, trauma and stress related disorders, dissociative disorders, conversion disorders, somatoform disorders among others. As ICD-10 and DSM-5 classifications are the most followed in India, they are discussed below:

ANXIETY DISORDERS IN ICD-10

In ICD-10, anxiety disorders are broadly

classified under two headings based on the circumstances or the situations in which anxiety is evoked:

F40: Phobic anxiety disorders

F41: Other anxiety disorders

F40: PHOBIC ANXIETY DISORDERS: anxiety is evoked only, or predominantly, by certain well-defined situations or objects (external to the individual)	
Agoraphobia	- With panic disorder - Without panic disorder
Social phobia	
Specific phobia	e.g.: acrophobia, animal phobia, claustrophobia, etc.
F41: OTHER ANXIETY DISORDERS: anxiety is not restricted to any particular environmental situation	
Panic disorder (episodic paroxysmal anxiety)	Includes panic attacks, panic states
Generalized anxiety disorder	
Mixed anxiety depression	Features of both anxiety and depression present in equal dominance
Other mixed anxiety disorders	Features of GAD plus disorders other than depression (OCD, dissociative disorders, etc.)
Anxiety disorder not specified	

Anxiety disorders arising secondary to substance use or other medical conditions are classified in those respective sections under ICD-10

ANXIETY DISORDERS IN DSM-5

1) Separation anxiety disorder
2) Selective mutism
3) Specific phobia
    - Animal
    - Natural environment
    - Blood-injection-injury
    - Situational
    - Other
4) Social anxiety disorder/ social phobia
5) Panic disorder
6) Agoraphobia
7) Generalized anxiety disorder
8) Anxiety disorder due to substance/ medication use
9) Anxiety disorder due to another medical condition
10) Other specified anxiety disorder
11) Unspecified anxiety disorder

DSM-5 diagnoses anxiety disorders which share features of excessive fear and anxiety and related behavioral disturbances. They are arranged developmentally: starting with anxiety disorders that begin in childhood such as separation anxiety disorder and so on. In contrast to ICD-10, anxiety disorders due to substance, medication or medical conditions are classified here itself.

SEPARATION ANXIETY DISORDER

6 year old Mr. A, started complaining of restlessness and anxiety when he started school, with excessive crying whenever he had to go to school. Even if his mother sat with him at school, he kept crying and insisted that he be taken home. He could not sleep alone at night always claiming to be scared. He would frequently follow his mother around everywhere the house. He was then taken to a psychiatrist and diagnosed with separation anxiety disorder and started on low dose clonazepam. He gradually improved and was comfortable attending school.

Separation anxiety is a normal phenomenon that everyone undergoes. Children experience it between 9 and 18 months when it peaks and diminishes by 2½ years. By then, children develop a sense of comfort to be away from parents. Anxiety may again resurface when children join school for the first time. Separation anxiety disorder is seen whenever an individual experiences excessive anxiety regarding separation from home and/or from people to whom the individual has a strong emotional attachment (e.g., a parent, caregiver, significant other or siblings). They also may have fear that they may be kidnapped. It needs to be present for at least 4 weeks in children and for 6 months in adults. Children may complain of fear of the dark, fear of monsters, they may make way into their parents'/ siblings' bed at night. They may show 'clinging' behavior (refusing to leave the attachment figure's side) or 'shadowing' (following them everywhere in their activities). Patient may seem demanding, intrusive and in need of constant attention. They may also experience school refusal, withdrawn behavior and depression. It has prevalence of 5% in school going children and 6% in adults. Environmental factors such as death/illness of a loved one, parental overprotection and intrusiveness can contribute to it (they reduce child autonomy).

As per DSM 5, any 3 of the following must be present:

1. Recurrent excessive distress when anticipating or experiencing separation from home or from major attachment figures
2. Persistent and excessive worry about losing major attachment figures or about possible harm to them, such as illness, injury, disasters or death
3. Persistent and excessive worry about experiencing an untoward event (e.g., getting lost, being kidnapped, having an accident, becoming ill) that causes separation from a major attachment figure
4. Persistent reluctance or refusal to go out, away from home, to school, to work, or elsewhere because of fear of separation
5. Persistent and excessive fear of or reluctance about being alone or without major attachment figures at home or in other settings
6. Persistent reluctance or refusal to sleep away from home or to go to sleep without being near a major attachment figure
7. Repeated nightmares involving the theme of separation
8. Repeated complaints of physical symptoms (e.g., headaches, stomachaches, nausea, vomiting) when separation from major attachment figures occurs or is anticipated

General management strategies are outlined at the end of the chapter. Apart from these, strategies also include gradual transitions from the attachment figure, parent child interaction therapy and group therapies.

SELECTIVE MUTISM

Ms. S, a 5 year old girl, presented with difficulty in talking with strangers. She would not interact in the school during group activities and used to speak only a few words with her friend. At home, she was seen to interact and talk with all the members. She seemed to freeze during class presentations and whenever attention was focused on her. Her mother is also on treatment for social anxiety disorder. She was referred to a psychiatrist, who through play therapy, was able to make her talk gradually.

Selective mutism, earlier known as Elective

Mutism is persistent failure to speak in one or more specific social situations, despite speaking in other situations. It is usually associated with social anxiety. It is seen in 0.3–1% of population and is common in 4-5 year old children. They may communicate with non-verbal cues or may take part in social interactions. This diagnosis is not diagnosed at 1st month of school. Oppositional defiant disorder, communication disorder, intellectual disability/ language barrier and speech and language delay must be ruled out in these children. Sometimes, these children may even seem 'overly talkative' at home. Mutism happens towards adults more than peers. Children may also talk inconsistently, or in low tone or with less words in other situations. Other associated features which can be seen are shyness, fear of social embarrassment, isolation, difficulty maintaining eye contact, blank expression and reluctance to smile or incessant smiling, difficulty expressing feelings, even to family members, tendency to worry more than most people of the same age, sensitivity to noise and crowds, withdrawn behavior, clinging behavior and compulsive traits. Family of social phobia is seen in 95% of the cases. Course of the illness is transient and spontaneous remission occurs in about 60% of the patients.

Management

No drug has been approved for selective mutism, but Selective Serotonin Reuptake Inhibitors (SSRIs) can be tried in severe cases. Non-pharmacological management strategies are more applicable. The following techniques can be tried:

- Self modelling: This therapy involves videotaping children answering questions with an adult the child is comfortable (parent) and same questions being asked by teacher/ someone else. The two videos are then compiled together and shown to the child. Positive reinforcement is given to the child every time the child sees himself verbally answering the teacher/ other adult.
- Mystery motivators: Child is shown an envelope with their name on it, which they have to ask for out loud in the class. It contains a desired reward predetermined by their parent.
- Stimulus fading: This involves interacting with the child in a controlled environment with someone with whom they are at ease and then gradually another individual is introduced (sliding-in technique)
- CBT/ Behavioral therapies
- Social skills training
- Relaxation
- Contingency management
- Play therapy
- Speech and language therapy

PANIC DISORDER

Miss M was waiting for her husband to come back home from office. Suddenly she started having palpitations, felt breathless and had a choking sensation. She developed chest pain and began perspiring. She also felt that she was about to faint and felt weak. She was very scared with the thought that something dreadful was happening to her. Her husband reached home and saw her condition. She was taken to a doctor who did all her workup, including an ECG. The ECG was normal. This was the third time that she was visiting the doctor after a similar episode. She was referred to a psychiatrist and was diagnosed to have panic disorder.

A panic attack is a sudden episode of intense anxiety consisting of physiological as well as psychological symptoms of anxiety and is accompanied by a feeling of impending doom.

The episode of anxiety usually lasts for a few minutes and subsides gradually on its own. In panic disorder panic attacks become recurrent. In between panic attacks there is 'anticipatory anxiety'. These panic attacks interfere with proper functioning of the individual.

Etiology

Biological Factors

- A dysregulation in noradrenergic system is a hypothesis explaining panic disorder. Autonomic nervous system of panic disorder patients shows an increased sympathetic tone, an excess response to moderate stimuli and slow adaptation of the sympathetic system to repeated stimuli.
- Serotonin receptor dysregulation is an important factor in the etiology of panic disorder. Decreased GABAergic inhibition in specific areas of brain such as amygdala, midbrain and hypothalamus can reduce anxiety features.
- $\alpha 2$ receptor antagonists like yohimbine induce panic attacks, thus underlying the role of adrenergic receptors in the etiology of panic disorders.
- Brainstem (locus ceruleus, median raphe nucleus), limbic system and the prefrontal cortex are implicated in panic disorders.
- There are some substances which can induce panic attacks and are called *panicogens*. Carbon dioxide, sodium lactate and bicarbonate cause shift in acid base balance and induce a panic attack. Substances acting on neurotransmitters e.g. $\alpha 2$ receptors inhibitor yohimbine, mCPP acting on serotonin receptors, GABA receptor inverse agonists like flumazenil, GABA receptor antagonist cholecystokinin, caffeine.
- Brain imaging- MRI studies have shown involvement of temporal lobes, particularly hippocampus and amygdala. PET studies have indicated a dysregulation in cerebral blood flow with cerebral vasoconstriction.
- Genetic factors- First degree relatives of patients with panic disorder are four to eight times more at risk of developing panic disorder.

Psychosocial Factors

It proposes panic attack as an unsuccessful defence against anxiety provoking impulses. Mild signal anxiety is perceived as severe signal anxiety accompanied by somatic symptoms resulting in a panic attack. Usually a psychological event which is stressful in nature precedes neurophysiological changes occurring before a panic attack. Separation from mother, childhood physical and sexual abuse predispose a female patient to develop panic attacks.

Clinical Features

The first panic attack occurs spontaneously in most cases. Sometimes it is precipitated after emotional trauma, physical exertion, and sexual activity. The panic attack lasts for about 20-30 minutes. During the attack patients find it difficult to speak and may have memory problems. They may experience depersonalisation. Patients focus on the bodily symptoms and get concerned about death or heart attack. They experience a feeling of impending doom. There is anticipatory anxiety that the attack will recur. Depression is the commonest comorbidity with panic disorder. Apart from that agoraphobia, social anxiety disorder, specific phobia, generalized anxiety disorder, PTSD and OCD can coexist with panic disorder.

DSM -5 proposes the following criteria for panic disorder:

1. Recurrent unexpected panic attacks. A panic attack is an abrupt surge of intense fear or intense discomfort that reaches a peak within minutes, and during which time-four (or more) of the following symptoms occur:
    - Palpitations, pounding heart, or accelerated heart rate
    - Sweating
    - Trembling or shaking
    - Sensations of shortness of breath or smothering
    - Feeling of choking
    - Chest pain or discomfort
    - Nausea or abdominal distress
    - Feeling dizzy, unsteady, light-headed, or faint
    - Chills or heat sensations
    - Paraesthesias (numbness or tingling sensations)
    - Derealization (feelings of unreality) or depersonalization (being detached from oneself)
    - Fear of losing control or "going crazy"
    - Fear of dying
2. One of the following must be present for at least 1 month:
    - Persistent concern or worry about additional panic attacks or their consequences (e.g., losing control, having a heart attack, "going crazy").
    - A significant maladaptive change in behavior related to the attacks (e.g., behaviors designed to avoid having panic attacks, such as avoidance of exercise or unfamiliar situations).
3. The above symptoms are not attributable to other psychiatric / medical disorder or the use of a substance.

Treatment

Patients show good improvement with treatment.

Pharmacotherapy- Alprazolam and Paroxetine are the two drugs approved by US food and drug administration for treatment of panic disorder. SSRIs and Clomipramine are preferred drugs followed by Venlafaxine and Buspirone. Alprazolam should be prescribed with caution because of its high abuse potential. It should be used briefly. Clonazepam can also be used for a short period. Imipramine also shows some improvement.

Psychotherapy- Cognitive behavior therapy is the mainstay of treatment in panic disorder along with pharmacotherapy.

SPECIFIC PHOBIA

Mrs. P, a 45 year old housewife was once bitten by a dog while she was coming back from the market. After that she started becoming scared of dogs. She used to avoid going from roads where she knew dogs would be or avoid meeting relatives who had dogs. Even when dogs would pass by, she would experience breathlessness, palpitations, and even had fainted once. On hearing dogs bark, she would usually get startled to the extent of becoming breathless. She avoided looking at dog photos and movies as well. She was then taken to a psychiatrist who started her on paroxetine tablet and taught her the technique of systematic desensitization. She gradually improved and can tolerate looking at or being near dogs, but still cannot touch one.

Specific phobia refers to fear of a specific object or situation. There is intense fear about the object or the situation even amounting to a panic attack. This fear leads to avoidance behavior. Specific phobia is one of the most common psychiatric disorders, but rarely presents to a psychiatrist since most people are able to avoid their phobic object/situation.

Etiology

1) Genetic – Specific phobia runs in families. The blood, injection, injury type of phobia is particularly heritable.
2) Psychoanalytic factors – It is believed to be fixed at phallic stage, when the child is trying to overcome the oedipal complex. Instead of overcoming it, it gets displaced to another object (animal, object), with him subsequently developing phobia.
3) Behavioral theories – phobias involve both: an element of classical conditioning (pairing of anxiety experienced after dog bite with the dog); and operant conditioning (relief in anxiety after avoiding dogs).

Clinical Features

A person with specific phobia experiences intense anxiety, even amounting to panic attacks. There is avoidance behavior seen in which anxiety provoking situations is actively avoided by the person and compensatory behavior develops. E. g. A person with fear of flying will try to travel by road or rail.

Broadly, there are **five** types of specific phobias:

1. *Natural/Environment Type*: e.g. a fear of thunder and lightning (astraphobia)
2. *Injury Type*: e.g. a fear of the dentist (dentophobia), or injections (trypanophobia)
3. *Animal Type:* e.g. dogs (cynophobia), snakes (ophidiophobia)
4. *Situational Type:* e.g. washing (ablutophobia) and enclosed spaces (claustrophobia)
5. *Others:* e.g. choking, vomiting etc.

The diagnostic criteria are as follows (DSM 5):

- The person exhibits excessive or unreasonable, persistent and intense fear triggered by a specific object or situation.
- The fear reaction must be out of proportion to the actual danger and appears almost instantaneously when presented with the object or situation.
- The sufferer goes out of her way to avoid the object or situation, or endures it with extreme distress.
- The phobia significantly impacts the sufferer's school, work, or personal life.
- In children and adults, the duration of symptoms must last for at least six months.
- Many anxiety disorders have similar symptoms. Therefore, your therapist must rule out other disorders before diagnosing a specific phobia

Treatment

Pharmacotherapy remains more or less the same as in panic disorder. SSRIs are the preferred medications.

The mainstay of treatment in phobia is psychotherapy.

1. Behavior therapy- in the form of a) Systematic desensitization, b) Implosion, 3) Flooding.
2. Insight oriented psychotherapy
3. Virtual therapy
4. Supportive psychotherapy
5. Hypnosis

SOCIAL PHOBIA/ SOCIAL ANXIETY DISORDER

Mr. B was a college student. He came to psychiatric outpatient clinic with complaints of fear of appearing for job interviews. He gave a history of being shy since childhood. In school he would never volunteer to answer questions in front of the class. As he entered college many of the boys got girlfriends, but he would feel extremely shy to approach a girl. He would be afraid that girls would laugh at him. He found it nearly impossible to participate in a seminar where he had to face the entire class and make a presentation which was to be evaluated by the teachers. He was good in studies. After college education he was looking for a job. He passed all the written tests. However when he went for a job interview he could not face the interview panel, would get extremely nervous, would develop dryness of mouth, palpitations, sweating and would not be able to answer any questions. He failed in a few interviews and then decided to seek help.

This is a classic case of social anxiety disorder. This involves fear of social situations where scrutiny or evaluation is possible. There is fear of facing strangers. It becomes apparent mostly in teen age.

Etiology

Genetic

First degree relatives of persons with social anxiety disorder are about three times more likely to be affected with social anxiety disorder than normal individuals.

Neurotransmitters

β–adrenergic receptor antagonists like propranolol improves performance anxiety e. g. In public speaking, hence adrenergic hypothesis of specific phobia has been proposed. Decreased dopaminergic activity has also been shown in specific anxiety disorder.

Psychological

Behavioral inhibition is the characteristic trait in social anxiety disorder. Children who show this trait tend to develop shyness as they grow up and have parents with panic disorder.

Clinical Features

Social anxiety disorder is characterized by a fear of being scrutinized, evaluated and examined. It includes fear of meeting strangers. The core feature is fear of *'being embarrassed'*. These patients may have fear in performing specific activities such as eating in public or public speaking.

DSM -5 has proposed the following criteria for the diagnosis of Social phobia:

- A persistent fear of one or more social or performance situations in which the person is exposed to unfamiliar people or to possible scrutiny by others. The individual fears that he or she will act in a way (or show anxiety symptoms) that will be embarrassing and humiliating.
- Exposure to the feared situation almost invariably provokes anxiety, which may take the form of a situationally bound or situationally pre-disposed Panic Attack.
- The person recognizes that this fear is unreasonable or excessive.
- The feared situations are avoided or else are endured with intense anxiety and distress.
- The avoidance, anxious anticipation, or distress in the feared social or performance situation(s) interferes significantly with the person's normal routine, occupational (academic) functioning, or social activities or relationships, or there is marked distress about having the phobia.
- In individuals under age 18 years, the duration is at least 6 months.

- The fear or avoidance is not due to direct physiological effects of a substance (e.g., drugs, medications) or a general medical condition not better accounted for by another mental disorder.

Treatment

Pharmacotherapy: Preferred medications are SSRIs, Venlafaxine, buspirone. Benzodiazepines may be given for a short duration. β –adrenergic receptor antagonists like propranolol are commonly prescribed to deal with performance anxiety.

Psychotherapy

1. Cognitive behavior therapy- cognitive training
2. Systematic desensitization.

AGORAPHOBIA

Mr. X, a 32 year old man, visited a hospital claiming to have sudden shortness of breath and feeling that he was dying, whenever he went shopping, since the last few months. These attacks typically lasted for 15-20 minutes and subsided on their own. All his routine investigations came back normal. After a few of these attacks, he stopped venturing out of his house and would often do so only if he had someone accompanying him. And in spite of that he experienced intense anxiety with restlessness. He avoided going to crowded places, movie theatres, malls, etc. He was diagnosed as Agoraphobia and was started on Paroxetine with progressive deep muscle relaxation and gradually improved.

Agoraphobia is a condition characterized by marked fear or anxiety about actual or anticipated exposure of public spaces. The term *agora* in Greek means market and was used to denote open public spaces. Patients typically experience anxiety in various scenarios such as public transportation, being in open spaces, being in closed spaces, standing in line or crowd, being alone outside home. It is any place from which person finds escape unlikely. The person typically avoids these situations and develops compensatory thoughts or behaviors if they know they will be exposed to it.

Etiology

Agoraphobia typically develops secondary to panic attacks when patients experience panic attacks in these situations and then avoids them (similar to the case). Sometimes they just think that they may experience panic attacks if they leave the comfort of their homes and hence avoid venturing outside. Similar to other psychiatric disorders, a combination of genetic and environmental factors are responsible for it. It could also happen secondary to substance use such as alcohol and benzodiazepines.

Epidemiology

Agoraphobia occurs about twice as commonly among women as it does in men. The gender difference may be attributable to several factors: sociocultural traditions that encourage, or permit, the greater expression of avoidance coping strategies by women (including dependent and helpless behaviors), women perhaps being more likely to seek help and therefore be diagnosed, and men being more likely to abuse alcohol in reaction to anxiety and be diagnosed as an alcoholic. About 1/3 of this population with panic disorder have comorbid agoraphobia. It is uncommon to have agoraphobia without panic attacks, with only 0.17% of people with agoraphobia not presenting panic disorders as well.

Clinical Features

There is marked anxiety or fear about the following situations:

- Public transportation
- Being in open spaces: marketplace, bridges, etc.
- Being in closed spaces: shops, theatres etc.
- Standing in line or being in a crowd
- Standing outside of the home alone

The individual avoids these places because escape from these places seems impossible, or they feel they will experience another panic attacks, if they have it secondary to panic attacks. They may be actively avoided or may require a companion. Symptoms typically must be present for 6 months. Certain medical disorders (mentioned earlier) can also cause similar symptoms, and hence must be excluded. Agoraphobia can still be present if these symptoms are in excess. Other psychiatric disorders such as depression, other anxiety disorders, paranoid personality disorder, avoidant personality disorder and schizophrenia may mimic agoraphobia and must be ruled out.

Management

When agoraphobia occurs with panic disorder, treatment of the underlying panic disorder helps in improving the condition. A combination of pharmacotherapy and psychotherapy is used.

Pharmacotherapy

i. Benzodiazepines: Lorazepam, Alprazolam and Clonazepam are the preferred drugs. They have rapid onset of action and are well tolerated.

ii. Selective Serotonin Reuptake Inhibitors (SSRIs): they are given in the same dose range as given for depression. They have added advantage of reducing further relapses and better side effect profile.

iii. Serotonin Norepinephrine Reuptake Inhibitors (SNRIs)

iv. Tricyclic Antidepressants (TCAs): these are superior to SSRIs in managing anxiety, but are usually 2nd line drugs due to their side effect profile.

Psychotherapy

i. Behavior therapy: Systematic desensitization, progressive relaxation, yoga, flooding etc.

ii. Supportive Psychotherapy: developing a therapeutic alliance and to promote adaptive coping.

iii. Insight-oriented Psychotherapy: this targets development of insight in to the conflicts.

iv. Cognitive Behavioral therapy

v. Virtual therapy: via computer programs, people learn to see themselves as avatars, which are placed in open and crowded places and gradually their anxiety is relieved.

GENERALIZED ANXIETY DISORDER

Mrs. V, was complaining of increased and excessive worrying over trivial issues: whether her children would reach school in time, whether they would come back home in time. She found it difficult to concentrate on her day to day work and would frequently make mistakes in her work. She would feel exhausted during the day and would find it difficult to fall asleep. Whenever she would have some work the next day, she would spend the previous day constantly worrying about it, and eventually would fail at it. This went on for 6-8 months and started getting depressed and staying aloof. She started being distant from her husband and children and was eventually brought to a psychiatrist.

Generalized anxiety disorder (GAD)in today's time has become more of a diagnosis of exclusion. These patients tend to have anxiety and 'worry' about everything, defined as excessive anxiety and worry about several events or activities for most days during a 6 month period. It is prevalent in 38% of the population, with M:F ratio of 1:2. Overall representation of GAD among various anxiety disorders.

Etiological Factors

- Neurochemical: dysfunction in glutamate/ GABA system, norepinephrine and cholecystokinin systems have been implicated
- Neuroanatomical: hyperactive amygdala with dysfunction in prefrontal cortex and hippocampus is suggested
- Physiological: autonomic hyperactivity and inflexibility
- Psychological: conflict between id and ego

Clinical Features

DSM 5 has the following criteria for diagnosis of GAD:

A. Excessive anxiety and worry (apprehensive expectation), occurring more days than not for at least 6 months, about a number of events or activities (such as work or school performance).

B. The individual finds it difficult to control the worry.

C. The anxiety and worry are associated with three (or more) of the following six symptoms (with at least some symptoms having been present for more days than not for the past 6 months);

   Note: Only one item is required in children.

   1. Restlessness or feeling keyed up or on edge.
   2. Being easily fatigued.
   3. Difficulty concentrating or mind going blank.
   4. Irritability.
   5. Muscle tension.
   6. Sleep disturbance (difficulty falling or staying asleep, or restless, unsatisfying sleep)

D. The anxiety, worry, or physical symptoms cause clinically significant distress or impairment in social, occupational, or other important areas of functioning.

E. The disturbance is not attributable to the physiological effects of a substance (e.g., a drug of abuse, a medication) or another medical condition (e.g., hyperthyroidism).

F. The disturbance is not better explained by another mental disorder

Management

Management strategies are same as those for other anxiety disorders. CBT and worry behavior prevention works best in GAD. Recent therapies best on mindfulness such as acceptance and commitment therapy are also implicated in GAD.

Non-pharmacological treatment modalities in GAD:

1. CBT
2. Relaxation therapies
3. Meditation
4. Exposure therapy
5. Worry behavior prevention
6. Acceptance and commitment therapy
7. Biofeedback

OTHER ANXIETY DISORDERS

1. **Anxiety disorder attributable to another medical condition**

   Many medical conditions are associated with anxiety symptoms. These disorders usually have symptoms similar to panic attacks and rarely manifest with social phobia or specific phobia. They improve when the medical condition improves and rarely require psychiatric management. Low dose benzodiazepines such as clonazepam or alprazolam can be used as symptomatic treatment. The following is a list of disorders associated with anxiety:

   1. Cardiovascular disorders, cardiac arrhythmias, anemia
   2. Endocrine disorders: Diabetes, thyroid disorders, adrenal dysfunction, pituitary dysfunction, parathyroid disorder.
   3. Respiratory disorders: chronic obstructive pulmonary disease (COPD) and asthma
   4. Substance/drug use
   5. Neurological disorders: epilepsy, migraine, encephalitis, MS, cerebrovascular disease
   6. Tumors: CNS neoplasms, carcinoid
   7. Inflammatory conditions: SLE, RA, polyarteritis nodosa
   8. Heavy metal toxicity
   9. Hypoglycemia, uremia, febrile illness

2. **Substance - induced anxiety disorder**

   It is seen secondary to chronic substance use. Anxiety symptoms are a part and parcel of intoxication and withdrawal syndromes related to several substances. The presentation may be complex and vary with type of substance use. Cognitive symptoms are predominant in such syndromes. Usually the anxiety symptoms abate with abstinence from the substance, unless permanent brain damage is present. Treatment is directed towards maintaining abstinence and managing the substance use disorder. If the symptoms are present in excess, use of benzodiazepines or SSRIs may be indicated. Substances most commonly implicated in anxiety are: alcohol, nicotine, cocaine and other stimulants, LSD, MDMA, caffeine, benzodiazepines and cannabis.

3. **Mixed Anxiety - Depressive Disorder**

   This condition is diagnosed when symptoms of both anxiety and depressive disorder are present, but criteria is not met for any one of them. Etiologically, dysfunction in HPA axis and serotonergic and noradrenergic systems is suggested. The course is usually complicated and patients experience symptoms of both on a daily basis. Management strategies include symptomatic management and course of drugs like SSRIs, SNRIs and TCAs can be tried.

MANAGEMENT STRATEGIES FOR ANXIETY DISORDERS

A variety of management strategies are available for anxiety disorders. In most cases, a combination of pharmacotherapy and psychotherapy is used in treatment. The treatment is tailored to the patient's complaints, history and examination findings. It is always advisable to take the patient into confidence and plan treatment deciding the goals of treatment agreed upon both by the patient and the therapist. Typically, treatment takes about 3-6 months for first episode, but may require a longer duration of treatment, especially in resistant cases and with multiple comorbidities. Patient should always be told about the probable duration of the treatment, expected improvement and posible side effects to watch for. This is especially important in anxiety disorders as patient feels more in control and is prepared for side effects and effects, and doesn't get anxious if anything untoward happens. The following tables outline the pharmacological and non-pharmacological therapies used in management of anxiety disorders.

A. PHARMACOLOGICAL STRATEGIES (Table 16.1)

Other drugs: these are not first line drugs, but can be used if above mentioned drugs fail.

- Mirtazapine
- Buspirone
- Bupropion
- Trazodone
- Vilazodone
- Vortioxetine
- β blockers (used in performance anxiety)
- Monoamine oxidase inhibitors (MAOI)
- Low dose antipsychotics

Table 16.1: Commonly used medications for anxiety disorders (Doses are in mg/day)

Class of drug	Common examples	Used in	Side effects
Selective Serotonin Reuptake Inhibitor (SSRI)	Fluoxetine (20–60 mg) Paroxetine (20–60 mg) Escitalopram (5–20 mg) Sertraline (50–200 mg) Fluvoxamine (100–200 mg; up to 300 mg for social anxiety disorder)	All anxiety disorders	Nausea, Vomiting, diarrhea, dizziness, sexual side-effects, agitation, sedation, bleeding tendencies, hyponatremia,
Serotonin Norepinephrine Reuptake Inhibitors (SNRI)	Venlafaxine (150–225 mg) Desvenlafaxine (50–100 mg) Duloxetine (20–60 mg) Milnacipran (30-200 mg)	All anxiety disorders	Dryness of mouth, Constipation, Hypotension, Sedation, GI distress, hypertension
Tricyclic Anti-depressants (TCA)	Amitriptyline (50–150 mg) Imipramine (50–150 mg) Nortriptyline (50–150 mg) Clomipramine (100–200 mg)	GAD Panic disorder Phobia	Sedation, weight gain, Dryness of mouth, blurred vision, constipation, hypotension, cardiac side effects
α **2** δ **ligands**	Pregabalin (150–600 mg) Gabapentin (300–900 mg)	All anxiety disorders	Sedation, dizziness, fatigue, agitation
Benzodiazepines	Clonazepam (0.5–2 mg) Lorazepam (2–6 mg) Diazepam (5–40 mg) Alprazolam (1–4 mg)	Used for immediate relief in all anxiety disorders	Sedation, disinhibition, ataxia, confusion, abuse potential on long term use.

B. NON- PHARMACOLOGICAL STRATEGIES (Table 16.2)

Table 16.2

Therapy	Mechanism involved	Remarks
Cognitive Behavior Therapy (CBT)	Targeting cognitive distortions, which will help in correcting faulty behavior.	Works well with comorbid depression. GAD may not respond to CBT due to metacognitions.
Systematic desensitization	Behavioral technique involving formulating a hierarchy of anxiety provoking situations and conditioning them with relaxation (from least anxiety provoking to most anxiety provoking)	Used most commonly in phobias. Has been shown to be beneficial in OCD as well.
Flooding	Involves exposure to anxiety providing situation directly without any intermittent systematic steps.	Used in phobias. Can be problematic if anxiety is severe
Progressive Muscle Relaxation	Progressively squeezing and relaxing groups of muscles	Patient has to be trained and taught the technique. Easy to use anywhere.
Other relaxation techniques	Body scanning, mental imagery, deep breathing, journaling, yoga etc.	
Mindfulness & Mentalization based therapy	Works on here and now and 'being in the present'	Techniques include: thought diffusion, self as context, acceptance and willingness
Biofeedback	Body parameters such as heart rate, blood pressure can be brought under voluntary control, leading to relaxation	Requires specialized equipment
Group therapy	Consists of a planned therapy with people diagnosed with a similar disorder, wherein they share their thoughts and feelings	Not commonly used in anxiety disorders. Self-help groups may help in some cases

BIBLIOGRAPHY

1. Kaplan HI, Sadock BJ, Grebb JA. Kaplan and Sadock's synopsis of psychiatry: Behavioral sciences, clinical psychiatry. Williams & Wilkins Co; 1994.
2. Gelder MG, Mayou R, Cowen P. Shorter Oxford textbook of psychiatry. Oxford: Oxford University Press; 2006 Jun 1.
3. Ahuja N, Ahuja S. A short textbook of psychiatry. New Delhi: Jaypee brothers; 2006 Jul 30.
4. American Psychiatric Association. Diagnostic and statistical manual of mental disorders (DSM-5®). American Psychiatric Pub; 2013 May 22.

Obsessive Compulsive and Related Disorders

17

Karishma Rupani • Avinash De Sousa

Obsessive–compulsive disorder (OCD) is a syndrome comprising a relatively diverse group of symptoms that include intrusive thoughts, rituals, preoccupations, and compulsions. OCD was included under the wide umbrella of Anxiety Disorders, until the DSMV; in which they constitute a new chapter. This is because OCD includes a whole gamete of heterogeneous symptom clusters which are diverse in phenomenological and psychobiological features compared to Anxiety Disorder in general and are now called Obsessive-Compulsive and Related Disorders (OCDRS); while the ICD 11 calls it a little different as Obsessive-Compulsive or Related Disorder

Now OCDRs constitute a new chapter in the DSM-5. This grouping of disorders includes obsessive-compulsive disorder (OCD), Body Dysmorphic Disorder (BDD), Hoarding Disorder (HD), trichotillomania (TTM) (hair-pulling disorder), and excoriation (skin-picking) disorder.

The DSM-5 and ICD 11 revision of introducing OCRDs emphasizes the importance of the diagnostic validity and clinical utility of these varied symptom clusters and serves the aim of improving the recognition and treatment of these underdiagnosed conditions.

OBSESSIVE COMPULSIVE DISORDER

Definition

OCD is characterized by the presence of obsessions and/or compulsions. Obsessions are intrusive and unwanted repetitive thoughts, urges, or impulses that often lead to a marked increase in anxiety or distress. Compulsions are repeated behaviors or mental acts that are done in response to obsessions, or in a rigid rule-bound way. Some patients may have only obsessions or only compulsions, but in most cases both obsessions and compulsions are present.

Specifically, a compulsion is a conscious, standardized, recurrent behavior, such as counting, checking or avoiding.

These recurrent obsessions or compulsions cause severe distress to the person. The obsessions or compulsions are time-consuming and interfere significantly with the person's normal routine, occupational functioning, usual social activities, or relationships. A patient with OCD may have an obsession, a compulsion or both.

Comparative Nosology

DSM-III provided operational criteria for OCD, defining obsessions and compulsions along the lines of the definition above. DSM-IV introduced the notion that compulsions can be mental acts. DSM V, introduced OCDR with an insight specifier.

The ICD 10 had a distinct section on Obsessive Compulsive Disorders, however Hair pulling and Skin excoriation were included in 'Habit and Impulse Control Disorders'. In the ICD 11 Obsessive-compulsive or related disorder. However the ICD 11 uses the term Body-focused repetitive behavior disorders for hair pulling and skin picking.

Another entity termed Olfactory Reference Syndrome (conviction about emitting a foul body odor) found its way under the umbrella of OCRDs in both DSM 5 and ICD 11. Its predecessor the DSM-IV mentioned such a condition under "delusional disorder, somatic type",

A. EPIDEMIOLOGY

The prevalence of OCD in India is 3.3%, with no gender difference in prevalence (males = 3.5%, females = 3.2%). But among adolescents, boys are more commonly affected than girls. The mean age of onset is about 19 years. Approximately one-quarter of cases have onset by age 10, with early onset more common in males. In other cases OCD may have a later onset. Onset after 30 is rare. *The* ***following Table gives the Obsessive–compulsive disorder – symptom profile in India.***

Obsessions	**%**
Contamination	18.8
Harming others	53.3
Symmetry	13.9
Hoarding	27.3

Compulsions	**%**
Cleaning	20.6
Checking	33.9
Symmetry	25.5
Hoarding	33.3
Mental acts	57.6

B. ETIOLOGY

GENETIC FACTORS

Twin studies

Twin studies and family studies have examined rates of concordant monozygotic twins versus discordant twins with OCD. These show data do support the notion that genetic factors are implicated in the etiology. However, as the concordance rate even in monozygotic twins is less than 100%, hence it is clear that environment also plays a role in the development of OCD. A review of twin studies reported heritability estimates of OCD symptoms ranging from 27% to 47%. However Child-onset cases have an even greater genetic loading 45–65%.

Pedigree analysis

Another approach to examining the role of genetics in OCD has been to investigate the rate of OCD in family members. OCD proband studies done show the rate of OCD in the relatives of OCD patients was about two times higher than in control samples, and rates in relatives of children and adolescent with OCD showed a tenfold increase.

Linkage studies

An attempt to identify chromosomal regions where genetic markers co-segregate with the disease. The first genome-wide study implicated chromosome 9p24. A second study produced evidence supporting chromosomes 3q, 7p, 1q, 15q, and 6q but the only one that has had significant peaks in more than one study is the Glutamate transporter gene (SLC1A1) on the chromosome 9p24 region.

Genome-Wide Association Studies

In the past few years, genome-wide association has been heralded as a powerful means of discovering susceptibility alleles. A meta-analysis (conducted for 20 polymorphisms that were examined in 5 or more datasets) indicated significant association between OCD and serotonin-related polymorphisms (5-HTTLPR and HTR2A) and, in males only, with polymorphisms in the genes involved in catecholamine modulation (COMT and MAOA).

NEUROBIOLOGICAL FACTORS

Neuroanatomical

These studies use two modalities of imaging; one structural and the other functional. Structural changes are seen using Computed Tomography and Magnetic Resonance imaging and functional changes are studied using positron emission tomography (PET), single photon emission computed tomography (SPECT), functional magnetic resonance imaging (fMRI), magnetic resonance spectroscopy (MRS), both have supported the central role of cortical-striatal-thalamic-cortical (CSTC) circuit in the pathophysiology of OCD.

Abnormalities in this circuit, specifically involving orbital frontal cortex (OFC) and Anterior cingulate cortex (ACC), as well as the striatum and medial thalamus. It is postulated that hyperactivity in the lateral-OFC may mediate obsessions while hypo activity in the medial-OFC may be related to the inability to extinguish the recall and this may result in compulsions and the inability to inhibit the compulsions.

Neurochemical Aspects

The hypothesis that OCD involves an abnormality in the serotonin neurotransmitter system has been called the serotonin hypothesis. Several different lines of investigation support this hypothesis: Several different lines of investigation support this hypothesis:

1. Therapeutic response of patients to chronic administration of serotonergic drugs and Serotonin Reuptake Inhibitors.
2. Measurements of central and peripheral neurotransmitter metabolite concentration (5 Hydroxy Indole Acetic Acid)
3. Measurement of serotonin receptor binding using radio ligands (Decreased levels of cerebrospinal 5-hydroxyindoleacetic acid)
4. Serotonin reuptake inhibition, have been correlated with clinical improvement after clomipramine treatment.

PSYCHOLOGICAL AND ENVIRONMENTAL FACTORS

Learning Theory

This is based on the psychological concept of conditioning and has been used to understand the development of obsessions and compulsions. Compulsions, whether mental or observable, usually decrease the anxiety engendered by obsessional thoughts. Thus, if a person is preoccupied with fears of contamination, repetitive hand washing usually decreases the anxiety caused by the obsessions. The compulsion becomes a conditioned response to anxiety. Because of the anxiety reducing aspect of the compulsion, this learned behavior becomes reinforced and eventually fixed.

Psychodynamic Theory

Psychodynamic understanding involves the interpersonal dimensions. Studies show that family members very often accommodate the patient through participation in rituals causing poor family functioning and non-resolution of the illness as this pattern of relatedness could become internalized and be recreated when the patient enters a treatment setting.

Sigmund Freud- OCD was termed *obsessive-compulsive neurosis* and was considered a regression from the oedipal phase (these are embedded in the unconscious) to the anal psychosexual phase of development.

Ambivalence

When patients with OCD feel threatened by anxiety about retaliation for unconscious impulses or by the loss of a significant objects love, they retreat from the oedipal position and regress to an intensely ambivalent emotional stage associated with the anal phase.

This unconscious conflict between passivity and aggression, or obedience and defiance leads to anxiety. The anxiety produced by these conflicts is hypothesized to lead to the formation of obsessions, compulsions and ambivalence (not in all cases) as well as the defences of reaction *formation*, isolation, and undoing.

C. DIAGNOSTIC CRITERIA

DSM-5 Diagnostic Criteria for OCD

Presence of obsessions, compulsions, or both:
Obsessions are defined by (1) and (2):

1. Recurrent and persistent thoughts, urges, or images that are experienced, at some point during the disturbance, as intrusive and unwanted, and that in most individuals cause marked anxiety or distress.
2. The individual attempts to ignore or suppress such thoughts, urges, or images, or to neutralize them with some other thought or action (i.e. by performing a compulsion).

A. *Compulsions as defined by (1) and (2):*

   1. Repetitive behaviors (e.g., hand washing, ordering, checking) or mental acts (e.g., praying, counting, repeating words silently) that the person feels driven to perform in response to an obsession or according to rules that must be applied rigidly.
   2. The behaviors or mental acts are aimed at preventing or reducing distress, or preventing some dreaded event or situation; however, these behaviors or mental acts either are not connected in a realistic way with what they are designed to neutralize or prevent, or are clearly excessive.

   Note: Young children may not be able to articulate the aims of these behaviors or mental acts.

B. The obsessions or compulsions are time-consuming (e.g., take more than 1 hour per day) or cause clinically significant distress or impairment in social, occupational, or other important areas of functioning.

C. The obsessive-compulsive symptoms are not attributable to the direct physiological effects of a substance (e.g., a drug of abuse, a medication) or another medical condition. Etiological substances/ medications include: intoxication with cocaine, amphetamines or other stimulants and exposure to heavy metals. Etiological medical conditions include: Sydenham chorea, medical conditions leading to striatal damage, such as cerebral infarction.

D. The disturbance is not better explained by the symptoms of another mental disorder (e.g., excessive worries, as in generalized anxiety disorder; preoccupation with appearance, as in body dysmorphic disorder; difficulty discarding or parting with possessions, as in hoarding disorder; hair pulling, as in trichotillomania [hair-pulling disorder]; skin picking, as in excoriation [skinpicking] disorder; stereotypnes, as in stereotypic movement disorder; ritualized eating behavior, as in an eating disorder; preoccupation with having an illness, as in illness anxiety disorder; sexual urges or fantasies, as in a paraphilic disorder; impulses, as in disruptive behavior disorders; guilty ruminations, as in major depressive disorder; thought insertion or delusional as in a psychotic disorder; or repetitive patterns of behavior, as in autism spectrum disorder.)

Specify **if:**

With good or fair insight: The individual recognizes that obsessive-compulsive disorder beliefs are definitely or probably not true or that they may not be true.

With poor insight: The individual thinks obsessive-compulsive disorder beliefs are probably true.

With absent insight/delusional: The individual is completely convinced that obsessive compulsive disorder beliefs are true.

Specify **if:**

Tic-related: The individual has a current or past history of a tic disorder.

In children and adolescents: In children with OCD, the aim of compulsions may not be easily articulated. In this age group it is crucial to differentiate normal developmental rituals from OCD and to assess the impact of OCD on developmental outcomes

The ICD 11

The ICD 11 and DSM 5 are at par where diagnosis is concerned, however the ICD 11 uses the term.

While the ICD 10 used the term 'Habit disorders' for recruitment hair pulling, nail biting; the ICD 11 includes the term Body-focused repetitive behaviour disorders for recurrent and habitual actions directed at the integument (e.g. hair-pulling, skin-picking, lip-biting), typically accompanied by unsuccessful attempts to decrease or stop the behavior involved, and which lead to dermatological sequelae (e.g., hairloss, skinlesions, lip abrasions).

One of the striking features of patients with OCD is the degree of intrusiveness of the obsession (image and or thought). This intrusive thought or image cause a sinking feeling of anxious dread that the patient tries to neutralize by the performance of the compulsion. Hence characteristic to this disorder is the compulsion, intended to reduce the anxiety associated with the obsession in not all but most cases. The patient recognizes the compulsion as being irrational and inappropriate that is **ego dystonic**, however yields into the compulsion nonetheless.

Magical Thinking

Inherent in magical thinking is omnipotence of thought. Persons believe that merely by thinking about an event in the external world they can cause the event to occur without intermediate physical actions. This feeling causes them to fear having e.g.; an aggressive thought, because for the patient it is as bad as having committed an aggressive act.

The DSM-5 self-rating questions assess the time occupied by symptoms, distress caused by the symptoms, difficulty in controlling the symptoms, avoidance caused by the symptoms, and interference associated with the symptoms. The Yale-Brown Obsessive-Compulsive Scale (Y-BOCS) is a clinician-rated instrument that assesses similar items, and that is commonly used as a primary outcome measure in clinical trials.

Case Vignette

Master X, a 17 year old child was brought with the complaints of irritability, sadness of mood and declining academic performance since a year and a half. On questioning, he mentioned that he was unable to complete homework, which was not like him. He said that he was not getting enough time for academics. On probing he reluctantly said that most of his time would squander because he needed to wash his hands 3 times before and after every meal, without which he claimed to feel dirty and turn around check whether or not he had dropped his belongings on the way while walking. He said that these activities consumed most of his time. His acts embarrassed him and so on several occasions he tried not to wash or check, because he realized the futility and of his behavior. But skipping the ritual caused tremendous anxiety, which was temporarily decreased by washing and checking, only to resurface again.

Co-Morbidities

Most frequently, individuals with OCD met criteria for depressive episodes, in 36–41%. Another DSM-5 also includes a tic-related specifier for OCD, as many patients with OCD have current or past history of tics. OCD with tics is more commonly seen in males, has an earlier age of onset. Comorbid anxiety disorders are also common in OCD. It is notable that substance use disorders are more common in community studies than in clinical studies of OCD.

Course and Prognosis

The course of OCD is generally chronic, and in the absence of intervention symptoms may persist for decades. Nevertheless, recent data emphasize that long-term outcomes can be positive. Thus patients should be encouraged to remain hopeful, and to try a range of different evidence based interventions over time.

Treatment

Pharmacotherapy

The "serotonin hypothesis" of OCD influenced a good deal of subsequent research on the said neurotransmitter for both OCD and OCRDs. In keeping with this, early studies reported that patients with OCD responded to Clomipramine, a relatively serotonergic tricyclic antidepressant. Thereafter randomized controlled trials showed that clomipramine was efficacious in both children/adolescents and adults with OCD, and that clomipramine was more effective than the relatively noradrenergic tricyclic antidepressant. The subsequent introduction of the SSRIs was important in that these provided a set of agents that was not only efficacious but also well tolerated The subsequent introduction of the SSRIs was important in that these provided a set of agents that was not only efficacious clomipramine, a relatively serotonergic tricyclic antidepressant, however head-to-head comparisons of clomipramine and SSRIs, there is equal efficacy,

Dose–response and time- response curve is steeper than that required for treating depression as meta-analysis indicates that higher doses of SRIs and at least 12 weeks are associated with better outcomes in OCD. Clinical guidelines therefore suggest increasing the dosage of SRIs over time in OCD to quite high ranges (e.g., escitalopram 30 mg, fluoxetine 80 mg, sertraline 200 mg). A general rule of thumb is that the dose required to obtain response should be continued for at least 1 to 2 years. Patients who fail to respond to one SRI may respond to another.

Augmenting Strategies

Evidence base comprising studies of low-dose dopamine receptor blockers in adult OCD is available. Some studies have indicated that these are particularly useful in patients with tics. Perhaps most promising are small studies which have indicated that certain glutamatergic agents, such as memantine, riluzole, ketamine, lamotrigine, and topiramate. Sometimes low doses of clomipramine are used to augment SSRIs, but careful electrocardiographic monitoring is required and vigilance to anticipate serotonin syndrome. D-cycloserine is a partial glutamatergic agonist that has been used to augment psychotherapy in OCD and anxiety disorders, but efficacy data in OCD are currently inconsistent.

Psychotherapy

Empirical research on the psychotherapy of OCD has emerged from behavioral and cognitive perspectives. In recent years, such approaches have been supplemented by the use of techniques from mindfulness. Exposure and response therapy is the gold standard as of now. This consists of making a hierarchy of gradual exposure to more distressing cues. The essential principle is to minimize avoidance of distressing cues, and instead to encourage in vivo exposure to feared situations. Systematic desensitization with imaginal exposure to feared consequences coupled with relaxation strategies. Early on, obsessive-compulsive symptoms were viewed from a psychodynamic perspective. However, there is no rigorous evidence that a psychodynamic approach is useful in the treatment of OCD.

The role of the family

Family sessions are an important component of psychotherapy, particularly in younger patients; families are likely to benefit from a better understanding of OCD, and of the principles of exposure and response prevention.

Somatic Therapies

Targeted neurosurgical lesions to CSTC tracts have been shown efficacious in a proportion of highly treatment-refractory patients. Initial work focused on stereotactic neurosurgical lesions, with subsequent work using radio surgical techniques. Deep brain stimulation (DBS)-nonablative surgical techniques involving indwelling electrodes in various basal ganglia nuclei are under investigation to treat both OCD and Tourette's disorder. DBS is performed using MRI-guided stereotactic techniques in which electrodes are implanted in the brain.

BODY DYSMORPHIC DISORDER

Definition

BDD is characterized by persistent preoccupations about one or more perceived defects or flaws in one's appearance. The defects or flaws appear slight or are not observable to others. In response to their appearance concerns, individuals with BDD demonstrate a range of mental acts or behaviors, including comparing themselves with others, checking in the mirror, or camouflaging their perceived flaws.

Epidemiology

The point prevalence estimates range from 1.7 to 2.4 percent; furthermore, studies have found high rates of BDD in cosmetic in dermatology clinics. Mean age of onset is in adolescence, and as in the case of OCD, community studies indicate a higher prevalence of females with BDD, while clinical reports indicate a roughly even male:female ratio.

Etiology

Family and twin data provide evidence for genetic susceptibility, however data on specific genetic variants underlying susceptibility to BDD is not known as of now. Functional brain imaging studies in BDD have shown involvement of the CSTC circuits that appear to play a role in OCD and neurocircuitry involved in visual processing. neuropsychological studies have suggested deficits in executive functioning and in visual processing. While childhood adversity, including history of teasing, has been associated with BDD without specificity.

Diagnosis and Clinical Features

The DSM-5 diagnostic criteria for BDD address the presence of appearance preoccupations, repetitive behaviors or mental acts in response to these preoccupations, the consequent distress and impairment, avoidance could range from minor social avoidance to being housebound and ideas of reference are not uncommon amongst them. Symptoms may focus on any area of the body, but they most commonly focus on the face and head, with concerns most often involving the skin, nose shape and size, and repetitive behaviors include comparing body parts with the same areas in others, checking body parts in the mirror or other reflective surfaces, grooming.

Of the various OCRDs, BDD is the one most associated with comorbid depression, with a lifetime rate of 75 percent and 80 percent having experienced suicidal ideation. Patients with BDD have less insight into the truth of their beliefs than those with OCD, and a first DSM-5 specifier for BDD addresses level of insight.

Assessment - The Yale-Brown Obsessive-Compulsive Scale (Y-BOCS) has been adapted for use in BDD, and the Brown Assessment of Beliefs Scale can be used to assess insight.

Only a quarter of BDD patients have fair or good insight, and around one-third have absent insight. The second specifier called muscle dysmorphia, in which patients focus on whether their body build is too small or not sufficiently muscular.

Course and Prognosis

The course of BDD is generally chronic, and in the absence of intervention symptoms may persist for decades.

Treatment

Clomipramine is more effective than the other TCAs, and data from randomized controlled trials indicate that SSRIs are efficacious in the treatment of BDD, including delusional BDD. Dopamine receptor blockers are not positive, but in clinical practice, addition of antipsychotics such as aripiprazole, and monotherapy with irreversible monoamine oxidase inhibitors are employed.

Psychotherapy

Cognitive restructuring and interventions to target visual processing abnormalities are employed. A combination of psycho and pharmacotherapy can be used judiciously.

HOARDING DISORDER (HD)

Definition

HD is characterized by the persistent and profound difficulty discarding with or parting from one's possessions. This in turn leads to significant congestion and clutter, and to substantive distress or impairment, so differentiating normal collecting from the clinical disorder.

Epidemiology

Point prevalence is 1.5 percent, male: female ratio is about 1. Unlike in most OCRDs, prevalence of hoarding increases with age. Hoarding symptoms often begin in childhood and adolescence, with diagnostic criteria met only in the 30s.

Etiology

Impairment in various neuropsychological domains including spatial planning, working memory, response inhibition, and set-shifting. Structural and functional brain imaging studies suggest the involvement of the ventromedial prefrontal and medial temporal regions in hoarding. A range of objects may be hoarded, but they are usually everyday items (e.g., newspapers, books, clothing), and the resulting clutter is usually highly disorganized.

Diagnosis and Clinical Features

DSM-5 diagnostic criteria for HD emphasize that individuals have difficulty discarding or parting with possessions, regardless of their actual value. This difficulty is due to a perceived need to save the items and to distress associated with discarding them, and results in congestion and clutter so that the use of living areas for their intended use is severely compromised. DSM-5 provides two specifiers for HD. Excessive acquisition is of items that are not needed or for which there is no available space and insight can be specified as good or fair, poor, or absent/delusional.

Treatment

Pharmacotherapy

Uncontrolled data indicate venlafaxine as efficacious and some case reports have noted a response to glutamate modulators.

Psychotherapy

Components include psychoeducation and goal setting, organization skills training, practice with resisting acquisition, and cognitive restructuring.

TRICHOTILLOMANIA (HAIR-PULLING DISORDER)

Definition

Trichotillomania (TTM) is characterized by pulling out of one's hair. This is not done for cosmetic reasons, but rather individuals often describe an irresistible urge to pull out their hair.

Epidemiology

1 to 3 percent meeting DSM-5 diagnostic criteria for TTM. Age of onset is typically at menarche, and female: male ratio is about 9:1.

Etiology

Deficits in working memory and visual spatial learning have been implicated. Structural and functional brain imaging studies suggest involvement of CSTC circuits relevant to habit learning and reward processing.

Diagnosis and Clinical Features

DSM-5 criteria refer to hair-pulling resulting in noticeable hair loss, repeated attempts to decrease or stop hair-pulling, clinically significant distress or impairment, with the hair-pulling or loss not attributable to another medical condition, nor better explained by the symptoms of another medical disorder. Hair-pulling may be from any area of the body, but is most commonly from scalp, eyebrows, and eyelashes. Hair-pulling may be triggered by states of both hyper arousal (e.g., stress) when the patient is aware of the urge to pull hair and hypo arousal, when the patient is less aware of hair pulling (e.g., boredom).

Associated Features

More than half of patients with TTM have comorbid psychiatric disorders. Depression or an anxiety disorder may be present in about 20–30% of individuals with TTM.

The most common comorbidity include body-focused repetitive behavior disorder (BFRBD) (classified in DSM-5 as Other Specified Obsessive–Compulsive and Related Disorder, and covering a range of symptoms such as nail-biting, lip-chewing, and cheek-biting).

Treatment

The largest positive clinical trial is with N-acetyl cysteine (NAC) (1,200 to 2,400 mg/day) that acts on the glutamatergic system, however it has not shown efficacy in pediatric populations. Trials of SSRIs and of venlafaxine in TTM have not consistently demonstrated efficacy.

Psychotherapy

Habit reversal therapy (HRT) is a set of cognitive behavioral techniques which include awareness training, competing response training (the patient substitutes hair-pulling with an incompatible action) and social support. Awareness training includes elements such as self-monitoring and collecting pulled hair.

EXCORIATION (SKIN-PICKING) DISORDER

Skin picking disorder (SPD) is characterized by the recurrent skin-picking, resulting in skin lesions. Individuals with skin-pulling attempt to decrease or stop skin picking, but are unable to do so and associated clinically significant distress or impairment.

Epidemiology

Prevalence studies show a point prevalence of 1.4 to 5.4 percent. The mean age is 12 years, coinciding with the onset of puberty and is more common in females.

Etiology

Family and twin studies provide evidence for genetic susceptibility with other BFRBDs and with a candidate gene SAPAP3. Brain imaging studies have suggested evidence of motor impulsivity.

Diagnosis and Clinical Features

DSM-5 diagnostic criteria for SPD refer to skin-picking resulting in skin lesions, repeated attempts to decrease or stop skin-picking, clinically significant distress or impairment, with the skin-picking not attributable to another medical disorder. Skin-picking may be from any area of the body, but is most commonly from the face, followed by the hands, fingers, arms, and legs. It has been suggested that there are two major kinds of skin-picking; focused and automatic as seen with TTM. A range of habits associated with the skin-picking can be seen such as stroking or playing with the skin, choosing a particular scab to pick, and mouthing the scab.

SPD should not be diagnosed when skin-picking occurs in response to obsessions about contamination, delusions or tactile hallucinations related to infestation (parasitosis), or may be induced by dopaminergic psychostimulants (e.g., cocaine). Skin picking may also be due to a factitious disorder (dermatitis artefacta).

Pharmacotherapy

There are data that NAC, a nutraceutical that acts on the glutamatergic system, and *low dose dopamine receptor blockers* may also be useful in SPD.

Psychotherapy

Components of Habit reversal training for SPD have included awareness training, competing response, training and self-monitoring.

OLFACTORY REFERENCE SYNDROME

Persistent (> six months), false belief that one emits an offensive odor, which is not perceived by others. There may be degrees of insight i.e. the belief may or may not be of delusional intensity inspite of which it now according to the classificatory system does not qualify for a delusional disorder.

This pre-occupation causes clinically significant distress (depression, anxiety, shame), social and occupational disability, or may be time-consuming.

The most common comorbidity is Major Depressive Disorder (upto 70%) and is treated in accordingly.

OCRD DUE TO ANOTHER MEDICAL DISORDER

This is a new category in DSM-5, to exclude conditions that are due to another medical disorder when OCRD symptoms are etiologically linked to another medical disorder with a temporal relationship

Obsessive-compulsive symptoms have been described in the context of various neurological lesions striatal pathologies post stroke and infection. An apt example of which is Pediatric neuropsychiatric disorders associated with Streptococcus (PANDAS) is a condition thought similar to Sydenham's chorea, in that a Streptococcal infection triggers an autoimmune reaction, resulting in sudden onset of obsessive-compulsive and other symptoms.

SUBSTANCE/MEDICATION-INDUCED OCRD

Skin-picking may be seen in patients with cocaine intoxication. This highlights the role of the dopaminergic system in OCRD.

OTHER SPECIFIED AND UNSPECIFIED OCRDS

DSM-5 notes a range of other specified and unspecified OCRDs, which include obsessional jealousy and cultural variants characterized by repeated concerns about body appearance for e.g. koro, which is characterized by concerns that the penis will recede into the body.

BIBLIOGRAPHY

1. Jaisoorya, *et al.*: Prevalence and correlates of OCD and subthreshold OCD in India Indian Journal of Psychiatry Volume 59, Issue 1, January-March 2017
2. Sadock, B. J., Sadock, V. A., & Ruiz, P. (2017) Kaplan and Sadock's Comprehensive Textbook of Psychiatry. *Obsessive Compulsive and Related Disorders.* (10th ed.). Wolters Kluwer. 1785-1798.
3. Tasman A. (2015). Obsessive–Compulsive and Related Disorders: Obsessive–Compulsive Disorder and Hoarding Disorder. (4th ed.). Wiley Blackwell. 1129-1139.

18 Stress and Trauma Related Disorders

Mansi Somaiya • Alka A. Subramanyam • Henal R. Shah

KEY POINTS

Acute stress disorder:

1. Severe acute stress reaction that occur in the initial month after a trauma
2. Trauma was defined on the basis of "actual or threatened death, serious injury or sexual violation
3. Intrusive symptoms, dissociative symptoms, mood disturbances and avoidance behavior, arousal symptoms
4. Management – psychotherapeutic approach – trauma focussed cognitive behavior therapy, management of anxiety and depression, relaxation, exposure therapy, cognitive therapy
5. Pharmacotherapy – Role of antidepressants, Benzodiazepines and propranolol

Post- traumatic stress disorder:

1. Severe stress reaction that occur within 6 months of the trauma
2. Recurrent intrusive symptoms – distressing memories, dreams, flashbacks, psychological distress with the exposure of internal and external cues , avoidance of stimuli that are associated with traumatic events, negative thoughts and emotional disturbances, disturbance in arousal and reactivity
3. Duration of more than a month is required
4. Management – psychotherapeutic approach – Trauma focused cognitive therapy, exposure therapy, cognitive therapy. EMDR (Eye Movement Desensitization and Reprocessing) technique has also been used.
5. Pharmacotherapy- Role of antidepressants and benzodiazepines

Adjustment disorder:

1. Behavioral and emotional symptoms which develop with a temporal relation with a stressor. It usually occurs within 3 months of the onset of the stressor.
2. It can be associated with:
   A. Depressed mood
   B. With anxiety
   C. With mixed anxiety and depressed mood
   D. With disturbance in conduct
   E. With mixed disturbance of emotions and conduct
3. It usually begins within 3 months of onset of a stressor but resolves within 6 months of termination of stressor.
4. Treatment: Psychotherapy – improvement of symptoms, mechanisms of coping and a support system. Brief psychotherapy, cognitive behavior therapy and interpersonal therapy and support groups.
5. Pharmacotherapy – antidepressants

Table 18.1: Differences between Acute Stress Disorder, Post-traumatic stress disorder, Adjustment disorder and depression

	Acute Stress Disorder	Post-traumatic stress disorder	Adjustment disorder	Depression
Stressor	Present Experiencing /witnessing actual or threatened death/ serious injury or sexual violation	Present Experiencing /witnessing actual or threatened death/ serious injury or sexual violation	Present	May or may not be present
Duration	3 days to 1 month of exposure to trauma	Usually begins within 3 to 6 months of exposure of trauma and lasts beyond a month	Symptoms occur within one month of stressor and do not last beyond 6 months	Can present in the presence or absence of a stressor. Duration of symptoms should be more than 2 weeks.
Symptoms	Intrusive symptoms (dreams/ memories/ thoughts); dissociative reactions, avoidance symptoms, negative thoughts and mood, alteration in arousal states	Intrusive symptoms (dreams/ memories/ thoughts); dissociative reactions, avoidance symptoms, negative thoughts and mood, alteration in arousal states	Emotional or behavioral symptoms in response an identifiable stressor with distress/ dysfunction	Persistent and pervasive sadness/ anhedonia/anergia/ appetite and weight changes/ sleep disturbance/ psychomotor activity changes/depressive cognitions/ decreased attention and concentration/suicidal ideas
Treatment	Trauma focussed Cognitive behavior therapy; medications	Exposure therapy, cognitive therapy, EMDR, pharmacotherapy	Psychotherapy, Antidepressants	Antidepressants, psychotherapy, somatic treatment – ECT

INTRODUCTION:

Most disorders in psychiatry are characterised by the nature of symptoms and the course it follows. However, some disorders in psychiatry are classified on the basis of causative influences which result in the symptomatology. The patients who have experienced or witnessed a life event – either a stressful life event that can threaten life or lead to harm can manifest an acute stress reaction or a significant life event leading to adjustment disorder. A less severe psychosocial stressor can result into an adjustment disorder.

Trauma and stress related disorder includes the disorders where there occurs the exposure to a traumatic or stressful event.

These include the:

1. Reactive attachment disorder
2. Disinhibited social engagement disorder
3. Post- traumatic stress disorder
4. Acute stress disorder
5. Adjustment disorder
6. Other specified trauma and stressor related disorder

The central issue in the two types of disorders is that they are precipitated by a stressor (traumatic or non-traumatic), which is the triggering event rather than a symptom/ phenomenon.

Some Essential Terms which are Required to be Understood:

Stressor- Any circumstance or personal state that threatens or is perceived to threaten one's well-being and thereby taxes one's coping abilities.

Types- Predisposing, Precipitating factor, Perpetuating factor

Predisposing factors- Those risk factors which act for a longer period of time or during an earlier part of life. Vulnerability factor. E.g. Family history of mental illness.

Precipitating factor- Those risk factors which operate immediately before the onset of illness and without which illness would not have had occurred. e.g. Child birth, divorce

Perpetuating factor- Which maintains or aggravates the illness. E.g. Interpersonal conflicts between the couple, alcohol use in spouse.

Case

ABC witnessed an accident a week ago. He can't help being preoccupied about it. He is reminded of the accident, the image of the person injured. The scene of the accident repeatedly plays on his mind. Last night he had a dream about car damaged in an accident. He gets startled when someone calls out to him. He has flashbacks of the event. He avoids going out, even looking at the road from the window. He appears anxious most part of the day. His sleep is disturbed. His friends and family often uplift him however, he remains dazed and his attention is difficult to arose. He decides to seek help. Can you help him?

Acute Stress Disorder

The Key Issues are

1. Severe acute stress reaction that occur in the initial month after a trauma
2. Trauma was defined on the basis of "actual or threatened death, serious injury or sexual violation

Conceptualisation

- Directly experiencing the traumatic event
- Witnessing in person the event[s] as it occurred
- Learning that the event[s](Events must be violent or accidental) occurred to a close family member or a close friend)
- Experiencing repeated or extreme exposure to aversive details of the traumatic event(s) (police officers repeatedly exposed to child abuse)

The presence of nine or more of the following symptoms out of fourteen from any of the categories of intrusion, negative mood, dissociation, avoidance and arousal, beginning or worsening after the traumatic event(s) occurred:

Intrusion Symptoms

- Recurrent, involuntary and intrusive distressing memories of the traumatic events.
- Recurrent distressing dreams in which the content and or effect of the dream are related to the events.
- Dissociative reactions (flashbacks) in which the individual feels or acts as if the traumatic events were recurring.
- Intense or prolonged psychological distress or marked physiological reactions in response to internal or external cues that symbolize or resemble an aspect of the traumatic event(s)

Negative Mood

- Persistent inability to experience positive emotions (e.g., Inability to experience happiness, satisfaction or loving feelings)

Dissociative Symptoms

- An altered sense of reality of one's surroundings or oneself (seeing oneself from another's perspective, being in a daze, time slowing)
- Inability to remember an important aspect of the traumatic event(s) (typically due to dissociative amnesia and not to the other factors such as head injury, alcohol or drugs)

Avoidance Symptoms

- Efforts to avoid distressing memories, thoughts or feelings or closely associated with the traumatic event(s)
- Efforts to avoid external reminders (people, places, conversations, activities, objects, situations) that arouse distressing memories, thoughts or feelings about or closely associated with the traumatic events.

Arousal Symptoms

- Sleep disturbance e.g. Difficulty falling or staying asleep, restless sleep
- Irritable behavior and angry outbursts (with little or no provocation), typically expressed as verbal or physical aggression toward people or objects.
- Hypervigilance.
- Problems with concentration.
- Exaggerated startle response.

Duration of the disturbance (symptoms in Criterion B) is 3 days to 1 month after trauma exposure.

Note: Symptoms typically begin immediately after the trauma, but persistence for at least 3 days and up to a month is needed to meet disorder criteria.

The disturbance causes clinically significant distress or impairment insocial, occupational, or other important areas of functioning.

The disturbance is not attributable to the physiological effects of a substance (e.g., medication or alcohol) or another medical condition (e.g., mild traumatic brain injury) and is not better explained by brief psychotic disorder.

Epidemiology

Prevalence of acute stress disorder varied from 7 to 59%, an average of 19% can be considered. In some studies, using the "subsyndromal" acute stress disorder criteria, prevalence ranging between 10 and 66% with an average of 26% was noted. In an Indian study, after a terror attack in Mumbai, India around 30% of victims who were brought in a public hospital, were observed to have acute stress disorder.

Risk Factors

- History of prior psychiatric disorder
- History of prior traumatic exposures
- Female gender
- Severe trauma
- High levels of neuroticism
- Avoidant coping style

Management

Management of acute stress disorder	
Trauma focussed cognitive behavioral therapy (CBT)	**Medications**
Psychoeducation	Antidepressants
Management of anxiety	Benzodiazepines
Exposure and cognitive restructuring	Propranolol

Trauma focussed cognitive behavioral therapy (CBT) is most extensively studied and can be considered first line treatment for patients with acute stress disorder.

Psychoeducation: It involves discussing the various symptoms, risk factors and management of the acute stress disorder. This enables to normalise the stress response, facilitate the recovery process.

Anxiety management: the goals involve reducing anxiety by various techniques

- Breathing retraining
- Relaxation skills
- Self - talk

Exposure Therapy

This involves the exposure to the event to the patient. The patient is asked to recall the traumatic event in the session. The patient is asked to describe the experience which includes the sensory symptoms, emotional changes and physiological symptoms

In vivo exposure: The patient is exposed to the feared stimuli in a graded manner. Initially, the patient is closely exposed to the minimally feared stimuli/reminders and later exposed to increasingly fearful situations. The patient is exposed to reminders till she/he is able to comfortably handle the feared stimuli.

Re-experiencing allows processing of emotions so that they can be less painful.

Cognitive restructuring: This involves the identifying the thoughts in relation to the traumatic event and triggers, the various thoughts about future negative events, trauma, somatic symptoms, autonomic symptoms and redirecting the thoughts enabling patient to generate alternate adaptive thoughts.

The above therapy has shown efficacy in acute stress disorder and reduces the likelihood of subsequent PTSD in patients with acute stress disorder.

COGNITIVE THERAPY

Only a sole approach in cognitive restructuring has also been used in acute stress disorder and prevention of PTSD on patients.

Pharmacological Approaches

Medications have been used to treat the symptoms of ASD. These include the Selective serotonin reuptake inhibitor (SSRI) and other anti depressants. Response with SSRIs have been noted in may trials. Other antidepressants such as Imipramine has been used with response.

Benzodiazepine are used to reduce anxiety, agitation and sleep disturbance that occurs after the event.

Propranolol– used in reduction of anxiety and autonomic symptoms.

Case

PQR, 16-year-old comes to your clinic along with her mother. Since the last 4 months the mother observed her withdrawn which was unlike her unusual self. Her sleep was disturbed and she began to avoid food. Mother asked her but she kept telling her it's study stress. PQR is unable to study. She gets startled when her father calls out her name. She avoids her father and any other male. She cries often. When you interview her in person, she confides being allegedly sexually abused by her 21-year-old boyfriend. She has flashbacks of "how he forced himself over me" and repeatedly has images and thoughts that come to her mind. She reports she could not have shared this with her mother as she feared what her parents would do. She avoids conversation with everyone. What is happening with PQR and can you help her?

Post-Traumatic Stress Disorder

This disorder dates back from the wartime era. The debilitating causes of war result in emotional, physiological and physical changes were witnessed in war victims. Studies reported 15 to 25% of persons exposed to trauma develop symptoms of post-traumatic stress disorder.

Risk Factors

Multiple factors have been implicated in the development of the disorder. It is linked to genetic, developmental, endocrine, neurobiological, cognitive and environmental factors and the interrelationship which results in symptoms.

Pre-existing Risk Factors

- Younger age
- Female gender
- Past psychiatric history
- Prior trauma/childhood abuse
- Lower socioeconomic status
- Low intelligence

Peritraumatic Risk Factors

- Intensity and frequency of trauma
- Distress and dissociation during trauma

Post Traumatic Risk Factors

- Lack of social support
- Ongoing stress / adverse life events
- Comorbid physical conditions
- Poor coping strategies

Biological Risk Factors

- Stress results in dysregulation of the hypothalamic pituitary adrenal axis
- Reduced levels of cortisol results and increased cortical sensitivity, increase in glucocorticoid receptors

NEUROBIOLOGY

Neuroimaging: Structural

Amygdala – important in the processing of fear and other emotions. Increased amygdala activity, size and function is seen in patients along with hyper responsiveness to a provocative stimulus. Also, a reduced pre-frontal size and function is seen in patients with PTSD. Prefrontal cortex functions in decision making, performance of executive functions such as planning, maintaining attention. Lower hippocampal volume has been reported too. On structural MRI, medial PFC which inhibits the amygdala is dysfunctional resulting in symptoms of fear.

Functional MRI – Symptom provocation studies resulted in higher amygdala response to general threat related stimuli and decrease in frontal regions.

SPECT: Symptom provocation studies: Exposure to audiotape of combat sounds reveals reduced regional blood flow in the caudate and superior frontal cortex and increased activation in the anterior cingulate and medial prefrontal cortex.

PET Scan: Increased blood flow in OFC, limbic regions, anterior cingulate gyrus and amygdala decreased flow in medial PFC.

Genetic Mechanisms

Genetic polymorphisms and epigenetic mechanisms affect gene expression, genes such as the receptor genes NR3C1, CRH type 1 receptor and FKBP5.

Mental Imagery

They are quasi perceptual experience which can be sensory images or abstract thoughts resulting in intrusive memories which results in emotional responses. Imageries can be in any modality e.g. Visual imagery which is linked to stimulation of visual cortex, middle frontal gyrus, ACC, hippocampus, amygdala. Mapping the neural process of imagery enables an understanding of the emotion processing and attention impairment. Hence imagery re- scripting can enable image transformation and reduction in distress due to intrusive memories.

Artificial Intelligence

With technological advancement, from computer or smart phone questionnaire to biometric data by testing sleep, heart rate variation and skin conductance an evaluation of PTSD, understanding the symptoms to severity can be carried out. Very recently, by means of speech analysis carried out by a computer software, the voices of persons with or without PTSD were diagnosed with almost 90% accuracy.

Clinical Features

In the diagnosis of PTSD, the patient presents with exposure to an actual or threatened death, serious injury and sexual violence in one or more of the ways:

- Directly experiencing the trauma.
- Witnessing a person undergoing the traumatic event.
- Learning about the event from a family member or close friend. In actual or threatened death of a family member or friend the event must be violent or accidental.
- Repeated exposure to aversive details of the traumatic event (first responders of collecting human remains, police officers repeated exposure to child abuse)

Additionally, the patient may have

intrusive symptoms associated with the traumatic event beginning after the traumatic events have occurred which includes the recurrent, involuntary and intrusive distressing memories of the traumatic event. In children, repeated play may be observed. Distressing dreams are related to the traumatic event. Dissociative reactions such as flashbacks in which an individual feels or acts as if the traumatic events were recurring. They also present with psychological distress and physiological reactions with cues in relation to the trauma. They may even have dissociative experiences and reactions in which the individual feels or acts as if the traumatic events may recur or are recurring such as flashbacks.

- Avoidance of or efforts to avoid distressing memories, thoughts or feelings about closely associated with the traumatic event.
- Avoidance of efforts / reminders which arouse memories, thoughts and feelings about the events.
- Negative thoughts about the trauma and the event which may present as inability to remember the events due to dissociative amnesia. Persistent and negative beliefs or expectations about oneself, others and the world.
- Persistent negative thoughts about the event.
- Decreased interest in significant activities
- Feelings of detachment or estrangement
- Inability to experience emotions
- There is marked alteration in arousal and reactivity which is associated with the traumatic event. Irritable and angry behavior, reckless behavior, hypervigilance, exaggerated startle response. Additionally, problems in concentration and sleep disturbance.
- The above symptoms lead to socio occupational dysfunction and causes distress. It is important to rule out any physiological effect of substance or medication or medical disorder attributing to the above symptoms.

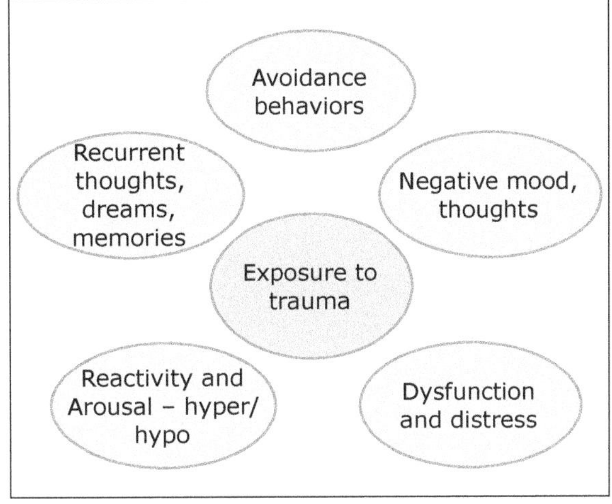

Fig. 18.1: Clinical features - Post-traumatic stress disorder.

Comorbid disorders

PTSD is associated with various psychiatric disorders which includes major depressive disorder, panic disorder and substance use disorder. They may also have sexual complaints and decreased libido leading to sexual dysfunction.

Early Intervention

The early intervention includes psychoeducation, normalization of responses and therapeutic management. It includes brief cognitive behavioral therapy: which is acute stress disorder which includes relaxation, psychoeducation, imaginal and in vivo exposure and cognitive restructuring.

TREATMENT GUIDELINES

Evidence based therapies and pharmacotherapy form the mainstay of treatment. There is evidence in the use of SSRIs selective serotonin reuptake inhibitors.

Psychotherapy

Trauma focussed therapy and stress inoculation therapies have been used in patients with PTSD.

Trauma focussed therapy: Refer to the principles mentioned in Acute stress disorder.

The evidence-based therapies used in PTSD are:

- Exposure therapy
- Cognitive therapy
- Eye movement desensitization and reprocessing

Exposure therapies such as prolonged exposure which involve a revisiting of the traumatic memory through imaginal exposure e.g. Retelling the story of the trauma or written or oral narratives. Cognitive therapies emphasize identifying core beliefs, maladaptive thought patterns and dysfunctional assumptions which are addressed through cognitive restructuring.

EMDR (Eye Movement Desensitization and Reprocessing)

It is a form of psychotherapy to address and process the traumatic life experiences and systematically facilitate adaptive responses. It involves guided lateral eye movements and substitute activities in the patient, so as to process the target picture, emotion, physical symptoms and thoughts. Once the process of desensitization is achieved a positive thought is paired with eye movement. The patient is asked to focus on the body and closure is brought about when the therapist debriefs the client.

Stress inoculation therapy is an important cognitive behavior therapy which focuses on the other symptom of PTSD such as anxiety, avoidance and trauma related cognitions.

Pharmacotherapy

Antidepressants such as SSRIs and Serotonin norepinephrine reuptake inhibitor have been used in patients with PTSD. They have proven efficacy in PTSD. Sertraline and Paroxetine are the only approved by the USFDA for the treatment of PTSD. Additionally, fluoxetine has also shown good results. Tricyclic antidepressants and mirtazapine have been tried and improvement was seen in patients with PTSD.

MANAGEMENT OF PTSD

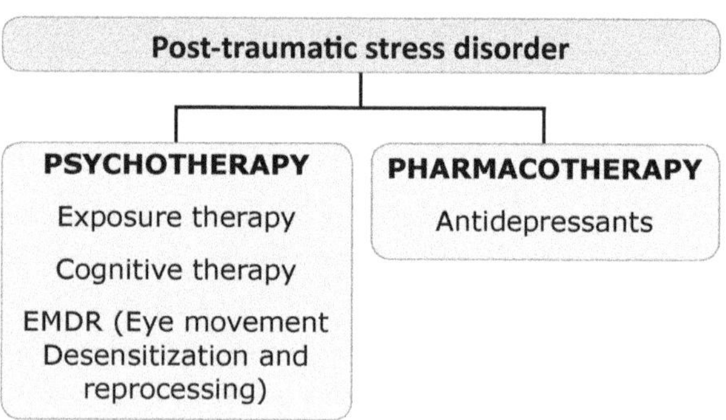

Case

XYZ lost her job recently because of the recession. Additionally, he had to make many changes such as shifting to smaller apartment, cutting down on his expenses. He would send half his salary home to his parents back home. After a few days, he managed to get a job however is earning 40% less then what he was earning. Making these changes, he would feel sad, preoccupied with his future, find it difficult to sleep. His appetite has been the same. He still maintains hope despite his worry. He finds it difficult to concentrate at times at work. He doubts his ability at times, not till the point of worthlessness. Denies suicidal ideas. He comes to you. What is happening to XYZ?

Adjustment Disorders

Before we understand the concept of adjustment disorders it is inevitable to understand the concept of stress. Stress is an etiological factor in adjustment disorder. It is also important to note that a life-threatening event is not required for the diagnosis. The meaning of stress is also affected by aspects such as resilience, support systems, coping mechanisms etc. Hence, a particular life event can serve as a stressor for one and not for the other.

Prevalence of Adjustment Disorder

The prevalence is variable. It may range from 5 to 20% in the outpatient psychiatric settings. In a study by Fabrega et al., 1987 women more than men were observed to have adjustment disorder.

Clinical Features

Behavioral and emotional symptoms which develop with a temporal relation with a stressor. It usually occurs within 3 months of the onset of the stressor.

The symptoms and behavior are significant and result in marked distress which is out of proportion to the severity and intensity of the stressor. Additionally, it results in social, occupational or other functional impairment.

It can be associated with:

- Depressed mood
- With anxiety
- With mixed anxiety and depressed mood
- With disturbance in conduct
- With mixed disturbance of emotions and conduct

Development, Course and Prognosis

It usually begins within 3 months of onset of a stressor but resolves within 6 months of termination of stressor. It is known to have a favourable prognosis and once the stressor is terminated the symptoms do not persist beyond 6 months (APA, 2000). The nature of the stressor too has an effect in the persistence of symptoms. If a stressor is acute such as loss of job, the symptoms may begin within a few days. If a stressor is ongoing, it also may result in persistence of symptoms.

Treatment

Psychotherapy

The therapeutic modalities focus on reduction of symptoms, improving mechanisms of coping, and a support system which enables resilience. Identify the distress and resultant dysfunction set in due to the stressor.

Eliciting the stressors allows identification of stressor which can be dealt with. Additionally, emotional disturbance in a patient may result in various harmful behaviors such as consumption of substance, self-harm or impulsive acts. It is important for the patient to discuss *adaptive coping strategies and gain a mastery* over the stressor. Also, *identify the meaning of the stressor for the patient*. The loss of relationship may result in the patient feeling rejected, leaving a patient with thoughts of, "I am not capable of sustaining a relationship." This thought may pervade across work, relationship with family, friends and social relations.

The Goals of Treatment

- Identifying maladaptive thoughts and distressing emotions

- Identify ways to reduce stress
- Enable patient to squarely perceive the stressor
- Find ways to healthy ways in coping
- Establish support for the patient

Brief Psychotherapy

The principal factor here is to identify the meaning of stressor and reframe the meaning of the stressor. However, in patients with persistent and ongoing stressor a more sustainable therapy may be required.

Cognitive Behavior Therapy

Identification of negative cognitions in relation to self, world and others and enabling a patient to find alternate healthy responses to the thoughts. It involves an assessment and understanding of dysfunctional assumptions and core beliefs. The alternate adaptive responses result in changes in emotional responses and thereby improve behavior and reduces distress.

Interpersonal Therapy

It involves the various principles which include

- Here and now framework
- Assessing from ***an interpersonal perspective and focused interpersonal areas***
- Alternatives and options to changing dysfunctional behavior patterns
- Systematic approach in formulation of the problem and treatment

Support Groups

Attending groups facilitate discussing coping strategies and modelling methods. Many studies have shown increased survival time, reduced distress level and enhanced quality of life.

Pharmacotherapy

Psychotherapy is the treatment preferred. However, in many cases due to emotional disturbances setting in, pharmacotherapeutic approaches have also been used.

Antidepressants improves emotional disturbance – depressed mood and anxiety and the overall psychosocial functioning. SSRIs, SNRIs and TCAs have been used with favourable outcome.

Treatment of Adjustment disorders	
Psychotherapy	**Pharmacotherapy**
Brief psychotherapy	Antidepressants in case of mood
Cognitive behavior therapy	disturbance /anxiety
Interpersonal therapy	
Support groups	

Other Specified Trauma – and Stressor – Related Disorder

This category includes the different presentations in which symptoms appear in relation to trauma or stressor resulting in distress and social, occupational or dysfunction in some other areas of functioning. It may not meet the criteria of adjustment disorder, acute stress disorder or post- traumatic stress disorder. The disorders included in the category include:

- Adjustment-like disorders with delayed onset of symptoms that occur more than 3 months after the stressor.
- Adjustment – like disorder with prolonged duration beyond 6 months even after the termination of the stressor.

- Ateque de nervios: Culture bound syndrome in the Latinos with acute emotional disturbances such as panic attacks, anxiety, cry spells, screaming spells, aggressive or suicidal behavior, dissociative experiences, precipitated by a sudden stressor such as death of a family member, sudden altercations with spouse or witnessing an accident of a family member.

Persistent Complex Bereavement Disorder (PCBD)

It is form of ***complicated grief where acute grief goes beyond the time frame that*** is ***considered culturally appropriate in the bereaved person's social network*** accompanied by ***complicating feelings, thoughts and behaviors***. In terms of severity it implies the extreme intensity of grief experienced by a person.

A typical grief scenario involves the distress experienced with loss which includes yearning, longing, searching; thoughts of the deceased with memories and on occasions perceptual disturbances may appear. A sense of loneliness, emptiness and anxiety, insecurity. Feelings of detachment from others and sense of deprivation. On occasions, regret, guilt or self -blame may emerge. Decreased motivation, self-confidence may also manifest in some patients.

Persistent complex bereavement disorder is a complex, disabling psychiatric disorder still considered a condition for further study in DSM 5.

A. The individual experienced the death of someone with whom they shared a close relationship

B. Since the death, atleast one of the following symptoms is experienced on more days than not and to clinically significant degree and has persisted for atleast 12 months after the death in the case of bereaved adults and 6 months for bereaved children:

1. Persistent yearning /longing for the deceased. In younger children, yearning may be expressed in play and behavior includes behavior after being separated from and also reuniting with a caregiver or other attachment figure.
2. Intense sorrow and emotional pain in response to death
3. Preoccupation with the deceased
4. Preoccupation with the circumstance of death. In children, it reflects in the play and behavior and may extend to preoccupation with possible death of others close to them.

C. Since the death, atleast six of the following are experienced which atleast last for 12 months and in children for 6 months:

Reactive distress to death:

1. Marked difficulty in accepting the death.
2. Emotional numbness and disbelief over the loss
3. Difficulty with positive reminiscing about the deceased
4. Bitterness and anger over the loss
5. Maladaptive appraisals about oneself in relation to the deceased or the death (e.g. Self -blame)
6. Excess avoidance of reminders of the loss such as avoidance of individuals, places and situations associated with deceased.

Social identity disruption:

1. A desire to die in order to be with the deceased
2. Difficulty trusting others since the death
3. Feeling alone or detached from other individuals since the death
4. Feeling that life is meaningless or empty without the deceased or the belief that one cannot function without the deceased
5. Confusion about one's role in life, diminished sense of one's identity (e.g., feeling that a part of oneself died with the deceased)
6. Difficulty or reluctance to pursue interests since the loss or to plan for the future such as family or friendships.

The disturbance causes clinically significant distress or impairment in social, occupational or other areas in life.

Traumatic Bereavement

Bereavement in case of suicide or homicide with distress regarding the nature of death, last moments, degree of suffering in relation to the mode of death.

Course and Prognosis

Usually the course is persistent and chronic.

Treatment of Complicated Grief

Complicated grief treatment involves **psychoeducation, self - regulation, rebuilding connections, aspirational goals, revisiting the death of the deceased, memories and thoughts.** The process involves acknowledging death and its consequences, revisiting mental representations of the deceased and redefining life goals and plans. It involves exposure of the patient to the situation of death and imagining the process of understanding and learning the death of the individual. This allows processing of emotions in relation to death, gradual reduction in the distress experienced and integration.

Trauma in children can particularly have deleterious effects in development. In children, trauma can affect the neurodevelopment – which implies the brain and CNS and can affect the social development such as attachment, character and personality, relationships with family, friends and others.

Treatment of Complicated grief:

1. Psychoeducation
2. Rebuild connections
3. Revisit the death, process emotions in relation to death, distress reductions

Reactive Attachment Disorder

Child caregiving and parenting are essential aspects in the development of secure attachments in the child. In children who have been neglected, various emotional and behavioral symptoms may present.

In reactive attachment disorder, the emotional and social needs are unmet due to neglect from parents, family or caregivers. As a result, there is a failure to achieve a secure relationship basis in relationships.

- A consistent pattern of inhibited, emotionally withdrawn behavior towards adult caregivers which is manifested by
- The child does not/ seek comfort when distressed
- Child does not respond to comfort with distress

- Minimal social and emotional responsiveness to others
- Limited emotional expression
- Experiences irritability, sadness and fearfulness even with non-threatening interactions with caregivers

In such children, history of failure/deprivation of meeting social, emotional and basic needs. Repeated changes of caregiver which affects the formation of stable attachments. It may also involve children who are reared in unusual settings such as foster care or institutional care. These symptoms present before 5 years of age.

Disinhibited Social Engagement Disorder

The children in this disorder actively approach unfamiliar adults, absence of inhibition and reticence, does not check back when venturing away looking for an adult, willingness to go with an unfamiliar adult. This behavior cannot be attributed to impulsivity. The grossly abnormal behavior is reflected in patients with severe neglect, institutional care. These symptoms usually develop in children less than 5 years of age.

Treatment Interventions

The treatment in the case of Reactive attachment disorder and Disinhibited social engagement disorder which is linked to trauma or neglect in childhood and psychiatric symptoms. The intervention made earlier can benefit the social and emotional development of an individual. Early intervention is supportive therapy for the mother which is provided. In foster homes, institutionalized children can result in maladaptive social skills. Therapy involves cognitive restructuring, re – parenting and trauma resolution. An intervention where a caregiving relationship is provided – emotionally available, sensitive and responsible and parental figure to which attachment can be developed. Additionally, also to enable the child to set attainable goals. Also, therapy for impulsivity, hyperactivity, anger management. The reactive attachment disorder intervention also involves placement in a secure and nurturing environment, parenting skills to the caregivers, family functioning and coping skills and interactions. Also, reducing contact with non-caregiving adults which may reduce signs of disorder. Psychopharmacological interventions are not indicated for the core features of Reactive Attachment Disorder and Disinhibited Social Engagement Disorder.

CONCLUSIONS

- Essential to remember there are varied reactions to a stressor or traumatic event.
- The clinician must assess symptoms and also look for psychosocial factors associated with resilience. This enables understanding of the progression of disorder.
- The disorders can be stressor related such as adjustment disorder or related to a life - threatening experience resulting in acute stress disorder or post traumatic disorder. It may result from loss of loved one resulting in persistent complex grief.
- In all the conditions, psychotherapy remains the mainstay of intervention. Pharmacological approaches have also been used for emotional disturbances.

BIBLIOGRAPHY

1. Casey PR, Strain JJ, editors. Trauma-and Stressor-related Disorders: A Handbook for Clinicians. American Psychiatric Pub; 2015 Dec 18.
2. Landolt MA, Cloitre M, Schnyder U, editors. Evidence-based treatments for trauma related

disorders in children and adolescents. Cham, CN: Springer; 2017 Feb 13.

3. King MC. Reactive Attachment Disorder: A Review. Journal of the Office of Graduate Studies at Lynchburg College. Lynchburg, VA. 2004.
4. Howlett JR, Stein MB. Prevention of trauma and stressor-related disorders: a review. Neuropsychopharmacology. 2016 Jan;41(1):357.

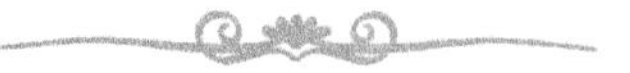

Substance Use Disorders 19

Atul Ambekar • Amit Singh • Rizwana Qureshi

SUBSTANCE USE DISORDERS: CLASSIFICATION AND DEFINITIONS

The commonest terms that one would associate with Drug use is "Drug Addiction" and "Drug Addict." These terms, however, have fallen to disrepute because of their pejorative and derogatory implications, and new terms like "Substance Use Disorder(s)" and "Substance User(s)" have taken their place.

Types of Drugs

A drug, broadly speaking, is any chemical substance that, when absorbed into the body of a living organism, alters normal bodily function. There is no single definition, as there are different meanings in medicine, government regulations, and colloquial usage.

In the area of substance use disorders, a drug or a substance is any chemical that, upon consumption, leads to changes in the functioning of human mind and more specifically leads to a state of intoxication. These drugs/substances are also referred to as – Psychoactive substances.[1]

Some of these Psychoactive substances, like Alcoholic beverages and Nicotine (Tobacco), are legally allowed for trade and consumption in most parts of India (albeit in a strictly regulated fashion) and have the status of Licit (or Legal) substances. The trade and consumption of many other substances are strictly prohibited and are therefore called Illicit (or Illegal) substances.

The World Health Organization (WHO) lists substance use disorders for the following classes of substances.

Substances listed by WHO

- Alcohol
- Opioids
- Cannabis and synthetic cannabinoids
- Sedative Hypnotics
- Cocaine
- Other stimulants, including caffeine
- Synthetic cathinones
- Hallucinogens and Dissociative drugs
- Nicotine (Tobacco)
- Volatile Inhalants

A brief description of common substances of use is as follows.

Alcohol

One of the oldest and most popular psychotropic substance/drug known to mankind is alcohol. In the ancient Indian texts one finds mention of *Madira* and *Sura*, which are believed to be alcoholic preparations. Ethyl alcohol (ethanol)

1 Throughout this unit, terms 'drug' and 'substance' have been used interchangeably

is the active ingredient. 'Distilled spirits' such as whisky, brandy, rum, vodka and gin contain 35% to 50% (usually about 42% in India) alcohol whereas beers ordinarily contain 4 to 8%. Wines usually contain approximately 12% alcohol. Due to these variations therefore, alcoholic drinks are measured in "Standard drinks", one standard drink of alcohol is 12.7 ml of alcohol by volume. The rule of thumb for comparison is, one Standard Drink = ½ bottle of Standard Beer = ¼ bottle of Strong Beer = 1 peg (30 ml.)Spirits = ½ packet of Arrack (i.e. country liquor) = 1 glass (125 ml.) of table wine. This helps in roughly estimating the magnitude of the drinking problem of a particular person.

The effects of alcohol on the user depends on the level of alcohol in the blood (called: blood alcohol concentration or BAC) and are as follows (**Table 19.1**).

Table 19.1

BAC in mg/dl	Effects
Around 40 to 80	Feeling of happiness, feeling of relaxation and talking freely, some clumsy movements of hands and legs, reduced alertness but user believes himself to be alert.
More than 80	Noisy, moody, impaired judgment, impaired driving ability.
At 100-200	Blurred vision, unsteady gait, talking loudly, slurred speech, quarrelsome, aggressive, gross motor in-coordination.
At 200-300	Inability to remember the experience – blackout.
More than 300	Coma and in higher levels even death.

Alcoholic drinks available in India can be divided into Indian Made Foreign Liquor (IMFL), which are drinks made in India according to specifications of International standards; Indian made country liquor (IMCL), which are drinks made in India with government license; and home brewed country liquor (HBCL), which may be illegally brewed. Most cases of toxicity develop due to other chemicals substances added to such home brewed liquor to make them stronger.

Cannabis

Cannabis is derived from the plant cannabis sativa, which grows in the wild all around the world including India. At low dose, cannabis causes a state of well-being (high) and a dreamy, state of enjoyment. This is generally followed by a period of drowsiness. Even relatively modest amounts of cannabis can impair coordination and make the operation of heavy machinery hazardous. Dexterity and hand steadiness are both adversely affected. At medium dose perceptual and sensory distortions occur. Capacity for depth perception declines and scenes appear to have greater depth. Sounds and colors may become more intense along with derealization (what is seen or heard has an air of unreality) and depersonalization (one's own body feels unreal). Subjective sense of time seems to be much slower than it actually is. Sometimes restlessness, fear and even panic may spoil the experience ("bad trip"). At higher doses delirium (confusion), psychosis and paranoid ideations (unwarranted suspicion) occur but are generally self-limited.

Cannabis is also available in various forms Viz: *Bhang*- paste of leaves of the plant or dried leaves, *Ganja* – dried flowering stem of the plant and *Charas* or hashish – extracted from the resin covering the plant. It can be smoked in cigarettes, or in clay pipes (most common method in religious settings and rural areas) or in water pipes like the traditional hookah or modern 'bong', where the smoke passes through water before being inhaled. Interestingly, though products of the same cannabis plant, *Bhang*, which is used in various religious festivals, is legal in India; while *Charas* and *Ganja* are illegal. There are synthetic preparations of cannabinoids many of which are generating research interest for their potential therapeutic use for a variety of health conditions.

Opioids

Opium is the prototype opioid which is derived from the poppy plant (Papaver somniferum). An opioid is any drug that acts like opium in the human body (as described below). There are three broad classes of opioids - Naturally occurring substances, such as morphine and codeine; semi-synthetics such as heroin, oxycodone that are produced by modifying natural substances and pure synthetics such as fentanyl and methadone that are not produced from opium but act just like opium on the human brain. When given to a subject who has not previously experienced the effects of the drug, opioids produce an unpleasant feeling. However on continued use, injecting heroin or morphine produces a short lived (less than a minute) intense experience - "rush". It is described as a state of profound happiness. There is also pain relief due to inability to feel any pain (opioids are used as medications for pain-relief for this property) and a dreamlike state characterized by decreased responsiveness to the environment.

Heroin, popularly called 'smack' or 'brown sugar' is one of the very common forms to be used. Heroin may be smoked, chased (inhaled) or injected (intramuscular or intravenous), however 'chasing' (inhaling the vapours emanating from a heated metallic foil) is the commonest mode of heroin use in India. Several other opioids that are used as medications (for pain relief) are also misused. Common among these are codeine cough syrups, morphine and pentazocine injections, and buprenorphine tablets/injections. Oral ingestion of opium as well as smoking through a special wooden pipe has been the traditional Indian method. "Khas" the seeds of poppy plant are non-narcotic and widely used in Indian cuisines.

Nicotine

Nicotine is the main active chemical in Tobacco, yet another legal and popular substance the world over. Nicotine generally causes heightened alertness and improved functioning in continuous repetitive tasks. Users also report relaxation and decrease in fatigue with smoking and irritability, restlessness, anger and frustration with difficulty in concentration and sleep while trying to leave.

Tobacco is the commonest substance of use in India, is legally and socially sanctioned and so used in a wide variety of ways including smoking, chewing, applying to gums, sucking and gargling. Beedi smoking is the most popular form of smoking in India, while cigarettes come second. Chewing paan (betel leaf) with tobacco is the major form of smokeless-tobacco use and peculiar to our region. Dry tobacco and areca nut preparations such as paan masala, gutka and mawa are also popular and highly addictive.

Sedative/Hypnotics

These are medications that are prescribed by doctors to reduce anxiety and produce sleep. They are also misused because of their easy availability and cheap price. Though detail discussion is outside the scope of this chapter, certain medications like Diazepam, Nitrazepam and Pheniramine are widely used. These may be used either in tablet preparation, as injections or as cough syrups.

Cocaine

A common substance in Americas and Europe, it is extracted from the leaves of Erythroxylon Coca, a plant that grows wildly in Latin American countries. As of now, it is not widely available in India. It is generally snorted, but can also be chewed and smoked. Its use cause a short lived sensation (7 to 10 minutes) of "rush" which is felt intensely pleasurable to the user. Therefore it is not generally taken continuously but in "binges" or "runs" where it is taken every thirty minutes to few hours for consecutive three to seven days.

Stimulants

These are a group of substances that cause activation of the brain thereby increasing alertness, producing euphoria, improving performance and decreasing fatigue. The prototype drug of this group is Amphetamine.

Hallucinogens

These are also called **Psychedelics**. These are a group of various drugs that have the common property to alter how a person sees or hears things (i.e. produce hallucinations). The classic example is LSD (Lysergic Acid Diethyamide), which has been described to make one see music and hear light. Other substances of this group include PCP (Phencyclidine) and Ecstasy.

Inhalants

These are substances that give vapors without heating. They are mostly petroleum products and are ubiquitous, present with glue, thinners, cleaners, solvents etc. The vapors are "huffed", sniffed or "Bagged" (re-breathing from a bag). Their use also produces a rush and sense of wellbeing and an urge to reuse after only five to six minutes. On regular use however they are associated with brain damage and multiple liver and lung problems.

Important Concepts/Definitions

Various terms have been used to describe the phenomenon of substance use. These include terms such as "Use", "Hazardous Use", "Harmful Use", "Dependence" etc. The following section describes the meaning of these terms.

Use

Use is simply the ingestion of alcohol or other drugs **without experiencing any negative consequences**. It may be **social use**, in parties and marriages; **recreational use, experimentation** and group activity by the youth, **dietary practice** or may be **religious ritual**.

Hazardous Use

A pattern of psychoactive substance use that significantly **increases the risk** of harmful physical or mental health consequences to the user or to others to an extent that warrants attention and advice from health professionals. However, no actual harm should have occurred.

Harmful Use

A single episode or a pattern of substance use that is causing damage to physical or mental health or has resulted in behavior leading to harm to the health of others. Harm to health of the individual may result from the behavior related to intoxication; direct or secondary toxic effects on body organs and systems; or a harmful route of administration. Harm to health of others includes any form of physical harm, including trauma, or mental disorder that is directly attributable to behavior due to substance intoxication.

Dependence

Substance Dependence is a "syndrome" rather than "disease". This implies that when a number of signs and symptoms are found in cluster in a substance user and a pattern of use becomes evident then the diagnosis of dependence is reached. The WHO defines Substance Dependence syndrome as "A cluster of physiological, behavioral and cognitive phenomena in which use of a substance or a class of substances takes on a much higher priority for a given individual than other behaviors that once had greater value". The complete WHO diagnostic guideline is given in the box below.

WHO Diagnostic guidelines for substance dependence

Substance dependence is a disorder of regulation of substance use arising from repeated or continuous use of substance. The characteristic feature is a **strong internal drive** to use substance, which is manifested by **impaired ability to control** use, **increasing priority** given to use over other activities and persistence of **use despite harm** or negative consequences. These experiences are often accompanied by a subjective sensation of **urge or craving** to use substance. Physiological features of dependence may also be present, including **tolerance** to the effects of substance, **withdrawal symptoms** following cessation or reduction in use of substance, or repeated use of substance or pharmacologically similar substances to prevent or alleviate withdrawal symptoms.

The features of dependence are usually evident over a period of at least 12 months but the diagnosis may be made if substance use is continuous (daily or almost daily) for at least 1 month.

Addiction

Addiction is an older term which has similar meaning as that of dependence. It is not favored in current diagnostic systems because of its derogatory connotation. However it is ingrained in literature and hence continues to be used.

EPIDEMIOLOGY OF SUBSTANCE USE IN INDIA

A substantial number of people use psycho-active substances in India, and substance use exists in all the population groups. Tobacco is the most commonly used psycho-active substance. The overall tobacco use prevalence in 15 years and older population as reported in the Global Adult Tobacco Survey (GATS) is 28.6%. Smokeless tobacco is a more commonly used form compared to smoking in India.

The recent report Magnitude of Substance Use in India (2019), provides the substance use prevalence estimates in 10-75 year population (Table 19.2) and indicates that there are wide variations in extent and prevalence of use across different states and between various substances.

Table 19.2: Substance use in India

Substances	Prevalence of current use (in %)	Prevalence of harmful and dependent use (in %)
Alcohol	14.6	5.20
Opioid	2.06	0.70
Cannabis	2.83	0.66
Sedatives	1.08	0.20
Inhalants	0.70	0.21
Cocaine	0.10	0.02
Amphetamine type stimulants	0.18	0.02
Hallucinogens	0.12	0.03

CAUSES OF SUBSTANCE USE DISORDERS

There is no simple answer to the question - "why people take drugs?" Many hypotheses exist to explain the occurrence of drug dependence. Some of these are moral model (use seen as sin, crime), characterological (use seen as a defect in personality), conditioning model (use as a result of learning new behavior) and biomedical model (genetic and physiological/ biological cause of SUD). However, it is not possible to explain the phenomenon of SUD based on one model exclusively. Currently SUDs are best conceptualized as bio-psycho-social in origin, i.e. a variety of factors interact with each other to result in substance use and dependence.

Substance Use: Biological Causes

Genetic

Substance use disorder has some heritable component, i.e. a person may be predisposed since birth to develop addiction. The offspring of alcoholic parents took to drinking more frequently, twins separated at birth showed similar drug use pattern later in life and children of non-alcoholic parents adopted by liberal alcoholic families were less susceptible to alcohol use! Indeed for alcoholism around 40 to 60 percent of the predisposition is actually heritable (runs in families). For other drugs too, genetic predisposition have been found, albeit to a lesser extent. Recent genome wide scans are trying to identify the genes implicated in development of drug dependence.

Neurobiological Mechanisms

Addictive substances lead to enhanced dopaminergic transmission in the mesolimbic pathway neurons (a component of medial forebrain bundle) projecting from ventral tegmental area to the nucleus accumbens. This leads to the perception of pleasure and reward. Thus the mesolimbic pathway, is also referred to as the reward pathway. Repeated exposure to substance leads to strengthened synaptic connections through long term potentiation. Over the course of development of addiction, relatively stable neuroplastic changes in various brain areas occur through altered expression of transcription factors and subsequent protein synthesis. Moreover, the brain areas (prefrontal cortex) associated with behavioral inhibition and control also started hypo-functioning. Thus, the 'impulsivity' associated with substance use goes uncontrolled due to loss of cortical function. With chronic substance use the recruitment of cortico-striatothalamocortical loop occurs leading to 'compulsive' use of substance.

Substance Use: Environmental Causes

Drug Related Factors

Availability and social sanction of drug use are the chief drug related factors that promote initiation and continuation of use. The very fact that socially sanctioned drugs like alcohol and tobacco are commonly used proves that availability plays major role in initiation. Studies have shown that for alcohol and tobacco, to certain extent, consumption has gone down whenever their price has increased. Availability also decides the pattern of drug use. When there was a sudden decrease in Indian market of heroin due to intensive law-enforcement, many heroin smokers shifted to injecting route of drug use (which was cheaper and easily available).

Additionally smoking a drug or injecting it into a vein increases its addictive potential, as compared to drinking it. Both smoked and injected drugs enter the brain within seconds, producing a powerful rush of pleasure. However, this intense "high" can fade within a few minutes, taking the user down to lower, more normal levels. It is a starkly felt contrast, and scientists believe that this low feeling drives individuals to repeated drug abuse in an attempt to recapture the high pleasurable state.

Worldwide observations have found that a sizable population of drug users reported onset of drug use while they were 'young'. Users generally started with "softer" drugs like Alcohol, Cannabis and then gradually graduated to "harder" drugs like opioids. These observations have given rise to the concept of **gateway hypothesis,** which says that drug use is a developmental sequence in which earlier drug use results in greater risk of use of later drugs. Nicotine and alcohol have been labeled as **gateway drugs** because they are socially sanctioned and provide the gateway of entry for a novice user to the world of drugs. However recent research supports a 'common liability to addiction' hypothesis more than the 'gateway hypothesis'.

Social/Cultural/Legal Factors

Environmental risk factors are characteristics in a person's surroundings that increase their likelihood of becoming addicted to drugs. A person may have many environments, or domains, of influence such as the community, family, school and friends. An individual's connection with the community in which they live plays a big part in their likelihood of using drugs. Statistics show that if a person's community has favorable attitudes toward drug use the risk of substance use is increased. Even religious proscriptions modify drug use as evidenced by the low use of alcohol in Islamic countries. The single biggest contributing factor to drug use risk is having friends (i.e. peer group) who engage in drug use. Family conflict and home management problems are contributing factors in drug abuse risk. If parents have favorable attitudes towards drug use or use drugs themselves, often their children will be more likely to use drugs. Conversely, a substance user is often in conflict with family and authority resulting in pushing him further to the accepting drug using peer group. Legal and policy issues not only govern the availability of drugs but also often result in incarceration of soft drug users who learn use of other and harder drugs in jail.

Substance Use: Psychological Causes

Concept of 'Self Medication'

It has been proposed that many drug users try to counteract their "painful feelings" by taking drugs. In this light, drug act as a kind of medication, helping the user to alleviate his emotional problems. By this principle chronic cannabis users may be seen as self-medicating for anxiety problems. Similarly, alcohol may be used to alleviate panic and anxiety. While such use may provide immediate relief of some symptoms, but in long term drug use may itself produce other psychiatric illness.

Psychologists also see substance use as a *learned behavior* picked up from parents and peers, and describe continued use as forms of classical and/or operant conditioning.

Personality Related Variables

Several common personality traits have been observed in people who take up and continue using drugs. "Low Frustration tolerance" and "Sensation Seeking" are by far the most studied of them. People with low frustration tolerance seek to avoid immediate pain at the cost of long-term stress and defeatism. They take to drugs to escape the simple and inevitable problems of daily life. Sensation seeking on other hand focuses on the need for new and varied experiences through risky behavior. Doing things at the spur of the moment without consideration of outcome (Impulsivity) and nonconformity to social rules and norms are integral part of their lives.

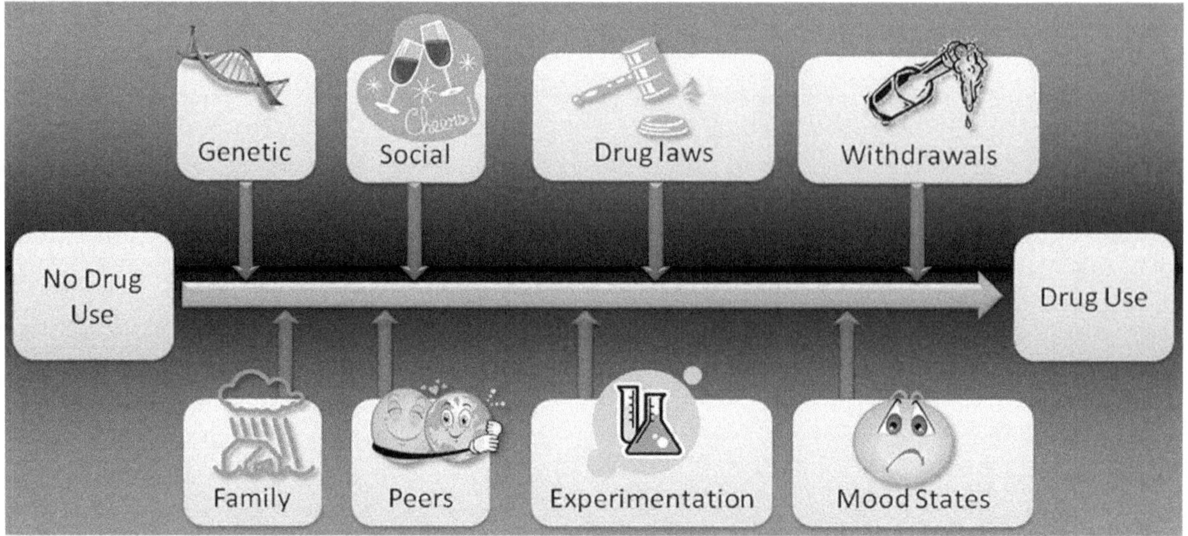

Fig. 19.1: Illustration showing various factors leading to substance use.

Many substance users also suffer from inability to experience pleasure from normal activities (Anhedonia) or understand their own emotions (Alexithymia) and therefore require a stronger high to feel pleasure. Such personality traits have been postulated to maintain substance use in affected persons.

These models of causation of SUD are not mutually exclusive and generally many factors overlap in every substance user to result in his/her dependence on substances. The simple illustration (**Fig. 19.1**) shows how various factors contribute to the phenomenon of substance use.

CONSEQUENCES OF SUBSTANCE USE

Physical Consequences

Physical complication of drug use are varied and numerous and differ from substance to substance. In general any drug harms the body in acute use by intoxication and by overdose toxicity. Acute alcohol overdose can cause fall, unconsciousness, severe vomiting, bleeding in stomach, and sedation, progressing to coma and ultimately death. Adulterants of alcohol can cause blindness, and even death. Opioids, cannabis and other drugs can cause various mental illnesses including the severe ones like psychosis in overdose. Chronic (long-term) use causes harm to almost all organ systems of the human body. Jaundice and liver-diseases (alcohol), dementia (alcohol), cardiac problems (alcohol), cancer (tobacco and alcohol), asthma (tobacco), viral hepatitis (IDU), HIV (IDU), psychiatric illness (most drugs) represent only a tiny fraction of the list. Even sudden stoppage of drugs by a dependent user can cause severe physical symptoms in the withdrawal state, which sometimes may be fatal. It is particularly important to find out what physical harm has actually occurred to the user, and show him the benefits he will have on leaving substance.

Social/Familial/Economic Consequences

Young adult males who are most productive members of any society are ironically most vulnerable to substance use disorders. Apart from the direct economic loss of money spent on substances, substance users face various indirect monetary loss due to loss in productivity, absenteeism from work, being expelled from job etc. Adolescent users drop out from school, thereby curtailing all future earning capabilities. Multiple physical complication and recurrent hospitalizations drain money. Stigma of substance use prevents them from getting job even when they are trying to quit substance.

Family members of substance users bear the major burden. Apart from money being diverted from family fund for sustaining substance use behavior, the whole family suffers from familial conflicts, stigma of drug use and discrimination.

The society at large suffers from loss of productivity and an increased burden to support and treat these potentially productive members. Crime rates rise, and rash behavior often cause accidents and destruction of properties.

Psychological Consequences

Psychological complications range from lack of wellbeing to frank depression. Substances like alcohol cause depression on long-term use and on trying to stop cause severe anxiety. Cannabis has been long associated with precipitation of the illness like schizophrenia. Opioids and amphetamines are known to cause psychosis. Any underlying mental illness is generally aggravated by substance use.

Legal Consequences

Substance users are usually at conflict with law. They are often incarcerated when caught with illicit substances and a life revolving in and out of jail follows, thereby severely hampering any gainful employment.

ASSESSMENT OF SUBSTANCE USE DISORDERS

Assessment forms the cornerstone in diagnosis and management of substance use disorders. A proper assessment is necessary for establishing a diagnosis, for planning treatment and for referral to a specialist for further treatment. Assessment however is not a one -time phenomenon. Generally it is done in the beginning to define the problem and formulate a treatment plan. It also needs to be repeated during treatment to monitor progress, and even after treatment to assess maintenance of abstinence status. In this section we look into various methods of assessment.

Clinical Interview and History

Clinical interview is performed to gather relevant and correct information quickly about various aspects of the problem. Interview should begin by asking open-ended questions, followed by the guiding questions to steer the conversation in meaningful direction. The guideline given below is meant to highlight important aspects of drug use that need to be evaluated.

Guidelines for taking history in a substance user:

1. Allow the patient to **settle down**, and ask about his **socio-demographic profile**
2. **Details of drug use** are then inquired into. This include
    a) age of **initiation**
    b) various **drugs** used
    c) **frequency** of use of those drugs
    d) quantity of drug taken usually (**usual dose**)
    e) time lag since the dose **last used**

f) if the patient has needed to increase the quantity of drug consumed in order to produce the same effect (**tolerance**)

g) if the patient has experienced any symptoms of **intoxication**

h) symptoms and signs when the particular drug is not taken or taken in reduced amounts (**withdrawals**), and

i) if patient feels compelling need/urge to take the substance (**craving**)

3. **Complications** associated with drug use should be inquired. These are the areas to be focused during rehabilitation. The areas probed are

   a) **Physical:** long term health hazards associated with drug use

   b) **Psychological:** chronic mental effects of continuous use of drug

   c) **Financial:** losses suffered/debts incurred

   d) **Occupational:** frequent absenteeism at work, constant change of job, memos issued, periods of unemployment

   e) **Familial/Social:** frequent fight with spouse or other family members, neglect of responsibility at home, social outcast

   f) **Legal:** involvement in illegal activities to sustain drug use, arrests/charges on account of drug use, caught driving under intoxicated state, drinking brawl.

   g) **High risk behaviors:** presence of injection use with needle sharing and unsafe sexual practices

4. **Past abstinence attempts:** herein inquiry should be made regarding

   a) **Number of attempts** made

   b) **Duration** of each attempt

   c) **Reason** for abstinence (why the patient wanted to quit)

   d) Whether **treatment** sought (what treatment worked or did not work before)

   e) **Nature of treatment sought:** pharmacological, psychological or combined

   f) **Reason for relapse**

5. **Reason for seeking treatment** and **motivation level** of individual: whether seeking treatment by self or brought forcibly by a family member. Assessing level of motivation would help the clinician decide the type of intervention needed.

6. **Co-morbid Psychiatric illnesses** such as a mood disorder, psychotic disorder and personality disorders need specialist care.

7. **Family history** of SUD, psychiatric illness and the current living arrangements. Extent of social support should be assessed.

Examination

General physical and systemic examination is important as it provides important clues regarding the type of substance used, phase at presentation (intoxication or withdrawal), extent of health impact, and often guides the treatment process. Some important findings of physical examination include

- Benzodiazepine, barbiturate, and alcohol withdrawal can present with tachycardia, psychomotor agitation, tremor, hypertension, seizures, and/or delirium.
- Smell of alcohol on the breath, slurred speech and other signs of intoxication indicate recent alcohol use. The excessive

alcohol consumption leading to liver failure or acute hepatotoxicity may manifest with jaundice, hepatomegaly, splenomegaly, portal hypertension, abdominal tenderness, weight loss, ascites, caput medusa, icteric sclerae, telangiectasia, parotid swelling and excoriations.

- Opioid overdose can present with constricted pupils, depressed respiration, and altered mental state. Whereas, opioid withdrawal can present with mydriasis, rhinorrhea, lacrimation, yawning, gastrointestinal distress, joint and body pain, anxiety, insomnia and restlessness.
- Needle track marks, thrombophlebitis, skin abscesses are indicative of injecting drug use.
- Methamphetamine and cocaine withdrawal can present with severe psychomotor retardation, cognitive deficits, depression and fatigue.
- Heavy tobacco use can present with stains on the fingers. Chronic airways limitation in smokers.
- Neurological exam should detail sensory abnormalities, nystagmus, motor weakness, abnormal reflexes, rigidity, bowel or bladder dysfunction, and any gait disturbance.
- Mental status exam:

  A detailed mental status examination should be conducted. Assessment should be done for anxiety, depression, suicidality, psychosis, neurocognitive deficits, and altered sensorium. Equally important is to assess the **motivational stage of the patient**.

Additionally laboratory assessment to confirm, corroborate drug use and to find the physical complications may be done in specialized treatment centers.

Use of Structured Tools for Assessment

Structured tools are **questionnaires** and **scales** that have been specifically developed to measure some aspect of substance use. They offer the advantage of being brief, easy and rapid to administer, and their results can be objectified and compared. However they are limited in their scope, and can augment but not replace the clinical interview.

Screening

Screening is usually applied to a large group of individuals and is very brief by nature. A number of instruments have been developed towards identification of a number of individuals with drug abuse problem in a relatively short period. Some frequently used instruments are–

1. **CAGE:** an acronym for 4 questions used to assess those with alcohol problem
2. **MAST:** Michigan Alcohol Screening Test
3. **DAST:** Drug Abuse Screening Test
4. **AUDIT:** Alcohol Use Disorder Identification Test

The CAGE questionnaire is given below in the box.

CAGE is a mnemonic for the following four questions:

1. Have you ever felt that you should **C**ut down on your drinking?
2. Have people **A**nnoyed you by criticizing your drinking?
3. Have you ever, felt bad or **G**uilty about your drinking?
4. Have you ever, had a drink first thing in the morning to steady your nerves or get rid of a hangover (i.e. drink as an **E**ye-opener)?

Interpretation of CAGE questions

Answering "*Yes*" to 2 questions – Strong Indication for alcohol dependence

Answering "*Yes*" to 3 questions – Confirms alcohol dependence

Severity

Commonly used tools for measuring severity include the **Addiction Severity Index (ASI)** and **Maudsley Addiction Profile (MAP)**. The ASI is an interview that assesses history, frequency, and consequences of alcohol and drug use, as well as five additional domains that are commonly associated with drug use: medical, legal, employment, social/family, and psychological functioning.

Motivation

The commonest questionnaire used to judge motivation is the **Readiness to Change Questionnaire (RTCQ)**. The RTCQ is a 12-item questionnaire, based on Prochaska and DiClemente's stages-of-change model, for assignment to Precontemplation, Contemplation, and Action stages.

TREATMENT OF SUBSTANCE USE DISORDERS

Goals of Treatment

Treatment goals differ from patient to patient and over time and may need to be reframed as the treatment progresses. Traditionally, the **primary goal** of treatment was to achieve permanent abstinence. However, this goal may remain elusive and alternate goals have to be pursued for some. In this subgroup, intervention is directed towards decreasing the harmful consequences of continued drug use. Such an effort is practical and attainable, and is called **"harm minimization"**. The other goals pursued are improvement of physical, psychosocial and occupational functioning.

Goals may also be classified as immediate, short-term and long-term goals. **Immediate goals** may be completion of detoxification (i.e. treatment of withdrawal symptoms) and intervention of psychosocial and medical crisis (crisis management). **Short-term goals** may include management of medical and psychiatric problems and re-integration with family. **Long-term goals** consist of prevention of relapse, re-integration into the society, occupational rehabilitation and improvement in overall quality of life.

Treatment Goals
Abstinence
Harm minimization
Improvement of health, social, occupational functioning
Improved quality of life

Phases of Treatment

Comprehensive treatment of substance use disorders comprises of initial, middle and late phases. The **initial phase** is of detoxification, which usually lasts for 2-4 weeks. Here efforts are made to free the person of all intoxicants, treat the symptoms of withdrawal (stopping the drugs) and attend to the immediate medical consequences of drug use. The **middle phase** is aimed at maintaining a drug free status (relapse prevention) and initiates the process of reintegration into the society. It may last for 3-6 months. During the **late phase**, adoption of a healthy life style and alternate coping strategies are promoted. Usually treatment is multimodal, which includes pharmacological and non-pharmacological treatment approaches.

Treatment Phases	
Initial	2 to 4 weeks
Middle Phase	3 to 6 months
Late Phase	> 6 months

Treatment Modalities

Certain basic principles of management are common, irrespective of the nature of substance being used. Broadly speaking, there are two modalities: **pharmacotherapy** and **psychosocial interventions**.

Goals of pharmacotherapy are–

- reversal of acute effects (intoxication and overdose),
- amelioration of withdrawal symptoms,
- decline of craving,
- prevention of relapse
- restoration of normal physiological functions.

Currently, various pharmacological agents are available for the above purposes.

Pharmacological Management

Alcohol use Disorder: Pharmacological Treatment

Alcohol intoxication rarely requires more than simple supportive measures, such as decreasing external stimuli and removing the source of alcohol. However, when respiration or other vital parameters are compromised by excessive alcohol intake, intensive care may be required. Treatment of alcohol withdrawal depends on the severity of withdrawal syndrome. The withdrawal symptoms typically follow the abrupt discontinuation of alcohol consumption. However, they can also develop when users simply reduce their usual high intake.

- Uncomplicated alcohol withdrawal begins 6–12 hours after the cessation of drinking and peaks at 24–48 hours, then subsides within 1-2 weeks, even without treatment. The symptoms include anxiety, tremors, nausea and vomiting, tachycardia and hypertension.
- Alcoholic withdrawal seizures usually begin within 8–24 hours after the cessation of drinking and peak between 24 and 48 hours. Usually, the seizures are of generalized tonic clonic type. Withdrawal seizures rarely evolve into status epilepticus.
- Alcohol withdrawal delirium (delirium tremens, or "DTs") occurs in about 5% of hospitalized alcoholic patients but in about one-third of those with withdrawal seizures. Symptoms include clouding of consciousness, hallucination, agitation, tremor and autonomic hyperarousal. The delirium begins 2–3 days after cessation of alcohol use and peaks 4 or 5 days later. Death is rare, although mortality rates of 10-20% were reported in the past.

The management of alcohol withdrawal consists of general support (i.e., adequate food and hydration, careful medical monitoring), nutritional supplementation, and the use of benzodiazepines. People with mild to moderate dependence and history of uncomplicated withdrawal can be managed as outpatients. Whereas, those with comorbidity, impaired ability to follow instructions, inadequate or absent social support, or a history of severe withdrawal symptoms will require careful monitoring and may need to be hospitalized.

Benzodiazepines are the mainstay of opioid withdrawal management. Long acting benzodiazepines such as chlordiazepoxide and diazepam are preferred agents because of their safety and cross-tolerance with alcohol. However, in individuals with hepatic dysfunction lorazepam and oxazepam are used because these benzodiazepines lack metabolites and are renally excreted. Patients should receive an adequate diet plus multivitamins including thiamine.

Thiamine should be given before any situation in which glucose loading is required, because glucose can deplete thiamine stores especially in malnourished individuals. This helps in preventing the development of Wernicke's-Korsakoff syndrome among chronic alcohol users.

Parenteral administration of rapid acting benzodiazepines such as diazepam and lorazepam interrupt withdrawal seizures. In addition, adequate withdrawal management with benzodiazepines prevents and ameliorates alcoholic hallucinosis. However, low dose of antipsychotics such as haloperidol or olanzapine can also be used for brief duration.

Management of delirium tremens usually requires frequent administration of intravenous benzodiazepines; thus, equipment for respiratory support should be available. The 10-item Clinical Institute Withdrawal Assessment (CIWA) Scale is an objective rating scale that can be used to monitor the withdrawal state and guide the benzodiazepine requirement.

Benzodiazepines continuation beyond treatment of the acute alcohol withdrawal syndrome has no role in management.

Several medications have been approved for the treatment of alcohol dependence and may be offered in combination with psychosocial treatment to prevent relapse. Disulfiram, acamprosate, naltrexone, and nalmefene have been approved for this purpose.

Disulfiram inhibits aldehyde dehydrogenase, an enzyme necessary for the metabolism of alcohol. This leads to the accumulation of acetaldehyde which is toxic, when alcohol is consumed over disulfiram. This disulfiram ethanol reaction is unpleasant and manifests as facial flushing, nausea, vomiting, palpitations, hypotension etc. Because patients taking disulfiram are aware of the potential adverse reaction, they are motivated to avoid alcohol.

Naltrexone and nalmefene are opioid antagonists, suggested to reduce the pleasurable effects of and craving for alcohol. Acamprosate, a glutamate receptor modulator, also reduces craving. These agents help patients to maintain abstinence, thereby reducing the risk of relapse.

Opioid use Disorder: Pharmacological Treatment

Opioid overdose syndrome is a medical emergency that can be fatal. It is characterized by the triad of altered mental status, miotic pupils and depressed respiration. Opioid antagonist naloxone is used as the specific antidote.

Among people affected by opioid use disorders, withdrawal symptoms and craving for the substance may be severe and extremely distressing. Various pharmacological options can be used to treat opioid withdrawal. Medications used for reducing the patient discomfort include

- Opioid medications: Long acting opioid medications such as buprenorphine and methadone

  Due to their agonistic action on opioid receptors, these medications reduce the severity of opioid withdrawals. The medication doses can subsequently be tapered down to stop after brief use or continued safely at adequate doses for long (months to years) to achieve abstinence from illicit opioids.

- Symptomatic treatments: Non-opioid alpha-adrenergic agonists such as clonidine and lofexidine suppress the autonomic signs of opioid withdrawal. Benzodiazepines can be used to treat mild cases of withdrawal and have the advantage of relieving anxiety and promoting needed sleep. Mild analgesics, such as the nonsteroidal anti-inflammatory drugs, can relieve muscle aches and pain. Gastrointestinal distress can be treated with dicyclomine.

Pharmacological agents that are used for the long-term treatment of opioid dependent individuals include:

- Opioid antagonist: Naltrexone
- Opioid agonists: buprenorphine and methadone

Opioid agonists used for maintenance treatment are effective agents in reducing the use of illicit opioids. The agonist dosages are such that they take care of withdrawals and cravings and block the euphoric effect produced by illicit opioid use.

Cannabis use Disorder: Pharmacological Treatment

When smoked, intoxication occurs within 10–30 minutes and can last 2–4 hours, depending on the dosage, although behavioral changes may continue for many hours. The undesired effects of cannabis intoxication includes impaired concentration, anterograde amnesia, motor incoordination, anxiety, paranoia, illusions. These adverse effects are usually self-limiting.

Symptoms of cannabis withdrawal are primarily psychological which includes irritability, anxiety and impaired sleep. No specific pharmacological agent is approved for management of cannabis dependence. Benzodiazepines (e.g., diazepam) may help to calm highly anxious users. The default management approach for cannabis withdrawal is supportive counselling, accurate information and appropriate planning.

Sedative, Hypnotic, and Anxiolytic use Disorder: Pharmacological Treatment

Sedative, hypnotic, and anxiolytic intoxication and withdrawal vary slightly from drug to drug. The withdrawal symptoms may be more intense with the shorter-acting drugs (e.g., alprazolam) and more prolonged with the longer-acting ones (e.g., diazepam).

Clinical features of intoxication include lethargy, impaired mental functioning, poor memory, irritability, self-neglect, emotional disinhibition, slurred speech, ataxia, and impaired coordination. With higher dosages, death can result from respiratory depression.

Abrupt drug discontinuation leads to emergence of withdrawals in the form of anxiety, restlessness, a feeling of apprehension, tremors, weakness, nausea and vomiting, orthostatic hypotension, sweating and other signs of autonomic hyperarousal. Seizures can develop in the course of withdrawal. Thus, withdrawal needs to be carefully monitored. Management consists of very slow taper of the drug over days or even weeks. Alternatively, patients are switched to long acting benzodiazepines such as diazepam, the dose of which can gradually be tapered.

Stimulant use Disorder: Pharmacological Treatment

Stimulants include dextroamphetamine, methylphenidate, methamphetamine, cocaine, and several other substances that share similar pharmacological activity.

Stimulant intoxication is characterized by autonomic hyperarousal, psychomotor agitation or retardation, muscular weakness, respiratory depression, chest pain or cardiac arrhythmias, confusion, seizures, dyskinesias, dystonias or paranoia. Cocaine intoxication also has the potential to induce tactile hallucinations (e.g., "coke bugs"). Serious medical complications include acute myocardial infarction due to coronary artery constriction and anoxic brain damage due to cocaine-induced seizures.

Because intoxication is generally self-limiting, no specific treatment is necessary. Benzodiazepines can be used to treat agitation or anxiety.

Cessation or reduction of a stimulant drug can lead to symptoms of withdrawal commonly referred to as a "crash." Symptoms include fatigue and depression, nightmares, headache, profuse sweating, muscle cramps, and hunger. Symptoms usually peak in 2–4 days. Intense dysphoria can occur, peaking between 48 and 72 hours after the last dose of the stimulant. Initial treatment is supportive and symptomatic management is done for withdrawal.

No medications have been shown to be consistently effective in treating stimulant dependence.

Hallucinogen-Related Disorders: Pharmacological Treatment

The clinical presentations of **hallucinogen** intoxication include problematic behavioral or psychological changes (e.g., marked anxiety or depression, ideas of reference, paranoid ideation, impaired judgment), disorientation, confusion, delusions, a catatonic-like syndrome, perceptual changes occurring in a state of full wakefulness and alertness (e.g., subjective intensification of perceptions, depersonalization, derealization, illusions, hallucinations, synesthesias) that developed during, or shortly after, hallucinogen use. "Bad trips" occasionally occur, in which patients become markedly anxious or paranoid. Features of autonomic hyperarousal may also be present. Another undesirable outcome is the flashback, a brief re-experiencing of the drug's effects in situations unrelated to taking the drug. The disorder is usually self-limiting, and treatment is generally supportive.

Although there is no known withdrawal syndrome for hallucinogens, benzodiazepines have been used to help calm users who experience an adverse reaction when "talking them down" (i.e., explaining that their reaction is due to the drug and providing reassurance) does not work.

Inhalant use Disorder: Pharmacological Treatment

Inhalants are CNS depressants and produce intoxication similar to that of alcohol but of shorter duration. Effects can last 5–45 minutes and include feelings of excitation, disinhibition, and euphoria. Adverse effects include dizziness, slurred speech, and ataxia. Inhalants also may induce an acute delirium characterized by impaired concentration and disorientation. Hallucinations and delusions have been reported with their use. Other effects include loss of appetite, lateral nystagmus, hypoactive reflexes, and double vision. At higher dosages, patients may become stuporous or comatose. Inhalants do not cause a specific withdrawal syndrome.

Tobacco (Nicotine) use Disorder: Pharmacological Treatment

Nicotine withdrawal usually begins within 1 hour after the last cigarette is smoked and peaks within 24 hours. Withdrawal may last weeks or months and consists of nicotine craving, irritability, anxiety, restlessness, and decreased heart rate. Weight gain and depression often follow smoking cessation.

Because the consequences of tobacco use are so potentially harmful, all physicians have a responsibility to urge their patients not to use tobacco products and to assist patients who do use them to quit.

Pharmacotherapies for smoking cessation include:

- Nicotine replacement therapy (NRT) in the form of nicotine transdermal patches and nicotine-containing gum, lozenges, sprays, sublingual strips and inhalers. The aim of NRT in those stopping smoking is to assist the transition from cigarette smoking to complete abstinence. This is achieved by temporarily replacing some of the nicotine obtained from tobacco cigarettes with NRT products and minimising nicotine withdrawal symptoms and the motivation to smoke.
- Antidepressants: Bupropion, nortriptyline
- Varenicline - It is a selective nicotinic acetylcholinergic receptor partial agonist and mimics the action of nicotine
- Others: clonidine

The combination of nicotine-replacement patches or gum with bupropion or varenicline may work even better.

While pharmacological treatment is mainstay of management of substance use disorders, addition of psychosocial therapies to medicines usually results in better outcome than medicines alone.

PSYCHOSOCIAL APPROACHES FOR TREATMENT

Psychosocial interventions are important aspects of addiction treatment, exercised to achieve various management goals such as termination or reduction of substance use, make personal and lifestyle changes, and engage in long-term recovery. The intervention type and intensity vary depending on the severity of the substance use problem and target behavior.

Structured brief advice and **Brief interventions** (BI) are used for hazardous or harmful substance use. BI assists in identification of a real or potential problem and motivate an individual to do something about it. It involves **motivational interviewing,** which is a non-judgmental and non-confrontational technique that attempts to address the specific issues that people are facing at any particular stage. The strategy seeks to prompt individuals to think differently about their use of substances and ultimately consider what might be gained through change.

The key features in Brief Intervention can be summarized using the acronym **FRAMES**:

Feedback: Personally relevant feedback after assessment such as on individual's drug use

Responsibility: Emphasis that it is the responsibility of the user to change

Advice: Non-judgmental advice on strategies for change

Menu of options: Alternate strategies and solutions available for each problem faced

Empathy: Warm, reflective and understanding approach

Self-efficacy: Encouraging the patient's confidence that change is possible

In tertiary care settings, more complex therapies like **family and marital therapy** and **network therapy** may be carried out to promote sobriety and drug free healthy life style. Other common tasks are building an improved client-counselor relationship, therapeutic alliance and improved communication with the patient and his/ her relatives. Such negotiated treatment to enhance motivation is very effective to improve treatment compliance.

Achieving permanent abstinence is a slow process. Patients go through short periods of abstinence and a reduction in drug consumption before becoming totally drug free. Considerable patience is required on part of the patient, family members and the treating team in the process of treatment.

Once the patient becomes drug free the goal shifts to maintaining the drug free status. **Relapse Prevention,** a psychological technique involves strategies, which help the patient to maintain the necessary changes in their drug free lives over time. The patient is made to understand that relapse is a process and lapsing to occasional drug use does not mean treatment failure. Family support is encouraged. Patient is also taught to identify high-risk relapse factors and social pressures of drug use, and trained to employ strategies to deal with them.

Psychotherapeutic interventions
- Motivational enhancement therapy
- Cognitive behavioral therapy/relapse prevention therapy
- Twelve-step facilitation therapy
- Network therapy
- Group and family therapies
- Contingency management

Other intervention modalities include **Self Help Approach**, where, people with similar problems unite to form "self help" groups for mutual help. These groups are voluntary and self-sufficient and provide mutual assistance to all its members. Self help groups like "Alcoholic Anonymous" (AA) and "Narcotic Anonymous" (NA) have congregations in most cities. Additionally, 'self-help' groups for family members, friends and children of drug and alcohol users have been developed. In **Social Correctional Approach**, drug and alcohol abuse is seen as a social deviance and residential programmes are offered as a correctional method. **Therapeutic Community** (TC) is the most well-known of the approaches offered under this concept. The effectiveness of Self Help Approaches or **Therapeutic Community** has not been conclusively demonstrated.

Basics in Psychosomatic Medicine 20

Elvin Lukose • Heena Merchant Pandit

PSYCHODYNAMIC THEORIES

Psycho analytic circles explained unexplained somatic or 'hysterical' symptoms as somatic equivalents or symbolic substitute for the expression of an unconscious conflict. Symptoms affect organs innervated by the voluntary motor or sensory nervous system act that as physiological channels to discharge the damned up psychic energy arising from the psychic tension.

Franz Alexander modified the idea by claiming symptoms to be the end result of certain specific unconscious conflicts driving its consequent behavior and perpetuating the accompanying characteristic physiological states.

Helen Dunbar and Meyer Freidman observed a relationship between personality traits and physical disorders like coronary heart disease.

The manifestation and choice of symptom by the underlying conflict could be the result of cultural influences on use of somatic language to express emotional distress defined as 'somatothymia'.

PSYCHOPHYSIOLOGICAL THEORIES

Walter Cannon and Harold Wolff scientifically demonstrated the physiological impact of emotions on the autonomic nervous system after studying the effect of emotional arousal on the gastric acid output. Hans Seyle provided the concept of 'General adaptation Syndrome' which elucidated the role of stress hormones in psychophysiological states. Following exposure to a chronic stressor

SYSTEMS THEORY

Georg Engel derived the *'biopsychosocial model'* and along with Zbigniew Lipowski formulated the causation of a psychosomatic illness as influenced by genetics, external (ecological, infectious, cultural, environmental), internal (emotional), somatic and constitutional factors.

TYPES OF CLINICAL PROBLEMS IN PSYCHOSOMATIC MEDICINE

- **Psychiatric symptoms secondary to a Medical condition**

  Delirium, Depression in SLE and Hypothyroidism etc.

- **Psychiatric symptoms as a reaction to medical condition or treatments**

  Pre-operative anxiety, depression secondary to amputation etc.

- **Psychiatric complications of medical conditions and treatments**

  Depression due to beta-blockers, psychotic features secondary to steroids etc.

- **Psychological factors precipitating medical symptoms**

  Somatoform disorders

- **Medical complications of psychiatric conditions or treatment**

  Serotonin Syndrome, Neuroleptic Malignant Syndrome etc.

- **Medical and Psychiatric disorders occurring independently in the same course**

  Wernicke's encephalopathy in Schizophrenia, Depression in transplant cases etc.

PSYCHOSOMATIC DISORDERS

1. Somatic Symptom Disorder
2. Illness Anxiety Disorder
3. Psychological factors affecting other Medical Conditions
4. Factitious Disorder

Somatic Symptom Disorder

Previously known as Hypochondriasis.
Somatic Symptom Disorder is characterized by preoccupation with the fears of suffering or holding a non-delusional idea of having a serious illness based on the patient's misinterpretation of somatic symptoms (one or more) for a duration of 6 or more months. Prevalence is 4-6 %.

Etiology

- Somatic symptom disorder consists of a heightened awareness of one's bodily sensations accompanied by anxiety regarding the same.
- Frequently seen as a part of somatic complaints in 80% of patients with depression and anxiety disorders.
- Psychodynamic explanations include experience of insurmountable conflicts and stress leading to diversion of psychic energy and displacement onto the body and developing a 'sick' role to avoid or escape the problematic situation or a method of 'atonement' for subconscious guilt.
- Patients are usually resistant to reassurances by doctors form clinical examination and laboratory investigations. Frequent engagement in multiple visits to doctors of different specialties and requesting unnecessary investigations and procedures is seen.
- The accompanying anxiety is often debilitating and interferes with socio-occupational functioning warranting psychiatric intervention. Must be differentiated from delusional disorder or other psychotic disorders wherein the patient may hold onto the idea of having an illness with a delusional intensity.

Treatment

- Antidepressants for underlying depressive or anxiety features.
- Psychotherapies (CBT) to identify maladaptive schemes and developing healthy cognitive schemes and minimal engagement in the 'sick role'.
- Education of treating physicians and nursing staff to avoid counter-transference and dismissal of patient's complaints.
- Doctors should not ignore any real objective evidence of an illness but at the same time, refrain from conducting unnecessary and ambiguous tests and procedures.

Illness Anxiety Disorder

Illness Anxiety Disorder is characterized by preoccupation with being sick or experience of some illness. Also includes patients with a particular illness, experiencing with fears or anxiety of complication or extreme outcomes, out of proportion to the illness. It differs from Somatic Symptom Disorder by the presence of few or no particular well-defined somatic symptoms.

Two variants include *Care-seeking* type and *Care-avoidant* type.

Etiology

- It is similar to Somatic Symptom Disorder in that there is history of insurmountable conflicts and stress leading to diversion of psychic energy and displacement onto the body and developing a 'sick' role to avoid or escape the problematic situation.
- Frequently seen after witnessing or hearing about death or occurrence of a major illness in family members, peers or neighborhood.
- The accompanying anxiety is often debilitating and interferes with socio-occupational functioning warranting psychiatric intervention.

Treatment

- Antidepressants for underlying depressive or anxiety features
- Psychotherapy to identify maladaptive schemes, developing healthy cognitive schemes, confronting inter-personal conflicts and encouraging healthy coping behavior.
- Education of treating physicians and nursing staff to avoid counter-transference and dismissal of patient's complaints.
- Doctors should not dismiss any real objective evidence of an illness but at the same time, refrain from conducting unnecessary and ambiguous tests and procedures.

Functional Neurological Symptom Disorder

Also known as Conversion Disorder, is characterized by the presence of deficits in voluntary motor and sensory functions which suggest another medical condition however, are triggered by stressors. Symptoms are not deliberate or feigned like in factitious disorder and malingering.

Prevalence rates vary from 11 to 300 in 100000 with female predominance (F:M=2:1).

Often seen as a comorbid illness to depression, anxiety disorders and schizophrenia. Personality disorders that frequently accompany conversion disorder include histrionic and passive-dependent type.

Etiology

- Excessive corticofugal output that causes a negative feedback to the brainstem reticular formation resulting in the inhibition of the patient's awareness of bodily sensations leading to neurological deficits observed clinically.
- *Motor symptoms* include involuntary movements like tremors and tics and deficit based symptoms like paralysis, aphonia, gait disturbances (astasia-abasia) etc.
- *Sensory symptoms* include blindness, visual field deficits, anesthesia and deafness. Some visceral symptoms include psychogenic vomiting, globus hystericus and autonomic symptoms like swooning and syncope.

Treatment

- Antidepressants for underlying depression or anxiety disorders.

- Encouraging patients to confront and handle the conflictual situation through psychotherapy can help in removal of secondary gains like relief from responsibilities or 'sick role' behavior.

Factitious Disorder

Historically known as *Munchhausen syndrome*, is characterized by deliberate attempts to simulate, exaggerate or induce symptoms in oneself or other with the motive of procuring medical attention to oneself or the other.

When symptoms are in the other, the disorder is known as *Factitious disorder by proxy*. Differs from malingering in the absence of a financial gain or evasion of responsibilities. Common signs and symptoms simulated include hemoptysis, hematuria, excoriations on the skin by self, ingestion of insulin or adrenaline to mimic hypoglycemia and hypertension, use of laxatives to induce diarrhea, use of anticoagulants to induce bleeding, use of fake blood to simulate vaginal trauma or hemorrhage, premature rupture of membranes etc.

Female predominance with F:M=3:1.

Etiology

- Psychosocial factors include past history of abuse, repeated or chronic hospitalization following which the admission into a hospital or the visit to the doctor is used as an escape from a traumatic experience or stressful home or familial conditions (rejecting/abusive parents).
- Every visit or admission to the hospitalization is seen as an attempt to recreate fulfilment of dependency needs and acceptance.
- An affinity for the care provided by the nursing staff, caretakers and attention provided by the doctors along with a sense of validation is noted as the core cognitive scheme in factitious disorder.
- Two clinical types are factitious disorder *with predominantly physical signs and symptoms* and one *with predominantly psychological signs and symptoms*. Clinically, a combination of both is also observed.
- *Factitious disorder imposed on the other (by proxy)* is where the patient produces signs and symptoms in another person who is either related to the patient or under the former's care. Most common situations involve a mother (patient) with a child (victim).
- Psychodynamic explanation in Factitious disorder imposed on the other (by proxy) include relief from the 'caretaker role' and assuming the 'sick role' through frequent hospitalizations.
- Psychometric testing on MMPI may show 'fake bad' wherein the patient deliberately provides false information about the severity of one's disturbance. Patients may have an associated personality disorder like histrionic and anti-social personality disorder. Patients with schizophrenia will hold delusional beliefs of being ill in the presence of other psychotic features like though disorder or hallucinations.

Treatment

- Active pursuit of a prompt risk to reduce mortality and morbidity; minimal use of tests and invasive procedures; education of staff about counter-transference and dismissal attitude towards patients; persuading for psychiatric intervention; diagnosis and management of underlying psychiatric diseases; appointment of a second party (guardian) for taking medical decisions.

- Child welfare services or legal intervention maybe required in case of victims who are in pediatric age group along with hospitalization for isolation and observation

PSYCHOLOGICAL FACTORS AFFECTING OTHER MEDICAL CONDITIONS

GASTRO-INTESTINAL SYSTEM

Functional Gastro-intestinal Disorders

- FGID includes an array of gastro-intestinal disorders that involve a close interplay of anxiety, stress and heightened physiological responsiveness of the gastro-intestinal tract.
- Role of the lateral hypothalamus, limbic system and downstream sympathetic and parasympathetic autonomic responses have been studied.
- Essentially, the limbic system and its modulation of the vagus are considered to be an emotions-gut pathway of response. Following are the various FGIDs

Functional Upper GID

a) Globus
b) Non-cardiac chest pain
c) Functional heart-burn
d) Functional dysphagia

Functional Gastro-duodenal Disorder

a) Functional Dyspepsia
b) Aerophagia
c) Functional Abdominal Pain
d) Functional biliary pain

Functional Bowel Disorder

a) Functional Diarrhea
b) Functional constipation
c) Irritable Bowel Syndrome
d) Functional Incontinence
e) Functional anorectal pain

Peptic Ulcer Disease

- PUD results in burning epigastric or gnawing pain 1-3 hours after meals and involves the stomach or the duodenum.
- Causation involves an imbalance between the aggravating factors (diet factors, smoking, alcohol etc.) and the mucosal defense barriers affecting the bicarbonate buffer thus culminating in excessive acid secretion and mucosal damage.
- The conflict between one's over-dependency and an overdriven competitive aggression motivated by a subconscious need for independence was hypothesised by Franz Alexander to be the starting point in the behavioral patterns that result in peptic ulcer disease.
- Psychological factors include stressful life events or maladaptive lifestyles that include erratic eating habits and substance abuse (smoking, alcohol etc.).

Ulcerative Colitis and Crohn's Disease

- UD and CD are inflammatory diseases affecting predominantly the large intestine and the small intestine respectively.
- Symptoms include diarrhea, abdominal pain and weight loss with extracolonic manifestations in UC being uveitis, skin diseases and biliary involvement (sclerosing cholangitis).
- Psychological factors include high dependency needs and some studies have shown a high rate of panic disorders preceding the GIT manifestations in cases of CD. However no correlation has been established successfully in cases of UC.

CARDIOVASCULAR SYSTEM

Coronary Artery Disease

- One of the leading causes of death in industrialised countries, coronary artery disease has been associated with risk factors like substance abuse, stress and maladaptive lifestyles.
- Meyer Friedman's *Type A (Coronary) personality* which includes low threshold for aggression-hostility and frustration, competitiveness, urgency and ambitious outlook has been observed to raise risk to twofold for CAD and its associated mortality.
- Of all the features, 'hostility' has shown to have the highest contribution to the mortality. Hostility results in a physiological state of increased peripheral catecholamines and reduced modulation of heart rate by the parasympathetic nervous system.
- Higher frequency of interpersonal conflicts and anger lead to an excess sympathetic overdrive that gradually down-regulates the adrenergic receptors through negative feedback.
- Increase in consumption of fat and fast foods coupled with reduced ambulation at work and substance abuse due to high work demands lead to a maladaptive lifestyle changes that lead down to metabolic dysregulation and hyperlipidemia thus increasing the risk of CAD.

Sudden Cardiac Death

- Acute emotional stress can precipitate or exaggerate an underlying cardiac arrhythmia and increase the risk of fatal cardiac events in known cases of CAD leading to sudden cardiac death.
- Depression and anxiety increase the risk of sudden cardiac death.
- Sinus Node Dysfunction and Atrio-Ventricular conduction disorders are more susceptible to emotional and sudden stressful influences.

RESPIRATORY SYSTEM

Bronchial Asthma

- Asthma is a chronic illness of the airways characterized by paroxysmal attacks of bronchial spasm and narrowing of the tracheo-bronchial tract clinically experienced as coughing, breathlessness and chest tightness and auscultatory findings of wheezing.
- The symptoms at its peak intensity can result in a *'fear of losing breath'* which further triggers asthmatic attacks and anxiety responsible for high rates of hospitalisation and asthma-associated mortality.
- Depending on the personality profiles, asthmatic patients show a differential use of medications and attitude towards treatment. Patients who show personality traits like high neuroticism, increased sensitivity to rejection and emotional lability lead to greater and faster escalation of doses and increased durations of hospitalisation.
- Approximately 30% of asthmatics have a comorbid panic disorder or agoraphobia with family members suffering from mood disorders, substance use and personality disorders.

Chronic Obstructive Pulmonary Disease

- COPD is characterized by chronic inflammation of the respiratory tract resulting in impaired compliance and progressive fibrosis of the lungs.

- Predominantly found in chronic smokers, COPD has high propensity towards lung cancer.
- Approximately, 16-34 % of patients with COPD have anxiety disorders with 8-24% suffering from panic disorder.
- Patients also experience a poor quality of life due to interference with sleep; chronicity of the illness and side effects of bronchodilators and adrenergic (α_2) agonists.

Hyperventilation Syndrome

- Hyperventilation syndrome consists of symptoms of rapid and deep breathing for several minutes gradually leading to secondary symptoms of tingling sensations in extremities, light-headedness and giddiness and in some cases, syncope.
- Excessive loss of CO_2 results in respiratory alkalosis and cerebral vasoconstriction.
- Hyperventilation may trigger or exacerbate attacks of asthma, chronic obstructive pulmonary disease, arrhythmia or ischemic heart disease, epilepsy, vocal dysfunction and musculoskeletal disorders.

ENDOCRINE SYSTEM

Hypothyroidism

- Hypothyroidism results from levels of thyroid hormones and elevated thyroid-stimulating hormone (TSH).
- Approximately 40% of clinically hypothyroid patients have significant signs and symptoms of depression like depressed mood, lethargy and impaired cognitive function.
- *Treatment-resistant depression* has been shown to respond to thyroid hormone supplementation without laboratory investigation revealing evidence of thyroid malfunction. Subclinical hypothyroidism in a patient with major depressive disorder is a frequent cause of refractoriness to antidepressant treatment.
- Cognitive decline due to thyroid deficiency may hint towards dementia and is one of the reversible causes of dementia.
- Myxedema madness or *myxedema psychosis* is a psychiatric syndrome of paranoia, auditory hallucinations and occasionally, thought disorders.
- Studies have shown that 5% to 15% of myxedematous patients have some form of psychosis.

Hyperthyroidism

- Hyperthyroidism results from excess synthesis of thyroid hormones.
- Physical symptoms of hyperthyroidism like increased heart-rate, palpitations, tremulousness, excessive sweating and elevated blood pressure can mimic anxiety attacks and misdiagnosed as a primary psychiatric disorder.
- Psychotic manifestations like paranoid ideation, auditory and visual hallucinations.
- Additional psychiatric features include nervousness, fatigue, dysphoria, hypomania and delirium.
- Due to the heightened psychomotor activity, presence of pressured speech, euphoria and mood lability, the mood features may frequently be misdiagnosed as mania although both can occur in the same patient.

- No sufficient correlation has been found between hyperthyroidism and manic episodes.

Diabetes Mellitus

- Diabetes Mellitus is a disorder of glucose metabolism and is associated with impaired metabolism of lipid and protein due to imbalance in insulin and glucose demands of the body.
- It can often occur secondary to use of atypical anti-psychotics in psychiatric disorders due to unknown mechanisms.
- Psychiatric symptoms occur either secondary to fluctuations in glucose levels or as a reaction to the complications of diabetes mellitus.
- Hypoglycemia causes anxiety like symptoms of palpitations, sweating, jitteriness and light-headedness and at extreme, causes confusion, aggression and delirium that may culminate in seizures.
- Hyperglycemia may result in mood lability, psychotic features and delirium.
- Difficulty to accept the long term treatment often results in poor treatment adherence and diabetes self-management. These psychosocial problems eventually develop into depressive or other psychological disorders that are associated with poor self-care behavior, poor metabolic outcomes, increased mortality, functional limitations, increased health-care cost, loss of productivity, and reduced quality of life.
- Distinct from clinical depression, *Diabetes distress (DD)* has been defined as the unique, often hidden, emotional burdens and worries that a patient experiences when they are managing diabetes.
- Emotional dysregulation and impulsivity may lead to over-eating or substance abuse leading to uncontrolled diabetes most commonly in Type 1 Diabetes.

Cushing's Syndrome

- Cushing's Syndrome arises from excessive adrenocortical activity either due to a primary adrenal secreting tumor or secondary to excessive stimulation by ACTH from the pituitary also known as *Cushing's disease*.
- Physical signs and symptoms of Cushing's syndrome include '*moon facies*', truncal obesity, osteoporosis, easy bruisability, gastritis, hypertension etc.
- Hypercortisolism shows mood features similar to depression in approximately 75% of the patient population with females more commonly affected than men.
- Additional features include emotional lability, irritability, anxiety attacks and hypersensitivity to stimuli.
- Truncal obesity and moon facies frequently lead to body image disturbances, social embarrassment and self esteem issues.
- Psychotic features may range from hyper vigilance to an extreme syndrome with paranoia and hallucinations in 5-15 % cases with greater frequency of psychosis and mania seen in iatrogenic hypercortisolism.
- Elevated cortisol leads to atrophy of the hippocampus and subsequent cognitive dysfunction presenting with concentration problems in 83% patients.
- Change in personality include elevation on Neuroticism dimension and is negatively correlated with improvement in cortisol levels.

Hyperprolactinemia

- Excess prolactin release could occur due to a pituitary tumor or secondary to use of certain medications and hypothyroidism.
- Elevated TSH in hypothyroidism increases release of prolactin while anti-psychotics decrease Dopamine's inhibitory influence on prolactin and result in hyperprolactinemia.
- Typical or first generation anti-psychotics and atypical anti-psychotics like Amisulpride, Risperidone and Paliperidone have more propensities to cause hyperprolactinemia. Other drugs that may cause hyperprolactinemia include certain antidepressants (SSRIs), OC pills, Propranolol and estrogens.

SKIN

Excoriation disorder

- Also known *Psychogenic pruritus*, excoriation disorder consists of lesions resulting from deliberate scratching or picking.
- Lesions may arise either on a fresh skin surface or at the edges of a pre-existing wound and are found in areas easily accessible and within the reach of the patient's hands.
- The behavior may result in response to an itch or an uncontrollable obsessive urge or tactile hallucinations.
- Some patients perceive tension relieving effects from deliberate excoriation.

Atopic Dermatitis

- Atopic dermatitis is a chronic skin disorder consisting of erythematous and maculopapular rash often exacerbated during anxious and depressed states due to heightened itch perception and amplification of urge to scratch.
- Children with behavioral disorders also show more severity compared to rest of the population.

Psoriasis

- Psoriasis is chronic skin disorder consisting of lesions with silver and glossy scales with underlying homogenous erythema.
- Stress especially arising from patient's interpersonal sensitivity is a well documented trigger of psoriatic exacerbations with each worsening leading to cosmetic disfigurement and decreased quality of life.
- Personality disorders associated with psoriasis include schizoid, avoidant and obsessive-compulsive personality disorders.
- Severity of illness has been correlated with patient's depressive symptoms and self-harm wishes. Alcohol dependence is a poor prognostic factor in the management of psoriasis.

Urticaria

- Urticaria or generalized itching has been seen to exacerbate during stressful life events.
- The vasodilation due to secretion of vasoactive intestinal peptide and substance P has been posited to be responsible for the development of wheals.

Hyperhidrosis

- Hyperhidrosis or excessive sweat secretion has been noted to be one of the somatic manifestations of anxiety resulting from an exaggerated arousal of the autonomic nervous system.

- Treatment with anti-depressants and adrenergic antagonists like beta-blockers, in addition to tropical applicants has shown improvement in the overall outcome.

MUSCULOSKELETAL SYSTEM

Sysytemic Lupus Erythematosus

- SLE is an autoimmune connective tissue disorder characterized by inflammation affecting multiple organ systems like skin, kidneys, joints, blood vessels and the central nervous system in a chronic fashion with acute exacerbations culminating in organ failure.
- Psychiatric manifestations consist predominantly of depression and psychosis.
- Depression may arise due to the chronicity and the lower quality of life due to the illness while psychosis usually implies CNS involvement or a reaction to the use of steroid in the treatment and management of episodes.

Rhematoid Arthritis

- RA is predominantly a disorder of the musculoskeletal system with inflammation of joints, disfigurement and chronic pain.
- Psychological triggers like stress impair the immune system resulting in worsening of symptoms.
- Most common psychiatric disorder associated with RA is depression occurring in almost 20% of the population and lowers the pain perception of patients leading to greater disability, frequent hospitalizations and lower quality of life.

Fibromyalgia

- Fibromyalgia is a musculoskeletal pain syndrome arising from stiffness in soft tissue like muscles, ligaments and tendons.
- Most affected region is the cervico-thoracic region with palpable nodes of localized tenderness termed as 'trigger points' over the trapezius and surrounding neck muscles.
- Pain and resultant fatigue can get severe enough to interfere with sleep, activities of daily living and impact efficiency at work. It also accompanies chronic fatigue syndrome and somatoform disorders.
- Psychiatric treatment with adrenergic tricyclic anti-depressants and sertraline has shown modest improvement in the overall pain perception and quality of life.

HEADACHE

Migraine

- Migraine is a vascular type of headache characterized by attacks of unilateral headache with throbbing quality associated with photophobia and phonophobia and nausea.
- Aura symptoms of scintillating scotoma, altered shape and size perceptions and fortification spectra may precede the attack especially in classical migraine.
- Additional features include giddiness, imbalance, and dysphoria and speech dysfluency during attacks.
- Role of CGRP (Calcitonin- G –related peptide) in the functional disturbance of cranial circulation has been suspected.
- Dysphoria ranging from emotional

irritability to rage can precede hours to days prior to an impending attack.

- Anxiety, depression and conflict situations causing high stress can trigger or worsen the episode.
- Personality profiles with high Neuroticism with more perfectionism and controlling behavior is seen more common in the suffering population.
- Psychiatric treatment with tricyclic anti-depressants and psychotherapy for controlling perception of stressful situations can help in reducing intensity and frequency of attacks.

Cluster Headache

- Similar in presentation to Migraine, it has additional features of unilateral ptosis, miosis, sweating and rhinorrhea.
- Because of the dermatomal nature of the symptoms, etiology of a trigeminal hypersensitivity has been suspected.
- Psychological triggers similar to migraine have been noted to apply in cluster headache.

Tension Headache

- Tension Headache is considered to be a muscular type of headache.
- It is seen due to prolonged contraction of muscles leading to altered cranial circulation and ischemia. Unlike migraine, tension headache is bilateral and has a dull quality.
- The patient often perceives a 'band tied around the head' kind of feeling with tenderness to touch and aggravation on placing the head on any surface.
- Around 80% of attacks are seen during periods of emotional stress and depression.
- Psychological triggers are similar to the ones noted in migraine and cluster headaches.

TREATMENT OF PSYCHOSOMATIC DISORDERS

Relaxation Therapy

- Relaxation therapy utilizes a wilful muscular relaxation to counter the physiological tension accompanying anxious somatic or painful states.
- The *Jacobson's method (JPMR)* involves training based on progressively tensing and relaxing groups of muscles in a controlled fashion to the point that the participant develops a 'muscle sense' and can efficiently put oneself in a 'relaxed' state when called for.
- Relaxation breathing exercises are useful for panic disorder, hyperventilation, performance anxiety and as a part of Lamaze method for women in labour.
- *Benson's concentration meditation* method is a variant of transcendental meditation that elicits the relaxation response– a state of reduced sympathetic arousal. An uncontrolled prospective study has shown a reduction in physician visits for patients with chronic pain.
- *Mindfulness meditation*, developed by Kabat-Zinn, is a nonjudgmental moment-to-moment awareness cultivated through sitting meditation and detachment from thoughts through an objective stance.

Biofeedback

- Biofeedback involves a bi-directional exercise by which the patient learns to control his physiological parameters like breathing rate, pulse, blood pressure, muscle tension, skin temperature etc. through a visual or auditory feedback from an array of instruments attached to the patient.

- Instruments used are electro-myogram (EMG), electro-cardiogram (ECG), electro-encephalogram (EEG), galvanic skin response (GSR) gauge, pulse oxymeter (pulse), blood pressure cuffs (BP) and thermistors for skin temperatures.
- Physiologically, there is lowering of sympathetic activation and self-regulation of arterial smooth muscle vasoconstriction activity. Hence, biofeedback has been seen promising in controlling migraine headaches, tension headaches and peripheral vascular phenomena (Raynaud's phenomenon).
- Combined with relaxation therapy, feedback helps in management of insomnia, anxiety and somatic symptom disorders.

Hypnosis

- Hypnosis is a therapeutic tool used in manipulating imagination, imagery and attention to induce a trance state wherein release of symptoms and acceptance of new thoughts and feelings are facilitated to facilitate improvement.
- PET studies on patients in a hypnotic trance state have shown a redirection of blood flow to different brain regions according to suggestions given to the patient that result in relief in symptoms.
- Common indications involve cessation of smoking, eating disorders, conversion symptoms and chronic pain.
- *Gut-directed hypnotherapy* has been attempted in the treatment and management of Irritable Bowel Syndrome with modest results.

Stress Management

Stress management involves a series of behaviors directed towards monitoring stressors and its effects on the body.

Self-observation involves the patient keeping a record of the stressful events and situations during the course of the day, the accompanying emotions and the somatic complaints experiences secondary to them. It increases awareness about the relationship between one's physiology and mental processes thus providing opportunities of problem-solving and better insight into one's somatic complaints. *Cognitive restructuring* is a part of Cognitive Behavioral Therapy where attempts are made to modify one's maladaptive schemes that are causing symptoms to occur and persist; replacing them with new cognitive schemes thus breaking the link between the symptom and the triggering thoughts.

Yoga

Yoga therapy utilizes a meta-cognitive approach in which, through a self regulated detachment, one gains a reliable control over one's physiological functioning bringing about an equilibrium in the somatopsychic functioning of the individual.

Yogic approaches have been successfully used in the management of bronchial asthma, essential hypertension, mucus colitis, peptic ulcer, cervical spondylosis, chronic sinusitis, gastritis and rheumatism.

BIBLIOGRAPHY

1. Sadock BJ, Sadock VA. *Kaplan and Sadock's synopsis of psychiatry: Behavioral sciences/*

clinical psychiatry. Eleventh Edition. Lippincott Williams & Wilkins; 2016.

2. Tasman, A. E., Kay, J. E., Lieberman, J. A., First, M. B., & Maj, M. E. *Psychiatry*, Vols. 1-2. Wiley Blackwell, 2015
3. Kalra S, Jena BN, Yeravdekar R. Emotional and psychological needs of people with diabetes. *Indian journal of endocrinology and metabolism*. 2018 Sep;22(5):696.
4. Singh, A. N. "Role of yoga therapies in psychosomatic disorders." *International Congress Series*. Vol. 1287. Elsevier, 2006.
5. Rashbaum, Ira G., and John E. Sarno. "Psychosomatic concepts in chronic pain." *Archives of physical medicine and rehabilitation* 84 (2003): S76-S80.

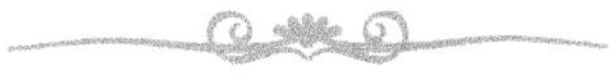

21 Personality Disorders

Chetan Vispute

INTRODUCTION AND DEFINITION:

Personality is defined as a complex pattern of deeply embedded psychological characteristics that are expressed by an individual in all the areas of psychological functioning and determines a person's behavior. The personality of a person allows the others to predict how this person would react, feel or think in a particular situation. The word **personality** is derived from the Latin term **persona,** originally representing the theatre mask used by ancient drama artist. Personality is often used interchangeably with words like character and temperament. **Character** refers to characteristics acquired during upbringing and nurturing. **Temperament,** on the other hand, refers to a basic biological (nature) predisposition toward certain behaviors. **Personality traits** are overt and highlighted aspects of personality. **Personality disorders** refer to maladaptive and dysfunctional personality traits leading to socio-occupational impairment and distress to individual and surroundings.

DSM 5 states the following about personality disorders:

- Impairment in personality (self and interpersonal) functioning.
- The presence of pathological personality traits.
- The impairment in personality functioning and personality trait expression are not better understood as normative for the individual's developmental stage or socio-cultural environment.
- The impairment in personality functioning and the personality trait expression are stable across time and consistent across situations.
- Significant impairment in self (identity or self-direction) and interpersonal (empathy or intimacy) functioning.

Not attributed to:

- Direct physiological effects of a substance (e.g., a drug of abuse, medication).
- General medical condition (e.g., severe head trauma).

DSM-5 Classification of Personality Disorder:

1. Cluster A: Paranoid, Schizoid, Schizotypal
2. Cluster B: Antisocial, borderline, histrionic, narcissistic
3. Cluster C: Avoidant, dependent, obsessive compulsive disorder

Personality disorders are quite common, chronic and enduring with prevalence rate of **10 to 20 percent** in general population. **50 percent** of patients suffering from psychiatric disorders have some personality disorder as a comorbidity. Personality disorders are

ego-syntonic (i.e. acceptable to ego) and **alloplastic** (i.e., adapt by trying to alter the external environment rather than themselves). A person cannot be strictly classified into one particular type of personality disorder but can have multiple traits or types simultaneously co-existing with each other.

ETIOLOGY

1. **Genetic**: The genetic heritability is high for personality disorders as the concordance rate for personality disorder was higher amongst monozygotic twins than dizygotic twins even if reared separately. Cluster A personality disorders specifically schizotypal are more common in first degree relative of patients with schizophrenia. Mood disorders are quite common with cluster B personality disorders. Substance use disorders are common with Anti-social personality disorder. Somatization disorders are commonly associated with histrionic personality disorders. Depression is often co-morbid with borderline personality disorder. Cluster C personality disorders are also associated with anxiety and depressive disorders.
2. **Biological**: High levels of testosterone, estrone and 17-oestradiol are associated with impulsivity seen in patient with borderline and antisocial personality disorders. Low level of serotonin metabolite 5-hydroxyindoleacetic acid (5-HIAA) is associated with low mood, self-harm, suicidal behavior in patients with borderline personality disorder.
3. People with personality disorder are more likely to have childhood neglect and history of sexual abuse and trauma. Punitive and aversive parenting styles with low attachment can lead to development of personality disorder in adulthood.
4. **Psycho-analytic:** Fixation into particular stage of Freud's psychosexual development.

PARANOID PERSONALITY DISORDER

Hallmark: lack of trust and extreme suspiciousness

Prevalence: 0.5-2.5% of general population. More common in males

Clinical Features

1. Tendency to bear grudges even with close aides and family members.
2. Unjustified doubts about loyalty or trustworthiness of friends or associates.
3. Hidden demeaning or threatening meanings read into benign remarks or events.
4. Suspicious towards spouse's fidelity
5. A combative and tenacious sense of personal 'right' and tendency to experience excessive self-importance.
6. Preoccupation with unsubstantiated 'conspiratorial' explanations of events.

Differential Diagnosis

1. Schizophrenia & delusional disorders: Patient with paranoid personality disorder do not have formal thought disorder or auditory hallucination
2. Schizoid personality disorder: A person suffering from schizoid personality disorder is aloof and withdrawn
3. Borderline personality disorder: suspiciousness is transient in borderline personality disorder unlike persistent and pervasive in paranoid personality disorder.

Course and Prognosis

Paranoid personality disorder has chronic course and poor prognosis. Multiple change of jobs, interpersonal and marital problems are commonly seen with paranoid personality disorder.

Treatment

Response to the treatment is usually poor.

1. Supportive Psychotherapy:
2. Cognitive Behavior therapy:
3. Pharmacotherapy: Antipsychotic medication can help control episodes of aggression and agitation. Benzodiazepines can be of help to control anxiety

SCHIZOID PERSONALITY DISORDER

Hallmark: alone, aloof and socially withdrawn

Prevalence: 0.5-1.5% of general population. More common in males

Clinical Features

1. Emotional coldness, detachment or flattened affectivity.
2. Limited capacity to express either warm, tender feeling or anger towards others.
3. Prefer solitude, have few friends, low interest in sexual relationship
4. Marked unintentional insensitivity to prevailing social norms

Differential Diagnosis

1. Schizotypal personality disorder: Oddities and eccentricities are more marked in thought, behavior, communication when compared with schizoid personality disorder
2. Paranoid personality disorder: are more resentful, expressive and can be engaged in communication.
3. Avoidant personality disorder: develop anxiety and have strong desire to participate in social activities
4. Pervasive developmental disorder: are more socially withdrawn and have stereotypical behaviors
5. Schizophrenia: Present with first rank psychotic symptoms, delusions and hallucinations.

Course and Prognosis

Onset is seen during adolescence. Schizoid disorder runs a stable long course. Schizoid personality disorder is commonly seen in the first degree relatives of schizophrenia

Treatment

Response to the treatment is usually poor.

1. Supportive Psychotherapy:
2. Individual Psychotherapy and Group Therapy
3. Pharmacotherapy: Antipsychotic and antidepressant have very limited role in treatment

SCHIZOTYPAL PERSONALITY DISORDER

Hallmark: odd eccentric behavior

Prevalence: 3% of general population. More common in males

Clinical Features

1. Odd bizarre beliefs and magical thinking present
2. Ideas of reference are present

3. Odd sensation, Unusual perceptions and experiences
4. Eccentric appearance.
5. Paranoia and constricted affect.
6. Social withdrawal and fewer relationships

Differential Diagnosis

1. Schizophrenia and other psychotic disorder: Persistent delusions, hallucination and disorganised speech are absent. Psychotic symptoms are brief and transient if they occur in schizotypal personality disorder.
2. Paranoid and Schizoid personality disorder: odd eccentric behavior is absent in paranoid and schizoid personality disorder
3. Autistic spectrum disorders

Course and Prognosis

Schizotypal personality disorder has a chronic course and is believed to be on the schizophrenia spectrum disorder. It is linked to dopaminergic dysregulation and commonly seen in the relatives of schizophrenia patient. It is associated with increased risk of schizophrenia.

Treatment

1. Social Skills training
2. Pharmacotherapy: Antipsychotic have shown modest improvement in ideas of reference and bizarre belief.
3. Supportive psychotherapy

BORDERLINE PERSONALITY DISORDER

It is also known as emotionally unstable personality disorder in ICD 11. Patients suffering from borderline personality disorder stand on the border between neurosis and psychosis. It is most widely studied personality disorder from biological perspective

Hallmark: Emotionally unstable and impulsive

Prevalence: 1-2% of general population. More common in females

Etiology

1. **Biological:** Person with borderline personality disorder demonstrate abnormal dexamethasone suppression test result, decreased REM latency, decreased thyrotropin response, abnormal sensitivity to amphetamine and decreased CSF 5 HIAA (a metabolite of serotonin) levels. Borderline Personality disorder is more common in first degree relatives of patients with depression.
2. **Defence Mechanism: Splitting** – Adopting a polarised or extreme view of the world where people are either all good or bad and fail to see that each person has good and bad aspects. **Projective identification** – the patient unconsciously project a figure onto the other people.
3. Past history of neglect, trauma, sexual abuse is commonly associated.
4. History of marital discord between parents and dysfunctional family is seen
5. Lack of attachment in childhood leading to defective mentalisation i.e. limited capacity to depict feelings and thoughts in self and other people

Clinical Features

1. Lability of mood with episodes of anger outburst
2. Chronic sense of boredom and emptiness
3. High rejection sensitivity

4. Difficulty in maintaining stable interpersonal relationship
5. Irritable and quarrelsome nature
6. Fear of abandonment by near and dear ones
7. Repeated acts of self-harm are common
8. Disturbances in and uncertainty about self-image, aims and internal preferences
9. Brief and transient psychotic symptoms associated during the period of severe stress.

Differential Diagnosis

1. **Dependent personality disorder:** are less chaotic in affect regulation and be less impulsive.
2. **Antisocial personality disorder:** are callous and lack empathy
3. **Histrionic personality disorder:** want to be the center of attention but usually demonstrate less affective dysregulation, impulsivity.
4. **Narcissistic personality disorder:** People with borderline personality disorder see rejection as abandonment. People with narcissistic personality disorder feel that they are entitled to special treatment because of their special status.
5. **Depressive disorder:** People with borderline personality disorder may present with depression but people with depressive disorder do not demonstrate primitive defence mechanisms such as splitting or projective identification.
6. **Schizophrenia**: both borderline personality disorder and schizophrenia may present with psychotic symptoms. People with borderline personality disorder present with transient psychosis, lack of first rank symptoms, perceptual disturbances and lack of negative symptoms.
7. **Bipolar disorder:** People with borderline personality disorder refer mood swings to fluctuations in mood from normal to irritability without hypomanic or manic features.

Course and Prognosis

Borderline personality disorder runs a chronic course with chaotic interpersonal relationship in personal and professional life. Depression and substance use disorders are comorbid with borderline personality disorder

Treatment

1. Psychotherapy
2. Dialectical behavior therapy: to reduce deliberate self-harm and regulate emotional instability
3. Pharmacotherapy: Antipsychotic, antidepressant and mood stabilizers are used to target specific clinical symptoms causing socio-occupational impairment

ANTI-SOCIAL PERSONALITY DISORDER

Hallmark: Impulsive, callous and disregards for social rules and regulation

Prevalence: 0.5-2.5% of general population. More common in males

Clinical Features

1. Very manipulative, deceitful and callous individuals
2. Lack of feeling, guilt and remorse and sometimes derive pleasure in others suffering

3. This type is synonymous with criminals and conmen who have disregard for societal rules and obligation
4. Impulsivity, mood fluctuation, and hostility is high
5. Very low frustration tolerance
6. Engage in high risk taking behaviors with disregard for safety of self and others
7. They often blame others for their impulsive acts and rationalise their reckless behavior.
8. High novelty seeking, low harm avoidance, low reward dependence

Differential Diagnosis

1. **Criminal behavior:** is associated with focal temporary illegal behavior for personal gain while other maladaptive patterns of antisocial personality disorder are absent.
2. **Bipolar Mood Disorder:** Hypomania and manic phases are absent
3. **Substance use disorder:** Can be a co-morbid condition with the Antisocial personality disorder

Course and Prognosis

Onset is usually seen adolescent age group with history of oppositional defiant and conduct traits. Depression and substance use disorders are associated throughout the course of disorder.

Treatment

1. Pharmacotherapy: Mood stabilizer to control impulsivity and mood swing. Antidepressant SSRI medication to treat co-morbid depression and anxiety. Stimulants are used to treat ADHD symptoms in adolescents and adults.
2. Cognitive and behavioral interventions to decrease high risk taking and impulsive behaviors.

HISTRIONIC PERSONALITY DISORDER

Hallmark: Flamboyant and attention seeking behavior

Prevalence: 2-3% of general population. Prevalence is equal in male and female population

Clinical Features

1. Feels uncomfortable and anxious if he/she is not the center of attention
2. Easily becomes irritable and throws tantrums if they are not center of attention
3. Over concerned about physical appearance and external characteristic
4. Both the sexes are over seductive, impressive and willing to give detail history to examiner
5. Highly suggestible and easily influenced by others.
6. Major defense mechanism used are repression and dissociation.
7. Self-dramatization and exaggerated emotional expression.
8. They seek instant gratification and approvals.
9. May act out impulsively and are gullible.
10. Depression and somatization are common comorbidities with histrionic personality disorder

Differential Diagnosis

1. **Bipolar Mood Disorder:** Manic symptoms are absent in histrionic personality disorder

2. **Somatization Disorder**
3. **Narcissistic personality disorder:** are very sensitive by humiliation when they are the center of attention.
4. **Borderline personality disorder:** Impulsive, rejection sensitive and sense of abandonment

Course and Prognosis

Onset is seen during late adolescence and youth. Symptom severity decreases with increase in age and maturity. They have less functional impairment when compared to other personality disorders.

Treatment

1. **Psychotherapy**: Psychoanalytically oriented psychotherapy is probably the treatment of choice for histrionic personality disorder to gain insight into inner (unaware) feelings.
2. **Pharmacotherapy**: Antidepressants for comorbid depression and somatic complaints, Benzodiazepines agents for anxiety, and antipsychotics for derealisation and illusions.

NARCISSISTIC PERSONALITY DISORDER

Hallmark: Grandiose sense of self importance

Prevalence: 0.4-0.8% of general population. More common in males

Clinical Features

1. Ideas of grandiosity and inflated sense of self importance with fantasies of unlimited success. The term is derived from the Greek myth of Narcissus who falls in love with his own reflection in a pool of water.
2. Attention seeking for admiration from others, dramatic behavior, needs constant praise, and unable to face criticism.
3. Self centered and lack of empathy with others, with exploitative behavior.
4. Shaky self-esteem, underlying sense of inferiority, easily depressed by minor events.
5. People with narcissistic personality disorder develops narcissism as a defence against awareness of low self-esteem.

Differential Diagnosis

1. Other cluster B personality disorders
2. Bipolar Mood Disorder.
3. Substance misuse.

Course and Prognosis

Narcissistic personality disorder is difficult to treat and runs a chronic course. They do not accept ageing in a healthy manner

Treatment

1. This patients are difficult to treat as they refuse the need to seek help. They feel that others need to change rather than undergoing it.
2. Psychodynamic psychotherapy is the preferred treatment in a psychologically-minded patient.
3. Pharmacotherapy: Antidepressants for treatment of depressive episodes. Mood stabilizers are prescribed for mood swings and impulsivity.

AVOIDANT PERSONALITY DISORDER

Hallmark: Inferiority Complex

Prevalence: 2-3% of general population. Equally common in males and females

Clinical Features

1. Persistent, pervasive tension and apprehension.
2. Avoidance of social or occupational activities involving significant interpersonal contact because of fear of criticism, disapproval or rejection
3. They express uncertainty and show a lack of self-confidence.
4. These persons enter relationships only when they are assured of uncritical acceptance.
5. Restricted lifestyle due to need for physical security.
6. Strong belief that one is socially inept, personally unappealing or inferior to others.

Differential Diagnosis

1. **Schizoid personality disorder:** are alone aloof and socially withdrawn
2. **Dependent personality disorder**: People with avoidant personality disorder avoid contact while people with dependent personality disorder focus on being cared for.
3. **Social phobia and depression**

Course and Prognosis

People suffering from Avoidant personality disorder are functioning well in protected environment in the vicinity of known people. They have a tendency to develop phobic anxiety and depression when their social support is taken off.

Treatment

1. **Cognitive behavior therapy**
2. **Assertiveness training**
3. **Social skills training**
4. **Pharmacotherapy:** Antidepressant, Benzodiazepines and beta-blockers are used in treatment of comorbid anxiety and depression

DEPENDANT PERSONALITY DISORDER:

Hallmark: Submissive and dependent

Prevalence: 0.3-0.6% of general population. Equally common in males and females

Clinical Features

1. Preoccupation with fears of being abandoned by a person with whom one has a close relationship
2. They require excessive amount of advice and reassurance from others to make everyday decisions.
3. Assumes subordinate roles even when offered leadership roles.
4. Encourages or allows others to make most of one's important life decisions.
5. Unwillingness to make even reasonable demands on the people one depends on
6. Feeling uncomfortable or helpless when alone without support. They urgently seek another relationship for care and support when a close relationship ends.

Differential Diagnosis

1. **Borderline personality disorder:** have chaotic relationships, impulsivity, and mood lability. People with dependent personality disorder want to be controlled but people with borderline personality disorder react strongly to the efforts to be controlled.
2. **Avoidant personality disorder:** People with avoidant personality disorder react

by avoiding while people with dependent personality disorder seek out for relationship

3. **Depression and social phobia**

Treatment

1. **Cognitive behavior therapy**
2. **Insight oriented therapies**
3. **Family therapies and group therapies**
4. **Pharmacotherapy:** Antidepressant, Benzodiazepines and beta-blockers are used in treatment of comorbid anxiety and depression

OBSESSIVE COMPULSIVE PERSONALITY DISORDER

Hallmark: pervasive pattern of perfectionism and inflexibility

Prevalence: 2- 8% of general population. More common in males. More common in first degree relative of people suffering from obsessive personality disorder

Clinical Features

1. Perfectionism that interferes with task completion affecting productivity
2. Excessive conscientiousness and scrupulousness
3. Excessive adherence societal norms, rule, orderliness, neatness and details
4. Rigidity and stubbornness.
5. Undue preoccupation with productivity to the exclusion of pleasure and interpersonal relationships.
6. They are inflexible and cannot delegate tasks to others unless done according to them
7. Feelings of excessive doubt and resist adaptability to new changes.
8. Psychodynamically, this disorder is believed to result from fixation at the anal sadistic phase, with the employment of reaction formation as a defense mechanism.

Differential Diagnosis

1. **Obsessive compulsive disorder:** Recurrent, repetitive and intrusive obsessions and compulsions are present.
2. **Generalized anxiety disorder:** Excessive day to day worries
3. **Schizoid personality disorder:** are aloof, alone and socially withdrawn

Treatment

Person suffering from obsessive compulsive disorder often seek help due to insight into their problems

1. **Cognitive behavior therapy**
2. **Group Therapy**
3. **Pharmacotherapy:** antidepressants (fluoxetine and clomipramine) and benzodiazepines are effective for breakthrough obsessive compulsive symptoms.

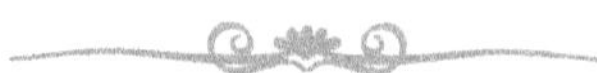

22 Psychocutaneous Disorders

Sayalee Daberao • Avinash De Sousa

INTRODUCTION

Psychocutaneous medicine or Psychodermatology deals with the disorders which lie on the boundary between psychiatry and dermatology. It is important for a dermatologist to recognize these disorders and manage the patients accordingly by a proper referral to a psychiatrist.

It is a well-known fact, that the patients with dermatological disorders worsen when they experience a stress or other psychiatric comorbidities. More than one third patients seeking treatment for dermatologic disorders. On the other hand, patients with chronic dermatological illness developing a psychiatric disorders like depression and anxiety are more than the general population or inpatients of general medicine. [(1)]

There are number of social and psychological sequelae of serious dermatological disease like acne, psoriasis, eczema, urticaria. The impact of cosmetic consequences are seen on the relationship, employment. The patients usually have lower self esteem because of the long standing and socially distressing illness. Minority of the cases, may experience ideas of self-harm or can attempt a complete suicide. [(2)]

PATHOGENESIS

The complex relationship between mind and skin has been studied extensively. The fact that both brain, nerves and skin are embryologically derived from the neural plate in ectoderm, suggest the same.

The neuro-immuno-cutaneous-endocrine model was proposed by O'Sullivan et al to explain mind and body relationship. This forms a basis of many inflammatory skin diseases, that are triggered or exacerbated with psychological factors.

Brain and skin share neuropeptides, cytokines, glucocorticoids and other important effector molecules.[3,4] Hypothalamic-pituitary axis (HPA) responds to psychologic stress, with upregulation of stress hormones like corticotropin-releasing hormone (CRH), adrenocorticotropin releasing hormone (ACTH), cortisol, prolactin. Sympathetic system gets activation leads to raised catecholamines and release neuropeptides and neuromediators like substance P. Mast cells are the main target for the stress hormones and their activation leads to immune dysregulation and various skin disorders.[5]

DELUSIONAL DISORDERS, SOMATIC TYPE

DELUSIONAL PARASITOSIS

The term ACAROPHOBIA (acaro: mite, phobia: fear) was first coined by G. Thibierge in 1890s. Delusional parasitosis (DP) is the condition in which there is a fixed belief that one has been infested with parasites. Other terms for DP are PARASITOPHOBIA, ENTOMOPHOBIA, MONOSYMPTOMATIC HYPOCHONDRIACAL PSYCHOSIS, EKBOM SYNDROME.

Clinical Features

- Patients with DP often describe the sensation of bugs crawling on or inside the skin.
- Some report seeing bugs or hearing buzzing sounds and some bring the parasite for further examination. This behavior is so characteristic that it has been referred to as "the matchbox sign".
- Often patients report some precipitant like history of a contagious infection or a real infection.
- They attempt self-treatment in the form of repeated excoriation of skin with needles, knives or fingernails, excessive use of insect repellent, repeated hand washing and checking.
- The fear of contaminating others is common.
- The delusion may be shared by relatives (folie a deux).
- Tend to visit dermatologists for the complaints.

Differential Diagnosis

1. Obsessive compulsive disorder: Repeated, intrusive thoughts of contamination (obsession) can produce the compulsive behavior like repeated hand washing, cleaning, checking to have relief from the obsessive thoughts.
2. Substance use: The similar sensation of bugs crawling under the skin (tactile hallucinations) can be seen in drug use like cocaine ("cocaine bugs") or amphetamines.

   In alcohol withdrawal the visual hallucinations consisting of the insects crawling over skin can be experienced (formication).
3. Schizophrenia: Tactile or visual hallucinations or the delusion of parasitosis itself can be a part of the symptoms of schizophrenia.
4. Major depressive disorder: Mood congruent psychotic features may involve hallucinations, which can mimic the condition.

Pathogenesis

There are three subgroups of DP:

1. Patients with *predominantly hypochondriacal traits,* who are convinced that they have some *incurable physical disease*. This is referred to as the hypochondriacal delusion of parasitosis or simply DP.
2. Patients *with paranoid delusions and without hypochondriacal traits*, who tend to fight against the parasite affecting their life, referred to as delusion of infestation.
3. Patients with hypochondriacal as well as paranoid delusions: referred as hypochondriacal delusion of infestation.

Treatment

a) Pharmacological:
   1. PIMOZIDE: most advocated antipsychotic. It is a potent opiate antagonist which has an antipruritic action
   2. Other antipsychotics: RISPERIDONE, HALOPERIDOL, TRIFLUOPERAZINE, CHLORPROMAZINE.
   3. NALTREXONE.

b) Psychotherapy has minimal efficacy in treatment of DP.

PRURITUS AND CHRONIC IDIOPATHIC PRURITUS

Pruritus is an unpleasant sensation that provoke the desire to scratch. In the brain, pruritus and psyche are intertwined in a complex manner. It is common observation that "itch" can be induced simply by thinking about it. Scratching provides immediate relief of discomfort and serves to reduce inner tension, this leads to conditioned scratching.

The vicious cycle of itch-and-scratch, if continued, can be perceived as loss of control helplessness and it is often accompanied by guilt.

Pathogenesis

- Multiple chemicals can provoke or enhance pruritus. The best-known are histamine, prostaglandins, prostaglandins, proteases, substance p, neuropeptides, cytokines (IL-2) and bile salts.
- Opioids, such as endorphin, met-encephalin, and leu-enkephalin, can play a role in causing itch.

Treatment

a) Pharmacological: DOXEPINE: effectively used antidepressant in chronic idiopathic pruritus.

b) Other antidepressants: SSRIs: PAROXETINE, SERTRALINE, FLUOXETINE, FLUOXEMINE, MIRTAZEPINE.

c) GABAPENTIN: structural analog of neurotransmitter GABA.

OBSESSIVE-COMPULSIVE AND RELATED DISORDERS: BODY FOCUSSED REPEATATIVE Behavior

1. Skin picking disorder (SPD)
2. Trichotillomania (TTM)
3. Body dysmorphic disorder (BDD)

1. SKIN PICKING DISORDER (SPD)

Erasmus Wilson first coined the term "neurotic excoriation" in 1889. Also known as, PATHOLOGICAL SKIN PICKING, DERMATELLOMANIA, PSYCHOGENIC EXCORIATION.

Clinical Features

- Excessive picking, scratching, digging, rubbing, gauging or squeezing the normal skin or previously diseased skin.
- Patients have irresistible urges to excoriate the normal looking skin or visible pre existing abnormalities like acne, papules or scabs.
- The lesions are characterized by clean, linear erosions, scabs and scars which could be hypopigmented or hyperpigmented.
- The distribution of lesions is confined to the accessible areas like face, arms and anterior thigh, sparing the middle and upper lateral back ("butterfly sign").
- Most commonly occurs in females.
- Associated with other psychiatric conditions like generalized anxiety disorder, OCD, trichotillomania, body dysmorphic disorder, compulsive nail biting, eating disorder, major depressive disorder, bipolar disorder.

Treatment

a) Pharmacological: FLUOXETINE is most studied SSRI in treatment of SPD.

b) Behavioral therapy: considered as first line treatment with potential for long term therapeutic effects.

2. TRICHOTILLOMANIA:

The term "Trichotillomania" is coined by Francois Hallopeau, from words tricho (hair), tillo (pull), mania (fury). Trichobezoar (hair ball in stomach) was first described in 18th century.

Subtypes

a) Focused pulling: Intentional hair pulling to control unpleasant personal experiences like urge, bodily sensation or thought. Patients resist the act of pulling and feel relieved after pulling.

b) Automatic pulling: This occurs outside the persons consciousness, most often during sedentary activities.

Clinical Features

- Patient presents with the areas of different hair lengths with blunt and tapered ends.
- Areas involved are typically scalp. Other common site are eyebrows and eyelashes.
- Areas of black dots on the surface of the scalp might also be noticed.
- The area around the hair loss is healthy.
- The hair does not pull out easily.
- Most commonly seen in women than in men.
- Comorbidly associated with mood, anxiety or eating disorders, personality disorders.
- Patients have family history of OCD or other anxiety disorder.

Treatment

a) Preschool children: In this age group TTM is most often automatic type; guiding the parents and raising their awareness is most effective in this age group.

b) Adolescents: Behavioral and reassurance that the hair can regrow if left alone.

c) Adult: Adult onset TTM is usually associated with psychiatric comorbidities and requires psychopharmacological and psychotherapy.

d) CLOMIPRAMINE was found to be effective in treating TTM, but with the better tolerability, the use of SSRIs remains the first-line medication for management of TTM.

e) Atypical antipsychotics (OLANZAPINE, RISPERIDONE, ARIPIPRAZOLE) can be used as an augmenting agent with SSRIs.

ONYCHOPHAGIA

This is a common behavior among children, beginning as early as 4 years of age with peak occurring during puberty. The condition consists of repetitive nail biting with experience of resistance for the act and relief after the act, like skin picking and hair pulling.

Patients with severe and chronic onychophagia experience hand infections, mandibular deformities. Its usually associated with stressful situations.

Behavioral therapy is most effective in treating the same.

3. BODY DYSMORPHIC DISORDER (BDD)

Patients with this condition experiences an excessive anxiety regarding their physical appearance.

Clinical Features

- Patient presents with imagined or slight flaw of one or many body areas, most commonly the facial skin (acne, wrinkles, scars, vascular markings), hair (thinning of hair, excessive body hair), nose (shape and size).

- Other body parts like genitals, buttocks, breast, abdomen, upper and lower extremities.
- History of multiple cosmetic surgeries.
- Behavior like repetitive checking in mirror, questioning, comparison of the defects of same body parts on others, reassurance.
- Manifests during adolescence.
- Equal sex distribution.
- Associated with suicidal ideas, major depressive disorder, anxiety, social isolation, problems at workplace.

Treatment

Patients with BDD can be challenging to engage in psychiatric treatment. SSRIs are the treatment of choice in treating patients of BDD. Cognitive Behavioral Therapy is also efficacious.

FACTITIOUS DISORDERS: FACTITIOUS DERMATITIS

Also known as *"dermatitis artefacta (DA)"*. Characterized by self inflicted injuries on skin, by using more elaborate methods than excoriating.

Clinical Features

- The lesions in DA imitate most cutaneous diseases. Presents as an aggravation of dermatosis like blisters, ulcers, erythema, edema, purpura and sinuses.
- The morphology of DA lesions is bizarre and linear with clear cut angulated or geometric edges.
- Dramatic dermal induration and necrosis occur from foreign body injection of milk, oil or grease into breasts, thighs and abdomen.
- The presence of completely normal looking skin surrounding the horrific looking lesions is a clue for the diagnosis of DA.
- The damage may involve a full thickness of the skin and severe scarring, requiring plastic surgery.
- Patient can not explain the details of history of appearance and evolution of the skin lesions.
- Usually the lesions are located in the areas which is easily accessible to the dominant hand
- Patient is unmoved by disfiguring painful lesions, and deny the self inflicting nature of the lesions.
- More commonly seen in females.
- Can present at any age group but most frequently seen in adolescents and young adults.
- The onset of the condition follows psychosocial stressor like relational disturbances, loss or threatened loss.
- Patients need to assume a sick role for gains like pursuit of sickness leaves or benefit.
- History of contact with multiple health services.
- Associated with comorbidities like borderline personality disorder, schizoaffective disorder, major depressive disorder, delusional parasitosis, Post Traumatic Stress Disorder, pathological intoxication with alcohol or LSD (Lysergic acid Diethylamide).

Treatment

Patients are resistant to accept a referral to psychiatrist, and direct confrontation may jeopardize the doctor-patient relationship. An empathetic relationship between the dermatologist and patient may help the patient to accept an appropriate therapeutic approach and psychiatric referral.

PSYCHOGENIC PURPURA

Psychogenic purpura (Gardener-Diamond syndrome) also known as auto erythrocyte sensitization syndrome, is extremely rare condition typically in female with psychiatric comorbidities.

Manifested as spontaneous development of painful erythematous lesions predominantly in extremities which can be isolated or multiple, progressing to ecchymosis over the next 24 hours. Hemostatic and coagulation tests reports no impairment (6).

BIBLIOGRAPHY

1. Jafferany M, Stoep AV, Dumitrescu A, Hornung RL. The knowledge, awareness, and practice patterns of dermatologists toward psychocutaneous disorders: results of a survey study. International journal of dermatology. 2010 Jul;49 (7):784-9.
2. Picardi A, Abeni D, Melchi CF, Puddu P, Pasquini P. Psychiatric morbidity in dermatological outpatients: an issue to be recognized. British Journal of dermatology. 2000 Nov;143 (5):983-91.
3. Arck PC, Slominski A, Theoharides TC, Peters EM, Paus R. Neuroimmunology of stress: skin takes center stage. Journal of Investigative Dermatology. 2006 Aug 1;126 (8):1697-704.
4. Slominski A, Pisarchik A, Zbytek B, Tobin DJ, Kauser S, Wortsman J. Functional activity of serotoninergic and melatoninergic systems expressed in the skin. Journal of cellular physiology. 2003 Jul;196 (1):144-53.
5. Yadav S, Narang T, Kumaran MS. Psychodermatology: A comprehensive review. Indian Journal of Dermatology, Venereology, and Leprology. 2013 Mar 1;79 (2):176.
6. Comprehencive textbook of psychiatry, vol. 2, pg 2332-2355.

Eating Disorders 23

Reetika Dikshit • Avinash De Sousa

ICD 10 Classification

F 50-59 : Behavioral Syndromes Associated with Psychological Disturbances and Physiological Factors

The disorders can broadly be classified into the following categories:

1. Eating Disorders
2. Sleep disorders
3. Sexual disorder and dysfunctions
4. Postpartum psychiatric disorders
5. Psychosomatic disorders

EATING DISORDERS

Eating disorders are characterized by clinical presentation primary focused on eating behavior. The following disorders are briefly discussed in the chapter:

1. Anorexia nervosa
2. Bulimia nervosa
3. Binge-eating disorder
4. Overeating disorder associated with other psychological disturbances
5. Vomiting associated with other psychological disturbances.

1. Anorexia Nervosa

Epidemiology

- Onset mostly in adolescents
- Mostly young adults; little later onset
- Excess in higher social class
- It occurs much more often in females as compared to the males. The common age of onset is adolescence (13-19 years of age).
- Genetic inheritance is noted.
- Anorexia nervosa: Monozygotes - 55% and Dizygotes - 5%
- A significant heritability exists for anorexia nervosa but not for bulimia nervosa.

Risk Factors

- Female sex, adolescence and early adulthood
- Western cultural adaptation
- Family history of ED, depression, substance misuse
- Adverse parenting (especially low contact, high expectations, parental discord)
- Childhood sexual abuse
- Critical comments about eating, shape, or weight from family and others
- Occupational and recreational pressure to be slim
- Low self esteem
- Perfectionism and obsessional personality traits

Criteria

According to ICD 10

- F50.0 Anorexia nervosa

A disorder characterized by deliberate weight loss, induced and sustained by the patient. It occurs most commonly in adolescent girls and young women, but adolescent boys and young men may also be affected, as may children approaching puberty and older women up to the menopause. The disorder is associated with a specific psychopathology whereby a dread of fatness and flabbiness of body contour persists as an intrusive overvalued idea, and the patients impose a low weight threshold on themselves. There is usually undernutrition of varying severity with secondary endocrine and metabolic changes and disturbances of bodily function. The symptoms include restricted dietary choice, excessive exercise, induced vomiting and purgation, and use of appetite suppressants and diuretics.

- F50.1 Atypical anorexia nervosa

  Disorders that fulfil some of the features of anorexia nervosa but in which the overall clinical picture does not justify that diagnosis. For instance, one of the key symptoms, such as amenorrhea or marked dread of being fat, may be absent in the presence of marked weight loss and weight-reducing behavior. This diagnosis should not be made in the presence of known physical disorders associated with weight loss.

According to DSM 5

- Restriction of food intake leading to weight loss or a failure to gain weight resulting in a "significantly low body weight" of what would be expected for someone's age, sex and height.
- Fear of becoming fat or gaining weight.
- Have a distorted view of themselves and of their condition. Examples of this might include the person thinking that he or she is overweight when they are actually underweighted or believing that they will gain weight from eating one meal. A person with anorexia might also not believe there is a problem with being at a low body weight. These thoughts are known to professionals as "distortions."
- Subcategories of anorexia nervosa:
  - Restricting Type: This is a subtype that is typically associated with the stereotypical view of anorexia nervosa. The person does not regularly engage in binge eating.
  - Binge-Eating/Purging Type: The person regularly engages in binge eating and purging behaviors, such as self-induced vomiting and/or the misuse of laxatives or diuretics. The binge eating/purging subtype is like bulimia nervosa; however, there is no weight-loss criterion for bulimia nervosa. As in previous editions of the DSM, anorexia nervosa "trumps" bulimia nervosa, meaning that if a person meets criteria for both anorexia nervosa and bulimia nervosa that anorexia nervosa (binge-eating/purging type) is diagnosed.
  - Specifier - partial remission or full remission (recovery)
  - Severity of the disorder based on BMI.

Clinical Features

Anorexia nervosa is an eating disorder characterized by the following prominent clinical features:

- There is an intense fear of becoming obese. This fear does not decrease even if body becomes very thin and underweight.
- There is often a body-image disturbance. The person is unable to perceive own body size accurately. However, body image disturbance may sometimes not be seen in

patients from non-Western cultural settings and several such cases have been described from India.

- There is a refusal to maintain the body weight above a minimum normal weight for that age, sex and height.
- Significant weight loss occurs, usually more than 25% of the original weight. The final weight is usually 15% less than the minimum limit of normal weight (for that age, sex and height) or a Quetelet's body-mass index (BMI) of 17.5 or less.
- No known medical illness, which can account for the weight loss, is present.
- Absence of any other primary psychiatric disorder.
- Amenorrhea, primary or secondary, is often present in females.
- In addition to these typical clinical features, other associated features are often present. The patient imposes dietary restrictions on self; can have peculiar patterns of handling food, such as breaking food into small bits, hiding food; and can engage in vigorous exercises.
- 'Anorexia' is a misnomer as there is never really a decrease in appetite, initially; in fact, patient is often preoccupied with food. A lot of time may be spent in collecting recipes and cooking food for significant others.
- Psychomotor activity is usually increased.
- Women with anorexia nervosa can present with poor sexual adjustment, with conflicts about being a woman and fear of pregnancy. Many patients are unconsciously unable to accept a 'female role'.
- A large number (up to 50%) of patients with anorexia nervosa also have bulimic episodes. These are characterized by rapid consumption of large amounts of food in a relatively short period of time, occurring usually when alone. This is known as eating binges or binge-eating. These binges are followed by intense guilt and attempts to remove eaten food, for example, by self-induced vomiting, laxative abuse, and/or diuretic abuse. If untreated, the weight loss can become marked.
- Death may occur due to hypokalemia (caused by self-induced vomiting), dehydration, malnutrition or congestive cardiac failure (caused by anemia).

Comorbidity

65% patients with anorexia have depression; 34% have social phobia while 26% have OCD

Obsessive-compulsive personality traits often accompany.

Differential Diagnosis

Anorexia nervosa should be differentiated from other conditions capable of causing significant weight loss.

Medical illnesses such as hypopituitarism, lateral hypothalamic lesion and debilitating systemic illnesses, e.g. disseminated tuberculosis.

Psychiatric disorders such as depressive disorder and schizophrenia.

Bulimia nervosa. Although bulimic episodes are common in anorexia nervosa (binge eating followed by vomiting), patients of bulimia nervosa usually maintain a near normal body weight (or are overweight), in sharp contrast to the patients with anorexia nervosa.

Treatment

The treatment of anorexia nervosa can be considered in two phases, which often merge into each other.

- Short-term treatment, to encourage weight gain and correct nutritional deficiencies, if any.

- Long-term treatment aimed at maintaining the near normal weight achieved in short-term treatment and preventing relapses. The various treatment modalities used can include:
  1. Behavior therapy (BT): Behavioral treatments are based on providing positive reinforcements (and at times, negative reinforcements) contingent on weight gain by the patient. A too rapid weight gain is not desirable or safe. The weight gain should not exceed 1.5 to 2 kg in a fortnight. As patients are usually unable to eat a large meal, especially in the initial part of treatment, it is advisable to suggest a greater number of meals (about six) per day. Occasionally, forceful Ryle's tube feeding may be needed initially, in resistant patients.
  2. Individual psychotherapy is often helpful in addition to supportive physical treatment. This could involve psychotherapy with a focus on cognitive behavior therapy, psychodynamic principles or supportive measures.
  3. Hospitalization, with adequate nursing care for food intake and weight gain, can be helpful in short-term treatment as well as prevention and/ or treatment of complications. However, hospitalization does not necessarily ensure long-term improvement. It is important to keep a close eye on water and electrolyte balance, need for supplementation with vitamins and minerals, and prevent osteoporosis.
  4. Drugs are an important adjunct to other modes of therapy. The drugs used can include:
     - i. Antipsychotics: Olanzapine has efficacy in improving weight gain, but it is important to be aware of possibility of prolongation of QTc particularly in patients with low BMI.
     - ii. Antidepressants (such as fluoxetine, clomipramine) for treatment of anorexia nervosa and/ or depression.
  5. Group therapy and family therapy can be helpful in psycho-education for the patient and carers/ family about nature of anorexia nervosa and its treatment. Psycho-education may also include discussion of current social norms of slimming and fitness, since there is evidence to suggest that anorexia nervosa is far more common in countries with social pressures for slimming, such as USA and UK. India is indeed quite fast catching up with similar social pressures. The prognosis is generally better if diagnosis is made early, absence of previous hospitalizations and absence of bulimic episodes. Weight gain and improvement in mental outlook often precede return of menstrual function.

2. Bulimia Nervosa

Epidemiology

- Mostly young adults; little later onset
- Even class distribution
- Substance use is increased in families of bulimic probands
- Bulimia nervosa: Monozygotes - 35% Dizygote - 30%

Risk Factors

- Female sex, adolescence and early adulthood
- Western cultural adaptation
- Family history of ED, depression, substance misuse, especially alcoholism, obesity

- Adverse parenting (especially low contact, high expectations, parental discord)
- Childhood sexual abuse
- Critical comments about eating, shape, or weight from family and others
- Occupational and recreational pressure to be slim
- Low self esteem
- History of being obese

Criteria

According to ICD 10

F50.2 Bulimia nervosa

A syndrome characterized by repeated bouts of overeating and an excessive preoccupation with the control of body weight, leading to a pattern of overeating followed by vomiting or use of purgatives. This disorder shares many psychological features with anorexia nervosa, including an overconcern with body shape and weight. Repeated vomiting is likely to give rise to disturbances of body electrolytes and physical complications. There is often, but not always, a history of an earlier episode of anorexia nervosa, the interval ranging from a few months to several years.

F50.3 Atypical bulimia nervosa

Disorders that fulfil some of the features of bulimia nervosa, but in which the overall clinical picture does not justify that diagnosis. For instance, there may be recurrent bouts of overeating and overuse of purgatives without significant weight change, or the typical overconcern about body shape and weight may be absent.

According to DSM 5

Recurrent episodes of binge eating. An episode of binge eating is characterized by both of the following:

- Eating, in a discrete period of time (e.g. within any 2-hour period), an amount of food that is definitely larger than most people would eat during a similar period of time and under similar circumstances.
- A sense of lack of control over eating during the episode (e.g. a feeling that one cannot stop eating or control what or how much one is eating).
- Recurrent inappropriate compensatory behavior in order to prevent weight gain, such as self-induced vomiting, misuse of laxatives, diuretics, or other medications, fasting, or excessive exercise.
- The binge eating and inappropriate compensatory behaviors both occur, on average, at least once a week for three months.
- Self-evaluation is unduly influenced by body shape and weight.
- The disturbance does not occur exclusively during episodes of Anorexia Nervosa.

Clinical Features

Bulimia nervosa is an eating disorder characterized by the following clinical features:

- There is an intense fear of becoming obese. There may be an earlier history of anorexia nervosa.
- There is usually body-image disturbance and the person are unable to perceive own body size accurately.
- There is a persistent preoccupation with eating, and an irresistible craving for food. There are episodes of overeating in which large amounts of food are consumed within short periods of time (eating binges).
- There are attempts to 'counteract' the effects of overeating by one or more of the following: self-induced vomiting, purgative

abuse, periods of starvation, and/or use of drugs such as appetite suppressants.

- No known medical illness is present which can account for the disorder.
- Absence of any other primary psychiatric disorder.

Treatment

The various treatment modalities that can be used include:

1. Behavior therapy: This is based on providing positive reinforcements (and at times negative reinforcements) contingent on the control of binge eating by the patient.
2. Individual psychotherapy: Antidepressant drugs are an important adjunct to other modes of therapy. A Selective serotonin uptake inhibitor (SSRI) such as Fluoxetine (in doses of 20-60 mg) is particularly useful as it can cause loss of appetite at least in the initial phase of treatment, along with its antidepressant effect. The drugs used in the past have included tricyclic antidepressants such as imipramine, though they are currently not widely used.
3. Group therapy and family therapy: These methods are used for psycho-education of patient and carers/family about nature of bulimia nervosa and its treatment.

3. Binge Eating Disorders

- Patients typically present in their 40s, with more males compared to other Eating disorders.
- In binge eating disorder, large amounts of food are consumed in a relatively short period, followed by severe discomfort and feelings of self-denigration. There is a sense of lack of control overeating during the episode. Additionally, there also may be eating of large amounts of food throughout the day with no planned mealtimes, eating alone because of being embarrassed, and/or feeling guilty and depressed after overeating. The disorder is not listed separately in ICD-10 and symptoms of binge eating are also seen in bulimia nervosa.
- It is characterized by recurrent episodes of binge eating in the absence of extreme weight-control behavior.
- An association with obesity is seen.
- Binge Eating Disorder is less common but much more severe than overeating. Binge Eating Disorder is associated with more subjective distress regarding the eating behavior, and commonly other co-occurring psychological problems.

Criteria

According to DSM 5

- Recurrent episodes of binge eating. An episode of binge eating is characterized by both of the following:
  - Eating, in a discrete period (e.g. within any 2-hour period), an amount of food that is definitely larger than most people would eat during a similar period of time and under similar circumstances.
  - A sense of lack of control overeating during the episode (e.g. a feeling that one cannot stop eating or control what or how much one is eating).
- The binge eating episodes are associated with three or more of the following:
  - eating much more rapidly than normal
  - eating until feeling uncomfortably full
  - eating large amounts of food when not feeling physically hungry
  - eating alone because of feeling embarrassed by how much one is eating

  - feeling disgusted with oneself, depressed or very guilty afterward
- Marked distress regarding binge eating is present
- Binge eating occurs, on average, at least once a week for three months
- Binge eating not associated with the recurrent use of inappropriate compensatory behaviors as in Bulimia Nervosa and does not occur exclusively during the course of Bulimia Nervosa, or Anorexia Nervosa methods to compensate for overeating, such as self-induced vomiting.

Treatment

- Self help group
- Weight loss programs
- CBT/IPT
- Role of drug is not very clear

PHYSICAL SIGNS AND SYMPTOMS OF EATING DISORDER

Physical Symptoms of EDs

- Increased sensitivity to cold
- Gastrointestinal symptoms—e.g., constipation, fullness after eating, bloated
- Dizziness and syncope
- Amenorrhea (in females not taking an oral contraceptive), low sexual appetite, infertility
- Poor sleep with early morning wakening

Physical Signs of EDs

- Emaciation; stunted growth and failure of breast development (if prepubertal onset)
- Dry skin; fine downy hair (lanugo) on the back, forearms, and side of the face; in patients with hypercarotenemia, orange discoloration of the skin
- Russel's sign –calluses in knuckles due to repeated vomit induction
- Swelling of parotid and submandibular glands (especially in bulimic patients)
- Erosion of inner surface of front teeth (perimylolysis) in those who vomit frequently
- Cold hands and feet; hypothermia
- Bradycardia (heart rate around 40 is common); orthostatic hypotension; cardiac arrhythmias (especially in underweight patients and those with electrolyte abnormalities). Systolic BP may drop up to 70 in the extremely starved.
- Dependent edema (complicating assessment of bodyweight)
- Weak proximal muscles (elicited as difficulty rising from a squatting position)

Abnormalities on Physical Investigation

Endocrine

- Low concentrations of luteinizing hormone, follicle stimulating hormone, and oestradiol
- Low T3, T4 in low normal range, normal concentrations of thyroid stimulating hormone (low T3 syndrome)
- Mild increase in plasma cortisol
- Raised growth hormone concentration
- Severe hypoglycemia (rare)
- Low leptin (but possibly higher than would be expected for bodyweight)

Cardiovascular

- ECG abnormalities (especially in those with electrolyte disturbance): conduction defects, especially prolongation of the Q-T interval, of major concern

- Ipecac (emetic substance) contains emetine an alkaloid that can cause myopathy and fatal cardiomyopathy which may be reversible in early stages.

Gastrointestinal

- Delayed gastric emptying
- Decreased colonic motility (secondary to chronic laxative misuse)
- Acute gastric dilatation (rare, secondary to binge eating or excessive re-feeding)

Hematological

- Moderate normocytic normochromic anemia
- Mild leucopenia with relative lymphocytosis
- Thrombocytopenia
- Other metabolic abnormalities
- Hypercholesterolemia
- Raised serum carotene
- Hypophosphatemia (exaggerated during refeeding)
- Dehydration
- Electrolyte disturbance (varied in form; present in those who vomit frequently or misuse large quantities of laxatives or diuretics): vomiting results in metabolic alkalosis and hypokalemia; laxative misuse results in metabolic acidosis, hyponatraemia, hypokalemia
- Other abnormalities
- Osteopenia and osteoporosis (with heightened fracture risk)
- Enlarged cerebral ventricles and external cerebrospinal fluid spaces (pseudoatrophy)

Effects on Pregnancy

- Decreased fertility –but regained near normally on complete recovery.
- May have more abortions
- Higher rates of hyperemesis gravidarum, anemia, impaired weight gain
- Compromised intrauterine fetal growth
- Premature delivery is more likely
- Rates of cesarean delivery are high
- Postnatal complications and post-partum depression are higher
- Associated with low birth weight, microcephaly, low APGAR scores.
- In actively anorexic mother, the neonate may have hypoglycemia

BIBLIOGRAPHY

1. World Health Organization (1992). The ICD 10 classification of mental and behavioral disorders. Clinical descriptions and diagnostic guidelines. Geneva: World health Organization.
2. Diagnostic and Statistical Manual of Mental Disorders (DSM–5): American Psychiatric Association.
3. Comprehensive textbook of Kaplan and Saddock.
4. RC Psych Royal College of Psychiatrists guidelines for eating disorder.

Factitious Disorder 24

Nahid Dave

DEFINITION

A condition in which the person wishes to attain a patient's role.[1] The patient may deliberately produce or exaggerate symptoms to achieve this role. Their sole motive is to get treatment not to seek attention or manipulating others.

At times the patient may inflict painful, deforming or life threatening injury on themselves for this goal. They fabricate their physical illness to gain admission and move from one hospital to another for the same.

EPIDEMIOLOGY

A majority of the patients go undiagnosed. Although it is a psychological disorder wherein the patient wants to seek treatment, the symptoms feigned are usually of physical illness. They may range from infections, repeated surgeries to self-inflicted injuries.[3]

According to a study conducted at NIMHANS hospital the Prevalence rate in India is 0.9 per 10,000 patients.[2]

Factitious disorder is seen more commonly among females in the age group of 20-40 years[2]. They usually have a history of education or employment in the health care system. This makes them well versed with diseases and treatment patterns

CO-MORBID

It has been found that it is not uncommon to have co-morbid psychiatric diagnosis like mood disorder, personality disorders or substance use disorders. Psychotic symptoms if present may indicate poor prognosis.

ETIOLOGY

1. Childhood Abuse or Deprivation

   History of frequent childhood abuse in the home setting and frequent hospital admissions. The hospital may be regarded as an escape from the hurtful environment at home. The patient may have found the hospital staff and doctors to be caring and loving in comparison to the absent father or rejecting mother. They tend to develop a compulsion to re-create the parent child role and need to seek acceptance and love.

2. Masochistic Personality Traits

   Some patients seek painful surgical procedures or invasive diagnostic method could have masochistic personality traits. The pain is perceived as punishment for past sins.

3. Identification

   Some patients wish to face the same pain and injury that a loved one has faced under the pretence of re-uniting with them magically.

4. Borderline Personality Traits

   If the patient is a health care professional, they are unable to differentiate between themselves and the patient they come in contact with.

TYPES

There are two types of factitious disorder:

A. Imposed on self

B. Imposed on Others

A. Imposed on self

1. Physical Symptoms only

Munchausen syndrome is described as a form of factitious disorder where only physical signs and symptoms are involved.[4] The syndrome was named after Baron Hieronymus Friedrich Freiherr von Munchausen (1720–1797), a German cavalry officer

They are able to misguide health care professionals with their sound knowledge in clinical presentations and diagnosis. They may even tamper with medical reports to build their case.

e.g.: Anticoagulants may be taken to fake bleeding disorders or insulin is taken to simulate hypoglycemia or fake a renal colic for narcotic medications.

They often insist on getting surgeries and may develop a gridiron or washboard like abdomen from multiple procedures.

Once admitted they make demands for particular treatment, medications and surgery

2. Psychological symptoms

Psychological symptoms of dementia, Grief, depression, psychosis, amnesia, eating disorder, dissociative identity make one simulated.

Patient may present with both physical and psychological symptoms as well

B. Imposed on Others

By proxy (Munchausen by proxy)

A patient of factitious disorder may produce signs and symptoms of physical illness in another person under their care.[6] The goal is to indirectly assume sick role. In the process they may even harm or hurt the person under their care, thus amounting to abuse.

It is seen very often in mothers who feign illness, lie about medical and surgical histories, alter laboratory samples or induce injury to the child to seek treatment.

Psychometric testing

MMPI or Minnesota Multiphasic Personality Inventory (MMPI) shows an invalid test profile as they try to exaggerate all their pain and symptoms and there is an elevation of all the scales. This falls under the category of 'Faking Bad' which means there is an attempt to appear more disturbed than reality.

They have been found to have normal or above average intellectual capacity as they have to be well prepared. There could be identity diffusion and also ambivalence regarding sexual identity.

Imposter Syndrome

Pseudologia Fantastica

A certain limited reality is blown out of proportion to enthral the listener. The truth is distorted and life stories are made more colorful. The interest that the listener develops in the stories reinforces the patient's conviction and creativity. They may claim to be war heroes or talk about loss of a loved one and build a fascinating tale around it.

DIAGNOSIS

There are a myriad of ways devised to understand factitious disorders.

e.g.: Patient may come with self-inflicted excoriations on the skin on the accessible parts of the body and more on the left side in a right handed person.

If there is Diarrhea by ingestion of castor oil or phenolphthalein, it can be understood by checking for laxatives in stool and increased stool weight.

They may warm the thermometer under a light bulb or hot liquid to fake having a fever.

If they feel it is possible they might get exposed they discharge themselves and carry on similar proceedings in another city and hospital.

DIFFERENTIAL

1. Conversion Disorder

   Patients of conversion disorder do not produce the symptoms consciously like factitious disorder. They are not usually aware of hospital proceedings, medical terminologies.

2. Hypochondriasis or Illness Anxiety disorder

   Hypochondriacs do not produce the symptoms deliberately and are not willing to undergo painful procedures like patients of factitious disorders.

3. Malingering

   Malingerers' goal for seeking treatment is very obvious environmental privileges e.g.: financial compensation, exemption from responsibilities, free services.

   They stop producing the symptoms when they no longer get the desired profit. In factitious disorder the aim is only to take treatment and stay in the sick role.

4. Schizophrenia

   A patient of schizophrenia may have a fixed delusion that they are actually ill and wish to seek treatment for the same. Factitious disorder patients are aware they are not ill and consciously feign symptoms.

5. Gansers syndrome

   This is a controversial illness seen amongst prison inmates and is classified under dissociative disorders or Conversion disorder.

   The inmate may give surprisingly approximate answers e.g. 2 plus 2 is 5. This results in averting punishment or pushing back responsibilities and so could be a variant of malingering as well.

   A patient of factitious disorder may intentionally give approximate answers in order to achieve sick role`

WARNING SIGNS[5]

- Changing medical history
- Vague symptoms which do not respond to treatment
- Relapses once the condition improves.
- Detailed information about medical disorders and hospital functioning
- Presence of many surgical scars
- Appearance of new symptoms if reports are negative

- Interest and demands for medical tests, diagnostic procedures and surgeries
- History of seeking treatment at many hospitals, clinics, and doctors' offices, possibly even in different cities
- Deny meeting of family members with treating doctors and previous health care professionals.
- Refusing psychological evaluation
- Illness increases when closer to discharge

COURSE AND PROGNOSIS

Illness begins during early adulthood, usually with a history of hospitalization for themselves or a loved one.

Severe trauma, repeated medications and surgeries are often detrimental to the patient's overall physical health. The need for repeated hospitalizations affects occupational and interpersonal life as well. The patients are admitted in the hospital alone and seek treatment and change hospitals by themselves. These patients are often undiagnosed. They may also have history of psychiatric admissions and short jail time for petty crimes. Patients are aware of the risks they subject themselves to but are unable to control their behavior.

Direct confrontation with the patient may result in the patient fleeing the hospital or a psychotic disintegration.

TREATMENT

It is paradoxical that patients wish to take treatment for feigned illnesses but refuse or flee when explained about having factitious disorder.

The treatment involves:

1. The primary goal is to address the emotional needs of the patient. Helping the patient understand the reasons for him seeking care and the adverse consequences on his physical health
2. It is also essential to reduce his physical morbidities by developing a strong alliance with the medical staff. They can be explained about his condition and even though he has fabricated his illness, he still suffers from factitious disorder.
3. Psychiatric treatment in a non- confrontational manner. He has to be managed with empathy and lack of aggression
4. Legal and ethical issues are of foremost importance. In case of Munchausen by proxy the relevant legal departments are to be notified.
5. The co-morbidities can be treated with pharmacotherapy.

DSM CRITERIA 300.19 (F68.10)

Factitious Disorder Imposed on Self

A. Falsification of physical or psychological signs or symptoms, or induction of injury or disease, associated with identified deception.

B. The individual presents himself or herself to others as ill, impaired or injured.

C. The deceptive behavior is evident even in the absence of obvious external rewards.

D. The behavior is not better explained by another mental disorder, such as delusional disorder or another psychotic disorder.

Specify:

Single Episode

Recurrent Episodes (two or more events of

falsification of illness and/or induction of injury)

Factitious Disorder Imposed on Another (Previously Factitious Disorder by Proxy)

A. Falsification of physical or psychological signs or symptoms, or induction of injury or disease, in another, associated with identified deception.

B. The individual presents another individual (victim) to others as ill, impaired or injured.

C. The deceptive behavior is evident even in the absence of obvious external rewards.

D. The behavior is not better explained by another mental disorder, such as delusional disorder or another psychotic disorder.

Note:

The perpetrator, not the victim, receives this diagnosis.

Specify:

Single Episode

Recurrent Episodes (two or more events of falsification of illness and/or induction of injury)

When an individual falsifies illness in another (e.g., children, adults, pets), the diagnosis is factitious disorder imposed on another. The perpetrator, not the victim, is given the diagnosis. The victim may be given an abuse diagnosis.

BIBLIOGRAPHY

1. Kanaan RA, Wessely SC. The origins of factitious disorder. History of the Human Sciences. 2010 Apr;23(2):68-85.
2. Dahale AB, Hatti S, Thippeswamy H, Chaturvedi SK. Factitious disorder-experience at a neuropsychiatric center in southern India. Indian journal of psychological medicine. 2014 Jan;36(1):62.
3. Bursten B. On Munchausen's syndrome. Archives of General Psychiatry. 1965 Sep 1;13(3):261-8.
4. Spiro HR. Chronic factitious illness: Munchausen's syndrome. Archives of General Psychiatry. 1968 May 1;18(5):569-79.
5. https://www.mayoclinic.org/diseases-conditions/factitious-disorder/symptoms-causes/syc-20356028
6. Meadow R. Different interpretations of Munchausen syndrome by proxy. Child abuse & neglect. 2002 May 1;26(5):501-8.

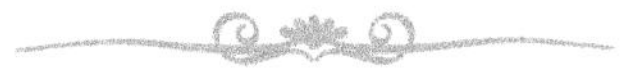

25 Sexual Disorders

Parag Shah

INTRODUCTION

Sexual Disorder refers to a problem during any phase of the sexual response cycle that prevents the individual or couple from experiencing satisfaction from the sexual activity. It is important to understand that sexual functioning is a complex bio-psycho-social process, coordinated by the neurological, vascular and endocrine systems.

While evaluating sexual functioning of an individual it is important to incorporate family, societal and religious beliefs, health status, personal experience, ethnicity and socio-demographic conditions, and psychological status of the person/couple. In addition, sexual activity incorporates interpersonal relationships, each partner bringing unique attitudes, needs and responses into the coupling. A breakdown in any of these areas may lead to sexual dysfunction.

To understand Sexual Dysfunction, it is necessary to understand some basic terminology related to sexual activity (**Table 25.1**) and also the normal human sexual response cycle as shown in **Fig. 25.1 & Table 25.2**.

The sexual response cycle is a model that describes the physiological responses that occur during sexual activity. This model was created by William Masters and Virginia Johnson.

Table 25.1: Basic Terminology related to Sexual Activity

Libido	**Feeling of sexual desire**
Orgasm	The peak of sexual arousal, when all the muscles that were tightened during sexual arousal relax, usually causes a very pleasurable feeling.
Intercourse	Sexual activity in which the penis goes into the vagina (vaginal intercourse) or the anus (anal intercourse).
Coitus	Sex in which the penis enters the vagina. Also called "vaginal sex" or "vaginal intercourse".
Masturbation	Touching one's own body/genitals for sexual pleasure.
Fantasy	A thought, idea, or daydream that causes sexual excitement.
Foreplay	Kissing, rubbing, stroking, and/or touching that leads to sex.

The sexual disorders may be classified as

- LIFELONG: The symptoms have been present since the individual became sexually active.
- ACQUIRED: The symptoms began after a period of relatively normal sexual function.
- GENERALIZED: The symptoms are not limited to certain types of stimulation, situations or partners.
- SITUATIONAL: The symptoms only occurs

with certain types of stimulation and situation (partner related, performance related & psychological distress or adjustment related)

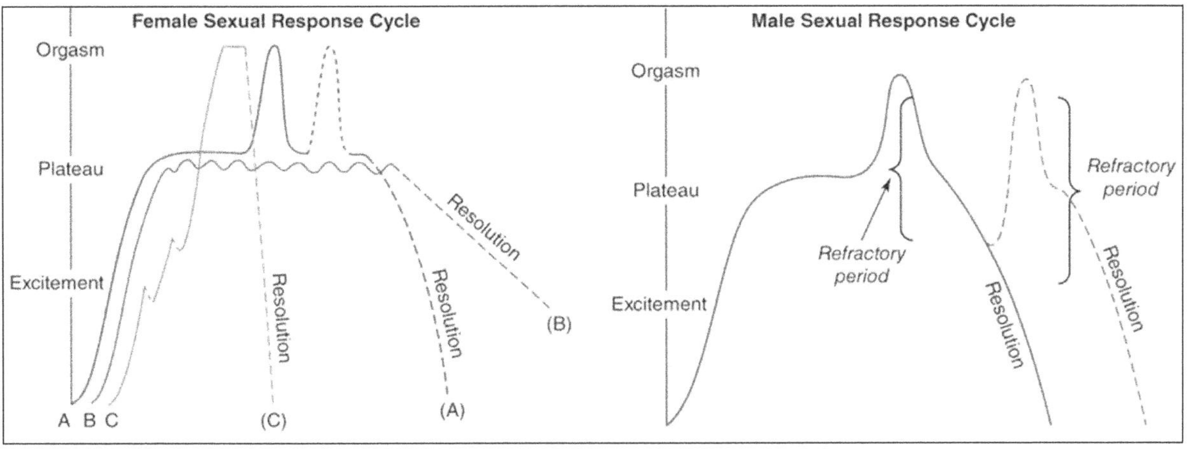

Fig. 25.1: Normal human sexual response cycle.

Table 25.2: Normal human sexual response cycle

Phases	Male	Female
Appetitive Phase	This phase is characterized by the sexual fantasies and the desire for sexual activity.	
Excitement Phase	This phase consists of a subjective sense of sexual pleasure & marks the beginning of the physiological responses to the sexual stimuli. Duration : several minutes to hours	
	• Penile erection due to vasocongestion of corpus cavernosa • Elevation of testes with scrotal sac	• Vaginal lubrication by transudation from vaginal wall due to vasocongestion • Lower 1/3 of vagina dilates • Erection of nipples • Clitoris becomes hard & turgid • Thickening of labia minora
Plateau Phase	This is a heightened state of excitement attained with continued stimulation.There is marked sexual tension in this phase, which sets the stage for the orgasm. Duration : 30 seconds to 3 minutes	
	• Sexual flush • Autonomic hyperactivity (tachycardia, tachypnea & increase in blood pressure) • Myotonia of facial & abdominal muscles • Elevation and enlargement of testes • Continued engorgement of penis • Cowper's gland secretion seen on glans penis which may contain viable sperm	• Sexual flush • Autonomic hyperactivity (tachycardia, tachypnea & increase in blood pressure) • Constriction of the lower 1/3 of vagina known as "orgasmic platform" develops • Retraction of clitoris behind the prepuce • Enlargement of breasts & labia minora • Drops of mucoid secretion of Bartholin's gland seen in vagina

(Continued)

<table>
<tr><th>Phases</th><th>Male</th><th>Female</th></tr>
<tr><td rowspan="2">Orgasmic Phase</td><td colspan="2">This is the phase with peak experience of pleasure out of sexual activity termed as Orgasm. There are rhythmic contractions of perineal muscles & reproductive organs with intense physical sensations & release of sexual tension.
Duration: 3-15 seconds</td></tr>
<tr><td>• 3 to 4 contractions at 0.8 seconds interval of vas deferens, seminal vesicles, and prostate.
• This contractions forces semen into bulb of urethra leading to 'Ejaculatory inevitability'
• Ejaculation-There are contractions of urethra and penis along with prostate leading to Ejaculatory spurt
• Autonomic hyperactivity becomes more marked
• Contractions of external & internal sphincters</td><td>• 3 to 15 contractions at 0.8 seconds interval in lower 1/3rd of vagina, cervix and uterus.
• A momentary sense of suspension, followed by intense pleasure starts at clitoris & spreads to whole of the pelvis.
• Genitals feel warm, electric and tingly
• This feeling spreads throughout the body
• Autonomic hyperactivity becomes more marked
• Contractions of external & internal sphincters</td></tr>
<tr><td rowspan="2">Resolution Phase</td><td colspan="2">• This is the phase when men and women return to the unaroused state.
• Anatomical & physiological changes reverse.
• Resolution brings in a sense of well-being & muscle relaxation.
Duration : 10 to 15 minutes</td></tr>
<tr><td>Refractory period which lasts for several minutes to hours in which men cannot be stimulated to further orgasm & ejaculation.</td><td>No refractory period seen</td></tr>
</table>

The sexual disorders can be classified on the basis of abnormality in any of the phases of the sexual response cycle including Sexual Pain Disorders **(Table 25.3)**.

Table 25.3. Sexual dysfunctions

<table>
<tr><th>Phases</th><th>Male</th><th>Female</th></tr>
<tr><td>Disorders of Appetitive Phase</td><td colspan="2">1. Hypoactive Sexual Desire Disorder
Persistently or recurrently deficient (or absent) sexual fantasies and desire for sexual activity.
2. Sexual Aversion Disorder
Persistent or recurrent extreme aversion to, and avoidance of, all (or almost all) genital sexual contact with a sexual partner.
3. Excessive Sexual Desire
Both men (Satyriasis) and women (Nymphomania) may occasionally complain of excessive sexual drive, usually during late teenage or early adulthood.</td></tr>
<tr><td>Disorders of Excitement Phase and Plateau Phase (Sexual Arousal Disorders)</td><td>Erectile Dysfunction
Persistent or recurrent inability to attain, or to maintain until completion of the sexual activity, an adequate erection.</td><td>Female Sexual Arousal Disorder
Persistent or recurrent inability to attain, or to maintain until completion of the sexual activity, an adequate lubrication-swelling response of sexual excitement.</td></tr>
</table>

(Continued)

Phases	Male	Female
Orgasmic Phase	**Male Anorgasmia** Persistent or recurrent delay in, or absence of, orgasm following a normal sexual excitement phase during sexual activity that the clinician, taking into account the person's age, judges to be adequate in focus, intensity, and duration. It often presents as **Delayed Ejaculation** Also known as retarded ejaculation. **Premature Ejaculation** Persistent or recurrent ejaculation with minimal sexual stimulation before, on, or shortly after penetration and before the person wishes it.	**Female Anorgasmia** Persistent or recurrent delay in, or absence of, orgasm following a normal sexual excitement phase. Women exhibit wide variability in the type or intensity of stimulation that triggers orgasm should be taken in account before diagnosing it.
Resolution Phase	**Priapism** It is a prolonged usually painful erection, unrelated to specific stimuli, occurs frequently due to medications such as intracavernosal injection of vasoactive substances, antihypertensives, anticoagulants, atypical antipsychotics or due to hematological disorders, perineal injury, spinal cord injury, penile malignant infiltration etc.	
OTHERS		
Sexual Pain Disorders	**Non Organic Dyspareunia:** Recurrent or persistent genital pain associated with sexual intercourse in a male.	**Non Organic Dyspareunia:** Recurrent or persistent genital pain associated with sexual intercourse in a female.
		Non Organic Vaginismus : Recurrent or persistent involuntary spasm of the musculature of the outer third of the vagina that interferes with sexual intercourse.

The most common sexual disorders are discussed here:

ERECTILE DYSFUNCTION

Several studies reported a prevalence of erectile dysfunction ranging from 6% to 64%.

It is defined as persistent or recurrent inability to attain, or to maintain an adequate penile erection until completion of the sexual activity.

It can be either Primary /Lifelong (no erectile function ever) or Secondary (onset after a period of normal functioning)

ED can be Generalized (generalized unresponsiveness and generalized inhibition) or Situational

Etiology – ED can occur due to psychological or non psychological (organic) factors or combination of both as below (**Table 25.4**).

Table 25.4

1. Psychogenic	• Inadequate sexual knowledge • Performance Anxiety • Interpersonal issues between sexual partners • Anxiety Disorder • Mood disorder • Sexual Phobias • Obsessive Compulsive Personality • Fear of the partner's genitals and intimacy • Fear of the pregnancy and sexually transmitted diseases • Belief in sexual myths (related to masturbation & Dhat Syndrome) • Sexual abuse in childhood • Environmental factors (lack of privacy)
2. Drugs	• Anti-hypertensives • Anti-cholinergics • Psychotropics • Estrogens and Anti-Androgens • Digoxin
3. Substance use	• Alcohol • Nicotine • Cannabis • Cocaine
4. Local Genital Disease	• Peyronie's • Priapism • Phimosis • Trauma • Hydrocele or varicocele
5. Endocrine Disorders	• Diabetes mellitus • Androgen deficiency (primary or secondary) • Hyperprolactinemia • Hyperthyroidism • Hypothyroidism
6. Neurological disorder	• Parkinson's Disease • Alzheimer's Disease • Spinal cord lesions (e.g. Transverse Myelitis) • Peripheral neuropathy, • Pudendal nerve injury
7. Vascular insufficiency	• Atherosclerosis • Penile Raynaud's
8. Systemic Illness	• Renal failure • Hypertension • Cancer • Postorgan transplant • Pelvic irradiation • COPD

Management

The alogorithm to be followed for evaluation and diagnosis of erectile dysfunction has been summarized in **Flowchart. 25.1**.

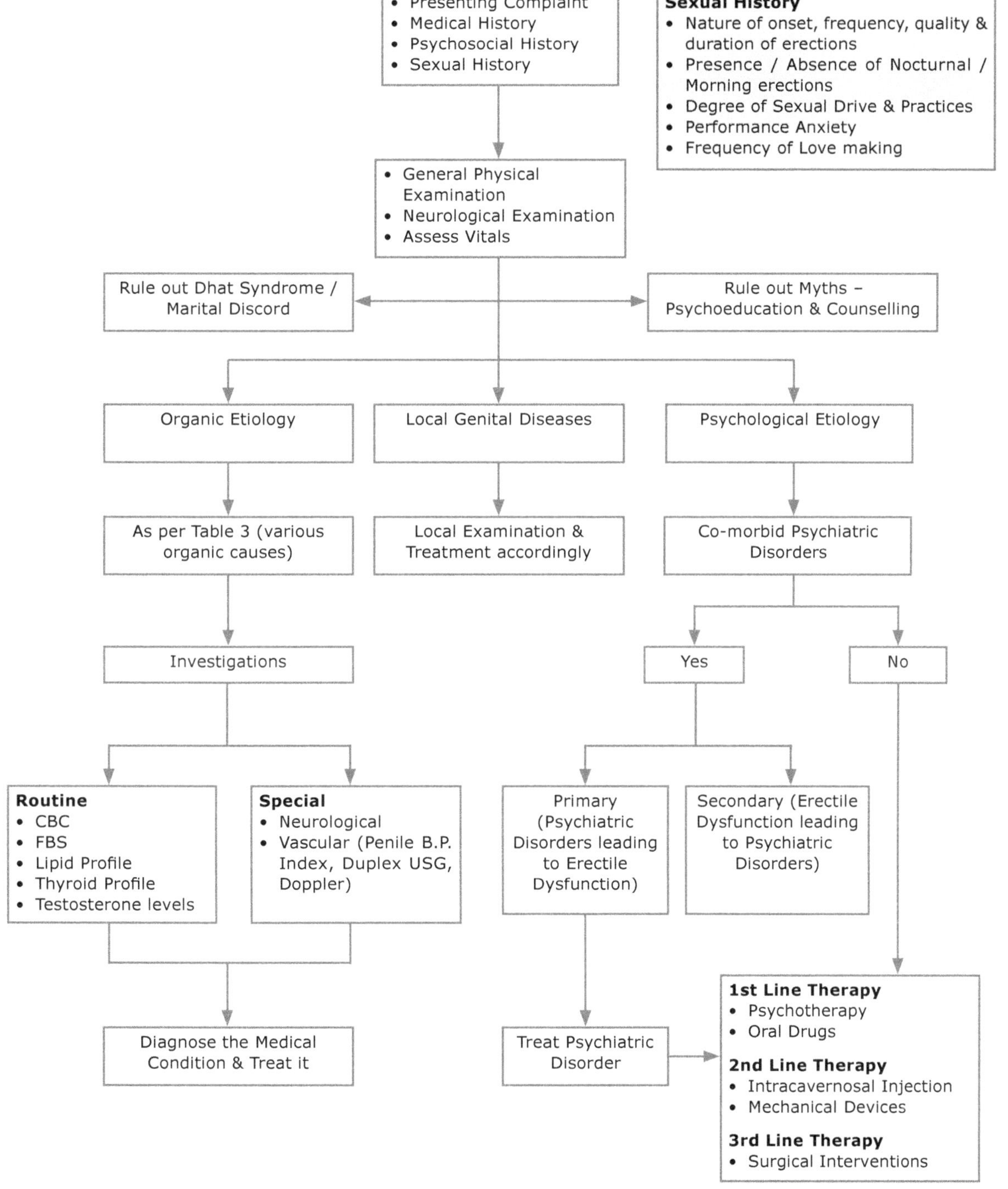

Flowchart. 25.1: Algorithm for evaluation & assessment of erectile dysfunction

In the absence of a specific correctable etiology, the management of erectile dysfunction is largely empirical and performed in a step-wise manner. That is, initial first line therapy is based on lifestyle modification, psychological intervention followed by pharmacotherapy using oral erectrogenic agents. Second-line therapies consist of an intraurethral suppository (IUS) of prostaglandin E1 (alprostadil) and intracavernosal injection (ICI) with vasoactive substances and mechanical erection devices. Surgical intervention is reserved as the final option after conservative options have been discussed or attempted.

Lifestyle Modification

Lifestyle modifications can have a major role in managing erectile dysfunction, especially in the younger patient.It includes :

- Eating a healthy diet
- Regular exercise
- Cessation of cigarette smoking

Psychological Intervention

As the most common etiology of erectile dysfunction is the psychogenic, so psychological intervention becomes the main stay of treatment.

It may be individual oriented dynamic approach, Couple therapy or group therapy.

The following are the main methods employed :

1. Psychoeducation: It provides a basic factually source of information, clarifies myths, misinformations & prejudices.
2. Behavior Therapy: They are aimed at modifying maladaptive negative cognitions leading to ED.

   The common behavior therapies include Relaxation and Desensitization, Operant Conditioning and Aversive Conditioning
3. Pyschosexual Psychotherapy : It is usually a dual sex therapy wherein both the partners are involved in therapy sessions. Therapists and patients discuss the psychological and physiological aspects of sexual functioning. Couples are suggested specific sexual activities to be followed in privacy at their home. The sensate focus therapy is specific for Erectile Dysfunction.

Sensate Focus Therapy

A cognitive behavioral approach is a programme of tasks, first described by Masters and Johnson The tasks involve the couple setting aside time to explore each other's bodies in turn by touching, stroking, caressing, and massaging— gradually introducing sensual, then erotic, and then sexual touch over a period of time. It consists of three stages: Non Genital Sensate focus, Genital Sensate focus and Vaginal Containment.

Non Genital Sensate Focus

In the first stage, the couple may touch each other's bodies excluding breasts and genitals. They are encouraged to enjoy and become increasingly aware of the warmth, texture and other qualities of their partner's skin. The aim here is to minimize pressure and expectations, and to appreciate new sensual possibilities.

Genital Sensate Focus

The second stage increases the touch options to include breasts. Sensation and gathering information about the partner's body is still encouraged and intercourse and touching of the genitals is still forbidden. The participants then use a technique of placing their hand over their partner's hand in order to show what they find pleasurable in terms of pace and pressure. Learning about the partner's body is still the goal rather than pleasure.

Vaginal Containment

The next step is containment without movement, allowing the penis to be accepted and contained by the vagina. Couples should progress at their preferred pace. Containment with gentle thrusting and rotating movement followed to orgasm.

Pharmacotherapy

The major drugs used for treatment of Erectile Dysfunction are described in **Table 25.5**.

Table 25.5

A. Oral Drugs	
1. Phosphodiesterae type 5 (PDE5) Inhibitors Mechanism: They competitively inhibit PDE5, leading to a build-up of cGMP upon NO release, initiating a cascade of events that lead to smooth muscle relaxation and promotion of an erection.	❖ The drug takes effect about 1 hour after ingestion, and its effect can last upto 4 hours. ❖ It is not effective in absence of sexual stimulation ❖ Common side effects : headache, flushing & dyspepsia ❖ Contraindication : persons taking Nitrates
Sildenafil	Dose: 50-100 mg orally to be taken an hour before intercourse
Tadalafil	Dose: 5-10 mg orally to be taken an hour before intercourse
Vardenafil	Dose: 5-20 mg orally to be taken an hour before intercourse
2. Others	
- Phentolamine	❖ Competitive alpha 1 and 2 inhibitor ❖ Reduces sympathetic tone and relaxes corporeal smooth muscle ❖ Side Effects : hypotension, tachycardia and dizziness
- Apomorphine	❖ Central dopamine receptor activator ❖ Its effect is mediated by the autonomic nervous system and results in vasodilatation resulting in blood flow to penis ❖ Side Effects : nausea and sweating
- Trazodone	❖ It is antidepressant that improves nocturnal erections. Dose: 50 to 100 mg per day in three divided dosages
- Yohimbine	❖ An alpha receptor antagonist
B. VasoactiveIntracavernosal Injections (ICI) They act locally on penis and can produce erections in the absence of sexual stimulation	
a) Papaverine	❖ A non- selective inhibitor of phosphodiesterase ❖ It acts by increasing cAMP thus decreasing intracellular smooth muscle. ❖ It is used in PIPE test (Papavarine induced Penile Erection) to distinguish between psychogenic and organic ED

(Continued)

b) Alprostadil	❖ It contains a naturally occurring form of Prostaglandin E, a vasoditing agent ❖ The erection occurs within 2-3 mins after administration and effect last as long as 1 hour. ❖ Side effects : penile bruising & altered liver function and serious adverse effect includes Priapism and sclerosis of the small veins

Mechanical Treatment

This includes

1. **Tension rings** – These are useful when an adequate erection can be obtained but not sustained. A tight rubber band at the base of the penis maintains an erection for up to 30 minutes.
2. **Vacuum Constriction Device** – It is a cylindrical mechanical device placed over the penis and then pumped, which creates a negative pressure vacuum to draw blood into the lacunar spaces within the corpora cavernosa of penis, causing tumescence. Devices are often used in conjunction with a tension ring that is placed at the base of the penis after tumescence is achieved, to prevent the backflow of blood.

Surgical Intervention

Surgical therapies are reserved for the subset of patients who have contraindications to the non-surgical interventions, those who experience adverse effects from (or are refractory to) the pharmacotherapy and those who also have penile fibrosis or penile vascular insufficiency.

1. **Penile Prosthesis** – There are 2 types of Prosthesis: a) A semi rigid rod prosthesis that produces a permanent erection that can be positioned close to the body for concealment and b) An inflatable type is implanted with its own reservoir and pump for inflation and deflation.
2. **Vascular Surgery** – When vascular insufficiency is present due to atherosclerosis or other blockage, bypass surgery of penile arteries can be attempted in selected cases.

PREMATURE EJACULATION

Premature ejaculation is the most common male sexual dysfunction. Several surveys among different populations estimate its prevalence at 29%, with a range between 1% and 75% depending on the population and criteria used to define the condition.

Definition: Persistent or recurrent ejaculation with minimal sexual stimulation before, on, or shortly after penetration and before the person wishes it.

The clinician must take into account factors that affect duration of the excitement phase, such as age, novelty of the sexual partner or situation, and recent frequency of sexual activity.

It can manifest as lifelong or acquired type, situational or generalized form and PME is primarily due to psychological factors or combined, i.e., psychological and organic factors.

Common etiological factors are given in **Table 25.6**.

Table 25.6

Psychogenic	• Neurotic personality • Anxiety • Depression • Interpersonal conflicts among sexual partners • Fear of an adverse health event during intercourse • Situational factors
Organic	• Physical illness • Physical injury • Increased central dopaminergic activity • Increased penile sensitivity

Management Algorithm – An Algorithm for diagnosis and evaluation of Premature Ejaculation is given in **Flowchart 25.2**.

Broadly management includes treatment of the basic cause like neurological, medical, psychiatric illness, teaching deficient skills, improvement in couple relationship, etc. The most common cause is psychogenic usually so specific intervention encompasses drug and psychosexual therapy.

Psychosocial Intervention: Psychoeducation &, Reassurance

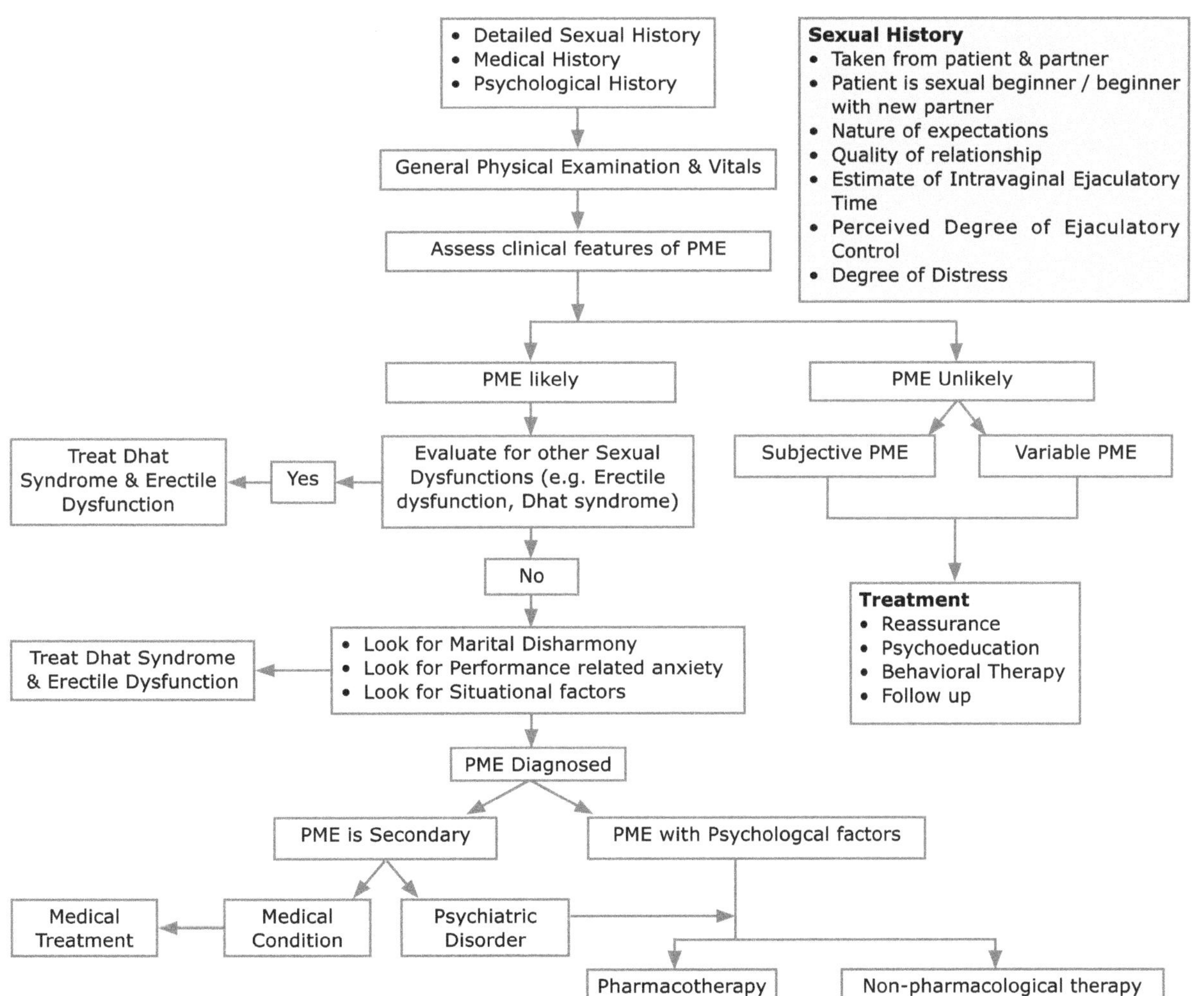

Flowchart. 25.2: Algorithm for evaluation & assessment of premature ejaculation (PME).

Non Pharmacological Treatment

It is considered that behavioral management should be the first line of therapy where ever possible. The most important being the psycho education to clarify the myths and the relaxation techniques to alleviate the anxiety related to performance. The specific behavioral techniques for PME involves stop start or squeeze techniques, which are usually introduced during genital sensate focus.

The **squeeze technique** was first developed by Semans in 1956, but was popularized by Masters and Johnson in 1970. The technique aims to increase the frequency of sexual contact and increase the sensory threshold of the penis. This technique is best carried out in the context of sensate focus exercises wherin a couple learns to pay attention to their body during foreplay, to communicate during genital stimulation about perceived excitement and to cooperate during intercourse.

The **stop-start technique** consists of the man focusing his attention fully on the sensation provided by the partner's stimulation of his penis. When he feels himself becoming highly aroused he should indicate this to her in pre-arranged manner at which point she should stop caressing and allow his arousal to subside. After a short delay this procedure is repeated twice more, following which the woman stimulates her partner to ejaculation.

The squeeze technique is an elaboration of the stop-start technique. The couple proceeds as with the stop-start procedure. When the man indicates he is becoming highly aroused his partner should apply a firm squeeze to his penis using the thumb and first two fingers at the place where the glans of penis joins the shaft for about 15-20 seconds. This inhibits the ejaculatory reflex. As with the stop-start technique this is repeated three times in a session and on the fourth occasion the man should ejaculate.

Pharmacotherapy

The major drugs used for treatment of Premature Ejaculation are described in **Table 25.7**.

Table 25.7: Drugs for premature ejaculation

DRUGS	
1. Antidepressants : Several studies have shown drugs that enhance central sertonergic transmission are effective for PME. Side Effects: nausea, perspiration, drowsiness and decreased libido	
Tricyclic Antidepressant-Clomipramine	❖ Dose: 25-50 mg/day ❖ Greatest increase in ejaculatory latency
SSRI	
Fluoxetine	❖ Dose: 5-20 mg/day ❖ Well tolerated ❖ Effective in treating men with severe PME who have never achieved intravaginal ejaculation & comorbid panic attacks.
Paroxetine	❖ Dose: 10-40 mg/day ❖ It is most potent ❖ Can be administered on 'on demand' basis 3-4 hours before intercourse also.
Sertraline	❖ Dose: 25 to 200 mg/day ❖ Better efficacy and safety
Dapoxetine 30mg - SOS	
2. Topical Anesthetics : They help by reducing the sensation to penis and hence help delay ejaculation. Side Effects: Temporary loss of sensitivity and decreased sexual pleasure in both the partners	
Lidocaine / prilocaine cream Or Lidocaine sprays	Lidocaine 2.5% 20-30 mins. prior to intercourse

HYPOACTIVE SEXUAL DESIRE DISORDER

The hypoactive sexual desire disorder is a highly prevalent disorder with prevalence rate upto15% and is more common in Females (previously called as frigidity) than in males.

HSD manifests as deficiency or absence of sexual fantasies and desire of sexual activity, with resultant marked distress or interpersonal difficulty.

Etiology

- Psychogenic
  - Boredom or unhappiness in a long-standing relationship
  - Marital discord leading to desire deficiency
  - Performance anxiety leading to excitement inhibition
- Psychiatric disorders
  - Depression
  - Stress and chronic anxiety
- Alcohol and substance misuse
- Secondary to poor sexual arousal and lack of orgasm
- Desynchronization of sexual aspiration and motivation
- CNS disease (partial epilepsy, Parkinson's, poststroke, adrenoleukodystrophy)
- Drugs
  - Antihypertensives
  - Psychotropics,
  - Dopamine blockers
  - Antiandrogens
- Gynecological & Obstetric Disorders causing pain on sexual intercourse
- Urological disorders causing pain on sexual intercourse
- Endocrine disorders - Androgen deficiency syndrome, Hyperprolactinemia
- Neurological disorders

Management (Flowchart 25.3)

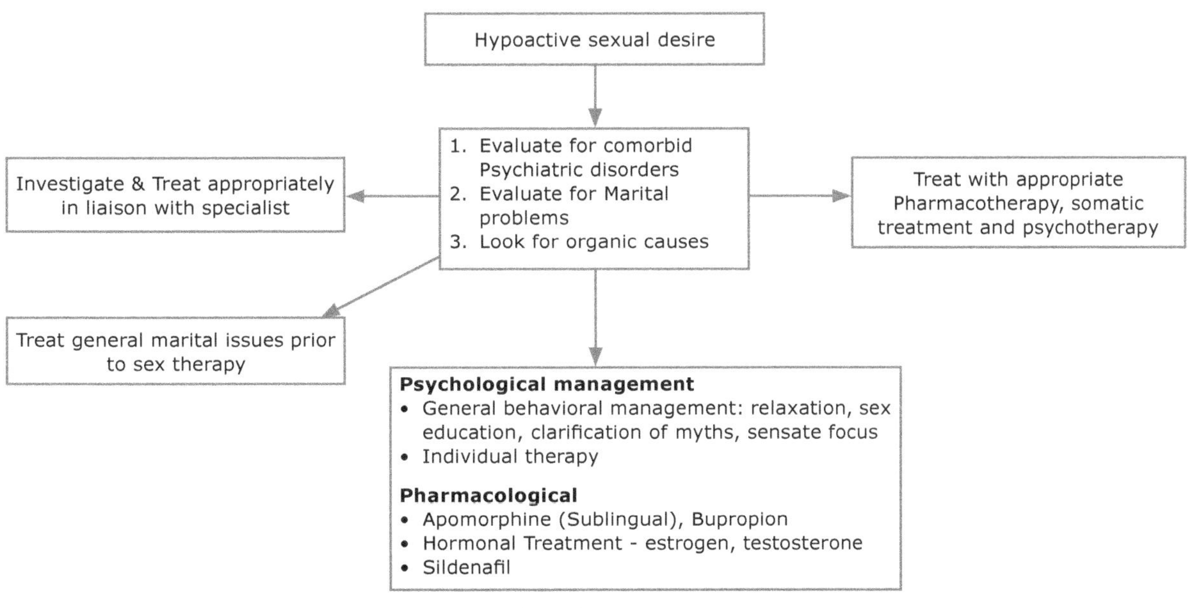

Flowchart. 25.3

CULTURE BOUND SYNDROME

Dhat Syndrome

Dhat Syndrome was first described in 1960 (Wig, 1960). It refers to a culture bound clinical condition characterized by guilt about loss of semen in young men, often leading to undue concern with its debilitating effect on physical and psychological health.

Patient presents with vague and multiple somatic and psychological symptoms like lack of physical strength, fatigue, listlessness, poor concentration, forgetfulness etc. The core feature is the undue concern with the passage of semen during micturition or while straining to pass stools, although there is no objective evidence of semen in urine or its passage otherwise.

There may be accompanying anxiety or depressive symptoms and the patient may present with or without sexual dysfunction and accordingly some researchers have described subgroups of Dhat syndrome, viz. Dhat syndrome alone, Dhat syndrome with anxiety or depressive symptoms and Dhat syndrome with sexual dysfunction.

Dhat syndrome has also been extended to include Indian women presenting with somatic symptoms associated with leucorrhea, and explained as due to loss of a 'vital fluid'.

Treatment

The most important aspect of treatment of Dhat syndrome is providing adequate sex knowledge and clarifying sexual myths. Sex education mainly focuses on anatomy and physiology of sexual organs and their functioning with reference to masturbation, semen formation, nocturnal emissions and their functioning with genitourinary system independent of gastro-intestinal tract etc. If there is the presence of associated anxiety or depressive symptoms that impede the process of therapy, anxiolytics or/ and antidepressants can be added for the least possible time and in the lowest possible doses.

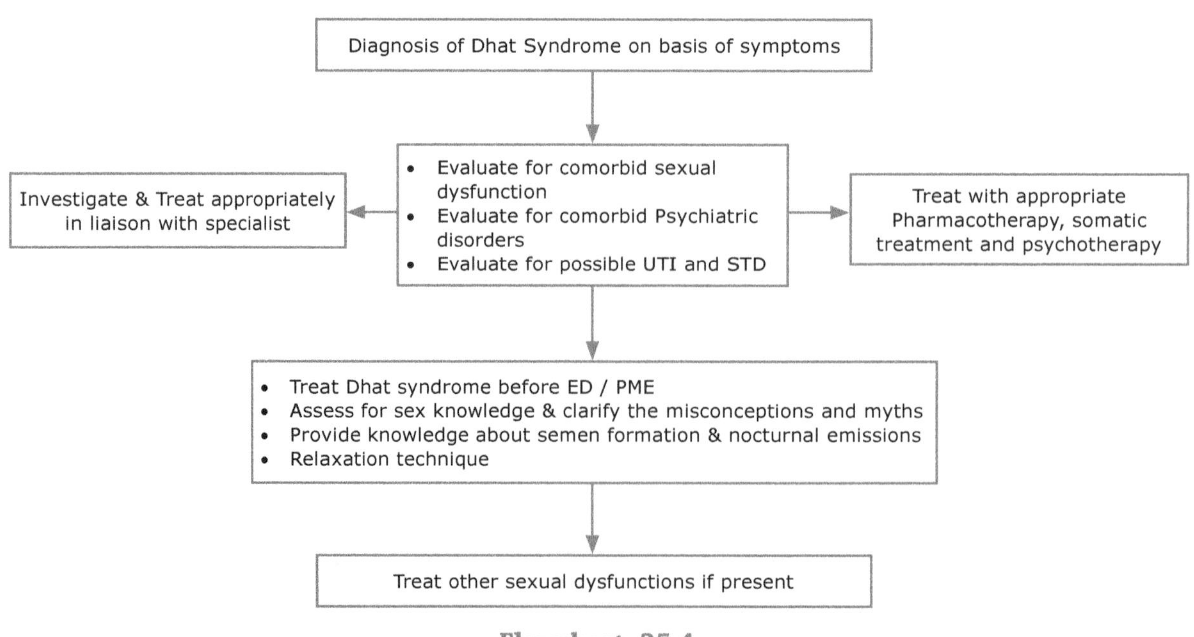

Flowchart. 25.4

COMMON SEXUAL MISCONCEPTIONS

Sexual misconceptions or myths are formed by the beliefs and assumptions prevalent in the native culture. This misconceptions arise from inadequate information, lack of awareness as well as sexual taboo prevalent in society. For some individuals, inappropriate sexual beliefs or myths can cause problems within a relationship. Some of the common myths and their clarification are as follows:

Table 25.8

Myths	Clarification
1. The man should be the sexual leader and always initiate sex.	By being the 'sexual leader' and taking responsibility for arousing both oneself and one's partner, not only they have the pressure of ensuring that the woman is satisfied, but they also miss out on the extra stimulation that could be given to them by their partner. Therefore, they have all of the pressure and less of the pleasure.
2. A woman should not initiate sex	It is important for a woman to be able to communicate her sexual needs and interests as well, rather than just waiting for her partner to initiate sex, or expecting her partner to know intuitively what specific sexual activities are enjoyable or desired on a particular occasion.
3. A woman should always have sex when her partner makes sexual approaches.	It is not a woman's 'duty' to have sex with her husband. A woman should feel able to say no to sex when she does not feel like it.
4. Formation of Semen : Semen is formed from blood and loss of it will lead to weakness.	Semen is a mixture of secretions from prostate, seminal vesicles and bulbuo-urethral glands plus sperms. Semen provides nutrition, helps motility and acts as a vehicle for the transport of sperms.
5. Masturbation is wrong. It is commonly believed that too much of masturbation is wrong and leads to mental illness, physical weakness and decreases potency. Masturbation is considered to be responsible for shrinkage or sideward curvature of penis and watery semen.	There is no scientific evidence to support this. The act of masturbation is as natural as making love, and, just like sexual intercourse it does not have any adverse effects on the health.
6. A 'respectable' woman should not enjoy sex too much and should certainly never masturbate.	Any woman of any age is a sexual being. She should feel free to experiment sexually in any way that feels comfortable. Enjoyment of sex is healthy, natural, and to be encouraged.

(Continued)

Myths	Clarification
7. Size of the penis. Very often males are preoccupied with the fact that larger penis are more effective.	This myth should be address by discussing about the size of normal penis in flaccid and erect position and the minimal length of penis required satisfying a female. The sensory endings are present only in the lower one third of vagina.
8. Circumcision and sexual performance: Many persons tend to belief that circumcision is helpful in prolonging coitus by delaying the ejaculation time.	No scientific evidence to support this.
9. Bending of Penis. Some males are very much distressed with the curvature of penis.	The slight curvature of the shaft of penis is perfectly normal and does not harm the sexual intercourse
10. Vasectomy/tubectomy decreases sexual potency.	The couple should be explained that use of contraception or such operations ensure prevention of fertilization and possible chance of pregnancy and hence allows them to enjoy sex more freely.
11. Drugs enhance sexual potency. It is a common belief that alcohol and/or Opioids or other drugs improve potency.	These drugs temporarily increase a men's sexual desire, but they definitely decrease the sexual performance.
12. Role of 'Physical strength' or 'Muscle power' in sexual performance. It is a common belief that muscular men can perform better than averagely built man.	There is no relation between muscle power and sexual performance and what matters is the motivation and proper knowledge about sex.
13. Sex happens automatically. This myth asserts that one should not have to learn about sex or ask the partner about what they like because sex is something one should instinctively know about.	Most of what people know about sex is learned from the media, parents, or friends. Much of this information promotes biased or unrealistic beliefs that may actually interfere with the enjoyment of sex. Good sex may involve re-learning much of what is known and assumed. However, with practice, this new knowledge will become natural and the sex lives and relationships will be enhanced.
14. Apprehension about potency : It is a common held belief in most of the Indian sub-cultures that masturbation and night emissions before marriage result in loss of potency in marital conjugal relations.	It is importsant to impart sex education at preliminary level so that the basic concepts related to sexual activity are clear.

SEXUAL HEALTH EDUCATION:

The first step in the treatment of any sexual dysfunction is education. The aims of education are to normalize the individual's experiences (i.e., help the individual realize that there are many others who have the same needs, problems, and experiences), reduce anxiety about sex by providing accurate information about arousal and normal sexual response, dispel sexual myths, dispel unrealistic expectations. Material used for the sex education should cover information about the anatomy of the sex organs, menstrual cycle, pregnancy, puberty, masturbation, formation of semen, night falls, types of sex, stages of sexual intercourse, normal male and female sexual response cycle.

BIBLIOGRAPHY

1. Comprehensive Textbook of Sexual Medicine 2005 by Nilamadhab Kar and Gopal Chandra Kar.
2. Clinical Practice Guidelines for Management of Sexual Dysfunction published by (Indian Psychiatric Society) by Dr. Ajit Avasthi, et al.
3. Fig. 25.1 – Human Sexual Response. Source: Masters, W.H. & Johnson, V.E. (1966).
4. Kaplan & Sadock's Synopsis of Psychiatry: Behavioral Sciences / Clinical Psychiatry (11th Edition).
5. Erectile Dysfunction: An article by Faysal A. Yafietal. Nat Reve Dis Primers;2:16003. doi:10.1038/nrdp.2016.3.

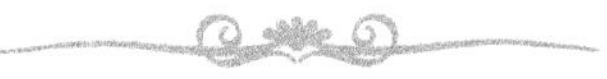

26 Gender Identity Disorder

Sagar Karia • Tejesvi Dave

DEFINITION

As per American Psychological Association Dictionary of Psychology, Gender is the condition of being male, female, or neuter. In a human context, the distinction between GENDER and SEX reflects the usage of these terms: Sex usually refers to the biological aspects of maleness or femaleness, whereas gender implies the psychological, behavioral, social and cultural aspects of being male or female (i.e., masculinity or femininity.)

Gender identity refers to a person's psychological identification as a man or a woman. It is one's sense of self or belief in being male or female. Gender identity can correlate with allotted sex at birth or can differ from it.

Early signs of gender dysphoria include that children may refuse to follow typical gender rules and expectations, adolescents may feel disgusted with the development of secondary sexual characteristics, and adults may feel trapped inside the body of opposite gender.

Terms Related to Gender and Sex

Let us have a look at few terminologies-

1. **Orientation:** It is a term used to refer to a person's emotional, romantic, and sexual attraction to individuals of a particular gender (male or female).

   Sexual orientation is usually divided into three categories:
   - Heterosexual: attracted to individuals of the opposite sex
   - Bisexual: attracted to members of either sex
   - Homosexual: attracted to individuals of one's own sex
2. **Natal Gender:** It refers to the gender allotted during the birth.
3. **Cisgender:** A person who's experienced gender and assigned gender is in alignment.
4. **Eunuch:** A eunuch is a male who is castrated. Castration is the process of removal of testicles.
5. **Transgender:** Transgender refers to the people whose gender identity does not match the sex they were assigned at birth.
6. **Transvestite:** It is commonly referred as Cross Dressing which involves experiencing pleasure and arousal from dressing like opposite gender.
7. **Transsexual:** Refers to an individual who wishes to undergo hormonal along with surgical procedures to alter the body so that it adapts to one's experienced gender.

HISTORY ABOUT GID

The term Gender identity was first invented by Robert Stoller in the mid-20th century. It signified one's inner belief of belonging to either the male or female gender category. Transgender is a term formulated by Virginia Prince in the early 1970s which referred to the people who lived as the opposite gender. Initially the gender change was combined with theory of homosexuality. Till the middle of the 20th century, some of the transgender presentations were usually classified as "psychopathological."

Lili Elbe was the first known recipient of male-to-female sex reassignment surgery, in Germany in 1930 wherein she underwent four surgeries: one each for orchiectomy, to transplant an ovary, for penectomy, and for vaginoplasty and a uterus transplant. But she died three months after her last operation. The option of changing genders gained popularity when American George Jorgensen went to Denmark as a man and returned to the United States in 1952 as transwoman Christine Jorgensen. The publicity around this transition led to an awareness around medical and non medical fields, after which concept emerged as gender identity.

Laura Dillon born as female was first person to undergo female-to-male sex reassignment surgery and become transman and called himself as Michael Dillon.

DSM and ICD

The previous editions of DSM and ICD did not have any gender dysphoria diagnosis. The diagnosis of Transsexual first appeared in ICD – 9 in 1975. Then in 1980, the latest edition of DSM – III offered a new diagnosis based on the growing research.

The **Table 26.1** below shows the emergence and journey of Gender Dysphoria.

Table 26.1

DSM / ICD	Parent Category	Diagnosis Name
DSM – III (1980)	Psychosexual disorders	Transsexualism
		Gender identity disorder of childhood
DSM – III – R (1987)	Disorders usually first evident in infancy, childhood, or adolescence	Transsexualism
		Gender identity disorder of childhood
		Gender identity disorder of adolescence and adulthood, nontranssexual type
ICD – 10 (1900)	Gender Identity Disorders	Transsexualism
		Dual-role transvestism
		Gender identity disorder of childhood
		Other gender identity disorders
		Gender identity disorder, unspecified
DSM – IV (1994)	Sexual and gender identity disorders	Gender identity disorder in adolescents or adults
		Gender identity disorder in children
DSM – IV – TR (2000)	Sexual and gender identity disorders	Gender identity disorder in adolescents or adults
		Gender identity disorder in children
DSM – 5 (2013)	Gender Dysphoria	Gender dysphoria in adolescents and adults
		Gender Dysphoria in Children
		Other specified gender dysphoria
		Unspecified gender dysphoria

DSM 5

DSM – 5 has revised the name from Gender Identity Disorder (GID) to Gender Dysphoria (GD) to reduce the patient's stress and make it less stigmatizing. The new term focuses on the Dysphoria and not on the Identity part of an individual.

Let's have a look at detailed Diagnostic Criteria of DSM – 5

Gender Dysphoria in Children 302.6 (F64.2)

A) A marked incongruence between one's experienced/expressed gender and assigned gender, of at least 6 months' duration, as manifested by at least six of the following (one of which must be Criterion A1):

1. A strong desire to be of the other gender or an insistence that one is the other gender (or some alternative gender different from one's assigned gender).
2. In boys (assigned gender), a strong preference for cross-dressing or simulating female attire: or in girls (assigned gender), a strong preference for wearing only typical masculine clothing and a strong resistance to the wearing of typical feminine clothing.
3. A strong preference for cross-gender roles in make-believe play or fantasy play.
4. A strong preference for the toys, games, or activities stereotypically used or engaged in by the other gender.
5. A strong preference for playmates of the other gender.
6. In boys (assigned gender), a strong rejection of typically masculine toys, games, and activities and a strong avoidance of rough-and-tumble play; or in girls (assigned gender), a strong rejection of typically feminine toys, games and activities.
7. A strong dislike of one's sexual anatomy.
8. A strong desire for the primary and/or secondary sex characteristics that match one's experienced gender.

B) The condition is associated with clinically significant distress or impairment in social, school or other important areas of functioning.

Gender Dysphoria in Adolescents and Adults 302.85 (F64.1)

A) A marked incongruence between one's experienced/expressed gender and assigned gender, of at least 6 months' duration, as manifested by at least two of the following:

1. A marked incongruence between one's experienced/expressed gender and primary and/or secondary sex characteristics (or in young adolescents, the anticipated secondary sex characteristics).
2. A strong desire to be rid of one's primary and/or secondary sex characteristics because of a marked incongruence with one's experienced/expressed gender (or in young adolescents, a desire to prevent the development of the anticipated secondary sex characteristics).
3. A strong desire for the primary and/or secondary sex characteristics of the other gender.

4. A strong desire to be of the other gender (or some alternative gender different from one's assigned gender).
5. A strong desire to be treated as the other gender (or some alternative gender different from one's assigned gender).
6. A strong conviction that one has the typical feelings and reactions of the other gender (or some alternative gender different from one's assigned gender).

B) The condition is associated with clinically significant distress or impairment in social, occupational or other important areas of functioning.

Other Specified Gender Dysphoria 302.6 (F64.8)

This category applies to presentations in which symptoms characteristic of gender dysphoria that cause clinically significant distress or impairment in social, occupational, or other important areas of functioning predominate but do not meet the full criteria for gender dysphoria. The other specified gender dysphoria category is used in situations in which the clinician chooses to communicate the specific reason that the presentation does not meet the criteria for gender dysphoria. This is done by recording "other specified gender dysphoria" followed by the specific reason (e.g., "brief gender dysphoria"). An example of a presentation that can be specified using the "other specified" designation is the following: The current disturbance meets symptom criteria for gender dysphoria, but the duration is less than 6 months.

Unspecified Gender Dysphoria 302.6 (F64.9)

This category applies to presentations in which symptoms characteristic of gender dysphoria that cause clinically significant distress or impairment in social, occupational, or other important areas of functioning predominate but do not meet the full criteria for gender dysphoria. The unspecified gender dysphoria category is used in situations in which the clinician chooses not to specify the reason that the criteria are not met for gender dysphoria, and includes presentations in which there is insufficient information to make a more specific diagnosis.

Etiology

The exact etiology is unclear but there exists a complex biopsychosocial link.

Biological Causes:

1. One of the well established biological links is explained via individuals born with androgen insensitivity syndrome or congenital adrenal hyperplasia. These children are usually brought up as girls even though they dress up and have innate sense of opposite gender.
2. In-utero exposure to phthalates in plastics and polychlorinated biphenyls are known to disrupt the regular endocrinology of sex determination before birth. Phthalates can lead to an increase in total fetal testosterone levels and thereby increasing chances of GID.
3. Neuroanatomical links have been found in certain studies like faulty neuronal development and differentiation in the hypothalamic links. Functional neuroimaging has shown variations in hemispheric ratios and amygdala connectivity according to gender.
4. Genetic association has also been identified for example some alleles like CYP17 T-34C, ERα, SRD5A2, and STS.

5. Exposure of certain hormones during development can alter some brain circuitry leading to development of GID.

Psychosocial Causes

- The inception of gender dysphoria was so often triggered by traumatic events, psychosis in the mother during pregnancy and childbirth, separation.
- Parenting also plays an important role. Labeling the child, non-verbal expressions like clothing, manners, style etc. For instance, a couple desiring boy and receiving a girl may decide to dress the girl as a boy and lay male gender expectations to the extent that this girl starts feeling uncomfortable with being a female.
- Problems during separation individuation process, for example son when separates from mother and identifies with father, during which he has bad experience with father or face rejection, he has no option but to reattach with mother for emotional security and males become aggressive/ sexual objects; thereby leading to GID.

Clinical features – Children, Adolescents, Adults

Children

Around 2–3 years of age, the concept of gender identity becomes clear and around the age of 5 years it solidifies. Once the child understands the fact that gender is constant, if gender dysphoria persists, it reflects. At this age the discomfort between natal gender and experienced gender surfaces.

Girls may express the wish to be a boy, or the desire to be a man once they grow up, would like to play with boys and prefer games like Cricket, Sports instead of conventional feminine toys like dolls and kitchen set. Girls with Gender dysphoria may connect more with boys and feel associated with them and would want to be like them. They would prefer to dress in pants and shirts / T-shirts than in frocks.

Boys with Gender Dysphoria may express the desire to be a girl or a woman once they grow up. Boys may not favor the games, dressing and lifestyle of a conventional male. They may admire and would want long hair, make up, fascination of doing household chores assuming it's a feminine task.

In some of the cases, boys may sit for urination while girls may stand to urinate

Boys and girls both may display opposite gender identification in role plays, dreams and fantasy

Adolescents

Adolescent phase represents the development of Secondary Sexual Characteristics. Adolescents with Gender Dysphoria would be uncomfortable with the development of these characteristics. Girls may feel disgusted with Menstruation cycle, development of breasts, widening of hips. Similarly boys may not be comfortable with enlargement of penis, growth spurt, nightfall.

Adults

Adults with Gender Dysphoria experience a lot of distress due to difference between the fully developed physical characteristics and experienced gender. Some of the adults express the desire to get rid of the primary and secondary sexual characteristics of the natal gender, while some of the adults may just struggle to accept the natal gender due to the society, culture and other external factors. Some of them may implement the life style of the experienced gender.

Comorbidity

An individuals with Gender Dysphoria show mild to moderate levels of anxiety and depression. This is due to number of factors like less acceptance or rejection from family and society, concerns about the future. Whether or not they decide to undergo the surgery, there is fear of unknown and how the life ahead be. Suicidal thoughts and/or attempt are higher as sometimes they feel that ending life is better than never ending struggle. In survey, adult transgenders around 25–43% have reported suicide attempts. Also a lot of individuals take shelter in the use of various types of substances as a temporary relief from the distress and discomfort that they experience. In clinically referred children with Gender Dysphoria, Journal of Psychosomatic Research states that 71% of the patients fulfilled the criteria for current and/or life time Axis 1 diagnosis. 42% of the patients were diagnosed with one or more Personality Disorders. The National Transgender Discrimination Survey reports the rate of HIV infection four times more than the national average. Autism spectrum disorder is dominant than in general masses. Also a lot of children/adolescents/adults face issues with controlling their impulsivity and anger. As per Psychiatry and Clinical Neurosciences 2010, adjustment disorder was 6.7%, anxiety disorder 3.6%, Mood disorder was 1.4%. A survey was conducted with a group of Psychiatrists regarding their experiences with treating and diagnosing individuals with Gender Dysphoria, they reported comorbidity with dissociative disorders by 26% and psychotic disorders by 24%.

Management

In the management of Gender Dysphoria, a core team consists of Psychiatrist, Psychologist, Endocrinologist, Plastic Surgeon and Gynecologist.

History Taking forms the base followed by physical and psychological evaluation. Once evaluated, hormonal and surgical procedures start depending on the patient's requirement.

History Taking

History taking is the base of this process. A good and detailed history of the patient is crucial.

Detailed history includes the following points:

- **Demographic Details**: Name, age, gender, education, occupation, area of residing, native.
- **Developmental Details**: Milestones, birth details, a mother experiencing trauma/mental illness during pregnancy and/or birth, substance use in the mother during pregnancy, alcohol use.
- **Family History:** Anyone in the family suffering or has suffered from any psychiatry illness, trauma, substance abuse, severe conflicts, alcohol use disorder.
- **Social History**: Childhood, academic record, inter-personal relationships, sexual relationships, social support.

  A lot of gender dysphoria symptoms are reflected from the childhood and prepuberty stage, hence it is important to focus little more in that phase.
- **Past Psychiatry Details**: Any psychiatry issues the patient is suffering or has suffered in the past. This would include - suicidal attempts, depression, anxiety, substance abuse, sexual abuse, violence, trauma, alcohol use.
- **Physical Examination**

  It is done to check for any genital anomalies or any other congenital deformities.

- **Psychological Intervention**

  Patients are counseled regarding the entire procedure of evaluation and further management.

  They are explained the need for cross dressing before actually undergoing Hormone Replacement Therapy or SRS.

  They are explained about irreversibility of the SRS procedures and also the fertility issues post surgery. For fertility preservation, sperms/ ova can be preserved and used later on in Invitro Fertilization procedure.

  They are explained the risks and benefits of hormonal treatment like venous thromboembolism, bone mineral density and pubertal suppression.

- **Hormonal Management**

  Gender affirming hormones are used for development of male/female secondary sexual characteristics.

  Hormones like estrogen is used in natal males to develop breasts, widen the hips, soften the hair, reducing facial and body hair and make the face feminine, while testosterone in natal females will allow for the muscle to increase its mass, slightly change the voice and make it deeper, stopping periods, increased sex drive, more facial and body hair. The use of both these hormones will affect an individual's emotions. Time taken to reflect the changes varies from individual to individual. The hormone therapy is started before the surgical procedures. Hormone therapy will start changing ones body from natal gender to experienced gender.

- **Surgical**

  Sex Reassignment Surgery (SRS) is also known as Gender Reassignment Surgery (GRS).

  Surgeries for Transmen (female to male) include:

  - Bilateral mastectomy (removal of both breasts)
  - Hysterectomy (removal of the womb)
  - Salpingo-oophorectomy (removal of the fallopian tubes and ovaries)
  - Phalloplasty (creation of a penis)
  - Scrotoplasty (creation of a scrotum)
  - Metoidioplasty (lengthening of clitoris)

  Surgeries for transwomen (male to female) include:

  - Orchidectomy (removal of the testes)
  - Penectomy (removal of the penis)
  - Vaginoplasty (construction of a vagina)
  - Vulvoplasty (construction of the vulva)
  - Clitoroplasty (construction of a clitoris with sensation)

Some individuals may need to have to go through various plastic surgeries to modify the appearance of the face, neck, or other regions of the body. A lot of transsexual individuals may not want to undergo all of these surgical procedures due to financial constraints or medical complications and warnings

Differential Diagnosis

Non-acceptance to conventional Gender characteristics: A lot of people do not follow the conventional gender roles laid by the society. E.g. A girl may not wanting to keep long hair but prefers boy cut hairstyle along with wearing jeans and a shirt, a man could be very comfortable taking care of his skin by using the cosmetic products. In both the above examples, the preference of lifestyle may not be conventional but the individuals are comfortable with the natal gender. A lot of males and females are more comfortable with atypical gender roles.

In the male dominated culture, especially in less developed area, child and adolescent girls often wish if they were a boy due to various reasons, e.g. freedom. As time passes and an individual grows, these aspects are often forgotten while the wish remains the same. While Case history taking, these areas have to be explored.

Clinical diagnosis as Gender Dysphoria should be given only if the client is distressed about the natal gender and is causing significant impairment.

Transvestic Disorder: Transvestic disorder is also referred as cross dressing. Here the individual gets sexual arousal from dressing as opposite gender. This behavior is displayed in heterosexual and homosexual adults. In this case an individual does not experience distress because of his natal gender; e.g.. A man is comfortable being a man and with the masculinity but experiences sexual arousal after wearing woman's clothing or fantasizing about it.

Psychosis: In psychosis, a person may have delusion of being opposite gender, thorough evaluation needs to be performed. Schizophrenia and Gender Dysphoria may co-occur.

BIBLIOGRAPHY

1. Coates S, Friedman RC, Wolfe S. The etiology of boyhood gender identity disorder: A model for integrating temperament, development, and psychodynamics. Psychoanalytic Dialogues. 1991 Jan 1;1(4):481-523.
2. Garg G, Marwaha R. Gender Dysphoria (Sexual Identity Disorders). InStatPearls [Internet] 2018 Oct 11. StatPearls Publishing.
3. American Psychiatric Association. Diagnostic and statistical manual of mental disorders (DSM-5®). American Psychiatric Pub; 2013 May 22.
4. Wallien MS, Swaab H, Cohen-Kettenis PT. Psychiatric comorbidity among children with gender identity disorder. Journal of the American Academy of Child & Adolescent Psychiatry. 2007 Oct 1;46(10):1307-14.
5. Hoshiai M, Matsumoto Y, Sato T, Ohnishi M, Okabe N, Kishimoto Y, Terada S, Kuroda S. Psychiatric comorbidity among patients with gender identity disorder. Psychiatry and Clinical Neurosciences. 2010 Oct;64(5):514-9.
6. Fenway Health. Glossary of gender and transgender terms.
7. Zucker KJ. Gender identity disorder in children and adolescents. Annu. Rev. Clin. Psychol.. 2005 Apr 27;1:467-92.
8. Selvaggi G, Ceulemans P, De Cuypere G, VanLanduyt K, Blondeel P, Hamdi M, Bowman C, Monstrey S. Gender identity disorder: general overview and surgical treatment for vaginoplasty in male-to-female transsexuals. Plastic and Reconstructive Surgery. 2005 Nov 1;116(6):135e-45e.
9. Unger CA. Hormone therapy for transgender patients. Translational andrology and urology. 2016 Dec;5(6):877.
10. Sutcliffe PA, Dixon S, Akehurst RL, Wilkinson A, Shippam A, White S, Richards R, Caddy CM. Evaluation of surgical procedures for sex reassignment: a systematic review. Journal of plastic, reconstructive & aesthetic surgery. 2009 Mar 1;62(3):294-306.
11. Benjamin J. Sadock, Virginia A. Sadock. Kaplan & Sadock's Comprehensive Textbook of Psychiatry. Philadelphia: Lippincott Williams & Wilkins, 2017.

27 Paraphilias

Sagar Karia • Tejesvi Dave

DEFINITION

The term paraphilia is derived from the Greek words 'para' means besides/faulty and 'philia' means love. Paraphilia thus refers to a love that is different from the accepted norm by the society.

Paraphilia is a disorder in which an individual is aroused, has sexual urges or behavior involving objects, minors or non - consenting adults, the suffering of oneself or partner.

A paraphilia can be so strong that a person may find it difficult to resist an impulse for such sexual act.

As per DSM 5, the term Paraphilic disorder is reserved for those cases in which a sexually deviant fantasy or impulse has been expressed behaviorally over a period of at least 6 months causing significant distress in the important areas of functioning.

Most of this sexual deviation occurs with men.

ETIOLOGY

The exact etiology of Paraphilia is unknown. Neuroanatomical and neuroimaging studies of sex offenders have shown that there may be congenital or acquired brain damage in this population. Studies have shown that defects of right amygdala and closely related structures may be involved in pedophilia. Neurologial theory proposes damage to frontal and or temporal lobe which translates into individual's inability to control sexual impulse and thereby leading to paraphilic behavior. Role of monoaminergic neurotransmitters have been proposed based on role of dopamine, norepinephrine and serotonin in human sexual motivation, appetite and consummatory behavior and pharmacological agents that affect monoamines have facilitative and inhibitory effects on sexual behavior.

TYPES OF PARAPHILIC DISORDERS

There are 8 types of Paraphilic disorders that would be included in this chapter, which are Voyeuristic Disorder, Exhibitionistic Disorder, Frotteuristic Disorder, Sexual Masochism Disorder, Sexual Sadism Disorder, Pedophilic Disorder, Fetishistic Disorder, Transvestic Disorder.

Let us have a detailed look at these different types of Paraphilic Disorders.

Voyeuristic Disorder

Voyeurism refers to the achievement of sexual gratification while spying on others performing sexual activities without their knowledge. An individual suffering from Voyeuristic disorder should atleast be 18 years of age who is sexually aroused from witnessing an unaware person naked, process of removing clothes or engaged in any sort of sexual activity. It is also called as "Peeping Tom".

Exhibitionistic Disorder

Exhibitionism means exposing the genitals. It is also known as "flashing". An individual (usually male) is sexually aroused by exposing his genitals to an unsuspecting, non-consenting strangers (usually children or females). It is usually followed by masturbation to achieve orgasm.

Frotteuristic Disorder

In this disorder, the sexual pleasure is derived by touching or rubbing against non consenting individual (usually of opposite sex). It usually occurs in crowded places, where the victim may not be in a position to react.

Sexual Sadism Disorder

In Sexual Sadism Disorder an individual receives sexual arousal and satisfaction at the cost of someone's pain and suffering. The sexual arousal occurs when the person (the 'sadist') causes physical and/or psychological humiliation, suffering or injury of the sexual partner (the 'victim'). Some of the acts include tying the partner, beating, and stabbing, forcing intercourse, cutting and even killing. In most of the cases, the other partner is likely to suffer from Sexual Masochism Disorder.

Sexual Masochism Disorder

In this disorder, sexual arousal and satisfaction is received from humiliation, beating or suffering. An individual (the 'masochist') gets aroused if someone tortures them as it would manifest in their fantasies. In a lot of cases, the other partner is the one suffering from Sexual Sadism Disorder.

Pedophilic Disorder

In Pedophilia, an individual is sexually attracted towards the children. An individual here engages himself in sexual activity with a prepubescent child or children of 13 years of age or younger. The individual is at least age 16 years and at least 5 years older than the child or children in Criterion.

Fetishistic Disorder

The term "fetishism" originates from the Portuguese word *feitico*, which means "obsessive fascination." The word fetish means magical, i.e. the nonliving object 'magically' becomes phallic for that person. The fetish objects may include shoes, gloves, bras, underpants, stockings, etc. Here the fascination is on the non-living objects or having a highly specific focus on non-genital body parts. It is not a fetishistic disorder if a person cross dresses or uses the devices meant for the purpose of tactile genital stimulation like vibrators.

Transvestic Disorder

In Transvestic disorder, an individual is sexually aroused only if he is dressed as an opposite gender. The individuals suffering from Transvestic disorder are heterosexual males. This disorder should not be confused with fetishishtic disorder where a man with fetishism for female undergarments, puts them on while masturbating.

Other Paraphilias

This include sexual arousal with urine (urophilia), feces (coprophilia), enemas (klismaphilia), corpses (necrophilia), etc. Zoophilia is also called as bestiality where a person has persistent and significant sexual interaction with animals.

DIFFERENTIAL DIAGNOSIS AND COMORBIDITY

Differential diagnosis and comorbidity may include conduct disorder, antisocial personality disorder, substance use disorder. Conditions that occur comorbidly with paraphilias include hypersexuality and other paraphilic disorders. Depressive, bipolar, anxiety, alcohol and substance use disorders; attention-deficit/hyperactivity disorder; and conduct disorder and antisocial personality disorder, obsessive compulsive disorder are also frequent co-morbid conditions.

MANAGEMENT

1. Pharmacology
2. Psychotherapy

Pharmacology

The 4 main class of drugs helpful in treatment of paraphilias include

1. **Selective Serotonin Reuptake Inhibitors (SSRIs):** Fluoxetine and sertraline have been used for treating paraphilias. SSRIs act by reducing sexual desire in patients by increasing levels of serotonin. Other actions which might help of SSRIs are control of impulsiveness, obsessive compulsive characteristics and indirect reduction of serum testosterone levels.
2. **Antiandrogens and hormonal treatment:** Various hormones that have been used are estrogen and medroxyprogesterone acetate. Cyproterone acetate is the antiandrogen blocking androgen receptors and causing reduction in all types of sexual behaviors. But need to be careful of these hormonal side effects.
3. **Luteinizing Hormone Releasing Hormone (LHRH) agonists:** They initially cause increase in Gonadotropin Releasing Hormone (GRH) secretion and then reduction to almost zero level. This leads to dropping in levels of circulating testosterone and dihydrotestosterone to castration levels. Examples of this category are leuprolide acetate and triptorelin.
4. **Other Psychotropics:** Primarily serotonergic tricyclic antidepressant Clomipramine has also been proved useful. Lithium Carbonate, antipsychotics (benperidol, thioridazine, haloperidol) and antiepileptics (carbamazpine) have also been used.

Psychotherapy

1. **Role Reversal:** This technique involves the therapist helping the client to realize that their behavior (i.e., exposing themselves, exhibiting sadist-type behaviors) is causing harm to someone. The goal of this approach is for the client to develop empathy towards the victims. If the client is able to develop sufficient empathy toward their victims, they may reduce or discontinue the behavior. Role reversal technique may be a useful treatment intervention for individuals with exhibitionism, frotteuristic, pedophilia, sexual sadism, and voyeurism.
2. **Covert Sensitization:** Covert sensitization involves eliminating the unwanted behavior by creating an association between the behavior and a highly disturbing "covert" (i.e., imagined) e.g.: electric shock, stimulus or consequence. Once the association is firmly established, engaging in the behavior is no longer appealing. In the case of paraphilias, the client is asked to imagine feeling shame when friends/family members observe him engaging in the behavior associated with the paraphilia or the client witnessing the loved one performing the similar act. This type of

intervention can be used with nearly all of the paraphilias and can help the client not engage in the behavior or to find the behavior less pleasurable.

3. **Orgasmic reconditioning:** Here the client is encouraged to engage in masturbation with his fantasy associated with paraphilia, but to complete the masturbation exercise (orgasm about to happen) while looking at an appropriate object (i.e., a picture of an adult partner) or performing a conventional behavior. It is a relearning process in which an individual associates sexual gratification with appropriate stimuli.
4. **Aversive Therapy:** Aversion therapy is a form of behavior therapy in which an aversive or a repulsive stimulus is paired with an undesirable behavior in order to reduce/eliminate that behavior. The pairing of deviant fantasies with unpleasant sensations is thought to decrease both fantasies and behaviors. For example, everytime a person engages in any behavior associated to paraphilia, he would be given electric shocks or grounded without food and water for 12 hours.
5. **Masturbatory Extinction:** In Masturbatory Extinction the client is encouraged to masturbate and orgasm to an appropriate fantasy. Then after orgasm (i.e., ejaculation) he is encouraged to continue masturbating but to the deviant sexual fantasy. This causes the appropriate fantasy to be reinforced with an orgasm but not the inappropriate fantasy (Plaud, 2007).
6. **Masturbatory Satiation:** In masturbatory satiation, the client is asked to masturbate with the deviant fantasy in mind even after reaching orgasm for one hour. The client may eventually lose interest in such fantasies as it does not end in reinforcing ejaculation (Plaud, 2007).
7. **Support Group:** Here the focus would be on taking responsibility for actions, victim impact and empathy, establishing family support, building relationship and social skills, and cognitive restructuring. The individual may lack social skills and have difficulty establishing relationships with others.

Paraphilia is the lesser spoke disorder. With proper diagnosis and treatment plan, an individual can be helped.

BIBLIOGRAPHY

1. American Psychiatric Association. Diagnostic and statistical manual of mental disorders (DSM-5®). American Psychiatric Pub; 2013 May 22.
2. Sadock BJ, Sadock VA. Kaplan and Sadock's synopsis of psychiatry: Behavioral sciences/ clinical psychiatry. Lippincott Williams & Wilkins; 2011 Dec 26.
3. Ahuja N, Ahuja S. A short textbook of psychiatry. New Delhi: Jaypee brothers; 2006 Jul 30.
4. Brad ford JM. The neurobiology, neuropharmacology, and pharmacological treatment of the paraphilias and compulsive sexual behavior. The Canadian Journal of Psychiatry. 2001 Feb;46(1):26-34.
5. Gijs L, Gooren L. Hormonal and psychopharmacological interventions in the treatment of paraphilias: An update. Journal of Sex Research. 1996 Jan 1;33(4):273-90.
6. Hill A, Briken P, Kraus C, Strohm K, Berner W. Differential pharmacological treatment of paraphilias and sex offenders. International Journal of Offender Therapy and Comparative Criminology. 2003 Aug;47(4):407-21.
7. Rösler A, Witztum E. Pharmacotherapy of paraphilias in the next millennium. Behavioral Sciences & the Law. 2000 Jan;18(1):43-56.

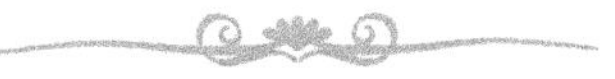

28 Psychiatric Aspects in LGBTQ+ Populations

Pragya Lodha • Avinash De Sousa

The LGBTQ+ community is a community that comprises of the sexual (and/gender) minorities identifying as lesbian, gay, bisexual, transgender, queer/questioning (abbreviated as LGBTQ+) and several others among the known 26 sexual identities. Though sexual minorities have always been a part of the society, the recent 2 decades have seen increasing public, social and scientific awareness towards the LGBTQ+ and their problems. It was the gay rights movement in 1970s and the advent of HIV/AIDS in the 1980s that brought about a sociocultural shift in garnering a larger attention towards sexual and gender identities. To understand clearly, sex refers to the biological genitalia that one is born with and gender is the psycho-social construct with which the person identifies with. Thus, gender and sexual identities are different.

Ever since history, homosexuality was disregarded as a part of the society, considered a crime/sin and was punished (though, the earliest understandings of homosexual relationships, dating back to Plato, were considered sacrosanct). In the history of psychiatry and mental health, homosexuality was earlier regarded as a mental illness. It was only in 1978, when the third edition of the Diagnostic and Statistical Manual of Mental Disorders (DSM-III) was published that homosexuality was freed from the status of being a mental illness. However, the diagnosis of Gender Identity Disorder continued to prevail and was abolished only in 2013 with the Diagnostic and Statistical Manual of Mental Disorders 5 coming in. It was only recently, in 2018, that homosexuality was decriminalised in India- this meant that if someone was found to be homosexual, they wouldn't be but behind prison (unlike before when homosexuality was considered a crime). However, though psycho-social movements have created a furore for acceptance and inclusion, there is still non-acceptance and discrimination. The LGBTQ+ population face discrimination which is the single most concerning reason for them to face problems in various sectors such as that of education, health care access, political inclusion, access to public spaces and overall inclusion.

National Mental Health Survey of India 2015-16 by National Institute of Mental Health and Neurosciences (NIMHANS) estimates that one in ten people in India experience mental illness in their lifetime. Though we don't have much research in the Indian context, the National Alliance of Mental Illnesses (NAMI) of the United States of America tells us that persons from the LGBTQIA+ community are three times more likely to have a mental health problem like depression and anxiety; they are four times more likely to feel suicidal and/or attempt suicide; and they are at a three-fold greater risk to develop substance misuse.

Some general facts about mental health challenges among the LGBTQ+:

- The stigma faced by the community is also double-edged due to their sexual/gender minority and mental health issues that they face.
- The prevalence of mental health problems is found to be 2-4 folds higher in the LGBTQ+ populations versus their heterosexual counterparts.
- The rates of suicide among the LGBTQ+ are also 3-4 times higher than in heterosexual population
- Among the LGBTQ+, lesbians and transgender have a 2 folds higher risk of discrimination and mental health challenges
- LGBTQ+ population face a 2-3 folds higher delay in receiving treatment.
- Due to the homophobic nature of the society, they often reach out for help also late due to the fear of being denied help or not being understood.

DEBUNKING MYTHS RELATED TO LGBTQ+ MENTAL HEALTH

Given that homosexuality is a topic discussed with stigma around it, its not uncommon to encounter myths with regards to the LGBTQIA+ community. Following are some essential myths debunked to better understand the community:

1. It is unnatural to be LGBTQIA+

   It is absolutely normal to choose any gender/sexual orientation that one may want to. It is a matter of choice for a person to conform or not conform to their assigned gender or expected orientation. Homosexuality being considered as an illness was a result of minority status, non-conformity and lack of awareness about alternate identities and sexualities- which no more prevails.

2. Homosexuality is a mental illness and can be "cured" by psychotherapy and or electroconvulsive therapy (ECT).

   Although homosexuality was once thought to be a mental illness, the American Psychiatric and Psychological Associations no longer consider it to be one. Psychiatric and psychological attempts to "cure" homosexual/queer persons have failed to change the sexual orientation/gender identity of the patient and have rather invoked emotional trauma.

3. LGBTQIA+ persons can be identified by certain mannerisms or physical characteristics.

   People who are queer come in as many different shapes, colors and sizes as do people who are heterosexual.

4. Early sexual experiences are indicative of one's sexual orientation as an adult.

   Many LGBTQIA+ persons have early heterosexual experiences, but are still lesbian, gay, bisexual or queer. Many heterosexuals have had sexual contact with members of their own sex, but are still heterosexual. Experimentation and exploration about one's orientation and identity is a part of healthy development.

5. We know what causes sexual orientation.

   Many queer persons know that who they are attracted to (members of their own sex) at an early age, sometimes as young as 6 or 7 years old. Others learn much later in life, in their 30's, 40's or 50's. Some research indicates that sexual orientation is determined between birth and age 3, but no one is sure what causes particular orientations. There is no confirmatory evidence with regard to hormonal surge/ imbalance or psychological factors that *determine* orientation.

6. Person with an LGBTQIA+ orientation cannot make good parents.

   This myth stems from the belief that sexual relationships are formed for procreation only. Although many heterosexuals decide to have children, many do not make the same decision or are unable to have children. On the other hand, many LGBTQIA+ people choose to have children or raise children with their partner. What is most important in a family is being loved and cared for.

7. People from the LGBTQIA+ community are more promiscuous than their heterosexual counterparts.

This is more of a stereotype. LGBTQIA+ individuals are equally capable of having stable, loyal and fulfilling relationships. Another related myth is that being LGBTQ+ is only about sex. They live full lives, which includes shopping for groceries, doing the laundry, raising children, planting a garden and going to work everyday. Being queer is about who you love emotionally, intellectually and sexually and how you identify yourself.

RISK FACTORS

We understand risk factors for the risk of mental illnesses among the LGBTQ+ in two approaches- one is the risk factors that hold for everyone in general and second approach is the LGBTQ+-specific factors like stigma and discrimination that compound the risk to developing mental illnesses among the community. The enlisted below are risk factors:

General risk factors:

1. A history of mental illness in the family, such as a parent or sibling
2. Stressful life situations, such as financial problems, a loved one's death or a divorce
3. An ongoing (chronic) medical condition
4. Brain damage as a result of a serious injury (traumatic brain injury), such as a violent blow to the head
5. Experiences of trauma
6. Use of alcohol or recreational drugs
7. A childhood history of abuse, bullying or neglect
8. Unhealthy relationships and/or environment
9. Social isolation
10. A history of mental illness

LBGTQ+ specific risk factors:

1. Stigma, prejudice and discrimination increases the prevalence of homophobia that further increases levels of isolation and hate towards the community
2. Non-acceptance/rejection by family and socially not accepted
3. Homelessness is one of the greatest risk factors
4. Poverty levels have been found to be higher among the LGBTQ+
5. Higher rates of engaging in prostitution also affects their sexual health
6. Biased based bullying
7. Lack of socio-political support

PSYCHIATRIC AND MENTAL HEALTH PROBLEMS

The following are the several mental health challenges faced by the LGBTQ+ population;

1. The prevalence of mental health problems among the LGBTQ+ is found to be 2-4 folds higher than their heterosexual counterparts. The delay in medical and mental health treatment has also found to be 2-3 folds higher.
2. Higher rates of major depression, generalized anxiety disorder and substance use or dependence have been reported.
3. Some psycho-social issues that also have mental health implications include: relationship violence, homelessness, social isolation, stigma & discrimination on the basis of sexual orientation and gender identity, self-esteem issues, coming out, bullying & cyber-bullying, lack of access to health care, transitioning and medical transitioning.
4. The process of coming out, by definition revealing one's sexual identity, is one that has seen decrease in age over the years, from the age of 20 in 1970s and 80s to the age of 14 in 2015. This poses psychological challenges as the younger cohort has lesser cognitive capability to deal with the societal stigma and discrimination which may be faced as a consequence to 'coming out'. There is a sense of loss that the LGBTQ+ report to experience socially and psychologically, which is clinically essential to evaluate as they raise the vulnerability to develop further mental health problems.
5. Being subject to homophobic attitudes and outright social distancing increases the risk for developing depression, anxiety and in many instances, increase the risk for suicide as well.
6. It is commonly found that severe psychiatric illnesses such as bipolar disorder, schizophrenia, psychosis, delusional disorder and substance use disorder are also prevalent. Among these, rates for higher substance use disorder have been highly reported.
7. Loss of self-esteem, lack of confidence and being at the receiving end of shame and prejudice also induces guilt and internalised homophobia among the LGBTQ+ pupil.
8. It is a misnomer and derogatory to affirm the sexual/gender orientation of a person being LGBTQ+ as a result of them having being (sexually) abused in their childhood. This has a direct negative effect on the mental health, sometimes leaving long-lasting impact and leading to greater risk to mental illnesses as well.
9. Suicidal ideation is found to be higher (2 folds) among the LGBTQ+ group as well which is very often linked with psychosocial factors like stigma, discrimination, familial and/or social rejection and bullying. Since the prevalence of mental illnesses is also found to be higher in the LGBTQ+ persons, rates of suicide also are seen to increase.
10. In the past, mental health issues for transgender people were narrowly viewed under the diagnosis of gender identity disorder. This led to pathologizing of the person's unique psychosocial experiences, therefore, limiting therapeutic responses and treatment options. The diagnosis of "trans-sexualism" first appeared in the International Statistical Classification of Diseases and Related Health Problems 9 in 1975 and, in 1980, in the Diagnostic and Statistical Manual of Mental Disorders III. However, recent research advancements (beginning since 2013) have confirmed that being transgender is not a mental illness. But in India, little medical research has been conducted on the issues of trans persons and the notion that being transgender is a mental illness continues.

11. Importance of informed consent, confidentiality and anonymity is equally important for everyone irrespective of their age, gender or any other socio-demographical feature. However, the larger clinical practice sees that though these norms are maintained for the heterosexual population, there is a compromise in following these ethical principles of practice when it comes to homosexuals or trans individuals as a consequence of the inherent bias that may be held against them.

12. Another concern that holds against trans patients is that there is greater stigma attached to approaching for help in a homophobic and transphobic society. Chances are less to find to a homosexual doctor or therapist as oppose to a greater chance of finding heterosexual professionals (though they may and most often, they do lack specialized care skills and knowledge to treat trans patients).

13. The assessment before the sex reassignment surgeries and accessing hormone treatment remain at the merciful approval of the practitioners, some of them who continue to give a diagnosis of Gender Identity Disorder (the revision of Gender Identity Disorder in DSM IV TR has evolved to that of Gender Dysphoria in DSM 5 which implies the treatment of distress, depression or anxiety due to the non-conformity to the gender and does not involve any techniques or therapies to dissuade the personal choice/preference of an individual to identifying with a gender). The process of pre-counselling before the sex reassignment surgery may miss the underlying emotional factors and many a times, involves dissuasion from the sex reassignment surgery in order to conform to the biological sex of the individual. Ethically, before the surgery, the individual is made to undergo various social norms and make lifestyle choices so as to prepare them for the post-surgery life.

14. Post-surgery and post hormone treatment care and counselling is missing, which is a crucial aspect in order to build and settle the transformations in the patient

15. One of other nuances that often go amiss is the difference between sexual orientation and gender identity. Though the two are inter-linked they are different concept in existence and understanding. Professionals must be clear and precise about making of note of the same. When talking about sex reassignment surgery, it is important to know the gender identity of the individual and not the sexual orientation.

16. Unrequired electroconvulsive therapy (ECT), tying the patients to beds and institutionalisation are resorted to for convincing patients about the 'consequences of sex change' and instead stand the chance of an ethical dilemma. Unfortunately, several practitioners resort to giving ECT in order to prevent the sex reassignment surgery for the individual thinking it is part of the treatment, however, one must be aware that this means is unethical and incorrect.

17. As a result of the apparent stressors, an increasing number of LGBTQ+ people are seeking therapy. However, therapists often lack the skills to work effectively with such patients and are often insensitive, ignorant and unaware regarding the several transgender issues. Many mental health professionals and medical practitioners lack an understanding of the LGBTQ+ spectrum health issues. Thus, an expertise to treat their concerns with an understanding of the ethical standpoints is missing.

18. Homophobia continues to prevail among mental health practitioners as well which becomes a barrier to providing healthcare services.
19. Counselling and psychotherapies also need a branch of specialisation in order to understand and appropriately address the concerns and mental health issues of the LGBTQ+ communities that are amplified due to multiple concerns.
20. After having recognised the 'non-binary' gender, the education and training centres fail to be inclusive in terms of providing the care for trans community.

STEPS TOWARDS BETTER CARE

1. Health care professionals must be educated and trained about the health challenges of LGBTQIA+ as part of their curriculum
2. Develop goals, policies, training modules, and other tools in close consultation with the community (LGBTQIA+) stakeholders, including community representatives, policy and research organizations and community health centers serving the community.
3. Encouragement of training programmes for mental health students and professionals.
4. Encouragement of liaison practice with mental health professionals along with allied professionals.
5. Working effectively with LGBTQ clients and family systems requires a re-examination of heterosexually-centric assumptions at personal, professional, societal and cultural levels.
6. Greater advocacy and more acceptance-based practices at educational levels are required to integrate the minority population and adequately realise their rights.
7. Access to mental health specialists and experts is a critical first step in treating people with mental health issues; increased numbers of psychiatrists, psychologists, and social workers are required per capita in the country. It is a known fact that greater number of mental health professionals typically result in lowered rates of suicide.
8. LGBTQ+ mental health professionals should be recruited as part of the service providing systems.
9. Should someone be looking for mental health services for queer persons, the referral must be made responsibly by first checking who is the referral being made to- one must check if the mental health practitioner is LGBTQIA+ friendly.

An important part of addressing mental health is also to inculcate the practice of self-care. It is important to take care of yourself first, it is not being selfish. If you are able to take care of yourself, you will be able to take care of other people too. Self-care is about taking active steps to deal with challenging situations and stressors. Self-care includes:

- Eating well-timed and balanced
- Sleeping at least 6-7 hours a day
- Making sure to spend time with people who value you
- Taking out some time in the day to do things you like/give you happiness
- Exercising/Walking
- Talking about your problems/feelings to someone you trust
- Taking steps to take care of your health

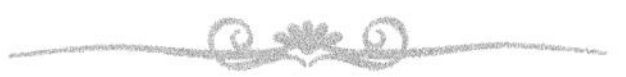

29 Sleep Disorders – an overview

Vijay Krishnan • Ravi Gupta

INTRODUCTION

Sleep and dreaming have fascinated poets, artists, scientists and doctors, probably since the very dawn of human self-awareness. It is a phenomenon that is at once essential to normal human existence, but whose purpose to physiology remains hard to completely define. However, at present we can be certain that sleep interacts with almost every other physiological system in the body: this may explain in part why disruptions of sleep are such a sensitive marker for many disorders. In the chapter that follows, we provide an overview of our current understanding of the process that undergird normal sleep, and provide a suggested approach to sleep disorders, based on the international classification of sleep disorders 3rd edition (ICSD-3).

WHAT IS SLEEP?

Sleep is best described as a state of disengagement to and from environmental stimuli. It is differentiated from other states of reduced alertness i.e., unconsciousness and coma by a number of characteristics.

1. The state is relative – beyond a certain threshold, internal and external stimuli do affect the sleeper's exteroceptive and interoceptive apparatus.
2. The state is fully reversible – contrary to coma, a complete reversal of all processes underlying sleep occurs spontaneously or in response to stimuli
3. It is associated with unresponsiveness – cognitive and motor responses to stimuli are altered in that they are restricted to simple instinctive responses

These characteristics are useful to differentiate sleep from other states of altered consciousness that may resemble it, and may occur either normally or as part of a disease process. Disorders of sleep itself, which may affect these characteristics, are described in detail in the chapter that follows.

HOW IS SLEEP STUDIED?

A comprehensive clinical assessment may be enough to make the diagnosis for a majority of sleep disorders. This assessment will have to include an assessment of all medical conditions that might affect sleep, as sleep may also commonly be disrupted as a consequence of any stressor. Such an assessment may be carried out as part of an clinical assessment, or may be made structured using questionnaires that have been developed to assess different aspects of sleep (**Table 29.1**). However, please note that questionnaires cannot replace a good clinical history obtained based on thorough knowledge of the topic.

Table 29.1: Selected Structured questionnaires for assessment of sleep and sleep disorders

Name	Purpose	Length of assessment	Method	Scoring
Sleep Diary	Structured	Every day	Self-reported	By the clinician
Epworth Sleepiness Scale	Daytime sleepiness	Not specified	Self-reported	>10 shows daytime sleepiness
Insomnia Severity Index	Severity of insomnia	Past 7 days	Self-reported	0-28, Classifies insomnia in mild, moderate and severe
Pittsburgh Sleep Quality Index	Overall Sleep Quality Assessment	10 minutes	Self-rated	0-21, > 5 indicate poor quality sleep
Berlin Questionnaire	Screen for obstructive sleep apnea	10 minutes	Self reported, available in Hindi	Indicates low risk and high risk for obstructive sleep apnea
RLS Diagnostic questionnaire for Indian population	Screen for RLS	10 min	Self reported	

Objectively sleep is assessed based upon physiological parameters. "Polysomnography" is a multi-modal assessment of diverse physiological parameters that are known to reflect normal and abnormal sleep physiology. The assessment commonly includes 6-channels of electroencephalographic (EEG) record to study brain electrophysiology; two channels of electro-oculogram that measures eye movements; electromyographic recording of submentalis and anterior tibialis muscles bilaterally; recording of body position; continuous monitoring of respiration- flow and effort; oxygen saturation; at least one lead of electrocardiogram and, synchronized video recording. These parameters are recorded through the period of wakefulness just before falling asleep, transition to sleep and during sleep during whole night. Additional optional parameters that may be measured include limb movements through actimeter, galvanic skin response, intra-esophageal pH and esophageal manometry. In cases of suspected sleep related seizures and parasomnia EEG channels are expanded. By comparing patterns of change in these parameters measured simultaneously, a wealth of information may be obtained about sleep physiology.

Typical polysomnographic changes may be seen in many sleep disorders, and are described in the appropriate sections. These may be necessary to make a positive diagnosis, or else may serve to confirm or support a differential diagnosis.

SLEEP ARCHITECTURE AND STAGES OF SLEEP

Normal sleep proceeds through a typical sequence of stages that are assessed through the measurement of various physiological parameters (see section on polysomnography). Broadly, two stages of sleep are clearly differentiated: rapid-eye-movement (REM) sleep and non-rapid eye-movement sleep

(NREM). Progression of these stages across night may be studies using a hypnogram (**Fig. 29.1**). In normal individuals, at the onset of sleep, wakefulness gives way to N1 stage, leading to a progression to N2 and N3, followed by a stage of REM; this is known as one sleep cycle that lasts for around 90 minutes, and is then repeated through the course of the night 4-5 times (**Fig. 29.1**).

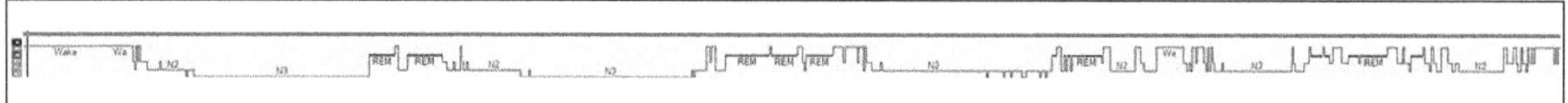

Fig. 29.1: Hypnogram showing sleep macro-architecture during night.

Wakefulness is characterized by mix frequency waves, saccadic eye movements, blink artefacts and high chin tone. When the person closes the eyes, alpha waves appear in occipital leads and eye movements become slower (**Fig. 29.2**).

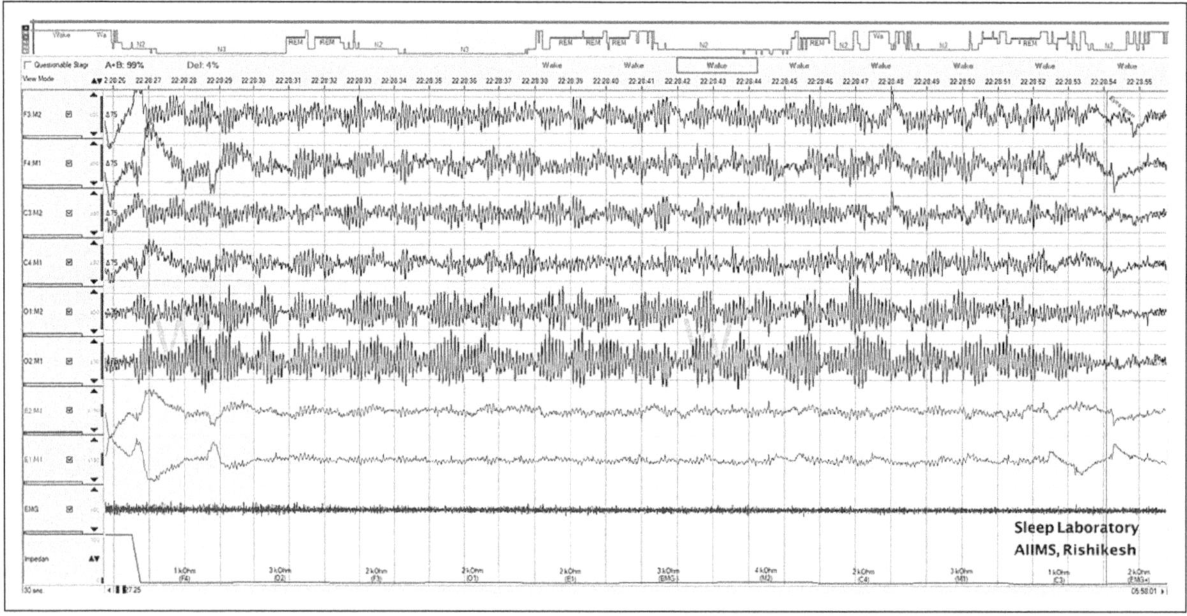

Fig. 29.2: 30 sec epoch showing alpha waves in posterior leads (O1:M2; O2:M1).

REM sleep is characterized by typical rapid eye movements along with reduced or absence of muscle tone in most of the skeletal muscles and low voltage mixed frequency waves on sleep EEG (**Fig. 29.3**).

The other stage ("non-REM" or NREM sleep) is further subdivided based on electrophysiological parameters into 3 stages (N1-N3). In general, these stages are differentiated by a progressive slowing of the background activity from the normal awake alpha rhythm (8-12 Hz) to slower theta (4-7 Hz) and delta (0.5-3 Hz) predominance. The depth of sleep (the degree of relative non-reactivity to stimuli) increases between stages 1 and 3. In addition, certain characteristic waveforms are also seen in EEG, especially during N2 sleep (**Fig. 29.5**).

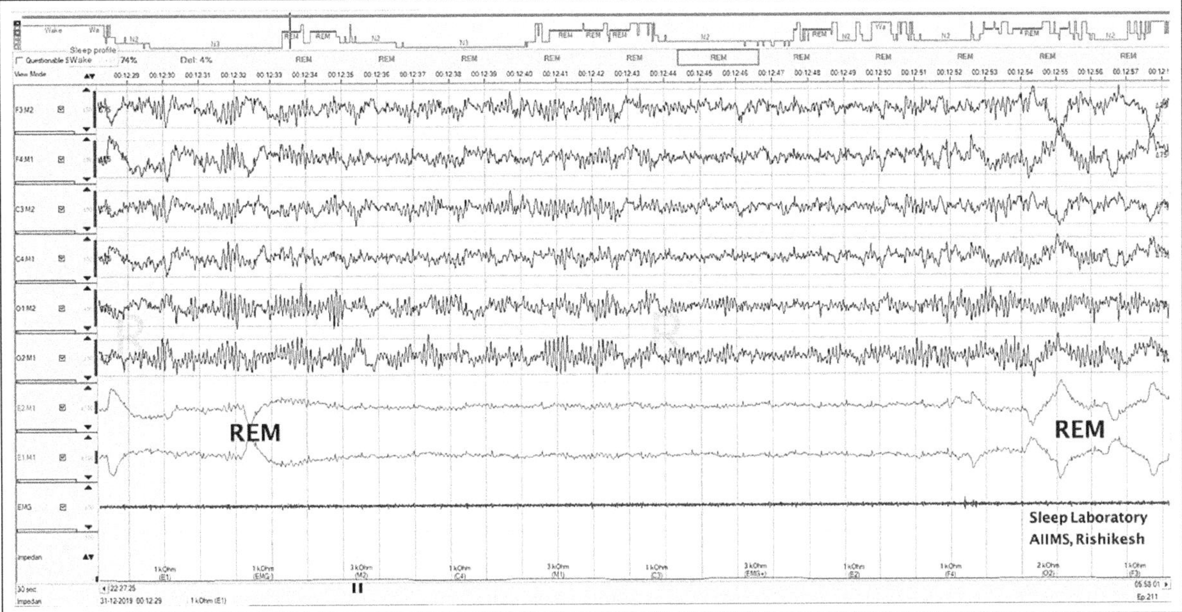

Fig. 29.3: 30 sec epoch showing REM sleep: Note low voltage mixed frequency activity in EEG, muscle atonia and rapid eye movements.

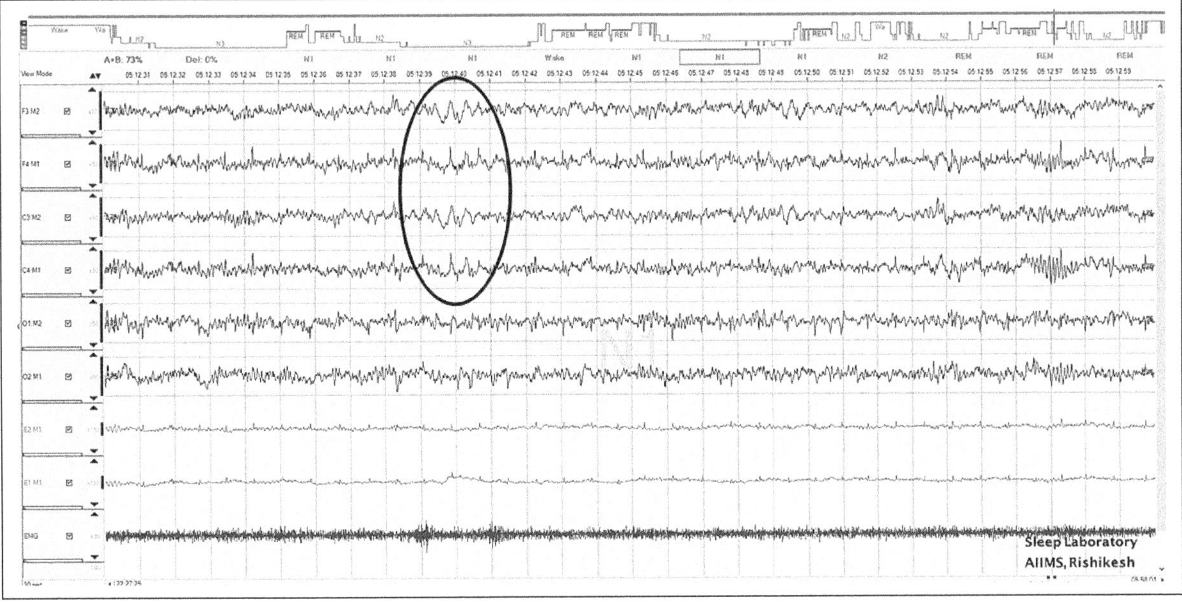

Fig. 29.4: 30 second epoch showing N1 sleep. Look at low voltage mixed frequency EEG activity, Vertex waves (in circle) with relatively high chin tone.

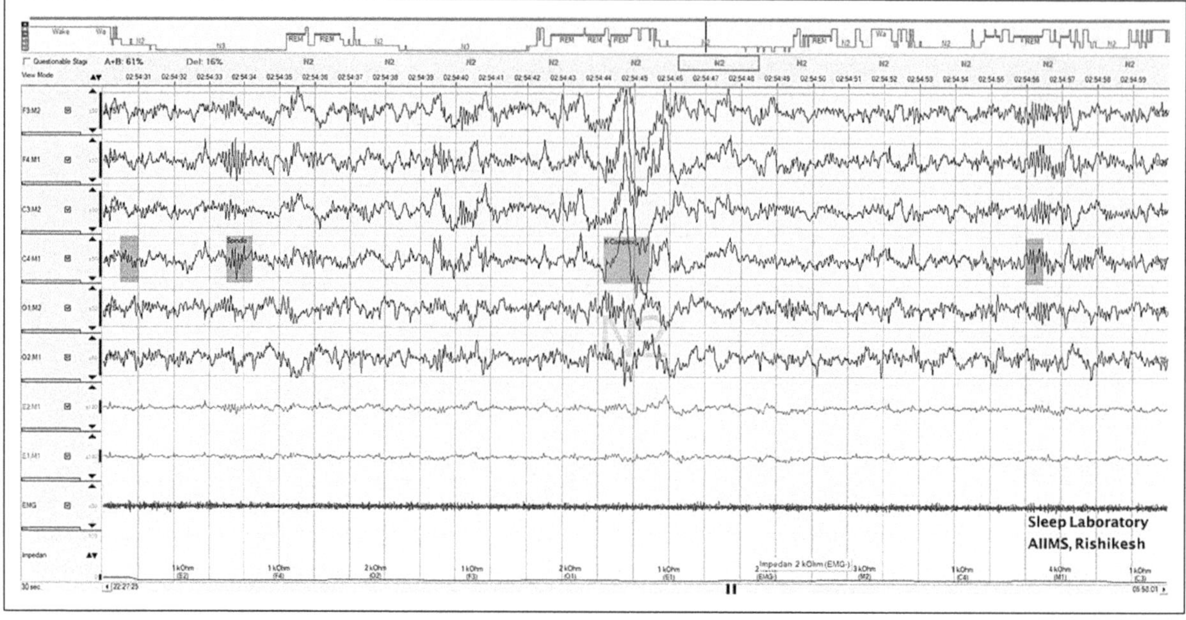

Fig. 29.5: 30 second epoch showing N2 sleep. Please appreciate spindles and K complexes.

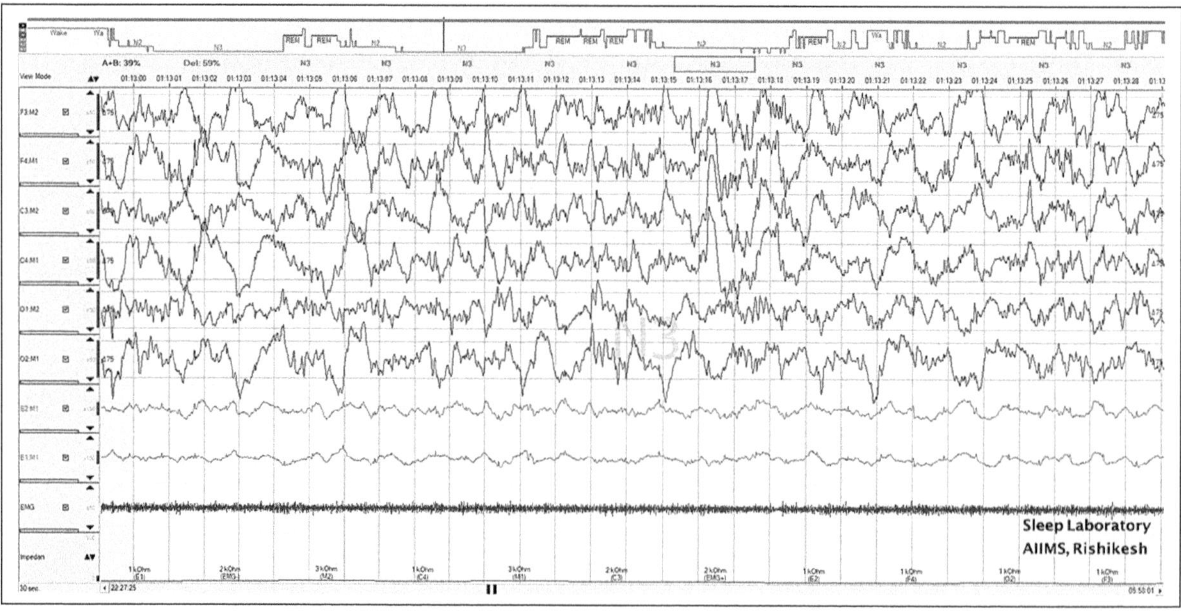

Fig. 29.6: 30 seconds epoch showing N3 sleep. Delta waves (>75 microV) can be seen in more than 20% of epoch.

Certain factors appear to have a role in determining the relative proportion of the various stages. N3 (deep) sleep varies depending upon how long the person has been awake prior to falling asleep. With a prolonged period of wakefulness prior to sleep onset, N3 sleep predominates in the early hours of sleep, and diminishes towards morning. On the other hand, REM is influenced by circadian rhythm and it predominantly appears towards morning.

BIOLOGY OF SLEEP

Two processes are differentiated in the normal cycle between sleep and wakefulness. The ***homeostatic* ("S")** and the ***circadian* ("C")** processes, which are governed by bodily and environmental/diurnal factors, respectively. Homeostatic process tries to make the body fall asleep in response to duration of wakefulness. As a person remains awake for longer, the "sleep pressure" builds up, which increases the probability of falling asleep. In healthy individuals, homeostatic process mainly regulates the proportion of deep sleep (N3 sleep). In other words, longer pre-sleep wakefulness, higher the proportion of N3.

Circadian process regulates the sleep-wake cycle in response to environmental timing. In other words, it sends signals to the brain in response to environmental light and dark cycle. For humans, light falls on the retina and a glutamatergic excitatory signal is sent to the suprachiasmatic nucleus of the hypothalamus. The action of this signal is to inhibit secretion of melatonin from the mammillary bodies. On the other hand, darkness promotes secretion of melatonin through pineal gland. Melatonin's physiological action is to promote sleep by stimulating acting on GABAergic neurons in ventro-lateral pre-optic nucleus of the Hypothalamaus and thereby inhibiting reticular activating system, which promotes wakefulness. Apart from light, other influences on melatonin levels include a variety of environmental influences, including food, exercise and social interaction. The overall effect of the circadian process is to "entrain" the sleep-wake cycle and maintain its synchronisation with the external cycle of light and dark.

The final common pathway governing the switch between wakefulness and sleep appears to the firing of GABA-ergic inhibitory neurons from the ventrolateral preoptic nucleus (VLPO) of the hypothalamus. When they are activated, they inhibit monoaminergic centers in the midbrain (including the serotonergic raphe nuclei, noradrenergic locus ceruleus, histaminergic tuberomamillary body, and the cholinergic basal forebrain nuclei), and facilitate a switch from wakefulness to sleep. You may recall that these monoaminergic neurons are part of reticular activating system which plays an important role in maintaining wakefulness and alertness.

Other physiological changes also occur under the influence of these transitions. Importantly, NREM sleep and REM sleep differ in terms of basal metabolic rate and patterns of blood supply. A number of hormones are known to have circadian patterns in their levels. Table 2 shows relative changes in physiological parameters during REM and NREM sleep.

Table 29.2: Comparison of physiological parameters during wakefulness, NREM and REM sleep

Parameter	Wakefulness	NREM	REM
Heart Rate	Irregular	Slow	Increased rate and variability
Blood Pressure	Higher than sleep	Decreased	Increased
Respiratory rate	Higher than sleep	Decreased	Increased, but with suppression of cough
Body Temperature	Higher than sleep	Regulated to a lower set-point	Reduced regulation - temperature resembles that of local environment
Muscle Tone	Higher	Lower than wakefulness	Lowest
Metabolic Rate	High	Lower	Higher than NREM
Hormones	----	Growth Hormone and Prolactin secreted during N3	-----

SLEEP DISORDERS

Disordered sleep may be developed by a number of different pathways. Characteristic patterns of sleep disruption are described for disorders such as mania (reduced *need* for sleep – i.e. a reduction in the absolute period of sleep without compensatory daytime somnolence or fatigue) and melancholic depression (an early morning awakening). Similarly endocrine disorders such as hyperthyroidism alter sleep architecture. Apart from these conditions, many other health conditions may prevent the transition into sleep by causing discomfort, or interrupt sleep. Under these heads would be conditions causing chronic pain or shortness of breath, seizure disorders, urinary symptoms or hypoglycemia occurring at night.

These conditions may feature prominently in the differential diagnosis of a patient who complains of problems with sleep. However, a comprehensive discussion of these conditions is outside the scope of this chapter. Here instead we will focus on those conditions which affect sleep as the predominant feature of the clinical picture. It occurs when physiology of sleep gets altered to generate symptoms. However, such differentiations in medical science are necessarily artificial, as sleep has a complex interaction with other bodily processes.

Largely, disorders may affect *how much* sleep a person is getting, how much *control* they have over staying awake or falling asleep at the time they wish to, or the *quality* of sleep is altered. At times, patients may present with deviations from normal behavior that is not expected during or around sleep. In the section that follows, certain selected conditions are described in terms of their most common presentation, pathophysiology, and management.

INSOMNIA

Insomnia is difficulty (or inability) in one or more of the following domains with frequent recurrence (> 3 nights a week):

- Falling asleep
- Staying asleep
- Waking up prior to the normal waking time.

Associated daytime dysfunction, along with night-time symptoms described above, in the form of headache, lethargy, daytime somnolence, poor attention, memory impairment or mood changes are also essential to the diagnosis of insomnia. Insomnia cannot be diagnosed in persons who do not have adequate opportunities to fall or stay asleep (e.g., due to long working hours or voluntary efforts to stay awake).

A duration of illness less than 3 months is called "short-term" insomnia, whereas persistence beyond this period indicates chronic insomnia.

Diagnosis is largely clinical, but supportive evidence may be obtained by the use of a sleep diary or Actigraphy. On a polysomnogram, sleep onset latency and/or proportion of N1 sleep may be increased. Sleep onset latency refers to time elapsed between lying on bed with intention to fall asleep and appearance of sleep. Usually sleep onset latency of less than 30 min is considered normal. Similarly, there might be frequent and prolonged nocturnal awakenings or early morning awakenings in sleep-diary (**Fig. 29.7**).

Insomnia affects 10-20% of the adult population, and affects older adults more frequently; it is also more common among women. Known risk factors include stressful life events, poor sleep habits, anxiety or worry

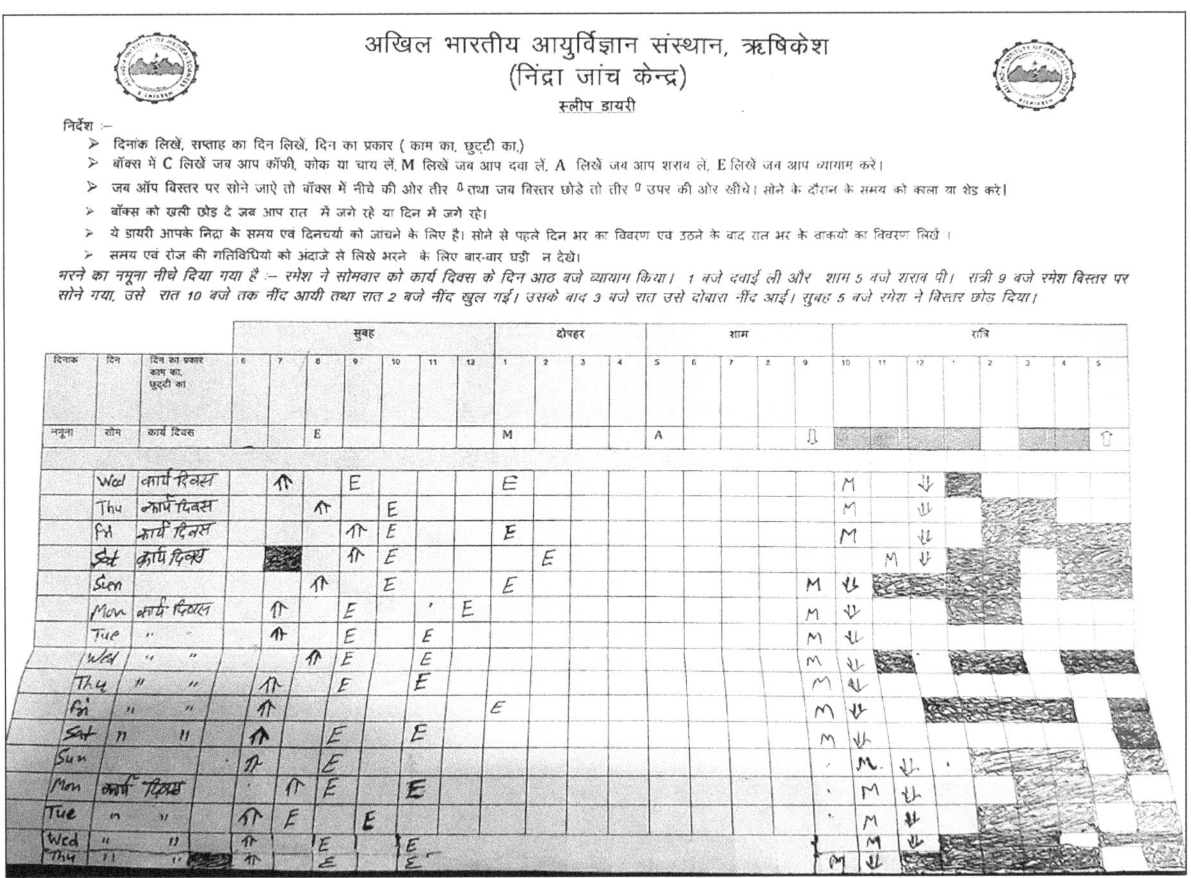

अखिल भारतीय आयुर्विज्ञान संस्थान, ऋषिकेश
(निंद्रा जांच केन्द्र)
स्लीप डायरी

निर्देश :–
- दिनांक लिखें, सप्ताह का दिन लिखें, दिन का प्रकार (काम का, छुट्टी का,)
- बॉक्स में C लिखें जब आप कॉफी, कोक या चाय लें, M लिखें जब आप दवा लें, A लिखें जब आप शराब लें, E लिखें जब आप व्यायाम करें।
- जब ऑप बिस्तर पर सोने जाऐ तो बॉक्स में नीचे की ओर तीर ⇩ तथा जब बिस्तर छोड़े तो तीर ⇧ उपर की ओर खींचे। सोने के दौरान के समय को काला या शेड करे।
- बॉक्स को खली छोड़ दे जब आप रात में जगे रहे या दिन में जगे रहे।
- ये डायरी आपके निंद्रा के समय एवं दिनचर्या को जांचने के लिए है। सोने से पहले दिन भर का विवरण एवं उठने के बाद रात भर के वाकयों का विवरण लिखें ।
- समय एवं रोज की गतिविधियो को अंदाजे से लिखे भरने के लिए बार-बार घड़ी न देखे।

भरने का नमूना नीचे दिया गया है :– रमेश ने सोमवार को कार्य दिवस के दिन आठ बजे व्यायाम किया। 1 बजे दवाई ली और शाम 5 बजे शराब पी। रात्री 9 बजे रमेश बिस्तर पर सोने गया, उसे रात 10 बजे तक नींद आयी तथा रात 2 बजे नींद खुल गई। उसके बाद 3 बजे रात उसे दोबारा नींद आई। सुबह 5 बजे रमेश ने बिस्तर छोड़ दिया।

			सुबह							दोपहर				शाम					रात्रि							
दिनांक	दिन	दिन का प्रकार काम का, छुट्टी का	6	7	8	9	10	11	12	1	2	3	4	5	6	7	8	9	10	11	12	1	2	3	4	5
नमूना	सोम	कार्य दिवस			E					M				A				⇩								⇧
	Wed	कार्य दिवस		↑		E				E									M		↓					
	Thu	कार्य दिवस			↑		E												M		↓					
	Fri	कार्य दिवस				↑	E			E									M		↓					
	Sat	कार्य दिवस				↑	E				E									M	↓					
	Sun				↑		E			E								M	↓							
	Mon	कार्य दिवस		↑		E		'	E									M	↓							
	Tue	" "		↑		E		E										M	↓							
	Wed	" "			↑	E		E										M	↓							
	Thu	" "		↑		E		E										M	↓							
	Fri	" "		↑						E								M	↓							
	Sat	" "		↑		E		E										M	↓							
	Sun			↑		E													M	↓						
	Mon	कार्य दिवस			↑	E		E											M	↓						
	Tue	" "		↑	E		E												M	↓						
	Wed	" "		↑		E		E											M	↓						
	Thu	" "		↑		E		E										M	↓							

Fig. 29.7: Sleep diary showing insomnia: Please look at increased sleep-onset latency (blank space between downward arrow and first shaded area) and prolonged midnight awakenings (blank spaces between shaded areas).

prone personalities. These factors do not induce insomnia among all persons exposed to these circumstances. Instead, these factors interact with genetic factors to uncover insomnia and this is why prevalence of insomnia is lesser than the proportion of people exposed to stressful events. Environmental factors (e.g., Noise, light, uncomfortable ambient temperatures) may also be important. In addition, other sleep-related disorders e.g., circadian rhythm sleep disorders, restless legs syndrome must be ruled out before a diagnosis of insomnia can be entertained.

Insomnia is currently understood to be a state of hyper-arousal, as evident in neuronal hyperactivity, sympathetic activity close to bedtime, and raised corticotropin releasing hormone (CRH) and cortisol.

Management of insomnia is necessarily multimodal. **Sleep Hygiene** refers to steps that a person may undertake to curtail the influence of external factors (such as light, noise, ambient temperature or posture), activity levels (exercise, stimulant or alcohol use) or routine. These are summarized in **Table 29.3**. While sleep hygiene may be sufficient in itself to manage a certain proportion of patients, it is an essential component for the education of all patients presenting with insomnia.

Medications are recommended for the management of short-term insomnia. A number of hypnotic medications are available, with benzodiazepines and so-called Z-drugs (Zolpidem, Zopiclone/ Eszopiclone) being the most commonly prescribed. The choice of medication for a particular individual depends on their symptom profile and other characteristics. In general, longer-acting agents are not preferred as they may produce daytime sedation, and contribute to ataxia, especially in the elderly. Shorter and faster-acting agents may be insufficient to sleep interruptions that occur later in the night, and in these situations longer acting hypnotics may be preferred. A number of non-benzodiazepine sedatives are also used frequently to provide sleep, including antidepressants (mirtazapine, trazodone, amitriptyline), antipsychotics (chlorpromazine), or antihistamines (promethazine). However, as of now scientific evidence are insufficient to advocate their use as hypnotic agents. The duration of prescription is usually limited to 1-2 weeks, however zolpidem has been found effective for as long as one year without development of tolerance or major side effects.

For chronic insomnia, cognitive-behavior therapy (CBT-I) has been shown to be effective. It is aimed to increase sleep-promoting

Table 29.3: Good Sleep Hygiene practices: Dos and Don'ts

Do	Don't
1. Maintain a regular sleep routine	1. stay in bed awake for more than 5-10 minutes
2. Regular Exercise (not to be done immediately before bedtime)	2. nap during the daytime
3. Ensure adequate exposure to natural light during the day time	3. have a heavy, spicy or fat-rich meal at bedtime
4. Establish a regular relaxing bedtime routine (e.g., warm bath, soft music, light stretching)	4. have stimulants (caffeine, nicotine, caffeinated colas) close to bedtime
5. Ensure a comfortable sleeping environment (light, temperature, noise levels)	

behaviors and reduce sleep-defeating behaviors in addition to cognitive restructuring. Components may include sleep hygiene and relaxation therapy that reduce behaviors that interfere with sleep; sleep restriction and stimulus control therapy may also promote night-time sleep with minimal daytime somnolence. Various components are tailored to the problems of the individual patient for maximal efficacy.

HYPERSOMNIA

As the name suggests, hypersomnia is associated with an increase in the total duration of sleep, or a loss of control over sleepiness for at least 3 months. A number of conditions may produce this clinical picture:

- In idiopathic hypersomnia, sleep duration is increased beyond 12-14 hours in a day; sleep onset latency is reduced (< 8 minutes during the day after a good sleep at night and in the absence of sleep deprivation). Patients have difficulty waking up in the morning despite effort; and have multiple non-refreshing naps during the day.
- In narcolepsy, the patient experiences irresistible urges to fall asleep during the day. Other symptoms may include a sudden loss of muscle tone in reaction of emotional stimuli (called cataplexy); sleep paralysis (waking up with transient inability to move any part of the body) and, hypnagogic or hypnopompic hallucinations (dream like imagery at the transition of sleep and wakefulness). Among these symptoms, cataplexy is observed only in Type 1 narcolepsy while other symptoms are seen in both type 1 and type 2 narcolepsy. Narcolepsy is diagnosed by a finding of REM at the onset of sleep (< 8 minutes latency with ≥ 2 sleep onset REM periods during multiple sleep latency test), or a reduction in cerebrospinal fluid hypcretin levels (<110 pg/ml). The condition has been associated with a destruction of orexin neurons, and thus a pathology in the transitions between sleep and wakefulness.
- Insufficient Sleep Syndrome: It is characterized by wishful curtailment of sleep which can be acute or chronic. Acute sleep deprivation is characterized by not sleeping for 1 or more nights while chronic sleep deprivation refers to partial curtailment of sleep every night over a long period. For example, to meet the pressure of work or because of other reasons people do not take adequate amount of sleep that is required to work optimally and to remain alert during the day. Because of homeostatic factors, such curtailment keeps on accumulating sleep pressure, resulting in increased pressure to fall asleep and thus, hypersomnia.
- Other causes of hypersomnolence include atypical depression, medication, substance use disorders, and other medical disorders.

The differential diagnosis includes atypical depression, dissociation, and sleep apnea. These conditions may be ruled out by the presence of their characteristic symptoms.

Treatment of hypersomnia includes the use of stimulants (e.g., Modafanil, methylphenidate) that reduce the total sleep time. SSRI antidepressants may control cataplexy occurring due to narcolepsy. Scheduled naps may also be useful to reduce daytime somnolence in narcolepsy. Gamma-hydroxybutyrate also known as sodium oxybate can improve all aspects of narcolepsy.

SLEEP RELATED BREATHING DISORDERS

Certain conditions may involve altered blood oxygenation during sleep, due to alterations of breathing patterns during sleep (known as Sleep Apnea). The most common of these is obstructive sleep apnea (OSA).

The pathophysiology of this condition is related to the reduced muscle tone during sleep. When this reduced tone affects pharynx, it can cause this part of the upper airway to collapse, leading to reduced air entry despite continuing respiratory efforts from chest and abdomen. Such a collapse is more likely when the airway is further narrowed by increased parapharyngeal fat (which is proportionate to body weight), or anatomical abnormalities of the upper airway (e.g., Macroglossia, retrognathia, retrusion of the maxilla, or adeno-tonsillar enlargement).

The presentation of OSA is highly variable. Symptoms include snoring, choking or snorting at night (as inspired air flows turbulently through the narrowed airway) or pauses in breathing (apnoeic spells) (**Fig. 29.8**). These symptoms may only be reported by the bed partner and patient may remain oblivious to them. Interruptions in breathing may lead to sleep interruptions, excessive daytime sleepiness; a host of other symptoms are reported, including nocturia, sleep-talking, poor memory and loss of libido by patients of OSA.

Risk factors of OSA include obesity, family history of OSA, conditions associated with dysmorphic facies (Down's Syndrome, Treacher-Collins Syndrome) and endocrinopathies like acromegaly.

Diagnosis is made on the basis of polysomnography, where obstructive respiratory events are identified, including

- Apnea: complete cessation of breathing for at least 10 seconds

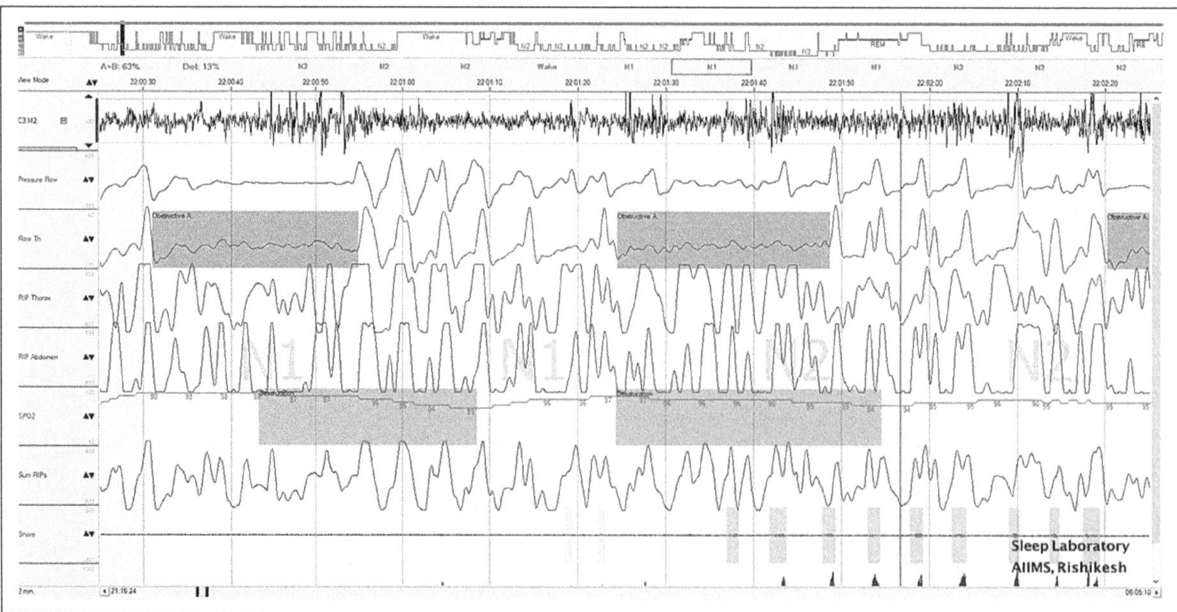

Fig. 29.8: 2 min epoch showing obstructive sleep apnea with cessation of airflow (> 10 seconds) and continuing efforts in thorax and abdominal channels.

- Hypopnea: At least 30% reduction in breathing amplitude leading to arousal or oxygen desaturation > 3%
- Respiratory event related arousal: progressively increasing respiratory effort culminating in arousal

To make a diagnosis of OSA among adults, at least 5 such events must be present in an hour.

OSA is a condition associated with significant complication rates. Untreated, the condition may lead to arrhythmias, coronary artery disease, hypertension or sudden cardiac death; pulmonary artery hypertension; metabolic syndrome and cognitive deficits. In addition, it also increases the risk for or at times mitigate depression, somatic symptoms disorder and fibromyalgia.

Treatment is multi-modal, and involves a programe of weight reduction where appropriate. Continuous Positive Airway Pressure (CPAP) provides air-splint and keeps the upper airway open against which a person can breath. This is most preferred therapy for treatment of obstructive sleep apnea. For anatomical abnormalities, appropriate surgical correction (by wedge glossectomy, adenotonsillectomy, uvulo-pharyngo-palatoplasty, or maxillary/mandibular advancement) may be therapeutic, however, soft tissue surgeries (wedge glossectomy, uvulo-pharyngo-palatoplasty and similar surgeries) have a high recurrence rates. The withdrawal of sedatives that reduce muscle tone further (e.g., Benzodiazepines) may also improve the condition.

SLEEP RELATED MOVEMENT DISORDERS

Restless Leg Syndrome (RLS; Also known as Willis-Ekbom Syndrome) is a distressing condition in which patients experience recurrent urges to move their legs. The condition is usually associated with a sense of unease (or “dysesthesia”) in the lower limbs, which are worse during rest, and improves with movement. These symptoms are circadian with appearance or worsening in the evening or in night. The usual presentation is with insomnia, due to the interference produced by these urges. RLS is more common in women; age of onset shows a bimodal pattern, with peaks in late adolescence, and in middle age.

RLS has shown associations with a number of other conditions that should be screened for in the assessment: these include iron deficiency anemia, rheumatoid arthritis, chronic kidney disease, pregnancy, psychotropic medications, etc. Other causes of pain or discomfort in the lower limbs e.g., arthralgia, pedal edema, or akathisia, are important differentials to rule out. Anxiety and depression may be associated with restlessness, that is differentiated by not having this typical circadian pattern, and by associated worrying or negative thoughts and symptoms of autonomic arousal.

Management involves the prescription of dopamine agonists (L-DOPA, Ropinarole, Pramipexole). Pregabalin or gabapentin are also effective.

PARASOMNIAS

Undesirable behaviors or experiences may also occur predominantly or exclusively during sleep. They typically occur episodically, and have been linked to particular stages of sleep. These are referred to as parasomnias, and are differentiated into NREM and REM parasomnias, which have certain shared characteristics (**Table 29.4**).

Table 29.4: Characteristics of NREM and REM sleep parasomnias

	NREM Parasomnias	REM Parasomnias
Spontaneous awakening from sleep due to event	Incomplete awakening	Common
Response to external efforts to awaken	Minimal	
Memory of event on awakening	Absent	Present
Association with dreams	Usually absent	Present
Key conditions	Sleepwalking, sleep terrors, confusional arousal	Nightmares, REM Sleep Behavior Disorder
Association with sleep onset		More common in the second half of the night

The presentation of parasomnias is variable. As some of these phenomena (nightmares, sleep talking) may occasionally occur without any dysfunction, the diagnosis of a disorder is reserved only when these abnormalities lead to distress or dysfunction. This may occur via different mechanisms: those associated with awakenings (e.g., nightmares and sleep terrors) present with sleep interruptions. Bed partners may be more aware of behavioral abnormalities, for example those due to sleep walking or REM behavioral disorders. Developmentally, sleep terrors may first present in early childhood—this has been related to the relative predominance of slow wave sleep at this age.

A video-synchronized polysomnography with extended EEG channels is helpful to identify parasomnias where there is clinical suspicion. They are helpful in making the diagnosis by relating the parasomnia episodes to the sleep stage at which they occur. The treatment of parasomnia involves identifying predisposing factors and managing them. NREM parasomnias may be treated using benzodiazepines. Clonazepam (0.5 to 2 mg at night) is effective in REM sleep behavior disorder.

SUMMARY

Sleep disorders are common, and may present with sleeplessness, poor quality of sleep or excessive daytime drowsiness/napping. Evaluation of such patients involves a careful assessment of their general health, as sleep disorders are a common manifestation of other conditions; in such cases, the primary focus of treatment is directed towards those other conditions, and may reduce comorbid sleep difficulties as well.

In the assessment of sleep disorders, difficulties with initiation (getting to sleep) or maintenance (staying asleep) may have different reasons. Pain, restlessness, worrying, arousal symptoms, shortness of breath or other causes of physical discomfort may be reported on clinical assessment. Partners may be an important source of information regarding abnormalities that the patient is unaware of, including snoring or unusual behavior. It is also important to consider that daytime sedation may be a manifestation of either an excessive drive for sleep, or the compensation for inadequate sleep duration or quality at the appropriate time (e.g., obstructive sleep apnea, circadian rhythm disturbances, or parasomnias).

Treatment of sleep disorders helps to ameliorate distress, reduce dysfunction, and also protects individuals from a host of documented long-term health consequences, including rates of cardiovascular illness, lowered immunity, and metabolic syndrome. Overnight video-synchronize attended polysomnography with manual scoring of data is currently the gold standard for diagnosis of sleep disorders, and is indicated in case of diagnostic uncertainty. Management is multimodal, and many patients may respond without pharmacological intervention by treating the cause. When indicated, a number of different classes of sedatives are available, but most must be used with caution due to the risk of dependence or limited efficacy in chronic sleep disorders.

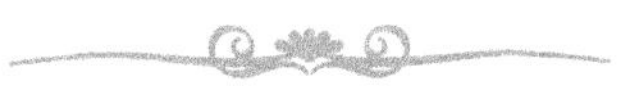

30 Overview of Child Psychiatric Disorders

Vishal Indla • Radhika M.S. • Manjiri Deshpande • V. Manasa Ram

INTRODUCTION

"How soon can a child go mad?" asked Henry Maudsley in his textbook the pathology of mind. Till the late 19th century, it was believed that children's minds were not developed enough and stable enough to show any significant pathology. Child and adolescent psychiatry has not been considered an established field till the early 1900s.[1] The establishment of world's first child psychiatry clinic by Leo Kanner and his work on autism spectrum disorder brought focus to child mental health issues. Understanding child psychiatry is interlocked with understanding child development, child rearing practices, and non-clinical aspects like child education and role of children in society across different cultures. This chapter tries to introduce undergraduates to this very nascent branch of psychiatry and help answer a few questions at the end, like–

a) Why is child psychiatry important

b) What disorders are seen in children?

c) How are they diagnosed and managed?

As per a review by Sharan and Sagar, worldwide prevalence rates for child and adolescent psychiatric disorders are 10 -20%.[2] In India, community studies show prevalence rates of 6.46% whereas school based studies show a prevalence rate of 23.33%.[3] According to this study out of 447 million of child and adolescent population in India, 29 million suffer from one or the other psychiatric illness at a given time.

CHILD DEVELOPMENT

Various theories of development like Sigmund Freud's stages of psychosexual development, Jean Piagets cognitive development theory, John Bowlbys attachment theory, Eric Eriksons psycho social development suggested how psychopathology in adults can occur due to childhood developmental disturbance

Important Milestones[4]

Receptive Language

- 12 months- responding to their name
- 18 months- pointing to body parts, pictures

Expressive Language

- 12 months- mama and papa, pointing out what they want
- 2 years- linking words; 3 years-repeats 3 words phrases

Social Emotional

- 3-6 months- eye contact
- 18-24 months- pretend play, joint referencing or shared interest.

Gross Motor

- 12-18 months- walking

Fine Motor

- 18 months- scribbles lines

Assessment and Interview[4]

Psychiatric interview is the basic fundamental tool in psychiatry, which is used both as a diagnostic and therapeutic tool. A thorough and detailed history is one of the most important tools that help the clinician in correctly diagnosing the patient.

In children less than 3 years of age, parents are the primary informants. In children going to school, a detailed account of teacher's observations should be obtained as child spends most of the time at school. In older children, information can be obtained directly from patients themselves.

History Should Include

History of presenting illness is elaboration of the presenting symptoms of illness from both the child and the parent.

Past history – H/o any medical or psychiatric comorbidities, h/o treatment should be recorded

Birth history – It includes details of consanguinity, mode of delivery – vaginal or c section or assisted, place of birth, weight at birth, any complications during child birth, order of birth, Apgar score, cry of the child, any NICU admissions, vaccination records

Development history – Age at specific milestones is assessed and any developmental delay should be recorded.

Family history – History of any psychiatric illnesses in the family.

Social and personal history – Regarding how child interacts with friends, his hobbies, habits

Educational history – Scholastic ability, behavior at school

In children, detailed assessment of *temperament* is essential. It includes Activity levels, Rhythmicity, adaptability, approach withdrawal, threshold level, and intensity of reaction, quality of mood, distractibility, persistence and attention span.

Parental functioning and type of parenting should be recorded.

Parenting styles can be classified as permissive, authoritarian and authoritative.

Mental Status Examination

Aspects of an MSE, which are unique to a child psychiatry patient, are discussed in this chapter.

Appearance of child – How they sit, dress, any mannerisms or abnormal movements

Relationship capacity - How the child is relating to the examiner; how the rapport is being established

Separation reaction - How the child is reacting to being separated from his parents during the interview; it is important to explain to the child that you would like to speak to them alone without their parent's presence

Psychomotor Activity

Affect – Whether the child is crying, smiling, anxious

Speech/language – Should also include reading and writing

Thought Content – Relationship with family members, peers, what child thinks of his presenting symptoms, should be assessed

Fantasy- A standard technique to explore the child's fantasy thinking is " the three wish test" the child is asked what they would wish for if a genie grants them three wishes. Sometimes underlying issues are exposed.

Ability to distinguish fantasy from reality should be assessed but this is slightly blurry in younger children and is a normal aspect.

Observation of play- It could be the only form of expression the child has. The form and content of play and accompanying fantasies provide a window into the child's psyche. It is also a useful indicator of the child's attention span, distractability, and frustration tolerance. Intellectual capacity-general knowledge, comprehension and calculating abilities must be assessed in all children as a rule during the examination.

The objectives of the psychiatric interview are

1) To arrive at a diagnosis and possible differential diagnoses
2) To identify the precipitating factors [what caused the problem]
3) To identify the perpetuating factors [maintenance factors]
4) To assess prognosis

It is difficult in the case of children to achieve the above objectives in a single session; multiple follow-ups may be needed in child psychiatry evaluation.

Physical examination of a child should never be ignored. It should be done to assess height, weight, hand preference, head circumference, and any suggestive body dysmorphic features. A systemic examination should be conducted esp. CNS – assess for motor problems, auditory, visual problems.

Psychological Assessment[4]

This includes the structured tools and rating scales, which help in confirming diagnosis and assessing severity of the disorder. We will briefly discuss a few scales, which are commonly used in India

Tests of Intelligence

For Infants

Developmental Screening Test- based on milestones especially that of language and speech. Developed by Dr. J Bharat Raj in 1983 at All India Institute of speech and Hearing, Mysore. *Applicable up to 15 years of age*. It gives mental age and a single IQ (DQ) score.

Vineland Social Maturity Scale- developed by Doll 1965, Indian adaptation by Malin 1972. This scale consists of 89 items arrange in age scales from birth to 15 years of age. The items mostly cover social milestones and hence the obtained age is called Social Age and the quotient as social quotient (SQ)

For Children

Seguin form board test - is valid up to *11 years of age*. Useful for children with speech and language disorders

Binet-Kamat test - Indian version of Stanford binet test.

Applicable from the ages of *5½ years to 18 years.*

Malins Intelligence Scale for Indian Children (*MISIC*) - Adaptation of *weschler* intelligence scale for children, from *6 to 15 years* of age. It has 11 scales- 6 verbal and 5 performance scales

Projective Tests

They are indirect measures of assessing a

child's personality and psychopathology. Based on psychoanalytic theory. In projective techniques, the situation is usually vague and open to various interpretations by children.

The Ones used in Children are–

Rorschach Ink Blot Test - This has a standard of 10 cards. It has 5 achromatic/black and white inkblots and 5 chromatic inkblots. While interpreting these inkblot designs, children tend to reveal their problem.

Children's Aperception test - Indian adaptation by Uma Chaudary. This test consists of ten animal pictures involved in activities such as eating, sleeping alone, toilet training and playing competitive games. The child is asked to narrate stories based on these images and often reveals their own feelings, struggles, aspirations and fears.

Draw a person Test, sentence completion test, rosenzweig picture are a few other projective tests used.

Scales for Specific Pathologies

ADHD	- Vanderbilt assessment scale
	Preschool ASRS
	Connors parent rating scale
SLD	- NIMHANS index of specific learning disability
Depression	- Children's depression inventory
	Children's depression rating scale
OCD	- Yale Brown obsessive compulsive scale
	Leyton obsessional inventory- child version
Anxiety	- Children's manifest anxiety scale
	Visual analog scale for anxiety
Phobia	- Revised fear survey schedule for children

CLASSIFICATION

DSM V and ICD 10 are currently used for classification and diagnosis of psychiatric disorders.

In ICD 10, childhood psychiatric disorders are found under the following categories

- F7 Mental Retardation
- F8 Disorders of psychological development (includes speech and language, learning disorders, motor, autism)
- F9 Behavioral and emotional disorders with onset usually occurring in childhood and adolescence (includes ADHD, conduct, separation anxiety, reactive attachment, tics, enuresis, encopresis, pica, feeding disorder, stereotyped movement, stuttering)

ICD 11 is more similar to DSM V and childhood disorders are classified in this way

Neurodevelopmental disorders (BlockL1-6A0)

- **6A00 Disorders of intellectual development**
- **6A01 Developmental speech or language disorders**
- **6A02 Autism spectrum disorder**
- **6A03 Developmental learning disorder**
- **6A04 Developmental motor coordination disorder**
- **6A05 Attention deficit hyperactivity disorder**
- **6A06 Stereotyped movement disorder**
- **6A0Y Other specified neurodevelopmental disorders**
- **6A0Z Neurodevelopmental disorders, unspecified**

Neurodevelopmental Disorders

These are disorders characterized by a delay or deviation in brain development, which manifest as developmental deficits leading to impairment in social, personal, educational and or occupational aspects of ones life. These are observed predominantly in early developmental age, before child goes to grade school

Table 30.1

Neurodevelopmental disorders in DSM V
Intellectual disability
Communication Disorders
Autism Spectrum Disorders
Attention deficit Hyperactivity Disorder
Specific learning disorder
Motor disorders

We will discuss these disorders comprehensively.

ADHD[5]

It is one of the most common psychiatric disorders seen in children with a worldwide prevalence rate of 5% in population less than 18 years of age.

Etiology – It is multifactorial with genetic and environmental components. It is estimated to be 76% heritable. Prematurity is a common risk factor.

Neurobiology – Existing data supports a catecholamine mediated fronto striatal dysfunction.

Clinical Features

It is characterized by inattention and or hyperactivity- impulsivity. Symptoms should have appeared prior to 12 years of age.

Inattention is characterized by difficulties initiating and completing a task, forgetfulness, easy distractibility, losing track of objects/ misplacing them, incomplete homework or class work in school going children.

Hyperactivity is characterized by excessive physical activity; children seem like they are always "on the go" as if run by a motor, fidgeting, talking too much, inability to remain still even when required. It can be seen as multiple complaints from teacher that child is wandering around in class, talks during class.

Impulsivity is the difficulty in delaying an action or response even when it's known that this will lead to negative consequences. It is observed as interrupting teacher while asking a question, blurting out wrong answer before teacher finishes the question, unable to wait for ones turn during playing.

ADHD Symptoms Across Different Age Groups (Table 30.2)

Diagnosis – It is either clinical based on DSM V or ICD 10. Structured assessments like VAS, pre school ASRS, Connors parent/teacher-rating scale can be used. ADHD could be

- Predominantly inattention type
- Predominantly hyperactivity type
- Combined type

Course – Growing evidence suggests that ADHD is chronic disorder whose symptoms often persist into adulthood. Patients with more severe symptoms and combined type are at higher risk for persistence

Comorbidity – Associated with externalizing disorders like ODD, conduct disorder. Risk of bipolar disorder, substance use disorder is seen

Table 30.2

	Pre school	**Primary school**	**adolescence**
Inattention	• Short play sequences (< 3 min) • Leaving activities incomplete • Not listening	• Brief activities (< 10 min) • Premature changes of activity • Forgetful; disorganized; distracted environment	• Less persistence than peers (< 30 min) • Lack of focus on the details of a task • Poor planning ahead
Hyperactivity	Whirlwind	Restless when calm expected	Fidgety
Impulsivity	Does not listen • No sense of danger (hard to distinguish from being disrespectful towards authority figures)	• Acting out of turn; interrupting other children and blurting out answers • Thoughtless rule- breaking • Intrusions on peers; accidents	Poor self-control • Reckless risk- taking

Treatment – pharmacotherapy is effective in most children. behavioral therapies are effective as both primary mode of treatment and adjunct based on the severity of symptoms. Non-pharmacological management is discussed towards the end of the chapter.

- *Medication* - medication is indicated as first line of therapy only in severe cases (e.g. those diagnosed as hyperkinetic disorder), and as second line when psychological approaches have not been successful within a reasonable time (e.g. 8 weeks) or are inappropriate.
- This can be divided into stimulant and non stimulant medication.
  - *Stimulant medication* consists of methylphenidate [trade name Inspiral in India, Ritalin -abroad] in various release forms like immediate release, sustained release and OROS-Osmotic Release Oral system [Concerta].

    Dexamphetamine [Adderal] is approved for treatment of ADHD in the United States but is prohibited from use in India due to its abuse potential[6]
  - *Non-stimulant medication* consists of atomoxetine, clonidine, modafinil.

Table 30.3

Medication	**Onset and duration**	**Dose**
Methylphenidate immediate release	Onset- 20 to 60 minutes Duration- 2 to 4 hours	Initially 5-10 mg daily, titrated up in weekly increments of 5 -10 mg up to a maximum of 2.1 kg per kg bd. wt
Methylphenidate sustained release	An afternoon dose of methylphenidate immediate release might be necessary to optimize treatment	
Concerta	Onset- 30 min–2 hours. Duration- 12 hours	Initially 18 mg per day can be titrated up to 54 mg per day. 18 mg= 15 mg of MPH immediate release

Atomoxetine is a noradrenaline reuptake inhibitor

Onset of action is 4–6 weeks. When switching from a stimulant, continue stimulant for first 4 weeks of therapy

For children < 70 kg: initially 0.5 mg/kg/day for 7 days, then increase according to response. Recommended maintenance dose 1.2 mg/kg/day (in single or divided doses) and up to 1.8-mg/kg/day, to a maximum of 120 mg daily if necessary

For children >70 kg: initially 40 mg daily for 7 days, then increase according to response. Recommended maintenance dose 80mg daily

SPECIFIC LEARNING DISORDER

Children with learning difficulties fall along a spectrum; some have less difficulty and others have more. Learning is supported by multiple core skills like reading, comprehension, writing, and calculations. Difficulties in learning can be seen with relation to any of these skills.

Learning disorders are characterized by persistent difficulty learning key academic skills in the formal schooling years. Key academic skills include reading of single words accurately and fluently, reading comprehension, written expression and spelling, arithmetic calculation, and mathematical reasoning (solving mathematical problems). In contrast to talking or walking, which are developmental milestones associated with brain maturation, learning skills have to be taught explicitly. Learning disorders can be seen specifically with (**Table 30.3**).

Etiology - it is multifactorial with high heritability. Prevalence is around 5% to 15%

Table 30.3

Impairment in reading [dyslexia]
Word reading accuracy
Reading rate or fluency
Reading comprehension
Impairment in written expression [dysgraphia]
Spelling accuracy
Grammar and punctuation accuracy
Clarity or organization of written expression
Impairment in mathematics: [dyscalculia]
Number sense
Memorization of arithmetic facts
Accurate or fluent calculation
Accurate math reasoning

Clinical features - poor scholastic performance, difficulty comprehension, multiple spelling mistakes, performing better in oral exams, writing mirror images of numbers, 'b, d' confusion, interchange of similar sounding words , difficulty with calculations, recognizing mathematical symbols like + or - difficulty following multiple instructions.

Diagnosis - in India, NIMHANS SLD index is commonly used. Two levels are available. SLD can only be diagnosed in children with average intelligence levels.

Course - it is initially diagnosed in elementary school years. It has a prolonged course and manifestation of symptoms change over age.

Comorbidity - associated with other neurodevelopmental disorders, anxiety and depression features

Management- SLDs mainstay of management is remediation-based therapy.

Medical management of possible comorbidities should be done.

Motor Disorders

The neurodevelopmental motor disorders include developmental coordination disorder, stereotypic movement disorder and tic disorders.

Prevalence of DCD is around 5-11%. In all motor disorders, males are more affected compared to females.

Etiology - it includes genetic and environmental factors.

Prematurity, hypoxia and low birth weight are risk factors.

Streptococcal infection in infants is an important risk factor.

Neurobiology

Cerebellum is the site of dysfunction in DCD, basal ganglia in stereotypic movement disorders, caudate nucleus in tic disorders.

Clinical Features

DCD is also called as clumsy child syndrome or developmental dyspraxia. It is characterized by balance problems, awkward gait, difficulty with sports, difficulty learning dressing skills like buttoning, zipping

- ***Stereotypic movements*** include a diverse range of repetitive behaviors that usually emerge in the early developmental period, appear to lack a clear function, and sometimes cause interruption in daily life. Often appear to be self-soothing or self- stimulating; however, they can result in self-injury in some cases. It should be remembered that up to 60 to 80 percent of normal toddlers show transient rhythmic activities that seem purposeful and comforting and tend to disappear by 4 years of age. These movements could be hand flapping, body rocking, head banging and self-biting.

Tic disorders are of 3 types based on the kind of tic and duration of the disorder.

- Tourette's disorder
- Persistent vocal or motor tic disorder
- Provisional tic disorder

A tic is a sudden, rapid, recurrent, non-rhythmic motor movement or vocalization. (DSM V). Tics can be vocal or motor, simple or complex.

Presence of both motor and vocal tics for more than one year is the hallmark of Tourette's disorder.

Maintaining age appropriate skills is difficult for people with tic disorders.

Course

Studies indicate that tic disorders tend to improve in late adolescence and early adulthood. Children with DCD remain clumsy well into their adolescence and adulthood.

Diagnosis - structured assesments helpful in diagnosis are–

- Developmental coordination disorder questionnaire
- Movement assessment battery
- Yale brown global tic severity scale
- The premonitory urge for tics scale

Comorbidity – motor disorders are commonly associated with other neurodevelopmental disorders like IDD, ADHD and ASD. Comorbid ADHD is a poor prognostic factor

Management

Non pharmacologic

Sensory integration therapy, neuromotor task training for DCD

Tic disorders - habit reversal or comprehensive behavioral intervention for tics

Exposure and response prevention is another promising behavioral therapy for tic disorders.

Pharmacologic

Pharmacologic treatment is advised if tics or stereotypic behaviors are causing pain or discomfort, leading to social stigmatization, self-injury and functional impairment.

Alpha 2 blockers – clonidine, guanafacine are used in tic disorders.

Favourable data from clinical trials is available for haloperidol, risperidone, pimozide and tiapride.

Use of botulinum toxin injections to temporarily weaken muscles associated with severe motor or vocal tics also appears effective

Communication Disorders

They include language disorder, speech sound disorder, social or pragmatic communication disorder and childhood onset fluency disorder.

- Language disorder affects vocabulary and grammar. Childs first words and phrases are often delayed. There may be problems with understanding synonyms, remembering new words, word finding. This manifests as inability to describe an event accurately and comprehensively.
- Children with speech production difficulties may experience difficulty with phonological knowledge of speech sounds or the ability to coordinate movements for speech in varying degrees
- **Childhood onset fluency disorder, also** known as stuttering is a commonly seen communication disorder. This could lead to self-esteem issues in child and give rise to anxiety. So early diagnosis and speech therapy is very essential. It is characterized by frequent repetitions or prolongations of sounds or syllables and by other types of speech dysfluencies, including broken words (e.g., pauses within a word), audible or silent blocking (i.e., filled or unfilled pauses in speech), circumlocutions (i.e., word substitutions to avoid problematic words), words produced with an excess of physical tension, and monosyllabic whole-word repetitions (e.g., "I-I-I-I see him") dysfluency is often not seen during oral presentations, singing, talking to inanimate objects. Fearful anticipation of the problem may arise. Child may avoid speaking or alter talking rate, becomes very deliberate
- Social (pragmatic) communication disorder is characterized by a primary difficulty with pragmatics, or the social use of language and communication, as manifested by deficits in understanding and following social rules of verbal and nonverbal communication in naturalistic contexts, changing language according to the needs of the listener or situation, and following rules for conversations and storytelling.

Childhood Schizophrenia[7]

Early-onset schizophrenia is defined as schizophrenia with onset of clear positive symptoms prior to 18 years of age. Schizophrenia with onset between ages 13 and

18 is also frequently referred to as adolescent onset. Onset of schizophrenia prior to age 13 is referred to as very early onset or childhood onset. Early-onset schizophrenia (EOS) arising in childhood and adolescence is now accepted to be clinically and biologically continuous with the adult-onset disorder

Etiology

- Genetic- Existing evidence suggests that the candidate genes originally implicated in adult onset cases (G72, DTNBP1, COMT, NRG1) may have a **higher penetrance** in EOS
- *Environmental*- advanced paternal age, pregnancy and birth complications, maternal intrauterine nutritional deficiency, childhood abuse and neglect
- *Neurobiology*- Brain changes reported in EOS appear to be very similar to those described in adult schizophrenia, supporting the idea of an underlying neurobiological continuity. Increased gyral curvature and a reduction in sulcal curvature along with sulcal thinning affecting frontal, temporal and parietal lobes is noted in EOS
- *Clinical phases*-
  - Premorbid social and developmental impairment are seen.
  - Prodrome- An insidious deterioration prior to onset of psychosis is typical of the presentation of schizophrenia in children and adolescents. Prodrome is characterized by nonspecific behavioral changes including social withdrawal, declining school performance, uncharacteristic and odd behavior and ideas, eccentric interests, change in affect, and unusual and bizarre perceptual experiences
  - At risk mental states-The presence of attenuated positive symptoms of schizophrenia, brief-limited intermittent psychotic symptoms (BLIPS), or a combination of familial risk indicators with recent functional deterioration
- *Clinical features*- Hallucinations are frequently multimodal, with the affected youth seeing, hearing, and/or feeling the hallucinated being. Frequently, youth with early-onset schizophrenia present with nonspecific symptoms such as poor attention or increased aggression. Children with schizophrenia also exhibit illogical thinking and speaking and tend to underuse self-initiated repair strategies to aid in their communication
- *Diagnosis*- the same DSM V and ICD 10 criteria as for adults apply.
  - A number of long-term follow-up studies of EOS describe a typically chronic, unremitting long-term course with severely impaired functioning in adult life
  - Treatment-Short-term use of benzodiazepines (e.g., lorazepam) is preferable to high-dose antipsychotics in the management of severe behavioral disturbance associated in acute psychosis.
  - The recommended order of treatment for first-episode schizophrenia in children and adolescents is: atypical antipsychotics as first line;
  - If inadequate response, change to a different atypical or conventional antipsychotic;
  - If response is still inadequate or side effects are intolerable, then initiate clozapine

- Antipsychotic medication is usually maintained for at least 2 years after a first episode of schizophrenia

Externalizing Disorders

Externalizing disorders are characterized by problematic behavior related to poor impulse-control, including rule breaking, aggression, and impulsivity.

Oppositional defiant disorder and Conduct disorder are considered externalizing disorders in children and adolescents.

ODD

It is characterized by enduring patterns of disobedient and hostile behaviors towards authority figures.

Prevalence is 2 to 16 percent. Seen more in boys than girls before puberty, equal prevalence after puberty.

Etiology –

Unresolved conflict; learning disruptive behaviors from environment.

Biological- associated with low serotonin levels

Clinical features- can be seen as angry/irritable mood; aggressive/defiant behavior; vindictiveness.

Deliberately annoys people and blames others, has low frustration tolerance, easily loses temper.

Is usually well behaved with strangers.

Management

Treatment is predominantly non pharmacological.

Multiple modalities like *parent training, anger management, functional family therapy, brief family therapy, multi systemic therapy and cognitive behavioral therapy are used.*

Conduct Disorder

Between 2 and 8% of children and adolescents have conduct disorder. More common in boys than girls. Ratio is 4-12:1

Conduct disorder occurs with greater frequency in the children of parents with antisocial personality disorder and alcohol dependence than in the general population. The prevalence of conduct disorder and antisocial behavior is associated with socioeconomic factors

Etiology

- The most-studied candidate gene in relation to conduct problems is the MAOA promoter polymorphism.
- Perinatal complications, smoking in pregnancy,
- Children with verbal deficits and executive dysfunction show higher risk of developing conduct disorder.
- Inconsistent parenting and physical abuse and child maltreatment are associated with conduct disorder.

Clinical Features

Excessive levels of fighting, bullying, lying, cruelty to animals, destruction of property, disregard for rules, fire setting, stealing, truancy from school, running away, unusual tantrum behavior and persistent severe disobedience.

Management

Pharmacological

- The best-studied pharmacological interventions for youth with conduct problems are psychostimulants (methylphenidate and dexamfetamine), used in children with co-morbid ADHD and conduct disorder

- Other pharmacological approaches for antisocial behavior targeted reactive aggression and over-arousal, primarily in highly aggressive and psychiatrically hospitalized youth. Medications used in these conditions include those purported to target affect dysregulation (e.g., buspirone, clonidine) and mood stabilizers (e.g., lithium, carbamazepine)
- In the last few years, the use of antipsychotics such as risperidone, and other drugs such as clonidine in outpatient settings has been increasing

Non pharmacological

- Fast track prevention intervention
- Kazdin's problem solving skills training
- Parent and teacher management program

Depression and Suicide

Major depression is an episodic, recurring disorder characterized by persistent and pervasive sadness or unhappiness, loss of enjoyment of everyday activities, irritability, and associated symptoms such as negative thinking, lack of energy, difficulty concentrating, and appetite and sleep disturbances. Manifestations can vary according to age, gender and educational and cultural background.

Most studies concur that about 1% to 2% of pre-pubertal children and about 5% of adolescents suffer from clinically significant depression at any one time.

The ratio of depression in males and females is similar in pre-pubertal children but becomes about twice as common among females compared with males during adolescence.

Etiology

Etiology of MDD is complex and multifactorial and a detailed discussion is beyond the scope of this textbook

It has genetic, neurobiological and environmental factors.

Environmental influences include children's family relationships, cognitive style—most depressed adolescents experience negative thoughts about self, the world and or the future; collectively known as *Becks triad* that seem to arise spontaneously (automatic thoughts), which contribute to a negative cognitive style—stressful life events and school and neighborhood characteristics.

Parental depression is the most consistently replicated risk factor for depression in the off spring.

Stressful life events—especially losses—may increase the risk for depression

Clinical Features

In children and adolescents it may not always be sadness, crying spells or suicidal ideas as seen in adults. Children may vocalize their feelings poorly. In the Table 30.4, we will see how symptoms of depression may present and differ across age groups.

Suicide

In many countries suicide is one of the leading causes of death among children and adolescents. Identifying young people at risk and offering effective treatment is a major concern of mental health policies. This chapter

Table 30.4

Pre-pubertal children	Adolescents	Adults
• Irritability (temper tantrums, non- compliance) • Affect is reactive* • Frequently comorbid with anxiety, behavior problems, and ADHD • Somatic complaints These are physical symptoms like headache, body pains etc.	• Irritability (grumpy, hostile, easily frustrated, angry outbursts) • Affect is reactive* • Hypersomnia • Increased appetite and weight gain • Somatic complaints • Extreme sensitivity to rejection (e.g., falsely perceived putdown or criticism) resulting, for example, in difficulties maintaining relationships	Anhedonia -loss of pleasure • Lack of affective reactivity • Psychomotor agitation or retardation • Diurnal variation of mood (worse in the morning) • Early morning waking

*Ability to be momentarily cheered up in response to positive events (e.g., visit by peers)

includes a review of suicidality in children and adolescents. Non-suicidal self-injury (NSSI) will also be addressed

Para suicide refers to a non-habitual, potentially life-threatening self- harming behavior which is performed without the intention to kill oneself. Because the behavior is non suicidal, most authors today prefer the term "non suicidal self-injury" (NSSI) (in this chapter the term non suicidal self-injury is used).

The terms "deliberate self-injury" or "deliberate self-harm" are typically used without distinguishing between NSSI and non-fatal suicide attempt

Suicide (from the Latin *sui caedere*, to kill oneself) means the act of a person intentionally causing his or her own death.

Suicide attempt

Denotes non-fatal acts or preparations intended to result in death. The suicidal act may have been abandoned, interrupted or was unsuccessful.

Suicidality refers to the cognitions and activities of persons seeking their own death, including thoughts, actions or omissions.

The key difference between deliberate self-injury and suicide attempt is in the *intent* to end one's life.

About 60% of depressed young people report having thought about suicide and 30% actually attempt suicide. Risk increases if:

- Suicides in the family
- Young person has attempted suicide previously
- Other comorbid psychiatric disorders (e.g., substance abuse), impulsivity and aggression
- Access to lethal means (e.g., firearms)
- Experienced negative events (e.g., disciplinary crises, physical or sexual abuse), among others.

Rating scales can be used to assess severity- *Hamilton rating scale for depression, childrens, depression rating scale.*

Treatment

Pharmacological

Antidepressants- SSRIS- citalopram, fluoxetine, sertraline

- Fluoxetine is the best studied and has the best evidence of effectiveness. Approved by the FDA for those aged 8 years or older.
- Escitalopram has been approved by the FDA for adolescent depression
- Sertraline, citalopram, escitalopram: less robust evidence of effectiveness, though they may be effective in patients who did not respond to Fluoxetine (Brent et al, 2008).

Psycho-social Interventions

- Cognitive behavioral therapy
- Interpersonal therapy
- Supportive family therapy

Separation Anxiety Disorder

Anxiety disorders are probably the most common psychopathology in youth, with prevalence estimates ranging from 5% to 25% worldwide, but a much lower percentage receive treatment (Boyd et al, 2000; Costello et al, 2003).

Separation anxiety disorder (SAD) accounts for approximately half of the referrals among all anxiety disorders

Most pediatric anxiety disorders have the same diagnostic criteria as those in adults except SAD, currently classified in DSM and ICD as one of the disorders usually diagnosed in infancy, childhood, or adolescence

SAD is characterized by an abnormal reactivity to real or imagined separation from attachment figures that significantly interferes with daily activities and developmental tasks

Clinical Features

- It is characterized by - Excessive and persistent fears or worries before and at the time of separation.
- Behavioral and somatic symptoms before, during and after the separation and
- Persistent avoidance or attempts to escape the separation situation.
- Child *worries* that something may happen to his parents (e.g., that they will disappear, get lost or forget about him) or that the child will get lost, kidnapped or killed if he is not near his parents. *Behavioral symptoms* include crying, clinging, complaining upon separation, and searching or calling for the parent after their departure.

Clinical presentation varies with age. Adolescents might complain of physical symptoms on school days.

- Separation anxiety symptoms usually peak between nine and 13 months of age and decrease usually after two years of age, with increasing levels of autonomy by the age of three. Separation anxiety symptoms may increase again by age four to five, usually when the child starts school.

Etiology

Neurobiology- The amygdala is one of the main areas implicated in anxiety.

Psychological- Fear conditioning is at the core of anxiety disorders.

Environmental- Low parental warmth, over protective parents, insecure attachment with mother, parental discord and early experiences like being involved in disaster or crime, exposure to family violence, birth of a sibling

Comorbidity- children with SAD also present with MDD, bipolar disorder and ADHD.

Rating scales should be applied to confirm diagnosis and assess severity.

Management- non-pharmacological management like cognitive behavioral therapy, psychoeducation and parent child interaction therapy is used.

Pharmacological- Medication should always be used *in addition* to behavioral or psychotherapeutic intervention. Medication is not generally recommended as a first line treatment for SAD.

However, it is a useful strategy when CBT achieves no response or partial response, or when the child is significantly impaired.

No medication has been specifically approved for SAD. However, various medications have been investigated for childhood anxiety disorders, such as selective serotonin reuptake inhibitors (SSRIs), tricyclic antidepressants (TCAs), benzodiazepines, buspirone, serotonin and noradrenaline reuptake inhibitors (SNRI), propranolol, clonidine, atypical antipsychotics, antihistamines and melatonin.

All medications should be started, stopped or adjusted under the supervision of a trained clinician.

Enuresis

Enuresis constitutes a very common group of disorders in childhood that occur worldwide at approximately the same rate. 10% of all 7-year-olds wet the bed at night and 2% to 3% during the day.

Despite a high remission rate, still 1% to 2% of all adolescents are affected by nocturnal enuresis and less than 1% by daytime wetting

Enuresis is defined by ICD 10 as involuntary (or even intentional) wetting in children 5 years of age or older after organic causes have been ruled out.

The wetting must have persisted for at least three months to be considered a disorder.

According to ICD-10, enuresis is diagnosed if wetting occurs two times a month in children under 7 years of age and once a month in children 7 years and older.

- Primary enuresis means that the child has been dry for less than 6 months (or not at all)
- Secondary enuresis means that a relapse after a dry period of at least 6 months has occurred

Clinical Features

- Deep sleep and difficult arousal, increased urine volume at night (polyuria) with large wetted volumes.
- The typical presentation is a child who is extremely difficult to wake and who wets the bed with large amount of urine.
- In contrast, bladder function during the day is completely normal.

Etiology

- It is genetically determined.
- 70% to 80% of all children with enuresis have affected relatives.
- The concordance rates are higher among mono- than di-zygotic twins

Comorbidity

ADHD is the most common comorbidity.

Externalizing disorders are also seen as comorbidities.

Management

Two main interventions are available: alarm treatment and pharmacotherapy

An alarm consists of a pad or a metal sensor, which is connected to a bell by a wire. Once the sensor becomes wet, an electric circuit is closed and the alarm is set off. Alarms are very simple devices; they can be cleaned and used by different children many times over. Sterilization is not required, as urine is per se a sterile fluid (unless UTI's are present), cleaning with a surface disinfectant is enough

After 14 consecutive dry nights, use of the alarm is discontinued and the child is considered to be dry.

Parents are advised to restart alarm treatment if a relapse (two wet nights per week) happens, this occurs in up to 30% of cases.

Pharmacotherapy- Indications for medication are:

- Unwillingness to undertake alarm treatment
- Lack of motivation in the children
- Family overwhelmed by demands such as a work situation, cramped housing, infants to care for, i.e., cooperation with alarm treatment is not possible
- Short-term dryness is required, e.g., for school outings.
- There are two groups of medication with a clear antienuretic effect: desmopressin and tricyclic antidepressants (TCAs). Although both are effective, desmopressin has less side-effects and is therefore the preferred substance
- Desmopressin is taken in tablet form in the evenings only. The oral dosage is 0.2 mg to 0.4 mg.
- TCAs such as imipramine are used

MANAGEMENT IN CHILD AND ADOLESCENT PSYCHIATRY [6]

Pharmacology

With the expansion of psychopharmacolgy in adults, increasing use of psychotropics is being seen in child and adolescent psychiatry.

As the etiology of many childhood psychiatric illnesses is not clear, treatment indications and targets remain empirical.

General Principles

- Start on a low dose and titrate slowly
- Use monotherapy as much as possible
- Identify the target symptom and treat the symptoms
- Individualize treatment protocol according to patient response.

Psychosocial Interventions[5]

General principles

- Be positive and encouraging to child and family.
- Provide support.
- Set boundaries; do not take over the role of parent
- Do not be authoritative or judgmental
- Be holistic; address not just the symptoms but also the social and emotional issues related to it.
- Prepare an individualized treatment plan
- There are no fixed treatment protocols

- Promote positive mental health
- We will discuss in brief a few widely used psychosocial interventions

Family Therapy

Parental skills training

- Know the child
- Improve listening skills
- Develop a positive, trusting relationship with the child
- Learn effective communication- it should be an open, free, two-way process. The child should be allowed to speak. Communicate without using negative, critical comments about the child.
- Control emotions; be consistent; be a role model.

Behavioral Therapy

Based on principles of classical and operant conditioning.

Used in ADHD, ASD, ODD, and other disorders. Aim of therapy is twofold-

- To strengthen, develop or maintain healthy behavior
- To reduce or eliminate unhealthy or maladaptive behavior

Techniques to Increase Positive Behavior

Reinforcement

- Giving reward for a positive desired behavior. Reinforcement can be tangible such as food; money or tokens ,which can later be exchanged for tangible rewards.

Modeling

- Learning through observing and modeling a certain behavior exhibited by adults.

Skills training

- Techniques to decrease maladaptive behavior-
- *Negative reinforcement and punishment-*
- Involves withdrawal of positive privileges like TV time or introducing aversive stimulus like scolding. Some procedures are

Time out

- Response cost
- Over correction

Play therapy

- It is a form of psychotherapy. Here, play is used as a means to explore, communicate and change. Play stimulates cognitive, affective and motor development in children. Playroom has to be set carefully. It needs to be a bright, open and quiet room. Toy material should include coloring material, dolls; stuffed human figures of both genders, toy vehicles, animals, jig saw puzzles, blocks, beads etc.

Sensory integration and occupational therapy

- Occupational therapy uses play activities in ways designed to change how the brain reacts to touch, sound, sight and movement. It is a combination of sensory experiences
- It is a planned and structured program
- Provides optimal arousal level
- Sensory input is used to excite or relax the child.

Topics Requiring Further Discussion

Internet addiction[8,5]

The Internet is without doubt one of the most popular mediums used by adults and children

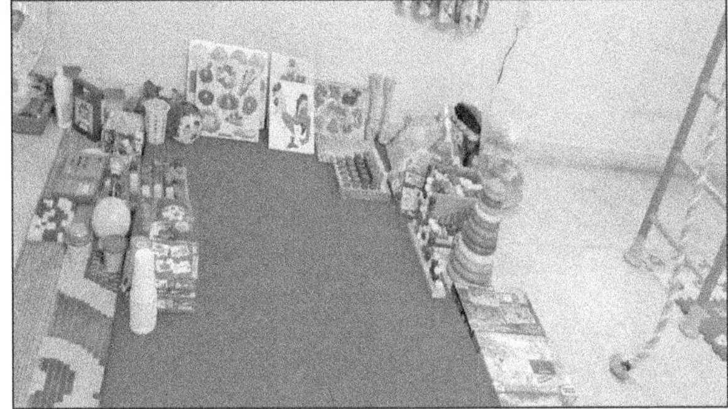

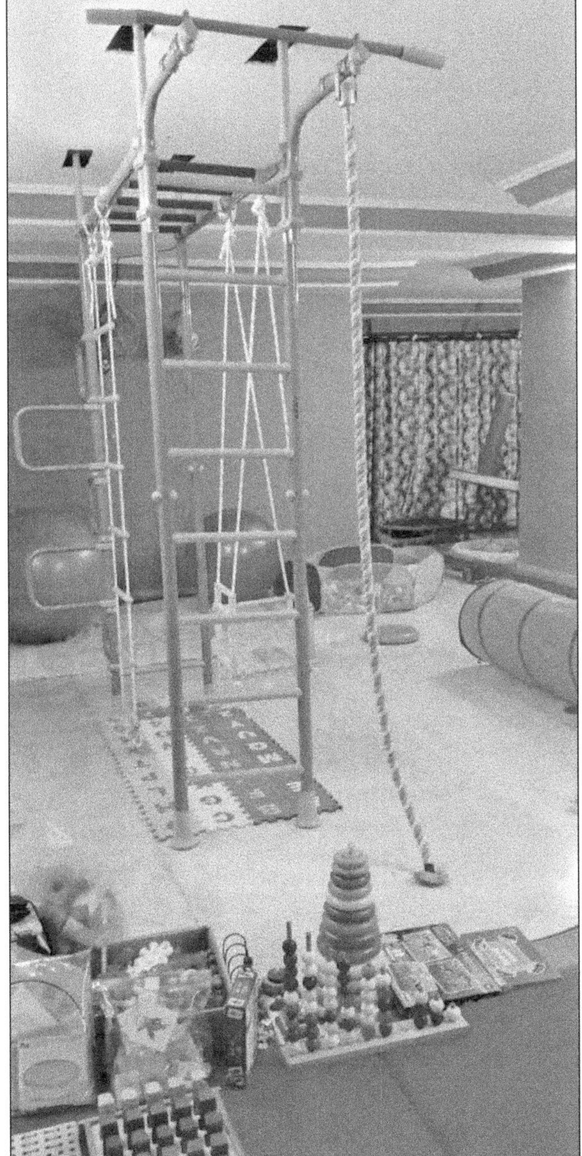

Fig. 30.2: Occupational therapy room (Courtesy of Indlas Child Guidance Clinic).

alike. Increasing availability of data services at low prices and increased number of electronic appliances like laptops, tablets, and smart phones has led to an explosive increase in Internet use in the last decade.

Children, as young as 2 years are spending more time on smart phones, at the cost of their social communication skills. Adolescents are finding it difficult to go through a day without using one of these apps like twitter, instagram, whatsApp, Facebook etc.

A negative correlation has been reported between time spent playing Internet games and academic performance, and a positive association between violent Internet game-playing and aggression

Not only does excessive Internet use has a negative impact on the mental and physical health of children and adolescents with Problematic Internet Usage, it might also increase risk of violence in this age group

Is it an illness?

Internet addiction has not been formally accepted as a disorder yet.
Block (2008) has recently highlighted the increasing incidence of Internet addiction and its high comorbidity with other psychiatric conditions.

Governments such as South Korea have declared Internet addiction a serious problem and a public health hazard (Block, 2008); Chinese psychologists also support Internet addiction to be recognized as a formal disorder by the World Health Organization (Flisher, 2010).

In DSM V, Internet gaming disorder has been classified under conditions for further study.

The DSM-5 work group reviewed more than 240 articles and found some behavioral similarities of Internet gaming to gambling disorder and to substance use disorders.

Internet gaming disorder is a pattern of excessive and prolonged Internet gaming that results in a cluster of cognitive and behavioral symptoms, including progressive loss of control over gaming, tolerance, and withdrawal symptoms, analogous to the symptoms of substance use disorders.

They typically devote 8–10 hours or more per day to this activity and at least 30 hours per week. If they are prevented from using a computer and returning to the game, they become agitated and angry.

There are currently no management plans for Internet addiction, as the diagnosis cannot be made.

Based on other comorbidities like anxiety, depression seen in excessive Internet use, this condition requires further investigation.

Child sexual abuse[9]

Child sexual abuse (CSA) is the involvement of children and adolescents in sexual activities (usually for adult sexual stimulation or gratification) that they cannot fully comprehend and to which they cannot consent as a fully equal, self-determining participant, because of their early stage of development

Nature or types of CSA

- Contact vs. non- contact- contact abuse entails touching of private parts of child or the abuser, fondling; non contact entails exposing oneself to the child, showing inappropriate pictures, or observing victim in various stages of undress.
- Penetrative vs. non penetrative
- Single vs. multiple episodes
- Known vs. unknown perpetrator
- Single vs. multiple perpetrators
- It is important to understand the nature and type of child sexual abuse as the severity of the impact of the abuse depends on not only on the type of abuse but also on the duration of the abuse and very importantly, whether the abuser is a known/trusted person or a stranger

CSA is not a clinical condition or diagnosis. It is important for the clinician to learn more about it so she or he is well equipped to identify a case and provide required support.

There are 3 contexts in which a child presents for consultation

1. CSA has already been established and child has been brought by agencies such as the police, child protection units or courts.
2. Child has reported CSA to parents but they have not reported to authorities and brought the child for consultation
3. When it is not (yet) known that he/she has been sexually abused; the child comes to the mental health system for some psychological or psychiatric manifestation, but upon enquiry and examination, CSA issues emerge in one of the following ways:
    - The child discloses or reports abuse.
    - An adolescent girl is found to be pregnant.
    - The child/caregivers report frequent urinary tract infections in the child and/or genital injuries in the child are reported/observed.
    - Emotional and behavioral issues that

are associated with anxiety, anger and depression

Index of suspicion in CSA

I.e. when to suspect child sexual abuse and how true one's suspicions likely to be.

High to Low Index Of Suspicion

- Disclosure by the child
- Detection of pregnancy, STDs and genital injuries
- Sexualized behavior, clear hints given by the child.
- Symptoms of depression or PTSD
- Sudden unexplained behavioral changes; school refusal and people avoidance
- Symptom patterns- sudden onset of bed-wetting, aches, pains, general ill health.

CSA Assessment and Inquiry

- Developmental assessment of child should be done.
- Inquiry regarding the details of CSA should be obtained in such a way that child doesn't undergo more unnecessary trauma.
- In younger children, dolls are used to help the child describe the traumatic experience.
- Questions can be open ended or leading questions depending on necessity
- All details are clearly documented.

Impact of CSA

Traumatic sexualisation- sexuality of the child is inappropriately shaped and developed. This is observed in child as precocious sexual behavior, promiscuity, and compulsive sexual behaviors.

Stigmatization- child forms negative opinions about him or herself- seen as guilt, shame, and low self-esteem.

Betrayal- due to child's immediate or delayed understanding that someone they trusted has betrayed them- seen as grief, depression, extreme dependency, mistrust, anger.

Powerlessness- child's agency is taken away from them; child experiences threat of injury- seen as anxiety, fear, need to control, and identification with aggressor.

Interventions for CSA

Medical Assistance- includes treatment of injuries, post exposure prophylaxis, pregnancy testing

Psychosocial and mental health interventions-

For the child-

Pharmacotherapy is used in case of severe anxiety, depression or Post Traumatic Stress Disorder.

First level Responses-

- Ensuring child's safety,
- Rest and recreation
- Relaxation exercises.
- Resuming daily routine and developmental activites.

Depth Therapeutic Inteventions- detailed discussion is beyond the scope of this chapter.

It consists of multiple techniques to improve positive mental health, self image and trust.

Providing emotional support for parents and psychoeducating them.

Medico Legal Assistance

POCSO ACT 2012- PREVENTION OF CHILD SEXUAL OFFENCES ACT

It provides guidelines on mandatory reporting and role of a mental health professional as expert witness.

CONCLUSION

Child psychiatry is a relatively new branch in the field of psychiatry. Due to various genetic and environmental reasons, there is an increasing incidence of neurodevelopmental disorders and behavioral disorders in children. But the availability of experts in the field of child psychiatry is nowhere near the required mandate. The number of child guidance clinics in India is very few and most of them are present only in the urban areas. This chapter hopes to improve the understanding undergraduates have about child psychiatry and kindle their interest and of course be useful for their examinations.

BIBLIOGRAPHY

1. Rey JM, Assumpção FB, Bernad CA, Çuhadaroğlu FC, Evans B, Fung D, Harper G, Loidreau L, Ono Y, Pūras D, Remschmidt H, Robertson B, Rusakoskaya OA, Schleimer K. History of child and adolescent psychiatry. In Rey JM (ed), *IACAPAP e-Textbook of Child and Adolescent Mental Health*. Geneva: International Association for Child and Adolescent Psychiatry and Allied Professions 2015
2. Sharan P, Sagar R: Mental health policy for children and adolescents in developing countries. J Indian Assoc Child Adolesc Ment Health 2007, 3:1–4.
3. Malhotra S, Patra BN. Prevalence of child and adolescent psychiatric disorders in India: a systematic review and meta-analysis.
4. Malhotra S. clinical assessment and management of childhood psychiatric disorders. Pub. CBS; 2013.
5. JM Rey's IACAPAP e-Textbook of Child and Adolescent Mental Health. Rey JM & Martin A (eds). Geneva: International Association for Child and Adolescent Psychiatry and Allied Professions, 2019
6. Taylor DM, Barnes TR, Young AH. The Maudsley prescribing guidelines in psychiatry. John Wiley & Sons; 2018 May 14.
7. Benjamin J. Sadock, Virginia A. Sadock. Kaplan & Sadock's comprehensive textbook of psychiatry. Philadelphia :Lippincott Williams & Wilkins,2017
8. Diagnostic and Statistical Manual of Mental Disorders: Diagnostic and Statistical Manual of Mental Disorders, Fifth Edition. Arlington, VA: American Psychiatric Association, 2013
9. Seshadri S, Ramaswamy S. Clinical practice guidelines for child sexual abuse. Indian J Psychiatry 2019;61, Suppl S2:317-32.

Autism Spectrum Disorders 31

Manjiri Deshpande Shenoy • V. Manasa Ram • Vishal Indla

Autism is a neuro-developmental disorder, with pervasive deficits in social communication and social interaction and of restrictive and stereotyped patterns of behavior, interests, or activities. Due to wide variation in the type and severity of symptoms experienced by people it is a "spectrum" disorder. Although ASD can be a lifelong disorder, pharmacological and non-pharmacological therapies can improve a person's symptoms and functional abilities.

Eugen Bleuler coined the term AUTISM (Greek. Autos=self) to describe active withdrawal into their own fantasy life seen in patients with schizophrenia. Leo Kanner first described 11 cases of children with autism with defects in communication and behavior in his paper "autistic disturbances of affective contact". He coined the term "Infantile autism". Other terminologies used previously are Kanner's autism, Infantile Schizophrenia, Early childhood psychosis", Symbiotic psychosis.

CLASSIFICATION

ICD-10 (World Health Organization, 1990) classifies autism under the *pervasive developmental disorders*, characterized by abnormalities in reciprocal social interaction, idiosyncratic patterns of communication and by a restricted, stereotyped, repetitive repertoire of interests and activities.

DSM-5 classifies autism under Autism Spectrum Disorder category, characterized by:

- Persistent deficits in social communication and social interaction across multiple contexts
- Restricted, repetitive patterns of behavior, interests or activities either current or elicited through the clinical history
- Clinically significant impairment in social, occupational, or other important areas of functioning
- Presence from early childhood (although it may not become fully manifest until social demands exceed the child's limited capacities), and
- Not explained better by intellectual disability or global developmental delay.

EPIDEMIOLOGY

Autism spectrum disorder (ASD) is an important cause of developmental disability worldwide. Its estimated prevalence is 1% in the United Kingdom and 1.5% in the United States. There have been various epidemiological surveys to determine the prevalence estimates of ASD during the past decade. The data based on these surveys showed an increase in the prevalence of ASD worldwide. The prevalence was estimated to be 61.9/10,000 globally in 2012.

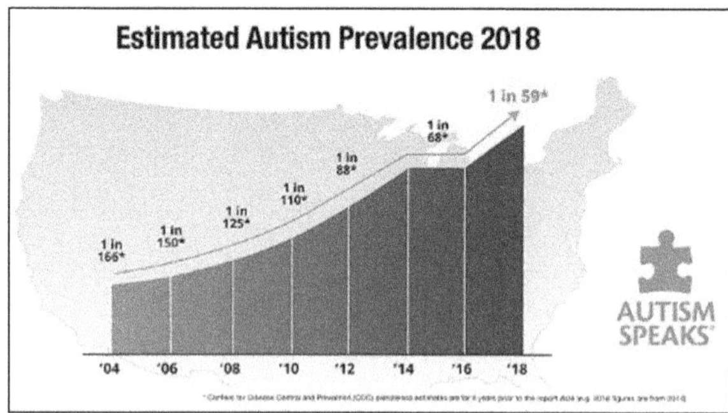

Fig. 31.1: Estimated austism prevalence 2018.

Center disease control (CDC), Atlanta determined that approximately 1 in 59 children is diagnosed with an autism spectrum disorder (ASD). Autism is 4 times more likely to be diagnosed in boys than girls. Most of the children are being diagnosed after age 4, though it can be reliably diagnosed as early as 2 years.

Intellectual disability ([IQ] < 70) is seen in about 31% of children with ASD, borderline range (IQ 71–85) is seen in about 25%, and IQ scores in the average to above average range (i.e., IQ > 85) is seen in about 44%. ASD occurs in all ethnic, racial, and economic groups. Minority groups tend to be diagnosed later and less often

Estimated prevalence of ASD in India ranges from 0.15% to 1.01%. In the INCLEN study, the prevalence of ASD (then termed as PDD) was 1 in 125 in children 3-6 years and 1 in 85 in children 6-9 years of age. The prevalence in rural areas was 0.90%, 0.6% in hilly regions, 1.01% in urban areas, 0.1% in tribal areas and 0.61% in the coastal regions.

ETIOLOGY AND RISK FACTORS

Genetic Factors

Genetic factors play a causative role in autism which is supported by twin and family studies. Siblings of autistic probands are 50 to 200 times, at risk for autism than general population. In monozygotic twins concordance rates for autism range from 36% to 96% but in dizygotic twins its only 0% to 27%.

Multiple genes seem to be involved. These genes are responsible for synaptic plasticity, synaptic scaffolding proteins, receptors, cell adhesion molecules or proteins that are involved in chromatin remodeling, transcription, protein synthesis or degradation, or actin cytoskeleton dynamics. For example, genes for neuroligins, SHANKs, CNTNAP2, FMR1 etc.

Neuroanatomic and Neuroimaging Findings

Neuroanatomic and neuroimaging findings, though not diagnostic, have consistently revealed increased cerebral volume which affects both grey and white matter, and also enlarged ventricles. Over growth of brain is observed in the first two years of life. Later during development, differences are observed in the function and structure of the 'empathy circuit' of the brain (amygdala, ventro-medial prefrontal cortex, temporo-parietal junction, orbito-frontal cortex, anterior cingulate, and other related brain regions). Abnormal connectivities are also found between frontal and parietal lobe functions that may cause disturbances in cognitive style, resulting in an over-reliance on processing details and a relative under-reliance on processing information as a whole.

On analysis of neuronal growth and pathways cortico-striato-thalamo-cortical circuits (for repetitive behaviors), ventral tegmental area connectivity to nucleus accumbens (for social interaction), and amygdala to ventral hippocampal connectivity (for social interactions) are areas of active interest and study. Excessive synapses are found due to a slow pruning process. However, diagnostic modalities to ascertain the same are yet awaited.

RISK FACTORS

The NICE guideline *Autism: Recognition, Referral and Diagnosis of Children and Young People on the Autism Spectrum*, while stressing the low quality of evidence found, lists the risk factors for ASDs that are clinically and statistically factors associated with an increased prevalence of autism.

- A sibling with autism.
- Birth defects associated with central nervous system malformation and/or dysfunction, including cerebral palsy.
- Maternal age > 40 yrs
- High Paternal age
- Gestational age less than 35 weeks.
- Parental schizophrenia-like psychosis, affective disorder or any psychiatric illness.
- Maternal use of sodium valproate, thalidomide in pregnancy.
- Low birth weight,
- Preterm delivery
- Birth asphyxia.
- Birth defects
- Admission into neonatal intensive care unit
- A learning (intellectual) disability.
- Attention deficit hyperactivity disorder.
- Neonatal physical illnesses such as post-encephalitic infections and sepsis
- Neonatal encephalopathy or epileptic encephalopathy, including infantile spasms.
- Autoimmune factors from reactions between maternal antibodies and the fetus

In relation to medical conditions associated with ASD, the NICE guideline lists the prevalence of ASDs in several medical conditions.

- Intellectual disability (8%-27.9%)
- Fragile X syndrome (24%-60%)
- Tuberous sclerosis (36%-79%)
- Neonatal encephalopathy/epileptic encephalopathy/infantile spasms(4%-14%)
- Cerebral palsy (15%)
- Down syndrome (6%-15%)
- Muscular dystrophy (3%-37%)
- Neurofibromatosis (4%-8%).

Future directions for genetic research in autism lie in identifying specific gene-environment interactions. Research must overcome the challenges of elucidating the roles of genetic heterogeneity, epigenetic mechanisms and environmental modifiers.

CLINICAL FEATURES

SOCIAL COMMUNICATION

Joint Attention

Deficits in joint attention include:

- Poor in orienting to people in a social environment,
- Low frequency of shared attention,
- Difficulty in monitoring of emotional states,
- Doesn't seek engagement and comfort from others,
- Poor in analysing other's intention and perspective.

Social Reciprocity

Deficits in social reciprocity include:

- Difficulty initiating and maintaining conversation,
- Limitations with maintaining turn-taking in interactions,
- Problems with providing random responses when conversation is initiated by others.

Social Cognition

It is related to person's ability to process, store, and apply information from people and social situations. It is the usage of cognitive processes during social interactions.

Deficits in social cognition include:

- Deficits in social and emotional learning including difficulty
- Managing emotions,
- Understanding others perspective
- Developing prosocial goals,
- Using interpersonal skills to handle developmentally appropriate tasks
- Inability in differentiating one's own feelings from the feelings of others
- Poor in understanding distinct information and construct meaning in a given context.

LANGUAGE AND RELATED COGNITIVE SKILLS

Deficits in language and related cognitive skills include:

- Impaired acquisition of words, word combinations, and syntax
- Initial words are often nouns and attributes, while words representing social stimuli, such as people's names (i.e., subjects) and actions (i.e., verbs), are delayed;
- The child loses words acquired previously;
- Use and understanding of nonverbal and verbal communication—
- Communication through facial expressions, body language, and gestures is delayed in the latter part of the first year of life and remain unconventional throughout development;
- Atypical gestures (e.g., pulling a caregiver's hand toward an item) emerge prior to more usual gestures (e.g., giving, pointing, and head nods/headshakes);
- Comprehending the gaze shifting, distal gestures, facial expressions, and rules of proximity and body language is limited;
- Receptive language appears more delayed than expressive;
- Echolalia and repetitions are observed;
- Vocal development deficits, including
- Unusual response to caregiver's vocalizations,
- Odd vocal productions beyond the first year of life,
- Peculiar prosody once speech emerges (speech may sound robotic);
- Symbolic play deficits, including
- Limited knowledge on functional and conventional use of objects,
- Repetitive, inflexible play,
- Restricted cooperative play in interactive situations;
- Conversation deficits, including
- Difficulty in understanding the social norms of conversation (e.g., balancing turns, speech volume, proximity, and conversational timing);
- Including inappropriate and unnecessary information in conversational contexts;
- Problems taking turns during conversation;
- Difficulty in initiating topics of common interests;
- Prefers to speak on topics of special interest;
- Difficulties in recognizing the need for clarification;

- Challenges adequately repairing miscommunications;
- Difficulty in understanding figurative language, like idioms, multiple meanings, and sarcasm;
- Literacy deficits, including
- Problems in reading for meaning (functional use of books),
- Difficulty in understanding narratives and expository text genres that require multiple perspectives (e.g., persuasive and comparative/contrastive),
- Poor in getting the main idea and summarizing,
- Inability to provide sufficient information for the reader when writing;
- Executive functioning deficits, including
- Lacking/limited flexibility,
- Poor problem solving,
- Poor planning and organization,
- Lack of inhibition.

Behavior and Emotional Regulation

Deficits in behavior and emotional regulation, including

- Difficulty in adjusting with changes in routine and/or moving from one activity to the next;
- Poor in generalizing learned skills;
- Using objects in odd ways and unusual attachment to objects;
- Difficulty sleeping;
- Crying, becoming angry, or laughing at inappropriate times with no obvious reasons.
- Social withdrawal and apprehension due to oddity in understanding of social events and inability to identify salient or irrelevant Information);
- Using early-developing and/or unconventional strategies for self-regulation (e.g., chewing on clothing, rocking, hand flapping, vocal play);
- Using unusual behavioral responses and emotional expressions (e.g., aggression, tantrums, bolting from situations);
- Restricted, repetitive patterns of behavior, interests, or activities (e.g., immediate echolalia and scripted language);
- Poor self-management skills.

Sensory and Feeding

Sensory and feeding challenges, include

- Over-responsiveness, under-responsiveness, or mixed responsiveness patterns to environmental stimuli, light, visual clutter, and social stimuli (e.g., social touch, proximity of others, voices) are seen as part of difficulties in sensory modality;
- More interested with sensory aspects of objects and events due to avoidance of social stimuli.
- Preference food based on manner of presentation or food texture;
- Restriction to variety of foods compared to other family members.

Sleep problems and irritability are common in ASD.

People with ASD may have savant abilities despite many challenges faced by them. The savant skills can be

- Extraordinary ability to learn things in detail and remember information for long periods of time

- Can be strong visual and auditory learners
- They can excel in math, science, music, or art.

Comorbid Medical & Mental Health Conditions

- Autism may be associated with many health problems across the life span
- Attention Deficit Hyperactivity Disorder (ADHD) – 30 to 61%
- Chronic sleep problems >50%
- Anxiety disorders – 11 to 40%
- Depression – 7% of children and 26% of adults.
- Chronic gastrointestinal disorders are 8 times more common in people wih autism
- Epilepsy (seizure disorder) – 30-35%
- Schizophrenia – 4 and 35% of adults with autism. (1.1 percent of the general population).
- Overweight and obesity are also common.

BENCHMARKS FOR SOCIAL COMMUNICATION

Birth- 12 Months

- Looks at human face and eyes;
- Turns to human voice;
- Searches for source of voice; can differentiate between tones of voice (angry, friendly)
- Can responds to caregiver with a smile;
- Follows caregiver's gaze and maintains eye contact
- Tries to engage caregiver in vocal turn-taking .
- Make sounds to get attention;
- shows joint attention skills (shares attention with care giver);
- Can make requests with non verbal commands ;
- Enjoys interactive games such as peek-a-boo.

12-18 Months

- Shows the objects to caregivers;
- Communicates his requirements by pointing and vocalizing;
- Says "bye" and other ritualized words;
- Conveys his disagreement by shaking head, saying "no";
- Tries to use verbal language rather than non verbal communication.
- Maintains eye contact to respond to others;
- Shows sympathy, empathy, and sharing .

18-24 Months

- Expresses his intention by single words;
- Can use phrases to command, indicate possession, express problems and gain attention;
- uses I, me, you, my and mine;
- Tries to participate in conversation by taking turns;

When the child is unable reach these bench marks, they can be at risk for AUTISM (RED FLAG SIGNS).

Treatment of Autism Spectrum Disorders

Despite the advances in early diagnosis and intervention, no therapy or medicine has been yet proven to completely reverse the core symptoms of autism.

A team of trained healthcare professionals such as developmental pediatrician, child psychiatrist, occupational therapist, behavioral therapist, speech and language therapist, child psychologist, special educator and social worker are necessary for the management of autism

The treatment involves psychoeducating the parents, pharmacotherapy and non-pharmacological methods

The pharmacotherapy of autism involves treatment of targeted behavioral symptoms rather than core autism features. Targets generally include hyperactivity, inattention, irritability, repetitive thoughts and behavior, self-injurious behavior, as well as aggression toward others or the environment

Antipsychotics have traditionally been shown to improve symptoms related to aggression, social withdrawal, hyperactivity, stereotypes, self-injurious behavior, and sleep disturbances. Although typical neuroleptics (first generation antipsychotics) such as pimozide and haloperidol, have been reported to be more effective in treating behavioral problems, the increased risk of tardive or withdrawal dyskinesia in a substantial proportion of children with autism continues to be a major concern (Campbell et al., 1997).

Risperidone and Aripiprazole (second generation antipsychotics) are the only two medications that have been approved by the US Food and Drug Administration (FDA) to treat patients with ASD

The indications for the use of these drugs include significant irritability and those displaying disruptive behaviors, aggression, self-injury and severe "tantrums" or "meltdowns" secondary to ASD, but as such these are not targeted for any of the core ASD symptoms. Although these medications have shown efficacy in reducing irritability, stereotype and hyperactivity with large effect sizes and high response rates, they have also demonstrated serious adverse effects, including dyslipidemia, hyperglycemia and weight gain (McCracken et al., 2002; McDougle et al., 2005; Owen et al., 2009; Findling et al., 2014) necessitating careful monitoring and appropriate intervention (Eapen et al., 2013).

Further, both drugs have not shown to be effective in improving communication or social deficits that are characteristic of ASD.

Risperidone was reported to improve self-injury, aggression, and agitation in 70% of the children and adolescents compared to the placebo response rate of 11.5%. More adverse effects, including increased appetite with associated weight gain, transient sedation, tremor, and drooling, were more common with risperidone than placebo. It is considered first line of medication for children and adolescents who display extreme irritability. Dose varies from 0.5 mg to 2 mg.

Studies utilizing aripiprazole in the treatment of tantrums, aggression, and self-injury in children and adolescents with autism found aripiprazole to be efficacious and safe. Doses ranged from 5 to 15 mg/kg.

Methylphenidate was found to be at least moderately efficacious at doses of 0.25–0.5 mg/kg for youth with ASD with attention deficit hyperactivity disorder. However, efficacy was lesser in this population than in those without ASD, and children with ASD developed more frequent side effects. Atomoxetine and clonidine have also found to be more effective than placebo.

Selective serotonin reuptake inhibitors, second generation antipsychotics and mood stabilizers such as valproate have been used for repetitive and stereotypic behavior.

Several randomized, placebo-controlled trials have examined the efficacy of naltrexone for core symptoms of autism, associated symptoms of hyperactivity and irritability. Overall, it appears naltrexone may have some benefits in reducing hyperactivity and impulsivity in children and adolescents with ASD, but core symptoms did not appear to improve with this medication.

Sleep is a major issue in autism. Upto 90% of children with autism have some form of sleep disturbance. The efficacy of melatonin for sleep disturbances in children and adolescents with ASD has been examined in multiple double-blind, placebo-controlled studies, making it one of the best-studied complementary alternative treatments used in ASD.

Other modalities used extensively with good results are sensory integration, occupational therapy, applied behavioral analysis, speech therapy, and remedial education. In case of all these therapies, earlier the intervention started, better is the outcome.

Applied behavioral analysis: ABA is short for Applied Behavioral Analysis, and it is often described as the "gold standard" for autism treatment. Applied Behavioral Analysis (ABA)is a system of autism treatment based on theories which state that desired behaviors can be taught through a system of rewards and consequences.

ABA is used to stop undesirable behaviors and teach desired behaviors and skills.

It works on a reward system and on the principle of positive and negative reinforcements.

Sensory integration therapy and occupational therapy: The idea of sensory integrative dysfunction was first proposed by A. Jean Ayres, an occupational therapist and educational psychologist, in the 1950s and 1960s. Symptoms of autism often include difficulty processing sensory information such as textures, sounds, smells, tastes, colors and movement. These difficulties can make ordinary situations feel overwhelming. A child may be hypo or hyper sensitive to one or more sensory pathways. Sensory integration therapy, as practiced by occupational therapists, uses play activities in ways designed to change how the brain reacts to touch, sound, sight and movement. Sensory integration therapy involves placing a child in a room specifically designed to stimulate and challenge all of the senses.' Successful sensory integration therapy decreases sensitivities to touch and other stimuli. The result is that the children are better able to play, learn, and interact with people and surroundings.

Speech and language therapy: Deficits in speech, language and communication are common in autism. Working with a speech therapist helps improve both nonverbal and verbal communication.

Newer techniques such as stem cell therapy and hyperbaric oxygenation are being tried, but there is no conclusive evidence for the same. Diets like gluten free, casein free (GFCF) diets have been tried, but lacks positive evidence.

Thus, treatment of autism requires a multimodal approach with a multidisciplinary team.

Flowchart 31.1

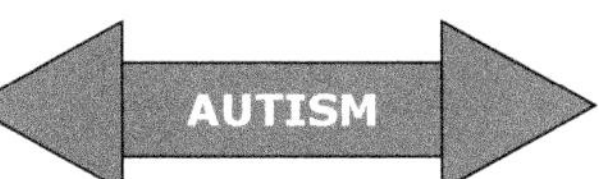

SOCIAL RELATIONSHIP AND RECIPROCITY
- Poor eye contact
- Lack social smile.
- Remain aloof
- Do not reach out to other persons
- Inability to relate to people
- Inability to respond to social/environmental cues
- Engage in solitary and repetitive play activities
- Inability to take turns in social interaction
- Do not maintain peer relationships
- Inappropriate emotional response.
- Show exaggerated emotions

EMOTIONAL RESPONSIVENESS
- Inappropriate emotional response
- Show exaggerated emotions
- Engage in self-stimulating emotions
- Lack fear of danger.
- Excited or agitated for no apparent reason

Behavior PATTERNS
- Engage in stereotyped and repetitive motormanners
- Show attachment to inanimate objects
- Show hyperactivity/restlessness
- Exhibit aggressive behavior.
- Throw temper tantrums
- Engage in self-injurious behavior
- Insist on sameness

SENSORY-ASPECTS
- Unusually sensitive to sensory stimuli
- Stare into space for long periods of time
- Difficulty in tracking objects
- Has unusual vision
- Insensitive to pain
- Respond to objects unusually by smelling, touching or tasting

SPEECH-LANGUAGE AND COMMUNICATION
- Acquired speech and lost it
- Difficulty in using non-verbal language or gestures to communicate
- Engage in stereotyped and repetitive use of language
- Engage in echolalic speech
- Produce infantile squeals or unusual noises
- Unable to initiate or sustain conversation with others
- Use jargon or meaningless words
- Uses pronoun reversals
- Unable to grasp pragmatics of communication (real meaning)

COGNITIVE COMPONENT
- Inconsistent attention and concentration
- Delayed response time
- Unusual memory
- Savant ability

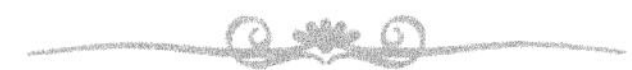

32 Intellectual Disability

Kalpana Pawar • Henal Shah

INTRODUCTION

Intelligence is the general mental capacity that involves reading, planning, problem solving, thinking abstractly, comprehending complex ideas, learning efficiently and learning from experiences. The distribution of intelligence in the community can be represented as a bell shaped Gaussian curve where the mean is 100 with a standard deviation of 15 (**Fig. 32.1**).

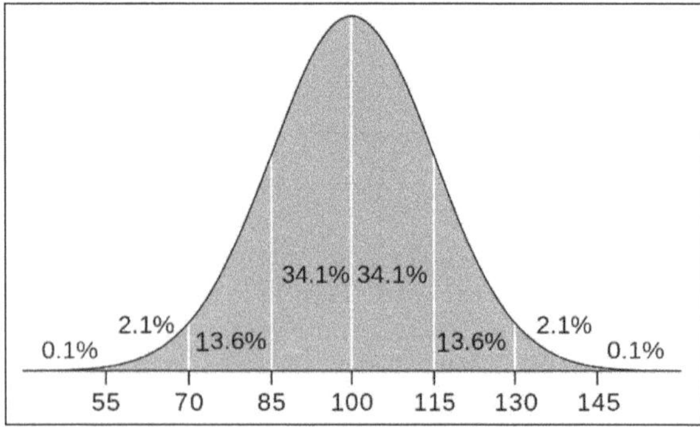

Fig. 32.1: Normal Gaussian distribution of intelligence.

Intellectual disability is arrested or incomplete development of mind of a person characterized by sub normality of intelligence (Indian PwD Act). Historically intellectual disability (previously termed as mental retardation) has been defined by significant cognitive deficits which has been established through standardized measures of intelligence in particular with an IQ score of below 70 and also by significant deficits in functional and adaptive skills. ID is designated when the measurement reveals an IQ two standard deviations below mean (100) of normal distribution of intelligence, i.e., below 70.

There are two different systems for classifying intellectual disability (ID): International Classification of Diseases 10 (ICD 10) and Diagnostic and Statistical manual of mental disorders 5th Edition (DSM-5). Both these system classify severity of ID according to the levels of support needed to achieve an individual's optimal personal functioning.

DSM-5 Defines intellectual disabilities as neurodevelopmental disorders that begin in developmental period that include both intellectual difficulties as well as difficulties in conceptual social and practical areas of living. DSM 5 has placed more emphasis on adaptive functioning and the performance of usual life skills.

3 areas of adaptive functioning are considered in DSM 5

1. **Conceptual:** Language, reading, writing, math, reasoning, knowledge, memory
2. **Social:** Empathy, social judgment, communication skills, the ability to follow rules and ability to make and sustain friendship
3. **Practical:** Personal care, job responsibilities, managing money, recreation and organizing social and work tasks.

DSM 5 Definition and Criteria

Intellectual disability is a disorder that includes both intellectual and adaptive functioning deficits in conceptual, social, and practical domains, which occur during the developmental period. Following three criteria must be met:

A. Deficits in intellectual functions such as reasoning, problem solving skills, learning from new experience, abstract thinking, planning, programming, judgment and academic skills which is confirmed by both clinical assessment and individualized, standardized intelligence testing

B. Deficits in adaptive functioning that result in failure to meet developmental and socio-cultural standards for personal, independent and social responsibility. These deficits limit functioning of an individual in one or more activities of daily life, such as communication, social participation, and independent living, across multiple environments such as home, school, work and community

C. Onset during the developmental period.

Specifiers for current severity

317 (F70) Mild

318 (F71) Moderate

318.1 (F72) Severe

318.2 (F73) Profound

International Classification of Diseases (ICD 10)

In ICD 10 Intellectual Disability is defined under the heading of Mental retardation.ICD 10 defines Mental retardation is a condition of arrested or incomplete development of the mind, which is especially characterized by impairment of skills manifested during the developmental period, which contribute to the overall level of intelligence, i.e. cognitive, language, motor, and social abilities. Retardation can occur with or without any other mental or physical disorder. ICD 10 classifies Intellectual Disability as following:

International Classification of Diseases (ICD 10)

In ICD 10 Intellectual Disability is defined under the heading of Mental retardation. ICD 10 defines Mental retardation is a condition of arrested or incomplete development of the mind, which is especially characterized by impairment of skills manifested during the developmental period, which contribute to the overall level of intelligence, i.e. cognitive, language, motor, and social abilities. Retardation can occur with or without any other mental or physical disorder. ICD 10 classifies Intellectual Disability as following:

ICD 10 Classification

F70	Mild mental retardation
F71	Moderate mental retardation
F72	Severe mental retardation
F73	Profound mental retardation
F78	Other mental retardation
F79	Unspecified mental retardation

Specifiers

F7x.0	No, or minimal, impairment of behavior
F7x.1	Significant impairment of behavior requiring attention or treatment
F7x.8	Other impairment of behavior
F7x.9	Without mention of impairment of behavior

PREVALENCE

Intellectual disability has an overall general population prevalence of approximately 1%, prevalence rates vary by age. Prevalence for severe intellectual disability is approximately 6 per 1,000 live births.

CLINICAL FEATURES OF INTELLECTUAL DISABILITY

Associated clinical features vary depending on several factors, most importantly the level of retardation. Persons with severe and profound ID come to diagnosis at a younger age, more often presented with related medical conditions, may present with dysmorphic features, and have a range of behavioral and psychiatric disturbances. In contrast, persons with mild ID often come to diagnosis much later (typically when academic demands become more prominent in school), are less likely to have medical conditions that could account for the ID, and usually are of normal appearance without any dysmorphic features (**Table 32.1**).

A) Mild Intellectual Disability(Mild ID)

Mild ID (IQ 55 to 70) characterizes the largest group of people with intellectual disability, possibly as many as 85 percent of all persons with ID. These individuals appear similar to unaffected individuals and often blend into the general population in the years before and after formal schooling. Many achieve academic skills at the sixth grade level or higher, and some graduate from high school. Usually their appearance is unremarkable and any sensory or motor deficits are slight. Most people in this group develop more or less normal language abilities and social behavior during the preschool years. As adults, many of these individuals hold jobs, marry and raise families; at times, however, they may appear slow or need extra help to negotiate life's problems and tasks.

B) Moderate Intellectual Disability (Moderate ID)

Moderate ID (IQ 40 to 55) is seen in approximately 10 percent of the population with ID and includes people with more impaired cognitive and adaptive functioning. Many persons with Down syndrome and fragile X syndrome often function in this range. Most children require special education services, achieving academic skills at the second to third grade level. Speech is usually relatively simple, and is often better understood by people who know the patient well. Activities of daily living such as dressing, feeding, and attention to hygiene can be acquired over time, but other activities of daily living, such as use

Table 32.1: Features of Mild, Moderate, Severe and profound Intellectual Disability

	Mild	**Moderate**	**Severe/ Profound**
IQ Range	69-50	49-35	<35
Percentage	85%	10%	5%
Ability of self-care	Independent	Need some help	Limited
Language	Reasonable	Limited	Basic or more
Reading and Writing	Reasonable	Basic	Minimal or more
Ability to work	Semiskilled	Unskilled, supervised	Supervised basic tasks
Social skills	Normal	Moderate	Few
Physical problems	Rare	Sometimes	Common

of money and road sense, generally require support. Needs for supportive services continue throughout life, and with proper supports, many live, work, and thrive in their local communities. Individuals in this range are employed in the competitive job market and need minimal job supervision, whereas others require more extensive supervision on the job and may work in sheltered workshops or other, more segregated settings.

C) **Severe Intellectual Disability (Severe ID)**

Severe ID (IQ 25 to 40) occurs in about 3 to 4 percent of the population of people with ID. Individuals at this level often have one or more medical causes for their delay, and many show concurrent motor, ambulatory, and neurological problems, as well as poorly developed communication skills. In the preschool years their development is usually greatly slowed. Most persons with severe ID require close supervision and specialized care throughout their lives. Some individuals learn to perform simple tasks or routines that facilitate their self-care or their ability to perform in a sheltered workshop or pre-workshop type of setting.

D) **Profound Intellectual Disability (Profound ID)**

Profound ID (IQ 25 and below) affects relatively few individuals (1 to 2 percent) and involves pervasive deficits in cognitive, motor and communicative functioning. Impairment in sensory-motor functioning are often seen from early childhood on, and most individuals require extensive training to complete even the most rudimentary aspects of self-care such as eating and toileting. The vast majorities of people with profound ID have identifiable organic causes for their delay, and most require total supervision and care throughout life.

ETIOLOGY

Etiological factors responsible for intellectual disability can be Genetic, developmental, environmental or combination of all. Intellectual abilities depend to a great degree on the integrity of the Central nervous system (CNS). A variety of biomedical causes can disrupt this integrity and starts the process leading to intellectual disability. But overall functioning of a person depends not only on CNS integrity but also on other factors such as patient's general state of health, associated disabilities, environmental factors (such as nurturing, learning opportunities, supports) etc. Thus, biomedical cause, whether genetic or acquire, may be a primary cause that will start the process of developmental delay but will not necessarily be the only factor responsible for the functional outcome, which will depend on the cumulative effects of all factors involved.

A. **Genetic:** Genetic factors include chromosomal and inherited conditions. Twin and adoption studies consistently indicate that intelligence in general population is moderately heritable (**Table 32.2**).

a. ***Chromosomal anomalies*** are variations from usual diploid set of chromosomes or segments of chromosomes.

Down's syndrome (trisomy 21) is the most common chromosomal anomaly causing ID, occurring in about 1.5 per 1000 pregnancies. The main features (**Fig. 32.2**) are upward slanted palpebral fissures, a low nasal bridge with epicanthal fold, flat nasal bridge, a small mouth and ears, a single palmar crease, short and wide palms. Considerable hypotonia and

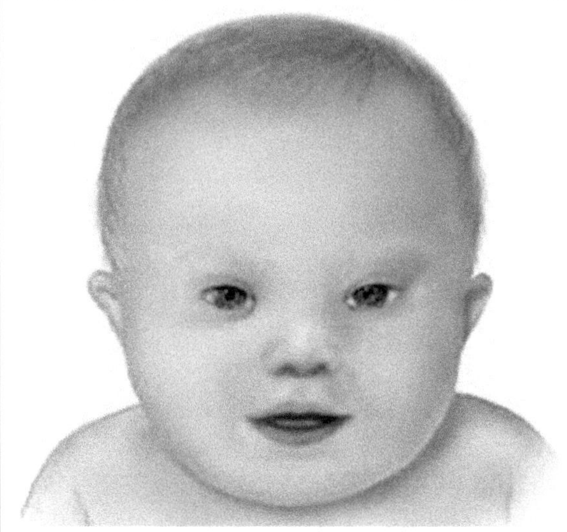

- Poor muscle tone
- Increased skin at nape of neck
- Flattened nose, upward slant of eyes
- Small ears and mouth, protruding tongue
- Epicanthic fold
- Brushfield spots on Iris
- Atlantoaxial instability
- Simian crease, clinodactyly, increased space between first two toes

Fig. 32.2: Characteristics of Downs Syndrome.

tendency towards respiratory problems are common. The degree of intellectual disability varies from severe to mild with a mean IQ of approximately 50. Incidence of Down syndrome increases significantly with maternal age 35 years and older. The incidence in women older than 40 years of age is approximately 1 in 40 live births.

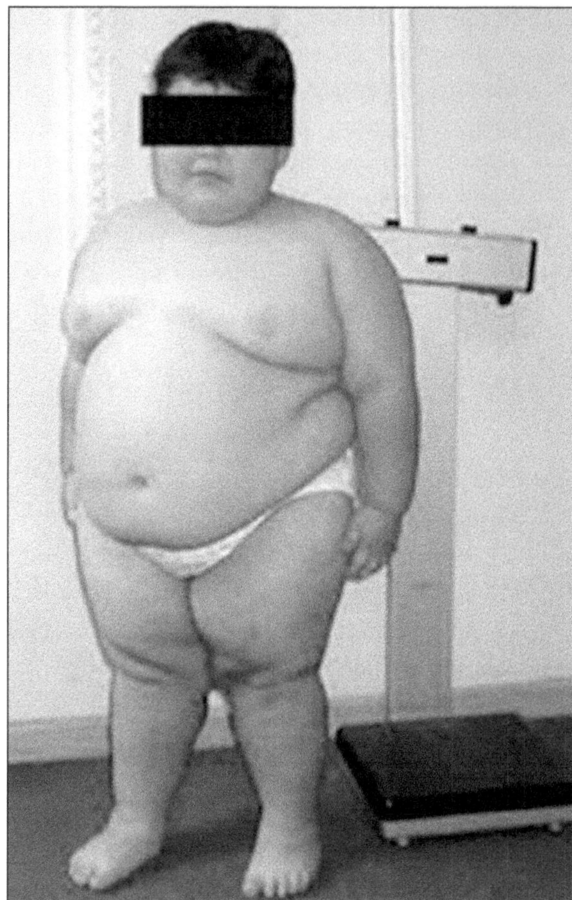

- hypotonic, feed poorly, and have small hands and feet.
- Later exhibit excessive appetite and hyperphagia that lead to severe obesity

Fig. 32.3: Characteristics of Prader-Willi Syndrome.

Malformation Syndromes due to Microdeletions: Microdeletions refer to loss of a few genes, that are not visible cytogenetically. Few examples of these microdeletions are *Prader–Willi syndrome* and *Angelman syndrome* in which deletions (microdeletions) of DNA have been reported in chromosome 15q11–13. In Prader–Willi syndrome, the paternally derived information at that site is usually absent, with Angelman syndrome, there is missing maternal information. Infants with Prader–Willi syndrome are generally hypotonic, feed poorly, and present with small hands and feet (**Fig. 32.3**). They later exhibit excessive appetite and hyperphagia that lead to severe obesity. Individuals with Angelman syndrome may present with moderate to profound intellectual disability, are nonverbal, ataxic, frequently laugh, and hold their arms flexed in such a manner to sometime be referred to as Happy Puppet syndrome.

b. Inherited conditions

Disorder of autosomal dominant inheritance: Tuberous sclerosis is an example of this disorder. It is caused by mutation in the gene affecting formation of ectodermal layer of the embryo. As skin and CNS develop from this layer, abnormality is seen in both.This disorder is characterized triad of Caf-au-lait spots or nonpigmented ash leaf-shaped areas, mental retardation and epilepsy and sometimes calcification of brain areas. It is a relatively rare disorder with a prevalence of 1 in 30,000 to 1 in 50,000 live births), but it may be found in about 0.5% of persons with severe intellectual disability.

Disorder of autosomal recessive inheritance: Most of the metabolic disorders belong to this category. Phenylketonuria is most common of the metabolic disorder with prevalence of about 1 in 10,000 live births. The enzymatic defect seen is diminished activity of phenylalanine hydroxylase, which leads to high phenylalanine level affecting myelination of the CNS. Common symptoms are mental retardation, seizure disorder, hypertonia, hyperreflexia with a musty odor in urine and sweat. The clinical symptom can be prevented by use of a low-phenylalanine diet soon after birth. Increasingly, a lifelong low-phenylalanine diet is recommended to prevent later deterioration in cognitive functions.

X-linked Intellectual disability: Fragile X syndrome is most *common inherited form of intellectual disability.* The characteristic phenotypical features include oblong face, prominent ears and jaws and macroorchidism, broad forehead, hyperextensible joints. Prepubertal boys with this syndrome appear quite normal. They are often restless and hyperactive and have short attention span. Approximately 25–35% of children with Fragile X syndrome, however, have been noted to meet diagnostic criteria for autism spectrum disorder.

A. *Developmental factors: Can be divided into prenatal, perinatal and postnatal causes*

Prenatal

a. **Maternal Infections:** Viral infections in the mother can interfere with organogenesis. ***Rubella infection*** during the first month of pregnancy affects the organogenesis of 50% of embryos. Infection in the third month of pregnancy disturbs the development of 15% of fetuses. Various systems are affected that may result in intellectual disability, microcephaly, hearing and vision impairment, congenital heart disease, and behavior problems. ***cytomegalovirus* (CMV)** infection may result in microcephaly, sensorineural hearing loss, and psychomotor retardation. ***Congenital toxoplasmosis*** may result in significant problems in about 20% of infected infants (hydrocephalus, microcephaly, and psychomotor retardation, visual and hearing impairment) and result in milder developmental problems later in life.

b. **Exposure to Toxic Substances:** Exposure to toxic substance like ethanol in the form of alcohol can cause development of fetal alcohol syndrome. Its occurrence in industrialized countries is estimated to be about one in 1,000 newborns. The child presents clinical features like notable dysmorphology including the presence of a smooth philtrum, thin vermilion, and short palpebral fissures.

c. **Toxemia of Pregnancy and Placental Insufficiency:** Intrauterine growth retardation (IUGR) occurs due to number of causes the most important being maternal toxemia which leads to placental insufficiency causing oxygen and nutritional deprivation which ultimately leads to prematurity and IUGR. Prematurity maybe of maternal or fetal origin.

Perinatal

Perinatal period refers to 1 week before birth to 4 weeks after birth. Any kind of brain insult during this period break CNS integrity and ultimately lead to intellectual disability **Infections**: Neonates infected with herpes simplex type 2 during a vaginal delivery may develop encephalitis within 2 weeks. Clinical features include microcephaly, profound intellectual disability, and Neurological deficits. Early treatment with acyclovir may alleviate the otherwise poor Outcome. Neonatal bacterial infections such as sepsis and meningitis also may have long-term consequences on developmental outcome.

Birth injuries and **asphyxia** due to any reason can also lead to some form of intellectual disability

Postnatal Causes

a. ***Infections:*** Bacterial and viral infections of the brain during childhood may cause meningitis and encephalitis and resulting significant neurological sequelae.

b. ***Toxic Substances:*** *Lead poisoning* is still an important cause of intellectual disability. The most frequent source of lead is pica—ingestion of flaking old lead-based paint of leaded gasoline for use in on-road vehicles. Gastrointestinal symptoms dominate in acute poisoning. Late manifestations include developmental delays and intellectual disability, ataxia, seizures and personality changes.

B. **Environmental factors:** A child needs good environmental stimulation for development of better physical and mental health. Certain environmental and psychological factors do affect the development of CNS during growing period of individual. Poverty is one of the important factors that predispose the child to many developmental risks such as teenage pregnancies, malnutrition, physical or sexual abuse, poor medical care etc. Severe maternal mental illness is another risk factor for developmental and behavioral problems. Children of mothers who have serious mental illness (SMI) including schizophrenia are at risk for the development of cognitive deficits, which may not be secondary to maternal illness but may represent genetically determined predisposition to schizophrenia.

Etiology of Intellectual Disability

Genetic
- **Chromosomal anomalies**
- Down's Syndrome
- Prader-Willi syndrome
- Angelmans Syndrome
- **Inherited condition**
- Tuberous sclerosis
- Phenylketonuria
- Fragile X syndrome

Developmental Factors
- **Prenatal**
- Maternal infections- Rubella, Cytomegalovirus (CMV), Congenital toxoplasmosis
- Fetal alcohol syndrome
- Toxemia of Pregnancy
- Placental insufficiency
- **Perinatal**
- Neonatal Herpes simplex encephalitis
- Neonatal bacterial infections
- Birth injuries
- Birth asphyxia

- **Postnatal**
- Meningitis, Encephalitis
- Pica

Environmental
- Poverty
- Teenage pregnancy
- Malnutrition
- Physical/ Sexual abuse
- Poor medical care
- Maternal chronic mental illness e.g. Schizophrenia

Table 32.2:Genetic disorders associated with Intellectual Disability

Disorder	**Etiology**	**Clinical features**
Down syndrome	Trisomy 21; 95% nondisjunction; 4% translocation; 1 in 1,000 live births	Hypotonia, upward-slanted palpebral fissures, midface depression, flat, wide nasal bridge, simian crease, short stature, thyroid abnormalities and congenital heart disease, mild to moderate ID
Fragile X syndrome	Inactivation of FMR1 gene at Xq27.3 due to CGG base repeats methylation Recessive 1 in 4,000 male births, 1 in 8,000 female births	Long face, large ears, midface hypoplasia, high, arched palate, short stature, macro-orchidism, mitral valve prolapse, joint laxity, strabismus, hyperactivity, inattention, anxiety, stereotypes, speech and language delays, Moderate to severe ID
Prader-Willi syndrome	Deletion in 15q12 (15q11–15q13) of paternal origin Dominant 1 per 10,000 live births	Hypotonia, failure to thrive in infancy, obesity, small hands and feet, micro-orchidism, crypto-orchidism, short stature, almond-shaped eyes, fair hair and light skin, flat face, scoliosis, orthopedic problems, prominent forehead and bitemporal narrowing, borderline to moderate ID
Angelman's syndrome	Deletion in 15q12 (15q11–15q13) of maternal origin; Dominant 1 per 20,000–30,000 live births	Fair hair and blue eye, dysmorphic faces including wide, smiling mouth, thin upper lip, and pointed chin, epilepsy, ataxia, small head circumference, microcephalic Happy Puppet syndrome; paroxysmal laughter, hand flapping, clapping, severe to profound ID
Williams' syndrome	Hemizygous deletion, which includes elastin locus; chromosome 7q11-23; Autosomal dominant 1 per 20,000 births;	Short stature, broad forehead, depressed nasal bridge, stellate pattern of the iris, widely spaced teeth; and full lips; "elfin-like" faces, Moderate ID

(Continued...)

Disorder	Etiology	Clinical features
Cri-du-chat syndrome	Partial deletion, 5p 1 per 20,000–50,000 live births	Round face with hypertelorism, epicanthal folds, micrognathia, Severe intellectual disability, infantile “catlike” cry, hyperactivity, stereotypes, self-injury, severe ID
Edwards’s syndrome	Trisomy 18	Growth deficiency, abnormal skull shape and facial features, clenched hands, rockerbottom feet, cardiac and renal abnormalities
Smith-Magenis syndrome	Complete or partial deletion of 17p11.2 1 per 25,000 live births;	Broad face, flat mid face, short, broad hands, small toes, and horse, deep voice, severe self-injurious behavior including hand biting, head banging, and pulling out finger and toe nails, stereotyped “self-hugging,” attention seeking, aggression, sleep disturbance (absent rapid eye movement)
Tuberous sclerosis complex (TSC) 1 and 2	Autosomal dominant 1 in 10,000 births; 50% TSC 1: 9q34 (hamartin); 50% TSC 2: 16p13 (tuberin	Epilepsy, autism, hyperactivity, impulsivity, aggression, spectrum of mental retardation from none (30%) to profound, self-injurious behaviors, sleep disturbances
Neurofibromatosis type 1 (NF1)	Autosomal dominant, But 50% of cases are spontaneous 1 in 2,500–4,000 live births	Café-au-lait spots, cutaneous neurofibromas, Lisch nodules, short stature and macrocephaly with moderate to profound ID 10%
Lesch-Nyhan syndrome	Defect in hypoxanthine guanine phosphoribosyltransferase Autosomal recessive rare (1 per 10,000–38,000)	Ataxia, chorea, kidney failure, gout Often severe self-biting behavior, aggression, anxiety, mild to moderate ID
Galactosemia	Defect in galactose-1-phosphate uridyl-transferase or galactokinase or empiramase, Autosomal recessive 1 per 62,000	Vomiting in early infancy, jaundice, hepatosplenomegaly, later cataracts, weight loss, food refusal, increased intracranial pressure and Possible ID
Phenylketonuria	Defect in phenylalanine hydroxylase (PAH) Autosomal recessive 1 per 11,500 births	Seizures (25% generalized), fair skin, blue eyes, blond hair, rash; when untreated: mild to profound ID

(Continued...)

Disorder	Etiology	Clinical features
Hurler's syndrome	Deficiency in α-L-iduronidase activity Autosomal recessive 1 per 100,000 live births	Early onset, short stature, hepatosplenomegaly, hirsutism, corneal clouding, death before 10 yrs old Moderate to severe ID
Hunter's syndrome	X-linked recessive iduronate sulfatase deficiency 1 per 100,000 live births	Normal infancy, symptom onset at 2–4 yrs old, flat nasal bridge, flaring nostrils, hearing loss, ataxia, hernia common, enlarged liver and spleen, joint stiffness, ID by 2 yrs, speech delay, loss of speech at 8–10 yrs old
Duchenne muscular dystrophy	X-linked recessive Dystrophin gene on Xp21	Males, progressive muscle weakness, including respiratory and cardiac muscles
Rett syndrome	MeCP2 gene mutation at Xq28 1 in 10,000 live births	Females affected (lethal in males), Epilepsy, compulsive hand-wringing movements, agitation, progressive ID

COMORBID CONDITIONS ASSOCIATED WITH INTELLECTUAL DISABILITY

Various physical, medical and mental disorders frequently co-occur in intellectual disability. These disorders can either co-occur with Intellectual disability or Intellectual disability can happen as a result of various medical illnesses.

A) Physical/ Medical Comorbidity:

It is common for individuals with intellectual disability to also have other medical, developmental, and behavioral issues.

a. Cerebral Palsy: Overall, approximately 20% of persons with intellectual disability also have CP, along with speech and language impairment. Various causes of CP include encephalopathy, hypoxic–ischemic events during labor and delivery, periventricular leukomalacia, perinatal hypoxic-ischemic encephalopathy, neonatal seizures etc. Individuals with CP may have cognitive skills within or above normal range, or may have intellectual disability ranging from mild to profound.

b. Seizures: Seizure disorder is more common in people with ID and is related to its severity, occurring in about 7% of children with mild ID versus 35% of severe ID. The type of seizure reflects etiological as well as prognostic information. For instance Infantile seizures are associated with conditions such as Tuberous Sclerosis. Myoclonic seizures, in turn, may be associated with metabolic disorders. Complex-partial seizures are associated with behavioral and sensory manifestations, including illusions, hallucinations, and alterations in consciousness and awareness. Interictal changes may include mood changes, anxiety, as well as fear, elation, or depression.

c. Sensory Impairment: Visual and Hearing impairment are fairly common in individual with ID although the prevalence data may vary. Hearing loss may be present with different genetic, metabolic, infectious, and acquired etiologies, and may be associated with intellectual disability. Visual impairment have been found to be as high as 50% in individuals with intellectual disability when strabismus and refractive errors are included.

B. **Psychiatric disorders among people with intellectual disability**

People with ID seem to be more vulnerable to emotional, behavioral disorders and psychopathology as compared to general population and rate of psychiatric illness is 3 to 4 times higher than people without ID. The etiology of psychiatric disorders in intellectual disability is similar to that in the general population, in that they result from a complex combination of biological, psychological, and social factors. However, there are some specific factors that add additional risk and complexity to the incidence and detection of psychiatric disorders in person with ID.

a. **Autism spectrum disorder and Attention-deficit hyperactivity disorder:** Studies in children with psychiatric disorders such as ASD & ADHD demonstrate a high prevalence of intellectual disability, with estimates that 50% of children with ASD and 15– 20% of children with ADHD having intellectual disability.

b. **Behavioral issues**: Thirty to forty percent of individuals with intellectual disability have been reported to present with some or other kind of behavioral abnormalities, particularly those with more severe intellectual disability, and individuals with autism and certain psychiatric disorders may present with Self Injurious Behavior. In few genetic syndromes certain behaviors might be unique: for example, extreme overeating and compulsivity in Prader–Willi syndrome, attentional and social problems in fragile X syndrome, inappropriate laughter in Angelman's syndrome, the unusual cry in 5p- syndrome, and the self-hug in Smith-Magenis syndrome or extreme self-mutilation by biting in Lesch–Nyhan syndromes.

c. **Psychotic disorders**: The epidemiological studies available suggest an increased prevalence of psychotic disorders among individuals with intellectual disability. Schizophrenia affects 3– 4% of people with intellectual disability, compared with less than 1% in the general population When IQ is less than 45, it is difficult to make the diagnosis with any certainty. The diagnosis of schizophrenia should be considered as one of several possibilities when intellectual or social functioning worsens without evidence of an organic cause, and especially if any new behavior is odd and out of keeping.

d. **Mood disorder**: The rate of depressive disorders is estimated to lie between 3% and 6%— slightly higher than that of the general population. However, people with intellectual disability are less likely to complain of mood changes or to express depressive ideation. Diagnosis has to be made mainly on the basis of an appearance of sadness, changes in appetite and sleep, and behavioral changes of retardation or agitation. Severely depressed patients with adequate verbal abilities may describe hallucinations or delusions. Mania has to be diagnosed on the basis of hyperactivity and behavioral signs of excitement, irritability, or nervousness. The rate of suicide in people with moderate and more severe intellectual disability is lower than in the general population.

e. **Anxiety disorders and related conditions**: Adjustment disorders are fairly common occurring when there are changes in the routine of their lives. Anxiety disorders are also frequent, especially at times of stress, and social anxiety is often common

f. **Obsessive– compulsive disorders** are also found at much higher rate than general population

g. **Somatoform disorders** and other causes of functional somatic symptoms can result in persistent requests for medical attention. Treatment is usually directed mainly to bringing about adjustments in the patient's environment, and reassurance. Counseling, at an appropriate level of complexity, can also be helpful.

h. **Eating disorders**: Overeating and unusual dietary preferences are frequent among people with intellectual disability. Abnormal eating behaviors, including pica are not uncommon, but classical eating disorders appear to be less common than in the general population.

i. **Personality disorder**: Personality disorder if co-occur is difficult to diagnose among people with intellectual disability. In the past, it has been assumed that persons with intellectual disability have a limited "personality" in common and some presumed traits e.g.; passivity, aggressiveness, attention getting, shyness, talkativeness, lack of sexual drive, and hyper or hypo sexuality. However, it is now more widely held that a full spectrum of personalities can occur in persons with intellectual disability, as in the general population. However certain characteristics such as low self image often related to their experiences of failure, perception that adults important to them (especially parents) are disappointed with them, and negative comparison between themselves and their age peers.

j. **Delirium and dementia:** Delirium in people with intellectual disability is more common in childhood and in old age than at other ages. Disturbed behavior due to delirium is sometimes the first indication of physical illness. Delirium may occur as a side effect of drugs (especially antiepileptic, antidepressants, and other psychotropic medication).**Dementia**: As the life expectancy of people with intellectual disability has increased in past few decades, dementia in later life has become more common. Alzheimer's disease is particularly common among people with Down's syndrome but dementia is also more common in other elderly intellectually disabled people, with a prevalence of 18.3% which is 2– 3 times more common in this population.

k. **Sleep disorders:** Impaired sleep is common in people with intellectual disability, with prevalence estimates ranging from 9% to 34%. Serious sleep difficulties, such as obstructive sleep apnea, excessive daytime sleepiness, and parasomnias, have a reported prevalence of 9%, and can be a source of considerable distress. Treatment follows the usual principles of identifying and treating underlying cause, and non-pharmacological interventions such as improving sleep hygiene Melatonin may have a role if medication is indicated.

l. **Motor speech disorders**: may coexist, affecting communications skills and speech intelligibility. Language disorders may occur in the context of cognitive and hearing impairment, as well as genetic disorders, brain injury, and other conditions that may affect neurological functioning.

Common Psychiatric disorders associated with Intellectual Disability

- Autism spectrum disorder
- Attention- deficit hyperactivity disorder (ADHD)
- Behavioral Issues
- Psychotic disorders(e.g. Schizophrenia)
- Mood disorders(e.g. Depression, Mania)
- Anxiety disorders
- Obsessive– compulsive disorders
- Somatoform disorders
- Eating disorders
- Personality disorder
- Delirium and dementia
- Sleep disorders

DIFFERENTIAL DIAGNOSIS

The diagnosis of ID is based on the appropriate assessment of cognitive abilities and adaptive skills; clinical assessment also includes a careful developmental and family history, physical examination, and laboratory studies as appropriate. As noted, the age of diagnosis often varies depending on the severity of the disability, so persons with more severe ID present for clinical assessment earlier than those with mild, or borderline, ID. Genetic syndrome associated with intellectual disability should be noted and kept as concurrent diagnosis with intellectual disability

a. **Autism spectrum disorder (ASD):** ASD can co-occur with intellectual disability. Diagnosis may be complicated by social and communication deficit in children with ASD which again can interfere with the understanding and complying with the psychological testing done for intellectual disability. Repetitive behaviors such as rocking or stereotypic hand movements may be seen in individuals either with significant intellectual disability or autism.

b. **Attention Deficit Hyperactive Disorder(ADHD):** High activity level and short attention span in a 6 year old with severe ID can be confused with ADHD. Can be differentiated from latter by presence of symptoms at two more settings.

c. **Sensory disabilities**: Deafness and blindness, can be mistaken for intellectual disability

d. **Major and mild neurocognitive disorders:** Intellectual disability is a neurodevelopmental disorder which is different from neurocognitive disorders characterized by loss of cognitive functioning. Technically Neurocognitive disorder can happen at any age or can also co-occur in ID (E.g. Individuals of Down's syndrome who develops Alzheimer's dementia in late life, or an individual with ID who loses further cognitive function following head injury). In such a case diagnosis of ID and neurocognitive disorder may both be given.

OVERALL GOALS OF PSYCHIATRIC TREATMENT OF PERSONS WITH INTELLECTUAL DISABILITY

The overall goal of all medical therapies, including psychiatric care of persons with intellectual disability, is to promote the optimal growth and development and ensure optimal physical, emotional, and social well-being of individuals concerned. Therefore multimodal approach is needed in the treatment of persons with intellectual disability. Following goals should be kept in mind:

a. Psychiatric treatment to minimize symptoms associated with a specific mental disorder
b. Prevent harmful behaviors (e.g., aggression, SIB)
c. Facilitate access to educational, social and community inclusion programs
d. Helping to facilitate improved functionality in educational, social and community settings
e. Improve the quality of life for the individual and the family

DIAGNOSING OF INTELLECTUAL DISABILITY:

The diagnostic process involves history taking, observation including medical examination, intellectual and adaptive assessment, identification of comorbid psychiatric condition and medical conditions and need based laboratory investigations

1. **History taking:**

   The purpose of detail history taking is to establish evidence for deficits in both intellectual functioning and adaptive behaviors that have an onset during the developmental period, and to know the possible etiology. Obtain birth and developmental details particularly related to motor, language and communication, self help skills, socioemotional skills, cognition and occupational skills and medical co morbidities. Also details about onset evolution and current level of functioning and any psychopathological disturbances should take into account. Along with this detail family history including three generation pedigree, consanguinity, family background, current living arrangements coping and adaptation by the family is also necessary.

2. **Physical examination:**

   Detail physical examination help to identify the etiology in a majority of cases. It consist of 3 parts, Anthropometry (To assess the nutritional status of individual), Dysmorphology examination (to identify anomaly) and examination of major organ systems (to rule out multiorgan involvement and comorbid medical conditions)

3. **Assessment of Intellectual functioning and adaptive behavior:**

   This step is to confirm clinical diagnosis and identify severity (mild, moderate, severe, profound) level of ID. Diagnosis can be confirmed by DSM 5 or ICD 10 diagnostic guidelines. Adaptive functioning is assessed using both individualized culturally appropriate measures. This information should be taken from parents, or other family members, teachers, counselors, care providers and from the patient to extent possible. For intellectual functioning IQ tests are used which measure human intelligence quotient as measured against an age-based average intelligence score. These IQ Tests measure and provide an intelligence quotient, which is score derived from standardized tests designed to access human intelligence (**Table 32.3**). Most IQ tests tend to measure both verbal and performance IQ. Verbal IQ is measured through both comprehension and working memory skills such as vocabulary and arithmetic. Performance IQ is measured through perception and processing skills such as matrix completion and symbol coding, all these measures and tasks are used to calculate person's IQ (**Table 32.4**).

4. **Laboratory Investigation:** Laboratory investigations are mainly done to find out the cause of ID. Causes can be treatable or non treatable.

Table 32.3: Psychological Testing for Intelligence Quotient (IQ) Assessment

Sr. No	IQ Test	Age limit for assessment	Content
1	Seguine Form Board Test	3.5 years onwards	Performance test
2	Binet Kamat Test	3 years to adulthood	Verbal and performance test
3	Standford Binet Test	3 years to adulthood	Verbal and performance test
4	Malin's Intelligence scale for Indian Children	6 to 15 years 11 months	Verbal and performance test
5	Vineland Social Maturity Scale (VSMS)	0 Onwards	Culturally appropriate adaptive behavioral skills
6	Bhatia's Battery of Performance	11 years 5 months and above	Performance test
7	Wechsler Intelligence Scale for Children (WISC)	5- 15 years 11 months	Verbal and performance test
8	Wechsler Adult Intelligence Scale (WAIS)	5- 15 years 11 months	Verbal and performance test
9	Wechsler Adult Performance Intelligence Scale(WAPIS)	5- 15 years 11 months	Performance test

Table 32.4: IQ range for severity of Intellectual disability

Severity	IQ Range (%)
Mild	50-69
Moderate	35-49
Severe	20-34
Profound	< 20

Chromosomal Studies: Chromosomal anomalies are the single most known common cause of ID. **Fluorescent in situ hybridization** (FISH) markers detects microscopic deletion in chromosomes. **Chorionic Villi Sampling(CVS)** done at 8 to 10 weeks of gestation is screening technique to determine chromosomal abnormalities.

Genetic studies have dramatically led to a better understanding of etiology of ID in the past decade, and for currently one can supply a molecular diagnosis for most patients with severe ID. The genetic heterogeneity of ID requires genome-wide approaches, and once genome sequencing is affordable and available it is probably likely to become the primary diagnostic test for ID.

Amniocentesis which is done at 15 weeks of gestation is useful in diagnosing chromosomal abnormalities prenatally.

Urine and Blood Analysis Enzymatic abnormalities in various chromosomal and metabolic abnormalities can be detected by urine and blood assay. E.g. Down's syndrome, Lysch Nyhan's syndrome, phenylketonuria.

Electroencephalography is considered when associated comorbidity of Seizure disorder.

Neuroimaging: CT and MRI have found high rates of abnormalities in case of seizure disorder, microcephaly, macrocephaly, cerebral palsy etc.

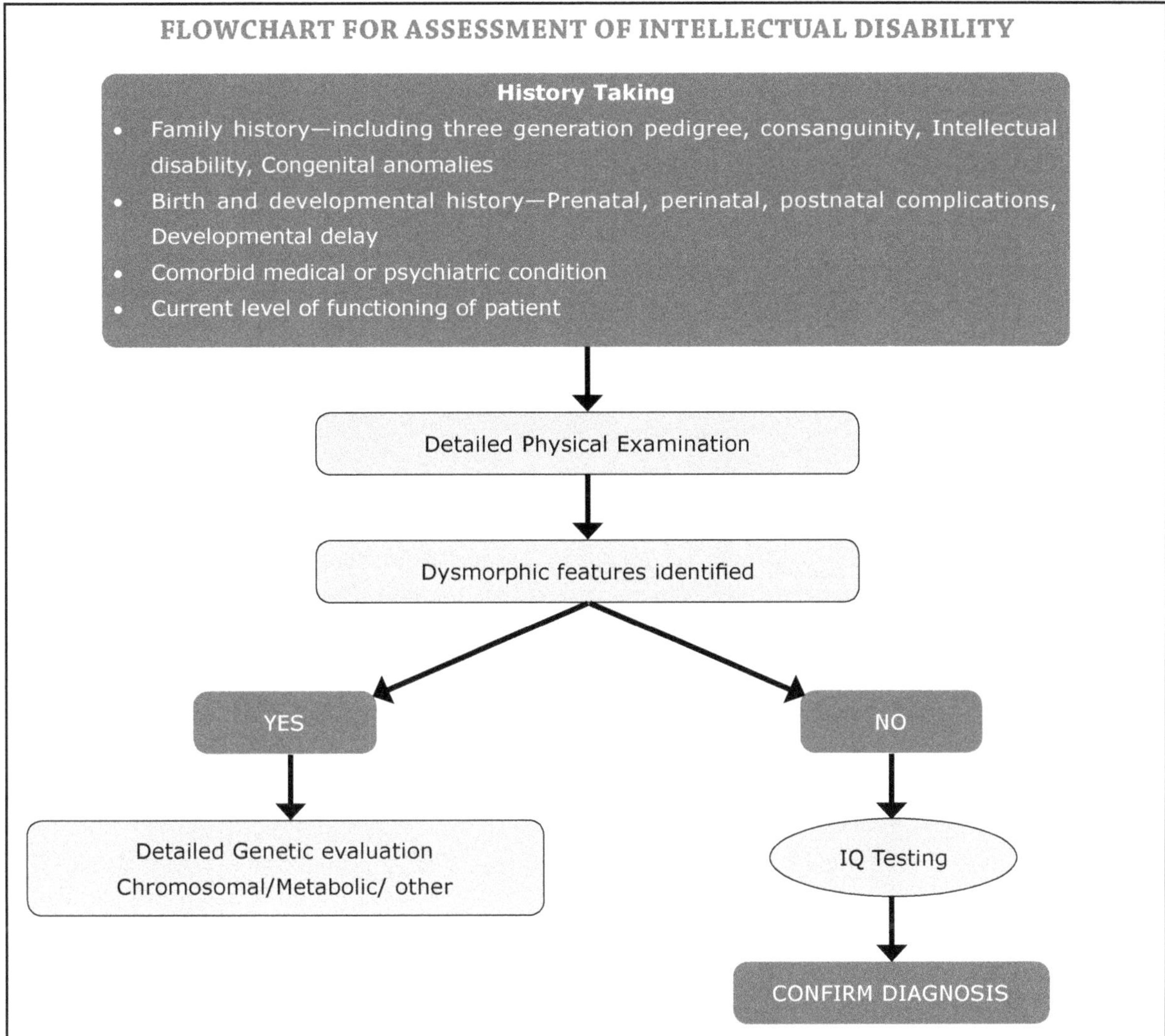

TREATMENT OF INTELLECTUAL DISABILITY

The overall goal of the treatment for ID is reduction or elimination of the disability, this can be achieved by

- Treatment of underlying medical condition that is causative of ID, e.g. Phenylketonuria
- Treatment of co morbid medical illnesses such as seizures, thyroid disorders.
- Treatment of co morbid psychiatric disorders. Psychiatric disorders require both medical and behavior therapy approaches. The children are prone to develop side effects and medications must be started low with a slow build up and as a part of a comprehensive plan. Antipsychotics, specifically Risperidone, has a role in decreasing problem behaviors in children with ID. The ADHD symptoms respond to methylphenidate. Atomoxetine and Amphetamine may also be useful. Aggression responds to Lithium. The use

of antiepileptic drugs, anxiolytics, and naltrexone for management of problem behaviors, but lacks enough evidence to back the use. Antidepressants do not reduce repetitive or stereotypic behaviors and are often poorly tolerated. Melatonin has promise in improving sleep. Behavior therapy works for temper tantrums, repetitive behavior, feeding problems and other issues. Cognitive behavior therapy is occasionally used for anxiety disorders and phobia.

- Interventions that are targeted for improving functioning of children with ID, such as educational, social, behavioral, family support etc. As far as possible mainstreaming (attending regular school) is preferred and child is sent to a special school only if he/she cannot be helped in a regular school. Alternate boards such as National Open school may be considered as they allow flexibility and choice of replacing subjects with vocational subjects. The Rights of persons with disability Act, 2017 mentions ID as a disability and outlines educational help that needs to be provided.
- Interdisciplinary approach which includes involvement of many specialists such as Social worker, Occupational Therapist , speech therapists and Physiotherapist
- Supporting and educating family as it is often seen that parents are confused and upset. Parental training in behavior management and mindfulness is useful.
- Helping in accessing rights of a disabled person, certification, guidance and advocacy. As per the Rights of persons with Disability, it is prescribed that a child can be assessed at any age and certified as disabled. Temporary certificate of disability is given for children less than 5 years, after that certificate needs to be renewed at 10 and 18 years of age and then permanent disability certificate is issued at age 18 years. This certificate helps in accessing provisions such as reservation in jobs and education.

PREVENTION OF INTELLECTUAL DISABILITY

1. **Primary Prevention**: It comprises actions taken to eliminate or reduce the factors responsible for Intellectual disability
   - Screening babies for phenylketonuria
   - Immunization to prevent Congenital rubella, measles and Rh mother –child incompatibility
   - Provision of prenatal Irons folic acid and vitamin supplementation to prevent neural tube defect
   - Genetic counseling
   - Psychoeducation of general public regarding various preventive measure
   - Continuing efforts of health professionals to ensure and upgrade public health policies
2. **Secondary and Tertiary Prevention:** Secondary prevention includes prompt attention and treatment of medical and psychiatric illnesses and associated complication. Tertiary prevention involves minimizing the sequelae or consequences of illness and improves quality of life. Treatment of comorbid disorders: Adequate control of seizure disorder with antiepileptic agents, Treatment of Psychotic disorders with antipsychotic agents like Haloperidol, Olanzapine Risperidone, Aripipraole etc. Risperidone has been proven to be better agent in case

of behavioral issues, disruptive behavior associated with ASD and explosive rage behavior. For ADHD Methylphenidate and Amphetamine- based preparations have been shown to be efficacious in treating ADHD. Selective Serotonin reuptake inhibitors (SSRI) e.g., Fluoxetine, paroxetine, sertraline are effective in the treatment of underlying depression and impulsivity.

Behavioral Interventions: Positive reinforcement for desired behavior and mild punishment for objectionable behavior helps to enhance social behavior and reduce aggression.

Educational intervention: Teaching academics for those individuals with ID who are teachable and training in adaptive skills, social skills and vocational skills for people who are trainable. Family Education: Education of the family regarding disability its course, ways to enhance competence and self esteem while maintaining realistic expectations

BIBLIOGRAPHY

1. American Psychiatric Association. Diagnostic And Statistical Manual Of Mental Disorders (DSM 5). American Psychiatric Pub; 2013.
2. Ji, N. Y., & Findling, R. L. (2016). Pharmacotherapy for mental health problems in people with intellectual disability. *Current opinion in psychiatry*, *29*(2), 103-125.
3. Martin A, Volkmar FR, Lewis M, editors. Lewis's child and adolescent psychiatry: a comprehensive textbook. Lippincott Williams & Wilkins; 2007(4th Edition).
4. Paul H, Cowen P, Tom B. Shorter Oxford Textbook of Psychiatry. Oxford: Oxford University Press (11th Edition)
5. Rights of person with disability Act, 2017 http://disabilityaffairs.gov.in/upload/uploadfiles/files/RPwD%20Act_enactment.pdf accessed on 4 January 2020.
6. Ruiz P. Comprehensive textbook of psychiatry. Sadock BJ, Sadock VA, editors. Philadelphia: lippincott Williams & Wilkins; 2000 (9th edition)
7. Rutter MJ, Bishop D, Pine D, Scott S, Stevenson JS, Taylor EA, Thapar A. Rutter's child and adolescent psychiatry. John Wiley & Sons; 2011(6th Edition)
8. Sadock BJ, Sadock VA. Kaplan and Sadock's Synopsis of Psychiatry: Behavioral Sciences/ Clinical Psychiatry. Lippincott Williams & Wilkins (10th edition)
9. Tasman A,Kay J, Liberman JA, Psychiatry Forth Edition. Wiley Blackwell.
10. Vissers, L. E., Gilissen, C., & Veltman, J. A. (2016). Genetic studies in intellectual disability and related disorders. *Nature Reviews Genetics*, *17*(1), 9.
11. World health organization. The ICD-10 Classification of mental and behavioral disorders; clinical description & diagnostic guidelines. Geneva: World health organization.

33 Learning Disability

Sheela Dang • Avinash De Sousa

Many children with learning disorders, also called learning disabilities, struggle in school long before being diagnosed. This can affect a child's self-esteem and motivation. Early intervention helps to reduce the issues faced by a student during their schooling years.

What is Learning Disability?

Learning disabilities, or learning disorders, are an umbrella term for a wide variety of learning problems. A learning disability is not a problem with intelligence or motivation. Kids with learning disabilities aren't lazy or dumb. In fact, most are just as smart as everyone else.

Learning disabilities are neurologically-based processing problems. These processing problems can interfere with learning basic skills such as reading, writing and/or math. They can also interfere with higher level skills such as organization, time planning, abstract reasoning, long or short-term memory and attention. It is important to realize that learning disabilities can affect an individual's life beyond academics and can impact relationships with family, friends and in the workplace.

Reading

Learning disorders in reading are usually based on difficulty perceiving a spoken word as a combination of distinct sounds. This can make it hard to understand how a letter or letters represent a sound and how letter combinations make a word.

Problems with working memory the ability to hold and manipulate information in the moment also can play a role.

When basic reading skills are mastered, children may have difficulty with the following skills:

- Reading at a typical pace
- Understanding what they read
- Recalling accurately what they read
- Making inferences based on their reading
- Spelling

A learning disorder in reading is usually called dyslexia, but some specialists may use the term to describe only some of the information-processing problems that can cause difficulty with reading.

Written expression

Writing requires complex visual, motor and information-processing skills. A learning disorder in written expression may cause the following:

- Slow and labour-intensive handwriting
- Handwriting that's hard to read
- Difficulty putting thoughts into writing
- Written text that's poorly organized or hard to understand

- Trouble with spelling, grammar and punctuation

Math

A learning disorder in math may cause problems with the following skills:

- Understanding how numbers work and relate to each other
- Calculating math problems
- Memorizing basic calculations
- Using math symbols
- Understanding word problems
- Organizing and recording information while solving a math problem

Nonverbal skills

A child with a learning disorder in nonverbal skills appears to develop good basic language skills and strong rote memorization skills early in childhood. Difficulties are present in visual-spatial skills, visual-motor skills, and other skills necessary in social or academic functioning.

A child with a learning disorder in nonverbal skills may have trouble with the following skills:

- Interpreting facial expressions and nonverbal cues in social interactions
- Using language appropriately in social situations
- Physical coordination
- Fine motor skills, such as writing
- Attention, planning and organizing

Specific Learning Disabilities

Auditory Processing Disorder (APD)

Also known as Central Auditory Processing Disorder, this is a condition that adversely affects how sound that travels unimpeded through the ear is processed or interpreted by the brain. Individuals with APD do not recognize subtle differences between sounds in words, even when the sounds are loud and clear enough to be heard. They can also find it difficult to tell where sounds are coming from, to make sense of the order of sounds, or to block out competing background noises.

Dyscalculia

A specific learning disability that affects a person's ability to understand numbers and learn math facts. Individuals with this type of LD may also have poor comprehension of math symbols, may struggle with memorizing and organizing numbers, have difficulty telling time, or have trouble with counting.

Dysgraphia

A specific learning disability that affects a person's handwriting ability and fine motor skills. Problems may include illegible handwriting, inconsistent spacing, poor spatial planning on paper, poor spelling, and difficulty composing writing as well as thinking and writing at the same time.

Dyslexia

A specific learning disability that affects reading and related language-based processing skills. The severity can differ in each individual but can affect reading fluency, decoding, reading comprehension, recall, writing, spelling and sometimes speech and can exist along with other related disorders. Dyslexia is sometimes referred to as a Language-Based Learning Disability.

Language Processing Disorder

A specific type of Auditory Processing Disorder (APD) in which there is difficulty attaching meaning to sound groups that form words, sentences and stories. While an APD affects the interpretation of all sounds coming into the brain, a Language Processing Disorder (LPD) relates only to the processing of language. LPD can affect expressive language and/or receptive language.

Non-Verbal Learning Disabilities

A disorder which is usually characterized by a significant discrepancy between higher verbal skills and weaker motor, visual-spatial and social skills. Typically, an individual with NLD (or NVLD) has trouble interpreting nonverbal cues like facial expressions or body language, and may have poor coordination.

Visual Perceptual/Visual Motor Deficit

A disorder that affects the understanding of information that a person sees, or the ability to draw or copy. A characteristic seen in people with learning disabilities such as Dysgraphia or Non-verbal LD, it can result in missing subtle differences in shapes or printed letters, losing place frequently, struggles with cutting, holding pencil too tightly, or poor eye/hand coordination.

What are the causes of Learning Disability?

Experts say that there is no single, specific cause for learning disabilities. However, there are some factors that could cause a learning disability:

- **Heredity:** It is observed that a child, whose parents have had a learning disability, is likely to develop the same disorder.
- **Illness during and after birth:** An illness or injury during or after birth may cause learning disabilities. Other possible factors could be drug or alcohol consumption during pregnancy, physical trauma, poor growth in the uterus, low birth weight, and premature or prolonged labour.
- **Stress during infancy:** A stressful incident after birth such as high fever, head injury, or poor nutrition.
- **Environment:** Increased exposure to toxins such as lead (in paint, ceramics, toys, etc.)
- **Comorbidity:** Children with learning disabilities are at a higher-than-average risk for attentional problems or disruptive behavior disorders. Up to 25 percent of children with reading disorder also have ADHD. Conversely, it is estimated that between 15 and 30 percent of children diagnosed with ADHD have a learning disorder.

What are the early signs of Learning Disability?

In the normal physiological development, the child is expected to acquire a certain set of basic cognition and motor skills. Any significant delay or gap in this development could be a sign of learning disability. A series of well-researched and proven tests and assessments have to be conducted before diagnosing the condition.

In general, 5 percent of school age children are affected by learning disabilities. Children with a learning disability may also have ADHD.

The signs of LD may vary slightly during each stage of childhood.

Preschool: The child may have some of these difficulties in preschool.

- Developing speaking skills at normal age (15-18 months) when speech typically develops in children

- Pronouncing simple words
- Recognizing letters and words
- Learning numbers, rhymes or songs
- Concentrating on tasks
- Following rules and directions
- Using fine/gross motor skills to do physical tasks.

Primary School: The child may have difficulty in:

- Connecting letters and sounds
- Differentiating between similar sounding words and rhyming words
- Reading, spelling, or writing accurately
- Distinguishing right from left, for example, confusing 25 with 52, "b" with "d," "on" with "no," "s" with "5"
- Recognizing letters of the alphabet
- Using correct mathematical symbols for doing maths problems
- Remembering numbers or facts
- Learning new skills; the child may be slower than other children of his or her age
- Memorizing poems or answers
- Understanding the concept of time
- Hand-to-eye coordination, being unable to gauge the distance or speed, thus leading to accidents
- Tasks involving fine motor skills: holding pencil, tying shoe lace, buttoning shirt and so on
- Keeping track of own possessions like stationery items

Middle School: The child may have difficulty in:

- Spelling similar words (sea/see, week/weak), usage of prefixes, suffixes
- Reading aloud, writing assignments, solving word problems in maths (the child may avoid doing tasks involving these skills)
- Handwriting (child may grip the pencil tightly)
- Memorizing or recalling facts
- Understanding body language and facial expressions
- Showing appropriate emotional reactions in a learning environment (the child may behave in an aggressive or rebellious way, and react with an excess of emotion)

High School: The child may have difficulty in:

- Spelling words accurately (the child may write the same word with different spellings in a single writing assignment)
- Reading and writing tasks
- Summarizing, paraphrasing, answering application problems or questions in tests
- Poor memory
- Adjusting to new surroundings
- Understanding abstract concepts
- Focusing consistently: the child may lack concentration on some tasks, while focusing excessively on others

While children with learning disabilities have difficulties in some areas of learning, they also have great aptitude, skill and talent in other areas of their interest. Most often, we focus on the disorder and neglect the child's talents or skills. It is important that parents and teachers recognize this hidden potential and encourage the child to pursue them.

Treatment options

If the child has a learning disorder, the child's doctor or school might recommend:

- Extra help: A reading specialist, math tutor

or other trained professional can teach your child techniques to improve his or her academic, organizational and study skills.

- Individualized education program (IEP): An individual education program for students who meet certain criteria for a learning disorder. The IEP sets learning goals and determines strategies and services to support the child's learning in school.
- Accommodations: Classroom accommodations might include more time to complete assignments or tests, being seated near the teacher to promote attention, use of computer applications that support writing, including fewer math problems in assignments, or providing audiobooks to supplement reading.
- Therapy: Some children benefit from therapy. Occupational therapy might improve the motor skills of a child who has writing problems. A speech-language therapist can help address language skills. Remedial Education would help to reduce the gap between what the child knows and what he is expected to know.
- Medication. The child's doctor might recommend medication to manage depression or severe anxiety. Medications for attention-deficit/hyperactivity disorder may improve a child's ability to concentrate in school.

Tips to manage academic concerns in a child with LD

Math

1. Use attractive material, however do not bombard in too much color.
2. Using different textures to teach numbers is a good option. Children learn well by the touch and feel method.
3. Allow the child to write numbers/letters in a salt tray, avoid sand as some may consume it.
4. Use real objects to introduce number value and counting.
5. Follow the right learning sequence, first 3D objects followed by flash cards or 2D material.
6. For the concept of greater and less than, make sure that the 2 examples you show are diverse. E.g. 2 and 10 and not 7 and 8
7. While teaching new concepts like addition and subtraction make sure there is a gap of a few days to avoid confusion.
8. While teaching fractions allow the child to cut a cake into slices or tear a tissue into pieces or cut a fruit. Only drawing in the note book may not help.
9. While teaching word problems make sure you have a clear list of mathematical operations, E.g.: sum, into and total, stand for addition.
10. If your child particularly has a difficulty in a subject or topic, mount a chart of it on a wall in your house.
11. Use the abacus or table board to teach math in an attractive manner.
12. If your child reverses a few numbers/letters make a list of them and practice them individually daily.

Reading

1. Start from big to small letters.
2. Introduce upper- and lower-case letters at the same time.
3. Teach the importance of the different punctuation marks while reading.
4. Teach sight words by sticking the word on the object itself.

5. If the child jumps between lines, place a ruler/scale or blank sheet of paper under each line that is being read.
6. Highlight words that he finds difficult to read or pronounce.
7. Encourage reading/memorizing one word from the dictionary daily.
8. E-flash apps is a good free app to teach all basic concepts. It mentions a word, says how to pronounce it and displays a picture too.
9. Encourage reading the newspaper headlines.
10. Encourage reading by introducing picture stories

Writing

1. To introduce writing use a thicker crayon or piece of chalk.
2. Use colorful pencils and pens to make writing more fun.
3. Use a gripper to improve the writing grip.
4. Write on sand or salt
5. Make a list of all the letters that are being reversed, omitted or substituted.
6. Use the wipe and right sheet to encourage to writing.
7. Join the dots, complete the maze and basic tracing activities.
8. Fine motor activities like beading, peg board games, building blocks and puzzles can help to improve writing and perceptual skills.

Procedure for Testing

- A letter is required from the school in which the child is studying.
- Certificate can be obtained from the LD Clinics of LTMG Hospital, Sion, Nair Hospital and K.E.M Hospital.
- A series of tests are conducted which may take between 2-4 months.
- A Special education/ Remedial educator, occupational therapist, physiotherapist, general physician, speech therapist and counsellor would assess the child.
- Ear and eye check-ups are mandatory too.
- A certificate thus obtained would help a child obtain an LD certificate or a Slow learner certificate.
- A child obtaining an LD certificate would thus avail certain concessions at school.
- A child obtaining a slow learner certificate would benefit best by following the NIOS curriculum.

Concessions provided for Learning Disability

SSC Board

- 25% Extra time
- Oral Test along with the written examination for Standard I to IX
- Promotion to next class on the basis of the average
- Writer/ typewriter
- Question papers to be read out
- Exemption from the Second and Third Language
- Physiology-Hygiene and Home Science in place of Science-Arithmetic
- Use of Calculator at Class X Examination
- Spelling errors and incorrect sentence construction to be ignored.
- Errors in respect of showing directions in Geography to be ignored.

- Students between Standard I & IX exempted from drawing diagrams, graphs, and charts.
- Marks for such questions proportionately distributed to the other questions or students to be provided with supplementary questions.
- 20% consolidated grace marks in one or more subjects
- Students are permitted to write in ordinary print
- Exempted from having to write answers in detail during exams
- A maximum of 20 marks should be given as grace marks for passing to those who have failed in the examination.
- SSC students are exempted from paper II in Mathematics (Algebra and Geometry). Students may take a vocational subject of 75 marks in lieu of Mathematics paper II.

Standard I to IV – errors of interchanging of computation signs and number reversal to be ignored

I. Arithmetic of Standard V in Standard V & VI

II. Arithmetic of Standard VI in Standard VII & VIII

III. Arithmetic of Standard VII in Standard IX & X

HSC

- HSC students may take a vocational subject instead of the second language.
- Students with any form of handicap (physical or mental) are also allowed writers
- Blind/deaf students are allowed to use tape-recorders in classrooms during lessons
- Cursive writing is not enforced

CBSE Board

- Exemption from studying third language up to middle school level (i.e. Class VIII)
- Permission to use an amanuensis.
- The amanuensis should be a student of class lower than the one for which the candidate will be taking the examination
- The candidate pays the fee as prescribed for use of the amanuensis to the Board. However, the Blind, Physically Handicapped or Spastic Candidates are being provided services of an amanuensis free of cost.
- The amanuensis is paid remuneration as prescribed from time to time by the Board.
- The candidate is permitted to use the services of an amanuensis in all or any of the papers. The same amanuensis is taken for all the papers.
- The candidates are being permitted to draw the diagrams etc. themselves, if desired by them
- Additional time as under is given in each paper:
  - **For paper of 3 hours duration 60 minutes**
  - **For paper of 2½ hours duration 50 minutes**
  - **For paper of 2 hours duration 40 minutes**
  - **For paper of 1½ hours duration 30 minutes**
- Alternative type questions are provided in lieu of questions having visual inputs for the blind candidates in English Communicative and Social Science for Class X and History, Geography and Economics for Class XII

- Separate question papers in enlarged print for Mathematics and Science & Technology in Class X are provided
- Blind candidates have the facility to use computer or a typewriter for writing answers
- Blind candidates have been permitted to offer subjects like Music, Home Science etc. which are not available in the school and to study these subjects privately as subjects of extended learning.

ICSE

In cases of candidates suffering from Dyslexia, Dysgraphia, Dyscalculia, Attention Deficit Hyperactivity Disorder (ADHD), certain concessions/support are admissible, depending on the nature and degree of the disability

The concessions/support available are: -

- Exemption from the requirement of the study of a second language in cases that warrant such an exemption because of the severe nature of the learning disability of the candidate.
- Allowance of additional time as specified above.
- Use of an/a Amanuensis/Reader/Reader-cum-Writer as specified above.
- The Question Paper may be read out, but not explained in any way to the candidate
- Casio fx-82 MS (Scientific Calculator) is to be used for Mathematical calculations only. Calculators of other makes with similar functions are also permitted.
- The use of a writer is allowed
- An additional hour is given for each paper
- One compulsory language as against two in addition to any four of the following subjects: math, science, social science, another language, music, painting and home science
- Leniency in paper assessment; spelling mistakes are overlooked for students with LD

34 Role of Parents and Teachers in Prevention of Child Abuse

Yusuf Matcheswalla • Avinash De Sousa

INTRODUCTION

Child abuse is an endemic mental health problem in India. Children who undergo abuse suffer from a variety of psychopathological outcomes in addition to the physical injuries they sustain as a result of the abuse. Children exposed to abuse are at greater risk for experiencing low self-esteem, lack of self-control, aggression and violence, academic problems, depressive features, alcohol dependence, interpersonal problems in relationships and also have increased chances of becoming an abuser themselves. The scars of child abuse continue way into adult life.

Early Indian child abuse research conducted by a Chennai based non-governmental organization (NGO) reported that 76% of the participants reported having experienced CSA once in their lifetime[1]. An epidemiological survey in a school in 2005 reported that 48% boys and 39% girls amongst 2211 participants had faced some form of CSA[2]. A report by the Ministry of Women and Child Welfare in 2007 stated that 57.3% boys and 42.7% girls in India, experience some form of abuse that includes physical abuse, sexual abuse, neglect, verbal abuse, emotional abuse and even two or more types together. These figures indicate alarming trends for India itself. Nearly more than half of the boys in India and half the girls aged 5-12 years had experienced at least one form of abuse in their lifetime[3]. In India, statistics reveal, that 1 in 10 children experience some form of CSA and 7000-7500 rapes in children occur on a yearly basis[4].

CSA is not a one off phenomenon but is rather multipronged, episodic and repetitive in nature. Community mental health experts must note that unlike communicable disease, where one may experience one episode or attack of an illness, CSA involves multiple episodes over months and years till the problem is detected or rather discovered. The psychological sequel and loss of self esteem caused by CSA is much more than many other psychiatric disorders[5]. The problem is hidden many a times when the perpetrator may be someone known to the child or may be a family member or neighbor[6]. In these cases, the child may have to live with the perpetrator even though abuse occurs and may not reveal any facts about the abuse, but rather may continue to be abused. In 70-85% instances of CSA, the perpetrator is someone already known to the child and the family[7]. It is often considered that only men are abusers while women do not abuse due to the maternal qualities they may possess. The fact remains that female child sexual abusers have been reported as well[8].

PARENTAL RISK FACTORS THAT MAY LEAD TO ABUSE

A multitude of factors increase the likelihood that parents will abuse their children which include the following –[9]

- Poverty, Unemployment, Lower levels of education, Poor family income.
- Teenage parenthood.
- Many children with inadequate spacing between them.
- Conflicts within the family domain.
- Unrealistic expectations about parenting and child development.
- Negative attitude towards one's child.
- Authoritarian parenting style.
- Physical punishment being a preferred method of behavior control.
- History of physical abuse or CSA in the parent.
- Presence of a psychiatric disorder or psychological problem in the parent.
- Substance abuse and drug use in the parents.
- Poor social support systems.

PARENT EDUCATION SHALL HELP REDUCE CHILD ABUSE[10-12]

Parent education programs can help reduce the likelihood that parents would abuse his or her children. There is a strong need to implement such programs in booth school and community settings to curb the problem of child sexual abuse or child abuse in general. The reasons for implementing such programs are highlighted below.

Parents will thus gain knowledge about parenting and child development

Many parents who may abuse their children are ignorant about how children develop and grow. Thus one must teach parents about child development in general and allay misconceptions that may be prevalent. Parents with a good understanding of child behavior across different ages likely to hold appropriate expectations from their children and thus are less likely to react to age appropriate situations than parents who may abuse their children. One must provide parents real life examples of child development and behavior patterns. Thus parent education must cater to newborns, toddlers, preschoolers, and school-age children and what parents need to expect at each of these stages.

Parents must also practice all that they have learned

The sessions must be interactive and must allow parents to share their views on a particular aspect of behavior and development. To achieve this objective, parents may describe several scenarios that they might encounter and must think about how their children might act in those situations. Debating and discussion on what is the appropriate approach in various situations can help parents anticipate their children's behaviors and respond in a manner conducive to positive child development.

Parents must be able to manage children without physical disciplining as far as possible

Having achieved an understanding of child development and behavior that may ensue, it becomes important for parents to learn important skills, such as child management technics in difficult situations so that at-risk parents can reduce the chances of abuse happening in their family situation. Many parents who abuse cite discipline as an excuse as they are unaware of how to deal with child misbehavior. It is often helpful for parents to role-play with each other and learn appropriate disciplining that may be verbal while being non abusive and non-physical in nature.

Parents need to learn stress management for their own well being

Stress is the biggest risk factor for child abuse and it is pivotal that parent education programs teach parents about means to manage stress in their daily lives. It is useful for parents to identify triggers or stressors and find ways to manage that stress. Some technics include participating in relaxation technics, adequate social support, exercising, rest, sleeping well and changing the attitude toward stress producing situations. Parents must also learn about childcare support or social services, which may help lessen some of their stress. This would in turn improve their quality of life and make them better parents in the long run.

Parents need to improve their relationships with others and amongst themselves

Parents with poor social support and relationship problems are at a higher risk for abusing their children. Parents thus need to learn and practice important communication skills, such as how to listen without interrupting, using "I messages" rather than "you-messages," and other soft skills technics. This may help reduce family conflict and improve relationships within their families and with other people. Forming supportive social networks shall bring a feeling of connectedness to others with higher levels of life satisfaction and thus shall help decrease the likelihood that they will abuse their children.

RECOGNIZING THE VARIOUS FORMS OF CHILD ABUSE

Signs that a child may be abused[13]

1. Aggression, oppositional and defiant behavior by the child.
2. The child shows a fear of certain adults.
3. The child may display disruptive behavior in the classroom.
4. Self destructive or self injurious behavior.
5. The child may come early to school, may not want to leave school indicating a fear of going home.
6. Risk taking behavior by the child.
7. Accident prone tendency as labeled by the parents.
8. The child may indulge in cheating, stealing or lying.
9. The child may be a low achiever in school.
10. Inability to form good peer relationships.
11. Clothing worn by the child may cover some body parts and may be inappropriate.
12. Regressive behavior by the child.
13. The child may move away from physical contact.

Physical Abuse

Physical abuse of children includes any non-accidental physical injury that sustained from burning, beating, kicking, punching and so on. While the injury cannot be labeled accidental there may not be intent of the child's caretaker to injure the child. Physical abuse is often quoted as being a form of discipline that is inappropriate for the child's age or condition and parent's may experience poor self-control due to stress, alcohol or drug use. Children with developmental disability and younger children are more susceptible to abuse than older children. Since children may injure themselves during play or while being active, the knees, elbows, forearms, or brows, are most likely to be injured. The soft tissue areas, such as the cheeks, hips, buttocks and thighs, are not normally injured in play and games. Bruises may have distinct shapes such as a hand mark, belt buckle marks or teeth and nail marks. Such bruises are indicative of physical abuse.[14-15]

Child Neglect

Neglect is often a type of maltreatment that has consequences that are just as serious as that of physical abuse. It is noted in nearly 50% of child maltreatment cases and is the leading cause of death due to child abuse. Living in poverty or poor shabby surroundings does not mean that a child is neglected. Neglect involves the care-giver's deliberate inattention to the basic needs of a child, such as food, clothing, shelter, love, warmth, medical care, and supervision. Neglectful families are often multi-problem families, though families with numerous problems are not always abusive in nature. These children may grow up believing that neglect is a normal way of parenting and will not seek assistance or help for the same.[16-17] Neglect also can be the result of extreme circumstances where leaving young children alone when the babysitter fails to show up happens because financial needs superseed basic needs and the job is the only means of income for the family.[18]

Some questions that teachers must ask and find answers to in child neglect

- Is the child looking for material gratification?
- Is the child stealing or lying consistently or occasionally?
- Is it necessary to look at the family in the context to provide any answers?
- Is the child-rearing practice followed a different lifestyle or true neglect?
- Does the parental behavior observed indicate the presence of abuse?
- Does the child display a lot of absenteesm from school?
- Is the child sleepy in school?
- Is the child inappropriately dressed for the day?
- Does the child exhibit poor hygiene?

Emotional Maltreatment and Abuse

Emotional maltreatment encompasses blaming, belittling, bullying or rejecting a child, constantly unequal treatment meted out to siblings and a persistent lack of concern by the parent. Emotional maltreatment when internalized can cause developmental delays, psychosomatic symptoms and other visible effects, such as speech disorders or selective mutism. The parents of an emotionally disturbed child generally accept the existence of a problem and are usually concerned about the child's welfare and seek help. On the other hand, parents of an emotionally maltreated child, blame the child for the problem and ignore or refuse all help being unconcerned about the child's wellbeing.[19]

Child Sexual Abuse

Child Sexual Abuse is defined as inappropriate adolescent or adult sexual behavior with a child. It includes fondling a child's genitals, making the child fondle the adult's genitals, intercourse, incest, rape, sodomy, exhibitionism, sexual exploitation or exposure to pornography. Sexual abuse may take place within the family (referred to as incest), by a parent's friend, neighbors or by caretakers or babysitter. Contrary to the myth of abuse often by strangers, most abusers are known to the child[20-21].

The Types of Perpetrators in Child Sexual Abuse[22]

A Known Adult

This type of abuser targets children outside the home and within the context of a trusted relationship. There have been cases of CSA where sports coaches, neighbors, group leaders, religious leaders and others known to the child may sexually assault them.

The Peer Adult

The sexual assault of a teen on a date or by a friend is under-reported as the teen often feels some level of self blame for the abuse. Engaging in sexual activity while dating is not new, but an acquaintance rape goes beyond repeated sexual requests in an effort to gain sexual compliance.

The Abuser who is a Stranger

Most victims know the individual who perpetrates sexual violence against them. There are cases, however of CSA being perpetrated by a total stranger. This can happen in the neighborhood, parks, playgrounds, malls and cinema halls.

Academic Clues to Child Abuse

Educational performance may provide a clue in child abuse. This is seen when there are sudden or extreme changes in academic performance. Studious children who suddenly seem disinterested in school or who are no longer prepared for class may be victims of CSA.[23]

Emotional Clues to Child Abuse

Teachers are typically sensitive to children who are "different" (e.g., physically or mentally challenged). One should be alert to children who are hostile and angry, those that avoid all who come in contact with them, or children who are passive, withdrawn, and uncommunicative. A sudden change in a child's emotional or psychological well-being may serve as clues to child abuse and neglect.[24]

Family Clues to Child Abuse

The teacher often has multiple chances to observe family dynamics. Normal interaction with the parents may indicate how they feel about the child.

There may be an increased risk of child abuse and neglect if the parents consistently reflect the following trends –

- Blaming or ridiculing the child.
- The child being negatively compared to siblings or peers.
- The child being viewed as bad or evil.
- Inability to see anything good in their own child.
- Reflecting unconcerned attitudes towards the child.
- Failure to keep appointments.
- Refusal to discuss problems of the child.

There may be times when the teacher is aware of a family in marital crisis or experiencing economic or emotional turmoil. This could be an indicator of probable child abuse.

Teacher's Checklist to determine Child Neglect

It is important for the teacher to note and observe the following in the child –

- The child often comes to school in dirty clothes or uniforms that are small or large for them or torn.
- The child seems inappropriately dressed for the weather.
- The child is always hungry and even at times stealing food.
- The child is tired with poor energy.
- The child shows poor hygiene or may have very bad breath or decaying teeth.
- The child seems malnourished.

- The child has unattended medical issues.
- The child shows stealing, vandalism, or other conduct related behaviors.
- The child shows frequent absences from school.
- The child demonstrates poor peer relationships.
- The child shows withdrawn and isolated behavior.
- The child is attention seeking and does anything to gain the same.
- The child shows aggressive and destructive behavior with no remorse over his or her actions.
- The child may have low self-esteem.
- The child has difficulty in problem solving or coping with stress.
- The child demonstrates a variety of academic/educational problems.
- The child's family is one where psychological problems are known.
- The child's parents are known to be callous and indifferent to the child.

Teacher's Checklist for Physical Abuse

The teacher must check whether the child demonstrates any of the following –

- The child shows extensive bruises in areas of the body that are not normally vulnerable and the bruises are of different colors indicating various stages of healing.
- The child shows frequent injuries around the head or face, the abdomen or midway between the wrist and elbow.
- The injury marks are in shapes such as handprints, hangar marks, or belt buckles.
- The marks indicate hard blows from an object such as whip-like object or cane.
- There is unexplained abdominal bleeding (i.e., caused by internal bleeding).
- There is a complaint of soreness and stiffness.

The child has some bald spots from severe hair pulling.

- The child shows human bite marks.
- The child is burnt from objects such as cigarettes, irons and other objects.
- The injury for which the explanation given is improper.

Teacher's checklist to look for Emotional Abuse

The teacher must observe whether the child sometimes exhibits –

- Inappropriate emotions such as jokes and laughing when in pain.
- Extreme behavior changes– happy or very depressed.
- Withdrawn attitude.
- Self injurious behavior like cutting oneself.
- Violence and aggressive behavior.
- Difficulty in attention and concentrating or learning new material.
- The child may show rocking movements and habit disorders like thumb sucking, head banging and nail biting.
- Enuresis (bed-wetting) or soiling (Encopresis) after an age when such behavior is not age appropriate.
- Frequent stomach aches or headaches.
- Delinquent behavior.

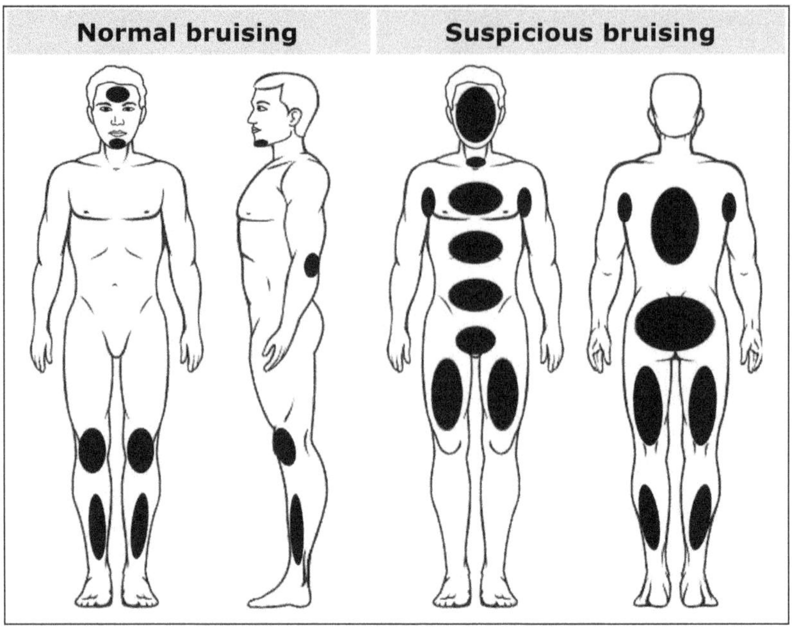

Teacher's checklist to identify Sexual Abuse

The teacher must check whether the child exhibits any of the following –

- Difficulties in walking or sitting in class.
- There is genital or anal itching, pain or bleeding.
- The child may frequently vomit without a reason.
- The child may have sexually transmitted diseases.
- The child demonstrates reserved behavior and secrecy.
- The child shows sexual knowledge which is more than what is age appropriate.
- The child engages in sexual play with peers.
- The child shows aggression.
- The child shows a fear of certain males or females.
- The child may exhibit seductive behavior.
- There is a sudden drop in school performance.
- The child has sleep problems, bad dreams and nightmares.
- The child cries without a reason.
- The child develops sudden phobic behavior.
- The child shows an older appearance than peers.
- The child talks of suicide wanting to kill himself.
- The child attempts to run away from home.
- The child may set things on fire and love watching them burn.
- Self-mutilation (cutting or scratching to draw blood).

Tips for teachers when talking to children who have been probably victims of abuse –

- Find a quiet, secure and private place to talk to the child.

- Listen intently to what is being told.
- Do not push the child to share more than he/she is willing to speak.
- The child needs warmth and acceptance.
- Ask only for information to assess the child's safety at first.
- Reassure the child that he/she has done the right thing by telling you.
- Acknowledge the difficulty of the decision and the personal strength shown.
- Make a clear distinction that the abuse or neglect is not the child's fault.
- Keep your own feelings under control.
- Be calm and non-judgmental.
- Tell the child you cannot promise not to tell.
- Tell the child that there is help available.
- Tell the truth.
- Be specific about what will happen next.
- Be supportive.
- Try to help the child regain control.
- Reassure the child that you will do your best to support him/her.
- Seek professional help and guidance in speaking to the child.
- Effective self-care is critical for the educator responding to abuse allegations.
- Do not express shock or disbelief while the child is talking.
- Do not ever try to talk a child out of what he/she is saying.
- If you are skeptical, do not express your doubts to the child.
- Do not try to determine for yourself if the allegation is valid or invalid.
- Do not correct or criticize the child's choice of words or language.
- Especially in sexual abuse cases, the child may use graphic language to disclose.
- Usually the perpetrator during the abuse has used this language.
- Do not ask a lot of questions.
- Do not conduct an investigation on your own.
- Document what the child said and let the investigators take over from there.
- In depth questioning jeopardizes the quality of information disclosed by the child.
- Do not call the child's parents.
- Do not promise confidentiality to the child.
- Do not convey anger or impatience if the child is not ready to discuss the abuse.
- Do not make negative comments about the perpetrator.
- Do not conduct a moral lecture about the incident.
- Refrain from judging the suspected perpetrator and his/her alleged actions.
- Do not disclose the information indiscriminately.
- Tell only those adults who need the information to protect and support the child.
- Do not stand over a child while he/she is disclosing abuse.
- Instead, place yourself physically on the child's eye level.
- Do not suggest to a child that you think he/she may have been abused.

TIPS FOR PARENTS WHEN DEALING WITH CHILD ABUSE

- Communication with children is not easy in areas as difficult as child abuse.
- Good communication with children will establish trust and help to reduce stress in your relationship.
- **Establish rapport :** Rapport comes from friendly and honest relations.
- Welcome the suggestions of children and enjoy their jokes.
- **Teach decision making :** Allow children to participate in decisions affecting their lives. Confidence in simple decision making in their lives will help to prepare them for the more difficult choices ahead.
- Whenever possible, join the group your kid joins or at least work closely with it.
- **Use peer pressure** - the influence of kids on other kids to help get your message across.
- **Explain consequences** - explain how your children's actions, such as ignoring family rules affects you.
- **Teach openness** - Explain the difference between good secrets such as a surprise party and secrets that make you feel bad.
- **Be the adult** - Children expect their parent's decisions to be fair, just and consistent.
- Create reasonable limits. Be aware of the capabilities of your children as they develop.
- Admit your own mistakes. Nobody is perfect.
- **Share your strategies** - Children often experience similar challenges to their parents. Share how you have overcome challenges like dealing with frustration, failure, fear, stress, loss and even success.
- **Smile, even if you don't feel like it** - Your body language speaks louder than your words and how you say them. Smiling can also help you to gain perspective.
- **Be curious** - Develop an insatiable curiosity about your children. Take a sincere interest in their views, their joys and their sorrows and their own identity.

TIPS FOR PARENTS TO TALK TO CHILDREN ABOUT SEXUAL ABUSE

- If you feel uncomfortable discussing sexual abuse with your children, let them know.
- Select words your child understands.
- One main concern of parents is finding words to explain sexual abuse. Most child abuse prevention experts believe that children should learn the proper names for their genitalia.
- Help your child to be comfortable with their bodies. An over-emphasis on privacy can make them uncomfortable.
- Provide the opportunity for your child to practice youth protection skills. Children learn better when they can practice the skills they are taught.
- Support your children in trusting their instincts - Don't make them kiss someone they feel uncomfortable with (even if they are a close family member).

BIBLIOGRAPHY

1. Aggarwal K, Dalwai S, Galagali P, Mishra D, Prasad C, Thadhani A. Recommendations on recognition and response to child abuse and neglect in the Indian setting. Indian Pediatr 2010;47(6):493-504.

2. Virani P. Bitter chocolate : Child Sexual Abuse in India. Penguin Books: India ; 2000.
3. Ministry of Women and Child Development. Report of the study on Child Abuse. Government of India ; 2007.
4. Finkelhor D, Korbin J. Child abuse as an international issue. Child Abuse Neglect 1988;12(1):3-23.
5. Collin-Vezina D, Daigneault I, Hebert M. Lessons learnt from child sexual abuse research : prevalence, outcomes and preventive strategies. Child Adolesc Psychiatry Mental Health 2013;7:22-8.
6. Behere PB, Sathyanarayana Rao TS, Mulmule AN. Sexual abuse in women with special reference to children: Barriers, boundaries and beyond. Indian J Psychiatry 2013;55:316–9.
7. Behere PB, Mulmule AN. Sexual abuse in an 8 year old child : where do we stand legally? Indian J Psychol Med 2013;13:203-5.
8. Doyle C. Child sexual abuse: a guide for health professionals (Vol. 44). Nelson Thornes ; 1994.
9. Wills DJ, Holden EW, Rosenberg M. Prevention of child maltreatment : developmental and ecological perspectives. New York: John Wiley & Sons ; 1992.
10. Daro D, McCurdy K. Preventing child abuse and neglect : programmatic interventions. Child Welfare 1994;73(5):403-31.
11. Cichetti D, Carlson V. Child maltreatment: theory and research on the causes and consequences of child abuse and neglect. New York: Cambridge University Press ; 1989.
12. Whipple EE, Wilson SR. Evaluation of a parent education program for families at a risk of child abuse. Families in Society 1996;77(4):227-39.
13. Kenny MC. Child abuse reporting: Teachers' perceived deterrents. Child Abuse Negl 2001;25(1):81-92.
14. Oates RK, Bross DC. What have we learned about treating child physical abuse? A literature review of the last decade. Child Abuse Negl 1995;19(4):463-73.
15. Kaplan SJ, Pelcovitz D, Labruna V. Child and adolescent abuse and neglect research: A review of the past 10 years. Part I: Physical and emotional abuse and neglect. J Am Acad Child Adolesc Psychiatry 1999;38(10):1214-22.
16. Hildyard KL, Wolfe DA. Child neglect: developmental issues and outcomes. Child Abuse Negl 2002;26(6):679-95.
17. Tanner K, Turney D. What do we know about child neglect? A critical review of the literature and its application to social work practice. Child Fam Soc Work 2003;8(1):25-34.
18. Connell-Carrick K. A critical review of the empirical literature: Identifying correlates of child neglect. Child Adolesc Soc Work J 2003;20(5):389-425.
19. Wolfe DA, McIsaac C. Distinguishing between poor/dysfunctional parenting and child emotional maltreatment. Child Abuse Negl 2011;35(10):802-13.
20. Putnam FW. Ten-year research update review: Child sexual abuse. J Am Acad Child Adolesc Psychiatry 2003;42(3):269-78.
21. Polusny MA, Follette VM. Long-term correlates of child sexual abuse: Theory and review of the empirical literature. Appl Prev Psychol 1995;4(3):143-66.
22. Glasser M, Kolvin I, Campbell D, Glasser A, Leitch I, Farrelly S. Cycle of child sexual abuse: Links between being a victim and becoming a perpetrator. Br J Psychiatry 2001;179(6):482-94.

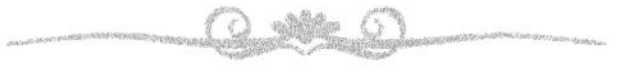

35 Child Sexual Abuse

Tejal Doshi • Avinash De Sousa

INTRODUCTION

The World Health Organization (1999) defines child abuse or maltreatment to constitute all forms of physical and/or emotional ill-treatment, sexual abuse, neglect or negligent treatment or commercial or other exploitation, resulting in actual or potential harm to the child's health, survival, development or dignity, in the context of a relationship of responsibility, trust or power.

Child sexual abuse is the involvement of a child in sexual activity that s/he does not fully comprehend, is unable to give informed consent to, or for which the child is not developmentally prepared and cannot give consent, or that violate the laws or social taboos of society. Child sexual abuse is evidenced by an activity between a child and an adult or another child who by age or development is in a relationship of responsibility, trust or power; the activity being intended to gratify or satisfy the needs of another person.

The term 'Child Sexual Abuse' has emanated much interest recently in India after the 82-page report presented by Human Rights Watch named "Breaking the Silence" on February 7th, 2013. It examines how current government responses are falling short, both in protecting children from sexual abuse and treating abuse and the alleged sexual misuse of children adopted from an orphanage in India. Many children are effectively mistreated a second time by traumatic medical examinations and by police and other authorities.

Child sexual abuse includes:

- Any sexual act between an adult and a minor, or between two minors, when one exerts power over the other.
- Forcing, coercing or persuading a child to engage in any sexual act.
- Non-contact acts such as exhibitionism, exposure to pornography, voyeurism, and communicating in a sexual manner by phone or Internet.

Mrazek (1980) proposed that any clinical working definition of Sexual Misuse must consider four factors:

1. An explicit description of what occurred including the nature of frequency of the act and threats involved
2. The mental age and emotional development of people involved
3. The quality of the relationship between them
4. The attitudes and involvement of other family members and the prevailing cultural attitudes.

THE VARIOUS FACES OF SEXUAL ABUSE

It is hard to decide under what legal statute,

a perpetrator of sexual misuse should be prosecuted, and it is indeed all the more made difficult to define sexual misuse, as sexual misuse has many faces. The following are the common ones encountered:

- Exhibitionism by the perpetrator
- Masturbation by the perpetrator in front of the victim
- Masturbation of the victim
- Sodomy
- Rape
- Incest
- Erotic stimulation (other than above)

Finkelhor mentioned that the commonest type of sexual misuse was some kind of genital fondling. Researchers have showed that intercourse occurred approximately in one-quarter of the reported cases, attempted intercourse in one-fifth, and oral-genital contact in one-quarter.

It is important that all Child Psychiatrists, Child Psychologists, Forensic Psychiatrists and Forensic Pathologists, and all those likely to come in contact with children who could have been sexually misused, should be ever mindful and aware of this possibility and make efforts to clearly evaluate and explore the possibility keeping in mind the fact that prevalence of sexual misuse in children is indeed very high.

PREVALENCE

Child sexual abuse is likely the most prevalent health problem children face with the most serious array of consequences. About 1 in 10 children will be sexually abused before their 18th birthday globally. About one in seven girls and one in 25 boys will be sexually abused before they turn 18. This year, there will be about 400,000* babies born in the U.S. that will become victims of child sexual abuse unless we do something to stop it.

The public is not fully aware of the magnitude of the problem. The primary reason is that only about 38% of child victims disclose the fact that they have been sexually abused. Some never disclose. There are also privacy issues surrounding cases of child sexual abuse. For instance, public police reports do not name the victim, and most media concerns have a policy that precludes naming victims.

Most people think of adult rape as a crime of great proportion and significance and are unaware that children are victimized at a much higher rate than adults. Nearly 70% of all reported sexual assaults (including assaults on adults) occur to children ages 17 and under. Youths have higher rates of sexual assault victimization than do adults. In 2000, the rate for youths aged 12 to 17 was 2.3 times higher than for adults. 44% of rapes with penetration occur to children under age 18. Victims younger than 12 accounted for 15% of those raped, and another 29% of rape victims were between 12 and 17.

Child sexual abuse is a dark reality in Indian society like in any other nation. 53% of our children are sexually abused, according to a statistic from a survey done by the Government of India. A 1985 study by the Tata Institute of Social Sciences reveals that one out of three girls and one out of 10 boys had been sexually abused as a child. 50% of child sexual abuse happens at home. In 1996, Samvada, a Bangalore-based NGO, conducted a study among 348 girls. Fifteen percent of girls were abused for masturbation, mostly by male relatives when they were less than ten years old; 75% of the abusers were adult family members.

Present day living seems to have made the problem indulged in from time immemorial:

1) The increasing sexual inadequacy of the adult due to psychopathology, sexual hang-ups, poor education, superstitious beliefs, and weird notions.
2) The greater degree of social isolation caused by modern day living in large cities which also causes anonymity.
3) Late marriages due to cultural bindings and economic conditions.
4) Martial disharmony due to incompatibility caused by psychopathology in the partners, in additions to the claim of equal rights and tending to be independent.
5) Increasing psychopathology per se as a result of the tempo and quality of life, causing individuals to move to children for sexual satisfaction.
6) Overcrowding in our cities that causes a loss of privacy, and seeking sexual outlets with children for the sake of convenience.

PROFILE OF THE SEXUAL MISUSER

Those who molest children look and act just like everyone else. Abusers can be neighbors, friends and family members. People who sexually abuse children can be found in families, schools, churches, recreation centers, youth sports leagues, and any other place children gather. Significantly, abusers can be and often are other children. About 90% of children who are victims of sexual abuse know their abuser. Only 10% of sexually abused children are abused by a stranger. The younger the victim, the more likely it is that the abuser is a family member. Of those molesting a child under six, 50% were family members. Family members also accounted for 23% of those abusing children ages 12 to 17. About 60% of children who are sexually abused are abused by people the family trusts. Homosexual individuals are no more likely to sexually abuse children than heterosexual individuals. Not everyone who sexually abuses children is a pedophile.

70% of child sex offenders have between one and nine victims, while 20% have 10 to 40 victims. Nearly 40% of sexually abused children are abused by older or more powerful children. The younger the child victim, the more likely it is that the perpetrator is a juvenile. Juveniles are the offenders in 43% of assaults on children under age six. Of these offenders, 14% are under age 12. Juveniles who commit sex offenses against other children are more likely than adult sex offenders to offend in groups, to offend at schools, and to have more male victims and younger victims. The number of youth coming to the attention of police for sex offenses increases sharply at age 12 and plateaus after age 14. Early adolescence is the peak age for youth offenses against younger children. A small number of juvenile offenders — one out of eight — are younger than age 12. Females constitute 7% of juveniles who commit sex offenses. Most adolescent sex offenders are not sexual predators and will not go on to become adult offenders. Most adolescent offenders do not meet the criteria for pedophilia and do not continue to exhibit sexually predatory behaviors. Adolescent sex offenders are more responsive to treatment than adults. They do not appear to continue to re-offend into adulthood, especially when provided with appropriate treatment.

Sexual Misusers seem to fall into certain categories depending on the variety of sexual misuse, but certain clear characteristics prevail in this group in general:

1) Unhappy childhood
2) An impaired relationship with parents, siblings and peers

3) Severe rejection by the parents during childhood

4) A faulty psychosexual development (in keeping with the Freudian theory which in turn was responsible for the type of sexual misuse)

5) School dropouts or peculiar educational accomplishments

6) A sexual life which was chaotic often competing for being designated as, Polymorphous Perverse

7) A history of psychiatric illness namely, Neurosis, Psychosis, Alcoholism, Drug Dependence, or Psychopathy

CLASSIFICATION OF SEXUAL MISUSERS OF CHILDREN

Perpetrators of sexual Misuse in the case of children though they might not show particular characteristics can be broadly classified as follows:

- Neurotics, where a neurotics conflict was the reason for sexual misuse in an attempt to bring about a resolution of or a solution to the conflict.
- Psychotics, where a psychosis that was functional was responsible for sexual misuses, which might be periodic and fluctuate with the periodicity of the psychosis and form of the psychotic picture.
- Organically based, where brain damage associated with dementia, a brain tumor, or as a result of their after-effects, or epilepsy (especially temporal lobe epilepsy) was responsible for sexual misuse of children.
- Mental Subnormality, where due to a deficiency of intellectual abilities, the perpetrators chose to move towards children for sexual satisfaction, as adults would not oblige or were not drawn towards them.
- The Psychopaths or Sociopaths, where sexual misuse of children was part of the general promiscuous antisocial tendency, which was extended to children who were used as a means of sexual satisfaction.
- The Sexual Deviants or Perverts, who as a result of a psychological make –up chose children for sexual satisfaction and abused them in various ways. These individuals could indeed be considered the true pedophiles though the word is indeed a misnomer and could instead be considered a form of hating children rather than loving children. Nevertheless, it must be remembered that certain pedophiles never harmed children in the process of these sexual exploits but on the other hand show them plenty of love which caused the children to be attracted to the pedophiles, again and again.
- The Sadists, whose sadistic tendencies were directed towards children and who obtained sexual pleasure out of making children suffer.
- The Alcoholics or Drugs Takers or individuals are dependent on alcohol or drugs, who sought children for Sexual Misuse under the influence of alcohol or drugs. These were indeed the latent pedophiles who needed alcohol or drugs to quieten their consciences and release their sexual tendencies.
- The Stress Misusers, who under stress conditions through their inability to get adult sexual satisfaction chose children.

Sexual Misuses of children is by no means a one-sided problem of only the perpetrators, though they carry the onus for the esteem to get some contributions from the victims as well. It is not every child becomes a victim of Sexual Misuse in spite of being available to the perpetrator, but it is well recorded that certain children seem to be predisposed.

UNDER WHAT CIRCUMSTANCES DOES CHILD SEXUAL ABUSE OCCUR?

Child sexual abuse often takes place under specific, often surprising circumstances. It is helpful to know these circumstances because it allows for the development of strategies to avoid child sexual abuse.

- 81% of child sexual abuse incidents for all ages occur in one-perpetrator/one-child circumstances. Six to 11-year-old children are most likely (23%) to be abused in multiple-victim circumstances.
- Most sexual abuse of children occurs in a residence, typically that of the victim or perpetrator – 84% for children under age 12, and 71% for children aged 12 to 17.
- Sexual assaults on children are most likely to occur at 8 a.m., 12 noon and between 3 and 4 p.m. For older children, aged 12 to 17, there is also a peak in assaults in the late evening hours.
- One in seven incidents of sexual assault perpetrated by juveniles occurs on school days in the after-school hours between 3 and 7 p.m., with a peak from 3 to 4 pm.
- FAC Commercial sexual exploitation and internet sex crimes against children are a small and yet significant part of the overall problem.

In 2006, arrests for online youth victim cases constituted only 1.2% of arrests for all sex crimes against children. There were 615 arrests for online cases vs. 49,345 arrests for all sex crimes against children. 9% of all 10 to 17 year olds receive unwanted sexual requests while on the Internet. Over a period of one year, one in 25 youth received an online sexual solicitation where the solicitor tried to make offline contact. 23% of all 10 to 17 year olds experience unwanted exposure to pornography. Child sexual abuse makes children more vulnerable to sexual exploitation. More than 90% of children who are commercially sexually exploited have been sexually abused in the past. About 75% of child pornography victims are living at home when they are photographed. Parents are often responsible. Abusers often form relationships with potential victims and their families prior to the abuse. This is called "grooming." Grooming is a process by which an offender gradually draws a victim into a sexual relationship and maintains that relationship in secrecy. At the same time, the offender may also fill roles within the victim's family that make the offender trusted and valued.

Grooming behaviors can include:

- Special attention, outings, and gifts
- Isolating the child from others
- Filling the child's unmet needs
- Filling needs and roles within the family
- Treating the child as if he or she is older
- Gradually crossing physical boundaries, and becoming increasingly intimate/sexual
- Use of secrecy, blame, and threats to maintain control

WHAT FACTORS INCREASE A CHILD'S RISK FOR SEXUAL ABUSE?

While no child is immune, there are child and family characteristics that significantly heighten or lower risk of sexual abuse.

The following risk factors are based on reported and identified cases of abuse:

- Family structure is the most important risk factor in child sexual abuse. Children who live with two married biological parents are at low risk for abuse. The risk increases when children live with step-parents or a single parent.
- Children living without either parent (foster children) are 10 times more likely to be sexually abused than children that live with both biological parents. Children who live with a single parent that has a live-in partner are at the highest risk: they are 20 times more likely to be victims of child sexual abuse than children living with both biological parents.
- Gender is also a major factor in sexual abuse. Females are five times more likely to be abused than males. The age of the male being abused also plays a part. 8% of victims aged 12 to 17 are male. 26% of victims under the age of 12 are male.
- Age is a significant factor in sexual abuse. While there is risk for children of all ages, children are most vulnerable to abuse between the ages of seven and 13. The median age for reported abuse is nine years old. However, more than 20% of children are sexually abused before the age of eight.
- Race and ethnicity are an important factor in identified sexual abuse. African American children have almost twice the risk of sexual abuse than white children. Children of Hispanic ethnicity have a slightly greater risk than non-Hispanic white children.
- The risk for sexual abuse is tripled for children whose parent(s) are not in the labor force.
- Children in low socioeconomic status households are three times as likely to be identified as a victim of child abuse.
- Children who live in rural areas are almost two times more likely to be identified as victims of child sexual abuse.
- Children who witness or are the victim of other crimes are significantly more likely to be sexually abused.

Family and acquaintance child sexual abuse perpetrators have reported that they look for specific characteristics in the children they choose to abuse. Perpetrators report that they look for passive, quiet, troubled, lonely children from single parent or broken homes. Perpetrators frequently seek out children who are particularly trusting. Find new victims and work proactively to establish a trusting relationship before abusing them. Not infrequently, this extends to establishing a trusting relationship with the victim's family as well.

PSYCHOPATHOLOGY OF THE VICTIMS OF SEXUAL MISUSE

The victim of Sexual Misuse has often been credited with certain characteristics that unhappy cause the victim to be drawn into an encounter with this particular type of sexual offender. Thus these children have been described as being hysterical, attention –seeking, provocative and seductive, that went out their way to draw attention to themselves from anyone who showed the slightest interest. The parents of such children unwittingly added to the confusion by dressing them up in a very attractive fashion. Mothers of such children were known to be hysterical themselves and fathers often had the same traits and were generally hysterical psychopaths or sociopaths. Godwin, Mc Carthy and Di Vasto found that 25% of mothers of sexually abused children reported a prior incest experience compared to 3% of controls. Those children who became the victims of sexual misuse had poor ties with the family members, including the sibling and even when a resemblance of closer ties existed the depth of these relationships are poor. Geiser (1979) felt that children who developed prolonged sexual relationships with adults outside their own families did so because of feeling unsupported, alienated and deprived within their families. These children had a peculiar inability to utilize their intelligence sufficiently in a given situation, and are often called stupid. Thus their reactions were generally wrong and their interactions with others faulty. These were often unstable, irrational, over-emotional and nervous. Goodwin, Simms and Bergman (1979) felt that victims of sexual misuse showed evidence of shyness, anxiety, depression and even felt like committing suicide after these exposures. Further, hysterical seizures and amnestic states were generally encountered in these victims, who exhibited an extreme degree of pseudomaturity. It would be interesting to note whether all this psychopathology was not already present even if in a minor degree before the child became a victim of Sexual Misuse.

All these traits add a new dimension to the act of Sexual Misuse bringing a dynamic factor that is emanating from the child-victim. Beyond doubt, Sexual Misuse serves to increase the tension in a family where the act is perpetrated, but in cases of Incest, it might serve to reduce the tension in a family. Here the child is very often collaborative and cooperates with the sexual offenders, generally the parent who seeks to have his sexual outlets within the family. Thus co-operation of the victim and the frequency of the attack are used to affect a classification of victims of Sexual Misuse.

Victims of Sexual Misuse have been classified as follows:

1. Accidental Victims, where the act occurs without co-operation of the victim and incidentally or accidentally as a result of the situation in which the victim happens to be placed.
2. Habitual Victims, where the victim is a party to the act and is repeatedly assisting the perpetrator in performing the act. At times, the co-operation of the victim may not be there, and in spite of the repetitive nature, the co-operation is obtained under threats of holding the victim to ransom.

Victims of Sexual Misuse have also been classified into:

1. Participant or Collaborative – Victims, where co-operation to the maximum is repeatedly given to perpetrate the sexual acts
2. Non- Participant or Non- Collaborative – victims, where the sexual act is a one-sided affair in which the victim does not only refuse to co-operate but also resists the act.

Whether co-operation exists or does not exist, and whether the act is thrust on the victim or performed gently the aftermath of Sexual Misuse of children has indeed far–reaching effects.

WHAT ARE THE IMMEDIATE CONSEQUENCES OF CHILD SEXUAL ABUSE?

Emotional and mental health problems are often the first consequence and sign of child sexual abuse.

- Children who are sexually abused are at significantly greater risk for later posttraumatic stress and other anxiety symptoms, depression and suicide attempts.

- These psychological problems can lead to significant disruptions in normal development and often have a lasting impact, leading to dysfunction and distress well into adulthood.
- Behavioral problems, including physical aggression, non-compliance, and oppositionality occur frequently among sexually abused children and adolescents.
- Child sexual abuse has been linked to higher levels of risk behaviors. Sexual behavior problems and over-sexualized behavior are a very common consequence of child sexual abuse. Age-inappropriate behavior can be a very important and telling sign that abuse is occurring. Children who have been sexually abused have over three times as many sexual behavior problems as children who have not been sexually abused.
- Victims of child sexual abuse are more likely to be sexually promiscuous.
- Academic problems in childhood are a common symptom of sexual abuse. Sexually abused children tended to perform lower on psychometric tests measuring cognitive ability, academic achievement, and memory assessments when compared to same-age non-sexually abused cohorts. Studies indicate that sexual abuse exposure among children and adolescents is associated with high school absentee rates, more grade retention, increased need for special education services and difficulty with school adaptation.

39% of 12-year-old girls with a history of child sexual abuse had academic difficulties. 7 to 12 year-old girls with a history of child sexual abuse were 50% more likely to display cognitive ability below the 25th percentile. 26% of 7 to 12 year-old girls with a history of child sexual abuse reported that their grades dropped after they were abused and 48% had below-average grades. A history of child sexual abuse significantly increases the chance of dropping out of school.

Substance abuse problems beginning in childhood or adolescence are some of the most common consequences of child sexual abuse. A number of studies have found that adolescents with a history of child sexual abuse demonstrate a three to fourfold increase in rates of substance abuse/dependence. Drug abuse is more common than alcohol abuse for adolescent child sexual abuse victims. Age of onset for non-experimental drug use was 14 years old for victims, compared to 15 years old for non-victimized youth. Adolescents were 2 to 3 times more likely to have an alcohol use/dependence problem than non-victims.

Delinquency and crime, often stemming from substance abuse, are more prevalent in adolescents with a history of child sexual abuse. Adolescents who were sexually abused have a 3 to 5-fold risk of delinquency. Behavioral problems, including physical aggression, non-compliance, and oppositionality occur frequently among sexually abused children and adolescents. These emotional and behavioral difficulties can lead to delinquency, poor school performance and dropping out of school. Adolescents that reported victimization (i.e., sexual abuse or physical abuse) were more likely to be arrested than their non-abused peers. Sexually abused children were nearly twice as likely to run away from home.

The risk of teen pregnancy is much higher for girls with a history of child sexual abuse. The increased risk for pregnancy at a young age is likely due to over-sexualized behavior, another common consequence of child sexual abuse. Girls who are sexually abused are 2.2 times as likely as non-abused peers to become teen mothers.[40,54] 45% of pregnant teens report a history of child sexual abuse. Males who are sexually abused are more likely than their non-abused peers to impregnate a teen. In fact, several studies indicate that the sexual abuse of boys is a stronger risk factor for teen pregnancy than the sexual abuse of girls. Most sexual abuse incidents reported by pregnant teens occurred well before the incident that resulted in pregnancy. Only 11 to 13% of pregnant girls with a history of child sexual abuse reported that they had become pregnant as a direct result of this abuse.

What are the long-term consequences of child sexual abuse?

Child sexual abuse has lasting consequences for victims. The real tragedy is that it robs children of their potential, setting into motion a chain of events and decisions that affect them throughout their lives.

Mental health problems are a common long-term consequence of child sexual abuse. Females who are sexually abused are three times more likely to develop psychiatric disorders than females who are not sexually abused.

- Substance abuse problems are a common consequence for adult survivors of child sexual abuse. Female adult survivors of child sexual abuse are nearly three times more likely to report substance use problems (40.5% versus 14% in general population). Male adult CSA victims are 2.6 times more likely to report substance use problems (65% versus 25% in general population).
- Adult women who were sexually abused as a child are more than twice as likely to suffer from depression as women who were not sexually abused. Adults with a history of child sexual abuse are more than twice as likely to report a suicide attempt.
- Among male survivors, more than 70% seek psychological treatment for issues such as substance abuse, suicidal thoughts and attempted suicide.
- Obesity and eating disorders are more common in women who have a history of child sexual abuse. 20–24 year-old women who were sexually abused as children were four times more likely than their non-abused peers to be diagnosed with an eating disorder. Middle-aged women who were sexually abused as children were twice as likely to be obese when compared with their non-abused peers.
- Child sexual abuse is also associated with physical health problems in adulthood. It is theorized that this is a consequence of the substance abuse, mental health issues and other consequences that survivors of child sexual abuse face.
- Generally, adult victims of child sexual abuse have higher rates of health care utilization and report significantly more health complaints compared to adults without a child sexual abuse history. This is true for both self-reported doctor's visits and objective examination of medical records. These health problems represent a burden both to the survivor and the healthcare system.
- Adult survivors of child sexual abuse are at greater risk of a wide range of conditions that are non-life threatening and are potentially psychosomatic in nature. These include fibromyalgia, severe premenstrual syndrome, chronic headaches, irritable bowel syndrome and a wide range of reproductive and sexual health complaints,

including excessive bleeding, amenorrhea, pain during intercourse and menstrual irregularity.

- Not only do survivors of child sexual abuse have more minor health conditions, but they are also at greater risk for more serious conditions as well. Adults with a history of child sexual abuse are 30% more likely than their non-abused peers to have a serious medical condition such as diabetes, cancer, heart problems, stroke or hypertension.[84]
- Male sexual abuse survivors have twice the HIV-infection rate of non-abused males. In a study of HIV-infected 12 to 20-year-olds, 41% reported a sexual abuse history.
- Adult survivors of child sexual abuse are more likely to become involved in crime, both as a perpetrator and as a victim. This is likely a product of a higher risk for substance abuse problems and associated lifestyle factors.
- Adult survivors are more than twice as likely to be arrested for a property offense than their non-abused peers (9.3% versus 4.4%). As adults, child sexual abuse victims were almost twice as likely to be arrested for a violent offense as the general population (20.4% versus 10.7%). Males who have been sexually abused are more likely to violently victimize others.

WARNING SIGNS IN CHILDREN AND ADOLESCENTS OF POSSIBLE CHILD SEXUAL ABUSE

Any one sign doesn't mean that a child was sexually abused, but the presence of several suggests that you begin asking questions and consider seeking help. Keep in mind that some of these signs can emerge at other times of stress such as:

- During a divorce
- Death of a family member or pet
- Problems at school or with friends
- Other anxiety-inducing or traumatic events

Behavior you may see in a child or adolescent:

- Has nightmares or other sleep problems without an explanation
- Seems distracted or distant at odd times
- Has a sudden change in eating habits
- Refuses to eat
- Loses or drastically increases appetite
- Has trouble swallowing
- Sudden mood swings: rage, fear, insecurity or withdrawal
- Leaves "clues" that seem likely to provoke a discussion about sexual issues
- Writes, draws, plays or dreams of sexual or frightening images
- Develops new or unusual fear of certain people or places
- Refuses to talk about a secret shared with an adult or older child
- Talks about a new older friend
- Suddenly has money, toys or other gifts without reason
- Thinks of self or body as repulsive, dirty or bad
- Exhibits adult-like sexual behaviors, language, and knowledge

Signs more typical of younger children:

- An older child behaving like a younger child (such as bed-wetting or thumb sucking)
- Has new words for private body parts
- Resists removing clothes when appropriate times (bath, bed, toileting, diapering)
- Asks other children to behave sexually or play sexual games

- Mimics adult-like sexual behaviors with toys or stuffed animal
- Wetting and soiling accidents unrelated to toilet training
- Signs more typical in adolescents:
- Self-injury (cutting, burning)
- Inadequate personal hygiene
- Drug and alcohol abuse
- Sexual promiscuity
- Running away from home
- Depression, anxiety
- Suicidal attempts
- Fear of intimacy or closeness
- Compulsive eating or dieting

Physical warning signs:

- Pain, discoloration, bleeding or discharges in genitals, anus or mouth
- Persistent or recurring pain during urination and bowel movements

REPORTING ABUSE

Every community has its own set of laws governing how, and to whom, a report regarding suspicion of child sexual abuse should be made. Most communities also have a mandatory reporting structure for professionals working with children and in many jurisdictions a failure to report child sexual abuse would constitute a crime. Typically, the reporting law leaves the final determination as to whether or not abuse occurred to the investigators, not the reporter.

It is important that health workers are aware of the laws governing the reporting of child sexual abuse as it applies in their own area. Not every community will have such legislation, and under these circumstances, the health professional will need to decide what will be the most effective course of action to take in order to try to protect the child from further abuse.

Researchers estimate that 38% of child victims disclose the fact that they have been sexually abused. Of these, 40% tell a close friend, rather than an adult or authority. These "friend-to-friend" disclosures do not always result in reports. This means that the vast majority of child sexual abuse incidents are never reported to authorities, though research suggests that disclosure rates to authorities may be increasing.

False reports of child sexual abuse made by children are rare. It is estimated that only 4 to 8% of child sexual abuse reports are fabricated. Most of the fabricated reports are made by adults involved in custody disputes or by adolescents.

ASSESSMENT AND EXAMINATION OF CHILDREN:

General Considerations

Whereas adult victims of sexual violence often present as a medical emergency, Children are brought to the attention of the health care professional through a variety of routes and circumstances

- A child sexual abuse allegation has been reported and there is a request for an examination by the child protection authorities and/or the police.
- A child is brought by a family member or referred by a health care professional because an allegation has been made but not reported to authorities.
- Behavioral or physical indicators have been identified (e.g. by a caregiver, health care professional, teacher) and a further evaluation has been requested. The timing

and extent of the physical examination depends on the nature of the presenting complaint, the availability of resources in the community, the need for forensic evidence, and the expertise and style of the health professional caring for the child . Decisions about the timing of the physical examination should be based on the length of time that has elapsed since the child last had contact with the alleged perpetrator.

As a Guiding Rule

- If last contact was more than 72 hours previously and the child has no medical symptoms, an examination is needed as soon as possible but not urgently.
- If last contact was within 72 hours and the child is complaining of symptoms (i.e. pain, bleeding, discharge), the child should be seen immediately; physical examination should be performed.
- Findings that may indicate sexual abuse include: abrasions or bruising of genitalia; tearing (new or healed) in the posterior aspect of the hymen; decreased hymenal tissue; injury to or scarring of the fourchette, fossa navicularis, or hymen; and anal lacerations or bruising. Physicians also should assess the child's sexual maturity and evaluate for signs of physical abuse, neglect, and self-injury.
- Abnormal findings, defensively incurred bruises on the arms and legs, and signs of trauma should be documented. Detailed records will be useful if legal action is taken.

The American Association of Pediatrics recommends testing for STDs depending on various factors (e.g., age, type of contact, signs or symptoms of the disease, community prevalence of disease). Gonorrhea, syphilis, human immunodeficiency virus infection, and Chlamydia trachomatis infection are diagnostic for sexual abuse and warrant a report to the appropriate agency. Trichomonas vaginalis is highly suspicious, and Chlamydia infection or herpes simplex virus lesions in the genital area also should be reported.

Children who have been sexually abused should be assessed by a physician and mental health professional. At follow-up examination, physicians should assess the healing of injuries, presence of STDs, and emotional recovery.

CHILD INTERVIEW

Child interview data may be gathered in one or more interviews, depending on the particular child, the professional conducting the interview, and the safety of the child's living arrangement. The interviewer must initially spend time getting to know the child. This allows the interviewer to learn about the child's life circumstances and possible context of abuse and to ascertain the child's developmental level, modes of communication, the child's affective or emotional state(s), and overall functioning, including the child's competency. With young children, this part of the assessment usually involves play activity with some questions. With older children, the interviewer is likely to rely primarily on talking to the child and asking questions. At this point, questions are usually about the child's life in general and are neutral. They might include queries about the child, as well as her/his school, friends, and family.

Either before, during, or following this general discussion, the interviewer speaks to the child about why she/he is being seen or how the information the child gives will be used. If the interview is to be taped or there are people behind the one-way mirror, the child should be informed. This material is communicated at the child's developmental level and varies with the circumstances of the case.

Information elicited, statements recorded, and behavior observed during this initial phase of the interview often lead naturally into a discussion of possible sexual abuse.

TECHNIQUES FOR INTERVIEWING THE CHILD

A variety of techniques can be used in trying to elicit information from the child. Appropriate questions and several types of media or props – anatomically explicit dolls, anatomical drawings, picture drawing, storytelling, and the doll house – are used.

Risk Assessment

If it is determined by law enforcement that a child has been sexually abused, the case is one of intrafamilial abuse, and the child is at home, then it is necessary to make a determination of risk to the child if she/he stays in that environment. Following are three types of potential risk:

- Risk of additional sexual abuse
- Risk of physical abuse
- Risk of emotional maltreatment

Types of Emotional Risk

In most instances, the child is at greater risk for emotional maltreatment than additional sexual abuse immediately after disclosure.

There are a variety of types of emotional abuse the victim may suffer:

- The child may be disbelieved by her/his mother, siblings, and/or extended family.
- The child may be blamed for the sexual abuse. She/he may be told she/he was seductive. The child may believe she/he allowed it because she/he got special favors from the offender.
- The child may be rejected by her/his family. Mother is angry at her/him. The child's siblings are angry because she/he has caused them embarrassment and loss of their father.
- The child may be blamed for the consequences of disclosure. Because she/he told, the father is going to have to leave the home, going to lose his job, going to jail. Now the mother will have to divorce the father. Now the family has to go on public assistance.
- The child may be pressured to recant.

Factors to Consider in Risk Assessment

If professionals determine that the child is at risk for future sexual, physical, or emotional maltreatment, then some plan should be made to protect her/him. Making a determination of risk is no easy task. Families may be quite secretive. Furthermore, decisions may need to be made on an emergency basis without complete information. Nevertheless, the following factors need to be considered:

1. Type(s) of sexual abuse:

   The more intrusive the sexual acts and the greater the number of types of sexual activities, riskier is the situation. However, risk in situations involving "just" fondling should not be minimized.

2. Characteristics of the abuse situation- Relevant characteristics are frequency of sexual activity, its duration, the presence or absence of force, and the use of threats. The more frequent and the longer the abuse has gone on, the harder it will be for the offender to refrain. The use of force and threats also signals increased risk. If the

threats are manipulative, such as "You'll break up the family if you tell," the risk is for emotional maltreatment. If the threats are of bodily harm, then the risk is for physical abuse.

3. Victim age- Generally, younger victims are more vulnerable than older ones.
4. Relationship between victim and offender- As a rule, the greater the degree of relatedness, the greater the risk, especially for emotional abuse. Further, an offender who lives with the family poses a greater threat for sexual and emotional abuse than one outside the family.
5. Number of victims- The more children the offender has sexually abused, the greater difficulty he will have controlling his sexual behavior.
6. Number of offenders- Multiple offenders, especially if they are all within the family, means that the family provides a very risky environment.
7. Reactions and functioning of the non-offending parent- As noted earlier, factors include the mother's reaction to knowledge of the sexual abuse, her relationship with the victim, and her level of dependency on the offender. If she disbelieves the child, is unwilling to attend to the child's best interest, has a poor relationship with the child, or is dependent on the offender, then the child is at risk for emotional abuse and perhaps additional sexual abuse in the home.
8. Reaction of the offender- As noted earlier, a confession, while unlikely, would mean less risk for the victim. Greater risk exists if the alleged offender denies the sexual abuse, especially if he blames the victim for disclosure. In either case, the offender's continued presence in the home poses a greater risk of abuse and emotional maltreatment.
9. The presence of other problems in family functioning- These problems might include substance abuse, family violence, both, spouse abuse and child abuse, mental illness, and mental retardation. Their effect depends on how many of these problems exist in the family, who has the problem, and the severity of the problem. However, their presence generally increases risk to the victim.
10. The choices are generally two – remove the offender or remove the victim. There is professional agreement that removal of the offender is preferable. Even though this strategy may not be as certain in preventing additional sexual, physical, and emotional abuse, it has the considerable advantage of providing a clear message to the victim, the offender, and the family that he is the person who has done something wrong and that this is serious.

If he denies the abuse, the offender's removal minimizes challenges to the child's sense of reality and anxiety about whether he/she or the offender will be believed. Even if the offender admits and is willing to seek treatment, he should be asked or ordered to leave until a clinical decision is made that he should return. This action decreases opportunities for the offender to minimize the abuse and to manipulate the child and other family members into feeling sorry for him, placing responsibility for his abusive behavior on others or circumstances, and minimizing the damage to himself.

However, an additional condition for keeping the victim in the home and removing the offender is the mother's support of the child, her ability to resist pressures from the offender, and her more general ability to handle stress related to sexual abuse and its disclosure. Finally, if the victim wants to be removed, this wish should be honoured.

TREATMENT OF VICTIMS OF SEXUAL ABUSE

Treatment of child sexual abuse is a complex process. Orchestration of treatment in the child's best interest is a genuine challenge. Moreover, it is often difficult to know how to proceed because there are so few outcome studies of treatment effectiveness.

Treat STDs with appropriate medications based on the infection and the child's age and weight. In post-menarchal children, consider the possibility of pregnancy.

Here, case management issues are discussed; the focus of the discussion is primarily on intra-familial.

CASE MANAGEMENT CONSIDERATIONS

The following issues are the most important:

- Separation of the child and/or the offender from the family,
- The role of the juvenile court,
- The role of the criminal court, the treatment plan for the family
- Visitation, and
- Family reunification.

The treating team meets periodically to assess progress and make future plans. Because of the complexity of case management decisions and the fact that a decision in one realm can have an impact on other aspects of the case, especially on treatment progress and outcome, multidisciplinary decision making is crucial. In the absence of a multidisciplinary team, such decisions should be made in consultation with other relevant professionals.

Before the implementation of the treatment plan, the following case management decisions should be addressed:

- Should the child remain a part of the family?
- Do the courts have a role in the case?
- Is there a question of visitation?

Should the Child Live with the Family?

The preferred outcome in cases of sexual abuse, as in other types of child maltreatment, is that after intervention the family will be intact. Generally, at the time of disclosure of the sexual abuse, the offender is not separated from the family. The victim may be removed if the mother is unable or unwilling to protect and support the victim or if the victim wishes to be removed. Many professionals advocate the removal of the offender even in circumstances in which the victim is removed.

After these initial decisions, a longer term plan must be made about whether the child should be a part of the family and, if so, whether or not that family should include both parents. This plan will be based on an assessment of each parent. Aspects of the functioning of both parents outlined previously in the discussion of risk assessment should be examined in deciding about the child's future living situation.

These include the following factors for the offender:

- The extent of the offender's sexually abusive behavior;
- The degree to which the offender takes responsibility for the sexual abuse;
- The number and severity of the offender's other problems, for example;

- Substance Abuse,
- Violent behavior,
- Mental illness, and
- Mental Retardation.

Regarding the non-offending parent, the following factors should be assessed:

- Reaction to knowledge about the sexual abuse,
- Quality of relationship with the victim,
- Level of dependency on the offender, and
- The number and severity of other problems.

Other possible problems are similar for the non-offending parent and the offending parent. However; the parents are usually more complex. Probably in the majority of cases, the parents present a mixed picture, rather than appearing to have either a very good or bad prognosis. Moreover, there may be gaps in information about the family when treatment planning is undertaken, and parental functioning is not static. Progress or lack of progress in treatment may result in reconsideration of the initial placement and treatment plan. Because of these complexities, most sexually abusive families should and do receive a trial of treatment. This generally entails individual treatment for all parties and the appropriate use of groups. Initial case decisions are periodically evaluated based on treatment outcome and reassessed accordingly.

There is also increasing consensus that criminal charges should be filed, even though the offender appears treatable. Some professionals feel that even treatable offenders should do some jail time, while others see the criminal process as a means of ensuring that the treatable offender will take responsibility for his behavior and/or enter into treatment.

In addition, factors related to the child should also be considered. These include the child's wishes. To be more precise, if the child does not wish for a reunified family, that desire should be given a great deal of weight. A child's wish for the offender not to leave home, however, should generally not be granted. In addition, some sexually abused children are so damaged, because of the abuse and other conditions, that they require specialized care outside the home.

ROLE OF THE COURTS

Two or three courts are potentially involved in a sexual abuse case—the Juvenile Court, responsible for child protection; the Criminal Court, responsible for offender prosecution; and the Divorce Court, if either parent decides to pursue divorce.

Court involvement can be either a help or a hindrance to therapeutic goals. The challenge is to integrate court involvement into the overall intervention. Early decisions about the role of the court can facilitate its role in the therapeutic process.

The court can be helpful in compelling family members, especially offenders, into treatment; in protecting victims and families from offenders; and in effecting alternative living situations for offenders (or victims, if necessary).

Court involvement can be problematic because legal safeguards for the defendant may prevent certain evidence from being admitted; because the adversarial process may interfere with the therapeutic process, including disruption of offender treatment by incarceration; and because it allows procedural delays that may prevent timely intervention.

Finally, testifying in court may have a positive or negative effect on the child. The effect, in part, depends on its outcome. That is, if the case is won, the impact of court testimony is more likely to be positive. Victims may gain a sense of mastery over the sexual abuse from testifying. On the other hand, victims may experience court testimony as additional trauma. Some are required to confront their abusers, endure lengthy cross-examination, and reveal shameful experiences to an audience. If possible, the courtroom should be cleared during the child's appearance.

TREATMENT MODALITIES

An approach to treatment that addresses prerequisite and contributing causes of sexual abuse and meets the treatment needs of the victim, family, and the offender must be multimodal. Ideally, individual, dyadic, family and group treatment modalities should be available, especially if reintegration of the offender and/or the victim into the family is planned. The types of treatment and their uses will be discussed as follows:

Group therapy is generally regarded as the treatment of choice for sexual abuse. However, usually groups are offered concurrent with other treatment modalities, and some clients may need individual treatment before they are ready for group therapy. Furthermore, there will be a few clients who are either too disturbed or too disruptive to be in group treatment.

Groups are appropriate for victims, siblings of victims, mothers of victims, offenders, and adult survivors of sexual abuse. In addition, "generic" groups that include offenders, parents of victims, and survivors of sexual abuse have been found to be very powerful and effective for all parties involved.

Groups may be time-limited, long-term, or open-ended. They may deal with specific issues (e.g., relapse prevention, sex education, or protection from future sexual abuse), or they may deal with a range of issues. Some programs have "orientation" groups for new clients, usually with separate groups for children and adults.

Victim's and offender's groups have been brought together for occasional sessions. Models that have concurrent groups for victims or children and their non-offending parents, where from time to time the two groups join for activities, are very productive.

Individual treatment is appropriate for the victim, offender, and mother of the victim (as well as for siblings of victims and survivors). As a rule, an initial function and a major one for individual treatment are alliance building. All parties have to learn to trust the therapist and come to believe that change is possible and desirable. The members of this triad may have different levels of commitment to therapy, with the victim usually the most invested and the offender the least.

Dyadic treatment is used to enhance and/or repair damage to the mother-daughter relationship, the husband-wife relationship, and the father-daughter relationship, as well as to deal with issues initially addressed in individual treatment.

Family therapy is the culmination of the treatment process and is usually not undertaken until there has been a determination that reunification is in the victim's best interest.

Multiple therapists can be very helpful. Such a complex series of interventions can rarely be provided by one individual. If possible, two therapists should be involved, even if it is only one person doing the group work and another individual, dyadic, and family work.

Sexually abusive families are very difficult to work with, and therapists need one another's support. Such families are crisis-ridden and multi-problem, making it very difficult for one person to have total responsibility for the family.

Assigning a different therapist to the victim and to the offender "recreates," although artificially, a family boundary that was crossed when the sexual abuse occurred. It also enhances a sense of privacy and safety for the victim—two elements violated by the offender.

In addition, co-therapy, using both a male and female therapist, has a considerable therapeutic advantage. It exposes family members to appropriate role models of both sexes. Co-therapy also enhances the ability of clinicians to effect change because of the leverage it allows, particularly in group therapy.

TREATMENT FOR EMOTIONAL REACTIONS TO SEXUAL ABUSE

Three common emotional consequences of sexual victimization:

Feeling responsible

An offender may make the victim feel responsible for the sexual abuse, for the offender's well-being, and/or for the consequences of disclosure. Victims may also feel guilty for not having stopped the sexual abuse as well as for any positive aspects of the abuse, such as physical pleasure, the special attention given by the offender, or an opportunity to have control over other family members because of "the secret."

The role of the clinician is to help the child understand intellectually and accept emotionally that the child was not responsible. The adult sexually abused the child; the child did not sexually abuse the adult. It was the adult's job – not the child's – to stop or prevent the abuse.

Altered Sense of Self

Guilt feelings, as well as the invasive and intrusive nature of the sexual activity, impact negatively on the child's sense of self and self-esteem. As Sgroi puts it, victims suffer from "damaged goods" syndrome. The effect is both physical, in that children have an altered sense of their bodies, and psychological, in that children may see themselves as markedly different from their peers.

The task of the therapist is to make victims feel whole and good about themselves again. Work, mentioned above, that addresses the issue of self-blame is helpful. However, so are interventions that help children view themselves as more than merely victims of sexual abuse. Normalizing and ego-enhancing activities, such as doing well in school, participating in sports, getting involved in scouts, or helping a younger victim, can be very important in victim recovery.

Anxiety and fear to be discussed here are related to the traumatic impact of the abuse per se on the child rather than environmental responses to it. The victim develops phobic reactions to the event, the offender, and to other aspects of the abuse. Experiences that evoke recollections of the abuse come to elicit anxiety. In some children, this anxiety and phobias become pervasive and crippling because of the level of avoidance they engage in to reduce their stress.

Before treating the child's fears and anxiety, the therapist must be sure the child is not being sexually abused or at risk for sexual abuse. Then the therapist engages the victim in a series of interventions that allow her/him to gradually deal with the abuse and related phobias and anxiety in ways that usually avoid excessive stress and allow mastery. These may include discussions, play therapy, or interventions in the child's environment. For example, the victim may be encouraged to ventilate by talking about the abuse and accompanying feelings, thereby reducing the level of distress related to it. Similarly, a child who is phobic about being left with a babysitter may be left with a relative first for short and then longer time periods, then with a babysitter for brief and then longer periods and thereby be desensitized to babysitting situations.

Additional emotional reactions may be found

Depending on the circumstances of the victimization and the child's personality, she/he may react with regression, anger, depression, revulsion, or posttraumatic stress disorder to sexual abuse. These emotional reactions are likely to manifest themselves in problematic behavior. These behavior's will be discussed in the next section.

TREATMENT FOR BehaviorAL REACTIONS TO SEXUAL ABUSE

Sexualized behavior

A serious reaction is sexualized behavior. Children who have been sexually victimized may masturbate excessively and openly or sexually interact with other people. Every act of sexualized behavior has the potential for increasing the probability of future acts. Not only is the activity likely to be physically pleasurable, but it may also enhance the child's view of her/himself as a sexually acting out person. Such acts may also stigmatize the child, which has a negative impact on the child's sense of self.

Clinicians should work to diminish and/or eliminate sexualized behavior through teaching behavioral controls. Sexual acting out may be controlled, for example, by teaching the child to masturbate privately. Behavior management techniques, which can involve rewarding "sex-free" days and using "time-out" for sexual acting out, can be taught to the child's caretaker. In addition, the child's energies that might have gone into sexual behavior can be channeled into more age-appropriate activities by having a caretaker monitor the child, interrupt any sexual acting out, and provide opportunities for positive alternative behaviors. These interventions are conducted with the child's caretaker and/or in dyadic work with child and caretaker.

One of the reasons treatment of sexualized behavior is so essential is because of a recently recognized phenomenon called the victim to offender cycle. Both male and female victims are at risk for this problem. Many offenders begin as victims, whose response to sexual abuse is to identify with the aggressor and to sexually act out in order to cope with their own sense of vulnerability and trauma. Professionals must recognize the potential danger of allowing sexualized behaviors to go untreated, which is that the child then is at risk for becoming first an adolescent offender and eventually an adult offender. The child not only damages him/herself but also may cause grave harm to many other children over the course of time.

Other behavior problems Other behavioral reactions to sexual abuse include such problems as aggression toward people and animals, running away, self-harm (cutting or burning), criminal activity, substance abuse, suicidal behavior, hyperactivity, sleep problems, eating problems, and toileting problems.

Some of these problems, for example, difficulties with sleep, eating, toileting, and being alone, may be acute after disclosure but diminish over time and eventually disappear. Short-term intervention, labeling the behavioral problems as common reactions and helping the victim resolve the underlying emotional or cognitive issues is generally helpful. Parents are encouraged to be understanding.

Treatment strategies for all behavioral problems include helping the victim understand the relationship between the behaviors' and the sexual abuse and emotional or cognitive reactions to it; helping the child develop insight into the self-destructive nature of some of these behaviors; assisting the victim in more appropriate expression of the emotions, for example, anger; and behavioral interventions to diminish and eliminate problematic behavior. With older children, group therapy is usually very useful in addressing these problems.

TREATMENT TO COGNITIVE REACTIONS TO SEXUAL ABUSE

An important part of treatment of victims of sexual abuse is to help them understand the meaning of the abuse. This includes learning what appropriate and inappropriate touching entails; what is wrong about sexual activity between adults and children, if they do not know this; why adults or a particular adult was sexual with them; and in some cases, why they were chosen as targets and what that means to them. How these issues are addressed will vary with the child's developmental stage. They may be more adequately dealt with in group treatment than individual therapy, and sometimes having the offender take full responsibility for the abuse in dyadic therapy with the victim is useful.

Moreover, an adequate explanation for a child at a young age may not be sufficient as she/he grows older. Thus, this particular issue will need to be addressed at a more sophisticated level as the child matures. This may be done by a parent but in some cases will need to be done by a therapist.

PROTECTION FROM FUTURE VICTIMIZATION

Treatment of victimized children needs to include strategies for future protection. Teaching children to say no and tell someone may be useful, especially if the material is presented in a group setting and there are opportunities to role play resisting sexual advances. Specific protective strategies involving family members and helping professionals need to be developed in intra-familial sexual abuse situations. Additionally, the therapist must appreciate that placing even partial responsibility for self-protection on the victim is potentially an overwhelming burden.

Treatment Issues for the Mother (Non-offending Parent)

Although the discussion that follows refers specifically to mothers as non-offending parents, much of the material is also applicable to non-offending fathers. Treatment issues for mothers of victims can be categorized under the following four general headings.

Issues related to the

- Sexual abuse,
- Mother-Victim Relationship

- Offender (spouse), and
- Other Personal Issues.

These issues are particularly relevant to cases involving mothers in intra-familial sexual abuse but also can be important when other persons are the abusers. Like victim treatment issues, they are interrelated, and there may be other issues that are salient in a given case. The relationship of the mother's treatment issues to factors to be assessed in making decisions about victim reunification with the family will become apparent.

Issues Related to the Sexual Abuse

It is difficult for most people, including mothers of victims, to understand why an adult might want to be sexual with a child. This is often the first issue that the clinician must address with the mother. This may be especially difficult for the mother to understand if the offender is her spouse or another close relative.

The therapist may offer professional understanding into the general causes of sexual abuse or those specific to the case. The parent might also be given material to read. However, group involvement, in either a generic sexual abuse or mothers' group, may be the most effective method for addressing this issue.

A related issue is that of believing the victim's disclosure of sexual abuse. Many parents will try to explain it away. As noted in the discussion of assessment of the nonoffending parent, coming to believe a victim is usually a process, rather than instantaneous.

The therapist may describe what in the child's disclosure makes her/him believe the child or speak generally about the conclusion that children rarely make false allegations and the reasons for that belief. However, group treatment, in which the mother is confronted by others who have also struggled with disbelief, is often the most effective mode for dealing with this issue.

Finally, the therapist will want to help the mother understand her role in the abuse, if she has had one. The nonoffending parent is not to blame for the victimization but in some instances may have contributed to risk of abuse or prolonged abuse, for example, by leaving the child for long periods of time with the offender or by discounting the child's early disclosures.

Interestingly, a good prognosis is suggested when a mother feels very guilty and the therapist must work to alleviate her sense of responsibility. Conversely, a poorer prognosis is indicated when the mother sees herself as absolutely blameless and the therapist has to point out things that the mother might have, done differently that could have prevented or minimized the abuse. As with other issues related to the abuse, this issue may be best dealt with in group therapy.

Issues Related to the Mother-Victim Relationship

Treatment of intrafamilial sexual abuse that results in successful reunification of the family rests upon the mother's relationship with the victim. This may be a very problematic relationship at the time of disclosure. The offender may have engaged in manipulations that have alienated mother and victim from one another. The victim may have developed problematic behaviors because of the abuse, which have damaged her relationship with the mother. The consequences of disclosure may be blamed on the victim, or the mother may never have related well to the victim (or other people).

This problem appears to be less severe with boy victims. Mothers are more likely to be supportive of them. In part, this is because when boys are sexually abused, the offender is more often, than with girls, someone outside the family. Moreover, when victimized within the family, boys tend to be abused along with their sisters, meaning the mother is less likely to regard a single child as to blame or as the source of her frustrations. However, this phenomenon may also relate to differences in role relationships between mothers and daughters and mothers and sons.

The therapist tries to enhance the mother-victim relationship by assisting the mother in developing empathy for the victim; by facilitating their communication; by helping them resolve on-going problems in their relationship, such as disputes regarding bedtime or chores; and by helping them develop opportunities for mutually enjoyable experiences. Initial work is usually done in individual treatment with the mother, and later within the mother-child dyad.

Improving the mother-child relationship is generally a prerequisite to assisting the mother in being protective of her child in the future. Although interventions are employed to help the offender control his behavior in the future, the major source of protection for the child is the mother.

Intervention to make the mother more protective is implemented in a variety of ways. If the mother has a more positive relationship with the child, she will be more predisposed to protect the child. Treatment to improve the mother-child communication should enhance the likelihood the child will tell mother. Moreover, the therapist usually works with both the child and the mother to encourage communication specifically about the child's safety.

Especially if the family has not been separated or, if separated, as the family is reunited, specific guidance should be given to the mother regarding safety. For example, she may be instructed not to leave the child alone with the offender, not to let the offender bathe the child, not to allow the offender any control over the child's activities, and/or not to give the offender the responsibility for disciplining the child. How long these protections remain in place will depend on the case.

Finally, the therapist usually helps the mother develop a specific plan in case the offender does reoffend. Her plan is communicated to the victim, the offender, and the rest of the family. It can often involve dissolving the marriage.

Issues Related to the Offender (Spouse)

In cases of intra-familial sexual abuse, the mother must decide whether she wants to sever her relationship with the offender or try to salvage the relationship. Some mothers decide at the time of disclosure to terminate the relationship or, alternatively, to work to preserve it.

For others, this decision takes time and observation of the offender's progress or lack thereof in treatment. Still others are indecisive and change their minds more than once.

The clinician may have an opinion about what the mother should do. However, it is wise to allow the mother to make her own decision. This does not preclude sharing opinions about the offender's treatability and the likelihood of the victim remaining or returning home should the mother choose to stay with an untreated or untreatable offender.

In cases in which the offender is the mother's partner, regardless of the decision to leave or to stay, the mother will need to address her relationships with men. The goal is to help her gain some insight into these relationships, including that with the offender, and to understand their problematic aspects. If she intends to stay with the offender, she must be assisted in changing that relationship. If she leaves him, the goal of insight is to help her in future relationships. Group treatment with other mothers is particularly useful in this work. Of course, if her intention is to preserve the relationship with the offender, dyadic work with the offender is necessary.

Often mothers are very dependent on the men who have abused their children. In most instances, it is important to help her become less dependent so that she will be better able to seek what is in her children's and her interest, should there be a conflict between the offender's interest and that of the rest of the family.

Independence may be fostered by involving the mother in activities outside the home, including therapy; enhancing her financial independence; encouraging her to do things without his assistance; and facilitating her assertiveness when they are in conflict. Opportunities for these types of interventions may present themselves quite naturally if the offender must leave the home at the time of disclosure of the sexual abuse. Because of the mother's need to function autonomously in his absence, he may return home to a situation quite different from the one he left.

Other Personal Issues

Most mothers must deal with other issues related to current functioning and past experiences in therapy. The most common issue regarding current functioning is low self-esteem. However, other issues, such as substance abuse, experiences of violence, dependency, and emotional problems, often need to be addressed as well.

The most common issue in terms of past trauma is having been sexually victimized themselves. Such an experience can have a variety of implications in terms of the mother's ability to deal with her children's sexual abuse. For example, at the time of disclosure, a mother may be so overwhelmed because of her own abuse that she cannot deal with her child's victimization. In such instances, her abuse may have to be addressed first. Her own victimization may have an impact on her willingness to believe the victim, her ability to discern risky situations (she may not note them), and her choices of partners, playing a role in her choosing someone who is sexual with children. In addition, it may cause her to mistakenly believe her children are being victimized.

Treatment Issues for the Father as the Offender
Although the following discussion will refer to the father as the offender, it is equally applicable to cases involving stepfathers and unmarried partners of mothers who are offenders. It is also relevant to some situations involving other intra-familial offenders. Treatment issues for the offending fathers can be broadly defined as falling into three categories, issues related to the:

- Father's past sexual victimization of children,
- Father's possible future victimization of children, and
- Other dysfunctional behaviors' and problems.

These broad categories tend to be overlapping.

Issues Related to the Father's Past Sexual Abuse of Children

In many cases, the first challenge for the clinician is obtaining a confession of the sexual offenses. Many fathers are too ashamed to admit what they have done. Others are reluctant to disclose their abuse during litigation because they are afraid of its impact on the outcome. They may be more willing once the court case is resolved. Others are ordered into treatment by the court while continuing to protest their innocence.

Operationally, confession means an admission to all of the acts the child has described. However, it is common for the child not to disclose all of the abuse; therefore, it is important for the offender's therapist to stay in touch with the victim's therapist in case there are additional disclosures. (In treating intra-familial sexual abuse, it is important for each family member to consent to share information with each therapist treating each family member.) To obtain a confession, the therapist actively confronts the father with the information on his offenses provided by the victim and others. In addition, group treatment, in which the father observes others confessing their victimizing behavior, can facilitate full disclosure.

With confession must come an acceptance of responsibility for the abusive acts. That is, the father must disvow any past excuses, such as his wife was not giving him sex or that he was drunk at the time. He must not minimize the behavior by saying, for example, "it only happened once," "there was no penetration involved," or "I stopped when she asked me to." As is probably apparent, it is extremely difficult to know when the offender has actually accepted responsibility rather than saying what he thinks the therapist wants to hear. Again, the use of group treatment can be especially helpful because other offenders may be more capable of discerning and confronting deception than a therapist.

A related task of treatment is for the father to appreciate the harm the abuse has caused the victim, his partner, and finally himself. There may be others affected as well, for example, siblings of the victim and the extended family. Some sort of communication from the victim and the offender's partner about the effects of the abuse on them can be useful. This may be in the form of a letter, a video or audiotape, or a face-to-face confrontation involving the therapist. Generic groups in which offenders are confronted by adult survivors and mothers of victims, other than the offender's own, can facilitate these insights. Written accounts, by victims, journalists, and professionals, of the impact on victims may be used, and offenders' groups can be the context for this work. As with the issue of responsibility, being sure the father is doing more than saying the right thing is a significant challenge.

At some point in treatment after the offender has confessed, taken responsibility, and come to appreciate the harm he has done, a series of apologies should be made. The offender must apologize to the victim, to his partner, and to the family in intra-familial cases. There may be others who have been affected and deserve an apology as well. This is a process, not a single act, usually conducted in the context of dyadic or family treatment. The fact that the offender apologizes does not imply that the victim and others need to forgive him. These interventions need to be carefully orchestrated and controlled by the therapist. Only after the offender has completed the process, demonstrating an appreciation of the harm done, should his return home be considered.

A final treatment issue related to past abuse has to do with prevention. In order to prevent future sexual abuse, it is important for the offender and the therapist to understand why the offender sexually abuses children. In this regard, the model presented earlier in this chapter is relevant.

Thus, the treatment process involves coming to understand the offender's arousal pattern and why he acts on the arousal. Then contributing factors are explored.

Sexual arousal to children. Arousal patterns vary. They may be conceptualized as follows:

Child is the offender's primary sexual object

Some offenders' sexual preference, sometimes exclusively, is for children. The term pedophile is generally used to refer to this type of offender. Often pedophiles not only prefer children, but children of a particular age and sex. Pedophiles tend to have multiple victims and actively seek opportunities whereby they can have sexual access to children, by choosing vocations and avocations that afford them contact with children. A contributing factor to this type of arousal pattern is often traumatic childhood sexual experience.

Child is one of multiple sexual objects

Other offenders have multiple paraphilias or aberrant sexual preferences and sometimes normal sexual preferences as well. The behavior of these offenders is characterized by sexual contact with children but may also include rape of adults, promiscuity with adults, exposure, voyeurism, sadomasochism, group sex, bestiality, and other sexual acts. The term sexual addict is often applied to this type of offender. The contributing factors or etiology of this pattern of sexuality appear to be a combination of childhood and adolescent experiences.

Child is a situational sexual object

Finally, there are offenders whose normal sexual orientation is toward peers but who become aroused by children under certain circumstances. Factors that contribute to such arousal may include the absence of other sexual outlets, stresses affecting normal marital and/or peer relations and communications, child pornography, and physical exposure or contact to children that is sexually stimulating. Although initial sexual contact involving this type of offender may be situationally induced, the experience may be very gratifying. Clinical experience indicates this is likely to result in an increased desire for and preference for sex with children.

As may be apparent from the last point, although these three arousal patterns are presented as though they are discrete, they probably are not. For example, it may be inappropriate to classify some offenders as having either a primary orientation to children or to adults.

Understanding the offender's arousal patterns may be done by having the offender describe what he experiences about his victims as arousing, having him discuss in detail his sexually abusive behavior, having him reveal his sexual fantasies, or measuring his erectile responses to various visual and auditory sexual stimuli using the penile plethysmograph. Treatment prognosis with pedophiles and sexual addicts is much poorer than for those who have situational sexual arousal to children.

The propensity to act on arousal

There is research that suggests that a substantial minority of the male population experiences sexual arousal to children. (Comparable research has not been conducted on women.) However, it appears that a great many more men experience these feelings than act on them. The willingness to act on these feelings appears to be related to one or in most cases more than one of the following deficits:

- pervasive superego deficits,
- circumscribed superego deficits,
- cognitive distortions,
- impulse control difficulties, and
- diminished capacity

Persons whose superego deficits are pervasive have little or no conscience. The term psychopath is often applied to them. This condition is thought to be a result of early traumatic life experiences. Those who have some superego deficits may experience an absence of conscience related specifically to sexual activity or sexual activity with children, or they may generally have a weak or impaired superego. Some combination of early experience, lifestyle, and cultural norms may create this sort of superego. Differing in degree is the offender who has cognitive distortions related to his sexual deviance. He will have persuaded himself that sexual abuse is not bad or not so bad by such rationalizations as "The child won't know what I'm doing so it's not harmful" or "Everyone needs sex; this is my way." After the initial act, distortions may be "The child didn't resist, so she must have liked it," "There was no penetration so it wasn't really sexual abuse," or "It's my wife's fault because she withheld sex from me." Some offenders appreciate that what they do is wrong, but they do it anyway because they have poor impulse control.

Finally, some offenders experience diminished capacity, which enhances propensity to act on arousal. Typically, this is a temporary condition, and its most common cause is substance abuse. Thus, the offender acts on his arousal because alcohol or drugs have decreased his ability to control his behavior. Initial instances of victimization when drunk may occur without a prior plan. However, subsequently, the offender may drink so that he will have an excuse to abuse. Furthermore, after the initial acts, the attraction of the behavior itself may increase and chemicals are less necessary to diminish control. There can be other causes of diminished capacity. Offenders may lack adequate ability in handling stress, depression, anxiety, and/or anger in healthy ways. In addition, some persons suffer from chronic diminished capacity as a result of mental retardation or organic brain syndrome. If they experience arousal to children, it will make them at ongoing risk for sexual abuse.
Contributing factors- Some factors that may enhance arousal or increase the propensity to abuse have been described above. There may be other factors that act on these prerequisites and ones that independently contribute to risk for sexual abuse, for example, child behaviors, mother behaviors, and opportunity to sexually abuse.

It is an important part of the treatment process to understand why the offender has sexually abused children so that he can be empowered to gain control over his arousal and propensity to act on arousal. Some of the intervention that addresses contributing factors may be initiated with the offender alone, but much is done in the treatment of other individuals in the family and in dyadic and family work.

ISSUES RELATED TO POSSIBLE FUTURE SEXUAL ABUSE

As noted in the previous section, preventing future sexual abuse relies on understanding what made the offender abuse in the first place. In this section, interventions that address arousal to children and propensity to act on arousal are discussed.

Sexual Arousal to Children

It has already been pointed out that sexual and other trauma during childhood may play a role in later sexual arousal to children. However, understanding the relationship of the offender's previous history to his arousal patterns is probably the least useful in prevention of future sexual abuse. In fact, often offenders manipulate the treatment process so that past history becomes an excuse for their offending. In spite of this risk, for some offenders, understanding the origins of previously incomprehensible behavior can render it manageable. Moreover, realizing that what the offender learned about sex roles as a child was wrong can lead to the development of more appropriate definitions of sex role behavior.

When deviant arousal patterns have been defined, the therapist will attempt to change these patterns. That is, the therapist will endeavour to decrease sexual arousal to children and increase arousal to appropriate sex objects. This is done through a variety of behavioral interventions that rely on both respondent and operant conditioning. These techniques include aversive conditioning, covert sensitization, thought stopping, masturbatory satiation, behavioral rehearsal, systematic desensitization, and masturbatory reconditioning. These techniques are often used in conjunction with social skills training, empathy training, and behavioral assignments.

Behavioral interventions are exacting, and some require a laboratory setting. They also require the full cooperation of the client if they are to be successful. Moreover, the changes they create are not assumed to be permanent (nor are those from other types of intervention), and clients may need booster sessions. Many mental health professionals are untrained in and uncomfortable with behavioral interventions. However, to date they are the only therapeutic techniques that have been found, based on empirical evidence, to decrease sexual arousal. It behoves every clinician treating offenders to be familiar with these techniques and use those that can be suitably employed in his/her agency.

The Propensity to Act on Arousal

Two approaches may be used to address propensity to act: techniques that enhance superego functioning by taking responsibility for sexual abuse and relapse prevention. Offenders whose propensity to act is based on pervasive superego deficits will probably not respond to treatment to reduce this propensity. However, those who have circumscribed superego deficits or are engaged in cognitive distortions probably will respond to interventions to address superego deficits. Treatment that is focused on getting the offender to take responsibility for his abusive behavior, to appreciate its harm, to acknowledge the feelings of traumatized parties, and to make amends or reparation is meant to enhance the offender's superego functioning and eliminate cognitive distortions, thus decreasing the probability of his acting on arousal in the future. Making amends or reparation usually involves a physical (e.g., community service) or monetary consequence that may serve to teach empathy and inhibit further abuse. In addition, when an offender lacks a strong internalized superego, the fact that there will be consequences for re-offense, such as prison or his wife leaving him, serves as an external superego. The strength of such interventions is in their deterrent effect.

In recent years, sex offender therapists have experienced success by using relapse prevention strategies, a technique borrowed from addiction treatment, in their intervention. Relapse prevention addresses propensity to act based on impulse control problems, reduced inhibition, and diminished capacity. Relapse prevention assumes that there are emotional states and behaviors on the offender's part that precede and ultimately precipitate the sexually abusive behavior. Often the offender is unaware of these factors and believes that his behavior is out of his control.

The clinician assists the offender in understanding these precursors and helps him develop a plan to manage such situations so that he does not reoffend. The clinician uses disclosures from the offender and others, including the victim, to obtain an accurate understanding of the circumstances that led to offending. Obviously such an intervention requires a candid and cooperative offender.

With some offenders, particularly those with cognitive limitations and difficulty being introspective, the clinician merely teaches the offender to anticipate, identify, and avoid risky situations. Thus, the offender may be instructed that he cannot assist at summer camp anymore or he cannot be left alone with his daughter.

With other offenders, the clinician helps him understand the chain of events, often seemingly unrelated to the sexual abuse that precedes the victimization. This might include a series of procedures, such as the grooming process an offender may employ in the seduction of his victim, or acts such as getting upset with his wife and getting drunk after she goes to bed as a prelude to going into the daughter's room to molest her. The therapist then teaches the offender to interrupt the chain of events rather early while he still has control of his behavior. Thus, the pedophile is instructed to avoid driving by playgrounds, and the offender whose abuse is precipitated by drunkenness is instructed to abstain completely. If he has a serious substance abuse problem, he is sent to a substance abuse treatment program, either before treatment of his sexually abusive behavior is begun or in conjunction with sexual abuse treatment.

The relapse prevention plan is usually written out, and the offender carries it with him so he can refer to it when he thinks he is in a high-risk situation.

Moreover, there are numerous other ways the family and others can be involved in helping the offender prevent a relapse. Because most offenders experience more than one deficit leading to propensity to act, interventions that focus both on his taking responsibility and on relapse prevention are advised.

Other Dysfunctional Behaviors and Problems

The offender may experience many other problems, and often these are contributing factors to the sexual abuse. Examples might be violent behavior, problems with the law, poor parenting skills, marital discord, poor social skills, low self-esteem, lack of education, and unemployment.

These are appropriate foci of treatment, and indeed it may be necessary to treat them because they increase the risk for future sexual abuse. Nevertheless, it is crucial that the clinician not allow him/herself to become side tracked into only dealing with these other problems. Distraction can occur more easily than one might think if the offender refuses to admit to the sexual abuse or is reluctant to focus on it in treatment, yet is more than willing to work on his other problems. This pitfall is usually avoided if group therapy, which forces the offender to deal with his abuse, is a major component of the intervention and/or if there are several therapists involved in the case.

Box 35.1: Contribution of child psychiatric teams

Child and family
- Treatment for symptomatic persons
- Links with adult and forensic services
- Assist with investigation

District level
- Liaison with children's homes etc.
- Training
- Research and development
- Area Child Protection Committees
- Strategic planning

Societal
- Public policy
- National strategy
- Research and teaching

PREVENTION

The first step to protecting children from sexual abuse is educating parents about the nature of the problem.

Awareness about child sexual abuse—what it is and who commits it—opens the door to some simple steps. Parents can take to protect children. No one has more at stake or a more vested interest in protecting children than the people who gave them life. Awareness, education, and responsible parenting give a child the best tools for her or his defence—and the child may be more likely to tell an adult if something happens. Parents bear the primary responsibility for the safety and well-being of their children.

Here are some practical actions that parents can take to help protect their children from sexual abuse:

1. By virtue of their physical size, adults have power over children—and that increases a child's vulnerability. For example, parents and other authority figures teach children to "obey adults." When children hear this message, they may interpret it to mean that all adults have the authority to tell all children what to do, all the time. If this is a child's interpretation, then the message has created additional vulnerability for the child. Yet, some simple, common sense steps can help minimize a child's vulnerability.

For example:

- Do NOT insist that children hug or kiss relatives or friends. Let children express affection on their own terms.
- Let children know that their feelings are important to you. Intervene if you notice that your child is uncomfortable doing something that another adult asks him or her to do. Let the child know that you will protect him or her from this discomfort. That doesn't necessarily mean that you should let children off the hook when it comes to doing their chores or cleaning up a mess they've made.

2. Learn to recognize and take advantage of teachable moments with children. Be willing to openly discuss sensitive issues. The American Academy of Pediatrics recommends the following age-appropriate conversations with children:

- From ages 18 months to 3 years—begin teaching children the proper names for all body parts.
- Ages 3 to 5 years—teach children about private body parts and how to say "no" to anyone who touches them in a way that makes them feel uncomfortable. Give them

direct answers to questions about sex.

- Ages 5 to 8 years—talk about good touches and bad touches, and safety away from home.
- Ages 8 to 12 years—focus on personal safety issues.
- Ages 13 to 18 years—discuss issues such as rape, date rape, HIV, other sexually transmitted diseases, and unintended pregnancy. There are also professionals in the community who can provide assistance with forming age-appropriate responses to children's questions and concerns. Remember, regardless of the child's age: Take advantage of teachable moments.

3. Games are a great way to reinforce the lessons you teach your children about safety issues.
4. Teach children to say, "Stop it," to instructions that might encourage them to do things that they really do not want to do. Reinforce the rule that children should say, "Stop it," to requests or demands that make them uncomfortable, even if they think they should obey. A discussion of these rules can teach a child that there are some times when it is okay to say, "Stop it," and other times when it is okay to go along with the instructions..
5. Know where children spend their time. Get to know the adults who show up at the various locations in the community where children gather and where they play together. Pay attention when an adult seems to single out on a particular child for a relationship or for special attention. Warning signs include treats, gifts, vacations, or other special favours offered only to one specific child.
6. Make unannounced visits to the child's nursery, babysitter, day care center, or school. When choosing a nursery, day care center, or school, make sure that there are no areas where children play or work that are "off limits" to parents.
7. Find out if the child's school or religious education programs include a sex abuse prevention curriculum. If not, volunteer to be on a committee to establish such a program. Work with teachers to review available programs and make recommendations to school administrators.

DON'Ts:

1. Do NOT allow a child to go alone on "vacation" with any adult other than the child's parent.
2. Do NOT allow a child to spend the night alone with any adult other than the child's parent or another safe adult.
3. Except in the case of a serious emergency, Do NOT allow a child to travel alone—even for a very short distance—with any adult other than the child's parent or another safe adult. You should also prohibit children from accepting expensive gifts from an adult, particularly if one child is singled out for special attention.

Parents can make an important difference. However, without a supporting organization to help bring together a community's resources, experts, and commitment, parents are limited in their ability to impact community-wide child abuse prevention. That's where we can help.

BIBLIOGRAPHY

1. Abel, G. G., Mittleman, M. S., & Becker, J. V. (1985). "Sex offenders: Results of assessment and recommendations for treatment." In M. H. Ben-Aron, S. J. Hucker, & C.D. Webster

(Eds.),*Clinical Criminology: The assessment and treatment of criminal behavior* (pp. 207–220).

2. Association for the Treatment of Sexual Abusers (ATSA). (2000). *The effective legal management of juvenile sex offender.*
3. Acierno, R., Kilpatrick, D. G., Resnick, H. S., Saunders, B., de Arellano, M. & Best, C. (2000). Assault, PTSD, family substance use, and depression as risk factors for cigarette use in youth: Findings from the national survey of adolescents. *Journal of Traumatic Stress*, 13, 381-396.
4. Arnow, B. A. (2004). Relationships between childhood maltreatment, adult health and psychiatric outcomes, and medical utilization. *Journal of Clinical Psychiatry, 65 [suppl 12],* 10 – 15.
5. Banyard, V. L., Williams, L. M., & Siegel, J. A. (2001). The long-term mental health consequences of child sexual abuse: An exploratory study of the impact of multiple traumas in a sample of women. *Journal of Traumatic Stress*, 14, 697 – 715.
6. Broman-Fulks, J. J., Ruggiero, K. J., Hanson, R. F., Smith, D. W., Resnick, H. S., Kilpatrick, D. G., & Saunders, B. E. (2007). Sexual assault disclosure in relation to adolescent mental health: Results from the National Survey of Adolescents. *Journal of Clinical Child and Adolescent Psychology*, 36, 260 – 266.
7. Briere, J., & Elliott, D.M. (2003). Prevalence and psychological sequelae of self-reported childhood physical and sexual abuse in a general population sample of men and women. *Child Abuse & Neglect, 27*(10), 1205-1222.
8. Carter, C. A., Bottoms, B. L., & Levine, M. (1996). Linguistic and socioemotional influences on the accuracy of children's reports. *Law and Human Behavior, 20*(3), 335-358
9. Cohen, E., Groves, B., & Kracke, K. (2009). Understanding children's exposure to violence. *The Safe Start Center Series on Children Exposed to Violence, 1,* 1-8.
10. Cyr, M., McDu_, P., & Wright, J. (2006). Prevalence and predictions of dating violence among adolescent female victims of child sexual abuse. *Journal of Interpersonal Violence*, *21*(8), 1000-1017.
11. De Bellis, M. D., Spratt, E. G., & Hooper, S. R. (2011). Neurodevelopmental biology associated with childhood sexual abuse. *Journal of Child Sexual Abuse*, *20*(5), 548-587.
12. Douglas, E., & Finkelhor, D. (2005). Childhood Sexual Abuse Fact Sheet. Crimes Against Children Center, University of New Hampshire.
13. Dube, S. A., Anda, R. F., Whitfield, C. L., Brown, D. W., Felitti, D. J., Dong, M., & Giles, W. (2005). Long-term consequences of childhood sexual abuse by gender of the victim. *American Journal of Preventive Medicine*, 28, 430 – 437.
14. Day, A., Thurlow, K., & Woolliscroft, J. (2003). Working with childhood sexual abuse: A survey of mental health professionals.*Child Abuse & Neglect*, 27 , 191-198.
15. Dekker, A. et. al. (1990). The incidence of sexual abuse in HIV infected adolescents and young adults. *Journal of Adolescent Health Care*. vol. 11, no. 3.
16. Daignault, I.V. & Hebert, M. (2009). Profiles of school adaptation: Social, behavioral, and academic functioning in sexually abused girls. *Child Abuse & Neglect*, 33, 102-115.
17. Elliott, M., Browne, K., & Kilcoyne, J. (1995). Child sexual abuse prevention: What offenders tell us. *Child Abuse & Neglect*, 5, 579-594.
18. Everson, M., and Boat, B. (1989). False allegations of sexual abuse by children and adolescents.*Journal of the American Academy of Child and Adolescent Psychiatry.* 28, 2:230-35.
19. Fang, X., Brown, D., Florence, C., Mercy, J. (2012) The economic burden of child maltreatment in the United States and implications for prevention. *Child Abuse & Neglect, 36*:2,156–165
20. Finkelhor, D. (2012). Characteristics of crimes against juveniles. Durham, NH: Crimes against Children Research Center.
21. Finkelhor, D., & Jones, L. (2012). Have sexual abuse and physical abuse declined since the 1990s? Durham, NH: Crimes against Children Research Center.
22. Finkelhor, D. (1994). Current information on the scope and nature of child sexual abuse. *The Future of Children*, Vol. 4, No. 2, *Sexual Abuse of Children*, pp. 31-53
23. Finkelhor, D., Ormrod,R., Chaffin, M. (2009) Juveniles who commit sex offenses against minors. Juvenile Justice Bulletin, OJJDP, Office

of Justice Programs

24. Finkelhor, D., Ormrod, R.K. & Turner, H.A. (2010). Poly-victimization in a national sample of children & youth. *American Journal of Preventive Medicine.*
25. Finkelhor, D., Ormrod, R., Turner, H. A., & Hamby, S. L. (2012). Child and youth victimization known to school, police, and medical officials in a national sample of children and youth. *Juvenile Justice Bulletin*, (No. NCJ 235394). Washington, DC: United States Department of Justice, Office of Juvenile Justice and Delinquency Prevention.
26. Finkelhor, D., & Ormrod, R. K. (1999). Reporting crimes against juveniles. *Juvenile Justice Bulletin*, (No. NCJ 178887). Washington, DC: United States Department of Justice, Office of Juvenile Justice and Delinquency Prevention.
27. Finkelhor, D., & Ormrod, R. (2001). Child Abuse Reported to the Police. *Juvenile Justice Bulletin*, (No. NCJ 187238). Washington, DC: United States Department of Justice, Office of Juvenile Justice and Delinquency Prevention.
28. Felitti, V.J., Anda, R.F., Nordenberg, D., Williamson, D., Spitz, A.M., Edwards, V., Koss, M., Marks, J.S., (1998) Relationship of childhood abuse and household dysfunction to many of the leading causes of death in adults: The adverse childhood experiences (ACE) study. *American Journal of Preventive Medicine* 14(4).
29. Friedrich, W.N., Fisher, J. L., Dittner, C.A., Acton, R, Berliner, L, Butler, J., Damon, L., Davies, W.H., Gray, A. & Wright, J. (2001). Child Sexual Behavior Inventory: Normative, psychiatric, and sexual abuse comparisons. *Child Maltreatment*, 6, 37-49.
30. Fuemmeler, B. F., Dedert, E., McClernon, F. J., & Beckham, J. C. (2009). Adverse childhood events are associated with obesity and disordered eating: Results from a U.S. population-based survey of young adults. *Journal of Traumatic Stress*, 22, 329 – 333.
31. Golding, J. M., Cooper, M. L., & George, L. K. (1997). Sexual assault history and health perceptions: Seven general population studies. *Health Psychology, 16,* 417 – 425.
32. Golding, J. M. (1996). Sexual assault history and women's reproductive and sexual health. *Psychology of Women Quarterly, 20,* 101 – 121.
33. Grossman, L. , Martis, B., Fichtner, C. (1999). Are sex offenders treatable? A research overview. *Psychiatric Services 50* (3): 349–361
34. Grayson, J. (2006). Maltreatment and its effects on early brain development. *Virginia Child Protection Newsletter,* 77, 1-16.
35. Girardet, R. G., Lahoti, S., Howard, L. A., Fajman, N. N., Sawyer, M. K., Driebe, E. M., et al. (2009). Epidemiology of sexually transmitted infections in suspected child victims of sexual assault. *Pediatrics*, 124, 79-84.
36. Greenfeld, L.A. (1997). Sex Offenses and Offenders An Analysis of Data on Rape and Sexual Assault. U.S. Department of Justice, Office of Justice Programs, Bureau of Justice Statistics, NCJ-163392
37. Herrenkohl, E. C., Herrenkohl, R. C., Egolf, B. P., & Russo, M. J. (1998). The relationship between early maltreatment and teenage parenthood. *Journal of Adolescence*, 21, 291-303.
38. Harrison, P. A., & Narayan, G. (2003). Differences in behavior, psychological factors, and environmental factors associated with participation in school sports and other activities in adolescence. *Journal of School Health, 73*(3), 113–120.
39. Jenny, Carole, Roesler, Thomas A. , Poyer, Kimberly L. (1994) Are children at risk for sexual abuse by homosexuals? *Pediatrics*, Vol. 94 No. 1, pp. 41-44.
40. Jones, L,. Mitchell, K., Finkelhor, D. (2012). Trends in youth internet victimization: Findings from three youth internet safety surveys 2000–2010, *Journal of Adolescent Health 50*: 179–186.
41. Kilpatrick, D. G., Ruggiero, K. J., Acierno, R., Saunders, B. E., Resnick, H. S., & Best, C. L. (2003). Violence and risk of PTSD, major depression, substance abuse/dependence, and comorbidity: Results from the National Survey of Adolescents. *Journal of Consulting and Clinical Psychology*, 71, 692-700.
42. Kellogg, N.D., Hoffman, T.J, & Taylor, E.R. (1999). Early sexual experience among pregnant and parenting adolescents. *Adolescence*, 43, 293-303.
43. Kendler, K., Bulik, C., Silberg, J., Hettema, J., Myers, J., & Prescott, C. (2000). Childhood sexual abuse and adult psychiatric and substance use disorders in women: An epidemiological and

Cotwin Control Analysis. *Archives of General Psychiatry*, 57, 953-959.

44. Kenny, M.C. (2004). Teachers' attitudes toward and knowledge of child maltreatment. *Child Abuse and Neglect, 28*, 1311-1319.
45. Leeb, R., Lewis, T., & Zolotor, A. J. (2011). A review of physical and mental health consequences of child abuse and neglect and implications for practice. *American Journal of Lifestyle Medicine, 5*(5), 454-468.
46. London, K., Bruck, M., Ceci, S., & Shuman, D. (2003) Disclosure of child sexual abuse: What does the research tell us about the ways that children tell? *Psychology, Public Policy, and Law, 11*(1), 194-226.
47. Lanier, P., Jonson-Reid, M., Stahlschmidt, M. J., Drake, B., & Constantino, J. (2010). Child maltreatment and pediatric health outcomes: A longitudinal study of low-income children. *Journal of Pediatric Psychology*, 35(5), 511-522.
48. McLeer, S. V., Dixon, J. F., Henry, D., Ruggiero, K., Escovitz, K., Niedda, T., & Scholle, R. (1998). Psychopathology in non-clinically referred sexually abused children. *Journal of the American Academy of Child and Adolescent Psychiatry*, 37, 1326 – 1333.
49. Mullers, E. S., & Dowling, M. (2008). Mental health consequences of child sexual abuse. *British Journal of Nursing, 17*(22), 1428-1433.
50. Moran, P. B., Vuchinich, S., & Hall, N. K. (2004). Associations between types of maltreatment and substance use during adolescence. *Child Abuse and Neglect, 28*(5), 565–574. doi:10.1016/j.chiabu.2003.12.002
51. Molnar, B. E., Buka, S. L., & Kessler, R. C. (2001). Child sexual abuse and subsequent psychopathology: Results from the National Comorbidity Survey. *American Journal of Public Health*, 91, 753 – 760.
52. National Crime Victimization Survey, Statistic calculated by staff at Crimes against Children Research Center. 2002.
53. National Institute of Justice. (2007). Commercial sexual exploitation of children: What do we know and what do we do about it? (Publication NCJ 215733). US Department of Justice. Office of Justice Programs.
54. Noll, J. G., Shenk, C. E., & Putnam, K. T. (2009). Childhood sexual abuse and adolescent pregnancy: A meta-analytic update. *Journal of Pediatric Psychology*, 34, 366-378.
55. Noll, J.G., Trickett, P.K., & Putnam, F.W. (2003). A prospective investigation of the impact of childhood sexual abuse on the development of sexuality. *Journal of Consulting and Clinical Psychology*, 71, 575-586.
56. Newman, M. G., Clayton, L., Zuellig, A., Cashman, L., Arnow, B., Dea, R., & Taylor, C. B. (2000). The relationship of childhood sexual abuse and depression with somatic symptoms and medical utilization. *Psychological Medicine, 30*, 1063 – 1077.
57. Olafson, E. (2011). Child sexual abuse: Demography, impact, and interventions. *Journal of Child & Adolescent Trauma*, *4*(1), 8-21.
58. Putnam, F. (2003). Ten-year research update review: Child sexual abuse. *Journal of the American Academy of Child and Adolescent Psychiatry*, 42 , 269-278.
59. Prevent Child Abuse America (2003). *Recognizing child abuse: What parents should know*. Chicago, IL. Retrieved 5-31-2013 from
60. Polusny, M. A., & Follette, V. M. (1995). Long-term correlates of child sexual abuse: theory and review of the empirical literature. *Applied and Preventive Psychology*, 4, 143 – 166.
61. Paolucci, E.O, Genuis, M.L, & Violato, C. (2001). A meta-analysis of the published research on the effects of child sexual abuse. *Journal of Psychology, 135*, 17-36.
62. Reyome, N.D. (1994). Teacher ratings of the academic achievement related classroom behaviors of maltreated and non-maltreated children. *Psychology in the Schools*, 31, 253-260
63. Rohde, P., Ichikawa, L., Simon, G. E., Ludman, E. J., Linde, J. A. Jeffery, R. W., & Operskalski, B. H. (2008). Associations of child sexual and physical abuse with obesity and depression in middle-aged women. *Child Abuse & Neglect*, 32, 878–887.
64. Raj, A., Silverman, J. G., & Amaro, H. (2000). The relationship between sexual abuse and sexual risk among high school students: Findings from the 1997 Massachusetts Youth Risk Behavior Survey. *Maternal & Child Health Journal*, 4(2), 125-134.
65. Rice, D. P., & Miller, L. S. (1996). The economic burden of schizophrenia: Conceptual and

methodological issues, and cost estimates. In M. Moscarelli, A. Rupp, & N. Sartorious (Eds.),*Handbook of mental health economics and health policy. Vol. 1: Schizophrenia* (pp. 321–324). New York: John Wiley and Sons.

66. Saewyc, E.M., Magee, L.L., & Pettingall, S.E. (2004). Teenage pregnancy and associated risk behavior among sexually abused adolescents. *Perspectives on Sexual and Reproductive Health* , 36(3), 98-105.
67. Sachs-Ericsson, N., Blazer, D., Plant, E. A., & Arnow, B. (2005). Childhood sexual and physical abuse and 1-year prevalence of medical problems in the National Comorbidity Survey. *Health Psychology*, 24, 32 – 40.
68. Saunders, B.E., Kilpatrick, D.G., Hanson, R.F., Resnick, H.S., & Walker, M. E. (1999). Prevalence, case characteristics, and long-term psychological correlates of child rape among women: A national survey. *Child Maltreatment*, 4, 187-200.
69. Siegal, J.A. & Williams, L.M. (2003). The relationship between child sexual abuse and female delinquency and crime: A prospective study. *Journal of Research in Crime and Delinquency*, 40, 71-94.
70. Simpson, T.L. & Miller, W.R. (2002). Concomitance between childhood sexual and physical abuse and substance use problems: A review. *Clinical Psychology Review*, 22, 27-77.
71. Smith, D. W., Letourneau, E. J., Saunders, B. E., Kilpatrick, D. G., Resnick, H. S., & Best, C. L. (2000). Delay in disclosure of childhood rape: Results from a national survey. *Child Abuse & Neglect*, 24, 273 – 287.
72. Snyder, H. N. (2000). Sexual assault of young children as reported to law enforcement: Victim, incident, and offender characteristics. Washington, DC: U.S. Department of Justice, Office of Justice Programs, Bureau of Justice Statistics.
73. Sedlak, A.J., Mettenburg, J., Basena, M., Petta, I., McPherson, K., Greene, A., and Li, S. (2010). Fourth National Incidence Study of Child Abuse and Neglect (NIS–4): Report to Congress, Executive Summary. Washington, DC: U.S. Department of Health and Human Services, Administration for Children and Families.
74. Stop It Now! (2013) *Warning signs in children and adolescents of possible child sexual abuse.* Northampton, MA.
75. Tebbutt, J., Swanston, H., Oates, R. K., O'Toole, B.I. (1997). Five years after child sexual abuse: Persisting dysfunction and problems of prediction. *Journal of the American Academy of Child & Adolescent Psychiatry, 36*, 330-339.
76. Townsend, C., & Rheingold, A.A., (2013). Estimating a child sexual abuse prevalence rate for practitioners: studies. Charleston, S.C
77. Townsend, C. (2013). Prevalence and consequences of child sexual abuse compared with other childhood experiences. Charleston, S.C.,
78. Ullman, S. E. (2007). Relationship to perpetrator, disclosure, social reactions, and PTSD symptoms in child sexual abuse survivors. *Journal of Child Sexual Abuse, 16*(1), 19-36.
79. Voeltanz, N., Wilsnack, S., Harris, R., Wilsnack, R., Wonderlich, S., Kristjanson, A. (1999). Prevalence and risk for childhood sexual abuse in women : National survey findings. *Child Abuse and Neglect*, 23, 579-592.
80. Wilson, H. & Widom, C.S. (2009). An examination of risky sexual behavior and HIV among victims of child abuse and neglect: A thirty-year follow-up. *Health Psychology, 27*, 14-158
81. Walker, E. A., Keegan, D., Gardner, G., Sullivan, M., Bernstein, D. & Katon, W. J. (1997). Psychosocial factors in fibromyalgia compared with rheumatoid arthritis: II. Sexual, physical, and emotional abuse and neglect. *Psychosomatic Medicine, 59*, 572 – 577.
82. Walrath, C., Ybarra, M., Holden, W., Liao, Q., Santiago, R., & Leaf, R. (2003). Children with reported histories of sexual abuse: Utilizing multiple perspectives to understand clinical and psychological profiles. *Child Abuse & Neglect*, 27, 509-524.
83. Widom, C.S. & Maxfield, M.G. (2001). An update on the "cycle of violence." Washington, DC: U.S. Department of Justice. National Institute of Justice.
84. Waldrop, A. E. Hanson, R. F., Resnick, H. S., Kilpatrick, D. G., Naugle, A. E., & Saunders, B. E. (2007). Risk factors for suicidal behavior among a national sample of adolescents: Implications for prevention. *Journal of Traumatic Stress*, 20,

869 – 879.

85. Wells, R., McCann, J., Adams, J., Voris, J., & Dahl, B. (1997). A validational study of the structured interview of symptoms associated with sexual abuse using three samples of sexually abused, allegedly abused, and nonabused boys. *Child Abuse & Neglect*, 21, 1159-1167.
86. Whealin, J. (2007-05-22). "Child Sexual Abuse". National Center for Post Traumatic Stress Disorder, US Department of Veterans Affairs.
87. Wolak, J., Finkelhor, D., Mitchell, K. (2006). Trends in arrests of online predators. Department of Justice, Office of Juvenile Justice and Delinquency Prevention Report. Crimes Against Children Research Center, University of New Hampshire.
88. Wolak, J., Finkelhor, D., Mitchell, K., Ybarra, M. (2008) " Online "Predators" and their Victims: Myths, Realities and Implications for Prevention and Treatment" published by *American Psychologist*, 63(2), 111-128
89. Walker, E.A. Gelfand, A., Katon, W.J., Koss, M.P, Con Korff, M., Bernstien, D., et al. (1999). Medical and psychiatric symptoms in women with children and sexual abuse. *Psychosomatic Medicine*, 54, 658-664.
90. Walsh, W.A., Jones, L., Cross, T.P., Lippert,T. (2008). Prosecuting child sexual abuse: The importance of evidence type. *Crime Delinquency OnlineFirst*,
91. Young, M. S., Harford, K., Kinder, B., & Savell, J. K. (2007). The relationship between childhood sexual abuse and adult mental health among undergraduates: Victim gender doesn't matter. *Journal of Interpersonal Violence*, 22, 1315 – 1331.
92. Yates, T. M. (2004). The developmental psychopathology of self-injurious behavior: Compensatory regulation in posttraumatic adaptation. *Clinical Psychology Review, 24*(1), 35-74.

Fussy Infants and Temper Tantrums

36

Dinesh Saroj

INTRODUCTION

Behavior problems are common in childhood. Periodically, all children have behavioral symptoms. Temper tantrums are among the most common childhood behavioral problems. They tend to decrease in frequency and intensity as the child grows older.

Temper tantrums are considered to be normal part of the natural course of child development and are rarely considered a serious emotional disturbance during this period.[1] Tantrums usually occur in the active, determined child who has abundant energy.

TEMPER TANTRUMS

Temper tantrums are defined as overt exhibition of behaviors in a severe, unpleasant and extreme manner which is also disproportionate to the prevailing situation and circumstance.[1] These may include varied presentation ranging from mild screaming or whining to severe head banging or breath holding for a short time.[2]

Common presentations include crying, screaming , pushing, pulling, biting, swinging the arms and legs with rage, throwing himself to the floor, kicking, throwing objects, banging one's head, hands, or feet against the wall or floor.[3,1] Temper tantrums are among the frequent reason for referral to a Developmental Pediatrician, Child Psychiatrist, Pediatric Neurologist or a Pediatric Behavioral Therapist.

PREVALENCE

10% to 15% of children develop behavioral problems that interfere with life adjustment.[4] Temper tantrums are commonly seen in the age group between 1 and 4 years; however, they occur most often between the ages of 2 and 3 years.[5]

Temper tantrums that persists beyond 5 years of age, lasting longer than 15 min in a go, or having frequency of more than five times a day, that are both frequent and disruptive are considered abnormal and are indicative of serious behavioral concern. Severe temper tantrums are seen in as many as 5%–20% of children.[6]

Tantrums that last at least 15 minutes & occurring at a frequency approximately three or more times per week are seen in approximately 5%–7% of children.[1] According to another study, at least one temper tantrum occurs every day in approximately 20% of 2-year-kids, 18% of 3-year-kids, and 10% of 4-year-kids.[7]

The tantrums tend to be more aggressive and frequent in children with behavioral disorders like Autism Spectrum Disorder or Language delays because of underlying frustration in difficulty to express themselves. The prevalence of temper tantrums do not differ by gender or race/ethnicity.[8]

Sometimes, tantrums are characterized by breath-holding spells and they affect 0.1 to 4.6% of otherwise healthy children having its onset between 6 and 18 months. They often occur between the age groups of six months and five years. They mostly subside by five years of age.[9]

Children exhibit tantrums when things do not go their way or they are denied access to something. Hunger, Illnesses, boredom, fatigue may act as precipitating factors. When children find it difficult to express themselves due to delayed language development, they often have tantrums. Tantrums also occur when there is discrepancy between child's needs and parental expectations and when the child needs attention.

Propensity for tantrums increase with rising level of insecurity amongst children. Overprotectiveness and excessive strictness on behalf of parents may also promote tantrum behavior.[10]

CHILD DEVELOPMENT

Understanding Child development is vital and preliminary step in managing temper tantrums successfully and effectively. Clinicians and caregivers can better devise appropriate management if they understand the developmental issues that give rise to tantrums.

An early child development is characterized by rapid formation of synaptic connections with simultaneous pruning of unused connections. Thus, an enriched environment ensures optimal growth and maintenance of synaptic connections in the developing infant brain.

A child, when born, exhibits biologic endowments that includes neurological, motor and sensory abilities (as mediated by vision, hearing, smell, touch, taste and position sense), that are utilized for integrating the experiences and interacting with the social environment. The complex interplay between genetic influences, caregiving and social factors modulate the brain architecture with resultant changes in growth, behavior and development.

The development progresses along these highly integrated multiple domains in the first two years of life helping child establish their autonomous identity in their social world. This is best explained by the transactional model of child development[11] which assumes that infants, caregivers, and their environment collectively determine the child's developmental and behavioral outcome, by a mutually dependent, bidirectional, complex and continuing process.[12] Thus, the child's family dynamics and sociocultural circumstances also tend to influence child's behavior.

Right from learning the concept of attachment/separation with the primary caregivers, to the attainment of autonomy/mastery, child goes through this bidirectional process of Mutual regulation. During this process, the child seems to exhibit varying degrees of presentations depending upon his physical, cognitive, neurologic status and temperamental characteristics.

Thus, Infants exhibit certain behaviors to shift themselves from one behavioral state to the other. Infant's capacity to regulate their behavioral state being immature, they rely upon the responses given by their caregiver.

A harmonious family environment, positive infant responses and co-operative parental attitude can have pleasurable experience in both the partners. On the other hand, a disturbed family environment, difficult infant's responses and non- co-operative parental attitude can disrupt the parent- child relationships.

TEMPERAMENT

The word temperament is derived from the Latin verb 'temperare', which means 'to mix'. Temperament is the behavioral style of an individual. The differences in the behavior of children to different stimuli under similar circumstances can be accounted by differences in their temperamental characteristics. The link between temperament and behavior continues to become complex as the child grows.

New York Longitudinal Study (NYLS) introduced the temperamental traits based on parental interviews and direct observations of child's behavior.

These include-

- Activity, Biologic Rhythmicity, Approach/ Withdrawal (initial reaction), Adaptability, Intensity, Mood, Persistence/ Attention span, Distractibility, and Sensory Threshold (sensitivity).
- These traits were further grouped into clusters – 'easy child' - about 40% kids, 'difficult child'- about 10% kids and 'slow-to-warm-up child' about 15% of the study population. However, it was concluded with further research that it is always better to discuss the child's individual traits with parents.[13]

Respective temperamental characteristics of children and their caregivers play a vital role in establishing mutual relationships, directing the same towards similarities leading to harmony and pleasure between child and his or her environment (Goodness of Fit) or differences producing conflicts and confusions (Poorness of Fit)

CLINICAL HISTORY

Atypical tantrums warranting timely referral to a specialist are important to be distinguished from typical ones. (See Table 1)[14]

Table 36.1: Normal and abnormal tantrums

	Normal temper tantrum	**Abnormal temper tantrum**
Age	12 months up to age 4.	Continuing past age 4.
Behavior during tantrum	Crying, flailing arms or legs, falling to the floor, pushing, pulling, or biting	Injury to themselves or others during the tantrum
Duration	Up to 15 min.	Lasting longer than 15 min
Frequency	Less than five times a day	More than five times a day
Mood	Should return to normal between tantrums	Persistent negative mood between tantrums

A thorough clinical history, beginning with an open-ended question such as, "tell me all about the tantrums" can definitely be of great value in understanding the developmental or psychological explanations for the tantrum(s). It should be inclusive of family history of behavioral and developmental disorders, social determinants of health and supported by formal developmental assessment. This can conveniently be administered during the well child visits at 12, 15, and 18 months and at two years of age when tantrums are frequent.[15] It helps developing a deeper insight into family and environmental dynamics which can then be modulated for the betterment of child's behavior.

It is recommended to keep a record of tantrums so as to elucidate improving or worsening pattern. Following questions can be administered to understand the preceding, during and after the event circumstances.[15]

1. At what times of the day do the tantrums occur?
2. Please specify the circumstances preceding the tantrums?
3. How long does the tantrums last during each single episode?
4. What behavior(s) does the child demonstrate during the tantrums?
5. How does usually the caregiver's react to or handle the tantrum (s)?
6. How does the child behave in between the tantrum episodes?
7. Have there been any recent changes to the child's environment (e.g at home or in school)?
8. Are there other behaviors that concern the caregiver like behavioral issues, anxiety or depression, sleep related issues?
9. Is the child witness to any family conflicts or any upsetting event in the family?
10. Are there other concerns that affect the child's functioning, such as loss of bladder control?

DISRUPTIVE MOOD DYSREGULATION DISORDER (DMDD)

Disruptive Mood Dysregulation Disorder (DMDD) is a newly annexed diagnostic entity in the depressive disorders' domain of the Diagnostic and Statistical Manual of Mental Disorders, 5th edition - DSM-5 (American Psychiatric Association, 2013).[16] It is characterized by persistent / non episodic negative mood and severe temper outbursts, which are disproportionate to the situation and the circumstances; manifesting anger and rages behaviorally and/or verbally; lasting more than one minute, but less than five minutes.[17]

Irritability being the core feature of DMDD, it is often the first reason for medical referral.[18] Irritability, in DMDD, is persistent and chronic (present in between temper tantrums), occurs across different settings (with peers, at school, at home,) for most of the time of the day & almost every day. Additional features include easy distractibility and inattention at school. According to a study conducted by Copeland et al., 2013, psychosocial impairment were noted significantly more in DMDD-affected youth than the unaffected ones.[19]

DIFFERENTIAL DIAGNOSIS

In case of atypical tantrums, it is imperative to consider other neuro-developmental and behavioral disorders like conduct disorders, oppositional defiant disorder, posttraumatic stress disorder, attention deficit hyperactivity disorder, autism, learning disabilities, and vision or hearing deficits, Disruptive Mood Dysregulation Disorder.[17,20,21]

PROGNOSIS

Typical tantrums usually keep excellent prognosis. Parents need to be reassured that the child is expected to outgrow tantrums with developing age.[8]

COMPLICATIONS

Tantrums usually tend to disrupt the family or classroom environment thereby aggravating anxiety of parents or caregiver. Otherwise, tantrums or breath-holding spells accompanying them, do not lead to developmental or cognitive issues in children.[9]

EVALUATION

Underlying Visual or Hearing deficits can precipitate frustration leading to tantrums. Hence, a vision and hearing screening is warranted. Laboratory tests are not indicated to diagnose and/or manage typical temper tantrums.[22]

There is no sufficient evidence to recommend use of instrument-based screening devices in children less than three years.[21] Screening for Lead intoxication is indicated at 12 months of age for children living in areas with high-risk for lead exposure.[22]

A detailed psycho-social evaluation of temper tantrums with standardized rating scales may be conducted by developmental pediatrician, child psychiatrist or psychologist. The Child Behavior Checklist can be administered with parents of children ages two to five years of age.[23]

MANAGEMENT

Physicians caring for the child are expected to counsel parents and the child intermittently, at regular intervals. At times, tantrums cannot be avoided but the accompanying stress can be minimized by following consistent management strategies. The best way to manage tantrum behavior would be to prevent antecedent factors. The common triggers include injury, fatigue, boredom, frustration, hunger and illness.[17]

Parent need to encourage children and help them learn to express their negative feelings in more acceptable ways and ensure to give them a patient listening. Younger children can be given option of depicting their feelings by use of facial expressions card like sad face, angry face, and happy face. Older children should be encouraged to express their feeling verbally. Parents should be taught to model their communication skills and avoid arguing in front of children.

They should help children develop decision making by offering choices that are acceptable to both of them and avoid using 'negatives' unless it pertains to a health or safety issue for the child himself or someone around. It is always advisable avoid saying ' no ' or using negative words while making an attempt to refrain kids from doing what parents don't want them to do. Child proofing the environment can avoid unwanted distractions towards unsafe objects or activities, thereby minimizing the usage of negative words and decreasing tantrums. It is highly imperative to ensure safety of the child and of someone around during a temper tantrum. The child can be moved to a safer place which brings down the risks and at the same time, helps bring down their anger.[10]

Parents should attempt to make daily chores (e.g. nap time or meal time) a routine. Also, they should prepare children with expectations when there is unexpected, sudden, unavoidable change in the activities. Ensure positive attention towards children by engaging them in constructive play activities. Child's exposure to crime scenes in television should be restricted as it predicts aggression in future.

Age appropriate and interest provoking tasks and play activities help bring down the tantrums by distracting kids. The tantrums must be handled calmly and patiently. Being consistent with their demands and expectations is highly desirable on behalf of parents. Attempt to negotiate or reason with child during a tantrum should be avoided. There's less chance for tantrums to recur once they are ignored and the child derives no benefit from it. Parents can be counseled that tantrums usually outgrow as the child matures and anger and frustration usually manifests in a different way with the growing age.

Child's frustration after repeated attempts to master a task go in vain, leads to tantrums. Bringing down the challenge and assisting accomplishing the task can help distract the child and thereby alleviate tantrums.

Parental attempt to regulate child's behavior is perceived as an attempt to restrict child autonomy. This leads to tantrum behavior. Parents should help facilitate self – control to kids by holding younger ones in arms and allowing older kids to remain alone in safe place- "time out procedure". There should not be a predefined time of isolation that is being imposed. Rather, the aim of this maneuver would be to help child develop self-regulation. Isolation time should cease with subsidence of tantrum and child should be praised for maintaining the quieter state. According to American Academy of Pediatrics, a 1-minute "time-out" is recommended for each year of the child's age.[8,17] However, there is always a possibility that child may get habituated to the 'Time –out procedure', if used too frequently. For this, they need repeated encouragement.

Striking an appropriate balance between the desired limits and child's desire for autonomy requires frequent negotiation. This should include more praise for a desired behavior ("time in") and apparent disapproval of an undesired behavior. At the same time, attempt should be made to keep these limits consistent, selective and firm. Parents should be helped choosing behaviors that are worth regulating. Breaking a child's will should not seem to be end of the battle.[12]

It is also important to offer nurturance to the child after the tantrum has subsided. Parents should be helped to keep realistic expectations by taking into consideration the stage, and not the age of child development. Although the child with tantrums is usually normal on physical examination, it is pertinent to look for mucosal pallor or tachycardia especially if the child has history of breath holding spells. A complete blood count may be obtained to assess for anemia. Iron supplementation is shown to reduce the frequency of breath holding spells.[17]

According to Belden et al, those children who are not able to calm themselves during tantrums or do self- injury or whose tantrums lasts for more than 25 minutes may be benefitted by a timely referral to developmental pediatrician, child psychologist, or child psychiatrist.[26] Consultation with an interprofessional team of specialists like developmental and behavioral pediatrician, child psychologist, or child psychiatrist can help improve outcome especially in case of atypical tantrums.

Parent-Child Interaction Therapy (P.C.I.T.) is an evidence based parent training program intended to train parents in skills that help manage challenging behavior in children between two to seven years of age.[17]

In case tantrums disrupt the decorum of the classroom, parents and the teachers need to jointly determine a plan for managing the challenging behavior. If the child self-injures during tantrum, a superficial wound needs a primary treatment with soap and water. In case of deep wounds, prophylaxis with broad spectrum Antibiotic like Amoxicillin-Clavulanate for three to five days is warranted along with close follow up. A timely referral may also be considered, if indicated. However, usually these wounds need not be closed or sutured, given the high risk for secondary infection.[8]

BIBLIOGRAPHY

1. McCurdy, M., Kunz, G. M., & Sheridan, S. M. (2006). Temper tantrums. In G. G. Bear & K. M. Minke (Eds.), Children's needs III: Development, prevention, and intervention (pp. 149–157).

Washington, DC: National Association of School Psychologists.

2. Mills, D., & Woodring, B. (2012). Growth and development of the toddler. In N. L. Potts & B. L. Mandleco (Eds.), Pediatric nursing: Caring for children and their families (pp. 273–305). New York: Delmar Cengage Learning
3. Kyle, T. (2008). Growth and development of the toddler. In T. Kyle (Ed.), Essentials of pediatric nursing (pp. 106–135). New York: Lippincott Williams & Wilkins.
4. Schmitt B D. PEDIATRIC COUNSELING. In: Carey WB, Elias ER, Coleman WL, Crocker AC, Feldman HM, editors. Developmental-Behavioral Pediatrics. Philadelphia: 2009; p. 846-55.
5. American Academy of Pediatrics. (2008). Temper tantrums: A normal part of growing up. Retrieved from http: https://www.nfaap.org/netforum/eweb
6. Goldson, E., & Reynolds, A. (2011). Child development and behavior. In J. M. Sondheimer, M. J. Levin, R. R. Deterding, & W. W. Hay (Eds.), Current diagnosis & treatment in pediatrics (pp. 64–103). Columbus, OH: The McGraw-Hill Companies.
7. Grover, G. (2008). Temper tantrums. In C. Berkowitz (Ed.), Pediatrics: A primary care approach. (pp. 199–201). Philadelphia, PA: W. B. Saunders.
8. Sisterhen L L; Soman-Faulkner K. Temper Tantrums. Treasure Island (FL): StatPearls Publishing; 2019.
9. Donahue SP, Ruben JB., American Academy of Ophthalmology. American Academy of Pediatrics, Ophthalmology Section. American Association for Pediatric Ophthalmology and Strabismus. Children's Eye Foundation. American Association of Certified Orthoptists. US Preventive Services Task Force vision screening recommendations. Pediatrics. 2011 Mar; 127(3):569-70. [PubMed: 21282266]
10. Wasserman Abby L. Common Behavioral Disorders of Childhood. In: Gottlieb M I, Williams JE, editors, Textbook of Developmental Pediatrics. 1 st edition, New York: Plenum; 1987. p. 241-42
11. Sameroff AJ, Chandler MJ: Reproductive risk and the continuum of caretaking causality. Rev Child Dev Res 4:187-244, 1974.
12. Augustyn, M, Frank D A, Zuckerman B S. Infancy and Toddler Years. In: Carey, Crocker, Coleman, Elias, Feldman, editors, Developmental – Behavioral Pediatrics. 4 th edition. Philadelphia: Saunders; 2009.p. 24-38.
13. Carey W B. Normal Individual Differences In Temperament And Behavioral Adjustment. In: Carey, Crocker, Coleman, Elias, Feldman, editors, Developmental – Behavioral Pediatrics. 4 th edition. Philadelphia: Saunders; 2009.p. 74-85.
14. Daniels E, Mandleco B, Karlen E. Assessment, management, and prevention of childhood temper tantrums. Journal of the American Academy of Nurse Practitioners 24 (2012) 569–573. Table 1, Normal and abnormal tantrums; p. 571
15. Daniels E, Mandleco B, Karlen E. Assessment, management, and prevention of childhood temper tantrums. Journal of the American Academy of Nurse Practitioners 24 (2012) 569–573.
16. Diagnostic and Statistical Manual of Mental Disorders, Fifth Edition. Arlington, VA, American Psychiatric Association, 2013.
17. Potegal, M., Kosorok, M.R., Davidson, R.J., 2003. Temper tantrums in young children: 2. Tantrum duration and temporal organization. J. Dev. Behav. Pediatr. 24, 148–154.
18. Yeh, M., Weisz, J.R., 2001. Why are we here at the clinic? Parent-child (dis)agreement on referral problems at outpatient treatment entry. J. Consult. Clin. Psychol. 69, 1018– 1025.http://dx.doi.org/10.1037/0022-006X.69.6.1018.
19. Copeland, W.E., Angold, A., Costello, E.J., Egger, H., 2013. Prevalence, comorbidity and correlates of DSM-5 proposed disruptive mood dysregulation disorder. Am. J. Psychiatry. 170, 173–179. https://doi.org/10.1176/appi.ajp.2012.12010132.
20. Harlor AD, Bower C., Committee on Practice and Ambulatory Medicine. Section on Otolaryngology-Head and Neck Surgery. Hearing assessment in infants and children: recommendations beyond neonatal screening. Pediatrics. 2009 Oct; 124(4):1252-63. [PubMed: 19786460]
21. US Preventive Services Task Force. Curry SJ, Krist AH, Owens DK, Barry MJ, Cabana M,

Caughey AB, Doubeni CA, Epling JW, Kemper AR, Kubik M, Landefeld CS, Mangione CM, Pbert L, Silverstein M, Simon MA, Tseng CW, Wong JB. Screening for Elevated Blood Lead Levels in Children and Pregnant Women: US Preventive Services Task Force Recommendation Statement. JAMA. 2019 Apr 16; 321(15):1502-1509. [PubMed: 30990556]

22. Egger HL, Erkanli A, Keeler G, Potts E, Walter BK, Angold A. Test-Retest Reliability of the Preschool Age Psychiatric Assessment (PAPA). J Am Acad Child Adolesc Psychiatry. 2006 May;45(5):538-49. [PubMed: 16601400]
23. Luby JL, Heffelfinger A, Koenig-McNaught AL, Brown K, Spitznagel E. ThePreschool Feelings Checklist: a brief and sensitive screening measure for depression in young children. J Am Acad Child Adolesc Psychiatry. 2004 Jun; 43(6):708-17. [PubMed: 15167087
24. Parladé MV, Weinstein A, Garcia D, Rowley AM, Ginn NC, Jent JF. Parent-Child Interaction Therapy for children with autism spectrum disorder and a matched case-control sample. Autism. 2019 Jun 12;:1362361319855851. [PubMed: 31187642]
25. Bruno A, Celebre L, Torre G, Pandolfo G, Mento C, Cedro C, Zoccali RA, Muscatello MRA. Focus on Disruptive Mood Dysregulation Disorder: A review of the literature. Psychiatry Res. 2019 Jun 01; [PubMed: 31164249]
26. Belden AC, Thomson NR, Luby JL. Temper tantrums in healthy versus depressed and disruptive preschoolers: defining tantrum behaviors associated with clinical problems. J. Pediatr. 2008 Jan; 152(1):117-22. [PMC free article: PMC2211733] [PubMed: 18154912]

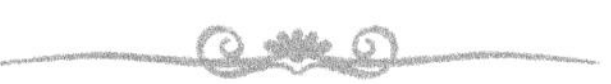

Organic Mental Disorders 37

G. Prasad Rao • Amulya Koneru • Sriramya Vemulakonda

INTRODUCTION

The term "organic disorders" refers to that category of mental disorders whose cause can be attributed to a specific systemic or neurological condition or illness, i.e. an organic condition as opposed to "functional disorders" for which there is no diagnosable organic condition.

This classification has been followed historically through the ages. However, many studies that have been done on "pure" psychiatric disorders such as schizophrenia, mood disorders, anxiety disorders etc. have shown that pathophysiology of these illnesses more often than not includes changes in biological factors such as structural changes in the brain, changes in connectivity between different regions of the brain, neurotransmitters, nerve growth factors, and even genetic changes. Genetic studies have shown that these diseases often run in the family with often variable phenotypic manifestations. Recently, a gut-brain axis has been found to be implicated in various neurological and psychiatric disorders. Further studies may reveal a broader understanding of psychiatric conditions leading to better diagnosis and outcome. This will warrant many changes to the classificatory system in the near future. It is not farfetched to imagine that treatment will become more tailored and "customised" to the individual based on various biological and psychological factors.

For now, we will follow the traditional classification of functional and organic disorders. This chapter will thus give a brief outline of psychiatric disorders that have a diagnosable cause.

CNS DISORDERS

Brain is the seat of consciousness in the body governing all the higher mental functions in the individual. Conditions affecting both gross and cellular structure of the brain cause a multitude of psychiatric symptoms. Sometimes, the presenting symptom is psychiatric in nature leading to a delay in diagnosis. A thorough history, physical examination, and mental status examination will guide us to the cause, course, early diagnosis, and management of the condition.

Traumatic Brain Injury

A traumatic brain injury (TBI) is defined as a blow to the head or a penetrating head injury that disrupts the normal function of the brain. Symptoms of a TBI can be mild, moderate, or severe, depending on extent of damage to the brain. Patient may experience symptoms like loss of consciousness (LOC), amnesia, disorientation, other signs of neurological injury, coma, and even death.

It has been estimated that nearly 1.5 to 2 million persons are injured and 1 million succumb to death every year in India. Highest occurrence of TBI is in the age group of 20-29, followed by 30-39 years. Male to female ratio was 1:0.3. Falls were more frequent in women, children, and elderly while road traffic accidents and violence were more common in men. Alcohol consumption has been found to be a major risk factor for TBI and has also been found to affect the prognosis. Recovery from TBI depends on various factors like severity and location of head injury, physiological and nutritional status, hospital interventions, and availability of rehabilitation services. TBI causes transient cell membrane disruptions leading to alteration of cell membrane potential due to redistribution of ions and neurotransmitters. There is increase in extracellular potassium levels and excessive glutamate release leading to depolarization of neurons followed by a hypermetabolic state. Intracellular increase in calcium levels leads to oxidative stress. Diffuse axonal injury happens when there is damage to the axolemma of axons due to the shearing and other forces. Calcium enters the cell leading to damage of cell structures. The β-amyloid precursor protein accumulates in the event of axonal injury and can be used as a marker for diffuse axonal injury. Post head-injury, there is decrease in dopamine and norepinephrine levels in the frontal lobes. Elevated levels of choline are found in CSF following injury. However in the long term, there is decrease in the cholinergic nuclei leading to reduced grey matter density of basal forebrain.

The course of recovery from TBI is variable. In mild TBI, the usual course in complete or near complete recovery in the symptoms. Cognitive symptoms have been found to improve at most by 3 months in most of the cases. Psychiatric symptoms like depression and irritability, and neurological symptoms like headache will usually take a few weeks to resolve. For moderate and severe TBI, there is often persistence of cognitive deficits, neurological symptoms like seizures, hyperacusis and photosensitivity, and psychiatric symptoms like depression, aggression, and apathy, all of which can lead to long term disability.

Post concussional syndrome: Symptoms of post concussional syndrome include headache, giddiness, fatiguability, photophobia, phonophobia, attention and concentration difficulties, and memory disturbances. Anxiety, sleep disturbances and irritability are also seen. Most of the symptoms subside by 3 months post injury but some symptoms often persist long term.

Acute effects include delirium, amnesia and agitation.

Post TBI cognitive deficits include impairment in attention, memory, learning, speech of information processing, speech, language and executive functioning.

Personality changes include impulsivity, recklessness, disinhibition, apathy, suspiciousness, and apathy.

Affective symptoms often seen post TBI are irritability, aggression, low tolerance to frustration, anxiety, emotional lability and depressive symptoms. PTSD and phobias are also encountered.

Substance use disorders have a unique role both in the causation and prognosis of TBI. Many accidents are frequently encountered under the influence of a substance – be it under intoxication, withdrawal, or any other illness attributable to substance use. Especially in the case of alcohol related disorders, TBI is frequent. Alcohol itself causes cognitive, mood, and other disturbances. Post TBI, in an individual already compromised due to the deleterious effects of alcohol, the structural damage will probably have a synergistic pathological effect leading to poor prognosis.

Common somatic symptoms include headaches (typically migraine, occipital neuralgia, or cervicogenic), fatigue, photosensivity, hyperacusis, insomnia and other sleep disturbances, drowsiness, dizziness, nausea and vomiting, vision difficulties, seizures, and balance problems.

Management

Imaging is the most commonly used investigation. CT may reveal contusions, sub arachnoid hemorrhage, and intra-cranial hemorrhage. MRI may reveal microhemorrhages as hyperintensities.

There is insufficient evidence for agents such as steroids, calcium channel blockers, mannitol, and magnesium as well as for interventions like hyperbaric oxygen and hyperventilation.

For the post TBI sequelae, treatment is usually symptomatic. Cognitive impairment is usually treated with stimulants like methylphenidate, amantadine, other drugs including donepezil. Cognitive rehabilitation is helpful as well as progressive physical exercise. Depression and anxiety are treated using SSRIS and other antidepressants and anti-anxiety drugs. Seizures are treated using anti-epileptics. Aggression and irritability can often be reduced using antipsychotics.

Stroke

Every year, about 16 million people worldwide have a first ever stroke. Of this population, about 5·7 million people die and another 5 million remain disabled. Post-stroke psychiatric disorders are very common in the population and distressing to both the patients and their caretakers. They often affect the prognosis and rehabilitation of stroke patients.

Depression occurs more frequently in patients after stroke than in the general population. Systemic reviews have found that 29%-33%of patients have depression up to 1 year after a stroke. Analyses of patients with long-term follow-up show that depression after stroke is often a chronic relapsing disorder. Treatment includes life style changes, psychological interventions, pharmacotherapy such as SSRIs and tricyclic antidepressants. When compared to depression, prevalence of mania is very low (<2%).

24% of stroke patients had anxiety symptoms post the event, and 18% had an anxiety disorder in the first 5 years after stroke. Depression had been correlated positively with anxiety. Treatment includes psychological interventions or antidepressants.

Post-stroke fatigue is often pathological where the weariness is constant, not related to previous level of exertion, and is often not attenuated following rest. The proportion of people with fatigue after stroke ranges from 23% to 75%. Fatigue has been found to persist in individual patients if it is present early after stroke and often has variable prognosis. There is some association with depression, sleep disturbances, and pain. There is insufficient evidence with regards to treatment and exercise and cognitive behavioral interventions might have some effect.

Apathy is a disorder of motivation both cognitively and behaviorally. A meta-analysis has reported prevalence of apathy to be around 35% post stroke. Remission rates of apathy have been found to range from 44-67%. Apathy was associated with lower levels of education, cognitive impairment, depression, and increased disability. It is associated with poorer prognosis. There is insufficient evidence for treatment of apathy. Nootropics may play a role in the management of apathy.

Emotional lability in patients as unstable emotional experiences and frequent mood changes, with emotions that are easily aroused, intense, or out of proportion to events and circumstances. Prevalence of emotional lability ranges from 8% to 32% in patients post stroke. Symptoms are thought to reduce in the 6 months after stroke. Antidepressants can be used to treat persistent symptoms.

Personality changes include impulsivity, recklessness, and disinhibition. Prevalence estimates for irritability vary from 12% to 53% of patients after stroke. Prevalence estimates for disinhibition vary from 6% to 76% of patients.

Prevalence of psychosis and single psychotic symptoms has been found to be very low post stroke. Symptomatology often depends on the area affected; e.g., visual hallucinations are more common in strokes affecting occipital lobe.

Malignancies

Brain tumors are relatively common with an annual incidence of 9 per 100000 for primary brain tumors and 8.3 per 100000 for metastatic brain tumors. Brain tumors may be classified based on their histopathological characteristics or location. Most common brain tumors are gliomas- accounting for 40-55% of the tumors. Secondaries are estimated to be 15-25% of the malignancies affecting brain. Psychiatric symptoms arising in malignancies include mood symptoms like depression and irritability, anxiety, memory impairment, personality changes, and psychotic symptoms. Often psychiatric symptoms maybe the presenting picture of a brain tumor.

Depression was found in 44% of all brain tumor patients, and was associated with cognitive dysfunction, impairment in functioning, reduced quality of life, and reduced rates of survival. Mania has also been found to be associated with tumors but to a lesser extent. Frontal lobe tumors are more commonly associated with mood symptoms.

Psychotic symptoms were found in 22% of patients. Pituitary gland tumors and temporal lobe tumors have been found to be most commonly associated with psychosis.

Frontal lobe lesions and ventricular cysts often manifest with personality changes. This may include disinhibition, inappropriate sexual behavior, recklessness and aggression.

Infections

HIV (Human Immunodeficiency Virus)

HIV belongs to the lentivirus subfamily of the retrovirus family. There are two forms of HIV virus – HIV-1 and HIV-2. HIV-1 is most commonly implicated in the causation of the illness in humans. It is an RNA virus that affects mainly macrophages and T lymphocytes – those that express CD4 receptors. HIV gains entry into the cells through co-receptors such as CXCR4 (on T cells) and CCR5 (on macrophages).

According to 2018 UN statistics, 37.9 million people are currently diagnosed with HIV globally. In them, children account for 1.7 million. In India, according to 2017 statistics, prevalence of HIV amongst adults is 0.2%. 2.1 million people are living with HIV in India. Women account for 41.9% of total HIV population. 69,000 people succumbed to AIDS(Acquired Immunodeficiency Syndrome) related illnesses. Psychiatry plays an intimate role in the epidemic of HIV. Psychiatric disorders are related to risk behaviors for infection, less access to medical and other forms of care, decreased adherence to management of both HIV and psychiatric illnesses, and increased physical comorbidities. Vice-versa, HIV/AIDS infection leads to causation of various psychiatric illnesses.

HIV-Associated Dementia

In HIV, the cause of neurocognitive impairment could be either directly due to HIV infection or due to opportunistic infections like cerebral toxoplasmosis, cryptococcal meningitis, progressive multifocal leukoencephalopathy, CMV (Cytomegalovirus) encephalitis, and CNS lymphoma. Before the era of antiretroviral therapy (ART), HIV dementia presented as subcortical dementia with impairment in cognitive skills, and motor skills rather than memory loss. Currently, patients show impairment in the domains of memory and executive functioning.

Mood Disorders

There is a 2 fold increase in the prevalence of depression in HIV patients when compared to the non-infected people. Depression and HIV have a reciprocal relationship in the course of either disease. Amongst the antiretroviral agents, efavirenz and raltigravir have been implicated in depression.

Typical presentation of mania can be seen in any period during the course of HIV infection in patients with premorbidly existing bipolar disorder. AIDS mania is the term given to mania which presents late in the infection or after the onset of AIDS. The predominant delusion the individual has is that they have been cured of HIV or that they have discovered the cure. Irritability, cognitive impairment, decreased psychomotor activity are seen alongside. The course is often protracted with poor recovery between the episodes.

Other Disorders

Antisocial personality disorder is the most common personality disorder associated with HIV. Psychosis in seen in 10% of those individuals affected with HIV.

Prevalence of substance use disorders ranges from 21% to 53%. Injectable drug use remains a huge risk factor in the incidence and spread of HIV infection due to usage of the same needle for drug intake by multiple people.

Delirium is seen in 43-65% of the patients affected with HIV. Mortality rate is often upto 20% in the population if not treated aggressively.

Other Infections

Lyme Disease

Lyme disease (caused by spirochaete Borrelia burgdorferi) has been reported to cause depression, other mood symptoms like irritability, mania, psychosis, and often dementia. The cognitive problems that have been reported include short term memory loss, impairment in verbal fluency and processing speed, word finding difficulties, and sleep disturbances. Less commonly, depersonalization phenomenon, OCD, panic disorder, and personality changes are seen.

Syphilis

Syphilis (caused by spirochaete Treponema pallidum) has 3 stages – primary, secondary, and tertiary syphilis. Nervous system is usually affected in tertiary syphilis that manifests months to years after the infection, though in the current era of antibiotics, neurosyphilis is rarely seen. Symptoms of encephalitis manifest as mood disturbances, sleep impairment, memory loss, and personality changes.

General paresis occurs 2 to 3 decades after the initial infection and primarily affects the frontal and temporal lobes. It presents with mood disturbances such as irritability and cognitive impairment such as poor attention and concentration, decreased motivation, memory loss, confabulation, anomia, apraxia, and pseudobulbar palsy. About 25% of the patients have depression, irritability, psychosis, paranoia and mania. Half of the patients will have cognitive disturbances that will often amount to dementia.

Non HIV viral infections:

Herpes simplex virus (HSV) encephalitis is often abrupt, manifesting with fever, altered mental status, headache, dysphasia, paresis, seizures, cognitive changes, hallucinations, memory loss, and other behavioral disturbances. HSV encephalitis may cause lesions in bilateral amygdala leading to Kluver Bucy syndrome which is characterized by hypersexuality, hyperorality, hypermetamorphosis (excessive exploration of the environment), placidity, visual agnosia, memory deficits, and inappropriate feeding behavior.

Ebstein-Barr virus (EBV) encephalitis presents with amnesia, cerebellar ataxia, seizures, coma, neurological deficits, psychosis, personality changes, perceptual distortions of size and space (known as Alice in Wonderland syndrome) and coma.

Rabies virus encephalitis leads to behavioral disturbances, agitation, extreme excitement, hallucinations and hydrophobia. It is invariably acute and fatal.

Subacute sclerosing panencephalitis (SSPE) is a very slow and progressive infection that usually occurs 7 to 12 years after the measles infection and is characterized by behavioral disturbances, personality changes, overall reduced school performance, hallucinations, apraxia, agnosia, movement disorders, and in later stages, mutism, dementia, stupor, coma, and death. Prognosis is usually poor.

Post group A Streptococcus infection, usually after 1 to 2 weeks, some children develop an abrupt onset of OCD and/or tics, movement disorders like chorea, sudden mood changes, deteriorating reading and calculation abilities, and enuresis. This is termed as PANDAS (pediatric autoimmune neuropsychiatric disorders associated with streptococcal infections). Another broader category with other etiological agents is termed as PANS (pediatric acute onset neuropsychiatric symptoms) that includes symptoms as such as OCD, restricted food consumption, sudden mood and behavioral changes like irritability, aggression, anxiety, depression, defiant behavior, deteriorating school performance, motor and sencory abnormalities, sleep disturbances, and enuresis and cannot be explained by Tourette disorder, Sydenham chorea, and systemic lupus erythematosus.

Epilepsy

According to International league against epilepsy (ILAE), a seizure is a transient occurrence of signs and/or symptoms due to abnormal excessive or synchronous neuronal activity in the brain. A person is considered to have epilepsy if there are at least 2 unprovoked (or reflex) seizures occurring more than 24 hours apart or 1 unprovoked (or reflex) seizure and a probability of further seizures similar to the general recurrence risk (at least 60%) after 2 unprovoked seizures, occurring over the next 10 years.

Prevalence of epilepsy is 0.63% globally. Prevalence of psychiatric conditions in patients with epilepsy ranges from 20 to 60%. There is a reciprocal relationship between epilepsy and psychiatric disorders. Epileptic patients are more prone to develop psychiatric conditions, especially depression as compared to general population while patients with depression and anxiety are more likely to develop epilepsy.

Depression is seen in 7.5 to 34% of patients with epilepsy. It is the most common psychiatric condition seen in association with epilepsy. Those with temporal lobe epilepsy and poor seizure control have a higher predilection to mood disorders.

The lifetime prevalence of psychosis in epilepsy ranges from 7 to 12%. Other disorders like anxiety disorders, personality disorders, suicidal behavior, and hyposexuality are more prevalent in people with epilepsy as compared to general population. Anxiety disorder is often a differential diagnosis to a seizure episode as often partial seizures can manifest as an anxiety or panic attack. Psychogenic nonepileptic seizures or dissociative convulsions are seen in 30% of patients with epilepsy.

Psychiatric behaviors are also seen in relation to the stage of the seizure. Depression, anxiety, recurrent intrusive thoughts can often occur either pre-ictally or ictally as a seizure episode. Post-ictally, there could be cognitive symptoms such as confusion, memory loss, and other cognitive changes.

Peri-ictal psychotic episodes are often severe and worsen with increasing episodes of seizures. Few patients show the phenomenon of forced normalization where psychotic symptoms worsen when they are seizure free. Inter-ictal psychosis often manifests as schizophreniform or schizophrenia like psychosis.

Gastaut-Geschwind syndrome: This is an uncommon type of personality change reported in epilepsy patients (esp. Temporal lobe epilepsy). Symptoms include hypergraphia, circumstantiality, interpersonal viscosity, hyperreligiosity, and hyposexuality. It is thought to be result of disrupted connectivity among cerebral areas.

Antiepileptics are the mainstay of treatment. Symptomatic treatment with SSRIs and antipsychotics often offer relief to the patients and psychological interventions like cognitive behavioral therapy are recommended in some patients.

Other Systems

Cardiovascular disease is known to increase the risk of depression and anxiety in predisposed individuals. Acute MI can often present with anxiety symptoms or a panic attack.

Amongst all the mental disorders to be associated with asthma, anxiety disorder is the most prevalent one. Specifically, panic disorder and post-traumatic stress disorder are more common. In patients with depression and COPD (chronic obstructive pulmonary disease), depression often leads to poor prognosis and quality of life.

Dermatological conditions often lead to disfigurement that is often visible and extensive. This leads to decreased self-esteem and body image issues. In chronic lesions affecting individuals in early childhood and adolescence, psychological development is affected and is often long-lasting. This leads to an increased vulnerability to psychiatric conditions, especially depressive, substance use and neurotic disorders.

Endocrinological Disorders

Thyroid Disorders

Thyroid disorders have long since been associated with psychiatric conditions. Hypothyroidism has a strong positive correlation with depression. In hypothyroidism, cognitive deficits include poor attention and concentration, and memory disturbances. Psychomotor retardation and easy fatiguability are seen. Often, hypothyroidism is a differential diagnosis for depression. Vice versa, patients with depression often have been found to have subclinical thyroid disease. In fact, triiodothyronine at the dose of 25-50 mcg is one of the second line drug choices in treatment of depression. It also has a role in rapid cycling of bipolar disorder. Hypothroidism has also been associated with anxiety and psychosis (myxedema madness).

Patients with hyperthyroidism often complain of restlessness, nervousness, irritability, and fatigue. Generalized anxiety disorder and panic disorder have been associated. Depression often presents with agitation. Cognitive impairment include distractibility, impairment in attention and concentration. Psychosis has a low correlation with hyperthyroidism. Often, thyroid crises have a presenting picture like that of delirium.

Parathyroid Disorders

The most common psychiatric association with hyperparathyroidism is depression with features of easy fatiguability in most patients, while irritability and anxiety have been found in a few patients. Memory impairment is seen but it has a slow progressive course. Acute delirious picture with hallucinations, delusions, and aggression has also been reported.

In hypoparathyroidism, emotional lability, nervousness, irritability, and impairment in intellectual functioning are seen. Anxiety disorders are a frequent accompaniment while mania and psychosis are rare.

Cushing's Syndrome

Major depressive disorder, mania, anxiety and cognitive impairment are the most important clinical abnormalities. Psychosis has also been frequently associated with endogenous Cushing's syndrome.

Addison's Disease

Depression, anxiety, easy fatiguability, emotional withdrawal, apathy, and loss of drive are seen. There are sudden mood fluctuations. Some patients show agitation, and suspiciousness, and often a dementia like picture is seen in few. Delirium with auditory and visual hallucinations has been reported in Addisonian crisis. Insomnia and other sleep disturbances have been reported.

Hyperaldosteronism

Depression, anxiety, OCD, panic disorder, and fatiguability have been associated with this condition. If left untreated, due to the resultant hypertension, vascular dementia can manifest.

Pheochromocytoma

Pheochromocytomas are tumors commonly originating from adrenal medulla that lead to increased production of catecholamines. Symptoms often appear paroxysmally and include headache, palpitations, sweating, tremors, chest and abdominal pain. Signs include autonomic disturbances such as hypertension or hypotension, tachycardia, pallor etc. Symptoms often present as an anxiety or panic attack. Sometimes, the anxiety will persist for a while.

Vitamin deficiencies (Table 37.1)

Table 37.1

Vitamin	Manifestations in deficiency	Neuropsychiatric manifestations in deficiency
Thiamine (B1)	Dry beri-beri – Cardiovascular system involvement leading to tachycardia, peripheral edema, congestive heart failure. Wet beri-beri – nervous system involvement leading to peripheral neuropathy, hyporeflexia, ophthalmoplegia	Memory impairment, irritability, other mood changes, fatigue, Wernicke's Korsakoff encephalopathy
Niacin (B3)	Pellagra : The four Ds Dermatitis Diarrhea Dementia Death	Apathy, neurasthenia, irritability, depression, dementia, seizures
Pyridoxine (B6)	Anemia, glossitis, peripheral neuropathy	Depression, irritability, confusion, lethargy
Folic acid (B9)	Megaloblastic anemia, glossitis, angular stomatitis, nausea, vomiting, hyperpigmentation of skin and mucosa	Depression, dementia, irritability, sleep disturbances,
Cobalamin (B12)	Pernicious anemia, megaloblastic anemia, ataxia, paresthesia, impaired proprioception and vibration senses, subacute combined degeneration of the cord	Irritability, psychosis, dementia

Metabolic Disturbances (Table 37.2)

Table 37.2

Metabolic disturbances	Symptoms
Hyponatremia	Nausea, vomiting, malaise, respiratory failure, encephalopathy, headache, confusion, delirium, mood changes
Hypernatremia	Dry mouth, lethargy, delirium, increased muscle tone, coma
Hypokalemia	Fatigue, myalgia, flaccid paralysis, apathy, depression, irritability, lethargy, anxiety, delirium
Hyperkalemia	Bradycardia, ventricular arrhythmia, muscle weakness, fatiguability,
Hypocalcemia	Seizures, carpopedal spasm, hyperreflexia, irritability, intellectual impairment
Hypercalcemia	Weakness, depression, irritability, psychosis, anxiety, altered mental status
Hypomagnesemia	Hyperreflexia, muscle cramps, seizures, ataxia, depression, irritability, chorea, athetosis, hemiparesis, confusion, delirium
Hypermagnesemia	Lethargy, confusion, flaccid paralysis, areflexia, coma
Hypophosphatemia	Irritability, anxiety, confusion, encephalopathy resembling Wernicke's, ataxia, myoclonus, weakness, syndrome resembling Guillain Barre, coma, seizures

Genetic Disorders

Genetic disorders often form a chunk of child and adolescent psychiatric cases. Early diagnosis and management is very important as delay often leads to further deterioration of the symptoms that could have been attenuated early on. The following diseases are a few examples of genetic illnesses that often can present with psychiatric symptoms.

Acute Porphyria

Porphyrias are a group of metabolic disorders that are due to mutations in the enzymes related to heme synthesis pathway. Acute porphyrias include acute intermittent porphyria, hereditary coproporphyria, variegate porphyria, and ALA dehydratase porphyria. Psychiatric symptoms in acute porphyrias are often manifold and varied. Symptoms include mood symptoms, sleep disturbances, anxiety symptoms, behavioral disturbances, and psychotic symptoms. Personality aspects often associated with porphyrias include neurotic personalities like anxiety and obsessive personalities. Other symptoms include mania and hypomania, catatonia, suicidal ideation, phobias, somatoform disorder, cognitive impairment, fatigue, and delirium. Treatment is usually symptomatic.

Wilson's Disease

Wilson disease is an autosomal recessive disorder caused by mutations in a copper transporting ATPase encoded by the ATP7B gene on chromosome 13q14.3. This disease affects liver, brain especially the basal ganglia, and the eyes. It can manifest clinically from first to fourth decade. Upto 70% of the patients present with psychiatric symptoms. These symptoms include behavioral changes, personality changes, aggression, disinhibition, and cognitive dysfunctioning. While presence of Kayser-Fleischer (KF) rings and low levels of ceruloplasmin in the serum offer clues to the diagnosis, gold standard test for Wilson's disease is liver biopsy with staining for copper. Treatment is usually with copper chelators such as d-penicillamine, trientine or ammonium tetrathiomolybdate. Symptoms often abate with this therapy over a period of 1 to 2 years.

Phenylketonuria

Phenylketonuria is an autosomal recessive disorder due to a mutation in the gene for phenylalanine hydroxylase on chromosome 12. This leads to accumulated levels of phenylalanine in the body which affects normal neural development. Treatment usually involves a diet that is low in phenylalanine and with tyrosine supplementation. If not treated early, affected children will develop mental retardation, developmental delay, anxiety, and other psychiatric disorders. Maintaining a strict diet is often hard and adults have been shown to have higher rates of psychiatric illnesses.

Heavy Metal Poisoning (Table 37.3)

Table 37.3

Metal	Effects due to toxicity
Lead	Abdominal pain, Anemia, Fanconi's syndrome, irritability, depression, cognitive impairment, lethargy, decreased libido, seizures
Mercury	Movement disorders like intentional tremor, cognitive impairment, irritability, sleep disturbances, confusion, delirium, erythism-socially anxious and timid, irritable; children may develop acrodynia or pink disease
Arsenic	Abdominal pain, diarrhea, nausea, vomiting, hyperpigmentation, ECG changes, Mees' line, polyneuritis, distal muscle weakness, delirium, seizures, coma, apathy, memory impairment, drowsiness

(Continued...)

Metal	Effects due to toxicity
Manganese	Headache, weakness, drowsiness, increased sleep, sudden and persistent laughing and crying episodes, impulsivity, irritability, cognitive impairment, Parkinsonism features
Thallium	Polyneuropathy, gastroenteritis, headache, anorexia, myalgia, movement disorders, lethargy, cognitive impairment, altered mental status, depression, dementia, psychosis, seizures
Bismuth	Movement disorders, gait disturbances, headache, sleep disturbances, apathy, mood lability, delirium, cognitive impairment, dementia

Medication-Induced Disorders

Chronic use of sedatives and anxiolytics such as benzodiazepines and Z drugs like zolpidem leads to mild cognitive impairment especially in the domains of memory and processing speed. Other medications associated with cognitive dysfunction include chemotherapeutic agents, steroids, nucleoside reverse transcriptase inhibitors, and anticholinergics.

Agents implicated in mood disorders include steroids, anti-parkinsonism drugs, anti-depressants themselves (causing antidepressant induced mania or hypomania), beta blockers, interferon alpha, vinca alkaloids, oral contraceptives etc.

Psychosis is often induced by anticholinergic agents, immunosuppressants, chemotherapeutic agents, steroids, disulfiram, antitubercular drugs and sympathomimetics.

Anxiety is known to be caused by stimulant drugs like methylphenidate, steroids, cardiovascular medications, withdrawal of anxiolytics, insulins, thyroid and caffeine preparations. Stimulants often cause OCD symptoms.

Drugs like cholinergic, adrenergic, dopaminergic, histaminergic and serotonergic agents, steroids, sympathomimetics, and thyroid preparations induce sleep disorders.

SSRIs, antipsychotics, antihypertensives, anticonvulsants are implicated in the cause of sexual dysfunction.

Management

The mainstay of management of organic disorders is the treatment of underlying cause. Early diagnosis is crucial and essential for good prognosis. History taking should include inquiries regarding past trauma, medication details, physical comorbidities, etc. Investigations should be done prudently but without hesitation in case of suspicion of an organic cause to the disorder. Liaison between various medical specialities is often the rule rather than being the exception for prompt treatment of organic disorders.

CONCLUSION

A comprehensive diagnostic and treatment formulation will help in prompt diagnosis and treatment of organicity. Ruling out organicity is a must before psychiatry referral as many neurological and other conditions often present with psychiatric symptoms. Treating doctors should have a good idea about the drug-drug interactions between other drugs and psychotropic drugs to prevent further complications.

Long term management includes physical rehabilitation in cases with neurological symptoms, psychological therapies such as supportive therapy, family therapy, and behavioral therapies.

Flowchart 37.1

History
- Past history of trauma
- Whether a case of DM/HTN/epilepsy/respiratory and cardiac disorders/TB/HIV/other infections
- H/o fever
- Occupational history
- Nutritional history
- Family h/o genetic disorders
- H/o medication use

Physical examination should include
- General examination
- Systemic examination
- Stigmata of nutritional, genetic and infectious disorders

Investigation
- Complete hemogram including peripheral smear
- Liver function, thyroid function, parathyroid function, renal function tests
- Serum electrolytes
- Vitamin levels wherever possible
- HIV testing
- Lumbar Puncture
- Chromosomal and genetic tests
- Imaging like CT or MRI
- Toxic screen panel
- Urine testing for porphobilinogen, catecholamine metabolites
- Levels of cortisol and other hormones like ACTH, FSH etc.

Treatment
- Treatment of underlying cause like stroke, head injury
- HAART
- Antibiotics, antivirals, NSAIDs
- Hormone supplementation
- Anti-thyroid drugs
- Vitamin supplementation
- Heavy metal chelators
- Withholding of suspected medication
- Symptomatic treatment with antipsychotics, SSRIs, NSAIDs, anxiolytics

BIBLIOGRAPHY

1. Sadock, B.J., Sadock,V.A., & Ruiz, P. (2017). *Comprehensive Textbook of Psychiatry.* (10th Ed.). Philadelphia : Wolters Kluwer.
2. David, D., Fleminger, S., Kopelman, M., Lovestone, S., Mellers, J. (2012). *Lishman's Organic Psychiatry.* (4th Ed.). New Jersey : Wiley Blackwell.
3. Gururaj, G. (2002) .Epidemiology of traumatic brain injuries: Indian scenario, *Neurological Research,* 24(1), 24-28. DOI: 10.1179/016164102101199503
4. Conner, S.H., & Solomon, S.S. (2017). Psychiatric Manifestations of Endocrine Disorders., J *Hum Endocrinol*, 2 (007).
5. Ferro, J., Caeiro, L. & Figueira, M. (2016). Neuropsychiatric sequelae of stroke, *Nat Rev Neurol,* 12, 269–280. (2016). doi:10.1038/nrneurol.2016.46
6. Dubé, B., Benton, T., Cruess, D. G., & Evans, D. L. (2005). Neuropsychiatric manifestations of HIV infection and AIDS. Journal of psychiatry & neuroscience : JPN, 30(4), 237–246.

Delirium 38

Sandeep Grover

INTRODUCTION

Delirium is an acute neuropsychiatric disorder, which is also referred with alternative terms like, Intensive care unit (ICU) psychosis, encephalopathy, acute confusional state, acute organic syndrome, acute brain failure, postoperative psychosis, toxic psychosis, cerebral insufficiency. It is a purely organic condition which is associated with one or more physiological and/or structural aberrations, affecting the brain. It is understood as a temporary state of brain failure. It is a condition, which is often seen in medical and surgical wards and intensive care setting. It is a medical-surgical emergency, which is often under-recognized and under-treated. Even after controlling for factors, such as severity and type of physical disease, it is often associated with increased risk of mortality, a significant increase in the length of hospital stay, treatment cost, functional decline and distress to the patient and the caregivers.

EPIDEMIOLOGY

Prevalence and incidence of delirium is influenced by the treatment setting. Usually, the prevalence and incidence of delirium is lower in the medical and surgical wards, when compared to the ICUs. Prevalence in medical inpatients ranges from 30-50% and is as high as 80% in patients admitted to the ICUs, with higher prevalence higher among patients on mechanical ventilation. It is seen in patients of all age groups, with higher prevalence among the elderly.

CLINICAL FEATURES OF DELIRIUM

The hallmark feature of delirium is an acute onset confusional state with impairment in attention and awareness being the core symptom of delirium. Its course is characterized by marked fluctuations, sometimes within the same day, with evening worsening of symptoms. It is usually short lasting. Other common clinical features of delirium are listed in Box 38.1.

Delirium can be further subtyped into as hyperactive, hypoactive and mixed subtype, based on the level of psychomotor activity. Hyperactive subtype of delirium is characterized by agitation, increased speech output, faster rate of speech and increased movements. Hypoactive delirium subtype is characterized by lower motor movements and reduced speech output. The patient often keeps on lying without much movement. Mixed subtype of delirium is characterized by symptoms of both hyperactive and hypoactive delirium. Among the various subtypes of delirium, hypoactive delirium is often missed and misdiagnosed.

Box 38.1: Clinical Features of Delirium

- **Acute onset:** Onset over hours to days, with a significant change from the baseline
- **Fluctuating course:** The symptoms of delirium fluctuate over time in terms of severity, and in between patient may have lucid intervals of normal functioning; diurnal pattern may also have been seen with worsening of symptoms at night (sun downing phenomenon)
- **Impaired attention:** Impaired capacity to direct, focus, sustain and shift attention. During examining this may manifest as forgetting instructions, distraction towards irrelevant stimuli, repeating the same question again and again
- **Reduced awareness:** Disorientation (time, place and person) in the form of misidentifying people around/familiar persons, behaving as if at home or workplace, talking about relatives who are not around, at times talking about dead relatives as if he is in the past
- **Disturbance of consciousness:** Patient may have altered level of consciousness. While reviewing the history, different caregivers, provide conflicting information with respect to the awake mental state of the patient over the time. During the Mental status examination patient may fall asleep in between and at other times appears to alert
- **Disruption of sleep and wakefulness:** Fragmented sleep, altered sleep-wake cycle (not able to sleep at night and daytime naps), experiencing vivid dreams and nightmares - difficulty distinguishing dreams from real perceptions
- **Emotional disturbance:** Frequent changes in the emotional state of the patient, varying from fearfulness to euphoria, anxiety and sadness/tearfulness during the same interview or over the multiple interactions in a day
- **Psychomotor disturbance:** Agitation (pulling out the tubes/drains/ catheters, frequently trying to get out of the bed, wander around in the ward/house, frequently changing the postures while in the bed) or Retardation (reduction in activity level, delay in responding to queries or not responding at all, marked reduction in verbal output, apathetic, withdrawn, low volume of the voice); patient may show both set of symptoms on the same day, sometimes, fluctuations may be very rapid, i.e., symptoms fluctuating over few minutes to hours
- **Disorders of thought:** Delusions (usually persecutory), disorganized speech, bizarre or illogical thinking, poor judgment and insight
- **Disorders of language:** Irrelevant and/or incoherent speech, un-understandable speech, slow and slurred speech, increased speech output with pressure of speech, difficulty in word-finding, difficulty in writing
- **Disorders of memory:** Difficulty in remembering about meals, intake of medications, visitors, *etc.;* inability to recollect things recently discussed/mentioned; However, patient can also have impairment of remote memory too
- **Perceptual disturbances:** Hallucinations (visual more common than auditory), illusions (may misinterpret wrinkles on the bed sheets/ blankets as animate objects with attempts to clean the bed sheet/blanket to remove the animate objects), misinterpretations (noise of hospital machines/ICU machines interpreted as gunshot, different alarms of a machine considered as police siren)
- **Visuospatial difficulties:** Difficulty or inability in constructing- drawing, copying, designs, copying 3D models (Constructional Apraxia); difficulty finding one's way in the environment (i.e., Topographical disorientation)

Risk Factors and Etiological Factors Associated With Delirium

As delirium is associated with multiple physical illnesses, multiple factors have been shown to be associated with the delirium. These factors have been variously classified and can be broadly grouped as predisposing/ precipitating factors and etiological factors

(Box 38.2). However, there is overlap between precipitating factors and etiological factors. Most of the patients have more than one etiological/precipitating factor associated with the emergence of delirium. The predisposing factors are further categorized as reversible and irreversible. Some of the irreversible factors associated with development of delirium include older age, male gender, etc. A simple pneumonic to remember the etiological factors associated with delirium is DELIRIUM [Drugs, Electrolyte Imbalance, Lack of Drugs (drug withdrawal), Infection, Reduced sensory Inputs (visual & hearing), Intracranial (e.g., CVA, subdural), Urinary retention/ fecal impaction and Myocardial/ Pulmonary].

Box 38.2: Risk factors for delirium

Predisposing factors

- Alcohol abuse
- Cognitive decline/dementia
- Co-morbid illnesses
- Elderly
- Male gender
- Poorer functional ability
- Sensory impairment- visual
- Severity of illness
- Treatment (prescribed drugs)
- Use of over the counter medication

Precipitating factors

- Iatrogenic events (surgery, any intervention)
- Indwelling catheter
- Malnutrition
- More than three medications
- Use of physical restraints

Etiological factors

- Acute Vascular lesions (Stroke, trauma)
- Endocrinopathies (Hypoglycemia, Diabetic ketoacidosis, Hypothyroidism, Hyperthyroidism, Cushing's syndrome)
- Hypoxia
- Infection (Sepsis, urinary tract infection, pneumonia)
- Intracranial pathology (Meningitis, encephalitis)
- Malignancies
- Metabolic disturbances (electrolyte imbalance, hypovolemia)
- Nutritional deficiencies
- Substance withdrawal (alcohol)
- Toxins
- Trauma
- Use of heavy metals
- Use of medications (anticholinergics)

Pathogenesis of Delirium

Although different hypotheses (Box 38.3) have been proposed for manifestation of delirium, neurotransmitter hypothesis is most popular and is considered to be involved in the final pathway of other hypotheses too. Among the various neurotransmitters which have been most closely linked with development of delirium include acetylcholine (reduction in levels) and dopamine (increase in the levels). Other neurotransmitters involved with development of delirium include gamma-aminobutyric acid (GABA), glutamate, norepinephrine, and serotonin.

Box 38.3: Etiopathogenesis of delirium

- Neuro-inflammatory hypothesis
- Neuronal aging hypothesis
- Oxidative stress hypothesis
- Neurotransmitter deficiency hypothesis
- Neuroendocrine hypothesis
- Diurnal dysregulation hypothesis
- Network disconnectivity hypothesis

Diagnosis

Diagnostic and Statistical Manual, Fifth Edition (DSM-5) includes delirium under the broad heading of Neurocognitive disorders which also include dementia, and mild cognitive impairment. Diagnosis of delirium as per the DSM-5 criteria requires presence of disturbance in attention, onset of symptom over a short period of time, disturbance in other domains of cognitive functions, symptoms not better explained by another pre-existing, established, or evolving neurocognitive disorder and do not occur in the context of a severely reduced level of arousal, such as coma. Further, there is evidence to suggest that the disturbance is a direct physiological consequence of another medical condition, substance intoxication or withdrawal (Box 38.4). Similarly, International Classification of Diseases, 11th revision (ICD-11), also classified delirium under the broad category of neurocognitive disorders (Block L1-6D7) and is coded as 6D70. According to ICD-11, delirium is characterized by disturbed attention (i.e, reduced ability to direct, focus, sustain and shift attention) and awareness, that tends to develop over a short period of time and tends to fluctuate during the course of the day, accompanied by other cognitive impairment such as memory deficit, disorientation, or impairment in language, visuospatial ability, or perception. Disturbance of sleep wake cycle (reduced arousal of acute onset or total sleep loss with reversal of sleep wake cycle) may also be present. The symptoms are attributed to a disorder or disease not classified under mental and behavioral disorders or to substance intoxication or withdrawal or to a medication. In terms of subtypes, ICD-11 categorised delirium into 4 subgroups, i.e, delirium due to disease classified elsewhere (6D70.0), delirium due to psychoactive substances including medications (6D70.1), delirium due to multiple etiological factors (6D70.2) and delirium due to unknown or unspecified etiological factors (6D70.3).

Box 38.4: Diagnostic Criteria for Delirium as per DSM-5

A. A disturbance in attention (i.e., reduced ability to direct, focus, sustain, and shift attention) and awareness (reduced orientation to the environment)

B. The disturbance develops over a short period (usually hours to a few days), represents a change from baseline attention and awareness and tends to fluctuate in severity during a day

C. An additional disturbance in cognition (e.g., memory deficit, disorientation, language, visuospatial ability, or perception)

D. The disturbances in Criteria A and C are not better explained by another pre-existing, established, or evolving neurocognitive disorder and do not occur in the context of a severely reduced level of arousal, such as coma

E. There is evidence from the history, physical examination, or laboratory findings that the disturbance is a direct physiological consequence of another medical condition, substance intoxication or withdrawal (i.e., due to a drug of abuse or to a medication), or exposure to a toxin, or is due to multiple etiologies.

How to Diagnose Delirium

DSM-5 or ICD-11 criteria can be used to diagnose delirium. However, often the non-mental health professionals are not very well versed with these criteria. Accordingly, screening for delirium in the hands of physicians, nurses and other staff, can be facilitated by using screening instruments like Confusion Assessment Method (CAM) and Confusion Assessment Method for the Intensive Care Unit (CAM-ICU). These instruments have been shown to have high sensitivity and specificity for diagnosing delirium.

Differential Diagnosis

As the symptoms of delirium overlap with other psychiatric conditions, it is important to distinguish it from other psychiatric conditions. The common differential diagnosis of delirium includes dementia, depression, and psychosis (Box 38.5). While evaluating for differential diagnosis, it is important to remember that many a times, delirium may get superimposed on these pre-existing psychiatric conditions, especially, dementia. Features, which distinguish delirium, from depression and psychosis include higher level of impairment in the cognitive functions. Patients of delirium often have evening worsening of symptoms. In contrast patients with depression usually have early morning worsening, and such diurnal variation does not occur in patients with psychosis. In terms of onset, delirium has acute onset, whereas patients with dementia usually have insidious onset of symptoms without much impairment in the level of consciousness till the late stages.

Assessment for Delirium

A thorough assessment of delirium involves making a correct diagnosis and identifying the underlying cause(s) (Box 38.6). It is important to remember that delirium is often multifactorial in origin. Assessment involves taking proper history, review of treatment chart, thorough physical examination, mental status examination and carrying out the required investigation. History taking should involve eliciting history in terms of duration of symptoms, type of onset, types of symptoms, course of the symptoms and temporal correlation with underlying medical illnesses, use of medications or substances, especially alcohol use should not be missed. A careful review of the medication chart can also help in identifying the causative or contributory factor. A thorough physical examination must be carried out to rule out all possible causes. Physical examination can often provide important hints about the underlying causes. All patients with delirium should undergo

Box 38.5: Differential Diagnosis of Delirium

Features	Delirium	Dementia	Depression	Schizophrenia
Onset	Acute	Insidious	Variable	Variable
Consciousness	Marked Fluctuations	Clear till late stages	Generally no impairment	Generally no impairment
Attention	Impaired	Impairment-late stages	Poor attention	Poor attention
Orientation	Disoriented	Disorientation is seen in later stages	Usually oriented	Usually oriented
Memory	Poor short-term memory	Poor short and Long-term memory	Usually intact	Usually intact
Fluctuation	Diurnal fluctuations are common	Diurnal fluctuations maybe present	Morning worsening of symptoms	Usually not seen
Psychotic Sx	Fleeting, simple	Less common	Less common	Persistent, complex
Hallucinations	Visual >Auditory; Tactile	Usually absent	If present, are auditory	Mostly auditory
Mood	Fluctuating	Flat, apathetic	Sadness	Apathy/flat

basic investigations. However, additional investigations must be carried out on the basis of leads obtained from history and examination to confirm possible underlying cause. Once identified, the abnormalities must be monitored closely, until the abnormality is corrected.

Box 38.6: Assessment for delirium

Proper history taking:

- Onset, type of symptoms, course of symptoms, diurnal variations, activity level, duration of symptoms, relationship with onset/worsening of medical condition or starting/increasing the dose of a medication or intoxication/withdrawal of substance or alcohol

Review Medication Chart:

- Look for the agents which can contribute to delirium (**ACUTE CHANGE IN M**ENTAL **S**TATE)
- **A**ntibiotics
- **C**ardiac Drugs
- **U**rinary Incontinence drugs
- **T**heophylline
- **E**thanol
- **C**orticosteroids
- **H_2** Blockers
- **A**ntiparkinsonian agents
- **N**arcotics
- **G**eriatric psychotropic agents
- **E**NT Drugs
- **I**nsomnia Drugs
- **N**on-Steroidal Anti-inflammatory Drugs (NSAIDs)
- **M**uscle relaxant
- **S**eizure medications

Thorough physical examination to identify the possible causes of delirium

- **Head:** look for evidence of head trauma
- **Pupil:** fixed & dilated (Intracranial insult or raised intracranial pressure), miosis (opioid toxicity), mydriasis (anticholinergic toxicity)
- **Fundus:** papilledema
- **Extraocular movements:** ophthalmoplegia (Wernicke's encephalopathy), nystagmus
- **Neck:** Thyromegaly, neck rigidity
- **Neurological examination:** focal deficits
- **Skin:** fever, dehydration, injection marks, marks of use of patches, evidence of liver dysfunction etc.
- **Lungs:** crepts, wheeze
- **Cardiac:** murmur
- **Abdomen:** mass, tenderness
- **Genitourinary:** urinary retention, local discharge
- **Rectum:** fecal mass, hemorrhoids etc.

(Continued)

Mental Status Examination:

- Attention, Orientation, Language, Visuospatial difficulties, Memory, Thinking, Perceptual disturbances

Investigations:

- Routine investigations- to rule out other causes
- Basic investigations like serum electrolytes, Renal Function Test, Liver function test, Hemogram, Arterial blood gas analysis are a must
- Other investigations – as indicated (Toxicology screen, Serological evaluation)
- If required – neuroimaging, electroencephalogram (EEG)

Consider differential diagnosis

- Depression, Dementia, Psychosis, Delirium superimposed on dementia

Confirm the diagnosis

- Use standardized diagnostic criteria for delirium

Management of Delirium

Once the diagnosis of delirium is made, treatment involves supportive care, correction of underlying cause(s), removal of un-necessary medications, use of non-pharmacological measures (Box 38.7) and the use of pharmacological treatments. As a higher number of medications are considered to a risk factor for delirium and some of the medications (Box 38.6) are known to cause delirium, medication chart should be reviewed. Effort must be made to stop the unnecessary medications, and medications considered to be possibly causative or contributory to development of delirium must be stopped. Reversible etiological factors should be corrected. Non-pharmacological measures are considered as first-line management of delirium and include supportive care, maintaining competence, ensuring good uninterrupted sleep, providing an unambiguous environment, communicate clearly and concisely, frequent reorientation, avoid physical restraints, assess and manage pain adequately and mobilise at the earliest (Box 38.7).

Box 38.7: Non-pharmacological management of delirium

Supportive Care

- Ensure safety of the patients
- Close observation and monitor the vital signs, temperature, oxygenation, hydration, electrolytes, glucose level, nutrition, input/output
- Prevent hypoxia, fluid and electrolyte balance
- Regularly evaluate the patients and take measure to avoid development of pressure sores
- Reduce immobility – encourage performance of self-care activities on their own, allow free movements
- Remove the catheter as soon as possible
- Monitor bladder and bowel habit and maintain normal elimination patterns

(Continued)

- Monitor the prescription with special focus on evaluation of potential adverse drug-drug interactions and drug-disease interactions
- Early mobilization

Maintaining competence

- Identify and correct sensory impairment: ensure patients have their glasses, hearing aid and dentures
- Consider an interpreter if needed
- Encourage self care and participation in treatment (for example have the patient give feedback on pain)

Ensure good uninterrupted sleep:

- Schedule treatment/interventions/ Intravenous fluids in such a way that patient can have maximum periods of uninterrupted sleep (use a sleep protocol to promote quiet hours)

Providing an unambiguous environment

- Removing unnecessary objects close to the patient's bed; allow adequate space between beds
- Consider using single rooms to aid rest and avoid extremes of sensory experience; disturbance caused by staff attending other patients in the same room should be minimized
- Do not frequently change the patient's bed location - frequent changes may increase disorientation
- Avoid using medical jargon in front of the patient as it may encourage paranoia
- Making eye contact, frequent touching, and using clear verbal instructions when talking to patients
- Encourage family and caregiver involvement- encourage family/caregivers to bring in client's personal and familiar objects
- Appropriate lighting– ensure that lighting is adequate; provide a 40–60 W night light to reduce misperceptions, windows with a view to outside, curtains and blinds open during the day, and minimal lighting at night may reduce disorientation
- Quiet environment especially at rest times – noise reduction strategies (e.g.: use of vibrating pagers/phones rather than call bells)
- Control sources of excess noise (such as staff, equipment, visitors): aim for < 45 decibels in the day and < 20 decibels at night
- Keep room temperature between 21°C and 23.8°C

Communicate clearly and concisely:

- Give repeated verbal reminders of the day, time and location, and identify key individuals, such as members of the treatment team and relatives
- Establishing proper eye contact, frequent touch, talk slowly but clearly and using clear verbal instructions while talking to patients

Frequent reorientation

- Provide clock and calendar that clients can see

(Continued)

Avoid physical restraints, if possible
Assess and Manage pain adequately
Mobilise at the earliest
Remove unnecessary medications
Prevent, detect and treat major postoperative complications

Box 38.8: Medications used for management of delirium

- **Antipsychotics: haloperidol, olanzapine, risperidone, quetiapine, etc.**
- **Benzodiazepine (only for alcohol withdrawal)**
- **Acetyl cholinesterase inhibitors: Donepezil, Physostigmine, rivastigmine**
- **Alpha-2 adrenergic receptor agonist (dexmedetomidine)**
- **Melatonin, Ramelteon**

Many pharmacological agents have been evaluated in the management of delirium (Box 38.8). Among these, antipsychotics remain the mainstay of treatment in all kind of delirium except for alcohol and benzodiazepine withdrawal delirium. Low dose haloperidol is the most commonly used antipsychotic for management of delirium. However, before starting the antipsychotics, benefits and risks must be weighed and baseline electrocardiogram (ECG) must be done to evaluate the QTc interval. Antipsychotics are usually considered in a patient who is agitated, restless has hallucination and delusions, and has lack of sleep. While using antipsychotics, monitor the symptoms and side effects. However, while using antipsychotics, it is important to remember that these should be used only for a shorter duration and in the lowest effective dose (Box 38.9). While using antipsychotics, it is important to monitor the ECG for any QTc prolongation.

In recent times, melatonin has emerged as a safe treatment option for management of delirium. Benzodiazepines are indicated for the management of delirium associated with alcohol and benzodiazepine withdrawal. Additionally, while managing patients with alcohol withdrawal, high doses of thiamine should be used to prevent development of Wernicke's encephalopathy.

Box 38.9: Antipsychotic doses used for management of delirium

Antipsychotics	The usual starting dose in patients with delirium
Haloperidol	0.25 to 0.5 mg Bid
Olanzapine	1.25 to 2.5 mg OD//Bid
Risperidone	0.25 to 0.5 mg OD/Bid
Quetiapine	6.25 to 12.5 mg OD/Bid

Outcome of Delirium

Delirium usually lasts for 3-10 days. If left untreated, it is often associated with increased mortality and prolongation of hospital stay. Adequate management can reduce the duration and severity of delirium.

Prevention of Delirium

As delirium is often associated with adverse outcome, best strategy of management is prevention of delirium. There is a significant overlap between the strategies used for prevention and treatment of delirium. Some of the important strategies include evaluation of cognitive functions at the baseline, evaluation for risk factors, modifying the reversible risk factors, removing the un-necessary medications and avoiding sensory deprivation (Box 38.9).

Box 38.9: Prevention of Delirium

- Evaluate the cognitive functions at the baseline
- Identify/evaluate for the risk factors for delirium
- Monitor cognitive functions on regular basis by using Mini Mental State Examination, Montreal Cognitive Assessment, Hindi Mental State Examination; In case there is a fall in 2 points on various cognitive function assessment instruments, screen the patient for delirium
- Minimize sensory deprivation (restoration of eyeglasses and hearing aids), Ensure proper sleep
- Stop unnecessary medications
- Minimize exposure to medications which have a high propensity to cause delirium (anticholinergic) and use alternative agents if possible
- Weigh the risk and benefit of use of medications with high anticholinergics properties, opioids and sedatives, especially among vulnerable elderly patients
- Avoid use of high doses of medications, especially while using polypharmacy
- Maintain adequate lighting of the area
- Take measures so that patient gets adequate sleep and encourage normalization of sleep–wake cycles
- Change of rooms must be kept to the minimum
- Frequent reorientation, Appropriate cognitive stimulation
- Adequate pain management
- Reduce immobility
- Avoid use of physical restraints
- Quiet environment: minimize or remove the unexpected & irritating noises (e.g., alarms)
- Minimise the use of indwelling urinary catheters

BIBLIOGRAPHY

1. Fabian, T. and Solai, L. (2018). Delirium. In: B. Sadock, V. Sadock, and P. Ruiz, ed., Comprehensive Textbook of Psychiatry, 10th ed. Philadephia: Wolters Kluwer.
2. Grover S, Avasthi A. Clinical Practice Guidelines for management of delirium in Elderly. Indian J Psychiatry 2018; 60 (Suppl 3): S329-S340.
3. Grover S, Kate N. Assessment scales for delirium: a review. World J Psychiatry 2012;2: 58-70.
4. Grover S, Kate N. Delirium Research: Contributions from India. In: Developments in Psychiatry in India: Clinical, Research and Policy Perspectives. Eds: Savita Malhotra, Subho Chakrabarti. Springer (India) Pvt. Ltd., 2015; pp 463-492.
5. Grover S, Mattoo SK, Gupta N. Usefulness of atypical antipsychotics and Cholin esterase inhibitors in delirium: A review. Pharmacopsychiatry, 2011; 44:43-54.
6. Maldonado JR. Acute Brain Failure: Pathophysiology, Diagnosis, Management, and Sequelae of Delirium. Crit Care Clin. 2017;33:461–519.
7. Mattoo SK, Grover S, Gupta N. Delirium in general practice. Indian Journal of Medical Research, 2010; 131: 387-398.
8. McNicoll L, Pisani MA, Zhang Y, Ely EW, Siegel MD, Inouye SK. Delirium in the Intensive Care Unit: Occurrence and Clinical Course in Older Patients. Journal of the American Geriatrics Society. 2003;51:591–8.

39 Dementia

Sandeep Grover • Swati Chaudhari

INTRODUCTION

Dementia refers to a disease process marked by progressive cognitive impairment in clear consciousness. These deficits represent a decline from a previous level of functioning as opposed to low intellectual functioning or intellectual disability which are developmental and static conditions. Cognitive deficits associated with other mental disorders (e.g. schizophrenia, bipolar disorder) are excluded from this category. Dementia is associated with significant impairment in functioning, quality of life, activities of daily living, dependency on the caregivers and caregiver burden.

Dementia is a fairly general syndrome with many causes, and hence a careful clinical workup of a patient with dementia is required to establish its cause. Approximately 15 percent of people with dementia have reversible illnesses, such as metabolic abnormalities (e.g., hypothyroidism), nutritional deficiencies (e.g., vitamin B12 or folate deficiencies), or dementia syndrome caused by depression, for which treatment needs to be initiated before irreversible damage takes place.

EPIDEMIOLOGY

The prevalence of dementia is rising with increasing life expectancy. The age-specific prevalence of dementia almost doubles every 5 years, from approximately 1.5% in persons aged 60–69 years to 40% among those above 90 years. The largest increase in absolute numbers of patients in dementia is occurring in developing countries.

HISTORICAL ASPECTS

Celsus first used the term dementia in the 1st century Anno Domini era, although one of the first attempts to describe an etiology beyond old age was in the 4th century Anno Domini era by Oribasius. It was not until the 19th century that the distinction between cognitive impairment due to dementia was separated from that caused by mental illness by Jean Etienne Dominique Esquirol, as described in his classic work Mental Maladies: A Treatise on Insanity. In 1845, Wilhelm Griesinger was the first to describe senile dementia as a disease of the cerebral arteries. However, it was one of Griesinger's students, Emil Kraeplin, who later narrowed the scope of dementia by differentiating senile dementia from psychoses with cerebral arteriosclerosis, which later came to be known as dementia precox and, finally, as schizophrenia. Also in the late 19th century, reports of plaques and atrophy in the brains of patients with memory deficits and mental confusion began to emerge. In 1907, Alois Alzheimer was the first to identify specific histopathological changes associated with progressive degenerative dementia. He described two cases of dementia characterized by symptoms of aphasia, apraxia, agnosia, and the histopathological finding of neurofibrillary tangles and milar foci (plaques) that distinguished it from dementia associated with cerebral arteriosclerosis. By the end of the

20th century, it was believed that dementia is a mixture of both Alzheimer disease (AD) and vascular dementia. In the 21st century, other types of dementia, distinct from Alzheimer and vascular dementia were identified but their causal etiology remains unclear and many hypotheses (theories) have been advanced but these are largely based on risk factors.

NOSOLOGY

The conceptualization of dementia has evolved through successive editions of the diagnostic and statistical manual (DSM). The DSM-5 utilizes the terms major neurocognitive disorder and mild neurocognitive disorder (**Table 39.1 & 39.2**), which broadly correspond with the commonly used terms of dementia and mild cognitive impairment (MCI), respectively. The term neurocognitive disorder is broader than "dementia"; it extends beyond late-life, to include neurocognitive impairment at all ages including, for example, those caused by traumatic brain injury or HIV infection. Major and mild neurocognitive disorders are the basic clinical syndromes; in a change from previous DSM editions, at the syndromic neurocognitive disorder level, memory does not have to be one of the impaired domains. DSM-5 provides further diagnostic criteria for the etiological subtyping of the syndromes.

International Classification of Diseases (ICD), 11th revision (ICD-11) describes neurocognitive disorders as acquired conditions characterized by primary clinical deficits in cognitive functioning, and include most conditions that are classified among ICD-10 organic, including symptomatic, mental disorders, i.e., delirium, mild neurocognitive disorder (called mild cognitive disorder in ICD-10), amnestic disorder, and dementia.

Etiology

The causes of dementia can be broadly divided into irreversible and reversible (**Table 39.3**). Patients, who have associated reversible causes of dementia usually, show improvement in the clinical picture with correction of the underlying etiology. Of all the subtypes of dementia, AD is the most common type, which constitutes 50 to 60% of the prevalence. The second most common type of dementia is vascular dementia which accounts for 15-30%. It is usually related to cerebrovascular diseases with hypertension being the most important risk factor. Other common causes of dementia, each representing 1 to 5 percent of all cases, include head trauma, alcohol-related dementias, and various movement disorder-related dementias, such as Huntington's disease and Parkinson's disease.

Alzheimer's Dementia (AD)

This is the commonest cause of dementia, and accounts for about 70% of all cases of dementia in United States. AD is characterized by insidious onset, progressive memory loss in the initial phase of the illness. Memory loss is usually followed by disturbances in the other cognitive functions such as language, executive functions, and visuospatial functions. As the severity of the illness increases, cognitive disturbances may be accompanied by behavioral and psychological symptoms and in the most advanced stage patients require assistance for basic activities of daily living, i.e. bathing, toileting, and dressing, and patients may not be able to communicate, recognize their family members, and become bed-bound.

There is some evidence to suggest that AD may have a genetic basis. High rates of positive family history and higher concordance rates in monozygotic as compared to dizygotic twins suggests genetic basis for the development of the disorder. AD has shown linkage to chromosomes 1, 14, and 21.

The most well established risk factors for

Table 39.1: DSM-5 Diagnostic Criteria for Major Neurocognitive Disorder

Major Neurocognitive Disorder

Diagnostic Criteria

A. Evidence of significant cognitive decline from a previous level of performance in one or more cognitive domains (complex attention, executive function, learning and memory, language, perceptual-motor, or social cognition) based on:
   1. Concern of the individual, a knowledgeable informant, or the clinician that there has been a significant decline in cognitive function; and
   2. A substantial impairment in cognitive performance, preferably documented by standardized neuropsychological testing or, in its absence, another quantified clinical assessment.

B. The cognitive deficits interfere with independence in everyday activities (i.e., at a minimum, requiring assistance with complex instrumental activities of daily living such as paying bills or managing medications).

C. The cognitive deficits do not occur exclusively in the context of a delirium.

D. The cognitive deficits are not better explained by another mental disorder (e.g., major depressive disorder, schizophrenia).

Specify whether due to:

- Alzheimer's disease
- Frontotemporal lobar degeneration
- Lewy body disease
- Vascular disease
- Traumatic brain injury
- Substance/medication use
- HIV infection
- Prion disease
- Parkinson's disease
- Huntington's disease
- Another medical condition
- Multiple etiologies
- Unspecified

Specify:

Without behavioral disturbance: If the cognitive disturbance is not accompanied by any clinically significant behavioral disturbance.

With behavioral disturbance (specify disturbance): If the cognitive disturbance is accompanied by a clinically significant behavioral disturbance (e.g., psychotic symptoms, mood disturbance, agitation, apathy or other behavioral symptoms).

Specify current severity:

Mild: Difficulties with instrumental activities of daily living (e.g., housework, managing money).

Moderate: Difficulties with basic activities of daily living (e.g., feeding, dressing).

Severe: Fully dependent.

Table 39.2: DSM-5 Diagnostic Criteria for Mild Neurocognitive Disorder

Mild Neurocognitive Disorder

Diagnostic Criteria

A. Evidence of modest cognitive decline from a previous level of performance in one or more cognitive domains (complex attention, executive function, learning and memory, language, perceptual motor, or social cognition) based on:
   1. Concern of the individual, a knowledgeable informant, or the clinician that there has been a mild decline in cognitive function; and
   2. A modest impairment in cognitive performance, preferably documented by standardized neuropsychological testing or, in its absence, another quantified clinical assessment.

B. The cognitive deficits do not interfere with capacity for independence in everyday activities (i.e., complex instrumental activities of daily living such as paying bills or managing medications are preserved, but greater effort, compensatory strategies, or accommodation may be required).

C. The cognitive deficits do not occur exclusively in the context of a delirium.

D. The cognitive deficits are not better explained by another mental disorder (e.g., major depressive disorder, schizophrenia).

Specify whether due to:

- Alzheimer's disease
- Frontotemporal lobar degeneration
- Lewy body disease
- Vascular disease
- Traumatic brain injury
- Substance/medication use
- HIV infection
- Prion disease
- Parkinson's disease
- Huntington's disease
- Another medical condition
- Multiple etiologies
- Unspecified

Specify:

Without behavioral disturbance: If the cognitive disturbance is not accompanied by any clinically significant behavioral disturbance.

With behavioral disturbance (specify disturbance): If the cognitive disturbance is accompanied by a clinically significant behavioral disturbance (e.g., psychotic symptoms, mood disturbance, agitation, apathy or other behavioral symptoms).

Table 39.3: Etiology of Dementia

IRREVERSIBLE DEMENTIAS
- Alzheimer's disease
- Frontotemporal dementia
- Vascular dementia
- Dementia with Lewy bodies
- Parkinson's dementia
- Huntington's disease
- Prion related dementia
- Down's syndrome

REVERSIBLE DEMENTIAS

Neurosurgical conditions
- Subdural hematoma
- Normal pressure hydrocephalus
- Intracranial tumors
- Intracranial empyema or abscess

Infections
- Meningitis (tubercular, fungal, malignant)
- HIV dementia
- Neurosyphilis
- Lyme's disease
- Whipple's disease
- Fungal/protozoal Intracranial abscess
- Neurocysticercosis

Inflammatory/autoimmune cause
- Sarcoidosis
- Multiple sclerosis
- Systemic lupus erythematosus
- Sjogren's syndrome
- Autoimmune limbic encephalitis

Metabolic conditions
- Hypo and hyperthyroidism
- Hashimotos encephalitis
- Hypo- and hyper- parahthyroidism
- Pituitary insufficiency
- Hypercalcemia
- Cushing's disease
- Addison's disease
- Hypoglycemia
- Wilson's disease
- Accidental hypothermia
- Electrolyte imbalance

Organ failure
- Chronic liver failure
- Hepatic encephalopathy
- Chronic respiratory failure
- Pulmonary insufficiency
- Chronic renal failure
- Uremic encephalopathy

Nutritional deficiencies:
- Vitamin deficiencies (A, B1, B6, B12 and folate)
- Iron deficiency

Psychiatric disorders
- Depression
- Substance use
- Alcohol abuse

Toxins/toxicity with metals
- Arsenic
- Mercury
- Aluminium
- Lithium

Medications/treatments
- Steroids
- Chemotherapy
- Radiotherapy
- Anticholinergic
- Anticonvulsants
- Chlorpheniramine
- Antibiotics
- Carbamazepine
- Phenytoin
- Valproate
- Antidepressants
- Antipsychotics
- Interleukin-2
- Antihypertensives

Traumatic head injury- usually due to falls, Concussions (skull fractures) or contusions (bruises) to the head

dementia and AD include old age and genetic susceptibility. Other risk factors include:

Vascular risk factors and disorders: Midlife high blood pressure, obesity, diabetes mellitus, cardiovascular disease, cerebrovascular disease, alcohol consumption, smoking, dietary and nutritional factors.

Psychosocial factors and lifestyles: Low education, poor social network, lesser engagement in mentally stimulating and physical activities.

Neurobiological findings: The classic gross neuroanatomical finding of a brain from a patient with AD is diffuse atrophy with flattened cortical sulci and enlarged cerebral ventricles. The classic and pathognomonic microscopic findings are senile plaques, neurofibrillary tangles, neuronal loss (particularly in the cortex and the hippocampus), synaptic loss (perhaps as much as 50 percent in the cortex), and granulovascular degeneration of the neurons. Neurofibrillary tangles and senile plaques are not seen exclusively seen in patients with AD. The β/A4 protein,which is a form of amyloid precursor protein and is yielded by the differential splicing, is the major constituent of senile plaques. The gene for amyloid precursor protein is on the long arm of chromosome 21. Whether the processing of abnormal amyloid precursor protein is of primary causative significance in AD is not known.

The neurotransmitters that are most often implicated in the development of AD include acetylcholine, norepinephrine, neuroactive peptides somatostatin and corticotropin; all of which are hypothesized to be hypoactive in AD.

Investigations: Routine clinical diagnostic testing includes the use of qualitative structural imaging (CT or MRI), largely to identify or exclude other causes of cognitive impairment. Quantification of change in global (whole brain and ventricles) and regional (entorhinal cortex, hippocampus, corpus callosum) volumes in patients with AD frequently demonstrate group differences in comparison to cognitively intact elderly patients, with MCI patients intermediate. The addition of SPECT or FDG-PET can increase the diagnostic accuracy of an expert evaluation, and can be particularly useful in differentiating individuals with AD from those with an FTD.

The absence of tracer retention during PET-amyloid imaging indicates that dementia is unlikely to be due to AD. Though not well standardized across laboratories, decreased cerebrospinal fluid levels of the 42 amino acid species of Aβ (Aβ1–42) is supportive of a diagnosis of AD as are elevated cerebrospinal fluid levels of total and phosphorylated tau protein. The genetic marker APOE4 can be of help as a diagnostic or predictive test in late onset AD.

Vascular Dementia

It is the second most common type of dementia seen worldwide. The primary cause of vascular dementia is presumed to be multiple areas of cerebral vascular disease. Vascular dementia is also referred to as 'multi infarct dementia', and is most commonly seen in those with preexisting hypertension or other cardiovascular risk factors. Hypertension leads to small- and medium-sized cerebral vessels infarction which produce multiple parenchymal lesions spread over wide areas of the brain. The clinical manifestations of vascular dementia are determined by the extent of blood vessel affected. The cognitive deficits in this condition largely depend on the site of the brain involved and memory may not be necessarily impaired. In contrast to other degenerative dementias,

Table 39.4: Diagnostic Criteria for Major or Mild Neurocognitive Disorder Due to Alzheimer's disease

Major or Mild Neurocognitive Disorder Due to Alzheimer's Disease

Diagnostic Criteria

A. The criteria are met for major or mild neurocognitive disorder.

B. There is insidious onset and gradual progression of impairment in one or more cognitive domains (for major neurocognitive disorder, at least two domains must be impaired).

C. Criteria are met for either probable or possible Alzheimer's disease as follows:

For major neurocognitive disorder:

Probable Alzheimer's disease is diagnosed if either of the following is present; otherwise, possible Alzheimer's disease should be diagnosed.

1. Evidence of a causative Alzheimer's disease genetic mutation from family history or genetic testing.
2. All three of the following are present:

a. Clear evidence of decline in memory and learning and at least one other cognitive domain (based on detailed history or serial neuropsychological testing).

b. Steadily progressive, gradual decline in cognition, without extended plateaus.

c. No evidence of mixed etiology (i.e., absence of other neurodegenerative or cerebrovascular disease, or another neurological, mental, or systemic disease or condition likely contributing to cognitive decline).

For mild neurocognitive disorder:

Probable Alzheimer's disease is diagnosed if there is evidence of a causative Alzheimer's disease genetic mutation from either genetic testing or family history.

Possible Alzheimer's disease is diagnosed if there is no evidence of a causative Alzheimer's disease genetic mutation from either genetic testing or family history, and all three of the following are present:

1. Clear evidence of decline in memory and learning.
2. Steadily progressive, gradual decline in cognition, without extended plateaus.
3. No evidence of mixed etiology (i.e., absence of other neurodegenerative or cerebrovascular disease, or another neurological or systemic disease or condition likely contributing to cognitive decline).

D. The disturbance is not better explained by cerebrovascular disease, another neurodegenerative disease, the effects of a substance, or another mental, neurological, or systemic disorder.

vascular dementia is characterized by abrupt onset and a step ladder deterioration. The patient often presents after a stroke with symptoms of confusion, disorientation, difficulty in speaking or understanding speech, and vision loss. The cognitive symptoms may be accompanied by focal neurological signs and symptoms. Risk factors for developing vascular dementia include hypertension, diabetes mellitus, dyslipidemia, metabolic syndrome, smoking, and use of estrogen in postmenopausal women. Other risk factors include increasing age, male gender, history of stroke, transient ischemic attacks, presence of cardiovascular disease, history of sleep apnea, history of depression, and family history of cardiovascular disease.

The causes of the infarctions can include occlusion of the vessels by plaques or thromboemboli from distant origins. Examination findings in these patients might include carotid bruits, fundoscopic abnormalities, or enlarged cardiac chambers.

Frontotemporal Dementia (Pick's disease)

Frontotemporal dementia (FTD) is also known as Pick's disease. FTD is characterized by atrophy in the frontotemporal regions. Pick's bodies, which are masses of cytoskeletal elements, are seen in these regions along with neuronal loss and gliosis. It constitutes approximately 5 percent of all irreversible dementias but cause is not known. Family history is positive in a small number of cases and these cases have an earlier onset.

It is characterized by deficits in behavior, language and executive functions that precede the development of memory deficits. It is also characterized by selective atrophy of frontal and temporal lobes and only in late stage, the structural and functional changes are diffuse. Features of Klüver-Bucy syndrome (e.g., hypersexuality, placidity, and hyperorality) are seen quite commonly in Pick's disease. Clinically, two different

Table 39.5: Diagnostic Criteria for Major or Mild Vascular Neurocognitive Disorder

Major or Mild Vascular Neurocognitive Disorder

Diagnostic Criteria

A. The criteria are met for major or mild neurocognitive disorder.

B. The clinical features are consistent with a vascular etiology, as suggested by either of the following:

1. Onset of the cognitive deficits is temporally related to one or more cerebrovascular events.
2. Evidence for decline is prominent in complex attention (including processing speed) and frontal-executive function.
3. There is evidence of the presence of cerebrovascular disease from history, physical examination, and/or neuroimaging considered sufficient to account for the neurocognitive deficits.

D. The symptoms are not better explained by another brain disease or systemic disorder.

Probable vascular neurocognitive disorder is diagnosed if one of the following is present; otherwise possible vascular neurocognitive disorder should be diagnosed:

1. Clinical criteria are supported by neuroimaging evidence of significant parenchymal injury attributed to cerebrovascular disease (neuroimaging-supported).
2. The neurocognitive syndrome is temporally related to one or more documented cerebrovascular events.
3. Both clinical and genetic (e.g., cerebral autosomal dominant arteriopathy with subcortical infarcts and leukoencephalopathy) evidence of cerebrovascular disease is present.

Possible vascular neurocognitive disorder is diagnosed if the clinical criteria are met but neuroimaging is not available and the temporal relationship of the neurocognitive syndrome with one or more cerebrovascular events is not established.

variants of FTD are described; these include behavior variant FTD (bvFTD) and primary progressive aphasia (PPA). The bvFTD is characterized by personality change which often leads to interpersonal problems. This subtype is characterized by atrophy of areas of the brain involved in conduct, judgment, empathy, and foresight. PPA subtype of FTD is characterized by problems of language, speaking, writing, and comprehension. PPA is further subdivided into semantic variant (i.e., characterized by difficulty in formulating spoken sentences), progressive nonfluent aphasia variant (i.e., hesitant, labored or ungrammatical speech), and logopenic progressive aphasia (characterized by difficulty in naming and retrieval of single words).

Lewy Body Dementia

Dementia of Lewy body (DLB) is an umbrella term for two related clinical diagnoses: "dementia with Lewy bodies" and "Parkinson's disease dementia." These disorders share the same underlying changes in the brain and very similar symptoms, but the symptoms appear in a different order depending on where the Lewy bodies first form.

Table 39.6: Diagnostic Criteria for Major or Mild Frontotemporal Neurocognitive Disorder

Major or Mild Frontotemporal Neurocognitive Disorder

Diagnostic Criteria

A. The criteria are met for major or mild neurocognitive disorder.
B. The disturbance has insidious onset and gradual progression.
C. Either (1) or (2);
   1. **Behavioral variant;**
      a. Three or more of the following behavioral symptoms:
         i. Behavioral disinhibition.
         ii. Apathy or inertia.
         iii. Loss of sympathy or empathy.
         iv. Perserevative, stereotyped or compulsive/ritualistic behavior.
         v. Hyper orality and dietary changes.
      b. Prominent decline in social cognition and/or executive abilities.
   2. **Language variant:**
      a. Prominent decline in language ability, in the form of speech production, word finding, object naming, grammar, or word comprehension.
D. Relative sparing of learning and memory and perceptual-motor function.
E. The disturbance is not better explained by cerebrovascular disease, another neurodegenerative disease, the effects of a substance, or another mental, neurological, or systemic disorder.

Probable frontotemporal neurocognitive disorder is diagnosed if either of the following is present; otherwise, possible frontotemporal neurocognitive disorder should be diagnosed:

1. Evidence of a causative frontotemporal neurocognitive disorder genetic mutation, from either family history or genetic testing.
2. Evidence of disproportionate frontal and/or temporal lobe involvement from neuroimaging.

DLB is characterized by hallucinations, parkinsonian features, and fluctuating level of attention and alertness. The central feature includes the presence of cognitive deficits, which typically involves attention and executive functions. Memory impairment may not be seen in the early stages, however, these emerge with the progression of dementia. The clinical features which are considered as suggestive of DLB include the presence of rapid eye movement sleep behavior disorder, severe neuroleptic sensitivity, and low dopamine transporter uptake in basal ganglia demonstrated by single-photon emission computed tomography or positron emission technique imaging. The supportive features of DLB include repeated falls and syncope (fainting), transient, unexplained loss of consciousness, presence of autonomic dysfunction, hallucinations in other modalities, visuospatial abnormalities and other psychiatric disturbances such as systematized delusions, aggression, and depression (**Table 39.7**). Lewy inclusion bodies (α-synuclein neuronal intracellular inclusions) are found in the cerebral cortex. Lewy body pathology can occur concurrently with AD, the amygdala is often the only region affected in these cases.

The distinguishing features of DLB and Parkinson's disease dementia are given in **Table 39.8**.

Parkinson's Dementia

Parkinson's disease is a disease of the basal ganglia and is commonly associated with dementia and depression. Around 20-30% of patients with Parkinson's disease go on to

Table 39.7: Diagnostic Criteria for Major or Mild Neurocognitive Disorder with Lewy bodies

Major or Mild Neurocognitive Disorder with Lewy Bodies

Diagnostic Criteria

A. The criteria are met for major or mild neurocognitive disorder.

B. The disorder has an insidious onset and gradual progression.

C. The disorder meets a combination of core diagnostic features and suggestive diagnostic features for either probable or possible neurocognitive disorder with Lewy bodies.

   For probable major or mild neurocognitive disorder with Lewy bodies, the individual has two core features, or one suggestive feature with one or more core features.

   For possible major or mild neurocognitive disorder with Lewy bodies, the individual has only one core feature, or one or more suggestive features.

   1. **Core diagnostic features:**
      a. Fluctuating cognition with pronounced variations in attention and alertness.
      b. Recurrent visual hallucinations that are well formed and detailed.
      c. Spontaneous features of parkinsonism, with onset subsequent to the development of cognitive decline.
   2. **Suggestive diagnostic features:**
      a. Meets criteria for rapid eye movement sleep behavior disorder.
      b. Severe neuroleptic sensitivity.

D. The disturbance is not better explained by cerebrovascular disease, another neurodegenerative disease, the effects of a substance, or another mental, neurological or systemic disorder.

Table 39.8: Differentiating features of DLB and Parkinson's disease dementia

Clinical feature	DLB	PDD
Cognitive impairment	Before or within one year of motor symptoms	Usually develops after 4-5 years (at least 1 year) of motor symptoms
Tremors	Less common	Common
Motor symptoms	Bilateral	Unilateral predominant
Axial predominant such as postural instability, gait difficulty	Common	Less common
Parkinsonism at dementia diagnosis	25-50%	100%
Response to levodopa	Poor	Good

develop dementia, while an additional 30 to 40 percent have measurable impairment in cognitive abilities. The slow movements of persons with Parkinson's disease are paralleled in the slow thinking of some affected patients, a feature that sometimes referred to as *bradyphrenia*. Usually, the cognitive symptoms in patients with Parkinson's disease develop after 4-5 years of the motoric symptoms. (**Table 39.9**).

Huntington's Disease

Huntington's disease is classically associated with the development of dementia. The dementia seen in this disease is characterized by more motor abnormalities and fewer language abnormalities than in the cortical type of dementia. The dementia of Huntington's disease exhibits psychomotor slowing and difficulty with complex tasks, but memory,

Table 39.9: Diagnostic Criteria for Major or Mild Neurocognitive Disorder Due to Parkinson's Disease

Major or Mild Neurocognitive Disorder Due to Parkinson's Disease

Diagnostic Criteria

A. The criteria are met for major or mild neurocognitive disorder.

B. The disturbance occurs in the setting of established Parkinson's disease.

C. There is insidious onset and gradual progression of impairment.

D. The neurocognitive disorder is not attributable to another medical condition and is not better explained by another mental disorder.

Major or mild neurocognitive disorder probably due to Parkinson's disease should be diagnosed if 1 and 2 are both met.

Major or mild neurocognitive disorder possibly due to Parkinson's disease should be diagnosed if 1 or 2 is met:

1. There is no evidence of mixed etiology (i.e., absence of other neurodegenerative or cerebrovascular disease or another neurological, mental, or systemic disease or condition likely contributing to cognitive decline).
2. The Parkinson's disease clearly precedes the onset of the neurocognitive disorder.

Table 39.10: Diagnostic Criteria for Major or Mild Neurocognitive Disorder Due to Huntington's Disease

Major or Mild Neurocognitive Disorder Due to Huntington's Disease
Diagnostic Criteria
A. The criteria are met for major or mild neurocognitive disorder.
B. There is insidious onset and gradual progression.
C. There is clinically established Huntington's disease, or risk for Huntington's disease based on family history or genetic testing.
D. The neurocognitive disorder is not attributable to another medical condition and is not better explained by another mental disorder.

language, and insight remain relatively intact till the late stage. It is associated with high incidence of depression and psychosis in addition to the classic Choreo athetoid movement disorder.

HIV-Related Dementia

About 50-70% of patients suffering from AIDS exhibit a triad of cognitive, behavioral and motoric deficits of *subcortical dementia* type and this is known as the AIDS-dementia complex (ADC) or HIV dementia (**Table 39.11**). Dementia can in fact be an initial presentation in about 25% cases of AIDS. As the AIDS virus (a lenti-virus, a type of retrovirus) is highly neurotropic and the virus crosses the blood-brain barrier early in the course of the disease cognitive impairment is nearly ubiquitous in AIDS. The development of dementia in people infected with HIV is often paralleled by the appearance of parenchymal abnormalities (white matter lesions) in MRI scans.

Other infectious dementias are caused by *Cryptococcus* or *Treponema pallidum*.

Head Trauma-Related Dementia

Dementia can be a sequalae of head trauma (**Table 39.12**). It has also been observed in professional football players or boxers (known as *Punch drunk syndrome*) who developed dementia after repeated head traumas over many years.

Table 39.11: Diagnostic Criteria for Major or Mild Neurocognitive Disorder Due to HIV Infection

Major or Mild Neurocognitive Disorder Due to HIV Infection
Diagnostic Criteria
A. The criteria are met for major or mild neurocognitive disorder.
B. There is documented infection with human immunodeficiency virus (HIV).
C. The neurocognitive disorder is not better explained by non-HIV conditions, including secondary brain diseases such as progressive multifocal leukoencephalopathy or cryptococcal meningitis.
D. The neurocognitive disorder is not attributable to another medical condition and is not better explained by a mental disorder.

Table 39.12: Diagnostic Criteria for Major or Mild Neurocognitive Disorder Due to Traumatic Brain Injury

Major or Mild Neurocognitive Disorder Due to Traumatic Brain Injury

Diagnostic Criteria

A. The criteria are met for major or mild neurocognitive disorder.

B. There is evidence of a traumatic brain injury—that is, an impact to the head or other mechanisms of rapid movement or displacement of the brain within the skull, with oneor more of the following:
   1. Loss of consciousness.
   2. Post-traumatic amnesia.
   3. Disorientation and confusion.
   4. Neurological signs (e.g., neuroimaging demonstrating injury; a new onset of seizures; a marked worsening of a preexisting seizure disorder; visual field cuts; anosmia; hemiparesis).

C. The neurocognitive disorder presents immediately after the occurrence of the traumatic brain injury or immediately after recovery of consciousness and persists past the acute post-injury period.

Substance/Medication-Induced Dementia

Substance/medication-induced major or mild NCD is characterized by neurocognitive impairment that persist beyond the usual duration of intoxication and acute withdrawal (**Table 39.13**). While nonspecific decrements in a range of cognitive abilities can occur with nearly any substance of abuse and a variety of medications, some patterns occur more frequently with selected drug classes. For example, dementia due to sedative, hypnotic, or anxiolytic drugs may show greater disturbances in memory than in other cognitive functions. Dementia induced by alcohol frequently manifests with a combination of impairment in executive-function and memory and learning domains. In alcohol-induced amnestic confabulatory (Korsakoff's) dementia, the features include prominent amnesia (severe difficulty learning new information with rapid forgetting) and a tendency to confabulate. These manifestations may co-occur with signs of thiamine encephalopathy (Wernicke's encephalopathy) with associated features such as nystagmus and ataxia. Ophthalmoplegia of Wernicke's encephalopathy is typically characterized by a lateral gaze paralysis.

Table 39.13: Diagnostic Criteria for Substance/Medication-Induced Major or Mild Neurocognitive Disorder

Substance/Medication-Induced Major or Mild Neurocognitive Disorder

Diagnostic Criteria

A. The criteria are met for major or mild neurocognitive disorder.

B. The neurocognitive impairment do not occur exclusively during the course of a delirium and persist beyond the usual duration of intoxication and acute withdrawal.

C. The involved substance or medication and duration and extent of use are capable of producing the neurocognitive impairment.

D. The temporal course of the neurocognitive deficits is consistent with the timing of substance or medication use and abstinence (e.g., the deficits remain stable or improve after a period of abstinence).

E. The neurocognitive disorder is not attributable to another medical condition or is not better explained by another mental disorder.

Prion Related Dementia

Prion diseases are a group of fatal neuro-degenerative conditions, which include Creutzfeldt-Jakob disease (CJD) and Gerstmann-Sträussler-Scheinker (GSS) in humans. These are different variants of CJD, based on the possible etiologies have been described, i.e., sporadic, genetic, and acquired. The sporadic variant accounts for 85% of cases of CJD and occurs due to posttranslational modification of native cellular prion protein into pathologic scrapie prion protein. The sporadic variant of CJD usually occurs at 60–65 years of age. The familial variant of CJD accounts for 10–15% of cases and results from genetic mutations of the prion protein gene (PRNP). Most of the cases of familial CJD are caused by autosomal dominant point mutations. The third variant acquired CJD, which contributes to 1% of CJD cases, occurs due to exposure to an external source of abnormal PRNP. GSS occurs due to PRNP mutations and is characterized by the long duration of illness, in contrast to the short duration of illness in CJD. CJD as an illness affects the gray matter and leads to neuronal loss, gliosis, and characteristic spongiform change. All prion diseases are characterized by cognitive impairment as the most common neuropsychiatric manifestation, followed by behavioral/personality changes, affective symptoms, psychotic symptoms and agitation. The cognitive symptoms include executive dysfunction, progressive loss of speech, visual symptoms, memory problems, parietal dysfunction, and a largely expressive dysphasia, with reduced motor speed. Patients with young onset sporadic CJD often present with affective symptoms. Electroencephalogram, cerebrospinal fluid analysis, and MRI of the brain show characteristic findings for CJD.

DIAGNOSIS AND CLINICAL FEATURES

DSM-5 makes a distinction between major and minor cognitive disorder based upon levels of functioning, but the underlying etiology is similar. The diagnosis of dementia is based on the clinical examination, including a mental status examination, and on information from the patient's family, friends, and employers. Clinicians should note patients' complaints about intellectual impairment and forgetfulness as well as evidence of patients' evasion, denial, or rationalization aimed at concealing cognitive deficits. Patients' appearance and behavior should be observed. Memory impairment is typically an early and prominent feature in dementia, especially in cortical dementias. Early in the course of dementia, memory impairment is mild and usually most marked for recent events. As the course of dementia progresses, memory impairment becomes severe, and only the earliest learned information is retained.

While history taking, a careful evaluation can guide the clinician to distinguish between cortical and subcortical dementia (**Table 39.14**).

Some patients with depression have symptoms of cognitive impairment, known as *pseudodementia or depression-related cognitive dysfunction,* which at times becomes difficult to distinguish from symptoms of dementia. Patients with depression-related cognitive dysfunction generally have prominent depressive symptoms, more insight into their symptoms than do demented patients, and often a history of depressive episodes (**Table 39.15**).

Assessment of Cognitive Functions

Diagnosis of dementia depends on the presence of cognitive impairment. Hence a proper and complete assessment of cognitive functions becomes mandatory. Some of the commonly used tests include Mini-Mental State Examination, Montreal Cognitive Assessment (MoCA), Clock drawing test, Mini-Cog, General Practitioner assessment of Cognition, Addenbrookes Cognitive Assessment, AD Assessment Scale – Cognitive section, Cambridge Assessment of Memory and Cognition which is the cognitive section of the comprehensive Cambridge Mental Disorders of the Elderly Examination (CAMDEX) assessment.

Table 39.14: Distinguishing Features of Cortical and Subcortical Dementia

Features	Cortical dementia	Subcorticaldementia
Site of lesion	Cortex (frontal and temporoparieto-occipital ganglia, and rostral brain stem)	Subcortical grey matter (thalamus and hippocampus)
Examples	Alzheimer's disease, Pick's disease	Huntington' chorea, Parkinson's disease, Progressive supranuclear palsy, Wilson's disease
Severity	Severe	Mild to moderate
Motor system	Usually normal	Dysarthria, flexed/extended posture, tremors, dystonia, chorea, ataxia, rigidity
Other features	Simple delusions; depression uncommon; severe aphasia, amnesia, agnosia, apraxia, acalculia, slowed cognitive speed (bradyphrenia)	Complex delusions; depression common, rarely mania
Memory deficit	Recall helped very little by cues	Recall partially helped by cues and (Short-term) recognition tasks

Table 39.15: Distinguishing features between Dementia vs Pseudodementia

Features	Dementia	Pseudodementia
Onset	Insidious	Rapid
Concurrent psychiatric symptoms	May be present	Always present, mostly of depressive nature
Duration of symptoms	Long term mostly	Short term
Course of symptoms	Slowly deteriorating	Rapidly progressive
Psychiatric history	Usually none	Usually present
Subjective complaints	Fewer	Describes in details about the cognitive deficits
Subjective response	Usually unconcerned	Expressed marked distress
Demeanor	Unconcerned, confabulations, has difficulty is carrying out the tasks, behavior in commensurate with the level of dysfunction	Distressed, emphasizes the deficits, makes little efforts, overall behavior incongruent with level of cognitive dysfunction
Mood/affect	Fluctuating	Consistently depressed
Reaction to deficits/failure	Tries to hide/conceal	Tries to highlight
Assessment	Makes efforts to answer to the questions	Does not make efforts
Answers to questions	Near-miss answers	Don't know
Type of memory loss	Recent more than remote	Both recent and remote memory equally impaired
Memory gaps	Memory gaps do not pertain to specific periods	Memory gaps of specific periods of life
Attention and concentration	Usually impaired	Usually preserved
Response to treatment	Deteriorating course	Usually improves

Physical Examination

A general physical examination is a routine component of the workup for dementia. It may reveal evidence of systemic diseases causing brain dysfunction or it may demonstrate systemic disease related to particular CNS processes. Focal neurological findings are seen more often in vascular dementia and frontal lobe signs and primitive reflexes occur in many disorders at later stages.

MANAGEMENT

Basic Investigations

A comprehensive laboratory workup must be performed as a first step, when evaluating a patient with dementia in order to detect reversible causes of dementia and reach a definitive diagnosis. The evaluation should be planned on the basis of clinical suspicion based on the history and physical and mental status examination results. An assessment of basic and instrumental activities of daily living is done to plan the management of deficits in any of the activity.

The list of investigations should include complete blood count, urinalysis, blood glucose, serum electrolytes, renal function tests, thyroid function tests, serum B_{12} and folate levels, serological tests for syphilis, arterial pO_2 and pCO_2, X-ray chest, ECG, X-ray skull, electroencephalogram,, lumbar puncture, CT scan/MRI scan of brain, neuropsychological tests, and drug screens. Other investigations may be guided by the history and physical examination findings.

The general treatment approach to patients with dementia is to provide supportive medical care; emotional support for the patients and their families; and pharmacological treatment for specific symptoms, including disruptive behavior.

Pharmacological

Pharmacological agents for management of dementia might include cholinesterase inhibitors like, donepezil, rivastigmine etc. These are used to treat mild to moderate cognitive impairment in AD. They potentiate the cholinergic neurotransmitter, which in turn produces a modest improvement in memory and goal-directed thought. None of these medications prevents the progressive neuronal degeneration of the disorder. Memantine protects neurons from excessive amounts of glutamate, which may be neurotoxic and has been seen to improve dementia.

Antihypertensive, anticoagulant, or antiplatelet agents may be used to treat vascular risk factors. Angiotensin-converting enzyme (ACE) inhibitors and diuretics are preferred as they lower blood pressure without affecting cerebral blood flow, and hence do not affect cognitive function adversely.

Other specific medications as per presenting symptoms can be prescribed; e.g., sedatives for insomnia and anxiety, antidepressants for depression and antipsychotic drugs for disruptive behavior/psychotic symptoms. Risk of polypharmacy and idiosyncratic drug effects in elderly should be kept in mind while prescribing.

Non Pharmacological

Psychosocial therapies are important in managing dementia as the deterioration of mental faculties has significant psychological meaning for patients as well as the family members. Many patients are quite distressed in initial stages when remote memory is preserved by clearly recalling how they used to function while observing their obvious deterioration. Emotional reactions ranging from depression to severe anxiety can originate

Table 39.16: Commonly used cognitive enhancers

Name of the Drug	Usual Starting dose in mg/day	Maximum recommended dose (mg/day)	Side effects
Cholinesterase Inhibitors			
Donepezil	5	10 Start with 5 mg once daily and increase to 10 mg once daily after 4 weeks if tolerability is good	Nausea, vomiting, diarrhea, insomnia, muscle cramps, anorexia, weight loss, bradycardia, syncope
Rivastigmine	3	12 Start with 1.5 mg twice daily and increase by 3 mg per day every 2 weeks till 6 mg twice daily	Similar side effects like Donepezil but slightly more severe gastrointestinal side effects
Galantamine	8	24 Start with 4 mg twice daily and increase by 8 mg every 4 weeks till 12 mg twice daily	Similar to Donepezil and Rivastigmine
Rivastigmine Transdermal patch	4.6 mg/ 24 hours patch	9.5 mg/24 hours patch Start with 4.6 mg/24 hours patch and increase to 9.5 mg/24 hours patch after 4 weeks if tolerability is good	Occasional Skin Irritation
Donepezil Extended Release	11.5	23 Titration to high dose Donepezil needs to be considered after at least 3 months maintenance with 10 mg Donepezil	More severe gastrointestinal side effects
NMDA antagonist			
Memantine	10	20 Start with 5 mg twice daily and increase by 5 mg every week and titrate to 10 mg twice daily	No significant adverse effects

from this realization. Patients may benefit from assistance in grieving and accepting the extent of their disability and from attention to self-esteem issues. Any areas of intact functioning should be maximized by helping patients identify activities in which successful functioning is possible.

Clinicians can help patients find ways to deal with the difficulties, such as keeping calendars for orientation problems, making schedules to help structure activities, and taking notes for memory problems. Cognitive rehabilitation can be attempted using restorative strategies (strengthening previously learned patterns of behavior through rehearsal), compensatory strategies (exploit intact strengths to substitute for impaired functions), adaptive strategies (adjusting to residual impairment through reappraisal) and enabling strategies (activity based treatments and exercise).

Clinicians can help caregivers understand the complex mixture of feelings like guilt, grief, anger etc., associated with seeing a loved one decline and can provide understanding to these feelings.

Course and Prognosis

The age of onset and the rapidity of deterioration vary among different types of dementia. The classic course of dementia is an onset in the patient's 50s or 60s, with gradual deterioration over 5 to 10 years, leading eventually to death. Patients with an early onset of dementia or with a family history of dementia tend to have a rapid progression. The most common course of dementia begins with a number of subtle signs which are often missed by the family members as well as clinicians. A gradual onset of symptoms is most commonly associated with dementia of the Alzheimer's type while the onset of dementia resulting from head trauma, cerebral hypoxia, or encephalitis can be sudden. In the terminal stages of dementia, patients become profoundly disoriented, incoherent, amnestic, and incontinent of urine and feces.

The course of the dementia varies from a steady progression (e.g. AD) to an incrementally worsening dementia (e.g. vascular dementia) to a stable dementia (e.g. dementia related to head trauma).

Symptom regression is certainly a possibility in reversible dementia after treatment is initiated.

Prevention of Dementia

Identification of risk and protective factors for dementia could provide potential for the prevention of the disease. At the moment, it seems possible to delineate two preventive strategies against dementia.

BIBLIOGRAPHY

1. Sadock B, Sadock V, and Ruiz P. Kaplan & Sadock's comprehensive textbook of psychiatry.
2. Husain M, Schott J. Oxford textbook of cognitive neurology and dementia.
3. Diagnostic and statistical manual of mental disorders, 5th ed. American Psychiatric Publishing; 2013.

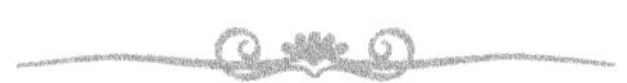

Geriatric Psychiatry 40

Alka A. Subramanyam • Nitin. B. Raut • Shipra Singh

INTRODUCTION

The size of geriatric population (persons > 60 yrs. of age) in India is growing rapidly and it constituted 7.4% of total at the end of this millennium. Mental health problems in elderly present unique challenges to health care professionals as well as the health care services due to social, psychological and physical changes in old age. Further the presence of medical comorbidities and cognitive dysfunction may affect the presentation, diagnosis and management of psychiatric disorders. To add to this, India looks at further rise in number and proportion of individuals in elderly age group in years to come, and its health care services are not equipped to deal with needs of this population. To diagnose psychiatric disorder in the elderly, the clinician must be able to gather information from a variety of sources, and produce a holistic management plan. This chapter provides a brief overview of common psychiatric disorders in elderly.

NORMAL AGING RELATED CHANGES

Biological Changes

As we grow old, the molecules, cells, tissues and our body parts undergo changes. The process of ageing is complex, and yet not fully understood. Though defining aging is debatable, it can be seen as the gradual accumulation of harmful biological changes associated with progressive loss of bodily functions. Together, these changes lead to a reduced physiological reserve and are commonly associated with increased morbidity and mortality. With increasing age there is decline in overall immune function putting them at increased risk of communicable diseases. There is increased risk of non-communicable diseases like diabetes mellitus, hypertension and coronary artery disease. The management of these disorders is further made challenging by the presence of more than one disorder and co-occurring sensory and motor disabilities (slowing of gait, balance problems, reduced reaction time etc.), as well as by an increased risk of side effects of medications.

Neurological Changes

Apart from gradual decline in brain weight, increasing age also results the ventricles to enlarge, and the meninges thicken. There is also loss of neuronal cells and their connections (synapses). There is also accumulation of aggregates of proteins i.e. senile plaques and neurofibrillary tangles, but with selective distribution and lesser amount than in Alzheimer's disease. There is also pruning of dendritic branches, white matter changes and gliosis etc. Aging is further associated with genomic changes like damage to DNA or changes in their expression, mitochondrial damage, and alterations in some growth factor and signaling pathways and so on.

Higher mental functions are also affected e.g. slowing of psychomotor functions and new information processing. Other functions like working memory, divided attention, and remote memory etc. also show some decline in elderly population. On the other hand, cognitive functions like verbal comprehension, problem solving & short-term memory remain un-affected. Despite this, there appears to be a balance between losses in some abilities and the benefits of gathered knowledge derived from life-time experience.

Level of certain neurotransmitters like dopamine and acetylcholine which play key roles in motor cognitive and emotional functions are also altered. However, certain factors may limit this age-related decline in cognition and other aspects of brain function and result in higher resilience; this includes cognitive stimulation, social and physical activity, and nutrition etc. Though exact mechanisms are not known for these changes, following ones are postulated:

- Oxidative damage to DNA, proteins, lipids.
- Mitochondrial damage
- Protein misfolding and their aggregation (e.g. tau protein, senile plaques, neuro-fibrillary tangles)
- Changes in hormonal level like estrogen, progesterone
- Reduction in transport across nerve cells & neurogenesis
- Reduced support from neurotropic factors

Psychological Changes

Old age is marked by variety of psychological changes. There is increased ability to control negative emotional states and increased expression of positive ones than younger population. There is also changes in personality and attitudes, such as increased cautiousness and rigidity. How elderly cope with stressful situations also changes. Coping refers to strategies that individuals use to manage stressful life situations by either reducing emotional distress or by using strategies to solve the problems. It is seen that elderly people use more of emotion-based strategies than younger population.

Old age also witnesses periods of psychological distress such as role transition after retirement and adjustment after death of spouse. Retirement has been found to be a significant stressor especially in persons from low income families, those facing unexpected retirement, people with health problems and certain types of personalities. Loss of spouse may be more stressful in elderly due to physical problems and general reduction in ability of stress management though long-term outcome has been found better than loss at younger age.

Though the stressors are often chronic and accumulative many elderly can face these challenges effectively. The phenomenon of *resilience* (the ability of maintaining adaptive behavior and positive emotions during stressful circumstances) has been offered as explanation.

Social Changes in Late Life

With age there is general reduction in number of social contacts and feelings of loneliness especially when co-occurring with other stressors such as death of loved ones, presence of psychiatric illnesses, physical or cognitive disability, institutionalization and financial dependency etc.

Other significant changes include change in family structure, children studying or working abroad, lack of useful resources to engage in after retirement. These changes have been found to be more marked with elderly above

85 years of age. All these factors have been found to be associated with depression as well as increased overall mortality in elderly.

Demographic Profile of Elderly Population

Reduction in fertility and mortality rates along with increasing survival in old age is contributing to population aging. Globally, the elderly population constitutes about 11.5 percent of the total population of 7 billion. By 2050, it is projected to rise to about 22 percent. The elderly constitutes the fastest growing age segment while the children and working age segments reduce gradually (**Fig. 40.1**). Similarly, the proportion of population over the age of 60 is expected to rise from 8 percent in 2015 to 19 percent in 2050 in India (**Fig. 40.2**). Elderly population is highly vulnerable to psychiatric and physical morbidities and loss of vital functions. This is complicated further by factors like breaking of family support system, non-availability of proper care and financial dependence. Urbanization increase in number of nuclear family, migration to cities and career-oriented lifestyle has led to neglect of our elderly population. This greatly impacts their mental status making them even more prone to psychiatric disorders.

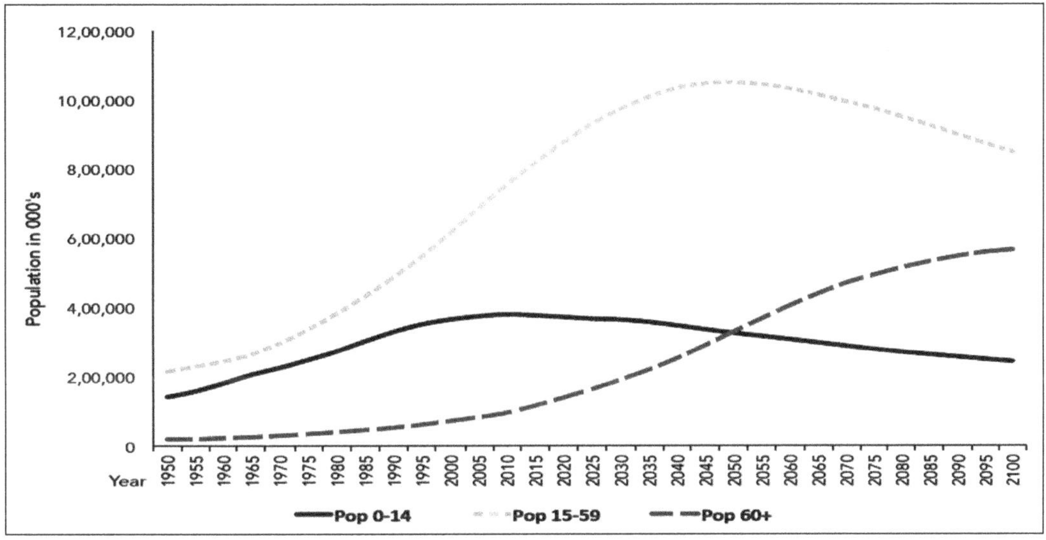

Fig. 40.1: World population by age category 1950-2100.

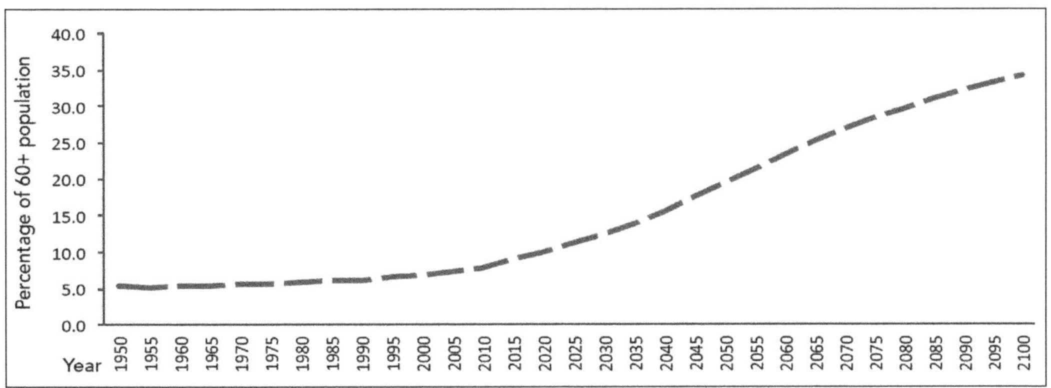

Fig. 40.2: Percentage of 60-plus population, India 1950-2100.

Epidemiology of Psychiatric Disorders in the Elderly

Psychiatric disorders in elderly contribute to significant morbidity. These disorders could be due to longstanding illnesses with onset in early life or having onset after the age of 60 years. The WHO conducted National Comorbidity Survey Replication (NCS-R) study reported lifetime prevalence of any psychiatric disorder to be 26.1 in which major Depression was most common disorder followed by specific and social phobia. While in India, the recent National Mental Health Survey, 2016, has reported lifetime prevalence of overall mental morbidity in people above 60 years of age to be around 15.1% (14.9%-15.3%). Table 40.1 shows prevalence of common mental disorders, severe mental disorders of individual disorders in elderly population, as per the NMHS 2016. (Is this in general or in the elderly?)

Assessment of Geriatric Patients

As the elderly patient has multiple co-existing health problems, a thorough evaluation of

Table 40.1: Prevalence (percentage) of common, severe mental disorders and of individual disorders in elderly population.

Disorder	Life-time prevalence	Point-prevalence	Comments
Common Mental Disorders	13.64	10.38	M > F 15.22 > 9.57
Severe Mental Morbidity	1.93	0.77	M > F 1.49 > 1.33
Dementia	----	5.6% -11.7%*	AD-50-75%, VD-20-30%, FTD-5-10%, DLB < 5% (of total cases)
Substance Use Disorder	27.78	4	26.34
Schizophrenia and other psychotic disorders	1.43 (1.37 - 1.48)	0.36 (0.33 - 0.39)	M > F,1.49 > 1.33
Mood Disorders	7.31	3.65	F > M
BPAD	0.56	0.3	M > F
Depressive disorder	6.93	3.53	F > M
Neurotic & stress related disorders overall	3.53	3.3	F > M
Phobic Anxiety	-	1.72	F > M
GAD	-	0.47	F > M
Suicide	10.6 (per lakh population)		M > F
Substance use disorders		Any substance-27.78% Alcohol 4.07% Other substances 0.56%	Tobacco use disorder 26.34%

*Reproduced from NMHS 2016, NIMHANS. * Prince MJ. The 10/66 dementia research group - 10 years on. Indian J Psychiatry. 2009;51 Suppl 1: S8–15.*

these problems becomes necessary as it would have a bearing on comprehensive management. Hence in addition to the routine psychiatric evaluation as in adults, many clinicians working with geriatric population recommend a Comprehensive Geriatric Evaluation, which is a process of evaluation of multiple problems of older persons, their resources and strengths, the need for services and development of an integrated plan of focussed intervention. Routine psychiatric evaluation is similar to that of adults and includes: -

- Presenting complaints and history of the presenting illness
- Past psychiatric and medical history
- Treatment history
- Family and Personal history (including *habits, nutrition, biological functions and lifestyle*). These assume more importance in the elderly, where social isolation, neglect and deprivation often go unrecognised.
- Premorbid personality
- Detailed Physical and Neurological examination
- Mental Status Examination

The goals of comprehensive assessment should be to help arrive at accurate diagnosis, to help select appropriate interventions, to recommend an optimal environment for care, to monitor condition and predict possible outcomes.

Figure 40.1 shows the components of **Comprehensive gero-psychiatric assessment.**

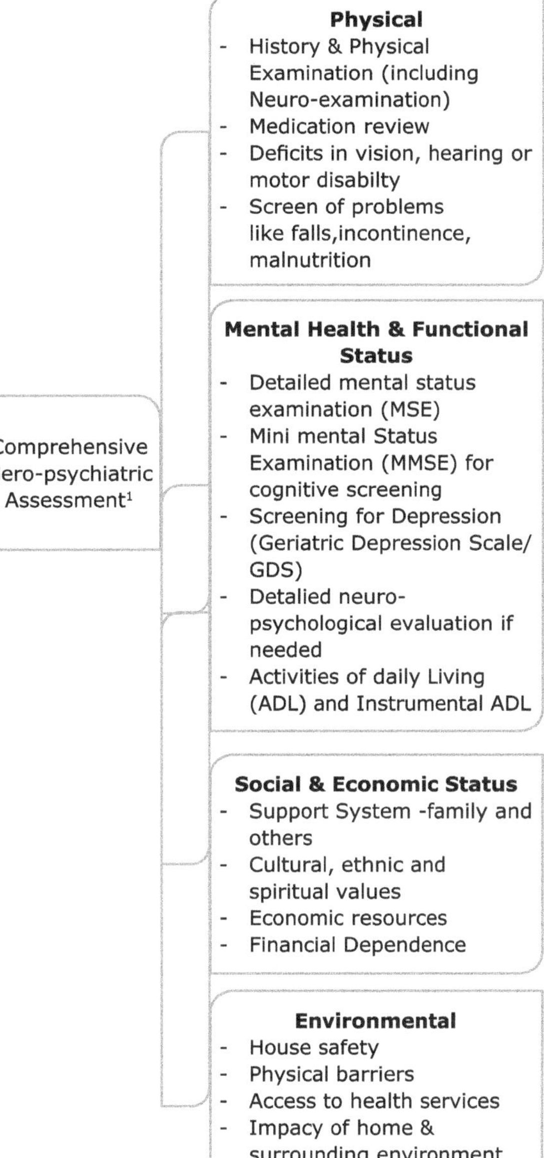

Fig. 40.3: Components of **Comprehensive psycho-geriatric assessment.** (Adapted from: Rubenstein, LZ: Geriatric assessment: An Overview of its Impacts. Clinics in Geriatric Medicine 3:1, pp1-15,1987.)

Assessment of Competence

Competence, which is in general, is the ability to act in the circumstances, including the ability to perform a job or occupation, or to reason or make decisions. Its assessment is of particular relevance in patients who have a cognitive dysfunction or are ill with a psychotic illness that makes it difficult for them to provide consent for treatment or legal procedures. Though *competency* per se is a legal terminology, it is task-specific and may vary for different circumstances. Some common procedures where assessment of competency is mandated are:

- Medical treatment and surgical procedures
- Power of attorney and will
- Consent by advance directives for research and withdrawal of life support systems

Laboratory Investigations- These be based on findings from history, examination, co-morbidities and probable diagnosis. Apart from relevant investigations following investigations (**Table 40.2**) may be done routinely to rule out common problems in elderly.

Examples of other optional investigations have been mentioned in **Table 40.3**.

Neuropsychological Testing

A neuropsychological profile includes testing the capacity of the higher functions of the individual which include overall cognition, memory, executive functioning, visuo-spatial orientation etc. to name a few.

These are helpful in evaluating an individual's overall cognitive and intellectual status and should be undertaken in patient suspected of having impairment even if the MMSE (Mini Mental State Examination) score is within normal limits. These tests allow differentiation of various cognitive deficits which will help knowing the type of dementia as well as for monitoring of progress or worsening. Some neuropsychological batteries available and

Table 40.3: Some examples of optional Investigations for elderly presenting with psychiatric symptoms

Investigations	Reason
Complete Blood Count	Anemia, Infections, Parasites
RFT, LFT, Electrolytes	Kidney, liver function
Thyroid status	Hypo/Hyperthyroidism, also for reversible cause of dementia/ depression
VDRL, HIV	Reversible causes of dementia
Sr. B-12, Folate, Vit. D	Deficiency, vascular
Imaging (CT /MRI)	For secondary causes, vascular, atrophy
ECG	Cardiac problems, vascular

Table 40.2: Routine Investigations for elderly presenting with psychiatric symptoms

Investigations	Reason
EEG	TLE, other brain dysfunction
Nerve conduction study	MND, Peripheral neuropathy
CSF	Infections, inflammation
VDRL, HIV	Reversible causes of dementia
Functional Imaging	Useful for diagnosing early Dementias, MCI
MR Angiography., Carotid Doppler	Carotid lesions, other vascular problems
Genetic Studies	For genetic variants of DEMENTIAS e.g. Apo-E. other genetic disorders

standardized for Indian population are the:

- Addenbrooke Cognitive Evaluation (ACE-R)
- Cognitive Screening Battery by Ganguli et al and the
- NIMHANS Neuropsychological Battery for the Elderly (NNB-E) etc.

Rating Scales and Standardised Instruments

Rating scales helps us not only for research purpose but also useful in clinical practice while dealing with elderly to identify specific problems, monitoring change and for teaching/ communication with colleague. These are usually for specific purpose like screening, diagnosis quantifying the severity etc. but should be translated & standardized for the population of practice. Some tests are enumerated below for specific disorders.

Brief Overview of Psychiatric Disorders in the Elderly

Dementia

Dementia as per ICD-10 is "a syndrome due to disease of the brain, usually of a chronic or progressive nature, in which there is disturbance of multiple higher cortical functions, including memory, thinking, orientation, comprehension, calculation, learning capacity, language, and judgment". Consciousness is usually preserved. These disturbances in brain functions are either accompanied, or preceded, by abnormalities of emotions, social behavior, or motivation. This syndrome is seen in Alzheimer's disease,

Table 40.4: Scales for assessment in Geriatric patients

Disorder/Domain	Scales/Instruments
Cognitive dysfunction/ Dementia	**For screening** - MMSE - Saint Louis University Mental Status (SLUMS) - Montreal Cognitive Assessment (MOCA) **For severity** - Clinical Dementia Rating (CDR) **For BPSD** - BEHAVE-AD - Neuro-Psychiatric Inventory (NPI) - Cornell Scale for Depression in Dementia
Activities of daily living	- Bristol Activities of Daily Living Scale - Everyday Abilities Scale for India (EASI) - Instrumental Activities of Daily Living Scale for Elderly (IADL-E)
Depression rating scales	- The Geriatric Depression Scale (GDS) - Hamilton Rating Scale for Depression (Ham-D) - Centre for Epidemiologic Studies Depression Scale (CES-D)
Psychosis	Brief Psychiatric Rating Scale
Interview schedules	Geriatric Mental State Examination (GMS)
Others	Anxiety Disorder-Geriatric Anxiety Inventory

in patients after stroke and in other conditions in which brain is primarily or secondarily affected.

The fifth edition of the Diagnostic and Statistical Manual of Mental Disorders (DSM-5) describes dementia, as **major neurocognitive disorder**. These impairment present as a decline from a previous level of functioning, thus differentiating it from mental retardation which is developmental and non-progressive. Although the course of dementia is often progressive, some forms of dementia can be reversible. Dementia is caused by a wide range of diseases, but most of the cases are due to Alzheimer's disease, which is the commonest cause, followed by vascular dementia and dementia with Lewy bodies. **Fig. 40.4** describes the general criterion of Demetia as per ICD-10 while **Table 40.5** shows criterion as per DSM 5.

G1. Evidence of each of the following:
(1) A decline in memory, which is most evident in the learning of new information, although in more severe cases, the recall of previously learned information may be also affected. The impairment applies to both verbal and non-verbal material. The decline should be objectively verified by obtaining a reliable history from an informant, supplemented, if possible, by neuropsychological tests or quantified cognitive assessments. The severity of the decline, with mild impairment as the threshold for diagnosis, should be assessed as follows:

Mild: A degree of memory loss sufficient to interfere with everyday activities, though not so severe as to be incompatible with independent living (see comment on cultural aspects of "independent living" on page 24). The main function affected is the learning of new material. For example, the individual has difficulty in registering, storing and recalling elements in daily living, such as where belongings have been put, social arrangements, or information recently imparted by family members.

Moderate: A degree of memory loss which represents a serious handicap to independent living. Only highly learned or very familiar material is retained. New information is retained only occasionally and very briefly. The individual is unable to recall basic information about where he lives, what he has recently been doing, or the names of familiar persons.

Severe: A degree of memory loss characterized by the complete inability to retain new information. Only fragments of previously learned information remain. The subject fails to recognize even close relatives.

(2) A decline in other cognitive abilities characterized by deterioration in judgment and thinking, such as planning and organizing, and in the general processing of information. Evidence for this should be obtained when possible from interviewing an informant, supplemented, if possible, by neuropsychological tests or quantified objective assessments. Deterioration from a previously higher level of performance should be established. The severity of the decline, with mild impairment as the threshold for diagnosis, should be assessed as follows:

Mild: The decline in cognitive abilities causes impaired performance in daily living, but not to a degree making the individual dependent on others. More complicated daily tasks or recreational activities cannot be undertaken.

Moderate: The decline in cognitive abilities makes the individual unable to function without the assistance of another in daily living, including shopping and handling money. Within the home, only simple chores are preserved. Activities are increasingly restricted and poorly sustained.

Severe: The decline is characterized by an absence, or virtual absence, of intelligible ideation. The overall severity of the dementia is best expressed as the level of decline in memory or other cognitive abilities, whichever is the more severe (e.g. mild decline in memory and moderate decline in cognitive abilities indicate a dementia of moderate severity).

G2. Preserved awarenenss of the environment (i.e. absence of clouding of consciousness (as defined in F05, criterion A)) during a period of time long enough to enable the unequivocal demonstration of G1. When there are superimposed episodes of delirium the diagnosis of dementia should be deferred.

G3. A decline in emotional control or motivation, or a change in social behavior, manifest as at least one of the following: (1) emotional lability; (2) irritability; (3) apathy; (4) coarsening of social behavior.

G4. For a confident clinical diagnosis, G1 should have been present for at least six months; if the period since the manifest onset is shorter, the diagnosis can only be tentative.

Comments: The diagnosis is further supported by evidence of damage to other higher cortical functions, such as aphasia, agnosia, apraxia.

Judgment about independent living or the development of dependence (upon others) need to take account of the cultural expectation and context. Dementia is specified here as having a minimum duration of six months to avoid confusion with reversible states with identical behavioral syndromes, such as traumatic subdural hemorrhage (S06.5), normal pressure hydrocephalus (G91.2) and diffuse or focal brain injury (S06.2 and S06.3).

Fig. 40.4: Diagnosis of dementia in general as per ICD-10. (Adapted from: The ICD-10, Classification of Mental and Behavioral Disorders, Clinical descriptions and diagnostic guidelines, WHO.)

Table 40.5: Major and Mild Neurocognitive Disorders as Diagnosed in DSM-5

Diagnostic Criteria	Major Neurocognitive Disorder	Mild Neurocognitive Disorder
A	Significant cognitive decline in one or more cognitive domains, based on:	Modest cognitive decline in one or more cognitive domains, based on:
	1. Concern about significant decline, expressed by individual or reliable informant, or observed by clinician.	1. Concern about mild decline, expressed by individual or reliable informant, or observed by clinician.
	2. Substantial impairment, documented by objective cognitive assessment.	2. Modest impairment, documented by objective cognitive assessment.
B	Interference with independence in everyday activities.	No interference with independence in everyday activities, although these activities may require more time and effort, accommodation, or compensatory strategies
C	Not exclusively during delirium.	
D	Not better explained by another mental disorder.	
E	Specify one or more etiologic subtypes, "due to"	
	• Alzheimer's disease • Cerebrovascular disease • Frontotemporal Neurocognitive Disorder • Dementia with Lewy Bodies • Parkinson's disease • Huntington's disease	• Traumatic Brain Injury • HIV Infection • Prion Disease • Another medical condition • Multiple etiologies

Adapted from: American Psychiatric Association: Diagnostic and Statistical Manual of Mental Disorders, Fifth Edition. Arlington, VA, American Psychiatric Association; 2013.

When the deficits are too mild and socio-occupational functioning is intact, the condition is then called mild cognitive impairment or mild neuro-cognitive disorder as per DSM 5.

Apart from these core symptoms other behavioral and psychological changes may be seen in majority of patients at some or other point during the course of illness which cause significant distress to the caregiver, and their management can be difficult. These are termed Behavioral and psychological symptoms of dementia (BPSD) (**Table 40.6**).

Table 40.6 various Behavioral and psychological symptoms of dementia (BPSD)

Behavioral symptoms (as observed by examiner)	Psychological symptoms (As per informants)
Agitation/ aggression	Anxiety symptoms
Shouting	Depressive symptoms
Restlessness	Apathy
Wandering behavior	Hallucinations and delusions
Abusive behavior	
Inappropriate sexual behavior	
Repetitive behavior	
Impaired sleep	

Differential Diagnosis

Common differentials which should be kept in

mind are: -

- Normal age-related cognitive decline- some decline in cognitive function is common in elderly however dementia is diagnosed only when the severity is sufficient to interfere with social and/or occupational functioning. The normal age-related cognitive impairment is called as **benign senescent forgetfulness.**
- Cognitive decline due to Depressive Disorder: It is the condition when cognitive symptoms in depression may mimic dementia clinically. Differentiation is very important as it is relatively easily treatable than dementia. Patients with cognitive decline due to depressive disorder often complain of memory impairment or poor attention/concentration, on the other hand the patients with dementia do not often complain and when confronted regarding any memory impairment, they often confabulate. As the two conditions often co-occur, clear differentiation often warrants a therapeutic trial with antidepressants.
- Delirium-As opposed to dementia there is acute onset and fluctuating course of symptoms characterized by impairment of consciousness and attention, global cognitive decline, psychomotor disturbances, impairment of sleep-wake cycle, and emotional disturbances. Though often delirium clouds or unmasks dementia and often has some underlying medical cause which can be managed.

Dementia is commonly classified either based on etiology or the predominant involvement of brain area i.e. cortical or subcortical though mixed picture is not uncommon. The important differences have been enumerated in **Table 40.7** while various etiologies have been listed in **Table 40.8**.

Differentiation between the four most common types of dementia is important and major difference in presentation, course, imaging findings etc. can help us differentiating between the group has been outlined in **Table 40.9**.

Basic Investigations

The history and assessment should be done as described before. The diagnostic tests are of great importance in finding the cause, or to exclude all other causes before diagnosing

Table 40.7: Cortical and Subcortical Dementia

Characteristics	Cortical Dementia	Sub-cortical Dementia
Location of involvement	Cortex (association areas between various lobes and hippocampus)	Subcortical grey matter (thalamus, basal ganglia, part of brain stem)
Examples	Alzheimer's disease, Fronto-temporal dementias	Dementia associated with Huntington's, Parkinson's disease, Focal thalamic and basal ganglia lesions and Multiple sclerosis
Prominent clinical presentation	- Prominent impairment of memory, word finding, or visuospatial abilities at least early in course - Severe language and memory impairment, agnosia, apraxia and acalculia - Usually no motor symptoms	- Slowness of thought, difficulty with complex sequential tasks, and disturbance of affect and personality - Prominent motor symptoms - Relative preservation of language, calculation, and learning

Table 40.8: Common Causes of Dementia as per etiology

• **Neuro-degenerative disease** Alzheimer's disease, Pick's disease, Parkinson's disease, Huntington's chorea, Lewy body dementia • **Vascular** Multi-infarct dementia, stroke, subdural hematoma • **Toxins** Alcohol, heavy metals, organic solvents, organophosphates • **Metabolic and endocrine causes** Renal failure, hepatic failure, hypothyroidism, Hyperthyroidism • **Inflammatory and autoimmune causes** Systemic lupus erythematosus, other forms of cerebral vasculitis, multiple sclerosis, Hashimoto's encephalopathy. • **Trauma** Severe head injury, repeated head trauma ('dementia pugilistica')	• **Infections** Creutzfeldt-Jacob disease, neurosyphilis, chronic meningitis, viral encephalitis, AIDS dementia, sub-acute sclerosing panencephalitis (SSPE) • **Vitamin and other nutritional deficiencies** Vitamin B12 deficiency, Pernicious anemia, pellagra, folic acid deficiency, thiamine deficiency • **Neoplastic causes** Intracranial malignancies, carcinomatous meningitis, paraneoplastic encephalitis • **Post-radiation** Acute and subacute radio-necrosis, radiation Thrombo-angiopathy • **Post-hypoxia** Severe anemia, post-surgery, CO poisoning, cardiac arrest, chronic respiratory failure

Table 40.9: Characteristics of Major types of Dementias

	Alzheimer's Disease	**Vascular dementia**	**Dementia Lewy Body**	**Fronto-temporal Dementia**
Course	Gradual onset progressive	– Variable presentation based on extent and location of vascular problems – Shows stepladder pattern	Gradual onset progressive	Gradual onset progressive
Presentation	– Memory impairment early in the course – Visuospatial & language difficulties as the disease progresses – Diagnosis is by excluding other causes	– Cognitive impairment onset after evidence of CVE – Presentation variable	– Early changes in attention and executive function & fluctuating – prominent visual hallucinations present early in the disease – Cognitive symptoms onset before or concurrently with motor symptoms	– Behavioral variant: Impaired executive abilities with Behavioral problems such as disinhibition, apathy, lack of empathy, and hyperorality – Language variant: Loss of semantic memory, including speech production, word – finding and comprehension, and grammar

(Continued...)

Table 40.9: Characteristics of Major types of Dementias (Continued)

	Alzheimer's Disease	Vascular dementia	Dementia Lewy Body	Fronto-temporal Dementia
Associated features	BPSD common - Early ones: Apathy, Depression - Moderate to severe: agitation, delusion, hallucinations and wandering wandering - Late: Seizures, Gait disturbance, incontinence,	- Risk factors like history of CVA or M.I. or T.I.A. are present	- Rapid eye movement sleep behavior disorder may be early sign1 - Nearly 50% have severe neuroleptic sensitivity - Falls, syncope and transient loss of consciousness are common - Autonomic dysfunction - Often a history of delirium during illness or surgery	- Extrapyramidal symptoms may be present - May Overlap with other Parkinson plus syndromes - Visual hallucinations may be present - Majority in sixth decade
Etiology/ risk factors	- Increasing age, genetics, Head injury, Family history	- Obesity, Hypertension, diabetes, smoking, hypercholesterolemia, hyper-homocysteinemia - Other risk factors thrombosis or hemorrhage	Genetic risk identified but no family history in most cases	- Up to 40% are familial - Present in up to 10% of patients with motor neuron disease - Cognitive assessments often normal
Imaging	Generalized atrophy (more in hippocampal and temporo-parietal region)	Evidence of ischemia or white matter hyper-intensities	Lewy bodies found primarily in the cortex - Medial temporal structures preserved	Pattern of brain atrophy dependent on subtype
pathology	amyloid Plaques and neurofibrillary tangles in cortex	- Cerebrovascular Disease - Single strategic Infarcts or diffuse in multi-infarct disease	Cortical Lewy Bodies (alpha-synuclein)	Damage/atrophy limited to Frontal and temporal lobes

Alzheimer's dementia. The list of investigations includes the ones described under assessment section. However Other relevant clinical, physical, neuro-psychological, laboratory or imaging investigations may be undertaken as suspected.

Treatment of the Underlying Cause

Some forms of dementia are treatable (reversible dementias). Treatment of such dementias is to manage the underlying condition like vitamin supplementation in dementia due to folate or B-12 deficiency or thyroxin supplementation in hypothyroid dementia, removal of the causative agent in toxic dementias and adequate treatment of Parkinsonism etc.

General Measures

- Coping skills training to deal with stress in daily activities.
- Treatment of medical co-morbidities, nutrition and hygiene.
- Supportive care for the patient and family/ carers.

Management of Behavioral and Psychological Symptoms of Dementia

Before initiating any treatment, careful assessment is required, and attention should be paid to:

- Contributory factors like UTI, pain of physical problems and constipation should be ruled out.
- BPSD may fluctuate and may last less than 3 months, hence any treatment should be done considering this fact and regular monitoring should be part of the management plan.
- BPSD are usually distressing for the carer than the patient should be kept in mind while making treatment decisions.

The first approach should be to treat any underlying reversible cause. If problems persist, next step is modification of patient's environment, living condition etc. or a behavioral or psychological intervention, as deemed appropriate. Medication should be used only when such approaches fail. Some non-pharmacological management approaches have been enumerated in (Table 40.10)

Table 40.10: Non-pharmacological interventions for behavioral and psychological symptoms of dementia

Sensory stimulation intervention	**Behavioral management technics**
– Music therapy (Most convincing evidence) – Aromatherapy – Bright light therapy – Massage – Dance therapy **Cognitive/ emotion-oriented interventions** – Cognitive stimulation – Reminiscence therapy **Miscellaneous** – Increasing social contact – Pet therapy	– Differential reinforcement – Stimulus control – Communication training – Token economy **Individualised care** – Exercise – Structured activity scheduling – Environmental modifications – Care-giver education and support

However, if non-pharmacological measures fail, medications may be required at least for short term.

Various drugs used to treat behavioral and psychological symptoms of dementia. However, side effects should be carefully monitored as elderly are more prone to develop adverse effects even at lower doses.

Table 40.11: Pharmacological management of BPSD

For mild to moderate agitation
– SSRIs, e.g. Escitalopram 5–20 mg, sertraline
– Benzodiazepines, e.g. lorazepam 0.5–4 mg/ oxazepam
– Trazodone 50–100 mg (also insomnia)
– Carbamazepine 100–300 mg
– Sodium valproate 250–1000 mg
For severe agitation with psychosis
– Olanzapine 2.5–10 mg
– Quetiapine 25–200 mg
– Risperidone 0.5–3 mg
– Aripiprazole 2-10 mg
For depression
– SSRI
– Mirtazapine 15–45 mg
For severe behavioral problems
– Haloperidol (0.5–4 mg)/Risperidone (0.5-3 mg)

Specific Drug Treatment of Various Dementias

- Drug treatment of Alzheimer's disease: Currently only two classes of drugs are approved for Alzheimer's disease: Donepezil (5-20 mg), rivastigmine (1-12 mg) and galantamine (16-24 mg/day) which are Cholinesterase inhibitors are approved in mild to moderate Alzheimer's disease, or memantine (5-20 mg) which is a NMDA antagonist is approved in moderate to severe Alzheimer's disease. Both these classes of drugs help only in slowing down the disease process but not halt it. Many novel treatments are underway; however, none has received approval till date.
- Frontotemporal dementia: No treatment has been approved for cognitive or behavioral symptoms; cholinesterase inhibitors may worsen the behavioral symptoms. Hence symptomatic management is advisable.
- Vascular dementia: Treatment of vascular dementia is currently limited to controlling risk factors, such as hyperlipidemia and blood pressure. Cholinesterase inhibitors and memantine though used commonly are not recommended for use.
- Dementia with Lewy bodies-Cholinesterase inhibitors have been found effective in dementia with Lewy bodies and in dementia associated with Parkinson's disease. Rivastigmine has been found most useful however memantine has been found to be ineffective.
- Dementia of Huntington's disease-though drugs are available for its psychiatric and motor symptoms, there is no approved treatment for cognitive symptoms.

Depressive Disorder in the Elderly

Though prevalence is described elsewhere, it is higher in certain populations like medical outpatients (5-10%), inpatients (10-12%), and residents in institutions (14-42%). Apart from major depressive disorder, adjustment disorder, dysthymia and depression secondary to medical conditions are included in this group.

Clinical presentation

Though the disorder itself is less prevalent than in the younger population, the sign/symptoms in the elderly are somewhat different than in younger adults. Most of elderly patients have either severe retardation or agitation. Sleep disturbances, fatigue, hopelessness, somatic and hypochondriac symptom are also more common. Psychotic symptoms frequently accompany severe depression in elderly mostly in form of somatic and hypochondriac delusions.

Cognitive Decline due to Depression

Some patients may present with cognitive decline in which they show difficulty with concentration and memory, but no objective findings. Differentiation from early dementia is important but difficult. Depression should be considered when patients themselves present with these symptoms and they have appeared after depressive symptoms.

Depression may be either under or over diagnosed in the presence of medical conditions that can cause fatigue, sleep/appetite disturbances and weight loss. So, attribution of these symptoms to the physical illness may cause underdiagnosis, and undermining physical illness can lead to overdiagnosis.

Suicide

Older adults are at significant risk of death by suicide, relative to younger adults. With age though the frequency reduces the lethality is higher. The risk factors for suicide in elderly include:

- Severity of depression- strongest predictor of suicidal ideation
- Psychotic depression
- Recent bereavement
- Chronic medical conditions or disability
- Loneliness and isolation associated with divorce or widowhood
- Cognitive difficulties
- Impulsivity and hopelessness

Etiology

The etiology of depressive disorders in elderly is similar to the etiology at younger ages, with biological, psychological, and social components. Some factors unique to old age are :

- Presence of physical illnesses, especially cardiac and neurological disorders.
- Psycho-social factors like loneliness, various dependencies, poor social contacts, lack of care and affection and stressful life events like death of spouse, retirement, changing family roles etc.
- Life-style related factors like irregular dietary habits, low physical activity, low spirituality and emotion focussed coping etc.

Apart from other psychiatric disorders like somatization disorder, Anxiety disorder and grief reaction the differential diagnosis include dementia when cognitive symptoms are prominent. Other common differentials are:

- Neurological disorders like stroke, multiple sclerosis
- Hematological issues like anemia, leukaemia.
- Chronic infections like HIV, Hepatitis
- Vitamin deficiencies B12, thiamine etc.
- Malignancies

Management

The principles of the treatment of depression in elderly are similar to that of younger adults.

- For mild to moderate cases psychotherapy should be considered if resources available.
- Risk of suicide should be monitored
- Any co-morbid physical disorder and medications if any.
- Monitoring side-effects

Psychological interventions have been proven effective in the elderly, but their availability is very limited especially in India. They are particularly useful in population having bereavement, having significant life stressors, poor social support, disabilities and poor coping strategies. They can also be helpful while awaiting the drug response or when patient is sensitive to biological modalities of treatment. Some evidence based Psychological Interventions for Depression in Late Life are:

- Behavioral therapy
- Cognitive Behavioral therapy
- Problem solving therapy
- Brief psychodynamic therapy
- Life review therapy

Other non-pharmacological treatments which are helpful include exercise, yoga, meditation etc.

Though the medications are as effective as in younger adults, they should be used cautiously, with the dictum 'start low, go slow' and hiking the doses after reviewing the side effects and response.

SSRIs are preferred to other classes because of their lower propensity to cause side effects and minimal drug-drug interactions. If patients do not respond to single drug a combination with another medication or other modality of treatment like psychotherapy or Electro-convulsive therapy should be considered. ECT can be considered in patients with severe agitation, suicidal ideations and attempts, depressive stupor or non-response to medications. After complete recovery, the same dose or combination should be maintained for at least 12 months for a first episode in the elderly, and longer in cases of recurrences or relapse.

Course and Outcome

Depression in elderly have been seen to follow the rule of threes: one third of them recover, a third remain the same, and a third deteriorate further. Some factors associated with good prognosis are relatively early onset (<70 yrs.), short duration, good pre-morbid functioning, no co-morbid physical conditions, good social support and religiosity to name a few.

Bipolar Disorder in the Elderly

Though the prevalence is lesser as compared to adult population, the clinical picture in both is similar. It is seen more commonly that depressive episode many times occur immediately after the manic episode also mixed episodes are more common than in younger population.

Occurrence of first episode of mania is common in elderly with history of recurrent episodes of depression. Like unipolar-depression, late-life Bipolar disorder is also usually associated with cognitive impairment (impairment in attention, memory and executive functions), higher medical comorbidity poor psycho-social support. These factors adversely affect outcome of BD.

The evaluation should focus on identifying any reversible medical conditions that may contribute to the mood symptoms. It should further include family history and details about prior mood episodes.

Due to significant overlap in clinical findings, delirium should be carefully differentiated by presence of fluctuating consciousness, disorientation, and memory and language impairment. BPSD can also be a differential diagnosis, especially when agitation and disinhibition is marked.

Management approach is similar to that of adults.

- **Acute mania** all atypical antipsychotics are approved except clozapine. However, choice should be based on all relevant details and medical condition. Among mood stabilizers Lithium is preferred only when there are minimal neurological and cognitive problems in classic euphoric mania. Valproate is also approved for acute episodes however hepatic complications, risk of encephalopathy should be kept in mind, along with close blood level monitoring for both these agents. Carbamazepine is another alternative. Start low and go slow should be the dictum adopted.

- Bipolar Depression - include drugs like Lamotrigine, Quetiapine and combination of olanzapine and fluoxetine like in younger adults. The role of anti-depressants is still controversial though very commonly used off-label.
- Maintenance treatment medications similar to that of adults are used however tolerability and efficacy has not been established in elderly especially of atypical antipsychotics.
- Psychosocial interventions include psychoeducation focussing on adherence and relapse prevention, social support and reduction of medical comorbidity. Common psychotherapies found useful in BD are Cognitive-Behavioral Therapy, interpersonal social rhythm therapy (IPSRT) and family-focused therapy.

Geriatric Anxiety Disorders

Anxiety is one of the most common symptoms with which elderly patients present. The commonest disorders seen are Generalized Anxiety Disorder (GAD) seen in (7.3%) followed by phobias (3.1%), panic disorder (1%) and OCD (0.6%). Further two more recent Indian studies have shown overall prevalence of anxiety disorders to 10.7-10.8%. With arrival of DSM 5 the classification of OCD is different from ICD 10 where it is included in anxiety disorders while in DSM 5 it has been separated. Apart from the aforementioned assessment, use of any concomitant medication use and presence of medical disorders which can be mistaken for anxiety disorders should be looked for and relevant investigations may also be undertaken.

Specific presentation of various anxiety disorders has been shown in **Table 40.12**. There are subtle differences in clinical presentation of anxiety disorders among young and elderly patients. GAD in elderly has similar features as that of younger adults. In Panic disorder, the severity of symptoms and overall distress is lower in elderly. While in OCD contamination and religious obsessions are more common as opposed to counting and symmetry in young people. Lastly in PTSD, elderly have more severe physical symptoms, social dysfunction and avoidance behavior while younger individuals have more psychological symptoms.

The focus of investigations should be to rule out secondary causes of anxiety using Hematological, biochemical or radiological investigations. Further quantification of symptom severity using appropriate scale. The Geriatric Anxiety Inventory has become the gold standard for assessment anxiety in elderly.

Some common differential diagnoses of Anxiety disorders in Elder individuals:

1. Side Effects of Medication use, including self-medication
2. Drug and alcohol use
3. Medical comorbidities
4. Other Psychiatric disorders (including cognitive disorders dementia)

However careful history, physical & mental

Table 40.12: Specific presentation of various anxiety disorders in elderly

Disorder	Specific Characteristics in the Elderly
Specific phobia	• Commonly seen but onset is usually early in life • Fear of falling is the commonest symptom'
Generalized Anxiety Disorder	• One of commonest disorders in elderly with onset in early life and chronic course • Sub-syndromic symptoms more common than disorder • Illness anxiety and health anxiety are commonest symptoms seen-
Social Phobia	• Again, usually early onset • May be difficult to diagnose due to poor socialization and isolation
Post-Traumatic Stress Disorder	• Subsyndromal PTSD is more common in older adults • Can be chronic • Best evidence seen in war veterans • In elder individuals-re-experience phenomenon are rare
Panic Attacks	• Uncommon than younger age group, unless pre-existing • Diagnosable panic disorder is rare • Overall functionality –less impeded than in younger adults
Obsessive Compulsive Disorder	• Onset after 55 years is very rare • Can be part of BPSD (Behavioral and Psychological Symptoms of Dementia) • Hoarding compulsions are unique to this age. Common in those with cognitive disorder, personality change or substance use.

status examination should help differentiate most of them.

Treatment

Elderly patients with Anxiety disorders rarely require in-patient care except when associated with severe depression or requires admission for separation from stressful situations or detailed evaluation.

Non-pharmacological Treatment

- Lifestyle modification involving sleep hygiene, exercise as feasible and dietary modification.
- Behavior therapies
  - Relaxation Therapy: Progressive muscle relaxation for anxiety. This can also be coupled with guided
  - Systemic desensitization: phobias and unspecified fears
  - Exposure and Response Prevention: For OCD
  - Eye Movement Desensitization and Reprocessing (EMDR): For PTSD.

Cognitive therapies: CBT as for anxiety disorders in adults

Some other therapies like mindfulness, yoga, art therapy, dance therapy have also been found useful.

Schizophrenia-like Disorders in the Elderly

Psychosis in simple terms is defined as presence of delusions and/or hallucinations and is relatively common in older adults. Etiology is varied as any neuro-pathological process at this age can present as psychosis. Late-onset schizophrenia (onset age 45 to 60) and very-late onset schizophrenia-like psychosis (onset over 60) have a somewhat different symptom profile and epidemiology from those of early-onset. Though psychosis can be either primary (due to primary psychiatric disorder) or secondary (to medical/neurological disorder) there are no reliable signs to distinguish between primary and secondary psychosis.

Schizophrenia and related disorders as per DSM include Schizophrenia, Schizoaffective disorder, Schizophreniform disorder, Delusional disorder and Brief psychotic disorder.

The precise etiology of late and very-late onset schizophrenia-like psychosis is largely unknown however it is postulated that schizophrenia with onset in early and middle age (45-60) is a neuro-developmental disorder, while the very late onset is neuro-degenerative in nature. Further familial and genetic causes of schizophrenia appear to be more important in early onset than later ones.

In clinical presentations early and late onset cases are similar, but the very late onset population differ slightly. They have a female preponderance, more paranoid and negative symptoms, more non-auditory hallucinations, higher cognitive dysfunction and more likely to show structural brain abnormalities.

Common differentials include delirium, dementia, or secondary psychosis due to a medical or neurological such as neurosyphilis, HIV, or neoplasm. As in younger population, schizophrenia must also be distinguished from other psychiatric disorders like delusional disorder and affective psychoses.

Though drug treatment is similar as that of young adults, late onset population require lower doses of medication and have high sensitivity to tardive dyskinesia. Further non-pharmacological measures like ECT, Psychoeducation and CBT etc. like younger adults, are also useful in elderly.

Data on delusional disorder in older adults is scarce. Delusional disorder generally presents in mid/ late adulthood with prevalence is 0.03% and shows female pre-ponderance while men experiencing more severe symptoms and worse outcomes. Risk factors for delusional disorder include a history of schizoid, avoidant, or paranoid personality disorder or schizophrenia in family. Treatment is similar to that of younger adult population.

Alcohol and Other Substance Use Disorder

Elder people with alcohol dependence usually present with history of excessive drinking that began in early adulthood. Common associated factors include medical illnesses, especially liver disease, are either divorced, widowed, or never married. Lot of them suffer from chronic illnesses like Wernicke's encephalopathy or Korsakoff's syndrome. Abuse of sedatives, hypnotics and analgesics is common in old age however substance-seeking behaviors and criminality is rarely associated.

The clinical presentation of alcohol and other substance use disorders mostly includes symptoms of confusion, poor self-care, associated mood or anxiety disorders, malnutrition and injuries due to falls.

Poor personal hygiene, depression, malnutrition, and the effects of exposure and falls. Delirium is also common during withdrawal phases in elderly.

Management focusses on dealing with co-morbid medical and psychiatric illnesses, adequate pain management etc.

Special Issues in Elderly

Apart from mental illnesses, a significant proportion of elderly population face are, negative expressed emotions, and various forms of abuse and /or neglect. In the recent nation-wide survey in India, one-fourth of elderly, irrespective of gender reported to be victims of some form of neglect or abuse. It can be defined as intended or un-intended actions by a caregiver or any trusted person resulting in harm or posing a serious risk of harm to an elderly person(abuse) or failure to satisfy basic needs/protect them from harm(neglect). Abuse can be physical, sexual, financial or psychological abuse or neglect. Neglect further can be of many types like emotional (failure/denial to provide love and affection), physical [failure/refusal to provide essential care (food, clothes, medical care) so as to seriously endanger the physical health] and /or financial (disregard towards financial obligations like rent, medical insurance, utility etc.). Risk of abuse/neglect is higher in elderly with mental health issues especially dementia, persons living in isolation or with other physical disabilities and found to exhibit increased mortality rate.

Though the awareness regarding need to identify and deal with elder abuse and respond to it, is on the rise, no specific interventions has been found useful. Thus, elder abuse is a huge un-identified health hazard which has not received enough attention, and requires joint efforts on part of society, government and NGOs using measures such as increasing social support, respite care, programes for carers and legal approaches etc. can be effective.

Ethical and Legal and Financial Issues in the Elderly

These are of special concern in elderly as

- Illnesses in elderly like dementia may compromises their capacity to make decisions and give consent for treatment, research etc.
- Issues such as testamentary capacity and advance directives also emerge in this age.
- Management of financial affairs like pension, property like and power of Attorney also require help.

Geriatric Mental Health Services in India

Major resources for dealing with mental health issues of elderly in India includes family as caregivers, Government and private psychiatric hospitals/nursing homes; and NGOs.

India has dearth of mental health professionals with only 4000 trained psychiatrists catering to 21 million elderly in need of mental health services. Similarly lack of access and underutilization of those services has also been reported. A study found that 46.3% had no knowledge of geriatric services nearby; and 96% had never utilised any geriatric service. A very few hospitals in India have dedicated geriatric units and most of them are available in cities at tertiary care hospitals. Only two centres in INDIA (NIMHANS Bengaluru & Geriatric Psychiatry Department at KGMC, Lucknow) provide specialized training in Geriatric psychiatry (Doctorate of Medicine{4} & Post-Doctoral Fellowships{3}).Further currently there are less than 25 geriatric psychiatrists in India, which is far from the number required to cater mental health needs of our elderly population. Other common concerns in government hospitals are lack manpower and infrastructure, inaccessibility and inequitable distribution; while private sector are dealing

Table 40.13: Some major government initiatives regarding care of elderly

Law/Scheme	Purpose/Benefits
Constitutional Provisions	Some provisions relate duty of government towards the elderly in the form of pension, social security, social insurance and economic and social support.
Hindu &Muslim law	– Legal obligations to both sons and daughters to maintain the basic needs of parents. – Though Christian & Parsi law do not have these elders can claim the same under Criminal Procedure Code, Section 125(1).
National Programe for the Health Care of the Elderly (NPHCE) 2010-2011.	– Objective is to strengthen social security provisions for pension, income tax benefits, provident fund gratuity, and medical assistance. – Capacity building for geriatric health care
Maintenance and Welfare of Parents and Senior Citizens Act, 2007	– Objective is to hasten the process of claim of monthly maintenance for parents and senior citizens – Specifies obligations on children and relatives to maintain their parents/grandparents or elderly dependent.

with high cost and poor quality of care. Recent MHCA 2017 also advocates "mental health establishment" i.e. provision of old age homes for older adults but, these services do not exist.

Elderly are also at risk of violation of their rights. The recently introduced MHCA 2017 focusses on protecting rights of mentally ill. Though some of the provisions such as mental capacity, Advanced Directive, and Nominated Representative are exclusive challenges related to elder mental health care, there is a need for more organised analysis of impact of MHCA 2017 on geriatric mental health care.

Apart from MHCA 2017, other major initiatives from government regarding care of elderly are listed in **Table 40.13**.

BIBLIOGRAPHY

1. Dening T and Thomas A (2013). Oxford Textbook of Old Age Psychiatry, 2nd edition. Oxford University Press, Oxford.
2. Gelder MG et al. (eds) (2009). Section 8: The psychiatry of old age. In: The New Oxford Textbook of Psychiatry. Oxford University Press, Oxford.
3. Harrison P, Cowen P, Burns T & Fazel M.(eds) 2018. Psychiatry of the elderly. In: The Shorter Oxford Textbook of Psychiatry. Oxford University Press, Oxford.
4. Sadock BJ, Sadock VA. Kaplan and Sadock's synopsis of psychiatry: Behavioral sciences/ clinical psychiatry. Lippincott Williams & Wilkins; 2011 Dec 26.
5. Varghese M, Dahale AB. The Geropsychiatric Interview-Assessment and Diagnosis. Indian journal of psychiatry. 2018 Feb;60(Suppl 3): S301.
6. Pinto C. The Geropsychiatric Interview, Assessment and Diagnosis. Clinical Practice Guidelines for Geriatric Psychiatry, Indian Psychiatric Society. 2007.
7. Shaji K S, Sivakumar P T, Rao G P, Paul N. Clinical practice guidelines for management of dementia. Indian J Psychiatry 2018;60, Suppl S3:312-28.
8. Subramanyam A, Kedare J, Singh O, Pinto C. Clinical Practice guidelines for geriatric anxiety disorders. Indian J Psychiatry. 2018;60(7), Suppl S3:312-28.

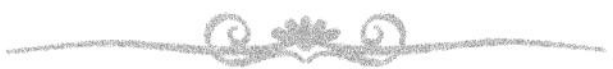

41 Suicide, Deliberate Self Harm (DSH) & Non-Suicidal Self Injury (NSSI)

Alka A. Subramanyam • Shipra Singh

INTRODUCTION

Suicide has been defined as "an act with a fatal outcome, deliberately initiated and performed in the knowledge or expectation of its fatal outcome". The word 'suicide' is derived from Latin words 'sui' and 'caedere', which together mean, "to kill oneself." There is a spectrum between thinking about self-harm to committing suicide. Stengel mentioned that a degree of suicidal intent was present in both suicide attempters and completers, and called the former group as 'failed suicide' group. Kessel and Grossman proposed that those 'attempted suicide' be replaced by 'deliberate self-poisoning' and 'deliberate self-injury'; Morgan suggested a single term 'deliberate self-harm' (DSH) including both. DSH thus is a willful self-inflicting of painful, destructive or injurious acts without intent to die.

HISTORICAL ASPECTS OF SUICIDE

The history of suicide dates back to ancient era, and has been glorified by some and deplored or condemned by others. Suicide in ancient India was essentially influenced by religious and socio-cultural beliefs, sacrificial motives and to sustain one's honor. After the death of Lord Rama, there was an epidemic of suicide in his kingdom. The Bhagavad Gita condemns suicide for its selfish reasons. Chandragupta Maurya ended his life by deliberate slow starvation in the orthodox Jain manner. Such death was linked to attainment of 'moksha'. Rajput women to avoid humiliation and enslavement by the invading foreign armies practiced 'Jauhar'. A similar practice of Sati involves a woman immolating herself on the pyre of her husband was practiced until recently in various parts of India.

EPIDEMIOLOGY

Suicide is one of the leading causes of death all around the world. As per Global Health Estimates by WHO, around 703,000 people died by suicide every year, suicide attempts are considered to be at least 25 times the suicide death rates. The important fact in these estimates is that 75% of these deaths happen in the developing countries. As per National Crime Records Bureau (NCRB), a total of 153,052 suicides were reported in 2020, which showed an increase of 10% compared to 2019. Maharashtra reported the majority of suicides (13%), followed by Tamil Nadu (11%) and Madhya Pradesh (9.5%). The rate of suicide, i.e. the number of suicide per lakh population, was 11.3 during the year 2020, with Andaman and Nicobar Islands having the highest rate, followed by Sikkim and Chhattisgarh. 'Family problems' and 'Illness' were the major causes of suicide, followed by drug abuse, marriage related issues, etc. The overall male: female ratio of suicide victims was 70.9:29.1. People aged 18-30 years and 30-45 years of age formed the most vulnerable groups resorting to suicides, accounting for 34.4% and 31.4% suicides respectively. Cases of mass or family suicides have also been reported.

Socially, for the sake of convenience, suicide may be understood pertaining to specific social group

- **Students**: Among all cases of suicide, percentage of students has increased from 5.5% in 2010, to 8.2 in 2020 (NCRB). Failure at examinations accounted for nearly a quarter of the cases. However, other reasons like peer pressure, over-expectation from parents and others, fear of failure, forcing courses and career choices, problems in relationships and increasing mental health issues in adolescents have also been indicated. The increasing number of suicides in students preparing for medical/engineering entrances in Kota (Rajasthan) is one such example.
- **Farmers**: India is an agrarian country and the trend of suicide in farmers is worrisome. NCRB mentions 7.0% of suicide victim belonged to farming sector. The reasons here are multifactorial-related to farming (failure of crops), financial (unable to repay loans, greater reliance on informal sources of credit) and political (inadequate and ineffective policies and resources).
- **Armed force personnel**: According to recent data, there were 891 deaths by suicide of members of the Indian armed forces between 2011 and 2018. The reasons range from occupational like long and continuous tenures of deployment at difficult posts to personal involving struggle with family issues, domestic problems and marital discord.
- **Suicides related to relationship issues**: Divorce, dowry and love affairs, cancellation or the inability to get married (according to the system of arranged marriages in India), and such conflicts relating to the issue of marriage, play a crucial role, particularly in the suicide of women in India.
- **Family/Mass suicides**: Mass suicide can be defined as the simultaneous suicide of members of a social group. It can be sub-divided further into: (a) hetero-induced, where in oppressed people may choose to kill themselves rather than submit to their oppressors, (b) self-induced, which is related to a distorted evaluation of reality, instead of an intolerable situation or a real risk of death. The history of mass suicide in India dates back to culture of 'Sati' or 'Jauhar' practiced by Rajput women to avoid capture and enslavement by invaders, to the death of 11 people from the same family as in 'Burari case'. During the year 2020, total of 121 cases of mass/family suicide waere reported, which involved 272 persons.

NOSOLOGY

According to ICD -10, 'purposely self-inflicted poisoning or injury' and 'suicide' are included under sub-section 'Intentional self-harm (X60-X84)' of Chapter XX- External causes of morbidity and mortality. However, DSM-5 has included and proposed criteria for 'Suicidal Behavior Disorder' and 'Non-suicidal self-injury' in the section of 'Conditions for further study".

Methods of Suicide

Varied methods have been adopted for suicide. Hanging and poisoning accounted for the highest numebers, i.e. 57.8% and 25.0% respectively, followed by drowning and self-immolation. Other measures were jumping from height, coming under moving vehicle, self-inflicting injuries and consuming sleeping pills. Considering means of suicide, the number of males was more for every method except fire/self-immolation, where number of female victims was more.

Risk Factors

I. DEMOGRAPHIC CHARACTERISTICS

a. Gender: Suicide is more common in men than in women, regardless of age or race; although rate of suicide attempt is 3-4 times more in women. Methods used for this are often different in both cases; men often commit suicide by hanging, firearms or jumping from high places, whereas women resort to poison or overdose of psychoactive substances/drugs.

b. Age: Suicide rates peak after age 45 in men and after 55 in women, midlife crisis playing an important role. Elderly attempt suicide less commonly than younger people, but have higher rates of completed suicide.

c. Religion: Protestants and Jews have had higher suicide rates compared to Catholics. Muslims have much lower rates. Literature from Hindu mythology including epics like Ramayana and Mahabharata has recorded instances of suicide.

d. Race: Suicide rates vary in races. Also, it is higher among immigrants than those in the native-born population.

e. Marital status: Being married, more so having children, reduces risk of suicide. Higher rates are seen in single, never married and divorced individuals.

f. Occupation: Work is protective against suicide; risk is higher in unemployed individuals. Suicide rates were found higher in women who work in arts, design, entertainment, sports and media; on the other hand, rates in men was higher those worked in construction and extraction. Rates are particularly higher in professions having access to lethal materials.

II. INDIVIDUAL FACTORS

a. Physical illness: Physical illness has an important link with suicide. History of seeking medical attention in last 6 months has been found in around one-third of the people who commit suicide. Disfigurement, especially in women, loss of mobility and chronic intractable pain are important contributors. Around one-fifth of all suicides were due to 'Illness' in 2020..

b. Mental illness: Patients with psychiatric illness are 3-12 times more at risk of committing suicide. Hospitalization in psychiatric facility appears contributory.

   i. Depressive disorder: Mood disorders are highly linked with suicide; around 60-70% of suicide victims had significant depressive symptoms. However, many Indian studies do not report this link as frequently as the Western literature.

   ii. Schizophrenia: Around 10% of patients having schizophrenia die because of suicide. Other risk factors in such patients include young age, male gender, unmarried, unemployed and recent discharge from hospital.

   iii. Substance Use Disorders: Drug users with easy availability, intravenous usage, chaotic lifestyle and personality disorders are at increased risk of suicide. Around 10-15% of patients with alcohol dependence commit suicide. Risk increases among those having physical complications, relationship or work-related issues.

iv. Personality disorder: Suicide rates are higher in various personality disorders. They play as predisposing factors for various mental disorders like depression, substance use, difficulties in relationships and coping with life stressors.

v. History of previous self-harm attempts

vi. Eating disorders: Anorexia nervosa, in particular, is a likely risk factor for suicide as well as being associated with an increased risk of mortality in general.

vii. Attention deficit hyperactivity disorder and suicidal behavior are found related in some studies.

III. PSYCHOSOCIAL FACTORS

These are often less apparent but important contributors to suicide act. Relationship problems like those pertaining to family, marital issues, love affairs; financial matters like bankruptcy/ indebtedness, property dispute; and other social problems like failure in examination, unemployment, professional/career problems, fall in social reputation, illicit relations etc. are found to be causative/contributory factors in suicide.

Etiology

I. SOCIOLOGICAL FACTORS:

According to Emile Durkheim, suicides can be classified into sub-types: altruistic, egoistic and anomic. Excessive integration into a group makes one susceptible to suicide as is seen in case of soldiers sacrificing their lives in battlefields, and is termed as altruistic suicide. On the other hand, egoistic suicide refers to those who are not strongly integrated into any social group, explaining the vulnerability of unmarried people. Anomic suicide is applicable where integration of individual into society is disturbed as in case of drastic change in economic situation or social instability; e.g., farmers' suicide. Instances where rules and regulations excessively regulate an individual and increase in social integration increases chances of suicide is termed as Fatalistic suicide (e.g. prison communities, slaves, cults etc.).

II. PSYCHOLOGICAL FACTORS

There are numerous theories proposed, ranging from aggression turned inwards to 'inverted homicide' or anger toward another person turned inward—but today with the advent of biological research, these theories have limited evidence.

III. BIOLOGICAL FACTORS

a. Neurotransmitter:

- Low concentrations of the serotonin metabolite 5-hydroxyindoleacetic acid (5-HIAA) in the cerebrospinal fluid (CSF) is found to be associated with suicidal behavior.
- Postmortem neurochemical studies have revealed decreases in serotonin or 5-HIAA in frontal cortex or brainstem of suicide victims. In addition, significant changes in presynaptic and postsynaptic serotonin binding sites is also noted.
- Decreased noradrenalin (NA) levels in brainstem and increased alpha2-adrenergic receptor densities

b. Genetic factors:

- In psychiatric patients, history of suicide in family increases the risk of attempted suicide and also of completed suicide.

- Monozygotic twins have a higher concordance rate for completed and attempted suicide than dizygotic twins as shown by twin studies.
- The genetics of suicide and self-harm behavior appears to be determined by two components: the heritability of psychiatric disorders, and of impulsive aggression or other personality traits.
- Short form of the 5-HTT gene might be associated with impulsive aggression and suicidal behavior.

Evaluation of Suicide Risk

It is very important that each medical student and practitioner be equipped to assess a patient with a potential for suicide.

Management of suicide is largely based on risk assessment and prevention on future suicide, and therefore requires comprehensive evaluation. Objectives of such assessments are:

1. Identification of the factors and features that are likely to enhance or attenuate the suicide risk or self harm behavior and which might be targeted for modification in both acute and long term interventions
2. To determine the appropriate treatment setting for the individual so as to ensure safety and prevent any further harm
3. Formulation of diagnosis (or differential diagnosis) over the multiaxial system, so as to develop management plan.

Table 41.1 presents important domains of a suicide assessment.

Irrespective of the patient expressing the same, it is always advisable to ask directly if the patient has ever had suicidal thoughts or attempted the same. Contrary to popular belief that this might seed a thought, it actually serves to help identify cases better.

Table 41.1: Evaluation of patients presenting with suicidal behavior

Current presentation (self-harm/suicidal behavior)
a. The circumstances and timing of the event
b. Method chosen for the suicide (availability and lethality of the method chosen)
c. Degree of intent
d. Presence of helplessness, hopelessness, worthlessness
e. Indicators of impulsivity
f. Patient's perception of death (including cultural/religious beliefs about death or suicide)
g. Feeling and reaction following the event
h. Reasons for dying/ reasons for living and plans for the future
i. Evidence of any current substance use
History
a. History of previous self harm behavior or suicide attempts
b. Evidence of an escalation in potential lethality of self-harm or suicidal behaviors
c. History suggestive of any psychiatric disorder (including personality disorders and substance use disorders)
d. Past history of psychiatric disorders and treatment received
e. Personality traits
Other relevant details
a. Previous or current medical diagnoses and treatments (especially enquiring about any chronic or debilitating illnesses)
b. Family history of suicide or suicide attempts, or of mental illness

(Continued...)

Psychosocial considerations

a. Presence of acute crises/stressful life situation
b. Presence of ongoing psychosocial stressors (including interpersonal issues or losses, recent separation, financial crisis, sudden change in socioeconomic status, history of abuse)
c. Employment status
d. Family support
e. Social relation and bonding
f. Coping skills
g. Past responses to stress

Management Approach

- Beginning with the initial encounter with the patient, attempt to build trust, establish mutual respect, and develop a therapeutic relationship with the patient.
- Attend to patient's safety and work to minimize self-endangering behaviors
- Identify appropriate setting (in-patient or out-patient) for the management, based on the risk assessment (**Fig. 41.1**).
- Develop a plan for treatment
- Treatment of any existing primary psychiatric illness or symptoms (like anxiety, agitation, insomnia). ECT is the treatment of choice for patients with major depression or psychotic disorders with suicidal risk.
- Plan for addressing personality disorders
- Addressing substance use disorder, in particular, given its high rates of among individuals with suicidal behaviors.

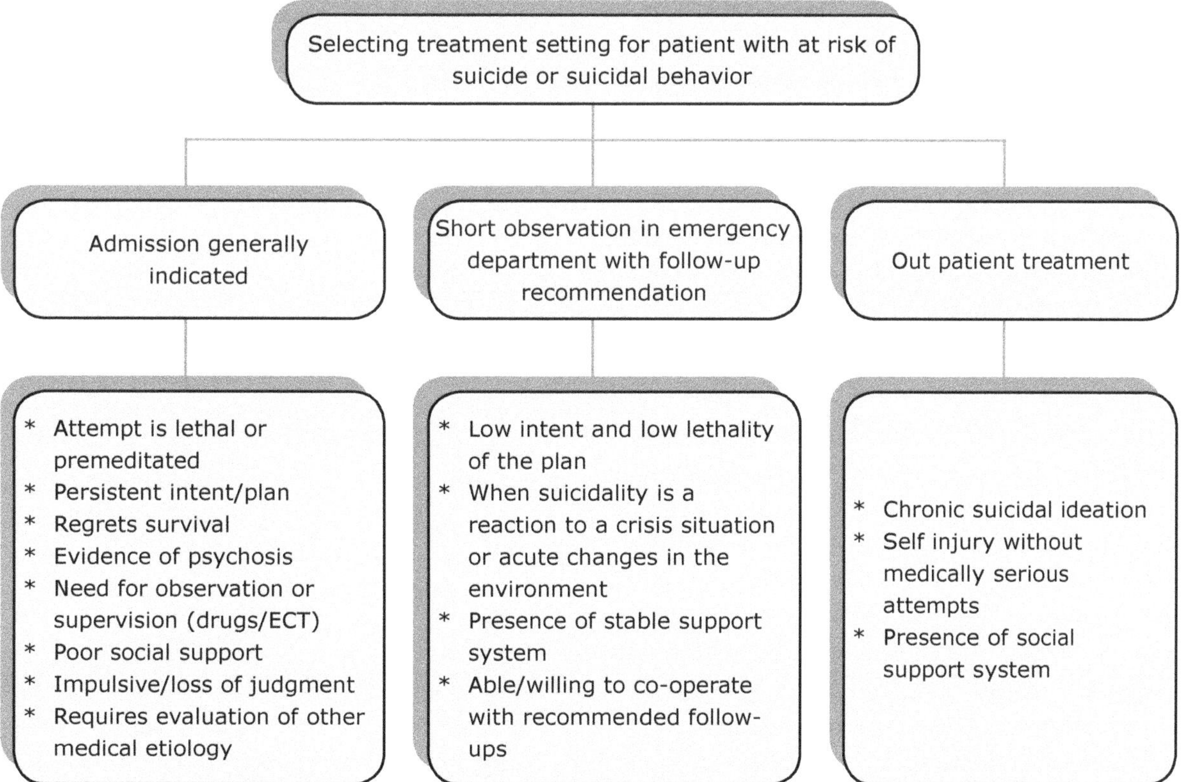

Fig. 41.1: Guidelines for Selecting a Treatment Setting for Patients at Risk for Suicide or Suicidal Behaviors.

- Medical disorders and their treatment
- Addressing psychological problems and stressors; enhance coping skills of individual
- Supportive psychotherapy may alleviate some of a patient's intense suffering
- Augment social support networks
- Optimal management requires multidisciplinary approach, which involves several mental health professionals (including psychiatrist, psychologist, psychiatric social worker, nurses) and primary care physicians, if patient is under treatment for other medical ailments.
- Promote adherence to treatment plan
- Providing education to family and patient about symptoms, disorders being treated, about the therapeutic approaches, how to identify early symptoms, such as insomnia, hopelessness, anxiety, or depression, that may herald a worsening of the patient's clinical condition, anniversary reactions, etc.
- Reassessment of safety and suicide risks (e.g. those suicidal patients recovering from depressive illness)

Legal Factors

According to the Section 309 of Indian Penal Code (IPC), suicide attempt was considered as an offence. However, the recent Mental Health Care Act, 2017 states that "any person who attempts to commit suicide shall be presumed, unless proved otherwise, to have severe stress and shall not be tried and punished under the said IPC Code. Also, the government shall have a duty to provide care, treatment and rehabilitation of such a person to reduce the risk of recurrence of suicide attempts." This might lead to subsequent enhanced reporting of suicides or self-harm attempts.

Thus suicide is no longer a reportable crime, but a medical condition requiring help and intervention.

Prevention

The management of suicide primarily lies in its prevention. To address this rapidly growing multifaceted issue, systematic, multipronged collaborative prevention strategies are required which involve intervention at every level in the community. Multiple preventive approaches have been applied and assessed for their impact.

I. TARGETING COMMUNITY

1. Suicide awareness program in community: Focused programs such as short talks, or dissemination of educational material through media, leaflets and placards can be the methods of spreading awareness in the community and have shown to contribute to identification of warning signs of suicide. Sharing of patient and suicide survivor experiences is also found useful.
2. Restriction of access to means: Legislative restrictions on availability and sales of firearms, access to pesticides and substituting lethal pesticides with less lethal compounds; constructing physical barriers at jumping hotspots; and using drugs which are safer in overdose in at risk individuals are some of the means to restrict access to means of self harm.
3. Media strategies for suicide prevention: Media influences perception and attitude of public, and therefore responsible reporting of suicide represents a population-level strategy for suicide prevention.

The Press Council of India has adopted guidelines (release dated September 13, 2019) on reporting on suicides, based on the WHO guidelines. In addition, Indian Psychiatric Society has provided suggestions for positive reporting. These guidelines would decrease the number of 'copycat suicides' and improve awareness about the issue in society.

Suicide and Social Media

- There has been increase in number of pro-suicide websites recently. These websites typically describe suicide methods (e.g., provide details of doses of medication that would be fatal in overdose) and provide social media forums for suicidal individuals. Sometimes these even normalize suicide or implicitly or explicitly encourage suicide pacts.
- There was a significant increase in adolescent suicides in U.S. after the recent Netflix series, '13 Reasons Why' which gives the narrative of a teenage girl who committed suicide in a great detail.
- Parental monitoring of the content that their children are viewing on various media sources is deemed necessary.

Targeting at-Risk Individuals

1. Suicide awareness program for medical and nursing professionals: Educating the primary care and emergency physicians in recognizing and responding to psychological distress and suicidal thoughts leads to early detection and thereby treatment of underlying psychiatric illness, if present. The Emergency Department assessment should incorporate assessment of suicide behavior and risk estimation.
2. Gatekeeper training: Gatekeeper implies to individuals who are engaged at places where they frequently interact with persons who can be potentially suicidal and could probably recognize the behavioral clues indicating elevated suicide risk. Potential gatekeepers would include teachers, peers, school support staff, colleagues, counselors at school or at workplace and employers. Gatekeepers would help in identifying the at-risk population from the community and making timely intervention. For student population, they can be trained to identify the risk factors, warning signs, support system available, and signs of depression, and can be imparted basic counseling skills to address at-risk population.
3. Suicide helplines: Suicide prevention helplines "provide phone-based services for individuals who are at risk of suicide or concerned about someone at risk of suicide." Some of the helplines in India are Sumaitri, Sanjeevni, Roshni and COOJ Mental Health Foundation, but their number is not adequate to cater the needs. The helplines generally have trained mental health professionals, who handle the acute suicidal crisis and make required referrals. The responder in helpline when having attitude of empathy, support, respect, and collaborative problem-solving has shown better outcomes.

II. TARGETING INDICATED POPULATION

1. Treatment of mental illness: In case of mentally ill patients, lithium, clozapine, olanzapine, antidepressants, and behavioral interventions such as dialectical behavior therapy have shown to have anti-suicidal effects.
2. Follow-up care: The risk of suicide in the period subsequent to discharge is quite high. Such patients can be provided various support and follow-up measures such as caring letters, postcards, frequent

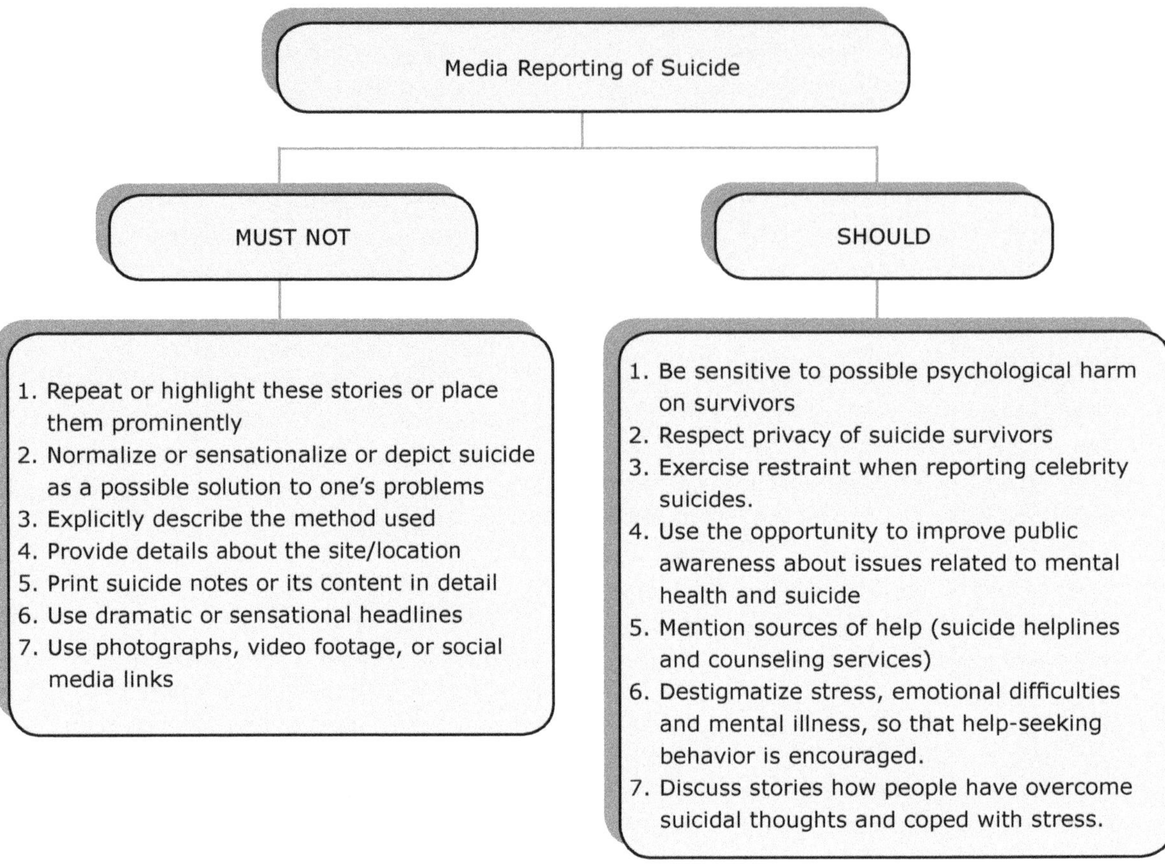

Fig. 41.2: Summary of recommendations for media reporting of suicide.

phone calls, text messaging, brief and regular sessions of supportive counseling, follow-up by mental health worker, and outreach programs.

NON-SUICIDAL SELF-INJURY

Non-Suicidal Self-Injury (NSSI) involves deliberate injury to one's body tissue without suicidal intent and for purposes not socially sanctioned. It is included in DSM-5 under 'Conditions for further study'. Proposed criteria for NSSI are listed in **Table 41.2**.

Clinical Features

NSSI most often starts in early teens and continues for many years. Prevalence of NSSI in adolescents is around 6.7%, in clinical populations ranges from 12% to more than 80% in psychiatric patients.

Hospitalization for NSSI reaches a peak at 20-29 years of age and then declines. This behavior is often learnt by observing or on recommendation of others.

Prevalence of NSSI is nearly similar in both genders. The essential feature of NSSI is repeated infliction of shallow yet painful injuries to the body surface, mostly for the purpose of reducing negative emotions or resolving interpersonal difficulties. The individual perceives an immediate sense of

Table 41.2: Proposed criteria for NSSI in DSM-5

A.	In the last year, the individual has, on 5 or more days, engaged in intentional self-inflicted damage to the surface of his or her body of a sort likely to induce bleeding, bruising, or pain (e.g., cutting, burning, stabbing, hitting, excessive rubbing), with the expectation that the injury will lead to only minor or moderate physical harm (i.e., there is no suicidal intent)
B.	The individual engages in the self-injurious behavior with one or more of the following expectations: 1. To obtain relief from a negative feeling or cognitive state 2. To resolve an interpersonal difficulty 3. To induce a positive feeling state
C.	The intentional self-injury is associated with at least one of the following: 1. Interpersonal difficulties or negative feelings or thoughts, such as depression, anxiety, tension, anger, generalized distress, or self-criticism, occurring in the period immediately prior to the self-injurious act 2. Prior to engaging in the act, a period of preoccupation with the intended behavior that is difficult to control 3. Thinking about self-injury that occurs frequently, even when it is not acted upon
D.	The behavior is not socially sanctioned (e.g., body piercing, tattooing, part of a religious or cultural ritual) and is not restricted to picking a scab or nail biting
E.	The behavior or its consequences cause: 1. Clinically significant distress 2. Interference in interpersonal functioning 3. Interference in academic functioning 4. Interference in other important areas of functioning
F.	The behavior does not occur exclusively during psychotic episodes, delirium, substance intoxication, or substance withdrawal. In individuals with a neurodevelopmental disorder, the behavior is not part of a pattern of repetitive stereotypes. The behavior is not better explained by another mental disorder or medical condition

relief with the process. Frequent such behavior can be associated with craving and urgency, resulting resemblance with addiction. Injury is commonly inflicted by a sharp object (knife, needle, razor) on front of thigh and forearms and is usually a series of superficial parallel cuts; or stabbing on the forearm. It might lead to blood borne disease transmission in certain cases. Other Common forms of NSSI include cutting, skin carving, biting, scratching, hitting, head banging, and interfering with wound healing. Males often use the methods of burning and self-hitting, while scratching and cutting are more common in females. Majority of individuals engaging in NSSI generally do not seek medical help.

Risk Factors

Adolescence is a vulnerable stage of development and NSSI is commonly found in this group. Severe childhood adversities like maltreatment (emotional/ physical/ sexual abuse or neglect) and mental health issues or substance use in parents are other identified risk factors. In addition, impulsivity in an individual may predispose to NSSI, as such individuals may act rashly at the time of distress and may be motivated to achieve immediate benefit of NSSI (e.g. managing affective dysregulation) rather than engaging in problem solving behaviors.

Etiology

I. Psychological theories

1. Affect regulation:
    a. NSSI helps to relieve intense distressing feelings such as sadness, guilt, flashbacks, or depersonalization
    b. To stop feeling numb or empty or an undesired emotional state
    c. To feel something, even if it is pain
    d. Distraction from the unwanted feelings through intense pain
2. Release of endogenous opiates through tissue damage in NSSI causes euphoria
3. A form of self-punishment
4. Interpersonal function: NSSI may serve a means to convey one's distress to others

II. Biological factors

1. Genetics: Genes involved in serotonergic neurotransmission, like 5-HTTLPR or TPH are implicated in deliberate self-harm. However, results are inconsistent.
2. Altered physiological reactivity: When imagining an act of NSSI, a decrease of physiological tension has been frequently reported.
3. Functional neuroimaging: Hyperactivation of limbic structures like amygdala and anterior cingulate cortex is seen in patients with deliberate self harm but are not specific to NSSI.
4. Neurotransmitters:
    a. Serotonin: Serotonin deficiency is proposed to be related to self harming behavior
    b. Cortisol: The HPA-axis interacts with endogenous opioids and serotonergic mechanisms. Adolescents who engage in NSSI have showed hyporesponsive HPA-axis, which in the event of stressful situations, compared to healthy controls.
    c. Endogenous opiate: Lower levels of endogenous opioids were found in individuals with NSSI repeatedly, which in the event of stressful situation gets restored by inflicting NSSI. Low opiod levels could also possibly explain an "addictive quality" of these behaviors.

Differential Diagnosis

NSSI has been long been regarded as a symptom of Borderline Personality Disorder. Although frequently associated, the latter is not invariably found in individuals with NSSI. Instead, most patients with NSSI meet criteria for other disorders like eating disorder or substance use disorder. The differential also includes 'Suicidal Behavior Disorder', wherein behavior is secondary to a wish to die, and not to experience relief or resolve conflicts.

Assessment and Management of NSSI

An overview of management of NSSI is given in **Fig. 41.3**. Various treatment approaches have been studied in NSSI. Dialectical behavior therapy has some evidence in reducing the frequency of self-injury; other modalities like emotion regulation group therapy, manual-assisted cognitive therapy, and dynamic deconstructive psychotherapy have also been studied. Atypical antipsychotics (aripiprazole), naltrexone, and selective serotonin reuptake inhibitors have also shown some benefits.

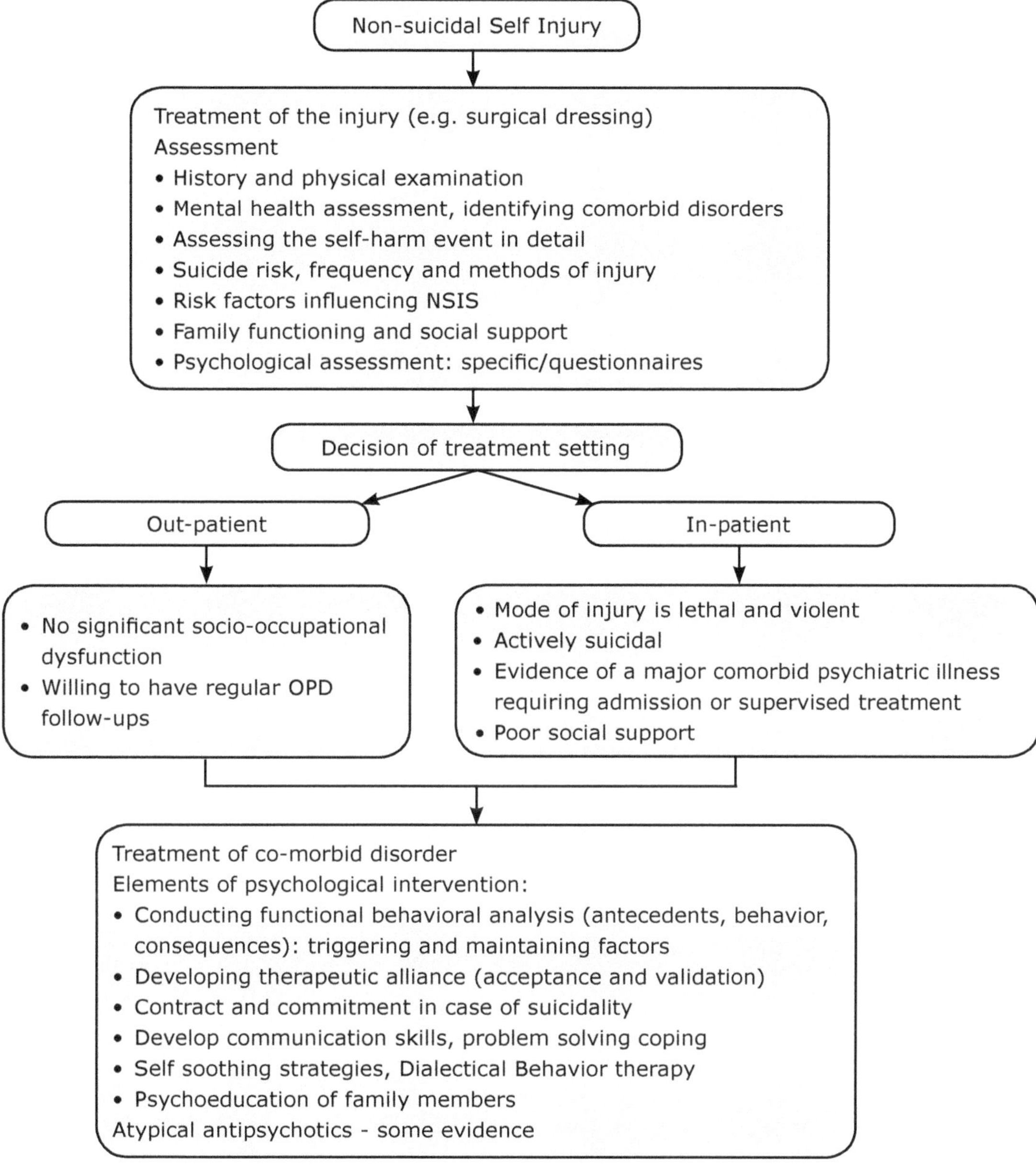

Fig. 41.3: Overview of assessment, selection of treatment setting and management of NSSI.

Suicide as an independent medical entity (with or without other psychiatric co-morbidity) is important to identify and intervene, for every astute clinician. There is now strong evidence to correlate at risk individuals for suicide, and identify high-risk behaviors in individuals prone to self-harm. Early identification can lead to accurate intervention, and prevention of loss of precious lives, to a large extent.

BIBLIOGRAPHY

1. Jacobs D, Brewer M. APA practice guideline provides recommendations for assessing and treating patients with suicidal behaviors.

Psychiatric Annals. 2004 May 1;34(5):373-80.
2. Cowen P, Harrison P, Burns T. Shorter Oxford textbook of psychiatry. Oxford University Press; 2012 Aug 9.
3. Sadock, B. J., & Sadock, V. A. (2007). Kaplan & Sadock's synopsis of psychiatry: Behavioral sciences/clinical psychiatry (10th ed.). Lippincott Williams & Wilkins Publishers.
4. Vijayakumar L. Media Matters in suicide–Indian guidelines on suicide reporting. Indian Journal of Psychiatry. 2019 Nov 1;61(6):549.
5. Accidental deaths and suicides in India. National Crime Records Bureau. Ministry of Home Affairs. Government of India. 2020.
6. American Psychiatric Association. Diagnostic and statistical manual of mental disorders (DSM-5®). American Psychiatric Pub; 2013 May 22.
7. Menon V, Subramanian K, Selvakumar N, Kattimani S. Suicide prevention strategies: An overview of current evidence and best practice elements. International Journal of Advanced Medical and Health Research. 2018 Jul 1;5(2):43.
8. National suicide prevention strategies: progress, examples and indicators. Geneva: World Health Organization; 2018. Licence: CC BY-NC-SA 3.0 IGO.
9. http://presscouncil.nic.in/WriteReadData/Pdf/PRtennineteentwenty.pdf

Psychiatric Emergencies 42

Harshal Sathe

INTRODUCTION

Psychiatric emergency is defined as an *acute disturbance of behavior, thought or mood of a patient which if untreated may lead to harm either to the individual or to others in the environment*. It has been observed that about a third of the cases visiting the emergency department has psychiatric symptoms. The developed countries have abundant financial as well as human resources for this subspecialty in psychiatry. However the services in developing countries such as India are inadequate for the needs of growing population of mentally ill people.

CLASSIFICATION OF PSYCHIATRIC EMERGENCIES

The psychiatric emergencies are classified into major emergencies, minor emergencies and medical emergencies in relation to psychiatric disorder or its treatment. The major conditions subsumed under these categories have been illustrated in **Table 41.1**. This chapter shall discuss the psychopathology and management of each of these conditions in emergency settings.

EPIDEMIOLOGY OF PSYCHIATRIC EMERGENCIES

Quantification of behavioral emergencies is the need of an hour given the size and catastrophic nature of the problem. However there are very few Indian studies which have assessed the epidemiological characteristics of psychiatric emergencies. According to the available information most of the patients referred to psychiatric emergency department belong to the age group of 17-25 years followed by those who are 26-40 years old. Males outnumber females by the ratio of 1.6:1 in the psychiatric

Table 41.1: Courtesy Sudarshan et al.

Major emergencies	Minor emergencies	Medical conditions with psychiatric symptoms
Suicidal behavior	Grief reaction	Delirium
Aggression and violent behavior	Trauma and stress related disorders	Neuroleptic malignant syndrome
	Panic attack	Serotonin syndrome
		Medication or psychoactive drug overdose

(Readers must take a note that discussion on Neuroleptic malignant syndrome, Serotonin syndrome, and medication or psychoactive drug overdose is beyond the scope of this chapter and that these topics shall be discussed in other relevant sections of the book)

emergency visits. Low socio-economic status, belonging to the rural background and backward caste were other demographic factors which significantly correlated with presentation of the patient in psychiatric emergency department.

Suicidal attempts, acute psychotic agitation, aggressive and violent behavior, substance intoxication and withdrawal, psychosomatic illnesses, neurological illnesses with behavioral alteration such as epilepsy, panic attacks, acute stress reactions and postpartum psychosis were among the most common psychiatric causes for patients to present at the emergency department. However a large group of patients visiting the emergency psychiatry department have psychological distress due to social problems which require supportive psychotherapy and problem solving.

SUICIDE AND PARASUICIDAL BEHAVIOR

The word suicide is derived from Latin word for self-murder. Suicide is defined as a *form of death in which a person ends his or her life intentionally and because of some specified or unspecified purpose*. Attempt to commit suicide is most common and severe among the psychiatric emergencies. Over 2 lakh people in India commit suicide every year. Although suicide is common in older people the number of young adults taking their lives is on a rise in the recent years.

4.1 Risk Factors for suicide

Gender: Although females are more likely to attempt suicide, completed suicides are more frequent in males. Men tend to use more lethal methods to commit suicide such as firearms and hanging whereas females generally tend to take over dose of medications or chemicals.

Age

Suicide is most common in men and women after the age of 45 years. However recent trends show that the prevalence is rising in the younger people.

Marital Status

Being single or divorced makes a person three times more likely to commit suicide than being married. Isolation and lack of family are known to significantly increase the suicide risk.

Occupation

Unemployed people commit suicide more often than the employed people. However some professionals such as doctors, lawyers, insurance agents are at the particular risk of suicide. Increasing professional stress, lack of future plans, feeling of isolation at workplace, low self-esteem are the factors associated with suicidality.

Physical Health Problems

Loss of mobility, disfigurement or chronic intractable pain which often accompany physical illnesses often prompt the person to end his or her life.

Mental Health Problems

95 percent of the people committing suicide suffer from severe form of mental illnesses such as depression (80%) and Schizophrenia (10%). The psychiatric patients are 3-12 times at a higher risk of suicide as compared to people who do not have a mental illness.

Etiology

The etiology of suicide has been subdivided into biological, psychological and sociological theories.

Biological Theories

Reduced Serotonin Levels

Reductions in the levels of serotonin or its metabolite 5-Hydroxyindole acetic acid (HIAA) in brainstem or prefrontal cortex have been found in various postmortem studies of the patients committing suicide. These studies also report significant changes in serotonin binding sites of presynaptic and postsynaptic receptors. Low concentrations of 5-HIAA in CSF has been shown to predict suicidal behavior.

Genetic Studies

In the molecular genetic studies, the Human Tryptophan Hydroxylase (TPH) gene polymorphisms have been linked with reduced serotonin levels in the brain. TPH is the rate limiting enzyme in the synthesis of serotonin.

Twin studies and adoption studies demonstrate heritability in attempted and as well as completed suicides. Hemingway family is a great example in this regard where members in more than four generations have consistently committed suicide.

Psychological Theories

Sigmund Freud believed that suicide happened because of anger turned inwards, towards an introjected cathected love object. *Karl Meninger* in his book Man against himself extended the Freudian belief and called suicide as a retroflexed murder or an inverted homicide. He put forth three components of hostility in suicide viz. wish to kill, the wish to be killed, and the wish to die. *Aaron Beck* in his work found hopelessness to be most closely related to suicidal behavior among all the thought patterns of depression. Nevertheless this is not the only factor. Affective excesses such as rage and guilt, identification with a suicide victim, or acting out on the suicidal fantasies are among the other psychological factors underlying suicide. Group dynamics have been theorized to underlie the mass suicides as has been seen in history.

Sociological Theories

Emil Durkheim at the end of 19th century theorized suicidal behavior on the difficulty in social integration of a person. Based on the pattern of social integration Durkheim suggested three types of suicides as follows:

1. Egoistic suicides: In this type there is lack of adequate social integration of an individual. The individual lacks social support and has intense feeling of loneliness. It explains why an unmarried person is more likely than a married person to commit suicide which is because of the lack of integration with the family.
2. Altruistic suicides: Here there is excessive integration of an individual with the society because of which social welfare occupies primacy over one's own life. Such individuals commit suicide for a social purpose. Self-immolation by monks for world peace is an example of altruistic suicide.
3. Anomic suicides: Disturbed social integration lies at the base of Anomie according to Durkheim. Anomie explains why sudden social or economic change makes a previously stable individual vulnerable for suicide.

Assessment of Suicidal Patient

While assessing a suicidal patient a detailed history along with a reliable informant is extremely important. The following factors should be included in the assessment of such a patient (as shown in Table 42.3)

Table 42.2: Assessment of suicidal patient

Areas of assessment of a suicidal patient
1. Socio-demographic data
a. Age
b. Gender (Risk increased in males)
c. Occupation (unemployment or work related stress)
d. Marital status (Single, divorced people are at increased risk)
2. Current problems
a. Significant loss (financial crisis, death of loved one, separation)
b. Acute or chronic health problems
c. Relationship instability
d. Mental illness such as depression, schizophrenia, bipolar mood disorder, etc.
e. Presence of Hopelessness
f. Personality disorders (risk is high in Borderline personality disorder)
3. Nature of suicidal thinking
a. Current ideation frequency, intensity and duration
b. Availability of means
c. Lethality of means
d. Preparatory behaviors such as suicide note
e. Active suicidal behaviors
4. Previous suicidal behaviors
5. Protective factors such as social support, problem solving skills, reality testing, etc.

Some psychometric tests such as Beck's Suicide Intent Scale proves to be worthwhile in measurement of suicidal behavior. SAD PERSONS scale developed by Peterson is a popular bedside instrument to assess the suicidal risk in a person.

Table 42.3: Sad persons scale for assessment of suicidal risk

Risk factors	High risk in	Score for high risk
S - Sex	Male	1
A - Age	<20 years, >45 years	1
D - Depression	Present	2
P - Psychiatric illness	Present	1
E - Excess drug use	Present	1
R - Rationality loss	Present	2
S - Separated	Yes	1
O - Organised plan	Plan for suicide present	2
N - No support	No social support	1
S - Sickness	Chronic illness	1

Scoring

0-4 indicates low risk, 5-6 medium risk and 7-10 high risk for committing suicide.

Management of Suicidal Patient

The management should begin with a thorough assessment of history and mental state of the patient as has been mentioned above. The patients who are actively suicidal, lack social support, have access to lethal means of killing themselves and have ongoing stressors in their life can be considered for temporary hospitalization till the suicidal ideation wanes off. Not all patients with suicidal ideation need to be admitted. However the patient should reach an agreement with the treating psychiatrist over notifying about suicidal thoughts coming to the mind so that the necessary timely action can be taken.

Pharmacological management

Patients who get diagnosed with psychiatric illnesses such as depression, schizophrenia or bipolar mood disorder according to the standard classification systems like ICD-10 or DSM-5 should be begun with corresponding medications to reduce the severity of illness. Selective serotonin reuptake inhibitors are used to treat depression and antipsychotic medications are used to treat schizophrenia and bipolar mood disorder to immediately control aggression, impulsivity and irritability. Lithium is a drug which has been shown to single handedly reduce suicidal ideation and should always be prescribed to acutely suicidal patients who are able to tolerate it.

Electroconvulsive Therapy

The depressed patients who are actively suicidal are found to benefit by electro-convulsive therapy (ECT). ECT is considered as a first line treatment in patients with severe depression who are suicidal as it is known to rapidly reverse the suicidal ideation.

Psychotherapy

Patients who have borderline personality disorder (BPD) have a high degree of suicidal ideation and repeated suicidal attempts. Dialectical Behavior therapy given by Marsha Linehan has been found to be effective in the treatment of BPD. Cognitive behavior therapy has already been proven to be effective in the patients of depression and other psychiatric disorders as well.

Other Important Points

Para Suicide

Para suicide is defined as a behavior in which the patient harms himself without intention to die. In the current version of Diagnostic and Statistical manual parasuicide has been renamed as Non Suicidal Self Injury. It is more common in females and psychiatric patients. Cutting of the skin is by far the most common form of self-mutilation and it is usually done over the wrist, forearm, abdomen commonly but other sites may also be involved. Patients with personality disorders such as borderline personality disorder and those with substance use disorders are more likely to indulge in self injurious behavior. Dialectical behavior therapy developed by Marsha Linehan has been found to be beneficial, particularly in reducing the self harming behavior in the patient.

Prevention of Suicide

Suicide is not an act of a free will but is an out product of mental illness. Hence improvement in identification and treatment of mental illness has been theorized to reduce the rate of suicides. The US based suicide prevention resource centre advocates the following strategies to prevent the suicides.

- Identification of the person at suicide risk
- Encourage the help seeking behavior when such a need is felt
- To ensure access to specialized mental health care and suicide prevention centre
- Responding effectively to individuals in crisis on a priority basis.
- Reducing access to the means of suicide
- Enhancement of life skills and resilience
- Promotion of social connectedness and support

Application of these strategies has shown to bring about a fall in the rate of completed suicides.

AGGRESSION AND VIOLENCE

Aggression and violence are the current areas of concern in psychiatry with increasing numbers of aggressive patients visiting emergency departments. The psychiatrists who are expected to assess the agitated patient in the hospital casualty are themselves at reasonable risk of being attacked. Hence it is challenging to create protocols for the management of violent presentations in the emergency section.

Risk factors for aggression and violence

Mentally ill patients are far more likely to demonstrate aggressive and violent behavior as compared to the general population. The risk is particularly high in the patients of psychosis and substance abuse. Violent behavior is also seen in various medical conditions such as traumatic brain injury, intracranial infections or cerebrovascular accidents. Male gender, low socio economic and educational status are the demographic risk factors associated with aggression.

Etiology of Aggression

Biological Factors

Genetics

Violence is polygenic phenomenon with various genes such as COMT, TPH acting in a coordinated fashion to produce the aggressive phenotype. Twin studies and adoption studies confirm the influence of heredity as well as the rearing environment in the development of aggressive behavior.

Neurotransmitters

The aggressive patients have been known to have lower levels of 5 hydroxy indole acetic acid levels in cerebrospinal fluid and higher dopamine secretion in the mesolimbic dopamine pathways in the brain. Similarly the disturbance in norepinephrine and Gamma aminobutyric acid levels in the brain are also known to contribute to this behavior.

Structural Changes

Various neuroimaging studies have demonstrated the role of prefrontal cortex and medial temporal lobe structures such as amygdala, hippocampus and basal ganglia in the regulation of various brain functions which get disturbed in aggression.

Psychosocial Factors

The psychodynamic theory incriminates the blockade of libidinal impulses and projection of self destructive instinct to the external object in the development of aggression.

The cognitive behavior therapy holds the cognitive distortions and dysfunctional assumptions in the interpersonal area at the root of violence.

When an individual views the violence and its positive reinforcement in the community he learns to behave in a violent fashion as per the social learning theory.

Assessment of an Aggressive Patient

The detailed assessment of an aggressive patient must include following points:

- Demographic factors such as age, gender and socioeconomic and educational status.
- A detailed history of the events surrounding the development of aggressive behavior which will also include overt stressors such as loss of a loved one or interpersonal conflict.
- Assess the thoughts, wishes and availability of means in relation to violent outbursts.
- Past and family history of aggressive behavior.

Managing the Aggressive Patient

Environmental Safety

The environmental modifications to control aggression include therapist factors such as friendly attitude, an expression of concern and soothing tone of voice. Removal of lethal weapons or articles, padded rooms, appropriate seclusion is the environmental factors which help to control aggression. It's important to avoid overcrowding and noisy surroundings during the management of aggression.

Restraint

Restraint is defined as "*the brief physical holding of an aggressive or agitated patient to effectively gain quick control of and minimize harm to the patient or others.*" Restraint involves the use of a physical intervention. The use of restraint in Indian setting is expected to be guided by the policy of coercion in mental healthcare act 2017. The section 97 of this act advice record keeping and monthly reporting to the review board of the restraint practices conducted in the mental health establishment.

The main indications of restraint are

1. To assume immediate control of a potentially threatening situation of angry and violent patient.
2. To limit the freedom of movement of a person, thereby preventing him from harming himself or others.

This procedure must be carried out in the mental health establishment which is equipped with appropriate tools and dedicated space to restrain along with trained staff including psychiatrists, psychologists, nursing staff and social workers. The mental healthcare act advice the formation of restrain committee in the establishment to record, supervise and report to the mental health review board on a monthly basis about the restraint procedures conducted there.

General guidelines for the use of restraints

- Ensure the safety of patient as well as the hospital staff.
- Use de-escalation techniques such as distraction or diversion of the patient prior to taking a final decision to restrain the patient.
- Restraint must be used when it's the only least restrictive alternative available to manage the patient.
- The actions taken by the restraining staff must be appropriate and proportional to patients behavior and the practice should be continued for minimum possible duration.
- Close monitoring of patient's physical condition must be carried out during the procedure.
- The procedure of restraint must be undertaken only by appropriately trained staff members.

Types of restraint procedures

There are various different types of restraint procedures as follows:

1. *Physical restraint*: This includes application of positive pressure against the resistance by staff to restrict the mobility and prevent the harmful behavior of an individual.
2. *Chemical restraint*: This involves the use of medications to control the undesirable behavior of the patient e.g. Haloperidol or lorazepam given by parenteral routes.
3. *Mechanical restraint*: It involves the use of protective devices such as leather belts, Geri chairs, Posey vests, mittens, belted

wheelchairs, sheeting, bed rails, protective helmet etc.

4. *Environmental restraint*: It deals with the building architecture and gadgetry so as to limit the freedom of movement of the patient.
5. *Psychological restraint*: This variety includes the use of psychological techniques such as instructions, suggestions about the appropriate behavior and deprivation from the resources necessary to engage in violence or leaving the premises.

Procedure of Restraint

- A thorough assessment of the patient should be done by an experienced professional and a provisional diagnosis must be made.
- Before deciding to use restraint procedures de escalation by the use of distraction or diversion should be tried.
- Prior to starting the restraint procedure a written order by psychiatrist specifying reason, type of restraint to be used, the positioning of the patient, plan of monitoring for safety, criteria for release of the restaurants and special precautions if necessary.
- Patient's clothes must be searched thoroughly for any potentially dangerous object so as to minimize the risk of injury to the staff members.
- Appropriate clothing should be provided, and no patient should be restrained in nude or semi nude state.
- It's important to inform the patient about reasons for restraint (legal guardians of patient should be called for if patient is a minor)
- Restrain using appropriate technique with intensity commensurate to the requirement.
- During the entire procedure the vitals of the patient must be monitored by a dedicated personnel.
- Patient's response to restraint must be documented and any changes or injuries must be duly noted.
- Release of the restraints must be in accordance with pre decided criteria or when the restrain ceases to be the least restrictive alternative.
- Debriefing the patient once he has been stabilized helps in prevention of further episodes of violence and aggression.
- Staff review of restraint practices helps in continuous improvement in service provision.

Psychotherapy

It is important that the therapist has necessary training and is able to maintain a safe environment while dealing with a violent patient. Development of therapeutic alliance and effective handling of negative countertransference reactions form the cornerstone of effective psychotherapeutic management of violence. The skill of self monitoring is indispensable for the therapist working in this area.

Various psychotherapeutic techniques can be used for control of violence and aggression. The behavioral techniques are based on contingency management principles and social skills training that shall help reinforce the desirable behavior and curb the unwanted one. The cognitive behavioral technic disputes the dysfunctional assumptions which underlie the escalation of anger and emotional distress which has contributed to violence. In group therapy, simulations of real world situations promote the patient to learn adaptive ways of responding to provocative situations.

Pharmacotherapy of Aggressive Behavior

Before considering administration of medications to manage aggressive behavior it is extremely important to do a detailed assessment so as to rule out any underlying medical conditions which may be responsible for the aggressive behavior. Psychiatric medications can be used only after ascertaining pure psychiatric origins of aggression. Antipsychotics are the most common drugs used for alleviation of aggressive symptoms. Although oral route is the first choice for giving the medicines in many cases use of parenteral route becomes necessary. 10 milligram of haloperidol is injected intramuscularly in the gluteal region and the dose is repeated after every 30 minutes till maximum of 60 milligrams. Parenteral administration of benzodiazepines such as lorazepam has shown to have comparable results to the use of haloperidol. If the aggression is secondary to manic symptoms or is happening in the absence of psychotic symptoms then mood stabilizers such as lithium and valproate may be helpful. Beta blockers such as propranolol have also been found to be useful in the management of aggression in a wide range of neuropsychiatric conditions.

TRAUMA RELATED STRESS DISORDERS

India, in the past few decades, has witnessed a large number of natural and man made disasters such as earthquakes, hurricanes, terrorist attacks etc. A large number of sufferers in these disasters experience emotional disturbances as well as behavioral alterations which are classified under the chapter for trauma related stress disorders in the fifth version of diagnostic and statistical manual. Acute stress reactions and post traumatic stress disorder are the two most common conditions found in this category. About 10 to 15 percent of people exposed to traumatic events are known to develop these conditions. Post traumatic stress is seen equally in both genders. The symptoms of acute stress reaction include two classes of symptoms as follows: 1. negative symptoms such as sadness, listlessness, anxiety and avoidance 2. The arousal symptoms such as flashbacks, nightmares, visual imagery. High intensity of perceived emotional pain, severe anxiety and panic states and suicidal ideation in these patients necessitate their inclusion in the current discussion.

The emergency management of acute stress reaction involves immediate removal of traumatic stimulus, reassurance and fulfilment of physical needs such as food and water. Pharmacological treatment options include the use of hypnotics such as benzodiazepines to control arousal symptoms and serotonergic medications (SSRIs) to heal the negative symptoms. Psychotherapeutic interventions of choice in trauma related disorders include trauma focussed cognitive behavior therapy (TF-CBT), biofeedback and mindfulness based treatment programs.

Sexual Assault

Patients with a history of sexual assault usually visit the emergency department in immediate post assault period. The doctor attending such a case requires sensitivity, compassion, communication skills and legal know how to manage these patients. In India more than 25000 rape cases are reported every year and it is estimated that this is not the true representation of the size of the problem as many cases go unreported.

Psychiatric Management of Sexual Assault Victims

Concurrent management of medical as well as psychiatric complications while maintaining the medico-legal requirements is needed in the case of sexual assault. It is important to screen all patients for medical problems through appropriate referral to concerned specialities before starting the psychological assessment. It is the best practice to place the patient in a safe and comfortable environment with a trusted relative. As per the policy adopted in ONE STOP CENTRE the patient stationed at one place is assessed by all the specialists at the same station so as to minimise the inconvenience and further aggravation of traumatic experience.

Clinical features

Sexual assault is a violation of most fiercely protected and private aspect of oneself. Most assault victims present with classic triad of signs such as intrusive recollections, increased arousal and numbing which is most often seen in post traumatic stress disorder. The sexual assault victim often passes through the emotional phases just like the sufferer of other life threatening traumatic conditions. These phases have been described in the following **Table 42.4**.

The victims of sexual assault are likely to develop mental illnesses such as anxiety and panic attacks, phobic avoidance of objects and situations which remind the patient of the assault, depression, sexual dysfunction, etc. Socio-occupational as well as psychological functioning of the patient is disturbed. Psychological recovery often takes longer than the socio-occupational adjustment. Characteristics of the sexual assault, personal characteristics of the patient and level of social support are the main factors which determine

Table 42.4: Emotional Phases in sexual assault

Phase	General description	Feelings experienced
Anticipatory phase	This phase begins prior to the assault when the threat is imminent. Victim tries to avoid the assault or plans coping strategies in unavoidable circumstances	Self blame and guilt gets developed
Impact phase	This phase lasts from actual assault for several days to weeks. Victim chooses to fight or surrender to the assailant depending on the situation	Patient experiences mental shock and fear of another attack. There is hyper vigilance, hyper alertness and disturbance in sleep.
Recoil phase	In this phase the victim tries to recover from the mental trauma and experiences intense emotions due to painful memories.	Victim experiences anger towards the incident, assailant or in general towards society
Resolution phase	The final phase in which the assault experience takes form of meaningful past which is expressed without emotional disturbance. It may take 6-24 months to develop.	Patient experiences relative calmness. The emotional disturbance gets limited to remembrance of the incident and the functioning in other spheres of life remains unaffected.

the severity of the post traumatic stress response in the patient.

Management of the victim of sexual assault

It is noteworthy that the person evaluating the victim is vigilant about his or her assumptions about the patient's needs. Non judgmental attitude, empathy are the desirable qualities in the medical staff handling the case of sexual assault. A female presenting with recent history of sexual assault shall require crisis intervention as a part of psychotherapeutic management. Crisis intervention in the sexual assault victim has been illustrated in the following table:

Table 42.5: Steps in Crisis Intervention

Crisis intervention steps
• The therapist should himself be calm and he must help victim to calm down • Ensure the safety of the victim • Ask whether any accommodation is required by the victim • Address the medical concerns of the victim • Address any other specific concerns • Discuss the option of legal reporting

The psychotherapeutic technique of choice depends on the presentation and psychopathology of the patient. Cognitive behavior therapy is helpful in cases of depression and anxiety whereas systematic desensitization shall be more helpful in the cases having features of post traumatic stress disorder. Group psychotherapy serves psychoeducational purpose as well as help the patient to get social support.

ANXIETY AND PANIC STATES

Experience of autonomic symptoms of anxiety such as sweating, palpitations, chest pains, sense of choking is often associated with catastrophic fear of death or insanity. According to the cognitive behavioral theory, in the panic attacks catastrophization is the underlying cognitive distortion. This catastrophic fear eventually drives the patient to the emergency room. The assessment of the patient with panic attacks start with the complete clinical evaluation and investigations to rule out medical comorbidities with similar presentation. Once the organic pathology is ruled out, the patient can be started on the antianxiety medications such as benzodiazepines, SSRIs etc. Cognitive behavior therapy has also been found to be useful in the treatment of panic states.

POSTPARTUM DEPRESSION OR PSYCHOSIS

The onset of depression or psychosis within 4 weeks of delivery in a mother often carries impending risk of poor self care and possible self harm or harm to the child. Lack of awareness about this condition leads to under recognition and inadequate treatment on an emergency basis. The prevalence of postpartum psychiatric disorders is estimated to be 19 to 22% in the females immediately after delivery. The acute nature of symptoms and potential harm posed to the infant and the patient herself make the emergency intervention necessary in the case of postpartum psychosis. Pharmacotherapy is the mainstay of management of postpartum psychosis. The treatment involves atypical antipsychotics and mood stabilizers. Supportive psychotherapy is the psychotherapeutic intervention that has been found to be effective.

DELIRIUM

Delirium is an acute and transient disturbance in mental functioning that is usually caused by organic dysfunction in the brain. The diagnostic and statistical manual criteria of delirium include acute onset and disturbance in attention and additional disturbance in other cognitive functions. The cause of delirium is either an organic illness or substance use. Incidence rate of delirium in the medical inpatient settings is between 5-10 percent. Psychiatric assessment is often summoned for whenever the case of delirium presents in casualty due to altered speech and behavior of the patient.

Management of Delirium

Management of delirium starts with finding the exact cause of the delirium and correction of the same. The patient is admitted to medical emergency unit and is provided supportive care along with the monitoring of vital signs and maintenance of fluid balance.

It must be noted that FDA has not approved any medication for the pharmacological management of delirium. The first as well as the second generation antipsychotics are most commonly used to manage delirious behavior of the patients. Studies show that drugs belonging to both these classes are equally efficacious and similarly tolerated in the delirious patients. Although recommended by the society of critical care medicine in 2002, there is still dearth of reliable literature proving the effectiveness of these medications in the treatment of delirium. Apart from antipsychotics, alpha-2 antagonist such as dexmedetomidine has been found to corrective as well as preventive role in delirium management in critically ill patients admitted to intensive care unit. Substitution strategies such as use of benzodiazepines in case of alcohol withdrawal delirium have been found to be effective in delirium secondary to the substance withdrawal.

INDIAN SCENARIO ON THE EMERGENCY PSYCHIATRY CARE

In India the emergency psychiatric services are inadequate to serve the needs of a growing number of mentally ill patients. The emergency psychiatry services include allocation of a separate space to handle psychiatric emergencies, ambulance services to transport uncooperative patient to the mental health facility and trained man power. Only a few regional centers in India such as karnataka state mental health authority have provided for these services with the assistance of various non government organizations (NGOs). In the rest of the country, the relatives of the mentally ill patient are responsible for his transfer to psychiatric facility which in many cases is done with the help of police. The relatives lodge a police complaint against the patient citing minor charges and then the police personnel escort the patient to the emergency department. This inhumane approach only increases the stigmatization of psychiatric problems in the community. Hence the policy makers and health care professionals should collaborate to solve this problem.

BIBLIOGRAPHY

1. Sudarsanan S, Chaudhury S, Pawar AA, Salujha SK, Srivastava K. Psychiatric Emergencies. *Med J Armed Forces India*. 2004 Jan;60(1):59-62. doi: 10.1016/S0377-1237(04)80162-X. Epub 2011 Jul 21. PMID: 27407580; PMCID: PMC4923517.
2. Saddichha S, Vibha P, Saxena MK, Methuku M. Behavioral emergencies in India: a population based epidemiological study. Social psychiatry and psychiatric epidemiology. 2010 May 1;45(5):589-93.
3. Raveesh BN, Lepping P. Restraint guidelines for mental health services in India. *Indian J Psychiatry*. 2019 Apr;61(Suppl 4):S698-S705. doi: 10.4103/psychiatry.IndianJPsychiatry_106_19. PMID: 31040460; PMCID: PMC6482694.
4. Moscarello R. Psychological management of victims of sexual assault. The Canadian Journal of Psychiatry. 1990 Feb;35(1):25-30.

Psychopharmacology 43

Akshay Chordia • Akanksha Sharma

OVERVIEW OF PSYCHOPHARMACOLOGY

Psychiatric medications have become among the most prescribed classes of pharmaceutical agents. Generally, the term 'Psychotropic drugs' is used to describe the drugs used for the treatment of psychiatric disorders. Traditionally these drugs include;

1. Antipsychotics or neuroleptics
2. Antidepressants
3. Mood stabilizers
4. Antianxiety or Anxiolytics
5. Anticraving agents or drugs for substance use disorders
6. Miscellaneous drugs, anticonvulsants, antiparkinsonian drugs, drugs for treatment of dementia, sedative, hypnotics, stimulants, Phosphodiesterase-5 inhibitors etc.

Pharmacodynamics

Psychotropics may act at several molecular sites by activating or inactivating receptors for a specific neurotransmitter (Dopamine antagonists, stimulants). Other drugs may prevent reuptake of a particular neurotransmitter into the presynaptic nerve ending by binding or blocking the reuptake transporters (SSRIs). Some drugs might act by blocking the passage of cation or anion in cellular membranes (calcium channel blockers). Some may bind to inhibit the catabolic enzymes that normally inhibit neurotransmitters, thereby increasing the availability of a specific neurotransmitter in the synaptic cleft (cholinesterase inhibitors). However several drugs have multiple sites of action, therapeutic relevance of which may remain unknown.

Drug Selection

The selection of a psychotropic drug for the treatment of a disorder depends on the various aspects of the drug and the patient's biology. The ability of drug to be effective is only partially predictable, as there is no psychotropic that is effective in all the cases of a given diagnosis. Three factors that should be kept in mind while selecting a drug are: 1. the pharmacology of drug, 2. the biology of patient and 3. The judgment of clinician.

The choice of drug also depends on the previous drug history which includes compliance, therapeutic response, the profile for adverse effects expected for the particular person.

Common Adverse Effects

Psychotropics may cause a wide range of adverse effects. The management includes dose titration, switching to another drug/class, and addition of another drug to prevent adverse effects.

Common adverse effects includes extrapyramidal reactions, weight gain, metabolic syndrome, sexual dysfunction, sedation, anxiety, agitation, akathisia, gastrointestinal upset, diarrhea, headache, dizziness, anorexia, dry mouth, orthostatic hypotension, constipation, blurred vision, urinary retention, etc. The further details of these adverse effects is described in each drug section.

History of Psychopharmacology

1869	Chloral hydrate in treatment of melancholia and mania
1903	Barbiturates use for sedation
1917	Malarial treatment of general paralysis of insane - Nobel prize to Julius von Wagner
1922	Barbiturate induced coma for treatment of psychosis – Jacob Klaesi
1927	Insulin coma treatment for Schizophrenia – Manfred Sakel
1934	Metrazol induced seizures for the treatment of psychosis – Laszlo von Meduna
1937	Dextroamphetamine used for behavioral symptoms in children – C Bradley
1938	Electroconvulsive Therapy for the treatment of psychosis – Ugo cerletti and Lucio Bini
1943	LSD synthesized – Albert Hoffman
1949	Lithium used in mania – John F Cade
1952	Introduction of Chlorpromazine – Jean Delay and Pierre Deniker
1954	Introduction of Meprobamate as an antianxiety Introduction of Reserpine
1958	First Tricyclic Antidepressant, Imipramine introduced for treatment of depression – Thomas Kuhn Iproniazid (MAOIs) introduced for the treatment of depression – Nathan Kline Haloperidol synthesized – Janssen
1960	First Benzodiazepine, Chlordiazepoxide introduced – Sternbach
1966	Valproate used in Bipolar disorder – Lambert
1967	Thioxanthenes and Haloperidol introduced Clomipramine used in OCD - Fernandez and Lopez-Ibor
1968	Pimozide used for treatment of Schizophrenia – Janssen
1970	Lithium, Carbamazepine and Valproic acid marketed in US
1971	Carbamazepine used inBipolar Disorder – Takezaki and Hanoaka
1982	Trazodone introduced
1988	First SSRI, Fluoxetine marketed
1989	Clozapine introduced for treatment resistant Schizophrenia – Kane et al
1994	First SNRI, Venlafaxine introduced First Non-Benzodiazepine for anxiety, Buspirone introduced
1996	Mirtazepine introduced
2006	First Transdermal antidepressant, Selegiline introduced

ANTIPSYCHOTIC AGENTS

Antipsychotics are derived from several classes of chemicals. Chlorpromazine was the first phenothiazine to be introduced in early 1950s. Several other classes including aliphatics, piperidines and piperazines commonly known as the first generation antipsychotics are associated with significant side effects, particularly extra pyramidal symptoms or Parkinsonism like symptoms and other movement disorder like Tardive dyskinesia. Because of these adverse effects at clinically effective dosage, first generation antipsychotics were gradually replaced by serotonin dopamine antagonists, known as second generation antipsychotics. SDAs have a lower propensity to cause extrapyramidal adverse effects. But these newer agents have other adverse effects, most notably sedation, weight gain, increase in blood sugars and serum lipid levels.

Indications

- Acute psychotic episode in schizophrenia
- Maintenance treatment in schizophrenia
- Acute and maintenance treatment in schizoaffective disorder
- Acute Mania
- Maintenance treatment of bipolar mood disorder
- Delusional disorder
- Major depressive disorder with psychotic symptoms
- Borderline personality disorder
- Substance induced psychotic disorder
- Mental disorders caused by medical condition
- Tourette's disorder
- Pervasive developmental disorders
- Huntington's disease
- Tic disorder
- Delirium (in low doses)

Mechanism of Action

Antipsychotic activity of these agents derives from inhibition of dopaminergic neurotransmission. One of the major mechanisms appears to be their capacity to block D2 dopamine receptors mainly present in the mesocortico-limbic, nigrostriatal and tubuloinfundibular pathway. The DRAs are effective when approximately 72 percent of the dopamine receptors are occupied. The clinical potency of a DRA matches closely with the propensity to block dopamine receptors.

The extrapyramidal side effects of antipsychotic agents are believed to be because of the blockade of D2 receptors in nigro-striatal pathway. Similarly, blockade of D2 receptors in tubuloinfundibular pathway may lead to hyperprolactinemia.

Second generation antipsychotics are known for its selective limbic dopamine blockade, D4 receptor blockade, or a combination of potent 5HT2 and weak D2 blockade. Hence these agents have a lesser propensity to cause extrapyramidal adverse effects. The effects of these agents seems to be because of their capacity to block mesolimbic dopamine receptors with lesser effect on nigrostriatal and tubuloinfundibular pathways.

Among second generation antipsychotics, clozapine in particular is effective in management of treatment resistant schizophrenia.

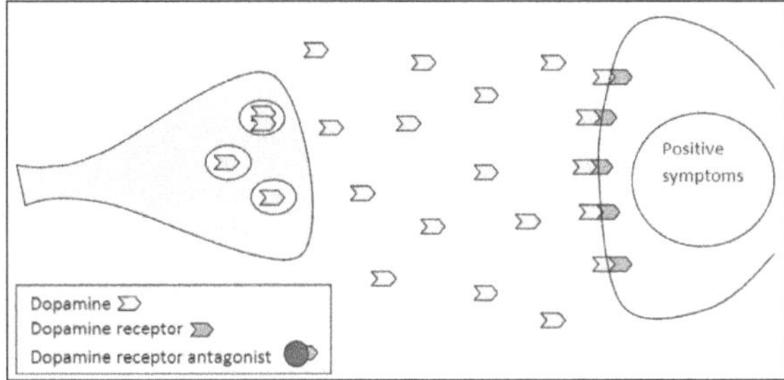

Fig. 43.1: Hyperactivity of dopaminergic neurons in the Mesolimbic pathway leading to the symptoms of psychosis.

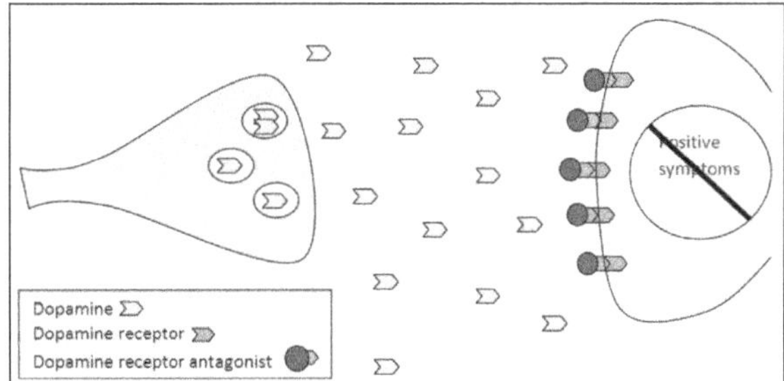

Fig. 43.2: Action of dopamine receptor antagonists on the post synaptic dopamine receptors leading to reduction in symptoms of psychosis.

Pharmacology

All DRAs are well absorbed orally with peak plasma concentration reaching usually 1-4 hours after oral administration and 30-60 mins after parenteral administration. The usual half life of these agents is approximately 24 hours.

Most of DRAs are highly lipophilic and highly protein bound. Parenteral administration results in more rapid and reliable onset of actions. Most are metabolized by cytochrome P450 CYP3a4 and 2D6 isoenzymes. Smoking, food, antacid and coffee interfere with the metabolism. Theoretically a single dose is sufficient to produce sustained therapeutic blood levels.

The main metabolic pathway is through liver. Oxidation and conjugation are most important methods of metabolism. The excretion of metabolites is through enterohepatic circulation.

Long Acting Injectables

Fluphenazine, flupenthixol, haloperidol, risperidone, paliperidone, Olanzapine and aripiprazole are available in long acting injectable formulations. These are useful for patients who refuse or forget to take oral medicines on a regular basis. One major drawback of injectable long acting form is that the side effects produced may continue for several weeks. So to begin with tolerance is checked with oral medicine and then switched to injectable long acting preparations.

Adverse Effects

Extrapyramidal Symptoms (EPS)

EPS consists of tremor, rigidity, akinesia, dystonias, dyskinesias and akathisia also sometimes called as pseudoparkinsonism. The tremor is usually coarse and affects daily activities when severe. Akinesia is paucity of motion and can be mistaken as psychomotor retardation seen in depression. The rigidity of EPS has a wooden quality and responds well with antiparkinsonian medications. Acute dystonias may appear with hours of starting treatment or increasing the dose. Dystonias are not life threatening but can frighten patients and the relatives because of its presentation. Torticollis (forced turning of neck), oculogyric crisis (upturning of eyes), rarely posturing (opisthotonus) may be painful sometimes.

EPS usually subsides quickly with anticholinergics such as benztropine, diphenhydramine and trihexyphenidyl. Prophylactic anticholinergic agents can be prescribed to prevent these adverse effects.

Akathisia is perceived as an inner sense of subjective severe restlessness and discomfort. These side effects usually results in poor adherence to the treatment.

Weight Effects

Most of the second generation antipsychotics can cause increase in appetite, reduced satiety, weight gain. Patient with antipsychotic medication suffer from increased rates of diabetes mellitus, hypercholesterolemia, atherosclerosis and cardiovascular problems. Aripiprazole and ziprasidone are realatively weight neutral.

Tardive Dyskinesias

TD is defined as involuntary choreiform, athetoid or rhythmic movement of tongue, jaw or extremities that occur is association with long term use of antipsychotics. Classic TD affects bucco-lingual muscles leading to in and out movements of tongue (fly catcher's sign), repeated pushing of tongue against the cheek (bonbon sign). Early sign of TD includes worm like movements of resting tongue.

Sedation

Patients generally accommodate to the sedative effects once stable dose is reached. Administering the medication at bed time sometimes help as day time dosing may interfere with daily activities. Sedation may lead to non adherence.

Anticholinergic Effects

Excessive anticholinergic activity may lead to dry mouth, blurred vision, constipation, urinary retention. It may lead to acute crisis in narrow angle glaucoma patients. Discontinuation of the anticholinergic agent is the best treatment.

Hypotension

Light headedness may occur with most of the low potency first generation antipsychotics. Among second generation, clozapine and quetiaeine are among the common agents causing orthostatic hypotension. Resulting sudden drop in blood pressure may lead to fall and injuries patients are advised to arise slowly and carefully to prevent sudden drop in blood pressure.

Sexual Side Effects

Blockade of dopamine often results in increased prolactin levels (dopamine inhibits prolactin release), which can result in low libido, delayed orgasm, gynecomastia in males, galactorrhea and menstrual irregularities in females. Thioridazone may lead to retrograde ejaculation.

Neuroleptic Malignant Syndrome

NMS is characterized by high fever, rigidity, autonomic instability and fluctuating consciousness. It is a life threatening condition. Whenever NMS is suspected, the offending agent should be immediately discontinued. Treatment of NMS aims at reduction of fever with tepid sponging or ice packs. Intravenous fluids are given and infection must be ruled out. In severe cases admission in intensive care unit is required. Bromocriptine and dantrolene sodium has been used with variable results.

Other adverse effects include reduction in seizure threshold, especially with higher doses of clozapine and chlorpromazine. Retinitis Pigmentosa has been seen with the use of thioridazone.

ANTIDEPRESSANTS

Antidepressants are those psychotropic drugs which are used for treatment of depressive disorders.

The first tricyclic antidepressant (TCA) *imipramine* was used in 1958 by Thomas Kuhn. It was different from phenothiazines by only a replacement of sulphur with an ethylene linkage. With this, imipramine was found not effective as an antipsychotic but instead quite beneficial in depressed patients. However it is to be noted that antidepressants have no euphoriant effect when administered to normal, non-depressed individuals.

Indications

Depression

1. Depressive episode (also called major depression, endogenous depression)
2. Secondary depression (e.g. in hypothyroidism, Cushing's syndrome)
3. Abnormal grief reaction

Child Psychiatric Disorders

1. Enuresis
2. Attention deficit disorder with hyperactivity
3. School phobia (sometimes, in low doses)
4. Separation anxiety disorder (in children)
5. Somnambulism
6. Night terrors

Table 43.1: Antipsychotic agents – classification and adverse effects

Generic Name	Starting dose	Usual dose	Maximum dose	Prominent side effects	Sedation	Extrapyramidal Effects	Orthostatic hypotension	Anticholinergic effects	Prodiabetes effects
Phenothiazines									
Chlorpromazine	150-400 mg	50 mg-1 g	1 g	Sedation, hypotension, shuffling gait	Severe	mild	Severe	Moderate	Moderate
fluphenazine	1 mg	1-10 mg	10 mg	EPS	Minimal	Severe	Minimal	Minimal	Minimal
Thioridazine	50 mg	50-800 mg	800 mg	Sedation, dry mouth, constipation	Severe	Minimal	Severe	Severe	Moderate
Trifluoperazine	2.5 mg	2.5-30 mg	30 mg	Hypotension, EPS	Mild	Moderate	Minimal	Minimal	Minimal
Perphenazine	16 mg	24-48 mg	64 mg	EPS, sedation	Moderate	Moderate	Minimal	Minimal	Moderate
Diphenylbutylpiperidine									
Pimozide	4 mg	4-10 mg	10 mg	EPS	Minimal	Severe	Minimal	Minimal	Unknown
Thioxanthenes									
Thiothexene	4 mg	4-24 mg	24 mg	Akathisia, EPS	Mild	Moderate	Mild	Mild	Minimal
Butyrophenones									
Haloperidol	1-2 mg	1-20 mg	20 mg	EPS, akathisia	Minimal	Severe	Minimal	Minimal	Minimal
Other first generation antipsychotics									
Loxapine	15 mg	15-225 mg	225 mg	EPS, sedation	Mild	Moderate	Mild	Mild	Unknown
Molindone	10 mg	10-100 mg	100 mg	EPS	Mild	Moderate	Mild	None	Unknown
Second generation antipsychotics									
Aripiprazole	2 mg	2-30 mg	30 mg	Akathisia, insomnia, agitation, anxiety	Minimal	Mild (moderate akathisia)	Minimal	Minimal	Minimal

(Continued...)

Generic Name	Starting dose	Usual dose	Maximum dose	Prominent side effects	Sedation	Extrapyramidal Effects	Orthostatic hypotension	Anticholinergic effects	Prodiabetes effects
Clozapine	50 mg	50-600mg	900 mg	Sedation, tachycardia, sialorrhea	Severe	Minimal	Severe	Severe	Severe
Olanzapine	5 mg	2-20 mg	20 mg	Weight gain, sedation, constipation	Moderate	Minimal	Mild	Mild	Moderate-severe
Paliperidone	3 mg	3-12 mg	12 mg	EPS	Mild	Moderate	Mild	Minimal	Moderate
Quetiapine	50 mg	50-800 mg	800 mg	Sedation	Moderate	Minimal	Moderate	Mild	Moderate
Risperidone	1 mg	1-10 mg	16 mg	EPS, hypotension,hyperprolactinemia	Minimal	Mild (<6mg) Moderate (>6mg)	Mild	None	Moderate
Ziprasidone	40 mg	40-200 mg	200 mg	Sedation, headache	Minimal	Mild Moderate akathisia	Minimal	Minimal	Minimal
Lurasidone	40 mg	40-160 mg	160 mg	Akathisia	Minimal	Mild Moderate akathisia	Minimal	Minimal	Minimal
Iloperidone	1 mg bid	6-12 mg bid	24 mg	Sedation, hypotension	Moderate	Minimal	Moderate	Minimal	Unknown
Asenapine	5 mg Sublingual	10 mg Sublingual	20 mg Sublingual	Sedation	Mild	Minimal	Minimla	Minimal	Unknown

Other Psychiatric Disorders

1. Panic attacks (e.g. SSRIs)
2. Agoraphobia and social phobia
3. Obsessive compulsive disorder
4. Cataplexy
5. Eating disorders
6. Borderline personality disorder
7. Trichotillomania
8. Depersonalisation syndrome
9. Post-traumatic stress disorder (PTSD)
10. Generalized anxiety disorder
11. Nicotine dependence
12. Alcohol dependence

Medical Disorders

1. Chronic pain
2. Migraine

Mechanism of Action

Antidepressants work primarily on monoamine neurotransmitters mainly on serotonin and monoamine oxidase A. This supports the monoamine hypothesis of depression as it suggests that depression is related to abnormal levels of monoamine neurotransmitters such as serotonin levels in the brain. By correcting the levels by administering it exogenously we can achieve therapeutic response to depression.

Classification of Antidepressants

1. Monoamine oxidase inhibitors (MAOI)
2. Tricyclic antidepressants (TCA)
3. Selective serotonin reuptake inhibitors (SSRIs)
4. Selective norepinephrine reuptake inhibitors (NRIs)
5. Serotonin norepinephrine reuptake inhibitor (SNRIs)
6. Mixed serotonin antagonist/reuptake inhibitor
7. Mixed serotonin/noradrenaline antagonist
8. Norepinephrine/dopamine reuptake inhibitor (NDRI)

MAO INHIBITORS

These act via inhibiting the activity of enzyme monoamine oxidase (MAO) the primary catabolic enzyme for monoamines. This in turn enhances the level of monoamines therefore achieving therapeutic levels for treatment of depression.

Owing to dietary restrictions associated with these, now not used for treatment.

E.g. Tranylcypromine

TRICYCLIC ANTIDEPRESSANTS (TCA)

1. Blocking reuptake of norepinephrine (NE), serotonin (5HT) and/or dopamine (DA) at the nerve terminals, thus increasing NE, 5HT and/or DA levels at the receptor site.
2. Down-regulation of the β-adrenergic receptors.

E.g. Imipramine, Amitryptiline

Dose range- 25-225mg/day in divided doses.

SELECTIVE SEROTONIN REUPTAKE INHIBITORS (SSRIs)

These act via inhibiting the synaptic reuptake of serotonin and hence facilitating the availability of serotonin. Most well tolerated, safe and efficacious antidepressants used in current times.

E.g. Escitalopram (10-20 mg/day), fluoxetine (20-80 mg/day), paroxetine (12.5-50 mg/day), sertraline (25-150 mg/day), fluvoxamine (50-200 mg/day)

SELECTIVE NOREPINEPHRINE REUPTAKE INHIBITORS (NRIs)

Like the SSRIs, medications in this class share a similar mechanism with the SSRIs, but act on the norepinephrine transporter and have little affinity for the serotonin transporter.

E.g. Reboxetine

SEROTONIN NOREPINEPHRINE REUPTAKE INHIBITORS (SNRIs)

Similar mechanism as SSRIs, but differ in the way that these have similar affinity towards serotonin and norepinephrine.

E.g. Venlafaxine (37.7-150 mg/day), duloxetine (20-80 mg/day)

MIXED SEROTONIN ANTAGONIST/ REUPTAKE INHIBITORS

These agents have multiple mechanisms of action, all of which appear to be of clinical importance. They have both serotonin (as well as norepinephrine) transporter inhibition as well as antagonism of 5-HT2A and alpha-1-receptors.

E.g. Trazodone (50-100 mg/day), nefazodone

MIXED SEROTONIN/NORADRENALINE ANTAGONISTS

These agents appear to work primarily through receptor blockade, specifically through blockade of the alpha-2-autoreceptors on presynaptic noradrenergic neurons, which enhances noradrenergic output. They may exert a similar effect toward autoreceptors on serotonin neurons. Antagonism of 5-HT2 and 5-HT3 receptors may also concentrate the effect of serotonin on 5-HT1A receptors.

E.g. Mirtazapine (7.5-45 mg/day)

NOREPINEPHRINE DOPAMINE REUPTAKE INHIBITOR (NDRI)

These agents inhibit the reuptake of norepinephrine and dopamine and hence facilitate their activity at synaptic level.

E.g. Bupropion (75-400 mg/day)

MOOD STABILIZERS

LITHIUM

Lithium is a monovalent ion, of group IA on the periodic table. Lithium exists in nature as both ^{6}Li and ^{7}Li. Around 1597 mg of lithium carbonate consists of 300 mg of lithium.

The use of lithium for the treatment of mania and the prophylaxis in bipolar mood disorder was first established by Austrian psychiatrist John F.J. Cade in 1949. Initially because of concerns regarding the toxicity, the use was limited. It gradually increased in late 1960s. In 1970, lithium was approved by U.S. FDA for the use in treatment of mania and later on for maintenance therapy in patients with history of mania.

Indication

- Bipolar I disorder
  - Manic episode
  - Bipolar depression
  - Maintenance therapy
- Major depressive disorder (as an adjuvant for refractory cases)
- Schizoaffective disorder and schizophrenia
- Cyclothymia
- Impulsivity and aggression
- Kleine Levin syndrome
- Pathological hypersexuality
- Periodic catatonia

Table 43.2: Selective Serotonin Reuptake Inhibitors (SSRIs)

Generic name	Starting dose	Usual dose	Maximum dose	Common adverse effects
Citalopram	10 mg	20-40 mg	40 mg	Nausea, insomnia, somnolence, sexual dysfunction, sweating
Escitalopram	5 mg	10-20 mg	20 mg	Nausea, headache, somnolence, sexual dysfunction
Fluvoxamine	50 mg	100-300 mg	300 mg	Nausea, insomnia, somnolence, sexual dysfunction, sweating Potent inhibitor of CYP 450 enzymes thus more prone to drug interactions
Fluoxetine	20 mg	20-80 mg	80 mg	Nausea, headache, akathisia, weight gain, weight loss, insomnia, sexual dysfunction, diarrhea
Paroxetine	12.5 mg	25-60 mg	60 mg	Sedation, nausea, headache, prone to withdrawal syndrome, diarrhea, sexual dysfunction
Sertraline	50 mg	50-200 mg	200 mg	Nausea, sexual dysfunction, akathisia, diarrhea, headache
Vilazodone	10 mg	10-40 mg	40 mg	Diarrhea, nausea, headache, insomnia

Table 43.3: Tricyclic Antidepressants (TCAs)

Generic name	Starting dose	Usual dose	Maximum dose	Common adverse effects
Amitriptyline	25 mg	100-250 mg	250 mg	Dry mouth, urinary retention, sedation, weight gain, constipation, orthostatic hypotension
Clomipramine	25 mg	150-250 mg	300 mg	Sedation, dry mouth, weight gain, constipation, urinary retention
Desipramine	25 mg	150-300 mg	300 mg	Dry mouth, urinary retention, sedation, weight gain, constipation, sweating
Imipramine	25 mg	150-300 mg	300 mg	Dry mouth, urinary retention, sedation, weight gain, constipation
Doxepin	25 mg	150-300 mg	300 mg	Dry mouth, urinary retention, sedation, weight gain, constipation
Nortriptyline	25 mg	50-150 mg	150 mg	Dry mouth, urinary retention, sedation, weight gain, constipation, orthostatic hypotension
Trimipramine	25 mg	150-300 mg	300 mg	Dry mouth, urinary retention, sedation, weight gain, constipation

Table 43.4: Other Antidepressants

Generic name and mechanism	Starting dose	Usual dose	Maximum dose	Common adverse effects
NDRI (Norepinephrine and dopamine reuptake inhibitor)				
Bupropion	75-150 mg	300-450 mg	450 mg	Insomnia, seizures, dry mouth, overstimulation
SNRI (Serotonin norepinephrine reuptake inhibitor)				
Venlafaxine	37.5 mg	75-150 mg	375 mg	Nausea, dry mouth, sexual dysfunction, hypertension
Desvenlafaxine	50 mg	100-200 mg	200 mg	Nausea, dry mouth, headache, insomnia, dizziness
Duloxetine	20 mg	30-60 mg	120 mg	Nausea, sexual dysfunction, hypertension
NaSSA (Noradrenergic and specific serotonergic antidepressant)				
Mirtazapine	15 mg	15-30 mg	45 mg	Sedation, weight gain, constipation, dry mouth, dizziness
SARI (Serotonin antagonist and reuptake inhibitor)				
Nefazodone	50-100 mg	300-600 mg	600 mg	Sedation, sexual dysfunction, hepatotoxicity
Trazodone	50 mg	300-600 mg	600 mg	Weight gain, sedation, priapism, hepatotoxicity
NSRE (Norepinephrine serotonin reuptake inhibitors)				
Tianeptine	12.5 mg	37.5 mg		Sedation, dryness of mouth, constipation
Tetracyclic antidepressant				
Amoxapine	100-150 mg	200-300 mg	400 mg	Nausea, Sedation, dry mouth, constipation, blurred vision
Maprotiline	25 mg	75-225 mg	225 mg	Dizziness, sedation, dry mouth, constipation, nausea, orthostatic hypotension
Mianserine	30 mg	60-120 mg	120 mg	Dizziness, sedation, dry mouth, constipation, nausea, tremors, headache, weakness

Table 43.5: Monoamine Oxidase Inhibitors (MOAs)

Generic name	Starting dose	Usual dose	Maximum dose	Common adverse effects
Phenelzine	15 mg	45-90 mg	90 mg	Weight gain, constipation, insomnia, hypersomnia, sexual dysfunction, orthostatic hypotension
Selegiline	6 mg	6-12 mg	24 mg	Available in patch form- skin irritation
Tranylcypromine	10 mg	30-60 mg	60 mg	Insomnia, hypertension, orthostatic hypotension (biphasic effect on blood pressure), cheese reaction
Isocarboxazid	10 mg	20-30 mg	60 mg	Weight gain, constipation, insomnia, hypersomnia, sexual dysfunction, orthostatic hypotension

Table 43.6: Antidepressants - Adverse effects and management

Category / side effects	Cause	M/C seen with	Management
Autonomic side effects			
Dry mouth	Muscarinic cholinergic blockade	Amitriptyline	None. Tolerance develops Pilocarpine 2%
Constipation	-same-	-same-	None. Tolerance develops. Laxatives
Mydriasis	-same-	-same-	None. Tolerance develops Pilocarpine 2%
Cycloplegia	-same-	-same-	None. Tolerance develops Pilocarpine 2%
Urinary retention	-same-	-same-	None. Tolerance develops Rule out BHP
Orthostatic hypotension	Alpha 1 adrenergic blockade	-same-	None. Tolerance develops Leg raising
Sexual side effects			
Impotence	Alpha 1 adrenergic blockade	Amitriptyline	
Delayed ejaculation	Alpha 1 adrenergic blockade	Amitriptyline Paroxetine	Cyproheptadine 1 hour before
Anorgasmia	5 HT Blockade	SSRI	
Priapism	Unknown	Unknown	Stop drug
CNS side effects			
Sedation	Alpha adrenergic blockade	Amitriptyline	Single dose at night
Jitteriness	Adrenergic:serotonergic	Fluoxetine	Add diazepam
Seizures	Decreased threshold	Buproprion	Change drug
Precipitation of mania	Sympathomimetic	TCA	Stop drug Add mood stabilizer
Cardiac side effects			
Tachycardia	Anticholinergic	Amitriptyline	Decrease dose
Hypertension	Noradrenergic	Venlafaxine	Close monitoring
Miscellenous side effects			
Bleeding	Decreased platelet Serotonin	SSRI	Change drug
Hyponatremia	SIADH	SSRI/SNRI	Change drug

Pharmacology

Lithium is rapidly and completely absorbed after oral administration with peak concentration occurring in 1-2 hours with standard preparation and 4-5 hours in slow release preparation. Plasma half life varies as per the duration of treatment; initially it is 1.3 days and is 2.4 days after a year of treatment. Blood brain barrier permits slow passage. Long term lithium toxicity is slow to resolve. Clearance of lithium is reduced in patients with renal insufficiency. The steady state is reached in 5 to 7 days of administration. Thyroid and renal concentration of lithium is higher than serum lithium levels.

The mood stabilizing property of lithium seems to be because of alterations of ion transport, effects on neurotransmitters and neuropeptides, signal transduction pathways and secondary messenger systems.

Adverse Effects

Neurologic

- Benign, non toxic – slowed reaction time, dysphoria, lack of spontaneity, memory difficulties, postural tremor.
- Toxic – coarse tremor, dysarthria, ataxia, seizures, neuromuscular irritability, coma, death
- Others- peripheral neuropathy, lowered seizure threshold

Cardiovascular

T wave flattening or inversion, episode of syncope, altered sinus node activity, sinus dysrhythmias

Renal

Morphologic changes, polyuria, nephrogenic diabetes insipidus, renal tubular acidosis, reduced GFR, nephrotic syndrome

Dermatological

Psoriasis, acne, hair loss, rash

Gastrointestinal

Loss of appetite, nausea, vomiting, diarrhea

Others

Weight gain, fluid retention, hypothyroidism, and hyperthyroidism

Lithium toxicity and over dose

- **Mild to moderate intoxication (lithium level, 1.5–2 mEq/L)**
  - GI – vomiting, abdominal pain, dryness of mouth
  - Neurologic – dizziness, ataxia, slurred speech, nystagmus and muscle weakness
- **Moderate to severe intoxication (lithium level, 2–2.5 mEq/L)**
  - GI – anorexia, nausea, vomiting
  - Neurologic – blurred vision, clonic movements of limb, muscle fasciculation, hyperactive deep tendon reflexes, delirium, syncope, convulsions, coma cardiac arrhythmias, hypotension, conduction and circulatory failure
- **Severe intoxication (lithium level, > 2.5 mEq/L)**

  Generalized convulsion, renal failure, death

VALPROATE

Valproate or valproic acid is one of the most widely prescribed mood stabilizers in psychiatry. It is a simple chain carboxylic acid. It is rapidly converted into acid form in stomach. Multiple formulations include:

- Valproic acid
- Divalproex sodium
- Enteric coated delayed release 1:1 mixture of valproic acid and sodium valproate

Pharmacology

It is rapidly and completely absorbed in 1-2 hours of oral administration. It takes 4-5 hours to achieve peak serum levels. Plasma half life is around 10-16 hours. The concentration for therapeutically effective free serum level is above 50-100 μg/ml. The extended release preparation can be taken once a day.

Postulated mechanism of action includes enhancement of GABA activity, modulation of voltage sensitive sodium channels, and action on extra-hypothalamic neuropeptides.

Indications

- ➢ Bipolar I disorder
    - Manic episode
    - Bipolar depression
    - Maintenance therapy
- ➢ Schizoaffective disorder and schizophrenia
- ➢ Impulse control disorder
- ➢ Behavioral agitation
- ➢ Borderline personality disorder
- ➢ Migraine
- ➢ Pain syndromes
- ➢ Seizure disorders

Adverse Effects

The common side effect of sodium valproate includes nausea, vomiting, sedation, tremor, ataxia, dysarthria, flushing, weight gain, hair loss, menstrual irregularities, polycystic ovaries and hyperandrogenism.

Serious side effects include hepatotoxicity, pancreatitis, hyperammonemia, teratogenicity, thrombocytopenia, Steven-Jhonson syndrome.

Drug Interactions

Other drugs used in psychiatric disorders may increase or decrease the serum levels of valproate. It includes commonly prescribed drug like lithium, clozapine carbamazepine, and fluoxetine. Perhaps the most important interaction to note is between lamotrigine and valproate. Valproate increases the serum levels of lamotrigine by more than double, increasing the chances of serious rash or Steven-Jhonson syndrome.

CARBAMAZEPINE AND OXCARBAZEPINE

Carbamazepine possesses some structural similarity with tricyclic antidepressant. It was first synthesized as a potential antidepressant. Later on because of its atypical profile it was approved for the treatment of trigeminal neuralgia and seizure disorders. It is now recognized as second line mood stabilizer.

Oxcarbazepine is an analog of carbamazepine. The usefulness of oxcarbazepine as a treatment for mania has not been established in controlled trials.

Indications

- ➢ Bipolar I disorder
    - Manic episode
    - Bipolar depression
    - Acute depression
- ➢ Acute alcohol withdrawal
- ➢ Impulse control disorders
- ➢ Psychosis with epilepsy
- ➢ Borderline personality disorder
- ➢ Pain syndromes – trigeminal neuralgia,

phantom limb pain, other neuralgias.

- Aggression in schizophrenia and schizoaffective disorders

Adverse Effects

Mild GI (nausea, vomiting, constipation, diarrhea and anorexia), CNS (ataxia, drowsiness, dizziness) are among the common side effects. More serious adverse effects include, blood dyscrasias, hepatit's, Steven-Jhonson syndrome, agranulocytosis, confusion.

In contrast to carbamazepine, oxcarbazepine does not have an increased risk for blood dyscrasias. The frequency of benign rash is also less with oxcarbazepine.

LAMOTRIGINE

Lamotrigine was developed as an antiepileptic drug and later on approved for maintenance treatment of bipolar I disorder. It has gained attention as a drug which maximally impact the depressive component and stabilizing mood from below.

Indications

- Bipolar I disorder
- Rapid cycling bipolar mood disorder (lengthening the intervals between depressive episodes)
- Borderline personality disorder
- Pain syndromes

Adverse Effects

It is generally well tolerated. It may cause dizziness, ataxia, headache, diplopia, nausea, blurred vision and somnolence. Rarely, it may cause development of a maculopapular rash which may lead to Stevens-Jhonson syndrome within first 4 months of starting treatment. Concomitant use of valproate increases the risk of adverse events and should be avoided if possible.

BENZODIAZEPINES

In 1959, chlordiazepoxide was first benzodiazepine to be introduced by Sternbach, which largely replaced the use of meprobamate for anxiety. Benzodiazepines are often highly effective in non specific anxiety and other anxiety disorders. They share a common effect on benzodiazepine receptor which in turn modulate ψ-aminobutyric acid (GABA) activity. Flumazenil is a benzodiazepine receptor antagonist used to reverse benzodiazepine over dosage.

Benzodiazepines activate all three specific GABA-benzodiazepine binding sites of $GABA_A$ receptor which opens chloride channels to reduce the rate of neuronal firing. Non-benzodiazepine hypnotics zolpidem, zaleplon, eszopiclone are selective to certain sub units of GABA receptor which accounts for their selective sedative effects and lack on anticonvulsant and muscle relaxant property.

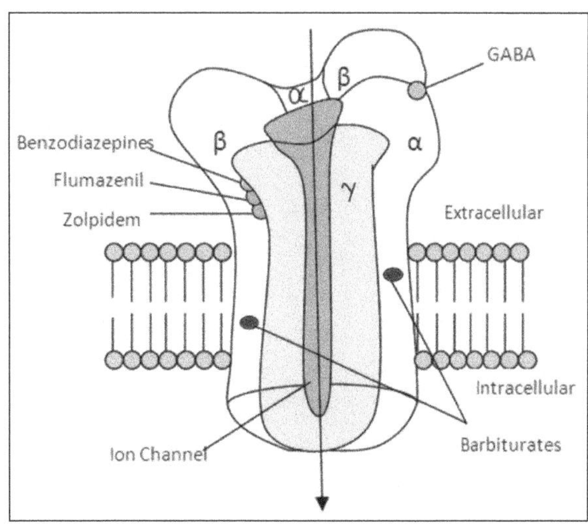

Fig. 43.3: GABA receptor.

Indication

- Short term treatment of Insomnia
- Non specific Anxiety
- Agitation
- Anxiety associated with psychiatric disorders
- Alcohol and other substance withdrawal
- Panic disorder
- Generalized anxiety disorder
- Emergency management of acute mania, acute psychosis
- Others – Anesthetics, Muscle relaxants, Anticonvulsants

Table 43.7: Benzodiazepines

Generic names	Half life (hours)	Starting dose (per day-mg)	Usual dose (per day-mg)	Maximum dose (per day-mg)	Common adverse effects
Anxiolytics					
Lorazepam	14±5	0.5	0.5-6	6	sedation, incoordination, confusion, addiction
Alprazolam	12±2	0.25	0.25-6	6	sedation, incoordination, confusion, physical dependence
Clonazepam	23±5	0.25	0.5-6	6	sedation, incoordination, confusion, physical dependence
Chlordiazepoxide	10±4	10	10-60	60	sedation, incoordination, confusion, physical dependence
Diazepam	14-19	5	5-10	30	sedation, incoordination, confusion, physical dependence
oxazepam	5-15	10	30-90	120	drowsiness, anterograde amnesia, dizziness, headache, paradoxical excitement
Hypnotics					
Estazolam	10-24	1	1-2	2	sedation, incoordination, confusion, physical dependence
Flurazepam	74±24	15	15-30	30	dizziness, day time drowsiness, ataxia, headache
Temazepam	11±6	15	15-30	30	dizziness, day time drowsiness, fatigue, headache
Quazepam	39	7.5	7.5-15	15	dizziness, day time drowsiness, ataxia, headache
Triazolam	2.9±1	0.125	0.125-0.5	0.5	dizziness, day time drowsiness, ataxia, fatigue, anterograde amnesia
Nitrazepam	20-60	2	2-10	20	sedation, incoordination, confusion, addiction

Table 43.8: Non-benzodiazepine anxiolytic and hypnotics

Generic name	Mechanism	half life (in hours)	starting dose	usual dose	Maximum dose	Common adverse effects
Anxiolytics						
Buspirone	5-HT_{1A} partial agonist	2.4±1.1	5 mg	15-30 mg bid	60 mg	Nausea, headache, dizziness
Propranolol	beta-blocker	3.9±0.4	10 mg	10-40 mg	120 mg	Bradycardia, hypotension
Hypnotics						
Zolpidem	selective binding of BZ_1 receptor	2.6±1.2	5 mg	5-10 mg	10 mg	Drowsiness, anterograde amnesia, dizziness, diarrhea
Eszopiclone	not known? interaction with GABA receptor	6	1 mg	2-3 mg	3 mg	Headache, drowsiness, dizziness, dry mouth, dysguisia
Trazodone	5-HT_{2A} partial agonist	3-6	25 mg	25-50 mg	600 mg	Drowsiness, priapism

DISULFIRAM AND ANTICRAVING AGENTS

Disulfiram

Disulfiram is used as a deterrent drug in the treatment for alcohol use disorder. It acts by blocking the enzyme aldehyde dehydrogenase, leading to the impaired metabolism of acetaldehyde which is the first metabolite of alcohol. Acetaldehyde accumulation after consumption of alcohol even in small amounts leads to various ill effects collectively known as disulfiram-ethanol reaction. Some patients continue consuming alcohol with dire consequences and some will stop taking it in order to return to drinking. Highly motivated patients and those who fear of the toxic effects are the candidates for its administration. These patients may still require the administration in supervision by a family member.

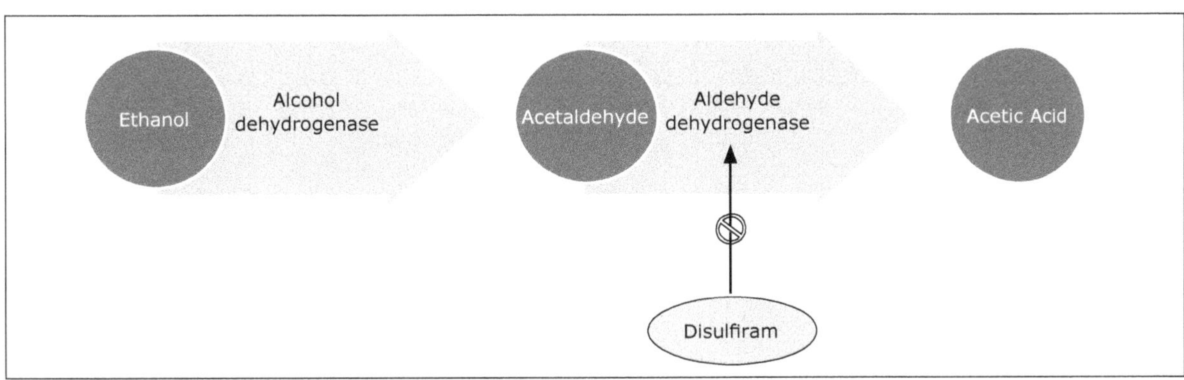

Fig. 43.4

ANTICRAVING AGENTS

Anticraving agents are used in substance use disorder cases to reduce the craving for the particular substance, promote abstinence and prevent relapse.

Table 43.9: Anticraving agents used for various substance uses.

Generic name	Mechanism of action	usual required dose	common adverse effects	Special mention
for Alcohol use				
Acamprosate	GABA analog	if weight < 60 kg - 1332 mg (4 tablets of 333 mg each in a day) if weight > 60 kg - 1998 mg (6 tablets of 333 mg each – 2 tablets TDS)	Nausea, diarrhea, vomiting, headache	to be avoided in patients with renal impairment
Baclofen	opiate receptor antagonist	30-90 mg	Weakness, dizziness, headache, fatigue, nausea, vomiting, euphoria	Discontinuation after long term use may be associated with a withdrawal syndrome.
Topiramate	$GABA_A$ receptor agonist	25-100 mg	Dizziness, weight loss, somnolence, nausea, diarrhea, disturbance in attention, fatigue	should be avoided in patients with history of nephrolithiasis
For Opioid use				
Naltrexone	predominantly mu-opioid receptor antagonist kappa and delta receptor antagonist to lesser extent	25-100 mg	Diarrhea, abdominal cramp, nausea, vomiting	should be started after several days of abstinence from opioids. (usually 7 to 11 days)
Methadone	mu-opioid receptor agonist	50-100 mg	sedation, diarrhea, constipation, sweating, dizziness, weakness, nausea, vomiting, dry mouth, headache	used for maintenance therapy to be legally obtained through licenced clinics withdrawal symptoms on discontinuation

(Continued...)

Generic name	Mechanism of action	usual required dose	common adverse effects	Special mention
Buprenorphine	mu-receptor partial agonist kappa-receptor antagonist	12-16 mg	dizziness, headache, orthostatic hypotension, respiratory depression, somnolence	Withdrawal symptoms on discontinuation is less severe
For Nicotine use				
Bupropion	Norepinephrine and dopamine reuptake inhibitor	100-300 mg	headache, insomnia, dry mouth, tremor, nausea risk of seizure with doses more than 400mg	used for smoking cessation in highly motivated patients along with nicotine replacement therapy
Nicotine	Nicotine replacement therapy	1,2,4 mg gum, lozenges 7,14,21 mg transdermal patch	dizziness, palpitations, jaw soreness, sweating and skin irritation in patch	Gum/lozenges to be chewed and parked/ tucked in between the cheek and gums.
Varenicline	$\alpha_4\beta_2$ nicotinic acetyl choline receptor partial agonist	0.5mg/d for 3 days, 0.5mg BD for next 3 days,1mg bd for next two weeks	nausea, headache, insomnia, nightmares, flatulence, constipation	reports of thoughts of suicide and occasional suicidal behavior (boxed warning)

CHOLINESTERASE INHIBITORS

Cholinesterase inhibitors like donepezil, rivastigmine and galantamine are used to treat mild to moderate cognitive impairment, particularly in Alzhiemer type. They act by inhibiting enzyme cholinesterase and reduce the inactivation of acetyl choline, thereby potentiating its neurotransmission. It produces modest improvement in memory.

Table 43.10: Cholinesterase inhibitors

Generic name	Usual dose	$T^{1/2}$	Common Adverse effects
Donepezil	5-23 mg	70 hours	Nausea, diarrhea, vomiting
Rivastigmine	3-12 mg	1 hour	Nausea, diarrhea, vomiting, headache, abdominal pain
Galantamine	8-24 mg	6 hours	Dizziness, headache, nausea, anorexia, diarrhea
Tacrine	No longer used	2-4 hours	Hepatotoxicity, nausea, vomiting, abdominal discomfort, myalgia

Table 43.11: Phosphodiesterase-5 inhibitors

Generic name	Usual Dose	Usual half life	Common adverse effects
Sildenafil	25-100 mg	3-4 hours	Headache, flushing, abdominal pain, vision problems, lower back pain, blue vision, nasal congestion, diarrhea, dizziness, rash Rarely-Myocardial infarction (contra-indicated in person taking amyl nitrate), Non Arteritic Anterior Ischemic Optic Neuropathy, Hearing loss
Tadalafil	2.5-20 mg	18 hours	same
Vardenafil	2.5-20 mg	3-4 hours	same

Memantine

Memantine is a non-cholinesterase inhibitor; it acts through blockade of N-methyl-D-aspartate receptors with low to moderate affinity. It may protect cells against excess glutamate by partially blocking NMDA receptors associated with abnormal transmission and allowing for physiological transmission. It is indicated in moderate to severe stage of Alzheimer dementia. In routine clinical practice, it is often combined with cholinesterase inhibitors for better response.

Adverse Effects

Memantine is well tolerated. The commonly seen adverse effects include dizziness, headache, constipation and confusion. It is contraindicated in patients with severe renal impairment. In cases of overdose, patients may experience restlessness, hallucinations, psychosis, stupor and loss of consciousness.

PHOSPHODIESTERASE-5 INHIBITORS

Phosphodiesterase-5 Inhibitors include drugs such as Sildenafil, and its congeners – Tadalafil and Vardenafil. These agents are mainly used to treat male erectile dysfunction.

They block subtype of enzyme Phosphodiesterase and prevent the inactivation of cyclic guanosine monophosphate (cGMP) which regulates blood flow in the penis. Increased level of cGMP smooth muscle relaxation (vasodialation) and increased inflow of blood in corpus cavernosum.

Indications

- Erectile dysfunction
  - Organic – Diabetes mellitus, hypertension, hypercholesterolemia, peripheral vascular disease, peripheral neuropathy, pelvic injury, Parkinson's disease, etc.
  - Psychogenic
  - Mixed
- SSRIs induced sexual dysfunction

BIBLIOGRAPHY

1. Kaplan and sadock's comprehensive textbook of Psychiatry.
2. Stahl's Essential Psychopharmacology.
3. Oxford textbook of Psychiatry.
4. KD Tripathi Essentials of Medical Pharmacology.
5. The Maudsley Prescribing Guideline in Psychiatry.
6. Goodman and Gilman's The Pharmacological Basis of Therapeutics.
7. A Short Textbook of Psychiatry – Niraj Ahuja.

Electroconvulsive Therapy and Brain Stimulation Therapies for Psychiatric Conditions

44

Shalini Naik • Preeti Sinha • Jagadisha Thirthalli

INTRODUCTION

Brain stimulation modalities are important treatment options for different psychiatric conditions. These are particularly useful when there is need for quick relief of symptoms and when patients do not tolerate or do not respond to other methods of treatment, including medications. Electroconvulsive therapy (ECT), Transcranial Magnetic Stimulation (TMS), Transcranial Direct Current Stimulation (tDCS), Vagal Nerve Stimulation (VNS), and Deep Brain Stimulation (DBS) are notable among brain stimulation modalities. ECT has a long history of use and is the most well-established among these. This chapter details various aspects of ECT and provides brief information about other brain stimulation treatments.

ELECTROCONVULSIVE THERAPY (ECT)

ECT is a procedure in which a precisely determined dose of electrical charge is delivered to the brain non-invasively through the scalp to induce generalized seizure lasting for a few seconds. The electrical charge is administered after the individual is anesthetized and after inducing relaxation of skeletal muscles.

Origin and Evolution of ECT

ECT is arguably the oldest surviving physical treatment for psychiatric disorders. While the psychotropic medications were developed based on serendipitous observations, 'convulsive therapies' had considerable theoretical rationale for their use. In the early years of the 20th century, Ladislas Joseph Von Meduna, a Hungarian psychiatrist and a neuropathologist, had theorized that psychosis and epilepsy were antagonistic to each other. He treated patients of psychosis by inducing seizures using chemicals such as camphor, strychnine, metrozol, etc. Seizure induction using chemicals was unpredictable and cumbersome. Ugo Cerletti and Lucio Bini, Italian neuropsychiatrists, discovered that seizures could be induced in animals using electricity and extrapolated it to humans in 1938. Across the globe, psychiatrists used Cerletti-Bini's 'electroconvulsive' treatment and observed considerable response in psychotic as well as mood disorders. Patients also experienced negative effects including pre-treatment apprehension about electric shock, impact on musculoskeletal system during convulsions and post-treatment cognitive disturbances. Progressive modifications in ECT administration have reduced these negative effects to a considerable extent. These modifications are summarized below:

A. Modified ECT

During the initial years, ECT was administered to patients while they were awake without muscle relaxants. This led to violent convulsions and consequent fractures, joint dislocations and tendon & ligament injuries. Use of muscle relaxants, which started in the 1950s, reduced the degree of convulsive movements. The practice of using anesthetic medication that had started in the 1940s now became essential, in order to avoid the extremely uncomfortable experience of inability to breath when muscle relaxants are used in conscious state. The use of anesthetic and muscle relaxing medications prior to the application of electrical stimulus came to be known as 'modified ECT' and this made ECT substantially safer and humane. Until recently, the practice of ECT without anesthesia and muscle relaxation (unmodified ECT) was in vogue in many centers in India. The Mental Health Care Act of 2017 has prohibited the use of unmodified ECT.

B. Electrical parameters

Earlier ECT devices used sine-wave electrical stimulus. A sine-wave (**Fig. 44.1a**) stimulus has gradual rise and fall of electrical current, with peak amplitude in the middle. Depolarization of neurons, which is necessary for the generation of seizures, happens only during the peak phase. The 1970s saw the development of next generation of devices, which used rectangular-shaped pulses of electrical stimulus (**Fig. 44.1b**), after removing the unrequired ascending and descending portions of the sine waves and retaining only the peak amplitude. These 'brief-pulses' have pulse widths of 0.5 - 2 milliseconds. Compared to ECT with traditional sine-wave stimulus, ECT with brief-pulse stimulus is associated with far less cognitive adverse effects. Minimum duration of electrical stimulation for the generation of action potential in neurons is about 0.2 milliseconds. Keeping with this, devices generating stimulus with pulse widths of < 0.5 milliseconds ('ultra-brief pulse') are gaining popularity. The benefit of ultra-brief pulse ECT over brief pulse ECT is not well established.

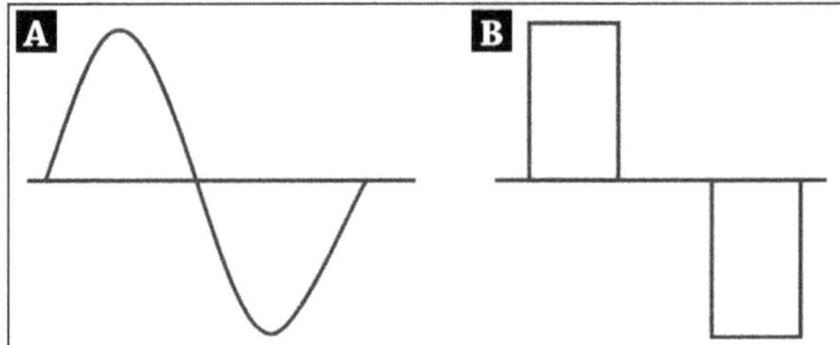

Fig. 44.1: (A) Sine wave; (B) Pulse wave.

In the beginning years, devices used constant voltage, wherein the total current administered was inversely proportional to the impedance of patient's head. With the advent of pulse-wave ECTs, most ECT devices are designed to keep the current constant – the devices adjust the voltage according to the impedance of the patient's head.

C. Electrode Placement

The site where pair of electrodes makes surface contact with the scalp to deliver electrical charge is called "electrode placement" or "electrode montage". Initially, electrodes were placed over temple regions on either side of the head ('bitemporal' electrode placement). Alternative electrode placements were designed later to reduce ECT-associated memory deficits by avoiding direct stimulation of the dominant temporal lobe.

Unilateral ECT

In 1949, right unilateral electrode [RUL] placement was introduced to avoid direct stimulation of the left temporal lobe. d'Elia RUL placement position, also known as temporoparietal right unilateral (TP-RUL) placement was proposed in 1970. It demonstrated fewer anterograde and retrograde memory disturbances in comparison to the frontotemporal right unilateral (FT-RUL) placement and became popular.

Bifrontal ECT

In Bifrontal ECT, electrodes are placed over the supraorbital ridge on both sides of the forehead. It was first reported in 1969 but, got popularized in 1990's. It probably has benefits of both 'efficacy' as that of bitemporal ECT and 'lesser cognitive adverse effects' as by RUL ECT.

Commonly used electrode placements described above are shown in **Fig. 44.2**.

D. Seizure monitoring

During initial years of ECT, seizure was monitored by observing generalized motor convulsions. Motor convulsions were absent or unreliable with the use of modified ECT. This necessitated alternative methods of monitoring seizures. In 1953, the 'cuff method' was introduced to isolate one limb from the effect of muscle relaxant and seizure was observed in this limb (Please see "ECT administration procedure" for more details). Monitoring of seizures using EEG became popular since the early 1980s. The cuff method is still in practice in situations where EEG monitoring is unavailable.

E. Formation of International professional bodies in ECT

Professional bodies have played a critical role in enhancing standards of ECT practice. The International Society for ECT and Neurostimulation (ISEN), was established in 1976 to promote the safe, ethical and effective use of ECT through education and research. The American Psychiatric Association (APA) and The Royal College of Psychiatrists (RCP), UK also established committees in 1978 and 1994 respectively to provide guidelines about legislative issues, indications and procedures for ECT; these bodies periodically update their guidelines and recommendations. The joint report of the American Psychiatric Association and the American College of Obstetricians and Gynecologists refers to carefully administered ECT as a safe and effective method to treat severe depression during pregnancy. American Academy of Child and Adolescent Psychiatry (AACAP) discusses the use of ECT in adolescents under certain circumstances. The views of the National Institute for health and Care Excellence

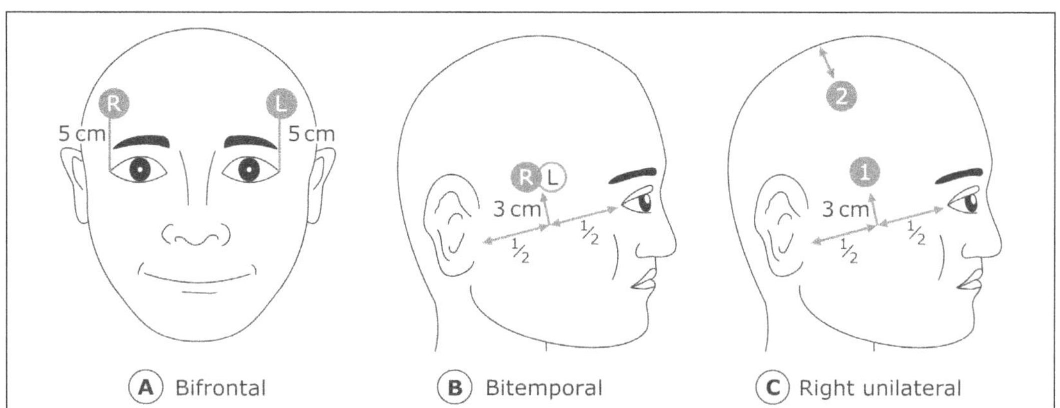

Fig. 44.2: Different Electrode placements in ECT.

(NICE) of the UK about the use of ECT in these special populations is similar to that of the American professional bodies.

F. Standardization of equipments and accreditation of ECT practice

ECT devices and services go through stringent regulatory and accreditation procedures in many countries. The Food and Drug Administration (FDA) of the USA granted pre-dated approval of ECT under class III category (i.e., devices with the greatest risk posed to the patients) in 1976. In 2018, it reclassified ECT devices to be under class II category (those with moderate to high risk), reflecting the current understanding of their safety. In the UK, the ECT Accreditation Service (ECTAS), works with ECT clinics to assure and improve the quality of administration of ECT. In India, ECT devices of contemporary standards have been indigenously developed through collaboration between the National Institute of Mental Health & Neurosciences (NIMHANS), Bengaluru and National Institution for Quality and Reliability (NIQR), an organization that sets standards for engineering ventures.

Clinical Indications

ECT has been used to treat several psychiatric disorders. Evidence for its use is well-established, through rigorously conducted randomized controlled trials, for depression including antidepressant non-responsive depression and depression as part of bipolar disorder. Several studies have indicated that ECT is highly effective in treating mania and schizophrenia as well, but the evidence-base for its use in these indications is considerably poorer compared to its use in depression. There are several case reports supporting its usefulness in treatment-refractory obsessive-compulsive disorder, severe noncognitive behavioral symptoms of different types of dementia and neurodevelopmental disorders. Across these conditions, ECT is commonly used in the following clinical situations:

1. Suicidal risk in the form of suicidal ideas, plans or attempts,
2. Catatonia
3. Refusal to eat food or drink fluids
4. Severe agitation and/or aggression
5. Severe depressive symptoms associated with psychotic symptoms
6. Intolerance to adverse effects of psychotropic medications or significant drug-drug interactions with medications used for co-morbid illnesses.
7. Poor response to pharmacotherapy and other treatments
8. Patient's preference for ECT

Note: ECT may be preferred in many of these situations due to rapid onset of its action.

ECT is used almost exclusively for depression in many North American and West European countries. The use of ECT for indications other than depression is commoner in India and other Asian countries. In some centers in these countries, ECT is used as commonly for schizophrenia as it is for depression. Commoner presentation of catatonic schizophrenia in these countries, and rapidity of improvement with ECT with consequent reduction of duration of hospitalization may be contributing to this practice.

ECT is rarely used in certain *neurological* conditions:

a. Neuroleptic Malignant Syndrome

b. Parkinson's disease (PD) with severe depression or psychosis. ECT has been observed to improve both psychiatric symptoms and motor symptoms, especially rigidity and bradykinesia.

c. Refractory status epilepticus.

Contraindications

There is no absolute contraindication to ECT. However, presence of a several conditions warrants specific precautions, intensive monitoring and consultation with medical specialist to avoid morbidity and mortality with ECT (See **Fig. 44.1**)

Fig. 44.1 Conditions that are associated with higher mortality and morbidity with ECT

Clinical conditions	Cause
Intracranial space occupying lesions	ECT induced seizures increases the intracranial pressure and predisposes to brain stem herniation
Intracerebral hemorrhage Unstable vascular aneurysms in the brain Retinal detachment	ECT causes considerable increase in blood pressure and predisposes to bleeding
Recent myocardial infarction (< 3 months) Moderate to severe hypertension, Uncontrolled cardiac arrhythmias Pheochromocytomas	Rapid fluctuations in cardiovascular function and increased cardiac load and oxygen demand during and immediately after ECT

Hemodynamic changes during ECT

The electrical stimulus leads to initial parasympathetic stimulation. Certain anesthetic agents like thiopentone and propofol may also contribute to hypotension during ECT. With the onset of generalized seizure, there is sympathetic surge, which overshadows the initial parasympathetic stimulation. Potential complications during the parasympathetic stimulation are hypotension, sinus bradycardia and vagal arrhythmias. Subsequent sympathetic activation causes tachycardia and systolic hypertension placing substantial demand on the heart. The sympathetic surge takes about 10-15 minutes to normalize after the cessation of seizure. Adequate ventilation shortens the duration of sympathetic hyperactivity. Continuous monitoring of vital parameters is essential during ECT procedure until the autonomic functions reach the baseline.

Anesthetic agents, muscle relaxants and pre-anesthetic medication

Anesthetic agent

An ideal anesthetic agent for ECT must have rapid onset of action, short duration of action with minimal effect on seizure threshold and hemodynamic system. Thiopentone (2–5 mg/kg) is the most commonly used intravenous anesthetic agent for ECT in developing countries. Methohexital (0.5–1 mg/kg) is preferred due to better hemodynamic profile, but it is expensive. Propofol and etomidate are preferred in patients with comorbid cardiovascular conditions.

Muscle relaxants

Muscle relaxant causes paralysis of all skeletal muscles including diaphragm and respiratory muscles. Therefore, positive pressure ventilation with 100% oxygen must be ensured during the procedure until the patient regains spontaneous breathing. Succinylcholine (0.5–1 mg/kg), a depolarizing neuromuscular blocker is the preferred muscle relaxant due to its rapid onset (30–60 seconds) and short duration of action (5–10 minutes). It is contraindicated in conditions prolonging its duration of action such as pseudo-cholinesterase deficiency, history of organophosphorus compound poisoning until serum pseudo-cholinesterase levels reach normal), potential risk of hyperkalemia (e.g. burns) and neuromuscular disease. The alternatives may be non-depolarizing muscle relaxants such as atracurium (0.3–0.5 mg/kg).

Pre-anesthetic medications

Anticholinergic agents are used to reduce the initial vagal effects of electrical stimulation on the heart, to prevent bradyarrhythmia. It is indicated often in the first ECT treatment session due to likelihood of repetitive electrical stimulation, and in sessions where beta-blockers or calcium channel blockers are concomitantly used. Atropine (0.6 mg IV) is used adjunctively with anesthetic agent while, glycopyrrolate (0.2–0.4 mg/kg IV) is administered 5 minutes prior to the anesthesia administration. The latter may be preferred due to its limited CNS and transplacental permeation.

Administration procedure

ECT requires a team of psychiatrists, anesthesiologists, psychiatric nurses, hospital assistants and/or technicians. The procedure involves pre-ECT measures, ECT treatment procedure and post-ECT care (see Fig. 44.2).

Monitoring of seizures

Cuff technic and EEG monitoring are two well-established methods for seizure monitoring in current practice.

Cuff technic

This procedure is performed before the administration of muscle relaxant. It involves placement of blood pressure cuff around the mid-calf on one side and inflation of cuff pressure to 50-80 mm of Hg above the systolic blood pressure of the patient. This ceases the arterial circulation distal to the cuff. After this, muscle relaxant (often succinylcholine) is delivered intravenously; succinylcholine induced fasciculations should be absent in the cuffed limb. Isolation of this limb enables the psychiatrist to observe convulsions after the electrical stimulus is applied. The cuff-method is contraindicated in patients with deep vein thrombosis and peripheral vascular disease (risk of pulmonary embolism due to dislodging of thrombus), sickle cell disease (risk of vaso-occlusive crisis), untreated hypocalcemia (risk of tetanic contraction of distal muscles) and major musculoskeletal injury distal to the cuff.

EEG monitoring

Epileptiform discharges generated during ECT may be monitored using electroencephalography (EEG). Typically, EEG seizures are usually 10-20 seconds longer than the motor seizures. There is greater likelihood of missing a seizure or of not identifying prolonged seizures if EEG monitoring is not used. Missing a seizure can lead to unwarranted repeat stimulation; prolonged seizure may cause cerebral hypoxia, post-ECT confusion and more cognitive impairment. For EEG monitoring, electrodes are placed in fronto-mastoid montage over scalp corresponding to Fp1 and Fp2 of the 10-20 international EEG system. They form 2 channels of EEG on either side of head with reference electrodes placed over mastoid.

EEG morphology during ECT (Fig. 44.2). Early phase of EEG includes rhythmic discharges of low amplitude in the alpha (8-13Hz) or beta (14-30 Hz) range. This is followed by moderate amplitude EEG with frequency of 6-10 Hz, and, later, by repetitive *spike and slow-wave complexes* with high amplitude and frequency of about 3 Hz. Typically, EEG seizure ends with abrupt cessation of these high-amplitude waves. This ‘post-ictal suppression’ lasts for several minutes.

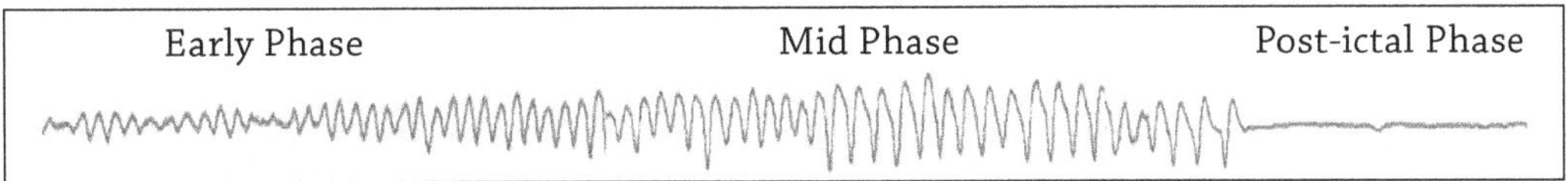

Fig. 44.3: Typical EEG morphology during an ECT-induced seizure.

Box. 44.1: ECT administration procedure.

Pre-ECT measures

- Written informed consent from the patient is sought. If patient is incompetent to decide about consent, it is sought from primary caregiver. If patient gains competency later, his consent is taken.
- Detailed medical and neurological examination is performed.
- Blood Investigations including complete hemogram, fasting sugar, electrolyte levels and creatinine are done along with ECG
- If intracranial pathology is suspected, CT scan or MRI brain is also done.
- Any solid food for at least 6 hours and clear fluid for at least 2 hours prior to the ECT session is avoided.
- Morning dose of antihypertensive medication (except beta-blockers) and Levo-thyroxine supplements are dispensed with a sip of water.
- Both oral and injectable hypoglycemic agents should be avoided.
- Hair should be kept clean and dry as damp hair and presence of oil/ cream may cause shorting of the current over scalp.
- If patient has dentures, jewellery, hair clips, contact lenses or hearing aids, they are removed.
- Before ECT administration, patient is encouraged to void urine.

ECT Treatment procedure

- The patient's feelings, apprehensions about the procedure are addressed.
- The patient is positioned in supine posture on a stretcher.
- It is ensured that dentures have been removed, and that there is no loose tooth or significant pathology in the oral cavity.
- Vital signs (heart rate, blood pressure, respiratory rate and oxygen saturation) are recorded.
- Intravenous line is secured on the side contralateral to that used for vital signs monitoring.
- One of the limbs is prepared for the cuff technic if monitoring of motor seizure is planned.
- Leads are placed over scalp for EEG monitoring of seizures.
- Stimulus parameters are set on the ECT device.
- After initial 100% oxygenation, anesthetic agent is administered intravenously.
- Once the patient is completely sedated, muscle relaxant is administered intravenously.
- The fasciculations appear during the initial activity of succinyl choline and disappear by the maximal state of relaxation in 1-3 minutes.
- Once fasciculations disappear, the bite block is placed between lower and upper rows of teeth pushing the tongue behind towards the center of oral cavity to prevent tongue bite
- Stimulus electrodes are placed over the head as per the plan of electrode placement.
- The decided electric stimulus is administered and the seizure duration is recorded as motor and/or EEG.
- If seizure duration is inadequate, a higher electric stimulus is administered.
- The BP cuff used for motor monitoring of seizure duration is deflated.
- Bite block is removed and 100% oxygenation is provided till the voluntary breathing starts.
- Oral cavity is checked and oral secretions are suctioned.
- Vital signs are monitored throughout the procedure.
- All medications, stimulus parameters, seizure response, and vital signs are documented.
- The patient is then shifted to the recovery area.

(Continued...)

Post-ECT care

- The level of consciousness and vital signs are here also serially monitored.
- The patient is watched for tardive/spontaneous or prolonged seizures, post-ictal agitation, confusion or delirium
- After the vitals have reached the baseline status and the patient has regained consciousness, he/she is shifted to the ward

Adequacy of seizures

Seizures with poor bilateral generalization are considered to be inadequate. Motor seizure of at least 15 seconds or EEG seizure, with morphology described above, of at least 20 seconds duration are regarded as adequate.

Prolonged Seizures

Different professional bodies have defined motor seizure lasting for more than 90 seconds or EEG seizure for more than 120 – 180 seconds as 'prolonged seizures'. Prolonged seizures must be aborted with intravenous bolus of short-acting benzodiazepines (lorazepam/midazolam) or low dose of anesthetic agents (thiopentone/ propofol). Instances of status epilepticus needing ICU care and parenteral antiepileptics are very rare.

Use of medications during ECT course

Patients are commonly initiated on ECT while they are receiving psychotropic medications. It is worthwhile being aware of the potential interactions between ECT and these medications.

- *Antidepressants* – Most anti-depressants are safe during ECT course. As tricyclic antidepressants have anti-cholinergic properties, it is important to monitor heart rate throughout the ECT procedure.
- *Antipsychotics* – Clozapine, at higher doses, lowers the seizure threshold. Hence, there is need to be cautious about prolonged duration of ECT-induced seizures or about the occurrence of spontaneous seizure after recovery from ECT-induced seizure (tardive seizures). Some antipsychotic medications including clozapine have significant anticholinergic properties and warrant monitoring of heart rate. Apart from these considerations, antipsychotics do not have any significant effect during ECT.
- *Anticholinergics* – Anticholinergic medication such as trihexyphenidyl, or agents with stronger anticholinergic properties can increase CNS related adverse events following ECT such as delirium and confusion.
- *Lithium* – It is believed that there is breach in the blood-brain barrier during seizures, leading to increased level of lithium in the CNS. Consequently, lithium may cause prolonged seizures, post-ECT delirium and significant memory impairment. It is advisable to either withhold or maintain serum lithium on the lower side of its therapeutic levels during the ECT course.
- *Antiepileptics* – Valproate, carbamazepine, lamotrigine and topiramate are commonly prescribed as psychotropics. They may raise the seizure threshold, leading to brief, partial, or missed seizures. If seizures cannot be elicited, then these medications may be reduced, or stopped.
- *Benzodiazepines* – These are usually prescribed for sleep problems, agitation or catatonia. They may increase seizure threshold, although to a much lesser extent than antiepileptics. If seizures cannot be elicited, then their dose may be reduced and long-acting benzodiazepine (e.g., clonazepam) may be replaced by short-acting ones (e.g., lorazepam).

Concomitant medications for other medical conditions

- As there is sympathetic surge for a brief period due to seizures, *antihypertensives* and *antianginal* agents prescribed by physician, must be administered with sips of water in the mornings before ECT.
- *Beta-blockers* should be avoided in the mornings before ECT, as they increase the risk of sinus bradycardia or asystole during initial parasympathetic surge.
- *Anti-diabetic medications* increase the risk of hypoglycemia and may cause tardive seizures or post-ictal delirium/ confusion. Hence, oral hypoglycemic agents and insulin must be administered after the ECT session.
- *Theophylline* may prolong the seizure duration and may lead to status epilepticus. An alternative anti-asthma agent should be considered.
- Hypothyroidism is associated with slower metabolism of anesthetic agents causing delayed recovery from anesthesia. Therefore, *Levo-thyroxine* supplementation must be administered with sips of water in the mornings before ECT.

Frequency of ECT Sessions

Commonly, ECTs are administered at frequencies of two or three sessions in a week. If there is need for faster clinical response, then *thrice weekly* schedule may be preferred. On the other hand, when cognitive adverse effects are of concern, *twice weekly* schedule is preferred.

Treatment Course

There is no fixed number of sessions of ECT. It is usually terminated either when patient recovers completely or when plateauing of clinical response is noted. Most patients receive 6 to 12 sessions of ECT. Patients with depression require lesser (around 6 to 8) number of treatments than those with schizophrenia (around 8 to 12 treatments).

Continuation and Maintenance ECT

In a subset of patients who do not tolerate or have inadequate response to conventional pharmacotherapy, ECTs may be administered beyond the index course at a frequency of once a week to once a month. These are called continuation or maintenance ECT. Continuation ECT generally lasts for six-month period; the focus is on prevention of exacerbation of symptoms of the same episode. ECT beyond six-month period to prevent recurrence of another episode is termed as maintenance ECT

Adverse Effects of ECT

ECT-associated adverse effects may broadly be classified into cognitive and non-cognitive effects.

Cognitive adverse Effects

Cognitive adverse effects are commonly reported with ECT and frequently limit initiation and completion of ECT course. On the contrary, pseudodementia, i.e., cognitive impairment seen in depression, particularly in the elderly, has been found to improve in response to ECT. ECT-associated cognitive impairment may be classified as post-ECT disorientation, memory and non-memory disturbances

- Almost all patients experience *post-ECT disorientation*, which lasts for a few minutes. Placing the patient in a calm environment usually suffices. If the patient gets agitated, short-acting benzodiazepines (e.g., midazolam/lorazepam) may be used. Patients often do not recollect this event.

- Severe post-ictal disorientation rarely progresses to *inter-ictal confusion or delirium*. Alcohol withdrawal, recent change in medication or metabolic status can precipitate it. This requires prompt evaluation and management.
- ECT related *memory impairment (amnesia)* is categorized as *retrograde* and *anterograde* amnesia. In the former, there is impairment in retrieving information learned before the commencement of ECT; in the latter, there is impairment in retaining information learnt after the start of ECT.
- Non-memory cognitive functions including concentration, working memory, spatial problem solving may get affected during ECT.

It is pertinent to note that deficits in cognitive abilities are not due to structural brain injury. Almost all ECT-associated cognitive impairment recover within 2-3 weeks from the day of termination of ECT course. Whether ECT causes long-term memory deficits is debatable. While occasional patients complain about such deficits, conclusive objective evidence for lasting memory deficits has remained elusive. Nonetheless, it is standard practice to perform subjective (i.e., report of patients /or their caregivers) and objective (i.e., standardized tests of cognitive functions) assessments before the start of ECT course and after every 2-3 ECT sessions. This helps in early detection of cognitive impairment and in carrying out one or more of the following strategies to address them:

- Change of electrode placement from bitemporal or bifrontal to right unilateral.
- Spacing out ECT sessions from thrice weekly to twice weekly or once weekly, and, if required, witholding ECT.
- Modifying electrical stimulus parameters, e.g., reducing the pulse width.
- Discontinuation or lowering the dose of offending drugs (e.g.,, lithium, anticholinergics)

Non-cognitive Adverse Effects

These range from common somatic complaints such as headache, nausea, vomiting, generalized muscle aches, and jaw pain, to serious life-threatening conditions such as cardiac arrest and status epilepticus (see under prolonged seizures above)

- *Headache* is commonly throbbing in nature, due to vasodilatation in electrode placement regions. It often subsides within a few minutes. If it is excruciating or persists longer, paracetamol or NSAIDs may be used.
- *Nausea* may cooccur with headache and it responds to antiemetics.
- *Vomiting* may be due to residual effects of anesthetic agents on peristaltic movements. Feeding must be initiated with fluids first and with solids later. If there is *projectile vomiting*, raised intracranial tension should be suspected and evaluated for.
- Cardiac complications include bradycardia, asystole during parasympathetic activation and tachycardia, atrial and ventricular arrhythmias, hypertension during activation of the sympathetic nervous system. Atropine can be given for the former condition and short acting beta-blockers such as esmolol is to be considered for the latter condition.

Mortality

With proper selection of patients and appropriate precautions, mortality can be minimized. Rate of deaths within 48 hours following ECT is around 1 per 10,000 patients or 2 per 100,000 sessions. This is comparable to that of general anesthesia for minor surgical procedures.

In summary, if standard methods are followed, adverse effects and mortality related to ECT can be minimized.

ECT in Special populations

Some patients need additional precautions during ECT, as they have accentuated risk for adverse events:

i. ***Pre-existing medical comorbidities***

Cardiovascular conditions

ECT causes transient but considerable stress on the cardiovascular system. Co-existing cardiovascular conditions amplify the risk of adverse cardiac events. These include recent myocardial infarction, unstable angina, post coronary artery bypass graft status, cardiac failure with ejection fraction< 50%, valvular heart disease and aortic stenosis. In these conditions, the initial vagal stimulation can precipitate sinus bradycardia, atrioventricular block or sinus arrest, leading to supraventricular tachyarrhythmias. Sympathetic surge due to seizures may cause ventricular tachycardia, premature contractions and fibrillation. Ventricular tachyarrhythmia and hypertension may synergistically increase myocardial oxygen demand in the compromised cardiac hypoperfusion status. In patients with cardiac risks, consultation with cardiologist should be done as a part of pre-ECT evaluation. Besides routine ECG, echocardiogram, cardiac stress test may be required in such cases. These patients require continuous monitoring besides routine ECG vital signs throughout the procedure till post-ECT recovery. Etomidate and remifentanil are safer anesthetic agents as they cause lesser hemodynamic fluctuations. For pre-medication glycopyrrolate may be preferred to atropine as it has lesser effect on heart rate. ECT can be safely conducted in those with implanted cardiac pacemakers as the electrical charge delivered via electrodes over skull does not get transmitted to the in-situ pacemaker. Fixed mode of pacemaker's activity is continued during ECT treatment as well.

Neurological conditions

ECT induced seizures increase cerebral flow by about 3 folds and oxygen demand by about 2 folds. These are of concern in patients with higher intracranial pressure, such as intracranial space occupying lesions, hemorrhagic cerebrovascular accidents and recent traumatic brain injury. In these conditions, both systemic hypertension as well as intracranial tension must be adequately controlled. Dexamethasone and nitroglycerine may be used for controlling increase in intracranial pressure. ECT is relatively safer in patients with ischemic cerebrovascular accidents. However, appropriate measures should be taken to avoid hypotension, which may cause hypoperfusion in ischemic brain regions. In patients with epilepsy, possibility of increase in seizure threshold due to anticonvulsants needs to be addressed without accentuating the risk of prolonged seizure during ECT.

Other medical conditions

In patients with myasthenia gravis, lower doses of muscle relaxants are used to avoid myasthenic crisis. In those with dyselectrolytemia, optimal correction of electrolytes should be ensured during ECT, as hyperkalemia may cause cardiac arrest and hypokalemia may prolong apnea time; hyponatremia may cause prolonged or tardive seizures and hypernatremia increases the seizure threshold.

ii. ***Extremes of age – Children, adolescents and elderly***

ECT is used far less often *in children and adolescents* due to several concerns. There is dearth of studies examining the effects of ECT on the developing brain. There are ethical and legal concerns as well – these are elaborated later in this chapter. Regardless of these concerns, ECT has been used in children to successfully treat severe psychiatric conditions, without apparent adverse effects. Children have lower seizure threshold and experience more instances of prolonged seizures. Hence, use of lower starting electrical dose, smaller dose increments and EEG monitoring are recommended in children.

In older adults, comorbid medical conditions and use of multiple medications are common. These may have complex interactions with ECT procedure. Further, age-related changes make their cerebral vasculature fragile. Rise in blood pressure during ECT aggravates the risk for the rupture of cerebral vessels. Therefore, there is greater emphasis on optimization of blood pressure in this population, even in the absence of pre-existing systemic hypertension. Elderly patients experience greater impairment in cognitive functions; modifications in ECT administration procedure are more often required in them to mitigate cognitive deficits. Due to decline in hepatic and renal functioning with age, relatively lower (50-80% of usual adult dose) dose of anesthetic agent and muscle relaxant may be required in this population.

iii. ***Pregnancy and lactation***

With appropriate measures, ECT can be carried out safely and effectively in all the three trimesters of *pregnancy*. Nevertheless, it is prudent to have liaison with an obstetrician prior to starting ECT. The electrical charge *per se* does not transmit to the uterus. Hence, there is no direct impact of electrical charge on the fetus. Thiopentone and succinylcholine, which are routinely used during ECT are too short-acting to have teratogenic effect. Glycopyrrolate may be preferred to atropine due to its lesser trans-placental permeability. Risk of abortion with ECT does not appear to be different from that for pregnant women with mental illness unexposed to ECT. After the first trimester, there is relaxation of esophageal sphincter, with increased risk of gastric reflux fluid aspiration under anesthesia. Proton pump inhibitors and prokinetic agents may be given intravenously 2-3 hours prior to ECT to prevent this. Fetal heart rate monitoring throughout the ECT procedure helps in quick detection of signs of fetal distress. After 20 weeks of pregnancy, the woman should rest in supine position with a lateral tilt of about 15-20 degrees angle with a wedge under the right hip. This prevents compression of large vessels. Convulsions *per se*, do not cause uterine contractions but the oxytocin release during seizure may precipitate uterine contractions. Tocolytics such as ritodrine or magnesium should be used if persistent uterine contractions are observed during or shortly after ECT. Presence of an obstetrician enhances the care of pregnant women during ECT.

ECT is safe during lactation. In fact, it is safer than psychiatric medications, which get expressed in the breastmilk.

Electrical aspects

Figure 44.3 depicts components of an ECT electrical train. These include amplitude (electrical current), pulse-width (time-period of each pulse) and pulse frequency (number of pulses per second, PPS), and train length

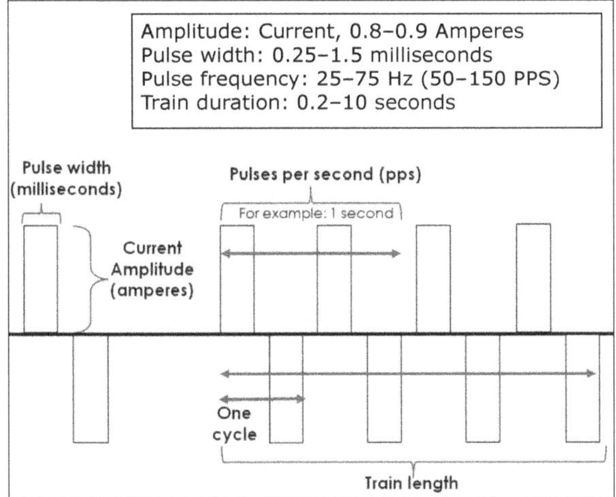

Fig. 44.4: Representative image of components of pulse waveform (Units and typical range of different components is shown in the textbox).

(stimulus duration). A pair of successive pulses in opposite directions constitutes one cycle; pulse frequency can also be mentioned as cycles per second (Hz; 1 Hz = 2 PPS). The charge is calculated by using the following formula:

Charge = current (in Amperes) × pulse width (in milliseconds) × pulse frequency (pps) × length of train (in seconds)

Stimulus Dosing Methods

Electrical charge to be used for a patient is determined in several ways. Empirical titration method is widely used. 'Seizure threshold' is the minimum electrical charge required to elicit a generalized seizure. In the titration method, seizure threshold is determined by starting with a low charge stimulus and up-titrating it gradually until a generalized seizure is elicited. In the subsequent sessions, the intensity would be 1.5 to 2.5 times suprathreshold for bilateral and 4 to 6 times suprathreshold for unilateral ECT. Seizure threshold depends on several factors. Factors associated with higher seizure threshold are:

- Age and sex: Older age, males
- Medications: Anticonvulsants, benzodiazepines
- Metabolic: Hypoxemia, hypercapnia, hypernatremia,
- ECT related: Bilateral electrode placement, later sessions in an ECT course

Mechanism of Action of ECT

Elicitation of seizure is necessary for the action of ECT. However, how seizure causes reduction of symptoms is not clear and is a subject of continued research in this field. Most research on the mechanism of action of ECT has been conducted in depression.

- A few consistent mechanistic findings are:
  - Neuroplasticity: ECT induces neuroplastic changes at synapse (synaptogenesis), neurons (neurogenesis), dendrites (dendrogenesis), vasculature (angiogenesis), as well as glial cells and their processes (gliogenesis)
  - Anticonvulsant theory – Seizures elicited during ECT get aborted spontaneously possibly due to the recruitment of GABA inhibitory neurons. Seizure threshold increases during the course of ECT, suggesting increased GABA-ergic tone.
- ECT seems to reduce the serum cortisol level and to normalize the dexamethasone suppression test. It is thus thought to bring down the hyperactivity of hypothalamo-pituitary-adrenal axis that is associated with depression. ECT perhaps also promotes neuroplasticity – there is evidence for increase in volume and neurogenesis of some regions of the brain such as the hippocampus and for ECT's influence on serum Brain Derived Neurotropic factor (BDNF). However, the precise nature of these and related changes is not yet known.

Trends in the Use of ECT

With the advent of antipsychotic and antidepressant medications in the 1950s and 1960s, the use of ECT has seen a downward trend globally. Nevertheless, substantial number of patients receive ECT across the globe for indications discussed above. It is estimated that about 100 – 500 individuals per million population receive ECT annually in different countries including advanced countries like USA, Australia, New Zealand, and European countries. In other words, about 1,00,000 and 1,30,000 individuals receive ECT annually in the USA and Europe respectively. In India and other Asian countries, about 10–20 percent of all psychiatric inpatients receive ECT; these figures are lower (about 1–5%) in advanced countries.

Public & Media Perspective, Myth & Concerns

Despite robust evidence for its efficacy and safety, the attitude of the public, patients, medical personnel and even the psychiatrists towards ECT is varied. Myths and misconceptions about its procedure, effects and adverse effects are widespread. Mass media have repeatedly showcased ECT as a brutal, punitive and non-consensual procedure for ambiguous indications and have demonstrated unrealistic portrayal of complete erasure of memories or dramatic change in personality with ECT. Transient cognitive effects are often misconstrued as deterioration in general intelligence. The importance of public and professionals having balanced view about ECT based on scientific evidence and without prejudices and misconceptions cannot be overemphasized.

ECT & the Law in India

ECT has specific mention in the latest mental health legislation of India. The Mental Health Care Act (MHCA) 2017 of India has prohibited the "use of ECT without the use of muscle relaxants and anesthesia". As per this law, use of ECT in patients aged less than 18 years can be done only with the informed consent of the guardian and with prior permission of the Mental Health Review Board (MHRB). Further, the Act specifically prohibits the use of ECT as an emergency procedure - this restrains the use of ECT without evaluation in a mental health establishment.

In the recent years, consent process for ECT has evolved as part of the legal and ethical expression of an individual's autonomy in his/her treatment-related decisions. Obtaining written informed consent from the patient is mandatory before starting ECT. If he/she has compromised capacity to make his/her treatment decisions secondary to his/her mental state, then, consent may be obtained from his/her nominated representative. In the latter case, one should obtain the patient's consent after he/she gains decision-making capacity. The crucial elements of an informed consent include the following: rationale for ECT, description of ECT procedure, discussion about the benefits and risks of ECT, alternatives to ECT and a statement that the consent may be withdrawn at any time and for any reason.

Transcranial Magnetic Stimulation (TMS)

Transcranial Magnetic Stimulation (TMS) involves stimulation of brain using magnetic pulses with coils held over the scalp. The device uses electrically insulated coils, through which electricity is passed rapidly. This creates a magnetic field, which passes through the scalp and, in turn, induces electrical impulses in the underlying neural tissue. Scalp and the skull offer considerable resistance to the passage of electricity for focal stimulation of the brain. TMS uses magnetic pulses, which easily pass through these structures and electrically stimulate the underlying part of the brain. TMS coils are of different shapes; the volume of brain stimulated depends on the shape of the coil. The area of brain stimulated by coils that are most commonly used in psychiatry is generally in the range of 2-3 cm^2.

Repetitive Transcranial Magnetic Stimulation (rTMS) uses trains of pulses. The influence of magnetic pulses on the underlying brain depends on the frequency and pattern of the pulses. rTMS with pulse frequency of 1 Hz or less and 5Hz or more, respectively, cause inhibition or excitement of the underlying brain. Based on the observation that patients with depressive disorder have reduced activity in the left dorsolateral prefrontal cortex and those with persistent auditory hallucinations have increased activity in the left temporoparietal junction, high frequency TMS is administered over the left dorsolateral prefrontal cortex and low frequency TMS over the left temporoparietal junction. Typically, rTMS is administered once a day for about 3 – 4 weeks. It has been used to treat a range of psychiatric conditions including depression, auditory hallucinations as part of schizophrenia, obsessive compulsive disorder, tic disorders, etc. The evidence for its use is the most convincing in the treatment of depression, including depression that has not responded to medications. TMS is well tolerated other than mild pain and twitching of the area of stimulation (due to stimulation of superficial nerves of the scalp). Chances of seizure due to rTMS are very remote if it is administered within the safety guidelines prescribed by professional bodies. Cochlear implants, intracranial electrodes for deep brain stimulation, aneurysmal clips, and intracardiac pacemakers are absolute contraindications for TMS. Past history of seizures and metallic implants in the brain are relative contraindications.

Magnetic Seizure Therapy (MST)

Magnetic Seizure Therapy (MST) is convulsive method of brain stimulation, performed under general anesthesia, using a modified TMS device that delivers very high-frequency (25–100 Hz) repetitive magnetic pulses to induce focal seizures. Compared to ECT, cortical region directly stimulated by MST is much less. The coil placement is highly precise during MST. MST has less impact on autonomic nervous system compared to ECT, and it is theorized to spare stimulation of hippocampus. Thus, it is associated with fewer memory deficits and rapid recovery from post-ictal disorientation and less hemodynamic changes. No study has compared MST and ECT.

Transcranial Direct Current Stimulation (tDCS)

Transcranial Direct Current Stimulation (tDCS) is a non-depolarizing, non-convulsive method of modulating brain excitability by applying low intensity, monophasic electric current (usually 1–2 mA) between anode and cathode electrodes placed over the scalp using a portable battery-operated device. It is expected to alter neuronal membrane potential through NMDAR mediated glutamatergic neurotransmission. It does not generate an action potential. Anodal tDCS facilitates *depolarization* of the resting membrane potential and results in enhanced excitability of the underlying cortical area. Cathodal tDCS facilitates *hyperpolarization* of the resting membrane potential and reduces excitability of the underlying cortical area. This property is made use of in treating conditions that are putatively associated with excessive activation or inhibition of certain cortical areas. For instance, application of cathodal tDCS over the left temporoparietal area and anodal stimulation over left dorsolateral prefrontal area has been successfully used to treat auditory hallucinations in schizophrenia and depression respectively. Different cortical areas are targeted for the treatment of obsessive compulsive disorder with tDCS. It is a relatively safe procedure with minor adverse events that are transient.

Vagus Nerve Stimulation (VNS)

VNS involves surgically enfolding of an electrode around the left vagal nerve in the neck; the electrode is connected to the pulse generator that is placed subcutaneously in the left subclavicular region. The left vagus nerve carries most of its afferent nerve fibers to the nucleus tractus solitarius that sends its projection fibers to cortical and limbic regions involved in depressive disorders. Intermittent left vagus nerve stimulation has been hypothesized to cause release of neurotransmitters like serotonin, norepinephrine and gamma amino butyric acid, which may have anti-depressant effects. It uses electrical pulses of 0.25- 1.5mA with pulse width of 0.15 to 0.25 milliseconds with a frequency of 15-20 Hz. VNS has acquired FDA approval for treatment resistant epilepsy and as an add-on treatment for chronic treatment resistant depressive disorder. Hoarseness of voice and cough are common side effects, while bradycardia or asystole are rare adverse events. Rare chances of vagal nerve injury, peri-operative infections, issues related to battery such as depletion, malfunction and replacement and high cost of the procedure and maintenance of VNS are the potential challenges associated with this treatment modality.

Deep Brain Stimulation (DBS)

In DBS, electrodes are implanted in localized brain regions using stereotactic surgical procedure; these electrodes are connected externally to a pacemaker that is surgically placed under the skin in the chest region. The pacemaker delivers continuous, high frequency electrical pulses of 60–130 Hz frequency, 0.06–0.2 milliseconds pulse width, using 2–10 volts batteries. These pulses modulate focal as well as distant connected brain regions. DBS does not cause lesion in implanted brain region. It is reversible, i.e., it can be removed if there is no response or any severe adverse event occurs. DBS is thus more advantageous than other neurosurgical procedures used to treat psychiatric conditions, such as capsulotomy, cingulotomy etc., wherein irreversible lesions are created. Its efficacy is being studied in severe, treatment refractory depression, obsessive compulsive disorder and Tourette syndrome. The subgenual part of cingulate cortex (Brodmann area-25) is the most commonly targeted site in depression; anterior limb of internal capsule is commonly targeted in obsessive compulsive disorder. Adverse effects are largely related to the surgical procedure or the device: peri-operative infection, lead misplacement, breaks in the connection of electrodes to the pacemaker may occur in about 5–10% of the cases; incidences of intracranial hemorrhage and seizure are very rare.

Box 44.2: Facts and Trivia about ECT

- Father of convulsive therapies – Ladislas J Meduna
- d'Elia electrode placement – Right unilateral temporo-parietal electrode placement
- Letemendia electrode placement – Bifrontal electrode placement
- Electricity used during ECT is approximately equivalent to the current used in lighting a 40 watt bulb for less than one second
- Anesthetic agent of choice for ECT in patients with severe cardiovascular comorbidities – Etomidate
- Anesthetic agent should be administered prior to muscle relaxants as patient must be

adequately anesthetized before diaphragmatic muscles start paralyzing. Intact awareness whilst diaphragm is relaxed can precipitate sense of breathlessness and apprehension related to the procedure.

- Addersely and Hamilton introduced the cuff method of seizure monitoring.
- During the cuff-method of monitoring seizures, the cuff must be placed on the right lower / upper limb for right unilateral ECT, in order to ascertain that the seizures are 'generalized' to the left cerebral hemisphere.
- For right unilateral ECT, if single channel EEG is used, it should be placed on the left side to ensure 'generalization' of seizure to the left cerebral hemisphere.
- Cardiovascular complication is the commonest cause of mortality with ECT
- Seizure threshold is estimated in dose titration method whereas it is predicted in age-based methods.
- Widely researched and biologically well implicated brain region in ECT – Hippocampus
- Depiction of ECT in some popular novels and movies (e.g., 'One Flew over the Cuckoo's Nest' 'Shock Corridor') has least resemblance to the contemporary practice of ECT, which is evidence-based, safe and ethical. However, these novels and movies have contributed much to the negative perception about ECT.
- Link to a short movie on ECT may be accessed here: https://www.youtube.com/watch?v=4X75S7yJvjA&list=PLYC2dpOdoBh1bURXLsK-zP38UCvf5U2iN

BIBLIOGRAPHY

1. Gangadhar BN et. al. (2013) ECT Administration Manual. Second Edition Bangalore. National Institute of Mental Health and Neuro Sciences (NIMHANS) Publication.
2. Gangadhar BN et. al. (2015) Handbook of Electroconvulsive therapy. Bangalore. National Institute of Mental Health and Neuro Sciences (NIMHANS) Publication.
3. Waite J and Easton A (2013) The ECT Handbook. Third Edition. London (GB) RCPsych Publications
4. Hussain MM, McClinctock SM and Croarkin PE. (2017) Electroconvulsive Therapy and Other Neurostimulation Treatments. In Kaplan and Sadock's Comprehensive Textbook of Psychiatry. Tenth Edition. Wolters Kluwer.

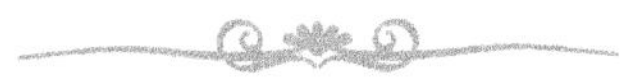

45 Surgeries for Psychiatric Conditions: a brief overview

Chetana Kishore • Janardhanan C. Narayanaswamy • Shyam Sundar Arumugham

The term "Psychosurgery" refers to the use of surgical technics for treatment mood, thoughts and behavioral impairment found in psychiatric disorders.

BACKGROUND

It is based on the premise that most psychiatric conditions have a biological basis. Although a "causative factor" has not been established for most psychiatric disorders, underlying mechanisms involving a combination of dysfunction of signaling, neurotransmission, up/downregulation of receptors and complex circuitry connecting cortical and sub cortical regions have been hypothesized to result in particular manifestation of behaviors. Most patients receive pharmacotherapy as the first line of treatment, with response rate varying between individual disorders. Psychological interventions are also helpful in certain conditions such as anxiety and mood disorders. Non-invasive brain stimulation treatments such as transcranial magnetic stimulation and transcranial direct current stimulation are other emerging treatments. A substantial minority of patients remain non-responders despite multiple treatment trials.

Treatment Resistance vs. Refractoriness

Treatment resistance in various psychiatric disorders such as schizophrenia, depression or Obsessive-compulsive disorder (OCD) is broadly defined as non-response to 2 or more classes of medications along with evidence based non pharmacological treatments, as applicable. The term "refractoriness" is generally used when a condition is non-responsive to all standard modalities of treatment. The clinical situation in such a scenario demands more innovative treatment options including surgical interventions.

HISTORY OF PSYCHOSURGERY

One of the earliest researchers who were noted to have performed the first modern psychosurgical operation was a Swiss psychiatrist Johann Gottlieb Burckhardt in the late 18th century on the basis that "disordered minds were a reflection of disordered brains". He excised various brain regions on patients with intractable illnesses and most of these patients experienced complications. Consequently, his approach was widely criticised.

Later in 1935, Antonio Egas Moniz a Portuguese neurologist conceived a treatment procedure he termed "leucotomy", which is known better today as "lobotomy". It awarded him the Nobel Prize in physiology/medicine in 1949. He is widely regarded as one of the founders of modern psychosurgery. It was part of a wave of new treatments for diseases of neurological/psychiatric origin which was emerging in the early 20th century. In research originating from primate studies, calming effects were observed following removal of frontal lobes. Similar observations were also made in behavior of soldiers who had frontal lobe injuries. This lead him to hypothesise that mental illnesses originated from "abnormal connections in the frontal lobe". Hence Dr. Moniz along with Almeida Lima, a neurosurgeon, developed a surgical treatment that involved disrupting white matter fibers. They initially used absolute alcohol to inject into the frontal lobe. Later they developed a needle like instrument with a retractable wire loop (which helped in separation of white matter fibers) called the "leucotome". The procedure became popularly referred to later as prefrontal leucotomy/ or simply as "Leucotomy". The treatment was considered "radical" and noted to lead to improvement in symptoms which outweighed the dysfunction due to illness and hence enjoyed popularity for few decades till later criticism ensued owing to enduring complications such as personality change and cognitive dysfunction.

The procedure was later popularised in the United States by Walter Jackson Freeman II and James W. Watts, who adopted a modified technic and renamed it "Prefrontal Lobotomy". Instead of the technic used by Moniz, this involved severing of connections between frontal lobe and thalamus. Later, Freeman further simplified it further by using metal pick to gain access to the brain through an orbital approach, which was known as trans-orbital lobotomy or simply known as "ice pick" lobotomy. The procedure was pursued overzealously with over 4000 surgeries performed. Consequently, it fell into disrepute due to the ensuing severe disability on patients and in some, even death. It was criticised by many as the most barbaric of treatments in modern era. The advent of chlorpromazine and other psychopharmacological interventions with its striking on psychiatric symptoms, lead to further decline in popularity of this procedure.

The development of stereotactic surgery (from the stereotactic method developed by Horsley and Clark) revolutionized the field. It makes use of three-dimensional coordinate system that permit the accurate positioning of probes inside the brain. It helps create discrete, subcortical lesions unlike the indiscriminate procedure of frontal leucotomy, which lead to its application in psychiatric disorders. Modern procedures have used computer based data management along with functional imaging and physiologic recording parameters. The main advantage was minimal disruption of brain tissue and accurate targeting leading to lesser side effects.

The first subcortical stereotactic surgery was performed in 1947 by Wycis and Spiegel. They performed dorso-medial (DM) thalamotomy, which is the model on which all modern psychiatric neurosurgical procedures are based.

Four of these stereotactic procedures became especially popular psychosurgical technics. They include cingulotomy, capsulotomy, subcaudate tractotomy and limbic leucotomy. These procedures aim to disrupt activity in the frontal, cingulate areas and their connections with the sub-cortical structures including thalamus. Most studies conducted on these procedures have always been methodically less rigorous. Nevertheless remains an option for severe cases. Ablative surgeries have evolved from crude "ice pick" technics, to the more precise thermo-coagulation, radiofrequency ablation and the markedly less invasive gamma knife technic which employs focused gamma radiation at discrete sites to create lesions.

Non-ablative surgeries include Deep brain stimulation a reversible neurosurgical procedure involving the placement of a medical device called a neuro-stimulator which sends electrical impulses, through implanted electrodes, to specific targets in the brain.

MAIN INDICATIONS

Due to the lack of high quality evidence and the invasive nature of the interventions, surgical interventions are recommended only in chronic, severe and treatment refractory psychiatric conditions. Current evidence supports the use of surgery as an experimental intervention for three main psychiatric indications, namely chronic, severe and refractory:

a) Depressive disorder
b) Obsessive-compulsive disorder (OCD)
c) Tourette syndrome

PROCEDURES

Ablative Procedures

a) CINGULOTOMY: Whitty developed cingulectomy, which was later modified by Ballantine (1962) into anterior cingulotomy which has been employed for treatment of depressive disorder, OCD and intractable pain. It involves creating a bilateral lesion in the anterior cingulate region including the adjacent cingulum bundle. The refinement of magnetic resonance imaging (MRI) has made improved the targeting. It is the commonly employed ablative procedure for the treatment of refractory depressive disorder. Repeat cingulotomy to extend the lesion or subcaudate tractotomy may be performed if there is inadequate response.

Targets: These lesions are expected to interrupt reciprocal connectivity from the dorsal anterior cingulate cortex (ACC) to the orbitofrontal cortex (OFC), amygdala, and hippocampus via the cingulum bundle, thereby affecting the cortico-striato-thalamo-cortical (CSTC) loop.

Adverse effects: No deaths have been reported. Intraoperative or post-operative seizures have been seen occasionally. Low rates of hemorrage and hydrocephalus have been reported, similar to other stereotactic procedures. Urinary incontinence, weight gain are other potential adverse effects. Long term behavioral or cognitive deficits have been rarely reported in psychiatric cingulotomy patients.

b) CAPSULOTOMY: Developed by Leksell and Talairach, it has been in use since 1949. Using radiofrequency or gamma radiation, centre of the anterior and middle third of the anterior limb of the internal capsule at approximately the level of the foramen of Monro is targeted. Magnetic responance guided focused ultrasound (MRgFUS) is another recent development. Recent evidence points to better response from ventral placement of lesions. It is commonly employed for treatment of refractory OCD.

Targets: The lesions are expected to interrupt the ventral fibers traversing the anterior internal capsule from the OFC and subgenual ACC to the thalamic nuclei. Thus, capsulotomy also possibly targets the frontal CSTC loops.

Adverse Effects: It is usually well-tolerated with no deaths directly attributed to the procedure. Transient headaches, confusion, disinhibition, urinary incontinence, weight gain, and lethargy have also been reported. Radiation necrosis and cyst have been reported following gamma knife surgery. Refinement in targeting has markedly decreased the incidence of cognitive and behavioral deficits.

c) SUBCAUDATE TRACTOTOMY: The lesion is placed in the region of substantia innominate inferior to the caudate nucleus. It is also known as Innominatomy, which again attempts to interrupt fibers from the cortex to the thalamus via striatum. It is used less commonly compared to other procedures.

Targets: This lesion interrupts connections between the OFC, subgenual ACC, striatum, thalamus and amygdala.

Adverse Effects: Transient headache and confusion may be seen. Seizures is another possible side effect, which might require anticonvulsants if there are recurrent attacks.

d) **LIMBIC LEUCOTOMY:** This was developed by Kelly and Richardson in the early 1970's. It targets a group of fibers from two distinct regions i.e. a combination of subcaudate tractotomy and cingulotomy. The procedure creates three 6-mm thermo-coagulative or cryogenic lesions in the lower medial quadrant of each frontal lobe (interrupting frontothalamic connections) and 6-mm lesions in the cingulum, bilaterally. One is hypothesized to involve the fronto-thalamic loop whereas the other involves part of the Papez circuit.

Adverse Effects include transient headache, confusion, amotivation, perseverative behavior, and incontinence. Concentration and memory are largely intact.

Non Ablative Procedures

a) **DEEP BRAIN STIMULATION (DBS)**

DBS is a neurosurgical procedure involving the placement of a neurostimulator (colloquially termed a brain 'pacemaker') which sends electrical impulses, through implanted electrodes, to specific targets in the subcortical structures. Although it was earlier developed for use in movement disorders and dystonia, the indications have expanded to include refractory psychiatric conditions including Tourette syndrome, OCD and depressive disorder.

Similar to a cardiac pacemaker, the equipment includes leads, extension cables and an implanted pulse generator (IPG). The IPG is generally placed subcutaneously below the clavicle and is connected to the lead (a coiled wire connected to four platinum-iridium electrodes) via extensions (insulated wire running through the brain to the IPG) and this is placed in different nuclei of the brain. The electrodes are placed surgically usually under local anesthesia using frame/frameless stereotactic procedure through a small burr hole. The electrical dosing is titrated in the IPG to provide a balance between control of symptoms and side effects.

Although the exact mechanisms remains elusive, various hypotheses have been suggested which include a) depolarization blockade at the output site b) synaptic inhibition c) modulating the abnormal oscillatory movements and d) Antidromic activation.

Common targets include the ventral capsule/ventral striatum region and subthalamic nucleus for treatment of OCD. Subcallosal cingulate, and anterior limb of internal capsule are the preferred targets for major depressive disorders. The antero-medial globus pallidus interna (amGPi) and the centromedian parafascicular nucleus (cmPf) of thalamus are the targets used for Tourette syndrome

b) **VAGUS NERVE STIMULATION (VNS)**

VNS started off in 1985 as an experimental procedure to treat epilepsy in dogs by Jacob Zabara. It was later applied in studying epilepsy in humans by Dean and Penry. Based on studies in late 1990s it was used in treating cases of treatment refractory depression after noticing beneficial effects on depressive symptoms in patients with epilepsy. Although the exact mechanism is unknown, it is believed that vagal projection into the solitary tract nucleus modulates various structures including amygdala and ventromedial prefrontal cortex leading to improvement in mood symptoms. Although immediate post-operative and short term follow up has shown low effectiveness, long-term studies have shown reduction of symptoms in a proportion of patients.

EFFICACY OF THE PROCEDURES

Barring a few randomized sham controlled trials (RCTs), especially on DBS, there is insufficient high quality evidence on these interventions. Hence psychosurgery is still considered an experimental treatment which may be attempted in refractory OCD, depression and Tourette syndrome. The available data suggest that most of these procedures are helpful in around half the subjects with the improvement occurring 6-12 months following the surgery. Like other functional neurosurgical procedures, psychosurgery aims at symptomatic improvement and is not curative. Pharmacological and psychological interventions may have to be continued following surgery to sustain improvement.

a) Depression:

Review of ablative surgeries showed varied response rates ranging from 44-92% for Cingulotomy, 60-100% for subcaudate tractomy and 30-78% for limbic leucotomy. Despite some inconsistent results, a recent meta-analysis of double blinded RCTs on DBS in depression showed significant reduction in depressive symptom scores with active DBS.

b) Obsessive Compulsive Disorder:

Review of ablative procedures in OCD revealed almost two thirds of patients undergoing capsulotomy showed response, with 30-60% response rates to Cingulotomy and 30-50% response rates for subcaudate tractomy. A meta-analysis conducted by Alonso et al on DBS in treatment refractory OCD patients identified response rates close to 60%. There are double blinded sham controlled trials demonstrating the efficacy of DBS in OCD. The US FDA has provided a humanitarian device exemption for use of DBS in refractory OCD.

c) Tourette syndrome:

DBS over amGPi and cmPf have been found to be helpful in refractory Tourette syndrome, with around 53% reduction in symptom severity. There is also some support from small RCTs to support its efficacy for this indicaton.

LEGAL SCENARIO IN INDIA

According to the latest Mental health care act 2017, mandates the approval of the state mental health review board before performing psychosurgery. This is in par with the practice worldwide, where a review by independent clinicians is generally obtained prior to performing surgery along with detailed informed consent.

SUMMARY

Surgical interventions are considered for chronic, severe and treatment refractory psychiatric conditions. Despite its chequered past, there has been re-emergence of interest in this field due to recent advancements in safety and precision of the interventions. Ablative procedures such as cingulotomy and capsulotomy have been found to be helpful in depressive disorder and OCD. There is an increased interest in DBS recently due to its reversibility, particularly for major depressive disorder, OCD and Tourette syndrome. Methodologically rigorous studies with greater number of subjects are required to advance our knowledge and improve our understanding on the role of surgical procedures in psychiatric practice.

BIBLIOGRAPHY

1. Alonso, P., Cuadras, D., Gabriëls, L., Denys, D., Goodman, W., Greenberg, B. D., ... & Nuttin, B. (2015). Deep brain stimulation for obsessive-compulsive disorder: a meta-analysis of treatment outcome and predictors of response. PloS one, 10(7), e0133591.
2. Aouizerate, B., Rotgé, J. Y., Martin-Guehl, C., Cuny, E., Rougier, A., Guehl, D., ... & Tignol, J. (2006). A systematic review of psychosurgical treatments for obsessive-compulsive disorder: does deep brain stimulation represent the future trend in psychosurgery. Clin Neuropsychiatry, 3(6), 391-403.
3. Andrade, P., Noblesse, L. H., Temel, Y., Ackermans, L., Lim, L. W., Steinbusch, H. W., & Visser-Vandewalle, V. (2010). Neurostimulatory and ablative treatment options in major depressive disorder: a systematic review. *Acta neurochirurgica*, *152*(4), 565-577.
4. Doshi, P. K., Arumugham, S. S., Bhide, A., Vaishya, S., Desai, A., Singh, O. P., ... & Srinivas, D. (2019). Indian guidelines on neurosurgical interventions in psychiatric disorders. *Indian journal of psychiatry*, *61*(1), 13.
5. Lakhan, S. E., & Callaway, E. (2010). Deep brain stimulation for obsessive-compulsive disorder and treatment-resistant depression: systematic review. BMC Research Notes, 3(1), 60.
6. Lapidus, K. A., Kopell, B. H., Ben-Haim, S., Rezai, A. R., & Goodman, W. K. (2013). History of psychosurgery: a psychiatrist's perspective. *World neurosurgery*, *80*(3-4), S27-e1.

46 Rehabilitation in Psychiatry

Kirti Yeshwant Tandel

INTRODUCTION

Rehabilitation in Psychiatry is a process, which delivers opportunities for persons with mental illnesses (PMI) to reach an optimum level of independent functioning in the community. By involving the patient's family and community, supported by a policy planner, the mental health professional often a Psychiatrist, develops an individualized program for the PMI. The goals of this program focus on maximizing the patient's resources and minimizing the disabilities in the socio-occupational domains, with an aim of mainstreaming the patient.

HISTORY OF PSYCHIATRIC REHABILITATION IN INDIA

1436 to 1469 A.D.	Mental hospital by Mohammad Khilji, at Dhar, near Mandu (Madhya Pradesh)
1858	The Indian Lunatic Asylum Act enacted by the British Government. The lunatic asylums were under the direct supervision of a medical officer.
1895	Dr. W. R. Rice, Surgeon general stressed the importance of Occupational Therapy for persons with mental illnesses as part of Psychiatric treatment
1870s to 1890s	Rehabilitation program for mentally ill at Mysore Lunatic Asylum called as 'Work Therapy', where persons with mental illnesses were involved in agricultural activities
1912	Indian Lunacy Act enacted by the British Government to develop conditions and functions of the lunatic asylums and improve the care of the mentally ill. The word 'Lunatic Asylum' was changed to 'Mental Hospital"
1929	Dr. Barkeley Hill founded 'The Indian Association for Mental Hygiene' which encouraged the study of mental health in the community.
1947	Indian Psychiatric Society was established
1950	Department of Occupational Therapy at Central Institute of Psychiatry, Ranchi
1954	Dr. Vidyasagar introduced the involvement of family in the psychiatric treatment at Amritsar Hospital, Punjab
1960	First Day Care centre for the mentally ill established at the All India Institute of Mental Health, Bangalore, which offered vocational training in carpentry, weaving, tailoring, candle making, etc.
1960s	Mental Health Center started at Christian Medical College Hospital, Vellore. Family members stayed along with patients. The patients engaged in tailoring, basket making, carpentry, etc.
1962	Day hospital started in Institute of Mental Health, Madras. It offered different vocational training.

(Continued...)

1964	First voluntary organization for the persons called Medico Pastoral Association (MPA) at Bangalore which organised counseling services and group activities.
1970s	Home based rehabilitation program for patients with Schizophrenia started by NIMHANS, Bangalore focusing on patients not able to avail the mental health facilities due to stigma, distance of the hospital from home, an poor drug compliance.
1972	First Halfway Home was established by Medico Pastoral Association (MPA)
1981	The International Year of Disabled celebrated by the United Nations in 1981, giving importance to the community based rehabilitation services for the people with disability.
1982	National Mental Health Programe (NMHP) was started by the Government of India three objectives, which emphasized on Psychiatric Rehabilitation for the mentally ill persons in the community
1983	Schizophrenia Care and Research Foundation (SCARF) was established by Dr. Saratha menon at Madras to provide various skills training for the mentally ill.
1986	World Association for Psychiatric Rehabilitation (Indian Chapter) (WAPR - IC) was established by Dr. sarada menon at Madras.
1987	Mental Health Act (MHA) established
2017	Mental Health Care Act (MHCA) passed. Emphasised on hospital and community based rehabilitation establishments and services, provision of half-way homes, sheltered accommodation, supported accommodation and provision for mental health services to support family of person with mental illness or home based rehabilitation

BASIC TERMINOLOGIES IN PSYCHIATRIC REHABILITATION

People with psychiatric disabilities have several complex factors that account for their life problems that make it difficult for the person to attain typical, age-appropriate goals for extended periods of time. These age-appropriate life goals may fall in the domains of economic, occupation, vocation, relationships, commitment, intimacy, family dynamics, physical and mental health, recreation and spirituality.

The psychiatric disabilities can be understood in the following four concepts:

1. **Diagnosis** – It's a representation of the collections of symptoms and dysfunctions that join together to form a meaningful syndrome. E.g. Schizophrenia, the mood disorders, anxiety disorders, obsessive–compulsive disorder (OCD). Substance use disorders and some personality disorders.
2. **Course** - Psychiatric syndromes not only vary among individuals in terms of the onset and course of the illness but also vary within the individual over time in terms of the severity of symptoms and the resulting dysfunctions.
3. **Co-morbidity** – It's very rare for Psychiatric illnesses to occur in isolation. This co-occurrence of other disorders significantly impedes the life goals; e.g. Substance use disorders frequently occur with psychiatric illnesses and further worsen the disease course.
4. **Disabilities** – This term refers to the inability of people with psychiatric illnesses to meet age and culture-appropriate life goals. These goals may range from acquiring a satisfactory job, managing one's physical and psychological health needs, enjoying life through leisure and spiritual pursuits, living

self-sufficiently or developing intimate and mature relationships. Handicap is a disadvantage from a disability that limits a role that can be performed by the individual.

RELATIONSHIP BETWEEN LIFE GOALS AND DISABILITIES

Disabilities are the absolute focus of Psychiatric Rehabilitation. Disabilities in mental health can be defined as those psychological phenomena that result from mental illnesses which block the attainment of goals and objectives in the majority of life domains. Thus the goal of Psychiatric Rehabilitation differs from other approaches in psychiatric care by helping people overcome their disabilities and enabling them to achieve their life goals.

What are Rehabilitation specific Life Goals?

Life goals are mostly age-defined and culturally influenced and serve as benchmarks for achievement. The rehabilitation program should take into consideration that the definitive definition of specific goals depends on people's understandings with their culture, ethos and their individual desires. The life goals can be categorized in following stages:

1. ***Finishing the required education and training to pursue one's vocation.***

   Education is the typical pathway most of us take to accomplish our work goals. It teaches the basic abilities that are required to be successful on the job. It provides work or vocation specific skills that are necessary for jobs e.g., computer skills needed in an information technology position. It also gives one a sense of mastery and competence. Work is the basis on which most people acquire an income to accomplish their independent living goals and thus acts like a source of identity. One's vocation provides a sense of position and recognition within the larger milieu of society. It defines a person's interpersonal association with the society he or she dwells in and gives a sense of belief of individuality and involvement in a personally meaningful industry.

2. ***Setting up an independent life style and managing household.***

   People with psychiatric disabilities need support to productively live in their own households. This also involves the decision about with whom the person resides like family members or alone, with friends or with work colleagues. Psychiatric Rehabilitation providers must assist people with the evolution of their independent living needs.

3. ***Acquire one's vocational goals.***

   Work has helpful effects on psychological wellness, helping an individual to feel productive. Through work an individual is able to develop vocational skills, connect to job services in the society, gets help with career planning and provides transportation aid.

4. ***Establishing an intimate and long-term relationship.***

   Adults change the form of interaction with their family of origin from a dependent pattern to an independent one. They seek a mutually loving relationship with siblings, parents and thereafter search for a significant other with whom they can develop an intimate long-standing relationship. Later on this relationship yields children and the family concept gives rise to challenges and responsibilities.

5. ***Addressing personal recreational and spiritual needs.***

   Work, relationships, health, and housing are only a part of adult life. Recreation offers a chance to widen one's interaction with the world. e.g.,hobbies. Religiousness can be a mean for people to around common ways of worshiping. Spirituality helps people to think about one's self as part of a larger force. Studies have shown that both religiousness and spirituality are linked with psychological well-being and less psychiatric symptoms.

Case 1: Mr. A is a 30-year-old man who had schizophrenia for the last ten years. After treatment and symptoms well under control, he goes back to his home and community. However he finds out that all his colleagues are now settled in their careers, some are even married and are doing well with their own families. His family wants him to work in a high paying job and stay occupied and support them. This confuses him and he feels lost and demoralized. But he is still capable enough to remember and use his skills and capabilities. Thus, it becomes very important that Mr. A receives the support of a mental health professional in assessing his changed circumstances. He needs assistance in deciding what skills he may be able to use, or what vocation he would like to choose. At the same time his family also needs to understand the situation and look at him as an individual and not his illness. This will certainly help Mr. A to acknowledge his own strengths and his aspirations.

Case 2: Ms B is a 22-year-old medical student diagnosed with bipolar mood disorder for which she was treated for the last 4 years. After treatment, she finds it difficult to get back to studies and complete the medical curriculum, which makes her think to do something else apart from medicine. However her family members are not supportive. They insist that she should finish her degree and at least start with general practice because anything less than that would be beneath their social status. Here, the family needs to be understanding and supportive towards Ms B and be empathetic towards their daughter's interests and capabilities which might have changed due to the previous illness.

WHAT IS REHABILITATION?

Rehabilitation is derived from the Roman Latin word 'habilitas' which means to reskill, to restore to a former capacity, to reinstate and to restore. It aims to prepare an individual to resume normal life after an illness or to restore to their former way of living. It is the process of helping people with mental health disorders to make the best use of their residual capabilities to function at an optimum level in as normal a context as possible.

What is Psychiatric Rehabilitation?

Psychiatric Rehabilitation is a process that helps an individual to recover from the difficulties of chronic mental health disorders. The Psychiatric Rehabilitation services help and support the individual who finds it difficult to cope with the everyday life or get on with other people in his socio-occupational domain. The different approaches in Psychiatric Rehabilitation helps the person to deal with problems, helps self-esteem to build up and get back their confidence back thus helping them to live an independent way of life.

GOALS OF PSYCHIATRIC REHABILITATION

The objectives of Psychiatric Rehabilitation revolves around enabling the person to perform their physical, emotional, social and intellectual skills which are required to live, work, learn and adapt in the society with the least amount of support necessary. The fundamental principle of the whole rehabilitation process is structured to improve the person's competencies and resilience and center on adjustment to everyday life. The broad process involves step-by-step assessment, training and amendment of living environments in different areas of the person's functioning relevant to individual and community life. These areas of functioning includes especially self-care, maintaining interpersonal relationships, peers and friendships, employment and vocational pursuits, financial management, residential living, food habits, transportation, etc. All the goals can be grouped under the following main categories:

1. ***To help person with mental illness to achieve recovery***

   The goal of recovery is a defining one in the process of rehabilitation. It is unique for each person with varying guidelines for achieving it.

2. ***To help person with mental illness to achieve maximum community integration***

   This goal helps the person to live with a degree of independence in the community and is one of the most consistent goals in the rehabilitation process. It helps the individual to achieve self-direction, rehabilitation and recovery.

3. ***To help person with mental illness to achieve highest possible Quality of Life***
   Regardless of the stage of the individual's illness and severity, all the importance should be given to achieve the highest quality of life possible. The concept of quality of life refers to an individual's subjective sense of life, for example, how he or she feels about the living arrangement and to the objective or goal e.g., annual income. It includes social support, food, shelter, companionship, employment, an active sex life etc.

VALUES OF PSYCHIATRIC REHABILITATION

1. **RIGHTS** - Everyone has the right of self-determination, including participation in all decisions that affect their lives
2. **DIGNITY** - Psychiatric Rehabilitation interventions respect and preserve the dignity and worth of every human being, regardless of the degree of impairment, disability, or handicap
3. **RECOVERY** - Optimism regarding the improvement and eventual recovery of persons with severe mental illness is a critical element of all services
4. **CAPABLE** - Everyone has the capacity to learn and grow
5. **SENSITIVE** - Psychiatric Rehabilitation services are sensitive to and respectful of the individual, cultural and ethnic differences of each consumer

GUIDING PRINCIPLES OF PSYCHIATRIC REHABILITATION

1. ***Individualization of All Services***
   - Responding to the individual needs and desires of the person.
   - allows each person to develop in the way he or she desires
2. ***Maximum Client Involvement, Preference, and Choice***
   - The rehabilitation module must be related to the very personal nature of individual's set of preferences, values, and aspirations.
3. ***Partnership between Service Provider and Service Recipient***
   - a positive connection between the service provider and the patient
   - Characterized by mutual respect and trust, working together to develop effective rehabilitation strategies.
   - Rehabilitation service providers bring specialized knowledge, skills, and technics whereas patients bring their experiences and understanding of their own needs and preferences

4. ***Normalized and Community-Based Services***
- In normalized residential settings, patients live in decent, harmless neighborhoods with equal access to transportation, shopping and other resources.
- They interact with neighbors with active participation in community activities unlike in a institutionalized settings where their social roles get restricted.

5. ***Strengths Focus***
- Recognition and building on an individual's strengths rather than weaknesses.
- Allowing patients and service providers to develop relationships around work and recreational activities.

6. **Situational Assessments**
- Focusing on the skills and modifications necessary for the patient to function effectively in the situations of his or her choice.
- Assessing their ability to meet the necessities of the chosen vocation by observing them completing necessary tasks in different environments.

7. ***Treatment/Rehabilitation Integration, Holistic Approach***
- Patients need knowledge and skills to comply with a treatment regimen along with monitoring the symptoms and side effects, thus helping them to communicate this to their doctor.
- Psychoeducation helps an individual to monitor and share the required information about symptoms, medications, side effects etc.
- Treatment and rehabilitation are complementary and interdependent.

8. ***Ongoing, Accessible, Coordinated Services***
- Services should be easily accessible, coordinated to ensure availability and avoid duplication and must be intended to accommodate the diverse and changing needs of individuals who may require different levels of services during different stages of their illness.
- Coordination of different services is also a vital aspect of successful community integration.

9. ***Vocational Focus***
- Work is a significant aspect of life and should be available to everyone who wants it.
- Assisting the individual to acquire the skills and resources necessary for successful independent life.

10. ***Skills Training***
- Helping individuals in recovery acquire the skills essential to function successfully in the surroundings of their choice.
- Identifying the skills needed to succeed and helping to acquire them.
- Using role play to teach the skills and provide opportunities for practice until the skill has been mastered

11. ***Environmental Modifications and Supports***
- Helping individuals with disabilities to access or negotiate the environmental modifications essential to function successfully, e.g., providing a ramp for someone with wheelchair

12. ***Partnership with the Family***
- Families are, the most vital and steady support system for people with mental illness.
- Inclusion of family members as partners whenever possible.
- Family psychoeducation, multiple family groups with the patient present is recognized as an evidence based practice.

13. *Evaluative, Assessment, Outcome-Oriented Focus*

- Periodic evaluation and assessment of the outcomes achieved and reviewing the quality of services on both an individual and a system-wide level.
- Identifying changes in the needs of the patients and modifying the programs accordingly

THE CONCEPTUAL FRAMEWORK OF REHABILITATION IN PSYCHIATRY

The loss or abnormality of psychological function in a mental health disorder limits the person's social and vocational roles in a community, which leads to significant disability. Disability as described earlier is a restriction to an individual's ability to perform a function. Unemployment resulting due to disability along with stigma and discrimination add to the overall problems that an individual with mental illness has to suffer in the community.

The Stress-vulnerability-protective factors model

Stress is often described to have a biopsychosocial basis. Chronic stress such as chronic work stress, interpersonal conflicts, marital problems, etc. can lead to mental health disorders. Genetic or biological predispositon is a known etiology for increasing vulnerability to psychiatric disorders. However, childhood trauma such as child abuse can also increase the vulnerability to psychiatric disorders leading to personality disorders and disturbed attachments. It is found that even low levels of stress may precipitate psychiatric illnesses in individuals with heightened vulnerability. Thus protective and precautionary factors such as the individual's resilience, effective coping mechanisms, social supports, adherence to treatment can help the person to prevent relapse and maintain remission. Rehabilitation and vocational programs developed on this model can act as a protective measure in preventing relapse and assisting recovery.

THE REHABILITATION TEAM

The basic Psychiatric Rehabilitation team includes the following:

1. Psychiatrists
2. Psychologists
3. Nurses
4. Occupational therapists
5. Social workers.

WHO NEEDS PSYCHIATRIC REHABILITATION SERVICES?

Person with mental illnesses may have difficulties in their socio-occupational domain at different stages of recovery. These difficulties may include:

1. Difficulty to organize and plan a daily routine and managing everyday activities like self-care, budgeting, shopping, cooking and money management.
2. Symptoms of psychiatric disorders such as Schizophrenia eg. auditory hallucinations which are distressing and which makes it difficult to communicate
3. Medicolegal implications due to behavior problems accompanying psychiatric illnesses especially in violent behavior which is found difficult or threatening
4. Co-morbid substance misuse which needs a systematic deaddiction plan
5. Being exploited or abused by others
6. Cognitive symptoms in psychiatric illnesses with difficulty in concentration, motivation and inability to organize oneself.
7. Poor response to pharmacological treatment options

8. Comorbid depression and anxiety with active suicidal ideations

THE REHABILITATION PROCESS

The Diagnosis–Planning–Intervention (DPI) Process of Psychiatric Rehabilitation

The rehabilitation process begins with the mental health professional, mostly the Psychiatrist, taking a detailed history of the patient regarding his strengths and interests. After the family understands the person's skills and limitations, it becomes easier for them to accept that their patient can lead a happy and satisfactory life according to his or her choices, that best suits the circumstances.

The psychiatrist builds a rapport with the patient with repeated engagements and tries to understand the problems that he may be facing as well as the family's perspective towards the illness. This helps the psychiatrist to make the person look forward to living an independent life in spite of the limitations posed by the illness.

The Diagnostic Phase

The Psychiatrist then helps the patient to self-determine readiness for rehabilitation and to develop readiness, if required. Then he helps the patient to set overall goals for rehabilitation and evaluate the skills and strengths related to them. The diagnostic information retrieved thereafter helps the psychiatrist to develop a rehabilitation plan for the planning phase.

The Planning Phase

In the rehabilitation plan, the goal of a treatment plan is focused mostly on reducing symptoms. It specifies how to develop the person's skills, strengths and supports in order to achieve the rehabilitation goals.

The Intervention Phase

In this phase, the plan is implemented to achieve the rehabilitation goals by altering the person

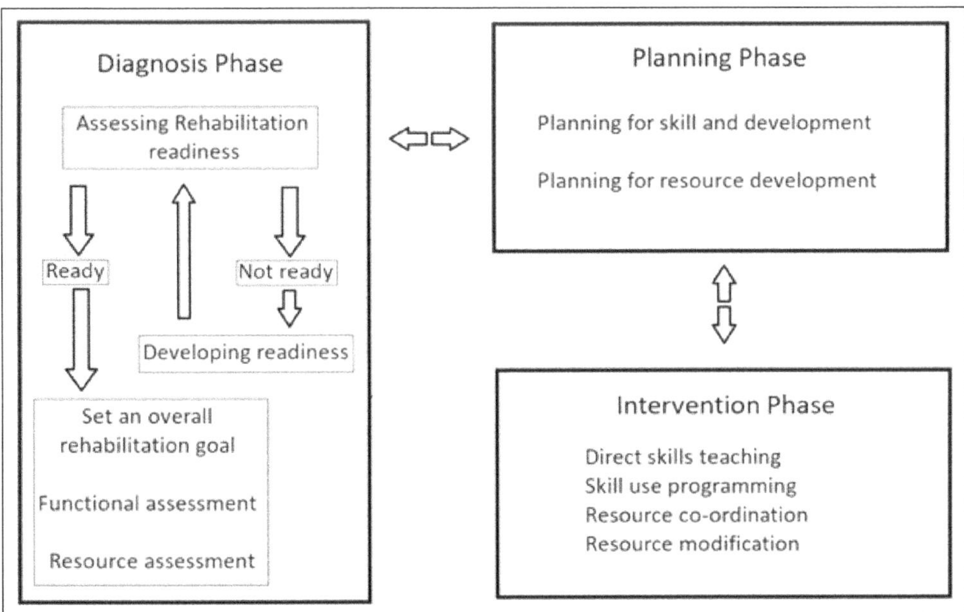

Fig. 46.1: An Overview of Diagnosis-Planning-Intervention Process of Psychiatric Rehabilitation.

and the surroundings, through developing the patient's skills and developing the environmental supports.

1. ASSESSMENTS

Clinical assessment is an integral component of understanding a case and subsequent treatment planning. Ongoing assessment and symptom monitoring help in titrating the degree of support required, taking early interventions to avoid a relapse, timing of new initiatives in the individual's life such as applying for a job and negotiating the termination of any support. Assessments help the service provider to assess the progress of the disorder.

- Assessments of Symptoms and Cognition
- Assessment of functioning and disability
- Assessment of Recovery, Strengths and Empowerment
- Assessment of Quality of Life

2. THERAPEUTIC SKILLS AND INTERVENTIONS

A. *SELF-MANAGEMENT OF PSYCHIATRIC ILLNESS*

An important goal of Psychiatric Rehabilitation is to help an individual to learn how to manage their psychiatric disabilities. This includes helping them to understand the nature and treatment of their illness and assisting them to develop strategies for minimizing their impact on their social lives. The person's ability to manage his or her own illness is an important step towards achieving a sense of personal wellness and control over one's own destiny because poor self-control over a psychiatric disorder can wreak havoc in the lives of these individuals as well as their caregivers

Self-management of one's psychiatric illness can be described as

- The ability to make informed treatment decisions,
- Reducing the impact of distressing or otherwise problematic symptoms
- Reducing relapses and rehospitalizations.
- To identify and pursue personal goals and to develop a physically and psychologically healthy lifestyle with hope, purpose and optimism

Approaches for illness self-management may also include:

- Shared decision making
- Psychoeducation (information about their psychiatric disabilities and the available treatments to make informed decisions)
- Enhancing adherence to medications with psychoeducation (both individual and family), motivational interviewing, behavioral tailoring and simplifying the medication regimen
- Relapse prevention training by educating people about nature of relapses, early warning signs of relapse, trigger identifications and establishing a relapse prevention plan
- Coping skills training and cognitive restructuring by helping people become more aware of their thoughts and beliefs in different situations and help to face them when they are associated with strong negative feelings.
- Self-help and peer support

B. *CASE MANAGEMENT*

Case management is defined as a process of accessing, coordinating and ensuring the receipt of services to assist individuals with psychiatric disabilities to meet their multiple and complex needs in an effective and efficient manner.

The major goals of case management are

- To maintain contact with the service providers
- To prevent aggravation of the illness to avoid hospitalization
- To reduce the duration of hospitalization
- To promote psychosocial functioning at the highest level during hospitalization
- To improve the quality of life for the individual and their family caregivers

There are different models described in case management. They are:

- Broker case management
- Clinical case management
- Strengths-based case management
- Rehabilitation case management
- Assertive community treatment
- Intensive case management

C. *MEDICATIONS AND PSYCHIATRIC REHABILITATION*

The rehabilitation process essentially includes learning to use medications effectively. However difficult it may seem, it requires a broader understanding of the medicines involved along with the responsibility to manage one's own illness. Psychiatrists often believe that "medication compliance" is very important and hence they encourage people to use their medications as prescribed. Yet it is a known fact that the patient often questions the need for medications, perceive a mixed picture of benefits and adverse effects related to medications and get information from many unreliable sources. Due to this they quietly experiment with their medications and make decisions on their own about how and when to take them often leading to misinformed decisions leading to relapse and rehospitalizations.

Psychoeducation and a trusting relationship with the doctor are core to a successful rehabilitation plan that mainly focuses on treatment adherence as a guiding principle. Psychiatric rehabilitation modules can work upon the following:

- Providing education and helping the person to communicate effectively
- Building a trusting relationship with the care provider,
- Overcoming concomitant substance abuse
- Developing personal strategies for using medications effectively.

D. *HOUSING*

Housing has a central role in psychiatric rehabilitation process. At an individual level, having a decent, safe place to live, physically as well as socially is basic to life satisfaction. The type of living arrangements influences other domains of living, including social integration. Similarly, unsatisfactory housing environment makes it difficult for the pursuit of recovery goals. Despite its central role in the rehabilitation process, housing has still not been given the priority it deserves. The types of housing accommodations in the rehabilitative process worldwide can be categorised as follows:

Homelessness

- Literally homeless (who lacks a fixed, regular, and adequate nighttime residence)
- Marginally homeless. (living in temporary settings such as emergency shelters).
- Functionally homeless. (living in

temporary and institution settings that are preceded by literally homelessness

Institutions/custodial care

- State psychiatric hospitals.
- Private psychiatric hospitals.
- General hospital psychiatric wards.
- Substance abuse hospitalization.
- Nursing homes or intermediate care facilities.
- Correctional facilities. (Jails, prisons, and other correctional facilities).
- Licensed Mental health Establishments (Structured, supervised group living arrangements provided as a short-term alternative to psychiatric hospitalization. Duration of stay is typically restricted to about 90 days

Independent Living

The factors that influence where a patient with mental illness stays are:

- Poverty
- Availabilty of housing
- Social security and safety
- Community acceptance
- Financial assistance
- Personal preferences

The objective of psychiatric rehabilitation should be to resettle chronically mentally ill patients from larger institutions to the normal community settings at the earliest which is called as deinstitutionalization. A residential continuum with different housing options includes round-the-clock staffed sheltered homes as well as independent and less staffed sheltered apartments which permit the patient to live independently in a community setting. Similarly, supported housing provides flexible and individualized services as per the person's requirements and demands. Other housing situations may include group homes, residential services, and apartments. A halfway home is an institution which allows patients to learn the necessary skills to re-integrate into the society and become self-dependent. Apart from serving as a residence it also provides medical, social, psychiatric and educational services. They are termed so because of them being halfway between a complete independent way of living on one hand to an in-patient or correctional facilities on the other where there is a high restriction in their behavior and freedom.

E. *EMPLOYMENT (VOCATIONAL REHABILITATION)*

The helpful effects of work for psychological wellbeing have been known for centuries. Thus, vocational rehabilitation has been an integral part of psychiatric rehabilitation modules since the beginning. The principle behind vocational rehabilitation is based on the fact that work improves activity, socialization, promotes gains in self-esteem and quality of life, helps the individual to lead a self-independent way of life. Thus, work indirectly improves adherence to rehabilitation in people with impaired insight by enhancing the self-esteem.

The vocational rehabilitation programs serve their purpose in stepwise manners as follows:

- **Brief and focused technics** used to teach how to find a job, filling out applications and appearing for interviews for less disabled persons
- **Transitional employment**

  It provides a temporary work

environment to teach vocational skills, enabling the affected person to move on to a more competitive employment.

- **Sheltered workshops**

  Provides pre-vocational training

- **Co-operative sectors**

  They employ disabled and non-disabled staff together on equal terms and sharing management, with mental health workers managing the cases in background and providing the necessary support. This helps in social integration of those who are under the process of rehabilitation.

- **Supported Employment**

  It is the most promising vocational rehabilitation model devised by Robert Drake and Deborah Becker. Research over the last three decades has pointed towards supported employment as an evidence-based approach to vocational services. It is based on the 'individual placement model' where people with disability are placed in competitive employment as per their likings as quickly as possible accompanied by an indefinite support needed to maintain their position. It also helps them to provide the training and supports required to succeed in that job. This is followed by an increase in the capacity to find and keep the job, improved self-esteem, social integration, better relationships maintenance, abstinence from substance misuse thus contributing to an improved cognition and quality of life with better symptom control. The goal of supported employment is to help patients find jobs that they are interested in and capable of, as early as possible. The characteristics of supported employment programs are:

  a. Quick job search and placement
  b. A competitive employment goal
  c. Selection of job according to individual preference, skills and experience of the person
  d. Follow-up employment consultant support maintained indefinitely
  e. Continuing case management structure
  f. Close co-ordination within all the mental health teams involved

F. *SOCIAL FUNCTIONING*

Social functioning can be defined as the quality and depth of an individual's interpersonal relationships, and the person's capacity to meet socially defined roles and expectations. It is a multifaceted concept whose nature can be best understood by considering several different life domains, that include

a. Role functioning

It is an individual's ability to meet socially and culturally defined roles such as student, employee, parent, homemaker or caregiver.

b. Social relationships

They involve the capability to have continued association with other people that are meaningful, pleasant and mutually rewarding.

c. Self-care and independent living skills

These include the person's ability to attend to grooming and hygiene, dress appropriately for the social situations, responding to health needs like visiting the doctor, taking medications and adhering to any dietary restrictions. They include a broader-range of abilities, such as cleaning and maintaining one's home, interacting appropriately with one's neighbors and landlord, doing laundry, financial management, cooking, shopping and using public transportation.

d. ***Leisure and recreational activities.***

These include activities that are meant for fun and entertaining pursuits, e.g. hobbies, sports, watching Television, going for movies, hiking and reading. They may also be included activities involving personal meaning, growth, fulfilment or health maintenance or improvement. Recreational activities such as keeping a journal, artistic expression, exercise, or spiritual enrichment also help in the long run.

e. ***Community reintegration.***

It can be explained as the extent to which a person with mental illness lives in the vicinity of those without any disability and how regularly they participate in the social activities in the community. This involves activities like attending social gatherings like school meetings, having regular communications with other people in the community, volunteering and taking participation in activities related to places of worship or even joining a local organization.

The different ways in which social functioning can be improved can be categorized as follows:

1. Improved management of the Psychiatric symptoms can help improve social functioning by minimizing relapses.
2. Using the principle of Social learning theory, social skills training (SST) is often used to break down complex skills into their component steps in order to teach more effective social behaviors.
3. Changes in the surroundings by creating more rewarding social or environmental settings, focusing on family psychoeducation and involving the patient in a setting that intends to provide more interpersonal contact.

Social Skills Training (SST)

Various researches over the last few decades have pointed out that SST improves social functioning by improving the social relationships and use of leisure time. Social skills are the behavioral components that help the patient to understand, learn and adapt to the social and environmental circumstances around him or her.

Social skills can be defined as those skills or abilities that

- Help the individual to recognize and reciprocate emotional cues from people around them,
- Facilitate interpersonal interactions
- Communicate with others in different social situations
- Create and maintain satisfying relationships in a community at large.

Persons with disabilities related to mental illness may experience social skills deficits in the form of inability to express their thoughts, feelings and emotions in a socially appropriate manner. This impairment in social skills may arise due to the primary pathophysiology of the mental illness or as a result of an early onset that may have restricted their opportunities for leaning new skills or impaired the use of those skills which they have already learned. Illness pathology often results in poor attention span, speech incoherence, learning difficulties, difficulties in retention, thus giving rise to cognitive deficits as a part of social skills impairment.

Thus, SST helps in the process of recovery and trains the individual to learn those specific skills required to learn, work in a community and live independently with minimum support and a functional way of life. This training is usually done in a stepwise manner, from simple to complex skills.

SST varies from individual to individual. These training modules are on the individual's:

- Level of functioning
- Level of skill deficits
- Requirements, demands or needs
- Premorbid personality

Table 46.2: Types of Social Skills in Psychiatric Rehabilitation

Verbal	**Form, structure, content, context and amount of speech**
Non-verbal	Eye-contact, facial expressions, posture and personal distance
Paralinguistic	Volume, pace, tone and pitch
Social perception	Processing of social information that helps in making appropriate decisions
Coversational skills	Initiating and maintaining a conversation
Expressions	Empathy, Sadness, Affection

Other important social skill trainings include:

- Greeting someone
- Requesting for something
- Negotiation skills
- Assertiveness
- Grooming
- Interaction skills with colleagues, etc.

Individualized and group trainings

SST can be done in both an individualized or a group setting. However, in India, an individualized module may work taking the diversity of culture and language into consideration. But in a rehabilitation center where the group is more or less homogeneous, a facilitator handling a group session is a more feasible option.

Family's Role

Family plays an important role in the Indian context. They are the first one to identify the deficits in social skills in their patients. Thus, a family member can be a close and effective therapeutic ally in the process of Social Skills training by ensuring a safe environment for the patient to apply the skills learned in an individual setting.

G. *COGNITIVE REHABILITATION*

The impairment in an individual's cognitive ability due to mental illness are largely ignored despite their significant impact on the individual's daily functioning. Cognitive rehabilitation, Cognitive remediation and Cognitive Retraining are the terms used interchangeably for all the researched and evidence based non-pharmacological interventions that help reduce the cognitive impairment and improve the functional behaviors in order to optimize the ultimate goal of improving the individual's quality of Life.

There are two basic models proposed in literature that are often used in combination in cognitive rehabilitation in psychiatric disorders:

1. ***Compensatory model***

   In this model, the deficits in the social skills are not addressed and are instead compensated for. This is done by utilising the intact cognitive abilities and environmental resources which help to optimise the daily functioning and ability to learn new skills. These include use of daily planners, reminder, writing a diary, making a to-do-list and strategy planning. These methods are often termed as prosthetic as they only help to address the residual deficits that are usually not responsive to change.

2. ***Restorative model***

   The basis of this model is the concept of neuroplasticity which states that the brain has the potential to learn throughout the life. The methods used are usually termed under 'cognitive enhancement' technics. There are two approaches used in this method.

   - The '***Bottoms Up***' approach focuses on the basic cognitive functions of perception and attention, often regarded as the building blocks. The development of higher-level functions are subsequently targeted on this base.
   - The '***Tops Down'*** approach targets on higher order executive functioning e.g., Problem solving and meta-cognition using paper-pencil tasks and computer based exercises. They resemble games that are appealing. They also reduce the need for specialist personnel to administer the exercises as they are often standardized. This approach is more popular as they are often self-administered. The other methods used are 'errorless learning', 'scaffolding', information processing technics such as –

o mnemonics,

o verbalization

o chunking

SUMMARY

- Rehabilitation in Psychiatry often uses approaches that are '***strength based'***. They build upon the assessed strengths of the individuals rather than their deficits or problems. The strengths are assessed as the basis for goals setting and targeting recovery. This is different from the traditional illness based approaches that focus more on problems and deficits of a person with mental health disorder.
- These approaches are often '***collaborative***'. They are individualized and person centered. They assist the person with mental illness in rediscovering self in the form of skills training and accessing the resources in the community they intend to live or work in. They help them to achieve an independent way of life successfully.
- Rehabilitation in Psychiatry helps the person to have a '***meaningful life'*** focused on the significant determinants of good mental health that involves vocation, education, social support, leisure, quality of life, wellness and leisure.
- The rehabilitation modules work in a way as to place the person in their '***chosen goal settings***' such as housing and jobs and helps them with the support system needed to sustain these goals for long. The Social skills training also take place in the individual's natural environments.
- The current methods used in rehabilitation in Psychiatry are '***evidence based'*** technics, such as supported employment and wellness programs, peer support programs.

BIBLIOGRAPHY

1. *Psychiatric Rehabilitation* by Nora M. Barrett,

Kenneth J. Gill, Carlos W. Pratt
2. *Manual of Psychosocial Rehabilitation* by Robert King, Chris Lloyd, Tom Meehan
3. *Principles and Practice of Psychiatric Rehabilitation: An Empirical Approach* by Patrick W. Corrigan, Kim T. Mueser, Gary R. Bond, Robert E. Drake, Phyllis Solomon
4. *Handbook of Psychosocial Rehabilitation* By Robert King, Chris Lloyd, Tom Meehan
5. *Community Mental Health in India* by BS Chavan, Nitin Gupta, Priti Arun, Ajeet Sidana, Sushrut Jadhav

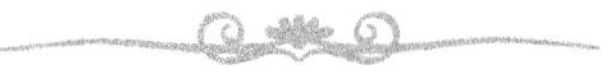

47 National Mental Health Programme

Delnaz Palsetia • Sagar Karia

INTRODUCTION

Mental health is an important component of health. World health organization defines the mental health as a state of well-being in which an individual realizes his or her own abilities, can cope with the normal stressors of life and can work productively and is able to make a contribution to his or her community. Mental health is the basis for well-being of an individual and the efficient functioning of the community. Mental health problems are increasing and the global burden of illness resulting from the psychiatric and behavioral disorders is significant·

It has been found in various community based surveys that prevalence of mental disorders in India is 6-7% for common mental disorders and 1-2% for severe mental disorders. Hence it becomes necessary to promote mental health services for the wellbeing of general population along with providing treatment for mental illnesses.

India was among the first few countries in the developing world to formulate a National Mental Health program (NMHP). NMHP was launched in 1982 with very comprehensive objectives. The basic aim of NMHP was to integrate the basic mental health care with general health services

The Government of India launched the National Mental Health Programe (NMHP) in 1982, with the following **objectives**:

- To ensure the availability and accessibility of minimum mental healthcare for all in the foreseeable future, especially to the most vulnerable and underprivileged sections of the population;
- To encourage the application of mental health knowledge in general healthcare and in social development; and
- To promote community participation in the mental health service development and to stimulate efforts towards self-help in the community.

Strategies

- Integration of mental health with primary health care through the NMHP
- Provision of tertiary care institutions for treatment of mental disorders.
- Eradicating stigmatization of mentally ill patients and protecting their rights through regulatory institutions like the Central Mental Health Authority (CMHA) and State Mental Health Authority (SMHA).

Specific Approaches

- Incorporating mental health skills to the periphery of health services
- Equitable and balanced distribution of resources.

- Integration of basic mental health care with general health services
- Linking it with community development

Service Component

The service component comprised of Treatment, Rehabilitation and Prevention.

Treatment

The treatment component was planned to be provided at various levels,

1. Village and sub-centre level: Multipurpose workers (MPW) and health supervisors (HS) under the supervision of Medical doctors (MO) were trained for:
   a. Management of psychiatric emergencies.
   b. Administration and supervision of maintenance treatment for chronic psychiatric disorders.
   c. Diagnosis and management of Grand –mal epilepsy.
   d. Liaison with local school teacher and parents regarding mental retardation and behavior problems in children.
   e. Counseling in problems related to alcohol and drug abuse.
2. Primary health centre (PHC): MO aided by health supervisor were trained for:
   a. Supervision of MPW"s performance.
   b. Elementary diagnosis.
   c. Treatment of functional psychosis.
   d. Treatment of uncomplicated cases of psychiatric disorders associated with physical diseases.
   e. Management of uncomplicated psychosocial problems.
   f. Epidemiological surveillance of mental morbidity.
3. District hospital: The district hospital to have 30-50 psychiatric beds and at least 1 psychiatrist attached to every district hospital. The psychiatrist was entrusted with the responsibility of clinical care of patients and training and supervision of non-specialist health workers.
4. Teaching psychiatric units and mental hospitals: Their desired role was:
   a. Providing help for difficult cases.
   b. Teaching.
   c. Specialized facilities such as occupational therapy units, psychotherapy, counseling and behavior therapy.

Rehabilitation

The subcomponents of rehabilitation include maintenance treatment of epileptics and psychotics at the community levels and development of rehabilitation centers at both the district level and the higher referral centers.

Prevention

This component was community based, with the initial focus on the prevention and control of alcohol related problems and later on other issues like addictions, juvenile delinquency and suicides.

Features of the NMHP

Decentralized and phased training courses were conducted for all the health personnel of the district so that they would deliver basic mental healthcare services to the needy.

- The services covered a population of 1.5 million distributed in seven talukas.
- A program officer for mental health was

appointed in the district health and family welfare office, WHO organized a mental health clinic in the premises and also toured the entire district in the premises to monitor the program.

- A simple recording and reporting system was developed. The district health officer monitored the progress every month during the monthly review meetings along with other health programs.
- Five essential drugs were made available for distribution in all the health centers in the district.
- During the first three years of the project (1985-88), 1200 patients with psychosis, 3525 patients with epilepsy, 750 patients with neurosis and 380 mentally retarded (learning disabled) persons were registered. Forty-two percent of patients with psychosis and 53% of those with epilepsy took treatment regularly and showed improvement. Seventy percent of patients came from places within a five-kilometre range of the health center. Thus, distance and availability of free care facilities appear to be important factors in good compliance.
- Good performers in the mental health care program of the system were good in all other health programs. Poor performers appeared to have had many personal and psychosocial problems which came in the way of their performance.
- As the mental health services became popular, patients reached the centers within a few days/ weeks of the onset of the illness and took a short and straight path instead of taking a long path by visiting various faith healers and other agencies.
- The district program gave professionals an idea as to how to organize services in a cost effective manner and maintain a reasonable quality.

The main strength of NMHP document drafted in 1982 was that it envisaged the integration of mental healthcare with the general primary healthcare.

On the other hand there was some inherent **weakness of this model** of care:

1. Emphasis was more on curative components rather than the preventive and promotive components;
2. Importance was not given to the role of support of families in the treatment of the patient.
3. Short term goals prioritized over the long term planning;
4. No clear outline regarding the administrative structure of the program;
5. Estimates of budgetary support were not made.

After initial implementation of NMHP; at the end of five years; it was observed that financial constraints limited its success. This gave rise to the concept of DMHP (District Mental Health Program) in 1996 and various changes were made in the consecutive five year plans. In the XIth plan an effort was made to address the main barrier in the mental health service provisions. In the XIIth plan the focus was on psychiatric problems to vulnerable sections of the population.

DISTRICT MENTAL HEALTH PROGRAM (DMHP)

NIMHANS (National Institute of Mental Health and Neurosciences) developed a program to operationalize and implement the NMHP in a district. DMHP was launched in 1996 with an aim to achieve the objectives of NMHP. Pilot of DMHP was done at Bellary district in Karnataka. Bellary is located about 350 kms away from Bangalore and the total population of Bellary was about 20 lakhs at that time.

The Main Components of the DMHP at Bellary were:

- Training for all primary care staff.
- Provision of 6 essential psychotropic and antiepileptic drugs (Chlorpromazine, amitryptiline, trihexyphenidyl, Injection fluphenazine decanoate, phenobarbitone and diphenylhydantoin) at all PHCs and sub centers.
- A system of simple mental health case records.
- A system of monthly reporting.
- Regular monitoring and feedback from the district level mental health team.

The Main Objectives of DMHP were:

- To provide sustainable basic mental health services in community and integration of these with other services.
- Early detection and treatment in community itself to ensure ease of care givers.
- To take pressure off mental hospitals.
- To reduce stigma, to rehabilitate patients within the community.
- To detect as well as manage and refer cases of epilepsy

Team of Bellary Model at District Level:

- Psychiatrist
- Clinical psychologist
- Psychiatric social worker
- Statistical clerk.

Role of Team Members

- At Primary Health Centers (PHC) and Secondary Centers (SC) health professionals were trained in managing common mental disorders.
- The medical officer at PHC was trained to diagnose and treat common mental disorders and refer the complex cases to district hospital.
- The psychiatrist at district hospital handled the mental health clinic and could admit 10 patients.
- Every month the program was reviewed by the district health officer with medical officers of all PHCs at Bellary district.

Conclusions of Bellary Model

- Mental healthcare delivery was made available in the primary healthcare setting.
- Provisions were made to adequately train primary care physicians to manage mental health issues.
- Supervision/support from the program officer/psychiatrist enabled the public healthcare system to provide adequate mental healthcare to the population.

Based on the assessment conducted by Indian Council of Marketing Research (ICMR) in 2008 and feedback obtained from various consultations DMHP had incorporated promotive and preventive activities for positive mental health that include:

- School mental health services: life skill education in schools, counseling.
- College counseling services: Through trained teachers/counselors.
- Work place stress management: Formal and informal sector, including farmers, women etc.

- Suicide prevention services: Counseling centre at district level, sensitization workshops, IEC, helpline

An effort is made to mainstream the components of NMHP under the National health mission so as to enable the states to plan the mental health services for their specific areas

NATIONAL MENTAL HEALTH PROGRAM IN THE XIITH PLAN

The National Mental Health Program in the XIIth plan(2012-2017), focussed on psychiatric problems in marginalized and neglected sections of the population.

Special issues

- Senior citizens suffering from severely disabling diseases such as depressions of late onset and other psycho geriatric disorders.
- Victims of child sexual abuse, marital/ domestic violence and dowry related ill-treatment, rape and incest.
- Children and adolescents affected by problems of maladjustment of other scholastic problems, depressions, psychosis of early onset, attention deficit hyperactivity disorders and suicidal behavior resulting from failure in examination or other environmental stressors.
- Victims of poverty, destitution and abandonment of such women thrown out of the marital home or old and infirm parents left to fend for themselves.
- Victims of natural or man-made disasters such as cyclones, earthquakes, famines, war, terrorism and communal/ ethnic strife, with special attention to the specific needs of children orphaned by such disasters.

DMHP IN XIITH FIVE YEAR PLAN

Goal

The goal of DMHP was to improve the health and social outcomes related to mental illness.

The key principles of DMHP in XIIth plan are:

- A life course perspective with attention to the children, adolescents and adults.
- A recovery perspective through continuous care provision and empowerment of people with mental illness and also their care givers.
- An equity perspective which includes specific attention to vulnerable groups and ensuring the geographical access to mental health services.
- An evidence based perspective by following the established guidelines for treatment and delivery model.
- A health system perspective defining clear roles and responsibilities for each level.
- A right based perspectives to ensure the protection of rights of persons with mental illness.

Primary objective

To reduce the distress, disability and premature mortality related to mental illness and enhance recovery from mental illness by ensuring the availability and accessibility to mental health care for all, particularly the most vulnerable and underprivileged sections of the population.

Secondary objectives

- To reduce stigma towards mental illness.
- To promote community participation in the mental health service development and to encourage efforts towards self help in the community.

- To increase access to preventive services to the population at risk, in particular, addressing the risk of suicide and attempted suicide.
- To inform the persons with mental illness, their care-givers, professionals and other stakeholders of the rights of persons with mental illness and ensure that rights are respected during the provision of care and services.
- To broad base mental health into other related programs
- To ensure a motivating and empowering work place for staff by allowing an opportunity to improve their skills and recognition of their work.
- To generate knowledge and evidence related to delivery of mental health care and services.
- To establish governance, administrative and accountability mechanisms to realize the above objectives.

During the XIIth five year plans:

- Extending the DMHP to the remaining 161-districts and the gains made in the previous plans consolidated.
- Up gradation of the remaining 39-Medical College Psychiatry Departments undertaken and 20-Mental Hospitals taken up for reconstruction.
- Central and state mental health authorities further reinforced and long term research projects initiated in selected institutions along with continuing support to community based research.
- Augmentation of IEC (Information Education and Communication) activities to cover all sections of the population covering entire country.
- Comprehensive assessment and performance appraisal done at the national and state level by independent agencies.

Ministry of Health & Family Welfare
Government of India

↓

Director General of Health Services
Joint Director-Mental Health
(Central monitoring agency for DMPH)

↓

Secretary
State Mental Health Authority
(State Monitoring Agency)
[Jt. Director-Mental Health;
Project Co-ordinator]

↓

District Project Officer
(District Level)

Fig. 47.1: Administrative levels of the NMHP.

BIBLIOGRAPHY

1. http://www.who.int/mediacentre/factsheets/fs220/en/. Mental health: strengthening our response, August 2014. Accessed on 15/5/2015.
2. Sixty sixth World Health Assembly, Comprehensive Mental Health Action Plan 2013-2020. Available at: apps.who.int/gb/ebwha/pdf_files/WHA66/A66_R8-en.pdf
3. Chandrashekhar CR. Community psychiatry (Chapter 25 from Handbook of psychiatry A South Asian Perspective Edited by Dinesh Bhugra, GopinathRanjith, Vikram Patel.) Byword Viva Publishers Pvt Ltd, New Delhi.
4. Ahuja N. Community Psychiatry (from A short Textbook of Psychiatry, Pg 236,7th Ed) Jaypee Brothers Medical Publishers (P) Ltd, New Delhi
5. Balamurugan G, Radhakrishnan G, Vijayarani M; Models and Roles in National Mental Health Programe; Indian Journal of Psychiatric Nursing 2019
6. Roy S, Rasheed N. The national mental health programe of India. Int J Curr Med Appl Sci. 2015;7:7-15.

48 Ethics in Psychiatry

Anup Subhash Bharati

The term 'Ethics' is described in multiple forms as per Merriam – Webster Dictionary,

a) As the discipline dealing with what is good and bad and with moral duty and obligation
b) A set or system of moral principles
c) A guiding philosophy
d) The principles of conduct governing an individual or a group

MEDICAL ETHICS

Medical ethics is a system of moral principles that apply values to the practice of medicine and medical research. It is based on a certain set of values and professionals can refer to it in case of any conflict. The core values include the respect for autonomy, non-maleficence, beneficence, and justice. There are several codes of conduct related to medical profession. 'The Hippocratic Oath' discusses basic principles and dates back to 5th century BCE. The Nuremberg Code (1947) and The Declaration of Helsinki (1964) are widely utilized documents related to medical ethics.

Tom Beauchamp and James Childress described common framework related to medical ethics and It recognizes four basic moral principles.

a) Respect for Autonomy – the patient has the right to take decisions about refusing or choosing their treatment.
b) beneficence – doctor should act in the best interest of the patient.
c) Non-maleficence – 'To Do No Harm' to patients.
d) Justice – distribution of health resources and treatment benefits on equal share, as per need, effort, contribution and merit of an individual.

Ethics and Psychiatry

Psychiatry deals with human behavior and emotions, thus ethical issues are much more relevant in psychiatry and they are sometimes complicated too. There are ethical dilemmas in drawing line of demarcation between normal and abnormal behavior, formulating psychiatric diagnosis and thus, treatment can be easily questioned. The dilemmas also pertain to individual freedom or autonomy, advance directives, confidentiality, cultural influences, doctor patient relation and many other domains.

The focus of understanding ethical issues in psychiatry started in 1970, when The American Psychiatric Association (APA) appointed a committee to develop a code of ethics. The World Psychiatric Association (WPA) developed a code of ethics in 1977.

IPS Code of Ethics - Indian Psychiatric Society (IPS) has recommended a code of ethics for psychiatrists in India in 1989, the principles are as follows:

a) Psychiatrist has a clear social responsibility
b) Psychiatrist must have high standards of professional competence and ensure continuing education
c) They will not violate ethical standards and when such violations come to their notice they will take steps to correct it
d) Benevolence and patient interest are important and should precede self interest
e) Psychiatrist must maintain high moral standards
f) Patient welfare is most important, treating with the best ability, not treating cases out of one's domain and termination of treatment when it is not helping the patient.
g) Confidentiality of records must be meticulously maintained to safeguard patients interests and protect them from discrimination, social stigma and harm
h) Psychiatry patients must be treated with dignity and respect, their human rights must be protected

MCI code of Medical Ethics

Medical council of India had formulated guidelines called as Indian Medical Council (Professional Conduct, Etiquettes and Ethics) Regulations 2002 amended up to 2016. This are applicable to all psychiatrist in India.

Cultural Influence

Due to the diversity across the globe, the ethical guidelines in medicine need to be broadly acceptable for everyone irrespective of ethnical, cultural and religious differences. There is ample evidence which shows that culture may influence the incidence, causes, manifestation, course and prognosis of various psychiatric illnesses. It also affects the presentation of psychiatric illness, development and expression of symptoms, experience of symptoms by individual, coping mechanisms and help seeking behavior. Cultural factors also play important role in doctor patient communication, prescribing patterns of doctor and the expectation of treatment by patients.

Confidentiality and Privacy

Every Physician needs to maintain complete confidentiality of the patients in most circumstances. In psychiatry, patient's often expresses their difficulties, their life stories, their fears and worries, sometimes very minute details which they might not have confessed to anyone as well as their sexual fantasies and desires too. Thus, it is unethical to share any information related to patient, their diagnosis and treatment to anyone without informed permission of the patient. If the confidentiality of the information not maintained, trust in the doctor-patient relationship would be breached and could negatively impact further treatment. So, it becomes responsibility of the treating psychiatrist to create a trusting environment.

There are some conditions where it becomes necessary to the psychiatrist to share some information related to the patient. For example, i) If any medical records of patients are to be produced in court or psychiatrist needs to testify in court related to the case, confidentiality is waived. ii) As per POCSO Act 2012, it is Mandatory for doctor to report cases of child sexual abuse. iii) In situations where a psychiatrist feels that a patient is in danger of harming self, confidentiality can be breached to ensure safety of the patient.

Informed Consent

Informed consent is the process in which doctor discloses appropriate information to a competent patient so that the patient can make voluntary decision to accept or refuse the treatment. It involves discussion of important points such as the nature of the treatment or procedure, any treatment alternatives, risks and benefits associated with it, assessment of patient's understanding. In order for the patient's consent to be valid, it should be voluntary and patient must be considered competent to make the decision. In psychiatry, this assessment of patient's capacity pertaining to treatment decisions is tricky as the mental illness many times hampers this capacity. With the enforcement of Mental Health care Act (MHCA) 2017, the advance directives of treatment need to be considered and can pose ethical issues in future. However, treatment can be started without consent in an emergency situation if the patient is potentially harmful to self or the others.

Doctor Patient Relationship / Boundary Violations

The therapeutic relationship between a doctor and the patient is established exclusively for the sole purpose of therapy and whenever this relationship deviates from its basic goal of treatment, it is called boundary violation and it becomes non-therapeutic. In psychiatry, the patient often shares and discusses personal and confidential matters, as well as many emotional aspects are involved in therapy sessions. Thus, the therapeutic relationship is often prolonged leading to development of strong emotional attachments on the part of patients. It is utmost important to have awareness of boundaries in a therapeutic relationship between a patient and a psychiatrist. Boundary violations is always harmful to patients, thus no gifts or any personal favors should be accepted from patients. Any sexual advances towards the patient or their caregivers is always unethical.

Involuntary / Supported Admission

May times, the patients suffering from mental illness have poor insight about their illness as well as due to the illness they lack ability to take treatment decisions. In this scenario, they might not agree for voluntary admission, and psychiatrist have to use involuntary hospitalization. Mental Health Care Act (MHCA) 2017, also have provision for emergency treatment and there is provision of supported admission.

Use of physical restraints must be minimal, under supervision, temporary period and has to be documented. The use of chaining is not allowed and unethical.

Ethical Issues in Psychiatry Research

Consent of the patient for research purpose should be voluntary and he/she can withdraw from the clinical or research trial at any point of time, this withdrawal should not hamper his/her further treatment options. While doing any research or clinical trial, it is mandatory to follow the Indian Council of Medical Research (ICMR) guidelines.

BIBLIOGRAPHY

1. Beauchamp TL, Childress JF. Principles of Biomedical Ethics. Oxford University Press, USA. 2001.
2. Agarwal A.K. Presidential address: Ethics in Psychiatry. Indian J. Psychiatry.1994;36(1):5-11
3. Agarwal AK, Gupta SC. Ethics in Psychiatry. In Vyas JN, Ahuja N, editors., Textbook of Postgraduate Psychiatry. JPB publishers,2003.
4. Ministry of Law and Justice. The Mental Healthcare Act; 2017. Gazette of India. Available from: http://www.egazette.nic.in/WriteReadData/2017/175248.pdf
5. The Medical Council of India. Code of medical ethics regulations, 2002 (Amended up to 8th October 2016). Available from: https://www.mciindia.org/CMS/rules-regulations/code-of-medical-ethics-regulations-2002
6. Wig NN. Ethical issues in psychiatry. Indian Journal of Medical Ethics 2004 1(3): 83-84.

Overview of Forensic Psychiatry 49

Prerna Khar • Disha Parikh

INTRODUCTION

Forensic psychiatry is a sub-speciality of psychiatry, where scientific and clinical expertise is applied to legal issues. It embraces civil, criminal, correctional or legislative matters and acts as an interface between law & psychiatry.

A landmark study done in India in 2011 by Math et al, on 5024 prisoners showed that 4002 (79.6%) individuals could be diagnosed as having a diagnosis of either mental illness/substance use. This highlights the need to be abreast with the various laws and legal aspects pertinent to the field of mental health.

CRIMINAL RESPONSIBILITY

As per law, crime is an offence for which one may be punished by law. For a crime to have occurred, there are 2 things which have to be proved in the court of law:

1. Actus rea: The individual committed the unlawful act.
2. Mens rea (Guilty mind): The individual acted upon his/her own free will, intentionally and with rational thinking.

Many individuals seek the insanity defense when accused of a crime. It is important to note that insanity has 2 components:

1. Medical insanity: Psychotic illness/severe illness that requires admission to a mental hospital.
2. Legal insanity/unsoundness of mind (SECTION 84 IPC): Incapable of knowing the nature of the act/act is wrong or that its against the law. Absence of a motive or forethought is considered one of the criteria for determining unsoundness of mind.

Historically the following tests were used to test unsoundness of mind: Right/wrong test, Wild beast test, the Insane Delusion test and the test of capacity to distinguish between right and wrong. These laid the foundation for the McNaughten's rule.

Mc Naughten's Rule

Daniel Mc 'Naughten, in 1843, tried to kill England's Prime Minister Sir Robert Peel. Mc Naughten thought Peel wanted to kill him (delusion of persecution) so he tried to shoot Peel, but instead shot and killed Peel's secretary, Edward Drummond. Medical experts testified that Mc Naughten was psychotic, and Mc Naughten was found not guilty by reason of insanity.

Section 84 Indian Penal Code (IPC) is based on Mc Naughten's Rule and has the following criteria:

Major criteria: Person must be suffering from mental illness during the commission of act.

Minor criteria: Indicate the person is:

a. Incapable of knowing the nature of the act or
b. Incapable of knowing his act is wrong or
c. Incapable of knowing it is contrary to law.

Mere abnormality of mind/partial delusion/ irresistible impulse/compulsive behavior of a psychopath affords no protection under Section 84 IPC.

Lucid interval: It is defined as a period of normalcy, during the course of an organic brain disorder. The individual can stand for a trial or testify for legal purposes. His/her testimony is accepted as evidence in the court of law, as the person is in full capacity of mental functioning. All crimes done under the period of lucid interval cannot seek the insanity defense. It is however important to note that it is difficult to ascertain the individual's state of mind at the time the crime was committed.

There are a few factors which indicate that the crime was done in a state of medical insanity which are:

- Lack of secrecy
- Use of unnecessary force
- No evident motive
- No accomplices
- No prior preparation
- Indifference to the crime

FITNESS TO STAND TRIAL

Assessment of the mental abilities of individuals to defend their case is called fitness to stand trial. In cases of fitness to plead, assessment is aimed at, whether a criminal defendant has sufficient ability to consult with his lawyer with a reasonable degree of rational understanding, and whether he has a rational as well as factual understanding of the proceedings against him.

Assessment is usually done by a forensic psychiatrist. Presence of a mental disorder is necessary but not sufficient condition to determine that a defendant is unfit. Even if a person is suffering from mental disorder, it should be assumed that he/she has the mental capacity to decide on various matters unless the contrary can be shown. Hence, it must be demonstrated that the mental disorder affects the defendant's performance on adjudicating process.

Assessment for fitness to plead or stand trial includes assessing the ability of the accused to understand the charges he/she has been accused of, ability to distinguish between a plea of guilty and not guilty, ability to instruct his/her lawyer and ability to follow the proceedings in the court. Positive symptoms of psychosis, especially thought disorder and delusions have been known to be associated with unfitness to plead.

The factors assessed are:

a) Comprehending the charges framed against them
b) Realizing the seriousness of the penalties if proven guilt
c) Following the proceedings of the court
d) Helping their lawyer to defend their case
e) Appropriate behavior in the court.

Hence, fitness to stand trial plays a crucial role in persons with mental illness or intellectual disability.

PSYCHIATRIST AS EXPERT WITNESS

Expert witness is someone who on account of his professional training is capable of deducing opinions and inferences from the facts observed by himself or noticed by others.

Any psychiatrist may become involved in legal proceedings as an expert. The expert witness must possess some special knowledge, skill training that helps in providing experience that lie beyond experience and general knowledge of judges.

Preparation of testimony as an expert witness

The preparation as an expert witness will primarily involve understanding what is expected through the testimony. The psychiatrist should collect and study all the relevant documents and should be prepared to differentiate between the facts of the case and derived opinions. There is also a need to anticipate likely questions and be prepared with the responses. Documents for presentation should include data given by the patient and caregivers, preferably verbatim, including the source of information, the details of investigations, joint consultations, referrals, serial mental status examination, ward observations, cognitive function testing, and so on, and opinion derived and the reasons of deriving the opinion.

If the doctor succumbs to the pressure and offers false expert advice, they can be implicated under:

1. Punishment for false evidence (IPC193)
2. False statement made in declaration which is by law receivable as evidence (IPC 199)
3. Causing disappearance of evidence of offense, or giving false information while screening the offender (IPC 201)
4. Destruction of document or electronic record to prevent its production as evidence (IPC 204).

MENTAL HEALTH CARE ACT, 2017 (MHCA)

This act came into force on 7thApril 2017. It replaced the earlier Mental Health Act 1948 and is aimed at providing good quality mental health care services to all individuals with mental illness. It brings about decriminalization of suicide, insurance coverage of mental health services, and ensures rights of people with mental illness are safeguarded. The Act comprises of 16 chapters and 126 sections.

Chapter I	: Preliminary
Chapter II	: Mental Illnesses and capacity to make mental health care decisions
Chapter III	: Advance Directive
Chapter IV	: Nominated representative
Chapter V	: Rights of persons with mental illness.
Chapter VI	: Duties of appropriate Government.
Chapter VII	: Central Mental Health Authority.
Chapter VIII	: State Mental Health Authority
Chapter IX	: Finance, accounts and audits.
Chapter X	: Mental health establishments
Chapter XI	: Mental Health Review Boards
Chapter XII	: Admission, Treatment and Discharge (sec 85 to 99)
Chapter XIII	: Responsibilities of other agencies.
Chapter XIV	: Restriction to discharge functions by professionals not covered by profession.
Chapter XV	: Offences and penalty.
Chapter XVI	: Miscellaneous.

We shall be discussing some of the important aspects of the Act:

1. *Mental Illness:* A substantial disorder of thinking, mood, perception, orientation or memory that grossly impairs judgment, behavior, capacity to recognize reality or

ability to meet the ordinary demands of life, mental conditions associated with the abuse of alcohol and drugs; but **does not include intellectual disability** which is a condition of arrested or incomplete development of mind of a person, specially characterized by sub-normality of intelligence.

2. *Capacity to make mental health care decisions/ treatment decisions:* Every person, including a person with mental illness shall be deemed to have capacity to make decisions regarding his/her mental healthcare or treatment if such person has the ability to-
   a) Understand the information that is relevant to take a decision on the treatment or admission or personal assistance; or
   b) Appreciate any reasonably foreseeable consequence of a decision or lack of decision on the treatment or admission or personal assistance; or
   c) Communicate the decision under sub-clause (a) by means of speech, expression, gesture or any other means.
3. *Advance Directive:* Every person, who is not a minor, has the right to make an advance directive in writing, specifying the way the person wishes to be cared for and treated for or not to be cared for and treated for a mental illness.
   - He/She also has a right to specify the individual or individuals, in order of preference, he wants to appoint as his nominated representative.
   - Every Board is to maintain an online register register of advance directives registered with it, which is to be invoked when the person ceases to have the capacity.
   - Psychiatrist in charge of treatment of the person with mental illness (PMI) is duty bound to follow the advance directive executed by the individual
   - Application to modify, alter or cancel the advance directive can be made to the Mental Health Review Board.
   - Advance directive is not applicable during emergency treatment, under sec 103.
   - In case of minors, legal guardians shall have right to make advance directive.
4. *Nominated Representative:* Every person, who is not a minor, has the right to appoint a nominated representative to discharge different functions assigned in the Act.
   - When no nominated representative has been appointed, persons are to be deemed as nominated representative in order of preference as given: relative, caregiver, *person appointed by the Board* or the *Director of department of social welfare*.
   - In case of minors, the legal guardians are to be their nominated representative, unless the concerned Board orders otherwise.
   - Nominated representative shall provide support to the PMI in making treatment decisions under sec 98 & 99 (supported admission).
5. *Rights of Persons with mental illness:* PMI have the following rights:
   - Right to equality and non-discrimination.
   - Right to protection from cruel, inhuman and degrading treatment.
   - Right to community living.
   - Right to a safe and hygienic living environment, with adequate provision of food, facilities for recreation and privacy.

- Right to confidentiality.
- Right to information.
- Right to access medical records. But, the psychiatrist may withhold information in case of likelihood of harm to the person with mental illness or to other persons.
- Right to personal contacts and communication.
- Right to legal aid.
- Right to make complaints about deficiencies in provisions of services.
- Non-discrimination in respect of medical insurance.
- Free and informed consent is required from them in case of research works. If unable to give free consent, permission to be obtained from the State mental health authority (SMHA)

6. *Duties of the Government:* Government is obliged to provide a range of services required by PMI- including mental health care and treatment, rehabilitation services, community living, entertainment services, occupational training without any discrimination and in all districts and to ensure that no one needs to travel for a long distance for these services. Duty has been assigned to the government to take measures to create awareness about mental health illness and to reduce stigma associated with mental illness.
7. *Mental health establishment (MHE):* Any establishment including Ayurveda, Yoga and Naturopathy, Unani, Siddha, and Homeopathic establishments, either wholly or partly meant for the care of the persons with mental illness, established, owned, controlled or maintained by the appropriate Government, local authority, trust, whether private or public, corporation, cooperative society, organization or any other entity or person, where persons with mental illness are admitted or reside at for care, treatment, convalescence and/or rehabilitation, either temporarily or otherwise and includes general hospital or general nursing home established and maintained by appropriate Government, local authority, trust, whether private or public, corporation, co-operative society, organization or any other entity or person. Does not include a family residential place if a person with mental illness resides with his relatives or friends.
8. *Functions of SMHA/Central Mental health authority (CMHA):*
   - To register MHEs
   - Make rules and regulations for registration of clinical psychologists, psychiatric social workers and mental health nurses and maintain a national/state register of them.
   - Train all relevant persons including law enforcing officials about the Act
   - Advise the Central/State Govt. on Mental Health matters
9. *Functions of the State mental health review boards (SMRB):*
   - To review supported admissions & admissions of minors
   - Registration of advance directives,
   - Hear applications to modify advance directives,
   - Appointment of nominated representatives in some cases
   - Approval of some types of treatments (e.g., ECTs in minors, emergency ECTs)
   - Hear applications regarding infringement of rights of PMI or non-disclosure of information or deficiencies of care and services.

- To visit and inspect prisons or jails
- To inspect mental health establishments in some cases

10. *Emergency treatment (section 94):* In case of emergency, medical treatment can be provide by any medical practitioner to a person with mental illness either at a health centre or in the community, subject to the informed consent of the nominated representative to prevent:
    - Death or irreversible harm to the person
    - The person inflicting harm to others or himself/herself
    - The person damaging property belonging to himself/herself or others
11. *Prohibited treatments:* The following are prohibited:
    - ECT without the use of muscle relaxants and anesthesia
    - ECT for minors. But may be given after informed consent of the guardian and approval of the Board.
    - Sterilization of men or women, when such sterilization is intended as a treatment for mental illness.
    - Chaining in any manner or form whatsoever.

The sections pertaining to admissions are not discussed as they are beyond the scope of this book.

NARCOTIC DRUGS AND PSYCHOTROPIC SUBSTANCES ACT (NDPSA), 1985

Narcotic Drugs and Psychotropic Substance Act was passed in 1985, amended in 1988, 2001 and 2014. It makes all drug offences non-bailable.

The Act is designed to fulfil India's treaty obligations under the following:

1) Single Convention on Narcotic Drugs,
2) Convention on Psychotropic Substances, and
3) United Nations Convention Against Illicit Traffic in Narcotic Drugs and Psychotropic Substances

The Act has 6 chapters and 83 sections

CHAPTER I: Definitions

- *Controlled substance*: Any substance which the Central Government may, having regard to the available information as to its possible use in the production or manufacture of narcotic drugs or psychotropic substances or to the provisions of any International Convention, by notification in the Official Gazette, declare to be a controlled substances.
- *Psychotropic substance*: Any substance, natural or synthetic, or any natural material or any salt or preparation of such substance or material included in the list of psychotropic substances specified in the Schedule. Around 76 substances have been included.
- *Narcotic substance:* Coca leaf, opium, poppy straw, cannabis includes all the manufactured drugs.
- *Manufactured drugs:* All coca derivatives, opium derivatives, medicinal cannabis, poppy straw concentrate, and any other notified narcotic substance or preparation. 88 have been included so far.

CHAPTER II: Deals with authorities and officers. The Central Government has set up the Narcotics Control Bureau with head quarters at New Delhi and zonal offices in Mumbai, Varanasi, Kolkata, Madras and Delhi.

CHAPTER III: Deals with prohibition, control and regulation

CHAPTER IV: Offenses and punishments

- Punishment for contravention in relation to poppy straw, coca plant and coca leaves, prepared opium, opium poppy and opium, embezzlement of opium by cultivator, cannabis other than ganja, manufactured drugs and preparations, psychotropic substances, illegal import into India, export from India or transshipment of narcotic drugs and psychotropic substances, external dealings in narcotic drugs and psychotropic substances, allowing premises to be used for an offence:
    - 1st offense: 10-20 years rigorous imprisonment, 1-2 L fine
    - 2nd and subsequent offenses: 15-30 years rigorous imprisonment, 1.5 to 3 L fine
- Punishment for contravention in relation to cannabis plant cultivation and cannabis (Ganja):
    - 1st offense: Rigorous imprisonment upto 5 years, fine upto 50,000
    - 2nd and subsequent offenses: Rigorous imprisonment upto 10 years, fine upto 1 lakh rupees (or even more)
- When the contravention involves a *small quantity*: Rigorous imprisonment for a term which may extend to 1 year, or with a fine which may extend to Rs. 10,000 or both;
- When the contravention involves a quantity *lesser than commercial quantity* but greater than a *small quantity*: Rigorous imprisonment for a term which may extend to 10 years and with fine which may extend to Rs. 1 lakh;
- When the contravention involves a *commercial quantity*: Rigorous imprisonment for a term which shall not be less than 10 years but which may extend to 20 years and also a fine which shall not be less than Rs. 1 lakh but which may extend to Rs. 2 lakh
- For the various substances, the quantities are defined in the below Table 49.1:

Table 49.1

Drug	Small quantity	Commercial quantity
Amphetamine	2 grams	50 grams
Charas	100 grams	1 kilogram
Cocaine	2 grams	100 grams
Ganja	1 kilogram	20 kilograms
Heroin	5 grams	250 grams
LSD	2 milligrams	100 milligrams
Methadone	2 grams	50 grams
Morphine	5 grams	250 grams
Opium	25 grams	2.5 kilograms
Tramadol *(2018 Notification)*	5 gms	250 gm

CHAPTER V: Procedures related to the Act

CHAPTER VI: Miscellaneous issues

PROTECTION OF CHILDREN FROM SEXUAL OFFENCES (POCSO) ACT

The POCSO Act was enacted on 14 November 2012 and amended in 2018. Prior to this Act, child sexual abuse was prosecuted under:

IPC 375- RAPE

IPC 354- Outraging the modesty of a woman.

IPC 377- Unnatural sexual offence

These Acts had their own disadvantages:

IPC 375 - Doesn't protect male victims or sexual acts other than peno-vaginal intercourse.

IPC 354 – has week penalty and does not protect the modesty of children.

IPC 377- Not designed to criminalize sexual abuse of children

The POCSO Act has 9 chapters and 46 sections. It defines child sexual abuse, lays down procedures for interviewing the child, court proceedings, fast tracking of cases, reporting of cases and punishments for various offences.

Definition: Child sexual abuse forms child abuse in which an adult or older adolescent uses a child for sexual stimulation. Forms of child sexual abuse include- engaging in sexual activities with the child (whether by asking or pressurizing, or by other means), indecent exposure(genitals), use of child in pornography.

Objectives of the Act:

- Ensure the process is child friendly: medical examination, recording the statement of the child by the Police and Magistrate, as well as examination of the child in court.
- Emergency medical care to be provided to the child within 24 hours
- To make arrangements to give the child such care and protection
- Punishment for offenders who commit sexual offences against children.

CHAPTER I: Preliminary clauses and definitions. Any individual below the age of 18 years is considered a child

CHAPTER II: *Sexual offences against children*

A) Penetrative sexual assault and punishment:

He penetrates his penis, to any extent, into the vagina, mouth, urethra or anus of a child or makes the child to do so with him or any other person.

B) Aggravated penetrative sexual assault and punishment:

The term "aggravated" in the act, refers to the following scenarios:

- When the abused child is mentally or physically disabled
- When the abuse is committed by a person in a position of trust or authority w.r.t. the child (police officer, member of the armed forces or security forces, public servant, management/staff of jail/remand home/place of custody or care, management/staff of an educational/religious institution)
- When done in gang, using deadly weapons/fire, causing grievous hurt or injury to sexual organs of child)
- When it causes the child to become mentally ill, causes pregnancy, inflicts diseases
- When done multiple times or child is below 12 yrs of age
- When done on a pregnant child, attempt to murder, during communal violence, or child made to parade/strip naked in public
- Assault committed during a natural calamity (2018 amendment)
- Administrating or help in administering any hormone or any chemical substance, to a child for the purpose of attaining early sexual maturity (2018 amendment)

C) Sexual assault and punishment:

Touching the vagina, penis, anus or breast of the child or making the child touch one or more of these parts of the accused or that of another adult or child, and doing so with a sexual intent.

D) Aggravated sexual assault and punishment

Status of the offender, status of the victim,

the impact on the victim, the nature of the assault makes it aggravated.

E) Sexual harassment and punishment. Includes any one or more of the following:

   1. Utters any word or makes any sound, or makes any gesture or exhibits any object or part of body with the intention that such word or sound shall be heard, or such gesture or object or part of body shall be seen by the child
   2. Makes a child exhibit his body or any part of his body so as it is seen by such person or any other person
   3. Shows any object to a child in any form or media for pornographic purposes

CHAPTER III: *Using child for pornographic purposes and punishment*

Whoever, uses a child in any form of media (including program or advertisement telecast by television channels or internet or any other electronic form or printed form, whether or not such program or advertisement is intended for personal use or for distribution), for the purposes of sexual gratification.

CHAPTER IV: *Abetment of and attempt to commit an offence*

CHAPTER V: *Procedure for reporting of cases*

- Reporting to be done to the Special Juvenile Police Unit or local police, who within 24 hrs, shall report to the Child Welfare Committee and the Special Court or Court of Session (where no Special court is designated)
- Obligation of media, studio or photographic facilities to report cases. Failing which, imprisonment upto 6 months or even 1 year (for head of the institution) or fine or both
- In case of a false complaint: to defame/extort/humiliate- 6 months imprisonment + fine

  By child – no punishment

  By adult to victimize child – 1 year + fine

Mandatory reporting: When a doctor has reason to suspect that a child has been or is being sexually abused, he/she is required to report this to the appropriate authorities (i.e. the police or the relevant person within his/her organization who will then have to report it to the police). Failure to do this would result in imprisonment of up to six months, with or without fine.

CHAPTER VI: *Procedures for recording statement of the child and Medical Examination*

It is preferable to record the statement at the child's residence or at a place where he/she usually resides or at the place of his/her choice and as far as possible by a woman police officer, not below the rank of sub-inspector. Child not to be called repeatedly to testify. There will be no aggressive questioning or character assassination of the child.

Medical Examination: All hospitals (govt, private or funded) must oblige for examination, without a charge to the victim (under CrPC, 1973). In case the victim is a girl child, the medical examination shall be conducted by a female doctor.

CHAPTER VII: *Special Courts*

CHAPTER VIII: *Procedure and powers of special courts and recording evidence*

For speedy trial, the evidence of the child is to be recorded within a period of 30 days. Also, the Special Court is to complete the trial within one year. Special courts to conduct the trial in-camera without revealing child's identity, whenever an in-Court trial is not possible.

Table 49.2

OFFENSE	MINIMUM TERM	MAXIMUM TERM	FINE
Penetrative Sexual Assault	10 years 20 years (If child is less than 16 years)	Life Imprisonment	Yes
Aggravated Penetrative Sexual Assault	20 years (Rigorous Imprisonment)	Life Imprisonment	Yes
Sexual Assault	3 years	5 years	Yes
Aggravated Sexual Assault	5 years	7years	Yes
Sexual Harassment		3 years	Yes
Use of child for pornographic purposes		5 years (first conviction) 7 years (second conviction)	Yes
a) Penetrative Sexual assault	10 years 20 years (If child is <16 years)	Life Imprisonment	Yes
b) Aggravated penetrative sexual assault	20 years	Life imprisonment	Yes
c) Sexual assault	6 years	8 years	Yes
d) Aggravated Sexual Assault	8 years	10 years	

CHAPTER IX: *Miscellaneous*

The Table 49.2 enlists the punishments for the various offenses, as per the 2018 amendment.

PROTECTION OF WOMEN FROM DOMESTIC VIOLENCE ACT, 2005

The Act is intended to protect women from being victims of domestic violence and to prevent the occurrence of domestic violence in the society. It aims to effectively protect rights of women. The Bill received the assent of the President of India in 2005.

The Act defines *Domestic incident report* as a report made in the prescribed form on receipt of complaint of domestic violence from an aggrieved person.

Respondent (Sec. 2(q)) It means any adult male person who is, or has been, in a domestic relationship with the aggrieved person and against whom the aggrieved person has sought any relief under this Act.

Aggrieved person (Sec. 2(a)) It means any woman who is, or has been, in a domestic relationship with the respondent who alleges to have been subjected to any act of domestic violence by the respondent.

Rights Granted To Women Under Domestic Violence Act, 2005

- The Domestic Violence Act '2005 secures a woman's right to reside in the matrimonial or shared household even if she has no title or rights in the household. A part of the house can be allotted to her for her personal use. A court can pass a residence order to secure her right of residence in the household.
- A woman who is victimized by acts of domestic violence will have the right

to obtain the services and assistance of Police Officers, Protection Officers, Service Providers, Shelter Homes and medical establishments as well as the right to simultaneously file her own complaint under Section 498 A of the Indian Penal Code for matrimonial cruelty

Liabilities And Restrictions Imposed Upon The Respondent

- He can be subjected to certain restrictions as contained in the Protection and Residence order issued against him.
- The Respondent can be made accountable for providing monetary relief to the aggrieved person and her children and pay compensation damages as directed in the Compensation order.
- He has to follow the arrangements made by the court regarding the custody of the child or children of the aggrieved person as specified in the Custody order.

Procedure

- The aggrieved person or any other witness of the offence on her behalf can approach a Police Officer, Protection Officer, or Service Provider and file a complaint with a Magistrate for obtaining orders or reliefs under the Domestic Violence Act, 2005.
- The court is required to take cognizance of the complaint by instituting a hearing within three days of the complaint being filed in the court.
- The Magistrate shall give a notice of the date of hearing to the Protection Officer to be served on the Respondent and such other persons as directed by the Magistrate, within a maximum period of 2 days or such further reasonable time as allowed by the Magistrate.
- The court is required to dispose of the case *within 60 days* of the first hearing.
- The court, to establish the offence by the Respondent can use the sole testimony of the aggrieved person. Upon finding the complaint genuine, the court can pass a Protection Order, which shall remain in force till the aggrieved person applies for discharge. If upon receipt of an application from the aggrieved person, the Magistrate is satisfied that the circumstances so require, he may alter, modify or revoke an order after recording the reasons in writing.

Penalty

For Respondent Sec. 31

The breach of Protection Order or interim protection order by the Respondent is a cognizable and non-bailable offence. It is punishable with imprisonment for a term, *which may extend to one year or with fine, which may extend to twenty thousand rupees or with both.* He can also be tried for offences under the Indian Penal Code and the Dowry Prohibition Act.

For Protection Officer Sec. 33

If he fails or does not discharge his duties as directed by the Magistrate without any sufficient cause, he will be liable for having committed an offence under the Domestic Violence Act '2005 with similar punishment. However, he cannot be penalized without the prior sanction of the state government. Moreover, the law protects him for all actions taken by him in good faith.

TESTAMENTARY CAPACITY

Testamentary capacity refers to person's full sense and mental sanity to have confirmed and signed the Will after understanding what his assets comprised and what he is doing by making a Will.

According to Indian Succession Act 1925, a person is said to have testamentary capacity only if he is in a sound disposing state of mind. It is essential that the testator should have sufficient capacity to comprehend perfectly the conditions of his property, his relations to the persons who were or should or might have been object of his bequest and the scope or the bearing of the provisions of his Will.

Testamentary capacity consists of:

- Understanding of the nature of the act (Will making) and its effects
- Knowledge of the nature and extent of one's assets
- Knowledge of persons who have a reasonable claim to be beneficiaries
- Understanding of the impact of the distribution of the assets of the estate
- A confirmation that the testator is free of any delusions that influence the disposition of the assets
- Ability to express wishes clearly and consistently in an orderly plan of disposition

Factors Affecting Testamentary Capacity:

1. Physical factors
2. Psychiatric disorders
3. Undue influence

The conditions discussed below may affect cognition, perception, which in turn may have effect on individual's ability to understand relevant facts related to testamentary capacity.

Factors which lead to brain dysfunction either due to certain diseases, trauma or medication may have an impact on the client's ability to think clearly.

Physical factors include a wide range of medical disorders, including head trauma, systemic diseases i.e. metabolic, endocrinal, infectious and other disorders that affect brain functioning and mental state. Certain drugs, alcohol may have effect on cognition and perception and hence may interfere in decision making.

Dementias such as Alzheimer's disease, Lewy body dementia, and vascular cognitive impairment are characterized by diffuse cognitive deficits. In cases of obvious and severe cognitive impairment, there will be little need for subtle interpretations of brain function, and the lawyers or the courts can assess the impact of the impairment without the help of experts. However, in many disputed cases, the level of cognitive impairment is relatively mild or subtle. Some individuals with dementia maintain their social graces and appear perfectly normal to a lay person. Therefore, probing and documentation of the rationale disposition, particularly in suspicious circumstances, are especially important to demonstrate that the individual is capable.

In dementia, executive impairment is particularly important, as it can affect insight, perception and judgment and impulse control. Mild forms of memory impairment can be associated with suspiciousness or even paranoid delusions as testators attempt to compensate for their memory deficits. In retrospective assessments, evidence for progression of dementia after the last Will was executed can help to support hypotheses about impaired thinking, perception, or judgment at the time of the execution of the Will.

Mood disorders, including depression and bipolar disorder, may produce cognitive distortions (delusions), compromise judgment, and cause irritability or impulsiveness. These acute and subacute changes may affect testamentary capacity and vulnerability to undue influence. Usually, these changes in mental state can be identified during a specific episode, but in some cases they can become chronic.

Delusions may be secondary to a number of clinical syndromes, including schizophrenia, delusional disorders, and other forms of neurological disease, such as dementia, delirium, acquired brain injury, and other brain lesions. According to the Banks v. Goodfellow criteria, the testator must be free of any delusions that directly affect the distribution of the estate. Changes made in the Will on the basis of false belief make the Will invalid. Even if such beliefs do not reach delusional intensity, they can make the testator vulnerable to undue influence.

Undue Influence

The lower the cognitive capacity of an individual, the lesser influence would be required to determine that the individual was incapable or unduly influenced. On the other hand, an individual with no cognitive impairment would have to be subjected to a severe level of influence to the point of coercion or containment before that influence would be considered undue. Undue influence has been defined by one of the courts as: "the opportunity of the beneficiary of the influenced bequest to mould the mind of the testator to suit his or her purpose.

MARRIAGE & MENTAL ILLNESS

Major mental health disorders may be the cause or effect of marital disharmony

Schizophrenia and Marriage

Marital status is significantly associated with first admission rates, age of onset, course and outcome of schizophrenia. Married men experienced a statistically significant delay (1-2 years) in the onset of psychotic symptoms compared with single men.

Depression and Marriage

Considerable interest has been there in the role of the marital status as a risk factor for depression. For men, it appears clear that those married have the lowest rate of depression. Separated or divorced men have the highest rate of major depression. In women, the association is slightly less.

Alcohol & Marriage

Marital and family tension is virtually inevitable in families with heavy drinkers. 60-80% of domestic violence is due to alcoholism. alcohol use disorder all that is dear to the spouse -family life, sexual relationship, economic resources, well-being of the children and status within the community.

Suicide

Compared with the general population, people who die by suicide are more likely to have been divorced, unemployed or living alone. Social isolation is a common factor among these associations. One-fourth of the persons committing suicide are unmarried. Suicide rate is highest in the first year of marriage. Higher rate of married women committing suicide may probably be due to marital disharmony, dowry or ill-treatment by the in-laws.

Special Marriage Act 1954

The Special Marriage Act is meant for any person in India and Indian nationals abroad, irrespective of the faith that the individual may profess. A marriage solemnized in any other form can be registered under this Act.

Conditions of Special Marriages 1. Monogamy

2. Mental soundness (Clause b) 3. Marital age 4. Relationship (Clause d) 5. Conditions of marriage in J&K (Clause)

Neither party: i) is incapable of giving a valid consent to it as a consequence of unsoundness of mind; or (ii) though capable of giving valid consent, has been suffering from mental disorder of such a kind or to such an extent as to be unfit for marriage and the procreation of children, or (iii) has been subject to recurrent attacks of insanity

Grounds For Divorce

The respondent, as per Clause (e), has been incurably of unsound mind or has been suffering continuously or intermittently from mental disorder of such a kind and to such an extent that the petitioner cannot reasonably be expected to live with the respondent.

Hindu Marriage Act

The Act of 1955 provided for four types of matrimonial relief: (i) Restitution of conjugal rights, (ii) Judicial separation, (iii) Declaration of nullity and annulment, and (iv) Divorce.

Ground for divorce are that the respondent has been incurably of unsound mind, or has been suffering continuously or intermittently from mental disorder of such a kind and to such an extent that the petitioner cannot reasonably be expected to live with the Respondent.

Muslim Law of Marriage And Divorce

A Muslim who is of sound mind and has attained puberty (presumed to have been attained on completion of 13 years, unless the contrary is proved) is qualified. A person of unsound mind cannot contract a marriage and such a marriage, if contracted, is void. However, if the guardian of the person of unsound mind considers such a marriage to be in his interest and in the interest of society and is willing to take up all the monetary obligations of the marriage, then such a marriage can be performed.

Divorce by recourse to court (judicial divorce): 1. Spouse has been insane for a period of 2 years. 2. Husband was impotent at the time of marriage and continues to be so. (Inability of the husband to consummate the marriage is one pattern of impotence.)

Parsi Marriage and Divorce Act, 1936 Amended In 1988

Unsoundness of mind is not a ground for annulment of marriage, Unless: 1. The plaintiff was ignorant of the fact at the time of the marriage, and 2. Has filed the suit within three years from the date of the marriage. 4. That the defendant has been incurably of unsound mind for a period of two years or upwards immediately preceding the filing of the suit.

Christian Law of Marriage And Divorce (1869)

In a Christian marriage unsoundness of mind is a ground for divorce on two conditions- - that is, it must be incurable and - it must be for at least two years immediately before the filing of the petition.

Role of Psychiatrist

Certificate given by the psychiatrist is only a statement of opinion. It attains the status of evidence only when its author undergoes cross examination.

Intention of law is to prevent the fracture of a family. If a hard decision is inevitable, it will be on a specific ground. Mental disorder is a ground for judicial separation. It is to be understood as the lack of a state of mind or capacity to understand one's affairs or marital obligations.

Mental illness is defined as a substantial disorder of thinking, mood, perception, orientation or memory that grossly impair judgment, behavior, capacity to recognise reality or ability to meet the ordinary demands of life, mental conditions associated with the abuse of alcohol and drugs. Medical evidence regarding the requisite degree of mental disorder is relevant, though not conclusive for divorce. Burden of proving the insanity of the respondent rests on the petitioner. It is the responsibility of the psychiatrist to keep the documents sound.

ADOPTION AND CHILD CUSTODY

In adoption cases, a psychiatrist may be asked to give an opinion about the suitability of the prospective adopting parents. According to the Hindu Adoptions and Maintenance Act, 1956, any Hindu male "who is of sound mind and is not a minor" can adopt a child, with the consent of his wife unless "she has been declared by a court to be of unsound mind". Similarly, any Hindu female "who is of sound mind", is not a minor, and is not married, can adopt a child. If she is married, then her husband should also be of sound mind. The person capable of giving in adoption should also be of sound mind.

Issues like suitability of a child for adoption may also need to be assessed, for example, physical and emotional needs of the child, and whether the proposed adopting parents would be able to fulfil those needs. Emotional stability and generally, resources of the couple planning to adopt the child also need to be assessed.

A psychiatrist may be requested by a court to give an opinion about which parent should be given custody in cases of divorce. In determining who should be given the custody of a child in cases of divorce, generally it is presumed that the welfare of a child of tender years is best served by maternal custody when the mother is a good and fit parent. However, there are several related issues, which may need to be looked into. The psychiatrist should take details of conflicts, if any, between parents, or between parents and grandparents, regarding the custody of the child. The issue of granting permission to the divorced father to visit the child with maternal custody also needs to be looked into, especially the frequency and duration of such visits.

There may be a situation where the mother due to mental illness is not able to take care of the child and the father is not available, and no alternative arrangements are possible within the family. In such a situation, the child may need to be placed in a foster agency.

THE JUVENILE JUSTICE ACT

The Juvenile Justice (Care and Protection of Children) Act, 2000 is the primary legal framework for juvenile justice. This law, brought in compliance of the 1989 UN Convention on the Rights of the Child (UNCRC). The Act provides for a special approach towards the treatment, prevention and rehabilitation of juvenile delinquency. It was further amended in 2006 & 2010.

It is an Act to consolidate and amend the law relating to children alleged & found to be either in conflict with law (JCL) or in need of care and protection.

JCL cases can only be heard in the juvenile justice board (JJB) and not by another court. The board must contain a Metropolitan or

Judicial magistrate (FC) and two social workers of whom at least one shall be a woman.

Objectives of the Act:

- To lay down a legal structure for the Juvenile Justice
- To provide a Special Approach To The Care And Protection Of Juveniles
- To outline the machinery and infrastructure
- To establish norms and standards for administration
- To establish linkages and co-ordination between the formal system of juvenile justice and voluntary efforts in the welfare of juveniles
- To constitute special offences in relation to juveniles and provide punishment

Orders That May Be Passed Juvenile has committed the offence:

- The Board may allow the juvenile to go home after advice or a counseling to the parent/guardian & juvenile.
- Direct the juvenile to participate in group counseling
- Order the juvenile to perform community service.
- Order the parent of the juvenile or the juvenile himself to pay a fine, if he/she over fourteen and earns money.
- Direct the juvenile to be released on probation of good conduct and placed under the care of any parent, guardian or other fit person executing a bond for good behavior & wellbeing of juvenile for a period not exceed 3 years.

Order That May Not Be Passed Against A Juvenile:

- No juvenile in conflict with law shall be sentenced to death or imprisonment for any term which may extend to imprisonment for life
- A juvenile cannot be committed to prison for inability to pay a fine or for not furnishing security.

Rehabilitation and Social Integration:

This section discusses certain non-institutional solutions (Chapter 7)

(i) Adoption

(ii) Foster care

(iii) Sponsorship

(iv) Sending child to an after care organization.

1. Orphaned and abandoned children are eligible for adoption.
2. *Foster care is used for temporary placement of children*
3. Sponsorship programs provide supplementary support to families, to children's homes and to special homes to meet educational, nutritional, medical and other needs of the children.
4. After-care organizations are set up to take care of children or juveniles after they leave special homes or children' homes.

CONCLUSION

Forensic psychiatry is an important upcoming field in our country. As a medical professional, it is essential to remain abreast with the latest laws and amendments, in order to serve our patients in the best possible manner and to ensure that individuals with mental illnesses get adequate care and justice, and are not abandoned in their journey.

BIBLIOGRAPHY

1. Chadda RK. Forensic evaluations in psychiatry. Indian journal of psychiatry. 2013 Oct;55(4):393.

2. Math SB, Murthy P, Parthasarthy R, Kumar CN, Madhusudhan S. Minds imprisoned: Mental health care in prisons. Bangalore: National Institute of Mental Health Neuro Sciences. 2011.
3. Basavaraju V, Enara A, Gowda GS, Harihara SN, Manjunatha N, Kumar CN, Math SB. Psychiatrist in court: Indian scenario. Indian journal of psychological medicine. 2019 Mar;41(2):126-34.
4. Agarwal S, Kumar N. Juvenile Justice (Care and Protection of Children) Act 2015: A Review. Space and Culture, India. 2016 Mar 26;3(3):5-9.
5. Jiloha RC. Mental capacity/testamentary capacity. Clinical Practice Guidelines of the Indian Psychiatric Society. Forensic Psychiatry. 2009:20-34.
6. "The Protection of Women From Domestic Violence Act, 2005"(PDF). Government of India Legislative Department. Retrieved 18 February 2021.
7. Math SB, Kumar CN, Moirangthem S. Insanity defense: Past, present, and future. Indian J Psychological Med 2015;37:381-7.
8. Nambi S. Forensic psychiatry revisited. Indian J Psychiatry 2010;52:S306-8.
9. Text book of postgraduate Psychiatry: Vyas, Ghimire. Forensic Psychiatry.
10. Forensic Psychiatry (Psychiatry and law): S Nambi. Chapter 13-Prison Psychiatry.
11. Insanity And Criminal Responsibility O Somasundaram. *Indian Journal of Psychiatry [Vol. VI, No. S]*1964
12. http://www.childlineindia.org.in/The-Protection-of-Children-from-Sexual-Offences-Act-2012.htm
13. The narcotic drugs and psychotropic substances act, 1985
14. The Mental Health Care Act 2017. Government of India. Available from: https://www.prsindia.org/uploads/media/Mental%20 Health/Mental%20 Healthcare%20Act,%20 2017.pdf.

50 Criminal Responsibility and Mental Illness

Sagar Karia

Criminal law holds the offender morally blame worthy and legally culpable for intentional and controllable wrong doings. The following two elements of crime are very important-

1. *Actus reus* (i.e. the guilty act which is against the criminal law).
2. *Mens rea* (i.e. the intent).

According to this, there must be a mind at fault to constitute a criminal act. Therefore, in court of law the plea of insanity defense is raised and the responsibility of psychiatrist comes into play.

McNAUGHTON RULES

Historically, **McNaughton case** is very important in relation to criminality and mental illness. Daniel McNaughton, 29 year old Scotsman was charged with the murder of Edward Drummond, secretary to the Prime Minister, Sir Robert Peel. Mistaking Drummond for Prime Minister, he shot him on 20th January 1843. At the time of the arrest, McNaughton said to the Police that "the Tories in the city were following me wherever I go and would persecute me. They have destroyed my peace of mind. In fact they wish to murder me". He was probably suffering from Paranoid Schizophrenia and had this delusion. The jury reached a verdict of not guilty by reason of insanity and he was sent to Bethlem Hospital for life.

Following the trial, there was a meeting at the House of Lords attended by fifteen judges in order to determine the standards for the insanity defense. **McNaughton Rules** came to existence on 19th June 1843. McNaughton Rules also known as the legal test states: to establish a defense on the ground of insanity, it must be clearly proved that at the time of committing the act, the party accused was laboring under such a defect to reason, from disease of the mind, as not to know the nature and the quality of the act he was doing or, if he did know it, that he did not know he was doing what was wrong or contrary to the law of the land.

Other historical rules include Durham Rule, American Law Institute's Test of Criminal Responsiblity, Irresistible Impulse Test, Policeman at the elbow test.

DURHAM RULE

The Durhman Rule was formulated in 1954 by the Judge David Bazelon in the Monte Durham vs United States, in the district of Columbia, USA. The rule, as stated that "an accused is not criminally responsible if his unlawful act was the product of mental disease or mental defect." Where in the mental disease refers to mental disorder and mental defect refers to mental retardation. However due to the confusion in these terms, the rule was discarded in United States vs Brawner case, 1972.

IRRESISTIBLE IMPULSE TEST OR THE NEW HAMPSHIRE DOCTRINE

This test was devised by Issac Ray and Judge Charles Doe in 1869 in New Hampshire, USA. Irresistible impulse can be pleaded only under defense of diminished responsibilty and not under insanity defense. Here it is difficult to check whether impulse was strong and irresistible or the offender was weak and was not able to resist the impulse voluntarily.

INDIAN LAW

Based on above various rules, in India we have Section 84 of Indian Penal Code (I.P.C.) which is applicable under insanity defense. Under the section 84 IPC, "nothing is an offence which is done by a person who, at the time of doing it, by reason of unsoundness of mind, is incapable of knowing the nature of an act, or that he is doing what is either wrong or contrary to the law." This concept of Insanity Defense is adopted from McNaughton rules. As per the law every man is assumed to be sane and burden of proof of insanity lies on the accused.

The Section 84 IPC can be divided into two broad categories of, major criteria (medical requirement of mental illness) and minor criteria (loss of reasoning requirement).

Major criteria (mental illness requirement) mean the person must be suffering from mental illness during the commission of act.

Minor criteria (loss of reasoning requirement) mean the person is:

a. Incapable of knowing the nature of the act or
b. Incapable of knowing his act is wrong or
c. Incapable of knowing it is contrary to law.

Both major (mental illness) and minor (loss of reasoning) criteria constitute legal insanity.

We should be aware of difference between "medical insanity" and "legal insanity". Medical insanity does not come under the Section 84 IPC. Any person, who is suffering from any kind of mental illness is called "medical insanity," however "legal insanity" means, person suffering from mental illness should also have a loss of reasoning power at the time of committing crime. Thus legal insanity is purely a legal concept and is unrelated to the various psychiatric diagnoses.

Intoxication: Section 85 and 86 of IPC states that an accused is not criminally responsible if the intoxicant was administered to him without his knowledge or against his will. If intoxication was due to voluntary consumption e.g. of alcohol or other drugs, it is no excuse for commitment of crime.

AUTOMATISM

An Automatic behavior is defined as "an apparently purposeful and complex behavior which occurs without conscious control and for which there is amnesia later." Some of the conditions in which automatism occurs include epilepsy, intoxication, concussion and hypoglycemia. The concept of automatism is vague and have no special provision in the Law.

COMPETENCY TO STAND TRIAL

A test of competence recognizes a criminal defendent as competent to stand trial if he "has rational and factual understanding of the proceedings against him". Some instruments and screening questionnaires used for assessment of mentally ill patients for fitness to stand trial include MacArthur Competence Assessment Tool- Criminal Adjudication (MacCAT-CA), Evaluation of Competency to Stand Trial- Revised (ECST-R).

SUICIDE

Under the Section 309 Indian Penal Code, if a person attempts to commit suicide or does any act towards the commission of such offence, can be imprisoned upto 1 year or charge a fine or both. The offence is bailable. However if Section 84 is applied, then mentally ill person is not held responsible.

In 1994, two judge bench of Supreme Court declared the offence void and Section 309, irrational and cruel stating that "under the Article 21, of the Constitution of India, the right to live can be said to bring in its trial the right not to live a forced life". In 1996, five judge Consitution Bench of Supreme Court set aside the earlier judgment and so the Section 309 IPC continues to be valid

CONSENT

Section 90 Indian Penal Code states that " A consent is not a consent if given by a person who has an unsound mind, is intoxicated, unable to understand the nature and consequence for which he has given the consent, or if the consent given by a person is under 12 years of age" .

The question of invalidity of consent may arise in rape, murder, grievous hurt and abetment to suicide.

Section 89 Indian Penal Code means any act which is done by a person in good faith for benefit of a child 12 years or below or an insane with the consent of his lawful incharge guardian will not be considered as an offence If the consent for sexual intercourse is given by a woman who has low intellectual capacity or any mental illness is of no purpose and the act will be counted as a rape

BIBLIOGRAPHY

1. Asokan TV. Forensic psychiatry in India: The road ahead. Indian journal of psychiatry. 2014 Apr;56(2):121.
2. Math SB, Kumar CN, Moirangthem S. Insanity defense: Past, present, and future. Indian journal of psychological medicine. 2015 Oct;37(4):381.
3. Vyas JN, Ghimire SR. Textbook of Postgraduate Psychiatry. Jaypee Brothers; 2016.

Family Psychoeducation in Psychiatry

51

Anil Dokhale • Omkar Nayak • Sushma Sonavane

INTRODUCTION

Family members play an important role in the lives of individuals affected with mental illnesses. They have to shoulder a major responsibility of taking care of these individuals, continuing their medications and being an effective support system for them. A variety of interventions referred to as 'family psychoeducation' programs are planned in patients suffering from major mental illnesses such as Schizophrenia. These programs are carried out as a part of an overall management plan, and while the main focus remains on the well-being and functioning of the patient, the family members also stand to benefit from the same.

DEFINITION

Term 'Psychoeducation' can be defined in relation to various psychiatric disorders. It is used to describe a therapeutic concept consisting of four elements, which include explaining to the patients about the various aspects of their illness, training in problem solving, training in communication, and training in self-assertiveness, wherein relatives are also included.

Psychoeducation, although not an independent therapeutic method, is a combination of several therapeutic elements contained within a complex psycho-social intervention.

1. The working group of 'psychoeducation of patients with schizophrenia' defined the term psychoeducation as a systemic, didactic psychotherapeutic intervention which is adequate for informing patients and their relative about the illness and its treatment facilitating both an understanding and personally responsible handling of the illness and supporting those afflicted in coping with the disorder.
2. Baeker defined it with a broader concept as: "a process of teaching clients with mental illness and their family members about the nature of illness including its etiology, progression, consequences, prognosis, treatment and alternatives.

MODELS OF PSYCHOEDUCATION

The aim of psychoeducation is to enable patients as well as patient's family members to deal, understand and cope up with the mental health disorder, to deal with severe and chronic psychiatric disorders. There are four psychoeducation models proposed and categorized by Zipple & Spanial in 1997.

1. Individual *Psychoeducation:*

   Individual psychoeducation can be more specific and focused and can cover information and content that is more relevant for an individual situation.

   It may be more suitable when group situations are not comfortable, as it has the safety and confidentiality of one to one interaction with the therapist.

2. *Family Psychoeducation:*

   It deals with creating mental health awareness, management of coping skills to prevent relapse, ensure compliance, strengthen psycho- social support, improve social and occupational functioning. In the long term it is beneficial for the patient and the patient's family.

   Further divided into:

   i. Single family psychoeducation group: In which members of a single family are involved in psychoeducation without the patient.

   ii. Multiple family psychoeducation group: In which family members of multiple families are involved in psychoeducation without the patients.

3. Mixed family psychoeducation group: In which family members are involved in psychoeducation with the patient.

   However, there are certain contraindications to family psychoeducation, which include relatives themselves having formal thought disorder, manic or elevated mood, schizophrenia or acute suicidality with generally decreased resilience to stress.

   Suppose, we are dealing with a patient of Schizophrenia, the family members may be integrated within the treatment as soon as they are capable of taking part in a group for a period of 60 minutes. Ideally only relatives of patients suffering from Schizophrenic psychosis should participate in the group so as not to evoke unnecessary confusion in the caregivers through the schizophrenia specific informational consent. Group sessions last for one hour, take place twice in a week and consist anywhere between 4 and 16 sessions.

3. *Group Psychoeducation:*

   It is a form of therapy in which patients and their family members share their experiences under guidance of a mental health professional. Group therapy helps people learn to improve their interpersonal relationships. Members may share their own problems, feelings, ideas and reactions. Members gain insight for themselves regarding their issues, they gain encouragement from other participants and provide support and direction to others struggling with issues they have faced in the past. Usually a typical session lasts for 70 –90 minutes.

4. *Community Psychoeducation:*

   It educates a large number of population which may be non –homogeneous , irrespective of illness or illness related risk status. Social media like whatsApp, facebook, newspaper, twitter, television show, have major role in facilitating the psychoeducation process.

THERAPEUTIC AND CRITICAL FACTORS IN PSYCHOEDUCATION

Psychoeducation can be seen to serve an interpreter function, which translates the complicated technical terms, into common everyday language which can be understood by the relatives and helps them to become experts of their illness. Relatives progress with the patient through each stage of treatment feeling encouraged and full of hope. Relatives are to increasingly gain access to positive thoughts and positive conceptualizations of themselves and their patients.

THE GOALS OF PSYCHOEDUCATION

Psychoeducation should ensure a comprehensive introduction into the realm of psychiatric illnesses for the family members of patients and also inform the recurrent patients of latest developments in terms of treatment options. The very strength of psychoeducation lies in the deliberate focus on the relatives attaining basic competence in handling psychiatric illness faced by their near and dear ones. The relatives of chronic patients can be sent a hope that they are not abandoned to their fate, through family psychoeducation.

BASIC COMPONENTS OF PSYCHOEDUCATION AS PER THE INDIAN PSYCHIATRIC SOCIETY GUIDELINES

1. Assessing the knowledge of the patient and caregivers about etiology, treatment and prognosis.
2. Introducing the diagnosis into discussion.
3. Discussing about various symptom dimensions.
4. Providing information about etiology.
5. Provide information about treatment in terms of available options, their effectiveness, side effects, duration of use.
6. Discussion about importance of medication and treatment compliance.
7. Providing information about possible course and long-term outcome.
8. Discussing about problems of substance use, marriage and other issues.
9. Discussing about relapse and how to identify early signs of relapse.
10. Dealing with day to day stress.
11. Improving expressed emotions and improving communications.
12. Enhancing adaptive coping to deal with persistent / residual symptoms.

CONCLUSION

Psychoeducation is thus primarily a form of therapy conveying reassurance and hope, with the aim of empowering those, whose close ones are affected using professional therapeutic technics in a working and therapeutic alliance. The take home message of psychoeducational programs must be that psychiatric illnesses are induced by biological factors in combination with psycho-social stress, therefore they must be treated with both medications and psychotherapeutic interventions.

BIBLIOGRAPHY

1. Desousa A, Kurvey A, Sonavane S. Family psychoeducation for schizophrenia: a clinical review. Malaysian Journal of Psychiatry. 2012 Aug 24;21(2).
2. Avasthi A. Preserve and strengthenthe family to promote mental health.Indian J Psychiatry 2010;52(2):113-126.
3. Awad AG, Voruganti LN. Theburden of schizophrenia oncaregivers : a review. Pharmacoeconomics 2008;26:149-162.
4. Srinivasan N. Families as partners incare : perspectives from AMEND.Indian J Soc Work 2000;61:352-365.
5. Murthy RS. Family interventions andempowerment as an approach toenhance mental health resources indeveloping countries. WorldPsychiatry 2003;2:35-37
6. Colom F.Keeping therapies simple: psychoeducation in the prevention of relapse in affective disorders. The British Journal of Psychiatry(2011) 198: 338-340.
7. Perry A, Tarrier N, Morris R, McCarthy E, Limb K. Randomised controlled trial of efficacy of teaching patients withbipolar disorder to identify early symptoms of relapse and obtain treatment. BMJ 1999; 318: 149– 53.
8. Colom F, Vieta E, Sánchez-Moreno J, Martinez-Aran A,Reinares M, Goikolea J, et al. Stabilizing the stabilizer: group psychoeducation enhances the stability of serum lithium levels. Bipolar Disord 2005; 7 (Suppl 5): 32– 6.

9. Bäuml J, Froböse T, Kraemer S, Rentrop M, Pitschel-Walz G. Psychoeducation: a basic psychotherapeutic intervention forpatients with schizophrenia and their families.Schizophr Bull. 2006 Oct;32Suppl 1:S1-9. Epub 2006 Aug 18.
10. Dixon, Lisa, Curtis Adams and Alicia Lucksted. "Update on Family Psychoeducation for Schizophrenia." Schizophrenia Bulletin 26, no. 1 (2000): 5-19.
11. Yadav S, Kumar S. Models of Psychoeducation: an Indian Perspective. Indian Journal of Applied Research. 2014;4(7).

52 Overview of Psychotherapy and the Psychotherapeutic Process

Janki Mehta • Avinash De Sousa

All human beings from all walks of life will face challenges, traumas or emotional stability. It is rare to not have conflicts. It is the living experience of this life that makes it unique. When faced with adversities, human being using the power of thinking will find solutions out of necessity or to avoid pain. Very often we may not be aware of the nuances that causes one to worry or feel pain. The role of the psychotherapist or trained psychologist is to make clients aware of their thoughts, emotions, behaviors that are causing them pain.

Psychologists/Psychotherapists are non-medical doctors licensed practitioners who have been trained with a minimum of a masters in psychology or applied psychology. The role could be to assess and evaluate using psychometric testing, mental status examination, case history and formulation, to do research, to build implement or execute intervention programs, to train others or offer psychotherapy at a personal, industrial or community level.

Counseling may often be used inter-changeably in the psychological setting and a mental health professional may mean psychotherapy when using the term counseling, but it is essential to differentiate the two. Counseling can be used in a variety of situations or sections imparting information or providing guidance/direction; e.g. a young student may visit a career fair and find themselves being given information by a college counselor who may or may not have a degree in psychology or a individual who may seek spiritual guidance from a religious leader may or may not have a background in psychology. Fundamentally both psychotherapy and counseling have the same 'talk' approach and that is the binding factor.

Psychotherapy refers to a model to help one overcome personal problems and be trained in a particular school or schools of therapy and may include undergoing therapy themselves to work through the personal neurosis, conflicts, defenses that one may be carrying. This enables them to be more empathetic caregivers. Psychotherapy as a term was historically used only for psychoanalysis but now used for the different approaches one may adopt in their clinical practice.

It addresses deep core issues that one may or may not be aware of. It works with the client's personality, their background, and their current circumstances to address the dysfunctional patterns of thought, feelings or behaviors. It focuses on the underlying unconscious layers that go beyond what is being said or the presenting problem that brought them into therapy and giving an opportunity to the client to truly liberate themselves from within rather than make superficial cosmetic changes to their lives. It appears like new age mumbo jumbo but psychotherapy is tried, tested and well researched. In its nascent roots psychotherapy was very closely associated to psychopathology thus in the atrium of only medical professionals dealing with extreme mental anguish, psychosis and distress. Psychotherapy helps clients see things in new light, it supports them through change and offers them a safe and non-judgmental space. The role of the therapist can be compared to that of a global positioning system or GPS helping the client who sits on the driver's seat, to navigate the realms of their own mind. One does not receive lectures, advice or discourses about the 'shoulds' and 'musts' of life rather the onus lies with the client to choose what they might want to work with

Therapists will be asked a lot of questions about therapy before an appointment is booked. One cannot blame clients for not knowing as therapy is often considered something only 'mad', 'crazy', 'mentally unstable' 'weak' or those who can't manage their lives do. It does not help either when mental health is not covered as an integral part of healthcare schemes or insurance policies in India. This is the unfortunate stigma and taboo that mental health has faced for years partly blamed by the portrayal of psychology in popular culture and the godmen that govern the magical cure, magical pill industry. Mis-information often causes more harm than lack of information. Poverty, lack of education and the struggles of daily life often keep people away from seeking help.

One gets asked how therapy works as all we will be doing is talking. In other words one cannot see anything concrete but can only think, feel or see the consequences of their actions in the form of behavior, so how does one know if it's real and not just something in their 'head'. Clients find it difficult to imagine or comprehend the complex entity called the mind – as it is not limited to a part of the body nor can it be seen on an X-ray, or like wound or infection. Clinical studies have shown that psychotherapy can be effective for of treatment for depression, marital dissatisfaction, health problems (such as eating disorders, pain, smoking) and substance abuse, obsessive-compulsive disorder, personality disorders, sexual dysfunction and posttraumatic stress disorder and with various populations, including children, adolescents, adults and elders (Chambless et al, 1998)

Psychotherapy is not merely 'talking' but the engagement, the observation of thoughts, emotions or the behavior and the process of change to overcome a problem, conflict or trauma that one suffers from in either or all of the three components. It is intentional and often there is a mutual agreement between client and therapist on goals or expectations of therapy.

Will the effects of therapy last? Enough research, enough studies show the long lasting effects of therapy, neuroscientists acknowledge that new pathways are created in the brain when one experiences a change. We also see certain lobes of the brain activate or deactivate after healing a trauma. Any change from within will most often be long lasting and permanent.

Ms. A. K. *(name changed)* came for therapy just about the time she had been diagnosed with depression by a psychiatrist. The doctor recognized the need for therapy along with medication. After a brief discussion over the phone an appointment was fixed. As a therapist one must ideally ask clients to come in only once the medication has had 15/20 days in their system. Experience often shows that it helps with the receptivity of therapy. Not that this is a thumb rule but in extreme cases it is always useful.

STAGES OF PSYCHOTHERAPY:

The psychotherapeutic process happens in different stages, these stages are fluid and do not have a script but seen as a framework to help both the therapist gain access to the client and give the counselee a broad idea of the psychotherapeutic process.

Ms. A. K. slid into Major depressive disorder after she lost her young husband at the age of 36, and with a young 3 year old. Ms. A.K. had been in much shock and grief that she needed to seek help with a psychiatrist. Her family reported that she had not slept for days, neither did she cry, just holding her baby and lying down. They say the toll it had started to take on her, her appetite was missing and she withdrew herself.

The phone conversation is often helpful in understanding the client's perspective. She was firm and clearly mentioned that therapy was something she was only coming for because her family has insisted.

At this stage it is not recommended that the therapist confront or argue, but respect the client's choice and let the session be the place for a deciding the course of action.

1) Rapport Building and Initial disclosure.
2) In-depth exploration.
3) Commitment to action/change.
4) Termination.

1) **Rapport Building:** Rapport building is a fundamental part of the psychotherapeutic process, as no individual will on face value feel safe, confident or sure enough to discuss the perils of their inner world to what might be a practical stranger. No amount of good standing as an expert, training or skill will be effective if the client does not feel like they can communicate with the therapist. It can be understood as the state of complete synergy between the client and therapist on communication. Each understands the other and working towards the greater good. Rapport is a observable form of communication in all aspects of life. A harmonious communication makes things easier and effective. It may include finding the middle ground or common ground and developing a mutually respectable bond.

The therapist may spend a couple of sessions developing this bond because only when trust is build deeper issues may start surfacing. This is an important factor that any good therapist will be working to build along with therapy to develop a mutually exclusive and respectable relationship.

There is no real checklist that one can tick to form a bond or therapeutic relationship with a client but one can always be certain that talking about their lives, name of client their significant others, pets, place where they live or grew up, their occupation, facts or obvious things you may have notice such as they are fond of a certain brand because they carry a bag with its name on it. Incidental information mentioned during their session can always add value to this working relationship. Therapist disclosure can also be used when appropriate. The therapist must remember that the client is the key focus and use rapport to maximize the therapy session not to have a casual conversation. Having built a rapport, it becomes easier for the client to trust the therapist and start speaking openly of the problems that brought them to seek help initially. Disclosure includes any known incident, trauma, event, person or circumstances, which made them uncomfortable or brought a change in their thought, emotion or behavior. It could also be the related to an unforeseen or assumed stress of the future. Anything that distresses the client can and will be discussed in a session. Therapist openness and genuine care will lead to client readiness to move to the next step of counseling which is in-depth exploration.

The first session with Ms. A.K. was silent, after her mother filled in with details; she spoke only of the fact that she needed to get back to work and care of their daughter. She found it difficult to sleep in at night and needed help to rectify that. The mother had disclosed that A.K. had lost her husband to suicide. He had taken some drastic steps in the middle of the night in the house and A.K. was the first person to find him like that in the bathroom. As a therapist, our duty was to give her space and time to open up. We spoke nothing about what had happened but gave her some basic behavior therapy and relaxation exercises so she could fall asleep. She diligently came back next week because in her words, ' I liked that I was not forced to speak about my husband,' my concern was genuinely not having enough rest and it hampered my functioning through the day.'

2) **In-depth exploration:** In-depth exploration can only occur once the initial hesitancies of the client are passed. In-depth exploration has primarily two goals—a) gain insight, b) use the insight to make change.

   So what does gain insight mean, it means to move beyond the names and information about the client or significant others or places in the clients life.

   a) It is the understanding of the significant events or people that have shaped the client's current personality or circumstances.
   b) The influence of the their socio-economic, religious, education, or biological factors on the opportunities that they could have had.
   c) The different problem-solving methods or skills that they may have adopted over time to cope with their life.
   d) Strengths that may be latent or unused.
   e) Feelings about themselves, their relationships, any unfinished business from the past.
   f) Goals they may have set or tried to achieve earlier but need help to execute.

This information gives the therapist a concrete picture and starts adding pieces to the puzzle. Having insight helps the therapist bring perspective to an issue that the client may not have noticed earlier. The role of the therapist here becomes particularly important, as human beings often can get entangled in their own emotions losing objectivity or clarity. The therapist helps the client to bring this to their attention by offering a newer perspective, supporting them through a particularly difficult revelation in therapy or literally zooming out and allowing for a macro view. This can also be a stage when deeper emotions will be explored, by that one means emotions that are misunderstood or emotions that have become habits over time that one does not even know they exist. These could be either positive or negative emotions.

Ms. A.K. took a few sessions to open up, she spoke of her plans to get back to work, her life before what had happened, her child and everything but the incident. One must understand life-changing traumas are extremely painful and the mind will often circumvent it to avoid any pain. It is natural and very common. On the fourth session, she spoke of the plans she had made with her husband to buy a small farmland and grow vegetables and have a lovely eco-lodge. As she started giving me details, she could not contain herself, the memories started building and she cried, she continued to bawl without understanding how much she had buried inside. The therapist space became a space where she found safety and comfort to allow this emotion, which was repressed for a long time. This session was a breakthrough one because it opened doors for healing to begin.

The therapist here may under no circumstance divert, distract or console the patient in a difficult revelation. The job of the therapist here is to allow the maximum release of emotions. Only thing one can do is offer some water and tissue. Not all sessions will have such dramatic breakthroughs but it is essential to be in tune with the client as small moments of insight or 'Aha' moments make place for action and change.

3) **Commitment to action/change:** In-depth exploration paves the way for the therapist to see the puzzles in totality. The dots often get connected and the client sees the cognitions, the feelings or behaviors that hold them back. They show the therapist the markers or flags that may have been causes, effects or roots of a certain problem. All human beings have blind spots and this phase helps one address them. Clients often have layers built as coping and the therapist helps uncover them or see them using probing questions, and possibly confrontation. Once the issue is opened up, many clients may face resistance, fear, may be in denial or cannot come to terms with their personal truths. The therapist provides time and space and helps address any concern and moves to help the client set a goal, work with the thoughts, feelings and behaviors to achieve the goal. It may include homework beyond sessions, journaling, dream exercises and many other technics subjective to the client and therapist training.

Ms. A.K. spoke of how she had lost her father at the age of 12 to suicide, he was an highly intelligent scientist and seeing her mother and her older sister go through difficult times made a strong and resilient person. She often was the doer in the family and everyone relied on her. She met her deceased husband in college and after a brief romance settled comfortably into a new life. She said she had only spoken of her father to him and he assured her he would always be there for her but life and fate served her the same card. She realized the initial shock and grief she felt had the same feel when she was a 12 year old and how her deepest issues with abandonment opened up yet again. She was angry at her father, her husband for leaving her, she was angry at herself for not looking out for her daughter and her mother for never talking to her. Each session gave her insight into her own world and helped her to work with the grief she was carrying all these years. We were able to change the feelings of abandonment and bring her to some peace and resolution which helped her talk to her mother and give her impetus to live life again for her daughter. She slowly found herself regain her jovial self back and we spoke about termination and smoothly transit back into her life.

4) **Termination:** Termination of therapy is often discussed in therapy when the therapist sees that a goal has been met,

or sufficient work has been done to resolve the problem when the client first entered therapy for. It is important to end therapy on a positive note. The role of the therapist is to ensure that they have provided enough resources to the client to take full responsibility and continue their life. It is generally mutually decided. One may have worked over one issue or multiple either way termination can be once if there was no time gap between sessions or multiple times if there was a time gap. Termination can happen when both the client and therapist believe that the client is ready to take on their newly acquired mastery in sessions can be applied in real life. Readiness to terminate can be discussed and often all worries and anxieties be addressed on termination. Abrupt termination is never recommended and it is a formal duty to provide important numbers, emails or resources beforehand. Therapists often leave the discretion of returning based on the therapeutic relationship shared.

CHARACTERISTICS OF AN EFFECTIVE PSYCHOTHERAPIST

When one thinks of a therapist, they may have caricature or threatening images of that shown in movies, very few people understand what entails to be a psychotherapist apart from years of studying and training and ability to be introspective. Over the years many have tried to identify the few characteristics that may make one an effective and good therapist. Most of these characteristics below were defined, mentioned and heavily relied upon in the Person/Client-Centered therapy school by Carl Rogers.

1) **Empathy:** Empathy very simply put is the therapist's ability to wear the client's shoes and see perspective from their lens. The ability to look at the problem from the individual's point of view rather than attempting to see it from their own. What empathy does it brings forth the ability for dialogue which sympathy may or may not bring. Empathy puts the therapist in the listener's chair than a chair of judgment or pity. Empathy helps one to understand the client's thought (cognition), emotions (affects), perceptions, motivations and behavior that may be causing distress. It requires an innate ability to attune into the inner workings of one's mind with utmost sensitivity and accuracy to work with the here and now.

   Carl Rogers who gave us person-centered/client-centered therapy approach once said (1959) "The state of empathy, or being empathic, is to perceive the internal frame of reference of another with accuracy and with the emotional components and meanings which pertain thereto as if one were the person, but without ever losing the 'as if' condition. Thus it means to sense the hurt or the pleasure of another as he senses it and to perceive the causes thereof as he perceives them, but without ever losing the recognition that it is as if I were hurt or pleased and so forth. If this 'as if' quality is lost, then the state is one of identification".

2) **Altruism:** Altruism is the ability to help or act out of a complete and genuine concern for the other individual. It refers to the therapist's motivation to help coming from a place of care rather than any ulterior motive and malice. This quality may not be written across textbooks around but it was an important characteristic that I was taught about at university because it was considered a valuable trait to be a good therapist. It takes one a long way into the helping profession.

3) **Unconditional Positive Regard:** Carl Rogers had a unique way at looking at human beings. He believed that we innately have the ability to understand ourselves, we have a large amount of untapped resources within us to help us facilitate change of our self-concept, our behaviors, our emotions but this may not be possible to tap into if the environment is conducive for change. One will not be able to both show their true selves and work through them if there is hostility or any perceived threat or fear. Thus, the role of the therapist is to create a place of absolute safety, where can be have a safe space to open up their vulnerabilities and without a hint of judgment regardless of the client's race, gender, sexual preference, ethnicity, disabilities, socio-economic background, religion or culture. It is absolutely necessary to have that for being a quality care provider.

4) **Congruency:** All human beings have an inner world and an outer world. The inner world is a private personal space that very few people may have access to, sometimes life circumstance or experiences may shut this inner world to our own selves as well. The external world is what we show/project to the external world. It is how we act, behave or portray ourselves as in front of others. This may or may not be fully aligned with our inner world. The therapist is expected to be as aligned, genuine and open about his or her own feelings and attitudes in the therapeutic relationship so as to help the client be open and authentic as well. The client can build a relationship of trust and knowing. The divide between the internal world and external is as minimal or nil for a good therapist. This is called genuineness or congruency.

5) **Active listening skills:** Active listening is a myriad of components that come together in a therapy session. The therapist will hear the content of what is being said, the feelings that may or may not have been said, the verbal cues, the non-verbal cues, gestures and body language. It is to be neutral and have no sign of judgment, paraphrase so the client can hear what they said and rectify if they need to. The therapist will clarify, question, reflect, summarizes and bring in their own unique observations. This may seem like a lot to do for many and often young therapists get nervous but with time and practice it comes as second nature.

ETHICS OF THE PSYCHOTHERAPEUTIC PRACTICE

Most therapists have a code of conduct and ethical guidelines to follow along with country based laws and regulations. It is very important to uphold these ethics as this leads to a safe and successful practice and respects the profession and clients who come with full faith and trust in the system. One cannot go into many details but some of the ethics that one must adhere to are:

1) **Confidentiality:** Confidentiality is the key to therapy. One must understand that the mind is a complex and fragile human entity. It holds possible all information that the client has experienced in their lifetime. This includes the good experiences, and the bad - the innermost fears, habits, fantasies and forbidden truths. The role here of the therapist is to be completely respectful of the client's wishes especially if they are consenting adults. The rules of confidentiality can only be broken under few circumstances, they are–

    a) Direct or implied threat to the client's life – or risk/self-harm reported by the client.

b) Direct or implied threat to the therapist or any other person.

c) Any known threat about violence, abuse or torture to the client or child's life – e.g. Sexual abuse, domestic violence.

In such circumstances it is necessary for the therapist to inform the concerned parties such as the family members, legal bodies, police, social workers, child protective services.

2) **Transference and Countertransference:**

Transference refers to the unconscious emotional bond and dependency that develops towards the therapist by the client. This very often has basis in the client's relationship outside of therapy with significant loved ones more often than not rooted in their relationship growing up with their primary caregivers or parents. This may lead to the client's unwillingness to move ahead, have regressed behavior and have unrealistic demands and expectations from the therapist. This can result in wanting more time, sexual longing especially if the client's sexual preference matches that of the therapist.

Countertransference refers to the bond that the therapist may develop. This is a slippery slope that a therapist can quickly go down if they are not careful. There could be possible misuse as due to the power dynamic between the client and therapist leading to abuse of role and opening more wounds to an already vulnerable client.

The codes of justice, benevolence, non-maleficence, fidelity – loyalty or promise keeping in this context have high value along with respect for complete autonomy for both the client and therapist.

APPROACHES TO THE SCHOOLS OF PSYCHOTHERAPY

The schools mentioned below are in a brief and condensed format to give one a glimpse and an overall sense of the vastness. Very often the saying 'all roads leads to Rome' comes to mind once one understands how therapy works. It means that the approach may be different but the end goal is the same, to help one to overcome and find solutions to their problems.

It is important to note that in the early 20th century there was only one form of psychotherapy – which was psychoanalytic psychotherapy but with time many schools were established moving away from the tradition of psychoanalysis. The term then took a generic format to explain the school the therapist may be trained in or the approach they use in their private practice.

I. **Psychoanalytic Approaches:** Psychoanalysis or psychoanalytic psychotherapy or psychodynamic schools as stem from the works of Sigmund Freud, the father of modern psychology. The lineage or torchbearers have a common consensus with the view that the human psyche is an independent entity called the human mind with its power dynamics, the complexities of the unconscious, the dreams, the symbolism and defense mechanisms all play a role in our lives especially the conflicts of early childhood. Sigmund Freud had an enormous influence in bringing therapy to mainstream.

Carl Jung a one time close associate of Sigmund Freud moved away from Freud after disagreeing that only childhood is the seat of all ill in latter life. He studied and was greatly influenced by anthropology, mythology, theology, alchemy and many disciplines giving a lot of weightage at seeing human beings in context to developmental, archetypal and traditional therapy with a spiritually oriented approach and as one collective organism.

Alfred Adler too was a colleague of Freud moved away after he felt differently giving human beings a more holistic approach looking at social, educational dimensions. He examined the family dynamics, birth order and been a respectable contributor to the field of psychology.

II. **Cognitive-Behavioral Approaches:** The premise for cognitive behavior approaches is simple; it does not look at the global factors or causes and works with specific strategies, behavior changes, or with the added step of dysfunctional cognitions. It hopes to reduce stress mediating the cognition the behavior in a verifiable manner using assessment, evaluation largely focusing on the present.

Behavior Therapy: One learns to deal with harm causing behaviors by identification, learn new coping styles using the created situations by the therapists. Systematic desensitization, exposure, response prevention are some of the technics used.

Rational Emotive Behavior Therapy (REBT) - Abert Ellis a clinical psychologist, came up with REBT formerly called rational and rational emotive therapy in an attempt to provide a present based approach and arguing that all our life events that cause distress come from irrational beliefs we hold and one can overcome them using a range of technics.

Cognitive Therapy: Aaron Beck developed Cognitive therapy to help work with thoughts that may cause us to have negative and positive moods. The approach is to catch and change, learn or understand the thought that has impact and its inferences we carry.

III. **Humanistic Approaches:** **Humanistic approaches mind together with the strong believe in the innate optimism and life-thriving determination of an individual. Thus the approach is to have a holistic approach to therapy.**

Person-Centered Therapy: Carl Rogers rejected the psychoanalytic ideas and based his work on the basis on human experience giving utmost importance to the core principles of empathy, unconditional positive regard, congruency to bridge the gap of the ideal and real self and see real change. He said these were the keys to successful personal growth.

IV. **Gestalt Therapy:** Fritz and Laura Perls devised Gestalt therapy after being influenced by the Gestalt work of Max Wertheimer, Wolfgang Köhler, and Kurt Koffka. Gestalt means whole or pattern in German and their approach was to see human life as a whole or greater than the sum of its parts. It looked at human beings in context to its entirety but highly focusing on the here and now giving importance to body language, language cues, stuck energy in the body and rejected intellectualizing therapy.

V. **Transactional Analysis:** Eric Berne moved away from Psychoanalytic tradition and focused on observable interpersonal interactions. He worked with the interaction of the private unconscious and the self-limiting drivers, injunctions, ego states, life scripts, games, rackets that we may adopt in our lifetime.

VI. **Existential Counseling:** A number of therapists moved away from the psychoanalytic traditions, it was also the world events that made individuals wanting to find meaning and purpose in life. They work with the inner challenges, dilemmas, morals, values, and principles to choices and commitment. It heavily drew inspiration from philosophy or life experiences such as that of Viktor Frankl who was a Holocaust Survivor himself. The belief is that finding purpose meaning through self-identification and responsibility can liberate man from their own inner conflicts.

NEWER APPROACHES

1) **Hypnotherapy:** Hypnosis had existed in various cultures throughout history but often associated with the dark arts/ occult sciences or a performance art like a circus. Rarely was it used in a channelized way till Joseph Breuer and his protégé Sigmund Freud experimented with it. It is successfully used in many phobias, fears or repressed memories work.
2) **Inner child work:** Inner child work helps individuals to access their own childhood conflicts that may be interfering with present life situations and work through them resolving conflicts of today.
3) **Neuro-linguistic programming:** NLP draws from strategies used by a community or important figures or successful heads of the fields by studying, observing, analyzing and applying them to reach a personal goal. It gives importance to the thoughts, patterns and language.

CONCLUSION

We have tried to cover a comprehensive idea of the psychotherapeutic practice. It is safe to say that one can now have a clearer understanding that we do not only talk but are engaging in a far more deeper dialogue with the client/ patients that come to us seeking solutions to their conflicts, problems or difficulty using the tools given to us through different therapeutic schools. Psychotherapy is a dynamic, ever improving and ever changing field, newer studies, newer research adds more to address and help more people than ever. Technology has made it possible to provide care in sometimes-remote parts of the world. There will always be critic claiming its ineffectiveness, its problems with misuse of power or exploitation. This particular field is far more satisfying than most others as the change seen and benefits from over a century old science is far more rewarding and has withstood the testimony of time.

Psychology - Basics 53

Pragya Lodha • Avinash De Sousa

WHAT IS PSYCHOLOGY?

Psychology is the scientific study mental processes and states and behaviors in human and animals. The focus of study is on human mind, its functions and human behavior in a given context. Though there does not exist unanimously agreed upon definition for psychology, it is understood as a discipline of soft-science that is heterogeneous with various interdisciplinary sub-fields also being a part of the field of psychology.

Specifically, psychology explores how people think, how they act, how they interact with their environment and with each other. Professionals who have done a Master of Arts (M.A.) or Master of Science (M.Sc.) degree in psychology are eligible to practice as psychologists. Psychologists all over the world are currently researching the scientific answers to fundamental questions such as how and why humans behave the way they do. This knowledge can then influence all aspects of public life such as health, education and social justice.

For most of the 20th century, psychological science consisted of a variety of specialized subfields with little interconnection. They ranged from clinical psychology to the study of individual differences and personality, to social psychology, to industrial-organizational psychology, to community psychology, to the experimental psychology and to physiological psychology. In the early years of the 21st century, psychology became an increasingly integrative science at the intersection of biology, neurology, economics, sociology, anthropology, law, sports, media and art.

PROFESSIONALS IN PSYCHOLOGY

There are different areas of psychology in which it is possible to practice and gain the title of a psychologist. This title is the benchmark of professional recognition, and reflects the highest standard of psychological knowledge and expertise. Some of the more well-known domains for psychologists are as follows:

- Clinical Psychology
- Counseling Psychology
- Educational Psychology
- Forensic Psychology
- Health Psychology
- Occupational Psychology
- Teaching and Research in Psychology
- Social Psychology
- Industrial-Organizational Psychology

Many people are often confused about the differences between psychology and psychiatry. In reality, both professions work with similar patients (particularly in hospitals and rehabilitation settings) but there are some critical and fundamental differences in their training and overall approach to mental health that distinguish them. Psychiatry is a specialisation of a medical degree meaning that all psychiatrists are trained doctors who have opted to specialise in the field of mental health. Due to this medical background, psychiatrists can prescribe medication whereas psychologists focus more or talk therapy as means for illness-management. Another difference of importance in clinical practices is to know between counseling psychologists and clinical psychologists.

DIFFERENCE BETWEEN A COUNSELING AND CLINICAL PSYCHOLOGIST

Professionals working as counseling psychologists are those who have completed their specialisation of M.A. or M.Sc. in Counseling psychology. As counseling psychologists, the focus is solely on therapeutic practice. They work closely with patients to look at mental health issues and explore the underlying problems that may have caused them. They work collaboratively with individuals to empower them to make decisions for themselves to improve their sense of personal wellbeing by making lifestyle changes, behavioral changes and imbibing the concept of self-determination (taking responsibility for their actions, thoughts and feelings).

Counseling psychologists work across a range of problems including bereavement, relationships, mental health issues and other significant life events. Counseling psychologists are generally trained in psychotherapy and may go ahead to further specialize in specific school(s) of psychotherapy. Counseling, which is different from psychotherapy is also a component of their practice. Where psychotherapy is more structured and model / school-specific practices to address mental illnesses, counseling is more unstructured and motivational in nature. They work in many places including industry, the prison service and in all levels of the education system. Primarily, counselors work in schools, colleges, private clinics or with organizations (NGOs, institutions and other organizations).

On the other hand, clinical psychologists are professionals have a specialization of M.A. or M.Sc. in Clinical Psychology. Though the aim of clinical psychologists is also to reduce the psychological distress and enhance psychological well-being, they deal with a number of mental and physical problems including anxiety, depression, addiction and relationship problems. The course teaching for clinical psychologists is more clinical in nature with regards to them covering greater number of clinical symptomatology and illnesses. Additional to psychotherapy, clinical psychologists also work with psychometric assessment. Though, counseling psychologists also carry out psychometric assessment, they are not holistically trained in all assessments. Clinical psychologists are holistically trained to carry out personality, intelligence and neuropsychological assessments. Clinical psychologists work in diverse settings from schools, educational set-ups, industries, private clinics, hospitals and prison services. Due to their role as a scientist-practitioner they are also involved heavily with research and in evaluation of current services to provide a strong evidence base for practice.

The focal difference between counseling and clinical psychology is their perspective and training. Where the focus for counseling psychologists is more on healthier, less pathological populations, clinical psychologists focus on individuals with more serious mental health issues.

Table 52.1: Difference between counseling and clinical psychologists

Counseling Psychologist	Clinical Psychologist
M.A. / M.Sc. in Counseling Psychology	M.A. / M.Sc. in Clinical Psychology
Works with less pathological, healthier population	Works with more pathological population
Psychotherapy is the primary medium of work	Psychotherapy and psychometric assessment are the primary media of work
Work more often in schools and educational settings	Work more often in hospital and clinical settings
Focus on research for evidence-based practice is less robust	Focus on research for evidence-based practice is heavily robust
Work more with adjustment-based issues	Work more with serious clinical issues

BIBLIOGRAPHY

1. Colman A. What is psychology? Routledge; 2016 Jan 28.
2. Foster J. Psychological therapies in primary care: Setting up a managed service. Routledge; 2018 Jun 27.
3. Kramer GP, Bernstein DA, Phares V. Introduction to clinical psychology. Cambridge University Press; 2019 Aug 22.
4. Murdoch DD, Gregory A, Eggleton JM. Why psychology? An investigation of the training in psychological literacy in nursing, medicine, social work, counseling psychology, and clinical psychology. Canadian Psychology/Psychologie canadienne. 2015 Feb;56(1):136.
5. Tribe R, Morrissey J, editors. Handbook of professional and ethical practice for psychologists, counsellors and psychotherapists. Routledge; 2015 Jan 30.

54 Cognitive Behaviour Therapy (CBT) & Rational Emotive Behaviour Therapy (REBT)

Heta N. Shah

Cognitive treatment systems can be used either alone or in combination with other theoretical approaches. Treatment that emphasizes on thoughts can make the counseling process more acceptable to people who are not used to sharing their emotions and thereby experiencing positive gains in treatment increases people's motivation and optimism which can then accelerate the course of treatment.

Cognitive therapy has grown rapidly over these years and is recognized as one of the major approaches to counseling and psychotherapy. Albert Ellis established the foundation of cognitive therapy but the work of Aaron T. Beck and his colleagues fueled the growth of this approach. Following Table 54.1 outlines the major differences between CBT and REBT –

Table 54.1

	CBT	**REBT**
Founded By	Aaron Beck in 1960s	Albert Ellis in 1950s
Theoretical Basis	Thoughts determine emotions & behavior	Irrational belief (B) system triggered by an activating event (A) cause the consequence (C) to the event
Aspects emphasized	Automatic thoughts, cognitive distortions & underlying beliefs and schemes	Irrational and rational beliefs
Modification	It is a therapy through which one's current negative behavior can be replaced with a positive and wholesome one	With this therapy, someone's deep-seated beliefs and notions can be uprooted
Focus	Its main focus is to change cognitive distortions	Its main focus is to change underlying beliefs which are irrational
Goal	Help people recognize and correct errors in information-processing systems	Help people to learn cognitive skills that promote rational thinking and lead to greater happiness and self-acceptance
Working Through	Cognitive Distortions*	Irrational Beliefs**
Process	Identification of both their immediate (automatic) and underlying (intermediate, core, scheme) thoughts and beliefs as well as associated emotions and behaviors; evaluating the validity of these thoughts and modifying them, if indicated	Identifying, assessing, disputing and modifying beliefs

(Continued...)

	CBT	REBT
Therapeutic Alliance	Collaborative relationship between therapist-client & therapist adopts Socratic approach	Collaborative relationship between therapist-client & therapist adopts philosophical approach
Strategies	Thought stopping, Diary writing, reframing situations by changing cognitive distortions, self-talk, positive imagery, etc.	Confronting irrational beliefs, worst scenario coping, accepting self & others as fallible beings, reframing situation by changing labels & beliefs, rational-emotive imagery, etc.

*__Cognitive Distortions__ – Cognitive distortions usually are negative thoughts about the self, reflecting guilt and low self-esteem, or negative thoughts about people's relationships and context that exaggerate the likelihood of undesirable events and behaviors. Few examples of cognitive distortions are –

- Overgeneralization: Drawing sweeping conclusions that are not justified by the evidence. E.g. "I am a failure as a parent because my son failed in exams.'
- Magnification/minimization: Making too much of the negative, devaluing positive information. E.g. "I got a B. This proves how inferior I am.
- Jumping to conclusions: Drawing hasty and unwarranted conclusions. E.g. "I know that person was angry onto me as he didn't smiled while talking to me."
- Tunnel vision: Focusing only on the negative aspects of a situation. E.g. "He just can't do anything right."

**__Irrational Beliefs:__ In REBT, irrational beliefs are defined as beliefs that are rigid, extreme and illogical (inconsistent with reality)/ Few examples of irrational beliefs are –

- I must do everything well, or I am incompetent.
- I must worry about anything fearful or risky.
- I must be loved by everyone, or I am not lovable.

Despite these differences between CBT & REBT, great overlap exists between them. Both of them can be easily integrated with other approaches to psychotherapy as it lays less focus on development of insight and exploration of client's background. Both the therapies has established effectiveness in treating a broad range of mental disorders, especially major depressive disorder and anxiety disorders. It could also be used as a form of individual, group and family therapy.

55 Family Therapy – An Overview of Key Constructs

Avinash De Sousa • Nilesh Shah

ABSTRACT

The aim of this chapter is to synthesize various family therapy concepts known and schools of thought available in a form that family therapists can use. There are multiple schools and concepts that have been used in family therapy. Family therapists, however, need an integrative concept that goes beyond the parent/child dyad. There is a need for understanding of concepts and a network of care which is made available for all family members of whatever age so that all family members feel secure enough to explore, in the knowledge that support is available if needed. Factors that contribute to the security or insecurity of the family base and critical family therapy foundations are outlined. The overall aim of family therapy is to establish a secure family base from which the family can explore new solutions to family problems both during and after therapy. The role of the therapist is to help to resolve conflicts that threaten relationships, and to explore relevant belief systems that may be contributing to a sense of insecurity. The conceptual framework presented allows for an integration of family therapy technics and ideas into a coherent whole. A new school of family therapy is not proposed but rather holistic integration of existent schools is sought.

Key words – concepts, Family therapy.

INTRODUCTION

Quite early in the development of family therapy some of the ideas of cybernetics were adopted by therapists trying to understand the fixed, but dysfunctional, processes occurring in many of the families they saw. The difficulties many families experienced when faced with the need to make changes were 'explained' by saying that the homeostatic mechanisms in the system tended to maintain the *status quo,* rather than permit needed changes to occur. In the present chapter we look at various concepts that have been central to the foundation of family therapy and their utility in clinical practice

SYSTEMS THEORY AND FAMILY THERAPY

General systems theory was proposed as a general theory of the organization of parts into wholes. A system was defined as 'a complex of interacting elements'. Some defined a ***system*** as 'a set of objects together with the relationships between the objects and between their attributes'. These definitions place no limits on what the 'parts' or 'objects' may be. They may thus be living or non-living. The theory is designed to cover physical phenomena and machines as well as biological systems (Goldenberg and Goldenberg, 2008). Authors also distinguished ***open from closed systems.*** Closed systems are those in which there is no interaction with the surrounding environment, as in a chemical or physical reaction in a closed container. Such systems obey rules different from those obeyed by open systems. Closed systems, for instance, show ***entropy,*** the tendency to reach the simplest, least ordered possible state from whatever may be the starting situation (Goldenberg and Goldenberg, 2008).

Open systems such as families do not show entropy. Instead there is a steady inflow and outflow of relevant information across the boundary of the system. If the characteristics of the boundary remain the same and the outside environment is also unchanged, a ***steady state*** is reached. The environment of most open systems is, however, liable to change. There may also be alterations in the characteristics of the boundary. These properties of open systems make change and evolution possible. To make things even more complicated, the individual family members may change (Sexton, Weeks and Robbins, 2003).

Systems theory itself consists of a complex of mathematical propositions about the properties of systems. Family therapists have not used the mathematical models, no doubt because the phenomena with which they deal cannot readily, if at all, be reduced to mathematical terms. For family therapy purposes, the term ***systems thinking*** is probably more appropriate than ***systems theory.*** The importance of systems theory to family therapy lies in the ideas and concepts it has brought to the field. These include the following: (Carr, 2008)

1. Families (and other social groups) are systems having properties which are more than the sum of the properties of their parts.
2. The operation of such systems is governed by certain general rules.
3. Every system has a boundary, the properties of which are important in understanding how the system works.
4. The boundaries are semi-permeable; that is to say some things can pass through them while others cannot. Moreover it is sometimes found that certain material can pass one way but not the other.
5. Family systems tend to reach relatively, but not totally, steady states. Growth and evolution are possible, indeed usual. Change can occur, or be stimulated, in various ways.
6. Communication and feedback mechanisms between the parts of a system are important in the functioning of the system.
7. Events such as the behavior of individuals in a family are better understood as examples of ***circular causality,*** rather than as being based on ***linear causality***
8. Family systems, like other open systems, appear to be purposeful.
9. Systems are made up of ***subsystems*** and themselves are parts of larger ***suprasystems.***

Systems thinking has more to offer family therapy than cybernetics, which is mainly concerned with feedback mechanisms. The idea of circular causality, as opposed to linear causality, as a basis for understanding the processes occurring in families, is however common to both. Linear causality describes the process whereby one event causes another (Ariel, 1999).

An important concept derived from systems theory is that of the relationship between systems, subsystems and suprasystems. All living systems are composed of subsystems. So if a family is the system under study, it will be found to consist of various individuals or groups of individuals which function as subsystems. Examples are parental, marital and child subsystems; there may also be boy and girl subsystems, or subsystems consisting of older and younger children. Such subsystems have their subsystems too; an individual human being is also made up of various systems, whether physical (renal, cardiovascular, nervous and so on) or psychological (ego, id, superego) (Becvar and Becvar, 2000).

Suprasystems to which families may belong include the extended family, the village, the neighborhood, the tribe, a church community and so on. These in turn are part of larger suprasystems, until we get to nations, groups of nations and planet earth itself. The earth, of course, is but part of a still larger celestial system. The system upon which family therapists usually concentrate is of course the family. Family therapists are interested also in the subsystems and, usually, the suprasystems of the families they are treating (Becvar, 2007).

Every system has a ***boundary,*** which marks it off from its surroundings. Living systems have readily identifiable physical boundaries, consisting of skin, mucus membranes, the bark of trees and so forth. The boundaries of emotional and psychological systems are not visible in the same way, but they are equally important. They control emotional interchanges, closeness and joint actions. The boundary between one subsystem and another is characterized by restricted emotional interchange, compared with that between those individuals within the one subsystem. Similar considerations apply to the boundaries between systems and their suprasystems (Becvar and Becvar, 2000).

The term ***'equifinality'*** describes the process whereby an open system maintains the same steady state with differing inputs. The chemistry of the body is a good example. The concentration of most electrolytes and other chemical compounds remains within narrow limits regardless of dietary intake. This is because of regulatory mechanisms involving the kidneys, lungs and other organs. Similarly families tend to have their set methods of functioning, regardless of what is happening around them, or what information or stimulation is coming in from outside. Although the principle of equifinality seems to have relevance to the way families function, the term is not nowadays much used in the family therapy literature (Coles, 2006).

COMMUNICATIONS THEORY

Communication within families has long interested family therapists, many of whom have developed theories about human communication, and how it may be modified when this is needed. There are three aspects of human communication viz. syntax, semantics and pragmatics (Goldenberg, 2002).

Syntax refers to the conventions used when words are put together in sentences and paragraphs to express meaning; it comprises the grammatical rules of the language.

Semantics is concerned with the meanings of words; it deals with the principles that govern the relationship between words or sentences and their meaning, the clarity of language and its use in particular situations. While the meanings of words may be defined in dictionaries, in practice people do not always stick to such definitions. In many families (and other settings) there are private languages and shared systems of communication which it is helpful for the therapist to understand.

Pragmatics is the study of the behavioral effects of communication. These are related as much, or perhaps even more, to the nonverbal behavior of those involved and to the context of the communication as they are to the semantic content of what is said (Ragg, 2006).

EPISTEMOLOGY

'Epistemology' is a term much used by family therapists. It refers to the theory on which a body of knowledge is based. It represents the underlying assumptions which people make when they seek to understand something. The search for new theoretical models for use in the treatment of families has thus involved the development of new epistemologies. Family therapy has needed a new theoretical basis, different from that traditionally used to understand individuals. This need led to the use of the term 'the new epistemology' by some therapists. It is however misleading because it suggests the existence of a specific, new, generally accepted way of thinking about and understanding families. No doubt many therapists have come to use new epistemologies, but the process is an evolutionary one. There is no one 'new epistemology/ and the evolutionary process has by no means come to an end. Indeed it is unlikely that it will ever do so (Berg, 1994).

COHERENCE

Coherence refers to one of the concepts that have emerged as part of the quest for new epistemologies by those who work with families. Authors define it as follows – "Coherence simply implies a congruent interdependence in functioning whereby all aspects of the system fit together. It would seem to be adequate for describing the behavior of a system-being-itself without inadvertently implying anything more than that" (Sprenkle and Moon, 1996).

VIRGINIA SATIR: COMMUNICATION AND FEELING

Virginia Satir, mainly through one book *Conjoint Family Therapy,* became one of the major forces in the field of family therapy. Over the past decade Virginia Satir has moved away from the world of therapy and into that of "growth potential," and has gone around the world helping people to communicate. As a result she has not made any further contribution to the field. Even so she is still widely read and influential among family therapists. The value in the book is mainly in the abundant illustrations she uses. Satir does not talk in abstractions but translates her basic philosophy into concrete examples (Satir, 1983).

In her writings she tends to allude more to others than developing basic theory. It is easier, therefore, in studying communication theory in family therapy, to see first the underlying concepts on which it is based, and then later to look at how these notions can be applied specifically.

In *Conjoint Family Therapy,* Satir states some basic premises and elaborates with case studies. The method has advantages and disadvantages. Positively, it helps the student see how, in practice, one might go about doing family therapy. Negatively, it also can produce a sense of frustration, leaving the student asking himself how Satir arrives at a particular statement. The usual devices used by theorists, that is citing authors, developing rational arguments for a position, and so on, are largely bypassed. However, when taken in conjunction with more theoretical positions, Satir's thinking fills up some of the *lacunae* that may exist in abstract thinking (Datillo, 1998).

Satir also brings a dimension of feeling to communicational theory that helps to counterbalance its obvious intellectual base. Satir exudes warmth and caring in her therapy. In the past few years she has moved off into the wider areas of the encounter and human potential growth movements. Of all the therapists studied, she is the one most involved in the emotional or the feeling level of people (Satir, 1983).

Satir emphasizes the feeling aspect of communication in the following remarks:

"There are four wrong ways people communicate. You can blame, you can placate, you can be irrelevant or you can be "reasonable." There's something incomplete about each way. The blamer leaves out what he feels about the other person, the placater leaves out what he feels about himself, the reasonable one leaves out what he feels about the subject being discussed and the irrelevant one leaves out everything" (Satir, 1967).

This is a good summary statement because she spells out what communication means: It is focused on feelings. It is not that cognition or control is unimportant but that feeling is central. The philosopher Descartes said: "I think, therefore, I am;" Satir says: "I feel, therefore, I am." It is a question of emphasis. The emphasis is on needs, but needs as related to emotional interchanges in the family system and not just material things. The family is the place where these kinds of needs are met. If they are not met, then symptoms begin to appear and are a clue to a disturbance in the system. The way to get to the disturbance, the underlying cause, is to attend to the here and now pain. Brains think and wills execute, but people feel pain in their emotional system. It is an obvious concept but perhaps so obvious that it is often overlooked. Satir begins with this level and proceeds to move into the family system, less in the role of expert therapist, and more as an empathic facilitator of communication (Shwab, 1990).

A basic concept for Satir is that of ***maturation.*** "The most important concept in therapy, because it is a touchstone for all the rest, is that of maturation. The state of maturation involves two basic levels of operation: (1) The mature person is fully in charge of himself; and (2) he is one who can make choices based on accurate perceptions about himself and others and is able to take responsibility for his decisions. The patterns of behavior that mark such a mature person will be: the ability to be in touch with his own feelings; the ability to communicate with others clearly; an acceptance of others as different from himself; and a willingness to see differentness as a chance to learn and explore rather than as a threat (Schwab, 1990).

Opposed to this picture of the functional person is the dysfunctional or inadequate person, one who cannot separate himself out of the family mass, and is unable to give or receive clear messages. The breakdown or impairment of communication is the sign that one has become dysfunctional. "We call an individual dysfunctional when he has not learned to communicate properly." What causes faulty communication? Satir states that it is linked to a person's self concept. If this is poor, and one has a low sense of self-esteem, the possibility of problems of communication is high. The poor self-image, the low esteem, in turn, is attributable to the early formative relations with the family structure, with the relation to mother and father. She suggests that the parents may have been poor models of communication, or the content of their communication may have been devaluating to the child, or the parental communication itself was disturbed. Also, in a more direct way, the child's self-esteem was impaired because his developmental steps in growth were not validated (Satir, 1983).

In her analysis of marital interaction, Satir ties in the fundamental concept of self-esteem which is basic to her system. She has observed that self-esteem and not sex is the basic drive in man. "From what I have observed, the sex drive is continually subordinate to and used for the purpose of enhancing self-esteem and defending against threats to self-esteem. "Self-esteem will operate at all levels of interaction. Therefore, it will be a force in the choice of marriage partner. If a man, for example, has a strong sense of self, then he will choose as a marital partner one who will enhance his self-esteem by complementing his personality and talents. However, if he has a low self-esteem, a poor self-image, he will reach out to the other not as a complement but as one who will supply what is missing in the "self" "... as an extension of self ..."

To relate to another, especially in as intimate and demanding a relationship as marriage, is to court disaster. Such a union will be dysfunctional by its very nature. This is so because both parties look to marriage as a place of getting rather than giving. Marriage is seen as a chance to do something about one's own inadequate personality. The only outcome of such a marriage is disillusionment and an increase in feelings of negative self-esteem. Logically, one might see divorce or separation as a way of terminating the mismatch. However, more often, the birth of a child is viewed as a means of attaining the desired self-esteem. The child is seen as a way of demonstrating to the community their worth to others, or esteem for themselves as parents, or as an extension of self (Satri, 1967, 1983).

What is important here is that the child is never seen in himself as a separate person with a value and worth apart from the parent's self-esteem. The child or children are thus given a load to carry which is most difficult and burdensome. They must literally live out parental fantasies. Success or failure then is always viewed from the vantage point of the parent. Individuality or difference in outlook gets translated as a lack of love, just as it does between the parents. In Satir's view the child is in an intolerable position as the third angle of the family triangle. Whichever way he or she turns, there is a problem. Since the parents are in conflict, any and all actions of the child will be interpreted as being for or against one or the other. This is further complicated in that by reason of sex the child is already identified with one or the other parent. "Given this state of affairs, if the child seems to side with one parent, he runs the risk of losing the other parent. Since he needs both parents, making such a choice inevitably hurts him." Not only does it hurt the child in the obvious sense of making him take sides but such a choice is deleterious to psychosexual development. A child needs a parent of the same sex to identify with and a parent of the opposite sex to be admired and sought as desirable. When a child, however, is forced to choose one or the other, psychosexual development is stunted or stifled (Schwab, 1990).

The final aspect to be looked at in Satir's system is the question of how one gets a sense of self-esteem. It occurs in the early development of the child and involves a variety of things. Besides the obvious physical needs, the child has need for a warm, ongoing, predictable relationship with another. There is also a need for an experience of mastery over his world. In addition, a validation of himself as a distinct and worthwhile person is needed. Finally, there is required a sense of what it is to be male or female and an acceptance of this. These qualities can be attained only in a relationship with the parents.

Satir implicitly has a value system which is related to the manner in which she does therapy. There are three primary beliefs about human nature: (Satir, 1983)

1. Every person is geared to survival, growth, and getting close to others. All behavior, however distorted, aims at implementing these.
2. That what society labels as sick or crazy is an attempt to signal that one is in distress.
3. Thought and feeling are bound together. A person can learn what he does not know and can change his way of interacting.

The model Satir is proposing is not the traditional medical model which sees an analogy between physical and mental health but what is called a *growth model*. In this model pathology is linked to the inability of a person to reach his potential for development. It has as an underlying premise the notion that human beings are geared toward fulfilment. Human nature is fundamentally good and not fundamentally evil. At the heart of her theory of doing therapy is a philosophical concept which determines the direction she will follow. The question of a value system is one which is critical in any kind of therapy (Schwab, 1990).

MURRAY BOWEN

The thinking of Murray Bowen has developed over the years through a process of refining basic concepts. Beginning with analysis, moving on to work with married couples, and finally to dealing with family systems, Bowen has traced his thought in a series of articles in professional journals and at various symposia on family therapy. This journey he called a process from couch to coach, from analysis to a system model (Bowen, 1978).

The initial working hypothesis of Bowen conceptualized schizophrenia as a "psychopathological entity in the patient which had been influenced to a principle degree by the mother. Bowen felt that an unresolved, symbiotic attachment to the mother was the basic problem of the patient. Then the role of the father was considered". Shortly thereafter, the hypothesis was extended, because of clinical observation, to the whole family. Bowen was now in the process of moving from the traditional intrapsychic approach toward a system analysis, going from the mother to the father to the whole family. Within a short time, Bowen added another dimension—the role of the grandparents: (Bowen, 1978)

"... the grandparents were relatively mature but their combined immaturities were acquired by one child who was most attached to the mother. When this child married a spouse with an equal degree of immaturity, and when the same process repeated itself in the third generation, it resulted in one child (the patient) with a high degree of immaturity, while the other siblings are much more mature".

Here, Bowen is saying that schizophrenia is not a disease entity as such, an isolated phenomenon, but the result of an ongoing process whose history can be traced. How does this process, begun with the grandparents, develop into an identified schizophrenic patient in the grandchildren? Bowen says it is caused by a bad relationship with the parents in the second generation. Clinically, he observes that the parents of schizophrenic offspring have poor marriages. They are characterized by a quality of interaction that Bowen labels as an "emotional divorce." This he describes as ... a marked emotional distance between the parents" (Kerr and Bowen, 1988).

Bowen believes the marital pair has picked up certain undesirable traits from their parents. They come into marriage themselves with unresolved conflicts. Marriage, and the intimacy it necessitates, make these conflicts more intense. The marital partners, unable to handle their feelings and problems, try to settle these by distancing from one another. Frequently, this gives a facade that the marriage is a happy one because it is not marked by open quarreling and dispute. Nevertheless, beneath the surface, there is a struggle. When a child is born into such a marital dyad, it becomes an interdependent triad. Bowen says that the child cannot escape from the triad so that the father, mother, and child are locked into the family oneness (Bowen, 1978).

Within this system there are a variety of combinations. Bowen observes that the most common pattern ". . . is one in which the mother. . . has the custody of the patient, while the father is distant and passive." Since the parents cannot relate in a meaningful way, the child gets "triangled" into the system. This means that the child becomes the focus of the relationship and therefore cannot escape. The child is locked into the system and finds it virtually impossible to leave the family. The therapist must strive to get the family to focus on itself as the problem rather than the identified patient and, hopefully, to get the members to work together (Kerr and Bowen, 1988).

From this work with schizophrenic families, Bowen draws two conclusions: first, the schizophrenic psychosis of the identified patient is only a symptom of a pathological family system; second, the identified patient's pathology can be seen and understood only in relation to the emotional system of which he is part. In other words, there is an emotional contagion in the family and the identified patient is the one who carries the label "sick," whereas, in fact, the emotional system itself is sick. What is significant about these observations is the transfer between schizophrenic families and other more "normal" kinds of families. Bowen maintains that the same factors are operating in all families, but to a lesser extent. Nevertheless, he would feel that his observations can be applied to any family system, and are of importance in our study of family therapy. He writes: "It was surprising to find that all the family dynamisms so striking in schizophrenia were also present in families with the least severe problems and even in "normal" or asymptomatic families" (Bowen, 1978).

The central concept in Bowen's theory is the "undifferentiated family-ego mass." By this he means a quality of "stuck togetherness" or fusion which is "... a conglomerate emotional oneness that exists in all levels of intensity." This quality of "stuck-togetherness" exists in families at varying degrees of intensity from extremely so to very slight. However, it is a characteristic that belongs to all families, which is why Bowen feels it is central. Time is an important dimension too. When stress and tension are at high levels the intensity of the "ego mass" may increase. Members of a family may even come to know feelings, fantasies, and dreams experienced by other members. The process then is cyclical having a series of phases in which the "ego mass" becomes more or less intense (Bowen, 1978).

How does the "family-ego mass" get started? What is the basic building block of Bowen's system? Bowen writes "... The basic building block of any emotional system is the 'triangle. He says that when the tension between two persons in the system goes beyond a certain point, the system "triangles" in a third person, in order that the tension shift within the system. Bowen holds that "An emotional system is composed of a series of interlocking triangles." The importance of "triangles" as building blocks will become clearer when we talk about the aims of family therapy. It is sufficient for now to observe that the family system, the "undifferentiated family-ego mass," gets built through an ongoing process of interlocking triangles (Kerr and Bowen, 1988).

A second theoretical concept has to do with the nuclear family emotional system and the outside emotional forces which affect it. These include the extended family, work situations, and social factors that chart the course of the process within the family-ego mass. These outside factors actually influence the intensity and the extent of the emotional process in the family-ego mass. The marital couple, in Bowen's experience, uses three major ways of controlling the intensity of the ego fusion within the family ego mass. The first is marital conflict. When this occurs, each spouse will fight for an equal share of the common self and neither will give in to the other. A second way of controlling intensity is a dysfunction in one of the spouses. This happens after conflict and one of the two will give in to the other. The one who gives in will then become very dependent on the other person, and often be labeled "sick," manifesting a variety of physical and emotional problems. The third way used is the transmission of the problem to one or more of the children. The child becomes the focal point of the problem and functions for a time but eventually breaks down under the burden of carrying the family (Papero, 1990).

This third way is so important and so common that Bowen says it exists in all families to some degree so that it is treated as a separate concept. It refers to how the parental undifferentiation is projected onto one or more children. The family projection process is the result of parental immaturity. The reason why this or that child is focused on in a given family is not always easily evident since the process may occur for a variety of reasons connected with the developmental stages of the marriage. But if one accepts a developmental notion in marriage, then the family projection process makes much more sense, so that the choice of a child is less capricious than at first glance. One might add further that clinically it is frequently observed that a child in a family not only is nominated for such a role but often "runs for the job," that is, actively seeks the role of scapegoat. Even though one can say that such behavior is self-defeating, nevertheless, the "victim" does get his strokes, albeit negative ones. From his point of view it may be better to be scapegoated than to be neglected (Rasheed, Rasheed and Marley, 2011).

The next concept is the multigenerational process by which transmission takes place. For example, a fairly extended period of time is needed for a person to arrive at the level of "no self" which characterizes the schizophrenic. It is a phenomenon that does not occur overnight. This concept is a natural corollary of concept one concerning the differentiation of self scale. The choice of a marriage partner is not accidental, but related to where one is on the scale. It has been noted that "The life style of a person at one level is so different from someone only a few points removed on the scale, they do not choose each other for personal relationships." Since it is out of personal relationships that marital partners are chosen, it follows that a spouse chooses more or less at his or her own level of differentiation. In practice, this means that a man less differentiated than his parents will choose a woman at his level. If their children do not reach their level of differentiation of self, the process moves further back down the scale. Obviously the process can go in the opposite direction as well so that movement in both directions is possible (Walsh and McGraw, 2002).

The practical aspect of this seemingly abstract concept can be seen in that the role of the grandparents is important in understanding current pathology in a grandchild. The process of moving up and down the scale accounts for the presence or absence of symptomatology. Health or sickness is not found in the study of a person in isolation but within the context of his family, and this includes the extended family reaching through several generations. Sibling position is a concept Bowen has borrowed from Walter Toman. The idea of birth position is not a new one. There is much folklore about it. For example, the oldest child is supposed to suffer from anxiety because he is the pace setter in the family; the youngest child is said to be spoiled; and then there is the "middle child syndrome." (Bowen, 1978).

In Bowen's thinking the sibling concept becomes much more sophisticated. It is related to concept three on family projection process. The child selected by the parents, the one who is most fused into the family system, will be the one who is the most infantile or immature regardless of chronology in the family. A knowledge of where a parent fitted into his own family of origin becomes important as to what is now going on within the current family system. The concept of triangle is " ... the basic building block or "molecule" of an emotional system," writes Bowen. This is true whether the system is family, social, or a work system. When a system involves four or more people, that system is made up of a series of interlocking triangles. (Kerr and Bowen, 1988).

As Bowen conceives interaction, when the relationship between two people in a system gets uncomfortable, one of them will triangle in a third party. This relieves the tension between the two. As we have just seen the building blocks of any emotional system are the interlocking triangles. Therefore, the process of differentiation involves a detriangling of the triangle. Bowen lists three specific ways this can be done. First, the best way is for a marital pair to do this in the presence of a potential triangle (the therapist) who remains emotionally detached. The couple cannot use or manipulate the therapist and make him part of the triangle by getting him on his or her side. A second way of doing this is to work alone with a therapist. At times, this may be the only possible way of doing therapy if other significant people in the system are unwilling or unable to be present. The third way occurs when the therapist acts as a coach from the sidelines. This is not as good because the impact of the triangle is lost, and the chances of bogging down are much greater. (Carr, 2008)

THEODORE LIDZ: MARITAL SCHISM AND SKEW

In the mid-fifties, Lidz and his associates at Yale University began a long and careful investigation of the relationship between schizophrenia and the family. What is significant about his research is that his conclusions are so similar to those of Wynne and his associates. Lidz observed general patterns of difficulty which seem to occur regularly in the relationship between the schizophrenic and his family. Among these patterns he sees three general areas of difficulty: (Hanna, 2007).

1. Deficiencies of paternal nurturance. This lack resulted in the patient's failure to achieve autonomy and an inability to function in a self-reliant way;
2. The failure of the family as a social institution, especially in its inability to provide the patient with adequate role models;
3. Failure to transmit the communicative and other basic instrumental technics of the culture to the child.

Lidz maintains that both a mother and a father are necessary if a child is to grow up in a reasonably successful way. A child must have a member of the same sex to identify with, and a member of the opposite sex who is seen as desirable. When the parents are divided and quarreling, the child cannot achieve this twofold goal. This cooperation between father and mother Lidz calls the parental coalition. It occurs when both are able to fulfill their respective roles as man and woman and as husband and wife (Marley, 2004).

In addition to the parental coalition, Lidz says that there must be a maintenance of generational boundaries between parents and children. He says that for the child's normal development, he must know that he cannot take one parent's place with the other, and that although he may identify with a parent, he does not become a parent figure in the familial home. Some marriages are either marked by a chronic failure to achieve a complementarity of purpose or role reciprocity or marked by excessive attachment to the parental home. Lidz labels such unions as marital schisms. Other marriages are characterized by one strong and one weak partner. In these unions the weak partner allows the stronger to dominate the relationship. These marriages are said to be skewed (Worden, 2003).

THE DOUBLE BIND

The key to understanding the double bind is to know the difference between a simple contradiction and a paradox. The former means that one has a choice of doing one thing or another and is a case of either/or. The latter, however, is defined as " . .a *contradiction that follows correct deduction from consistent premises.*" (Nichols, 1984)

1. Antinomies are statements which are contradictory but provable and found in logical and mathematical systems.
2. Semantic antinomies are those arising out of hidden inconsistencies in the level structure of thought and language.
3. Pragmatic paradoxes are divided into paradoxical predictions and paradoxical injunctions. These grow out of antinomies and semantic antinomies and are relevant here because they come out of ongoing interactions and determine behavior. The double bind is an example of a paradoxical injunction.

However, for double binding to take place there must be several conditions present over a period of time. First, there must be two or more persons present, one of whom is designated a "victim." Second, the experience must be reinforced by repetition. Therapists postulate that a single traumatic experience would not be sufficient. Third, a primary negative injunction must be present. The victim is told, "Do not do so and so, or I will punish you," or he is told, "If you do not do so and so, I will punish you." Fourth, a secondary injunction conflicting with the first at a more abstract level, and like the first, enforced by punishments or signals which threaten survival. This injunction is commonly communicated on a nonverbal level. Finally, a third negative injunction is imposed, prohibiting the "victim" from escaping from the field (Nichols, 1984).

What is so significant about the double bind is that it is not confined to schizophrenic families alone but occurs in mitigated form in a large number of so-called normal families. What does the "victim" do in a double bind? Jackson and his associates suggest three possibilities. First, one concludes the "victim" is overlooking something in the situation. He searches and searches but the more he tries to understand, the more confused he becomes. A second possibility is to become absolutely literal and follow each and every injunction to the letter. The basic premise underlying this approach is that things do not make sense anyhow so why worry. Anyone familiar with institutional living, for example, the army, will recognize this response. A third option is to withdraw from human involvement so that all incoming material is blocked out. The "victim" is caught because he cannot discuss the message with an outside party. He cannot metacommunicate, that is, talk about his communication and thus escape his field. The "victim" therefore remains trapped and unable to escape (Marley, 2004).

The concept of the double bind is important because it has survived in family therapy and has led to some important developments in the decade following its introduction. Like any good idea the double bind theory has been productive beyond its original conception. The therapist faced with repetitive patterns in a family wonders what he can do to break into the seemingly closed system (Marley, 2004).

PSEUDOMUTUALITY

The concept of pseudomutuality, first introduced by Wynne in 1958, developed throughout the following decade. Additional work done in the 1960s on the thought patterns of schizophrenics produced some refinements. Along with this research Wynne and his associates were also incorporating their findings into therapeutic strategies devised to deal with family systems (Carr, 2008).

A person seems to have two needs which bring him into conflict. On the one hand, he has a need to develop a sense of personal identity, and on the other, a need to relate to others. In terms of the family, the former need is centrifugal driving one outside its boundaries and is involved in the important psychic process of separation. The latter need, however, is centripetal driving a person back into the family system and is involved with the psychic process of striving for closeness. In a healthily functioning person these two needs are balanced. One is able to relate to others, to get close, and does not lose his sense of self and become absorbed in the other. He can move within the family system and can be himself. In a person who is having difficulty in functioning, however, a situation exists in which the person is often uncertain about his boundaries, and he has a real fear of losing his identity (Barker, 1998).

Wynne feels there are three options: (1) Mutuality, which is characterized by a divergence of self-interests; (2) Nonmutuality, which is found, for example, in the relationship of a customer and a sales clerk; (3) Pseudomutuality, which is "a predominant absorption in fitting together at the expense of the differentiation of the identities of the persons in the relation." (Walsh and McGraw, 2002)

PSEUDOHOSTILITY

Having introduced the concept of pseudomutuality Wynne developed one of pseudohostility.

This concept refers to a split or alienation which remains limited to a surface level. Beneath that surface, Wynne suggests pseudohostility like its counterpart, pseudomutuality, covers a need for intimacy and affection as well as the more obvious destructive element. Dynamically, pseudohostility and pseudomutuality are very close. They both cover more positive aspects and feelings which seem to get conveyed in diffuse ways (Hanna, 2007).

The two terms are ways of dealing with the observable phenomenon of alignments and splits that exist in families. An alignment is defined as the experience of common interest, attitude, or set of values among two or more persons in the family. A split is the comparable experience of opposition, estrangement, and difference. A combination of the two tells us the kind of emotional system we have (Hanna, 2007).

NATHAN ACKERMAN

Nathan Ackerman in writing about the family made the observation that it was a unit in itself, having its own psychological and social life. In the same article he makes two other observations. One is that the family unit is not static but is dynamic and changes at different times because of internal and external pressures. The other is that the family is an exchange medium and the values exchanged are love and material goods. In a sense Ackerman's fundamental approach to therapy is contained in the notion that there is a constant interchange occurring between the person, his family, and society. To fully understand how a person functions, it is necessary to see him in all these aspects. They are not isolated components, they are in constant interaction, the one influencing the other (Wise, 2005).

Nearly fifty years later, these concepts seem less striking than when first written. However, the shift in perception away from an almost exclusive orientation toward the intrapsychic to an interpersonal and especially to a family concept is mostly attributed to the writings of Ackerman. His task for over 30 years was to elaborate on the seminal notions just mentioned (Wise, 2005).

Ackerman stands as a bridge between the individual (intrapsychic) approach to pathology and the system approach, as seen in the communicational theorists. Trained as a psychiatrist and psychoanalyst, but also influenced by social psychology, Ackerman tried to combine both strains in his theorizing: "My personal synthesis of personality theory makes use of Freudian dynamics for understanding the internal mental processes but emphasizes the adaptational view of personality, man in society." Ackerman's basic stance is that there is a continuing dialogue going on between heredity and environment. He would maintain that neither can be considered apart from the other (Carr, 2008).

The key concept for Ackerman, among various hypotheses, is that of social role. "As a bridge between the processes of intrapsychic life and those of social participation, it is useful to employ the concept of social role." Ackerman defines social role as " ... the adaptational unit of personality in action," and for practical purposes regards it as synonymous with the concept of "social self." Ackerman sees social role as a semipermeable membrane in that it permits a limited penetration in both directions, that is, between the environment and the self. In actual practice Ackerman was always thinking in terms of roles. What does it mean to be a mother or father? How do you want \ our child to act in this instance? What are the expectations established in this family? Unless the roles are clearly delineated and more or less agreed on. the transactions within the family will not go smoothly. Focusing on these areas of conflict enabled Ackerman to narrow down the complaints within the family and to help the people work on certain issues. It is a technic for getting at the specific problems that exist. This is another area in which Ackerman would part company with some of the communication theorists. He feels that clarity of communication and understanding the other is not enough. It is not just the process of communicating that is important but the content, as well. He feels this is, to a large extent, ignored by many in the field. He writes: "It (therapy) must be oriented not only toward the aim of freedom from but also toward the further aim of freedom for a set of positive goals in life" (Anderson and Sabatelli, 2003).

One might make the observation that to work on roles or to seek a clarification of how people relate is a part of any kind of therapy and not exclusive to family therapy. However, what makes it different theoretically is that the roles are seen as part of a wider system of interaction. Ackerman, like all family therapists, ascribes to the concept of family balance or family homeostasis. The concept of homeostasis is a central one to family therapists of whatever school. Ackerman points out that homeostasis is not just limited to the family but applies to society, as well. He makes the point that the homeostasis of the person is dependent on that of the family, which, in turn, is contingent on that of the society. "These relations do not move in one direction only; they are, of course, circular and convoluted." With this notion we have come to the heart of Ackerman[1] s theory. The chain of events that link the individual member to his family and to society, although able to be conceptualized separately, in reality, are interrelated. Therefore, pathology or illness at any one level necessarily means illness at all levels, since we are talking not about individual parts, but a totality. Furthermore, Ackerman states there are three components of psychiatric illness: the intrapsychic, the interpersonal, and the psychosocial pattern of the family unit. No one element can be looked at apart from its relationship to the others. Ackerman sees individual therapy related to family therapy as one part to another part, albeit a larger one (Hanna, 2007).

Ackerman lists two core concepts by which the psychosocial dynamics of family life can be operationally defined. The first is psychological identity which subsumes strivings, expectations, and values. The second is stability of behavior, specifically in (1) continuity of identity in time, (2) control of conflict, and (3) adaptability and complementarity in new role relationships, that is, the capacity to grow and learn (Ragg, 2006).

The concept of psychological identity is the answer to the question "Who are we?" that the family must ask. The concept is an attempt to explain why a given family is what it is. For Ackerman the question of identity of self and that of the family are inextricably woven. One depends on the other; one influences the other. Although they may be separated and examined apart from each other, diagnostically, this cannot be done. Ackerman writes: "The image of self and image of family are reciprocally interdependent. At each stage of development, personal identity is linked to and differentiated from the identity of parents and family in a special way. " The second core concept is that of stability of behavior. It must be considered together with psychological identity. The sense of identity can only come about if there is a stability of behavior so that the two concepts are interrelated. Ackerman is saying that the family has to keep a sense of self in the midst of conflict, and yet, allow for growth and change. The old must be preserved but the new welcomed. Again we are back to the importance of role relations in Ackerman's theoretical notions. Flexibility and adaptability of role is essential if the family's behavior is to be stable. Therefore, the role relations must allow for developmental stages in the life of the family, especially for the maturing autonomy of the children. When the family roles "fit," when the people are flexible, the behavior remains stable and a sense of shared identity is forged. When there is rigidity in the roles, or disagreement about the definition of them, there is difficulty (Carr, 2008; Nichols, 1984).

CONCLUSIONS

This chapter has looked at the key concepts in family therapy without touching upon any specific approach but rather focusing on concepts that are vital to the everyday clinical practice of family therapy. Clinical work with families warrants diversification and knowledge from various schools of counseling and psychotherapy in order to understand families in a truly holistic perspective.

BIBLIOGRAPHY

1. Anderson, S.A., & Sabatelli, R.M. (2003). *Family integration: a multigenerational developmental perspective.* Boston MA, Pearson Education.
2. Ariel, S. (1999). *Culturally competent family therapy.* Westport CT, Greenwood.
3. Barker, P. (1998). *Basic Family Therapy.* Blackwell Publishing, UK.
4. Becvar, D.S., & Becvar, R.J. (2000). *Family therapy: a systematic integration.* Needham Heights MA, Pearson Education.
5. Becvar, D.S. (2007). *Families that flourish.* New York, Norton Press.
6. Berg, I. (1994). *Family based services: a solution focused approach.* New York, Norton.
7. Bowen, M. (1978). *Family therapy in Clinical Practice.* New York, Jason Arons.
8. Carr, A. (2008). *Family therapy: concepts, process and practice.* Wiley Blackwell, UK.
9. Coles, R.A. (2006). *Race and family: a structural approach.* Thousand Oaks CA, Sage.
10. Dattilo, F. (1998). *Case studies in clinical family therapy: a systems and cognitive approach.* New York, Guilford Press.
11. Goldenberg, H. (2007). *Counseling today's families.* Pacific Grove, CA.
12. Goldenberg, H., & Goldenberg, I. (2008). *Family therapy: an overview.* Belmont CA: Thomson.
13. Hanna, S.M. (2007). *The practice of family therapy: key elements across models.* Belmont CA: Thomson Brooks, Cole.
14. Kerr, M.E., & Bowen, M. (1988). *Family evaluation: an appraisal based on Bowen's theory.* New York: Norton.
15. Marley, J.A. (2004). *Family involvement in schizophrenia: models, essential skills and the process.* New York, Howarth Press.
16. Nichols, M.P. (1984). *Family therapy: concepts and methods.* New York: Gardner Press.
17. Papero, D.V. (1990). *Bowen's Family Systems Therapy.* Boston MA, Allyn and Bacon.
18. Ragg, D.M. (2006). *Building family practice skills: methods, strategies and tools.* Belmont CA: Thomson.
19. Rasheed, J.M., Rasheed, M.N., & Marley, J.A. (2011). *Family therapy: models and technics.* Sage Publications, UK.
20. Satir, V. (1983). *Conjoint Family Therapy.* Palo Alto CA, Science and Behavior Books.
21. Schwab, D. (1990). *A resource handbook for Satir's conjoint family therapy.* Palo Alto CA, Science and Behavior Books.
22. Sexton, T.L., Weeks, G.R., & Robbins, M.S. (2003). *Handbook of family therapy.* New York.
23. Sprenkle, D., & Moon, S. (1996). *Research methods in family therapy.* New York, Guilford Press.
24. Walsh, W.M., & McGraw, J.A. (2002). *Essential Family Therapy.* Denver CO, Love.
25. Wise, J.B. (2005). *Empowering practice with families in distress.* New York, Cambridge University Press.
26. Worden, M. (2003). *Family therapy basics.* Pacific Grove CA, Brooks & Cole.

Behaviour Therapy 56

Sushma Sonavane • Avinash De Sousa

Behavior modification is based on the principles of operant conditioning, which were developed by American behaviorist B. F. Skinner (1904-1990). Skinner formulated the concept of operant conditioning, through which behavior could be shaped by reinforcement or lack of it. Skinner considered his concept applicable to a wide range of both human and animal behaviors and introduced operant conditioning to the general public in his 1938 book, The Behavior of Organisms.

Behavioral therapy is an umbrella term for types of therapy that treat mental health disorders. This form of therapy seeks to identify and help change potentially self-destructive or unhealthy behaviors. It functions on the idea that all behaviors are learned and that unhealthy behaviors can be changed. The focus of treatment is often on current problems and how to change them.

Behavioral therapies (also called behavior modification) are based on the theories of classical and operant conditioning. The premise is that all behavior is learned; faulty learning (i.e. conditioning) is the cause of abnormal behavior. Therefore, the individual has to learn the correct or acceptable behavior.

An important feature of behavioral therapy is its focus on current problems and behavior, and on attempts to remove behavior the patient finds troublesome.

Behavioral therapy can benefit people with a wide range of disorders. Unlike other forms of therapy that look at the past, this type of therapy focuses on the present and looks at current problems the individual is experiencing and what to do about them.

There are several different conditions that behavioral therapy can help to treat. Some of these include depression and anxiety, panic disorders, and anger issues. Things like eating disorders, PTSD, ADHD, and phobias are also possible, among a range of other mental health disorders. Most types of behavioral and mental health disorders can be helped and treated through some form of behavioral therapy, though the specifics may change from one type of condition to another. They may also change from one specific individual to another. Therapies also work differently with different types of people, such as some being better for adults and some being intended solely for children. Finding the right type of therapy is going to be a combination of the therapist's thoughts and your own as well as a little trial and error to decide what works best for you specifically.

Operant Conditioning

Operant conditioning (instrumental conditioning) is a method of learning that occurs through rewards and punishments for behavior. Through operant conditioning, an association is made between a behavior and a consequence for that behavior. For example, when a lab rat presses a blue button, he receives a food pellet as a reward, but when he presses the red button, he receives a mild electric shock. As a result, he learns to press the blue button but avoid the red button. Operant conditioning is not just something that takes place in experimental settings while training lab animals; it also plays a powerful role in everyday learning. Reinforcement and punishment take place almost every day in natural settings as well as in more structured settings such as the classroom or therapy sessions.

Types of Behaviors

Skinner distinguished between two different types of behaviors:

- Respondent behaviors are those that occur automatically and reflexively, such as pulling your hand back from a hot stove or jerking your leg when the doctor taps on your knee. You don't have to learn these behaviors; they simply occur automatically and involuntarily.
- Operant behaviors, on the other hand, are those under our conscious control. Some may occur spontaneously and others purposely, but it is the consequences of these actions that then influence whether or not they occur again in the future. Our actions on the environment and the consequences of that action make up an important part of the learning process.

Schedules of reinforcement that impact the operant conditioning process:

- Continuous reinforcement involves delivering a reinforcement every time a response occurs. Learning tends to occur relatively quickly, yet the response rate is quite low. Extinction also occurs very quickly once reinforcement is halted.
- Fixed-ratio schedules are a type of partial reinforcement. Responses are reinforced only after a specific number of responses have occurred. This typically leads to a fairly steady response rate.
- Fixed-interval schedules are another form of partial reinforcement. Reinforcement occurs only after a certain interval of time has elapsed. Response rates remain fairly steady and start to increase as the reinforcement time draws near, but slow immediately after the reinforcement has been delivered.
- Variable-ratio schedules are also a type of partial reinforcement that involve reinforcing behavior after a varied number of responses. This leads to both a high response rate and slow extinction rates.
- Variable-interval schedules are the final form of partial reinforcement Skinner described. This schedule involves delivering reinforcement after a variable amount of time has elapsed. This also tends to lead to a fast response rate and slow extinction rate.

Types of Behavior therapy

Cognitive Behavioral Therapy

It is focused on your thoughts and beliefs. It attempts to change the way that you think. The idea is that your thoughts are unhealthy and that by changing them it will be possible for you to change more than just your perception, but the way that you interact with the world. It can help to guide individuals who are generally cynical or low on motivation.

Cognitive Behavioral Play Therapy

For children, play therapy is a great way to help them with any problems that they may be facing. Play therapy helps children develop insight. Play has no rules. It helps children overcome introversion or PTSD.

System Desensitization

It successfully helps to overcome phobias by gradually getting an individual to become more comfortable with their fears or phobias. E.g.: If a person is scared of butterflies. He is first shown a picture of a butterfly in a book, then he is asked to touch the picture, later he is shown videos of the same. The last step would be taking a person near a butterfly, from a distance. The phase at which this moves, depends totally on the comfort level of the client. During these stages the client is taught various relaxation and calming exercises too.

Classical Conditioning

The theory of classical conditioning suggests a response is learned and repeated through immediate association. Behavioral therapies based on classical conditioning aim to break the association between stimulus and undesired response (E.g.: phobia, anxiety).

Aversion Therapy

This process pairs undesirable behavior with some form of aversive stimulus with the aim of reducing unwanted behavior. E.g. For alcoholics aversion therapy involves associating drinking with a very unpleasant unconditioned stimulus, such as an electric shock. The client thus learns to associate the undesirable behavior with the electric shock, and a link is formed between the undesirable behavior and the reflex response to an electric shock.

In the case of alcoholism, what is often done is to require the client to take a sip of alcohol while under the effect of a nausea-inducing drug. Sipping the drink is followed almost at once by vomiting. In future the smell of alcohol produces a memory of vomiting and should stop the patient wanting a drink.

Flooding

Flooding (also known as implosion therapy) works by exposing the patient directly to their worst fears. E.g. A claustrophobic will be locked in a closet for 4 hours or an individual with a fear of balloons would be locked in a room full of them. What flooding aims to do is expose the sufferer to the phobic object or situation for an extended period of time in a safe and controlled environment.

Prolonged intense exposure eventually creates a new association between the feared object and something positive (e.g. a sense of calm and lack of anxiety). It also prevents reinforcement of phobia through escape or avoidance behaviors.

Operant conditioning is a method of learning that occurs through rewards and punishments for behavior. Through operant conditioning, an individual makes an association between a particular behavior and a consequence (Skinner, 1938). Examples of therapies using the principles of operant conditioning include:

Token Economy

Token economy is a system in which targeted behaviors are reinforced with tokens (secondary reinforcers) and later exchanged for rewards (primary reinforcers). Tokens can be in the form of fake money, buttons, poker chips, stickers, etc. While the rewards can range anywhere from snacks to privileges or activities. For example, teachers use token economy at primary school by giving young children stickers to reward good behavior.

Positive Reinforcement

Positive reinforcement is pairing a positive stimulus to a behavior. A good example of this is when teachers reward their students for getting a good grade with stickers. Positive reinforcement is also often used in training dogs.

Negative reinforcement

Negative reinforcement is the opposite and is the pairing of a behavior to the removal of a negative stimulus. A child that throws a tantrum because he or she doesn't want to eat vegetables and has his or her vegetables are taken away.

Punishment

Punishment is designed to weaken behaviors by pairing an unpleasant stimulus to a behavior. E.g.: Receiving a detention for bad behavior or being grounded for aggressive bouts and temper.

Shaping

The technics used in shaping are very similar to systematic desensitization. The main aim is to reduce phobias, fears or anxieties. E.g.: If a person is scared of dogs, the therapist would first ask the client to look at a picture of it. Later on, try to hold a stuffed animal prototype. The methods used are to desensitize the phobic individual.

Fading

The process of gradually withdrawing the reinforcement that was initially provided is called fading. E.g.: A student ought to work hard in an examination without being bribed about what he would he if he does well.

Chaining

Chaining refers to as forming a pattern of sequences to establish a goal. E.g.: A behavior chain for forming a habit of going to the gym might include steps like sign up for gym membership, purchase or gather workout clothes, pack gym bag, fill water bottle, drive to the gym, check in, do 15 minutes of cardio, spend 15 minutes on weight training.

Extinction

Extinction refers to a procedure used in Applied Behavioral Analysis (ABA) in which reinforcement that is provided for problem behavior (often unintentionally) is discontinued in order to decrease or eliminate occurrences of

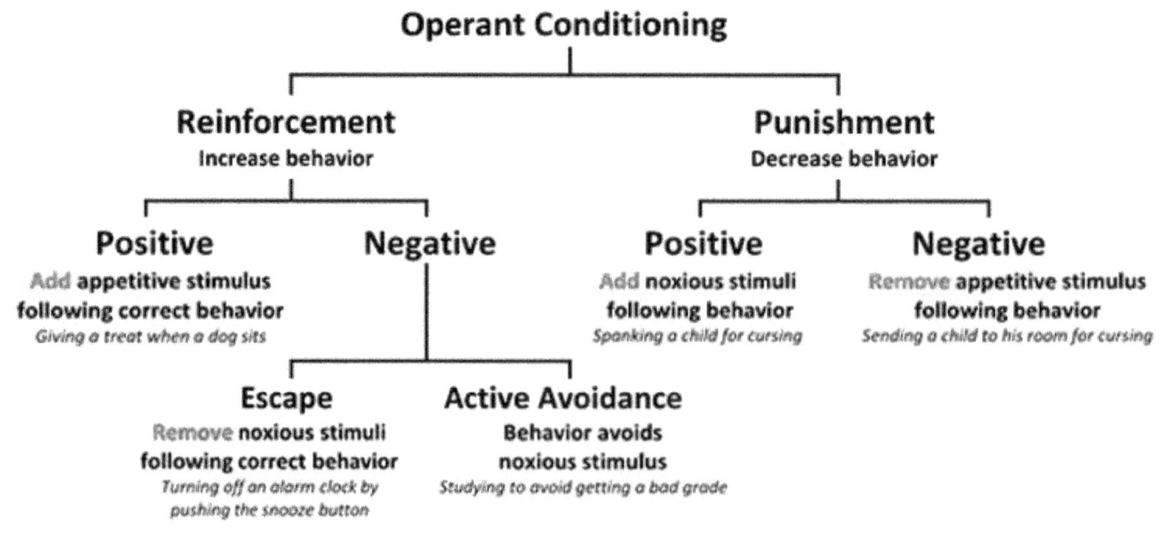

Fig. 56.1

these types of negative (or problem) behaviors. While this procedure is most commonly used in children with Autism and Down Syndrome, it can also be used very successfully to address a broader array of problem behaviors, including those exhibited by individuals without developmental disabilities.

Examples of Operant Conditioning

- If your child acts out during a shopping trip, you might give him a treat to get him to be quiet. Because you have positively reinforced the misbehavior, he will probably be more likely to act out again in the future in order to receive another treat.
- After performing in a community theatre play, you receive applause from the audience. This acts as a positive reinforcer inspiring you to try out for more performance roles.
- You train your dog to fetch by offering him praise and a pat on the head whenever he performs the behavior correctly.
- A professor tells students that if they have perfect attendance all semester, then they do not have to take the final comprehensive exam. By removing an unpleasant stimulus (the final test) students are negatively reinforced to attend class regularly.
- If you fail to hand in a project on time, your boss becomes angry and berates your performance in front of your co-workers. This acts as a positive punisher making it less likely that you will finish projects late in the future.
- A teen girl does not clean up her room as she was asked, so her parents take away her phone for the rest of the day. This is an example of a negative punishment in which a positive stimulus is taken away.

Behavioral therapy is an important treatment process for people who are suffering from certain behavioral problems, i.e. bad habits that are harmful to the person's welfare and health. The goal of the therapy is to help and better equip the patient to cope with different challenges without turning to negative habits as a coping mechanism.

Some examples of disorders that can be treated using Behavioral therapy:

- Anxiety disorders
- Obsessive compulsive disorder (OCD)
- Post-traumatic stress disorder (PTSD)
- Social phobia
- Bipolar disorder
- Schizophrenia
- Depression
- Personality disorders
- Eating disorders
- Attention deficiency hyperactivity disorder (ADHD)

Behavioral therapy is also useful for those suffering from:

- Autism
- Substance abuse i.e. drug or alcohol abuse
- Chronic pain, such as that caused by an existing disease or ongoing treatment for another condition
- Emotional distress

Technics used in Behavior Modification

- Development of coping mechanisms
- Role playing
- Relaxation methods, i.e. breathing exercises
- Positive reinforcement
- Journal writing

- Training in social skills
- Response modification
- Virtual reality therapy
- Contingency contracting
- Response costs
- Token economies
- Biofeedback
- Shaping and grading task assignments
- Habit reversal training

Common changes seen in most patients include:

- Better social skills
- Better emotional expressions
- Better management of pain
- Reduction in self-destructive incidents or actions
- Better adjustment and response to unfamiliar situations
- Fewer outbursts

Behavioral therapy has very minimal risks while most of the complications are emotional in nature, such as uncontrolled bursts of anger, pain, and crying as a response to the therapy sessions where patients are required to explore their thoughts and feelings. But while emotional, such as bursts of sudden feelings, can bring physical exhaustion as an aftermath.

For individuals experiencing different mental health disorders or who are struggling even more in life it is important to seek out for professional help and behavioral therapy can be one of the best ways to do it. A person gains insight if they are struggling with anxiety disorders, stress, bulimia, anger problems, depression or substance abuse, especially, this type of therapy has shown even better results.

Children also show great results from this type of therapy and the play therapy that they engage in, allows them to express things that they otherwise may feel uncomfortable or unable to express. This can help a child understand how to respond to situations and even help with learning and developing an understanding of good and bad behavior and how to interact with others. This can be especially helpful for children who have autism or ADHD. It can allow a child to learn how to interact positively with the people around him, including family, friends, and peers.

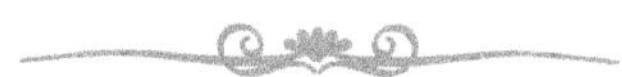

Psychiatric Aspects of TB and HIV

57

Maithili Umate • Varun Mehta

INTRODUCTION

Since the emergence of HIV 30 years ago, the role of neurological aspects has been recognized. However the psychiatric aspects of HIV have not received the due attention that they deserve. Psychiatric illness with high comorbidity with HIV not only cause their own independent substantial health burden but also complicate the course of the illness with impediment to care.

India has the world's largest tuberculosis (TB) epidemic with 2.2 million new cases and more than 300000 deaths every year contributing to an economic loss of $23bn from TB. Tuberculosis is a relatively common condition among patients with psychiatric disorders and vice-a-versa but the link between tuberculosis and mental illness is complex.

ETIOLOGY OF MENTAL ILLNESS IN HIV/ AIDS AND TUBERCULOSIS

HIV infection gradually depletes the immune system. Though in initial stages of disease the body produces more CD4 cells but gradually the virus disrupts the immune mechanism of the host through several specific mechanisms and producing large number of mutant strains while it is transcribed. HIV infects cells expressing CD4 surface protein and destroys T4 helper cells or CD4 cells critical in cell mediated immunity gradually leading to an immunocompromised state.

It has been postulated that neuronal loss occurs due to inflammation through action of macrophages and microglial cells or through activation of cytokines and chemokines that trigger abnormal neuronal pruning. A complex relationship between HIV, neuroinflammation and psychiatric and neurological comorbidities have emerged in recent research. Psychiatric illness may emerge as a consequence of HIV infection. Psychiatric illnesses are also a risk factor for HIV exposure and can further complicate the course and treatment of the disease after seroconversion.

HIV crosses blood brain barrier and causes immune activation in the brain and CNS. The inflammatory response to HIV infection leads to elevated cytokine levels, including IL-6 and TNF-α which can trigger a chain reaction involving tryptophan depletion and increased Kynurenine and its metabolites. It is possible that chronic inflammation and tryptophan depletion contribute to the deleterious effects of depression on medical outcomes. Apart from direct effect of HIV on CNS, opportunistic illness and their treatment as well as ART can precipitate psychiatric illness.

Tuberculosis is a classic example of a disease with both medical and social dimensions, characterized by its close relation to poor socioeconomic conditions. The increased risk of acquiring active disease occurs with alcoholism, smoking, intravenous drug abuse, diabetes mellitus, HIV infection, and other factors. The above-mentioned risk factors are very prevalent in psychiatric populations and increase risk of progression from latent TB to active TB. The occurrence of neuropsychiatric disorders as adverse events to antitubercular treatment has been the other plausible explanation for both occurring together. Further, the stigma and the social isolation with the diagnosis of TB is also considered another important contributory factor.

EPIDEMIOLOGY

Burden Of Psychiatric Illness

The rates of mental illness are higher among those with physical illness than in the general population and much higher still in those individuals with a diagnosis of tuberculosis and HIV/AIDS. Psychiatric disorders including substance use disorders are the top contributor to number of years lived with disability and is associated with shortened life span. Psychiatric illnesses play a critical role in HIV acquisition with 4-10 times increased risk. The heightened risk can be due to high risk sexual behavior like inconsistent condom use, having multiple sexual partners, trading sex and drinking alcohol before sex or other high risk behaviors like sharing IV needles during drug use. The risk is compounded by multiple co-occurring mental health conditions. Screening and treatment of mental health issues will be necessary to prevent vulnerable population from acquiring HIV. Psychiatric conditions are associated with poor outcomes and higher mortality, partly due to poor medication adherence.

Statistics

UN AIDS fact sheet 2019 shows that 37.9 - 44 million people are infected with HIV though new infections are down from 3.1 million in 2001 to 1.7 million in 2018 but only 62% were accessing Anti-Retroviral Therapy (ART). The prevalence of HIV is 0.22% in India in 2017 with high rates in Mizoram followed by Manipur and Nagaland. Of the estimated 21.4 lakh PLWH (Persons Living with HIV), Maharashtra has the highest number contributing to 15%. The incidence of HIV has gradually declined from 0.64 in 1995 to 0.07 with 87.58 thousand People being newly infected in 2017.

The prevalence of psychiatric illness such as substance abuse, depression, PTSD, sleep disorders, and psychosis are 1.5-8 times higher in persons with HIV. The prevalence rates of various psychiatric illness associated with HIV vary with contributions by substance use disorders (40-74%), depression (22-50%), anxiety disorders (2-40%), PRSD (30%), sleep disorders (10-50%) and severe mental illness (0.2-15%). In Africa where the prevalence of HIV is high, prevalence of serious mental illnesses among PLWH is 11-27%.

The prevalence of mental disorders, including depression and anxiety disorders, among people with TB is estimated to be between 40% and 70%. Depression is considered to be an invisible burden for people with TB. The co-infection with HIV may significantly increase the risk of depression alone by up to 70%. On the other hand, there may be lower rates of detection of tuberculosis in patients with co-morbid mental illness.

PSYCHOLOGICAL REACTION TO DIAGNOSIS

The diagnosis of HIV leads to different emotions and expectancies. The prospect of real and anticipated losses, the fear of physical decline and death, worsening quality of life and facing an uncertain future are the different psychological challenges faced by an individual. HIV being both infectious and potentially fatal and with the stigma surrounding it leads to an attenuation of the psychological reaction.

Individuals may experience guilt for having acquired the infection. It is important that the treating physician should have a supportive non-judgmental stance and anticipate the wide range of psychological reactions like shock, disbelief, panic, fear, guilt, anger, despair, hopelessness or numbness. Since many people struggle with disclosing their HIV status with others, it is important to discuss safer behaviors to prevent transmission and cope.

Pre-test counseling includes information on aspects of both negative and positive test, risk reduction interventions and window period. Post-test counseling includes helping them cope with the diagnosis, psychoeducational interventions, recommendation for treatment and risk reduction behaviors.

A transient HIV associated Acute Stress Reaction appears in some individuals who are recently informed about their seropositive status. It may also occur in those the disease spreads to AIDS. Some patients have preoccupation with thoughts or brood regarding the future, the uncertainties, the risk of them infecting others including their loved ones and fear of death. It generally remits in a few days but in severe cases may present with social isolation, rage, desperation, behavioral changes and suicidal thoughts and attempt.

The diagnosis of tuberculosis has been a cause of lot of fear and anxiety since thousands of years. This has persisted in spite of the advances in treatment as the misconceptions about tuberculosis still persist. Even now tuberculosis is thought to be an incurable disease, and a lot of stigma is associated with it. A mere diagnosis of tuberculosis can be a psychological trauma for a person with repercussions such as setback in occupation, social isolation with damaged status, lowered self-esteem, fear of spreading the illness to others and resultant helplessness.

PSYCHIATRIC SIDE EFFECTS OF ART

HAART (Highly Active Anti-Retroviral Therapy) and CART (Combined Anti-Retroviral Therapy) have dramatically reduced viral load and often result in increase in CD4 count. However anti-retroviral drugs are variably associated with neuropsychiatric adverse effects. These adverse effects are exacerbated by concomitant use of medication with similar toxicities, comorbid conditions, drug interactions and genetic factors.

Non-Nucleoside Reverse Transcriptase Inhibitors (NNRTI's) have known psychiatric adverse effects. Efavirenz is most often associated with emergence of depressive symptoms. Dizziness, abnormal dreams and suicidal ideation have been reported. These side effects occur more in those with pre-existing psychiatric illness and often subside within 2-4 weeks. Some patients may develop frank psychosis causing its discontinuation. Rilpirine is associated with depression, suicidality and sleep disturbances. Doravirine is associated with dizziness, sleep disturbances, altered sensorium, depression and suicidality. Nucleoside Reverse Transcriptase Inhibitors (NRTI), particularly zidovudine and abacavir can cause mania and psychosis. Integrase Strand Transferase Inhibitors (INSTI) like Raltegravir are associated with insomnia, depression and suicidality especially in those with psychiatric illness.

Didanosine, ganciclovir and stavudine are associated with development of mania. Least neuropsychiatric manifestations are seen in HIV integrase inhibitors, C-C chemokine receptor type 5 inhibitors and fusion inhibitors.

A number of other medicines (excluding Anti-Retroviral Drugs) used in treatment of HIV like interferon, metoclopramide, clonidine, propranolol, sulphonamides, muscle relaxants can cause Major Depression or similar syndromes. Ganciclovir and steroids are associated with mania.

PSYCHIATRIC SIDE EFFECTS OF ATT

Psychiatric adverse effects are well recognised in the treatment of tuberculosis since the 1950s. The risk of adverse reactions increases with age, malnutrition, and history of hepatitis and human immunodeficiency virus infection. Isoniazid (INH), the first line drug in the treatment of tuberculosis is associated with various neuropsychiatric adverse effects. These include perceived cognitive impairment and lethargy (the most common), headaches, blurred vision, peripheral neuropathy, sleep disturbance, and depression. Other uncommon but severe neuropsychiatric disturbances include generalized convulsions and psychosis. Usually the onset of psychotic symptoms varies from days to months, with few weeks being the most common time period since its initiation. The treatment for isoniazid-induced psychosis includes discontinuation of isoniazid, addition of an antipsychotic or a combination of both. A more troubling fact is the increased propensity to develop psychotic symptoms to other medication as well after initial episode. Psychosis in tuberculosis can also be uncommonly seen with ethambutol and rifampicin. Cycloserine, used in the treatment of MDR-TB, has reported rates of psychiatric side-effects of 20–33%. The reported side-effects include mania, insomnia and anxiety.

PSYCHIATRIC DISORDERS ASSOCIATED WITH HIV/AIDS

Delirium

Delirium is a state of global derangement of cerebral function and is characterized by inattention, confusion and fluctuating consciousness. Emotional changes are seen with delusions and hallucinations. It frequently occurs in medically ill or metabolically unstable patients. It occurs in 43-65% of HIV infected persons. It has an acute or subacute onset with high mortality rate of 20%. The first line of treatment is to find and treat the underlying cause. Reorientation of the patient should be done by maintaining diurnal variation of light cycle, providing orienting stimuli like calendars, clocks and active reengagement and reorientation by staff and family. Atypical antipsychotics or low dose high potency antipsychotics can be used to treat psychosis or behavioral problems.

HIV associated Neurocognitive Disorder (HAND)

It is divided into three classes according to symptom severity to Asymptomatic Neurocognitive Impairment, Mild neurocognitive Disorder and HIV associated Dementia. The risk factors for development of HAND are low CD4 cell count, Historical CD4 nadir, viral load, detectable virus in CNS, opportunistic infections and higher medical comorbidity.

With the advent of HAART and CART, there is a marked improvement in complications and survival rates. Though the prevalence of HIV associated dementia has dropped, the prevalence of mild to moderate HAND has remained unchanged due to increased life expectancy.

HIV associated dementia

It has an insidious onset. Before the advent of ART, it rapidly progressed to a severe subcortical dementia which culminated in death. With widespread Treatment with ART the prevalence of HIV associated Dementia. Early cognitive symptoms include forgetfulness, loss of concentration and mental slowing. Behavioral symptoms include apathy, decreased emotional reciprocity and social withdrawal. Depression, emotional lability, agitation and psychotic symptoms may occur. Fine motor coordination, clumsiness, leg weakness are seen in early stages of disease. Gradually symptoms worsen with tremors, ataxia, dysarthria and frontal release signs may be seen. Severe psychomotor retardation, paraparesis, incontinence and seizures may occur in late stages. Neurocognitive testing can help in diagnosis or early stages of disease and help in differentiating from Pseudodementia due to depression.

CT and MRI brain usually reveals cerebral atrophy, widened cortical sulci and enlarged ventricles. High intensity signal abnormalities are often seen on T2 weighted MRI images. CSF studies can be done to rule out CNS infections. Increase in total proteins and IgG fraction and index is a common finding on CSF study. A mononuclear leucocytosis may occur with detection of HIV core antigen p24 though it is not very specific. Management includes HAART which can slow the disease progression. MAO inhibitor deprenyl and peptide T has shown some beneficial effect. Memantine, nitroglycerin, nimodipine, pentoxifylline and lexipafant have shown some effect. Comorbid psychotic or depressive symptoms can be treated with antipsychotics and antidepressants. Psychosocial interventions include maintenance of daily schedule.

Depression

Depressive symptoms are the most common emergent psychiatric illness in Persons with HIV. The psychological impact of the diagnosis and the neurotropism of the virus causing changes in deep grey structures can give rise to depressive symptoms. Feeling blue, low, sad or feeling empty or devoid of emotions is often reported. Some depressive features are common in Depression and HIV like insomnia, loss of appetite and weight, fatigue, lack of energy, retardation and difficulty in concentration.

Lack of pleasure in previously enjoyable activities is a cardinal symptom of depression. Persistent low mood, suicidal thoughts and marked feelings of hopelessness, guilt and self-reproach are indicative of depression. Neurovegetative symptoms commonly seen are difficulties with sleep, appetite, concentration and memory. Early morning awakening with difficulty in falling back asleep is a characteristic feature.

Depression may precede or follow HIV infection. Depression is more common with PLWH with shared risk factors like MSM, transgenders and IV drug users. The stigma associated with HIV and especially the social isolation and the lack of support can trigger depression. Chronicity of the illness, emergence of comorbid and opportunistic infection and adverse effects of ART can contribute towards depression. Suicidality may occur in depression.

Antidepressant medication are the mainstay of treatment. It is advisable to start at low doses and titrate slowly and take optimal dose for adequate period. Augmentation or alternate class of antidepressant should be considered for those with partial or no improvement. Other treatments include mood stabilizer, benzodiazepine, Trazodone, thyroid preparations, atypical antipsychotic and low dose methylphenidate. Psychotherapy is an integral part of treatment of Major Depression and it reported that medications with Psychotherapy yields better result than either modality alone. Interpersonal therapy, Cognitive Behavior Therapy and Group therapy yields good results. Patients with partial response to treatment should be started on augmentation strategy or alternative treatment. Other medications include thyroid preparations, atypical neuroleptics, mood stabilizers, methylphenidate and benzodiazepines have shown benefit in some patients.

Bipolar mood Disorder

The treatment of mania in HIV infected persons is similar to those without. Mood stabilizers and atypical antipsychotics are often used in treatment but care has to be taken to prevent drug interactions. Manic episode can increase the risk of acquiring infection and transmission of the illness due to impaired judgment and increased risk taking behaviors.

AIDS mania occurs in late stages of the disease and is often associated with cognitive impairment and absence of family history of mental illness. AIDS mania is quite severe in its presentation and runs a malignant course with irritable mood and psychomotor slowing with cognitive slowing. The prevalence of AIDS mania has decreased since the advent of ART. It is treated with antipsychotics and mood stabilizers and atypical neuroleptics are preferred as patients are prone to developing Extrapyramidal symptoms.

Anxiety disorders

Anxiety disorders may precede HIV infection or can be triggered by HIV diagnosis. PLWH are vulnerable to anxiety due to long course of the illness with unpredictable future, stigma, fear of disclosure, social isolation and fear of death. Lack of family support, being single or unemployed are significantly associated with anxiety disorders. Generalized anxiety disorder is a common reported type of anxiety disorder with free floating anxiety, apprehension about daily events and muscle tension. PTSD has a higher prevalence in PWLH and has a complex relation with HIV. Presence of anxiety disorders can impair concentration and are associated with poor adherence, avoidant coping and substance use. Anxiolytics and antidepressants especially SSRI's have shown to be of benefit.

Schizophrenia and psychotic disorders

There is no evidence that HIV infection causes schizophrenia but schizophrenia contributes to behaviors that can cause HIV infection. Unsafe sex, multiple sex partners, sex while under influence of intoxicant or trading sex for money contribute as a sexual risk factor. Development of psychotic illness causes complex diagnostic and management problem. Comorbid substance abuse, side effects of ART, CNS infections may also contribute to development of psychosis. Antipsychotics are drug of choice but development of extrapyramidal side effects is common in those with AIDS.

Personality disorders

High rates of personality disorders are seen in persons with HIV as compared to general population. Antisocial Personality Disorder is the most common diagnosis and is a risk factor for HIV infection due to high rates of substance abuse, IV drug use, high number of lifetime sexual partners, unprotected anal sex and sharing IV needles. Personality characteristics like unstable extroverts and stable extroverts have been found to be high in PWLH in some studies.

Substance use disorders

Substance abuse is a vector for spread of HIV. The impact is not only through IV drug use but also impulsive and unsafe sexual practices that occur due to intoxication. Persons with HIV may be demoralized and are more likely to use drugs engage in high risk behaviors. Unsafe sexual practices are often seen in persons with substance abuse with trading sex for drugs or casual sexual encounters.

Substance abuse can increase the likelihood of HIV exposure and infection due to IV drug use or risky sexual behavior. Recent research suggests that HIV infection itself can cause increased drug seeking behavior and relapse. This is attributed to increases in proinflammatory cytokines and alterations in neural reward circuitry that may be due to residual production of nonstructural viral proteins.

Decreased levels of methadone may occur in those receiving rifampin, ritonavir, nelfinavir, efavirenz, fosemprenavir and nevirapine necissicitating dosage adjustments. Non adherence is a risk if opioid withdrawal occurs due to concomitant ART use.

Sedative Hypnotics and alcohol are detoxified with use of long acting benzodiazepine like diazepam or chlordiazepoxide. Lorazepam and oxazepam is used in those with liver disease. Detoxification of opiates is done with gradual tapering of sublingual buprenorphine or oral methadone. Adjunctive treatments can be given for symptomatic relief like clonidine, loperamide and ibuprofen.

PSYCHIATRIC DISORDERS ASSOCIATED WITH TUBERCULOSIS

Depression

A study conducted in Vellore, south India has shown that about one-fifth of the tuberculosis patient suffer from some psychiatric comorbidity, depression being the commonest. Clinical depression often under-recognized when comorbid with TB, can reduce the quality of life and increase mortality. Similar to depression in the context of HIV/AIDS, depression has the potential to impair adherence to complex TB medication regimens, contribute to multidrug resistance and potentiate community transmission. The patients with depression are less likely to be adherent to treatment due to feelings of hopelessness about therapeutic regimen, lack of social support, energy or memory. Tuberculosis and Depression have a bidirectional complex relationship. Depression may increase risk of TB reactivation, and/or inhibit the response to anti-tuberculosis treatment because of poverty, undernutrition, immunosuppression, and substance abuse. Tuberculous infection and/or disease reactivation may precipitate depression as a result of the inflammatory response and/or dysregulation of the hypothalamic-pituitary-adrenal axis.

Suicide

There is an increased risk of suicide behavior among individuals infected with tuberculosis who are females, being retreated for TB, misusing alcohol, with previous psychological distress or post-traumatic stress disorders. Though the exact reason is unclear, the comorbidity with HIV/AIDS likely increases the risk of suicidal ideation and attempts. Every individual receiving medical care should be asked about suicide symptoms as talking about it does not increase the risk of completing a suicide but rather helps in catharsis and finding solutions.

COMORBIDITY AND SHARED RISK FACTORS

HIV and mental illness has high comorbidity as well as shared risk factors. Vulnerable population like MSM (men having sex with men), transgenders, sex worker and people who use drugs, ethnic and racial minorities experience high perceived stigma and discrimination. This negatively affects their mental health and is further compounded by the stigma of mental illness and HIV. Factors like poverty, low education, unstable housing, lack of safety, violence, wars and disasters are among the shared risk factors.

Persons with untreated Mental Illness are vulnerable to nonadherence to treatment and indulge in high risk behaviors like unsafe sex and substance use. Thus they are at higher risk of contracting HIV infection, being nonadherent to treatment and hence have higher viral load and become more immunocompromised and have increased risk of infecting others.

The interplay of personality Disorders, substance use and affective disorders is complex and is a risk factor for contracting HIV infection. Once the disease is contracted decreased access to care, poor adherence to treatment leading to further progress of the disease and poor outcomes are sometimes seen. Unsafe sex and sharing IV needles leads to further spread of the disease. This has led some authors to say that HIV is a psychiatric epidemic.

Depression and HIV have a complex relationship with major depression being a risk factor for HIV infection due to its impact on behavior with increased substance abuse, self-destructive behaviors and promotion of poor partner choice. Both depression and HIV are seen at higher rates in homosexual men and persons with substance abuse disorders. The MACS study (Multicenter AIDS Cohort Study) showed increase rate of depression as CD4 levels fall below 200. Additionally it is seen that treatment of depression improves outcome of HIV treatment. Hence mental health care has an important role in HIV treatment and prevention.

CHALLENGES TO DIAGNOSIS

Mental health impairment due to psychiatric illness or severe distress can interfere with regular HIV testing and delayed diagnosis of HIV. This has a negative impact with delayed access to cART and increased risk of transmission to others.

The emergence of psychiatric illness in PLWH is complicated with similar symptoms in HIV, its associated comorbid conditions and mental illness. HIV associated dementia and other CNS condition can produce a flat apathetic state which can be mistaken for depression.

In patients with tuberculosis, functionality may be severely impaired due to chronic psychogenic and somatic pain, frequent hospital admissions, and dependency from medical and nursing personnel. For diagnostic purposes, it is often difficult to determine if the vegetative symptoms of depression or somatic symptoms of anxiety are evidences of the psychiatric disorder or symptoms of tuberculosis, or both. Further, depression is often dismissed as a normative reaction to situational stress.

CHALLENGES TO TREATMENT

Ensuring compliance to cART remains a challenge during prolonged treatment in HIV. Different psychiatric illnesses have been associated with non-adherence to treatment and elevated viremia, though Depression has the strongest correlation. The UNAIDS goals of 90-90-90 call for 90% of PLWH of initiating cART to sustain viral suppression by adhering to treatment. Psychiatric illness including substance use is among the most significant barrier to achieving these goals. These exacerbate the many social and economic barriers to accessing adequate and sustained health care. Targeting mental health issues should be integrated into care for HIV as treatment of comorbid psychiatric conditions is associated with better adherence and outcomes.

People living with TB and mental disorders are less likely to seek health care and may be less adherent to treatment. The non-compliance to treatment has widespread public health consequences. Despite the mental disorders being commonly comorbid among patients with TB, they are not easily recognised by health workers and treating physicians. At the public health level, the National Mental Health Programe and National Strategic Plan for Tuberculosis Elimination 2017–2025 work independently and have no integration to cater to the mental health needs of individuals with TB.

CONCLUSION

It is a known fact that HIV promotes the progression of latent tuberculosis infection (LTBI) to disease, and tuberculosis (TB) accelerates the progression of HIV disease. Independently, the psychiatric illnesses are also common in PLWH, TB and contribute to HIV/TB acquisition and poor outcomes. The shared risk factors among them increases their vulnerability. The significant mental and substance use problems are among the most significant barriers to achieving the downsizing of the HIV/TB epidemic. In the general population, mental and substance use disorders are the number one contributors to number of years lived with disability. This necessitates an obvious need for universal mental health screening and the provision of mental health treatment integrated into ongoing HIV/TB care. The lack of mental health services, adequate health care professionals and funding remain the major shortcomings in the effective implementation.

BIBLIOGRAPHY

1. Remein RH, Stiratt MJ, Nguyen N, Robbins RN, Pala AN, Mellins CA. Mental Health and HIV/AIDS The need for an integrated response *AIDS*: July 2019; Vol 33 (9): 1411-20.
2. Nedelcovych MT, Manning AA, Semenova S, Gamaldo C, Haughey NJ, and Slusher BS. The Psychiatric Impact of HIV *ACS Chem Neurosci.* 2017: 8(7): 1432-34.
3. Doherty AM, Kelly J, McDonald C, O'Dywer AM, Keane J, Cooney J. A Review of the Interplay Between Tuberculosis and Mental Health *Gen Hosp Psychiatry*. 2013:35(4): 398-406.

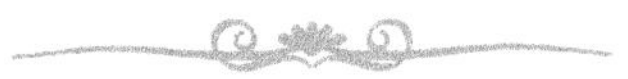

58 Psychiatric Aspects of Epilepsy

Sarika Dakshikar • Poornima Rao • Poornima Khadanga

INTRODUCTION

Epilepsy is a disorder of the brain characterized by an enduring predisposition to generate epileptic seizures. Epilepsy has biologic, cognitive, psychological, and social consequences which greatly affect quality of life of the patient. Manifestation of type of epilepsy and behavioral issues is vastly reflected through its anatomical and neurobiological correlates.

Antiepileptic drugs (AEDs) can play a role in the genesis of psychiatric symptoms. On the other hand, some psychotropic medications can lower the seizure threshold and provoke epileptic seizures.[1] Hence, this complex relation of epilepsy and psychiatric manifestation needs to be understood in depth.

DEFINITIONS

Seizure - A transient occurrence of signs and/or symptoms due to abnormal excessive or synchronous neuronal activity in the brain.[2]

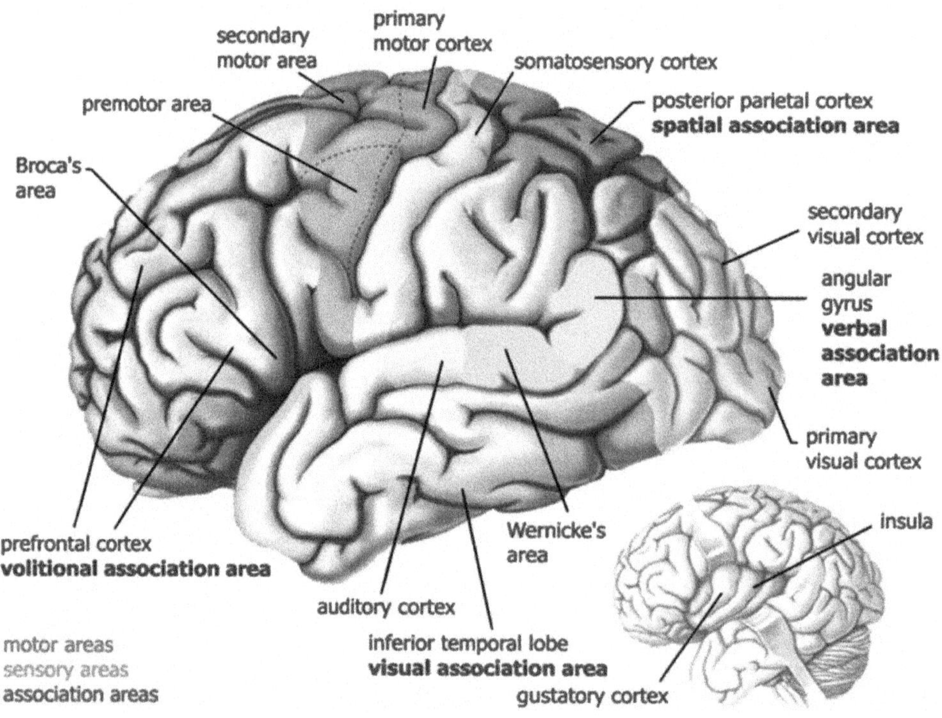

Fig. 58.1

Epilepsy – A disorder of the brain defined by any of the following conditions:

1. At least two unprovoked (or reflex) seizures occurring > 24 h apart;
2. One unprovoked (or reflex) seizure and a probability of further seizures similar to the general recurrence risk (at least 60%) after two unprovoked seizures, occurring over the next 10 years;
3. Diagnosis of an epilepsy syndrome.

Epilepsy is considered to be resolved for individuals who had an age-dependent epilepsy syndrome but are now past the applicable age or those who have remained seizure free for the last 10 years, with no antiseizure medicines for the last 5 years.[3]

CLASSIFICATION OF EPILEPSY[4]

ILAE 2017 Classification of Seizure Types Expanded Version

Focal Onset		Generalized Onset	Unknown Onset
Aware	Impaired Awareness	**Motor** Tonic-clonic Clonic Tonic Myoclonic Myoclonic-tonic-clonic Myoclonic-atonic Atonic Epileptic spasms **Nonmotor (absence)** Typical Atypical Myoclonic Eyelid myoconia	**Motor** Tonic-clonic epileptic spasms **Nonmotor** Behavior arrest
Motor Onset automatisms Atonic Clonic Epileptic spasms Hyperkinetic Myoclonic Tonic **Nonmotor Onset** Autonomic Behavior arrest Cognitive Emotional Sensory			Unclassified
Focal to bilateral tonic-clonic			

AURA OF EPILEPSY

An 'aura' is the term that some people use to describe the 'warning' they feel before they have a seizure. It acts as an alarming sign and patient can find a safe place or inform people in the vicinity so that he/ she won't get hurt during the seizure episode.

Aura typically lasts from few seconds to hours. It is still unclear if few auras are type of focal awake seizures.[5]

- a 'rising' feeling in the stomach or déjà vu (feeling like you've 'been here before')
- getting an unusual smell or taste (olfactory or gustatory)
- a sudden intense feeling of fear or joy
- a strange feeling like a 'wave' going through the head
- stiffness or twitching in part of the body (such as an arm or hand)
- a feeling of numbness or tingling (paresthesia)
- a sensation that an arm or leg feels bigger or smaller than it actually is (kinesthetic) or
- visual disturbances such as colored or flashing lights or hallucinations (seeing something that isn't actually there)

Many patients report extreme irritability, feeling of something going wrong, aggression, feeling on the edge, disturbed sleep before episode of seizure. Whether these symptoms can be called psychological aura is still debatable.

Temporal lobe epilepsy (TLE)

Most notable seizure type with psychiatric manifestations is temporal lobe epilepsy. Temporal lobe is a seat of primary auditory cortex and speech areas along with important secondary functions like processing of visual stimulus, memory and emotion. This neuro-anatomical peculiarity causes epilepsy involving temporal lobe to present with symptoms which appear as psychiatric symptoms like auditory and visual hallucinations, fear, déjà vu, euphoria lasting for few seconds up to 2 minutes. Speech disturbances are also notable during this phase. Phenomenon of aura is most commonly observed in TLE.

Temporal lobe seizures are also known as focal seizures with impaired awareness. Some people remain aware of what's happening, but during more-intense seizures, patient might look awake but be unresponsive. Repetitive purposeless movements of hands and lips are observed frequently during the episode of TLE.[6]

Exact cause of temporal lobe epilepsy is not known but sometimes it is attributed to scarring or anatomical defect in temporal area.

Characteristic signs and symptoms include:

- Loss of awareness of surroundings
- Staring
- Lip smacking
- Repeated swallowing or chewing
- Unusual finger movements, such as picking motions

After a temporal lobe seizure, one may have:

- A period of confusion and difficulty speaking
- Inability to recall what occurred during the seizure
- Unawareness of having had a seizure
- Extreme sleepiness

In extreme cases, what starts as a temporal lobe seizure evolves into a generalized tonic-clonic (grand mal) seizure — featuring convulsions and loss of consciousness.

PSYCHIATRIC MANIFESTATIONS IN EPILEPSY:

Prevalence of psychiatric problems – 20-60%

Most common psychiatric disorders observed with epilepsy are as follows:

- Psychosis,
- Mood disorder- Major Depressive Disorder and Bipolar Mood Disorder,
- Anxiety disorder,
- Cognitive Deficits,
- Intellectual disability,
- Epilepsy syndromes.

They can be seen during any of the phases of seizure:

1. **Ictal** – Symptoms during ictal phase i.e. during the episode of seizure, are short lasting and may not need separate treatment with psychotropic medications.
2. **Peri-ictal** – Peri-ictal psychiatric symptoms appear pre and post episode of seizure. Diagnosis of Peri-ictal psychiatric symptoms demands clinical expertise of evaluation and causality assessment. Thorough investigations like MRI of brain, video EEG definitely help in the diagnosis. Many a times, modification in antiepileptic medications or addition of benzodiazepine help the patients in resolving peri-ictal symptoms
3. **Interictal** - Inter-ictal psychiatric symptoms, however, warrants use of long-term use of psychotropic medications.

Clinical features vary on the type and phase of seizure along with type of psychiatric morbidity.

A. PSYCHOSIS AND EPILEPSY

Psychosis is a disorder which has been most clearly associated with epilepsy.

Lifelong prevalence - 7 to 12 percent.

Temporal lobe epilepsy and Psychosis – Prevalence – 7%

There is a five- to eight-fold greater risk of psychosis for epileptic patients than for the general population. Twice as many patients with left temporal lesions have psychosis. Temporal lobe epilepsy and psychosis have more severe grey matter loss in an entire temporal lobe as well as in the left hippocampus, insulae, anterior cingulum, and left inferior parietal lobule and predominant left temporal hypometabolism.[7]

Common Symptoms and Signs

1) Hallucinations – auditory, visual, olfactory, gustatory are most common. E.g. – Person far away speaks to patient without any communication device or Patient sees God or unpleasant smell or taste of familiar objects.
2) Delusions- referential ideation, paranoia frequently reported where patient feels people are talking about him/her or passing comments or plotting against them.
3) Decreased sleep- these hallucinations and delusion may evoke intense fear in patients causing sleep disturbances. Decreased sleep may start vicious cycle of seizure due to sleep deprivation. Hence, it needs to be asked while taking history.
4) Decreased self-care where patient needs to be coaxed for having meals on time, taking bath etc.

Treatment of Psychosis

- A long-term treatment extending from months to year is required.[8]
- Collateral psychotherapy in the form of psychoeducation, family therapy, self-help and reframing to be carried on.
- Episodes of aggression and violent behavior which is a common accompaniment in these patients can be treated with involuntary hospitalization and adequate usage of sedatives. Electro-Convulsive Therapy (ECT) have found to be effective on long term.[9] It is interesting to know that although ECT acts on the principle of seizure induction, it raises seizure threshold in epilepsy.

Pharmacotherapy of Psychosis

- A start low and go-slow strategy to be applied.
- Pharmacodynamic interactions should be kept in mind while initiating a treatment but these are not generally clinically significant.[8]
- Oral Benzodiazepines- diazepam, lorazepam, clonazepam
- Oral Benzodiazepines + antipsychotics (olanzapine, risperidone, quetiapine, chlorpromazine)
- Intramuscular administration of potent dopamine blocker like haloperidol
- Common side effects of antipsychotic medications may mimic symptoms of anxiety like restlessness, panic like symptoms. These need to be differentiated from core symptoms of epilepsy and aura. Treatment of side effect of antipsychotic medications include lowering the dose of antipsychotic medications or replacing it with another suitable molecule.
- Metabolic syndromes like weight gain, elevation in lipid and sugar levels caused by second generation antipsychotics is escalated by certain antiepileptic medications like Sodium Valproate and oxcarbazepine needs to be considered before initiating treatment.
- Clozapine is known to reduce seizure threshold. Hence, it's better avoided.

B. DEPRESSION IN EPILEPSY

Prevalence of lifetime depression in epilepsy was 12% (13–20%), higher than that of general population.[10]

Pathophysiology of Depression in Epilepsy: Bidirectional in nature.

1. Chronic stress exposure, the uncertainty and unpredictability of seizures may induce learned helplessness.[11]
2. Conversely, depression may facilitate the development of epileptic activity; proposed mechanisms of action for this association include hyperactivity of the hypothalamic-pituitary-adrenal (HPA) axis and disturbances of glutamate and γ-aminobutyric acid neurotransmitters.[12]
3. Social factors, such as a lack of occupational attainment, social engagement, or social support, may also influence the relationship between epilepsy and depression.[13]

Variables indicated in pathogenesis of depression in epilepsy[14]

Table 58.1

Patient related	Premorbid personality Temperament Gender differences
Antiepileptic drug related	GABA augmentation
Epilepsy related	Psychological Illness presentation Coping Mechanism Stigmatization Low expectancy of achievement Biological Hippocampal shrinking, Amygdala hypertrophy, Head injury Neurotransmitter abnormalities

Common Symptoms and Signs

Presentation is similar to features of Major depressive episode associated with–

1. Persistent and pervasive sadness of mood
2. Reduced energy leading to increased and easy fatiguability
3. Loss of interest and enjoyment in daily activities
4. Reduced self-esteem and self confidence
5. Ideas of hopelessness, helplessness and worthlessness
6. Wishes to die, suicidal ideas and attempt
7. Disturbed sleep
8. Decreased appetite

Episodic mood disturbances, often with agitation, suicidal behavior, and psychotic symptoms like delusion of guilt, may occur with increasing seizure activity.

Treatment of Depression[14]

First and foremost is optimising epilepsy treatment by improving seizure control, improving tolerability of anti-epileptic treatments, and balancing between both.

Antidepressant drug treatment, especially with SSRIs such as sertraline, citalopram and paroxetine, can be safely used in subjects with epilepsy.

The most concerned issue for antidepressants in epilepsy is the seizure threshold lowering property. Overdose and intoxication of tricyclic (TCA) and tetracyclic antidepressants (TeCA), SSRI, and serotonin norepinephrine reuptake inhibitor (SNRI) have been well documented as one of the potential causes of seizure.

C. MANIA /BIPOLAR DISORDER

Mood disorder due to epilepsy with manic features or with mixed features is much rarer than mood disorder due to epilepsy with depressive features or with major depressive-like features. Rarely, manic symptoms may emerge with an increase in seizure frequency or after seizure control.[15]

Prevalence: 1.5% in those with temporal lobe epilepsy[16]

Common symptoms and signs

1. increased energy
2. irritable and expansive i.e. unusually happy mood
3. increased activity which is goal directed in nature like spending spree
4. decreased need for sleep
5. grandiosity like making tall claims, having enormous power or wealth
6. pressure of speech presenting as increased talkativeness

Although a right temporal focus is a possible source of mania in epilepsy, this laterality is not well established.

Treatment

- Anti-Epileptic Drugs have become the mainstay of treatment for the manic phase of BAD, especially in patients with "mixed" states and/or rapid cycling.[17]
- lithium is effective in the prophylaxis of BAD and decreases the risk of suicide in this population by more than eightfold.[18]

D. ANXIETY AND EPILEPSY

Anxiety can occur as a reaction to the diagnosis, a symptom of seizures, or even a side effect of some anti-seizure medications

Prevalence of anxiety disorders in epileptic patients may be as high as 30 percent. These spectrums of disorders including generalized anxiety disorder (GAD), panic disorder, obsessive compulsive disorder (OCD), Post traumatic stress disorder (PTSD), phobia and social anxiety disorder are the second most common psychiatric comorbidities in patients with epilepsy after depressive disorders.[19]

Common symptoms and sign

- Palpitations, tremulousness of hands, sweating
- Shortness of breath, choking sensation
- Feeling dizzy, lightheaded
- Paresthesia
- Sense of impending doom, loss of control over self
- Apprehension about future
- Repetitive checking behavior, cleaning, repetitive thoughts and images
- Fear of specific object, animal and situation especially crowded places or closed spaces
- Fear and avoidance of social situations
- Re-experiencing traumatic events, emotional numbness, flashbacks and nightmares

Most frequently, anxiety appears after the diagnosis of epilepsy or after the first seizure and can involve the fear of having another event.

The symptoms manifesting during interictal phase must be distinguished from simple partial seizures which may mimic anxiety or panic attack.

Treatment

Treatment should be similar to the treatment of anxiety disorders in the general population and should focus on the following key areas: psychoeducation, relaxation, Cognitive Behavioral Therapy and anxiolytic medication. A detailed history about the ongoing medication is to be sought before initiating treatment.[20]

Table 58.2

	Disorder	Acute treatment	Long-term treatment
1.	Panic disorder	First choice: SSRIs* (any) + CBT+BZD+ Second Choice: TCAs# (any) + CBT	SSRIs (any) + CBT or CBT alone
2.	Generalized anxiety disorder	First choice: pregabalin Second choice: paroxetine, venlafaxine, imipramine	First choice: pregabalin Second choice: paroxetine, venlafaxine, imipramine
3.	Social anxiety disorder	First choice: SSRIs (sertraline, escitalopram, paroxetine) + BZD	First choice: SSRIs (sertraline, escitalopram, paroxetine)
4.	Posttraumatic stress disorder	First choice: SSRIs (sertraline, paroxetine)	First choice: SSRIs (sertraline, paroxetine)
5.	Obsessive-compulsive disorder	First choice: CBT Second choice: CBT + sertraline Third choice: CBT + clomipramine	First choice: CBT Second choice: CBT + sertraline Third choice: CBT + clomipramine

* SSRIs (Selective Serotonin Reuptake Inhibitor)- Citalopram, Escitalopram, Sertraline, Paroxetine, Fluoxetine, Fluvoxamine)

+ BZD (Benzodiazepines)-Clonazepam, Lorazepam,Diazepam

TCA (Tricyclic Antidepressants)- Imipramine, Clomipramine, Amitriptyline

Acute Treatment: 8-12 weeks

Functional Non-Epileptic Fits (Pseudo seizures)

These are a diverse group of disorders in which paroxysmal events (fits or 'funny turns') may be mistaken for epilepsy, but are not caused by epilepsy (no seizures or epileptiform activity in the brain). They are either physiological (about 10–20%) or psychogenic (about 80–90%) in origin. Diagnosis can be particularly difficult and requires specialist assessment. Hence

Table 58.3

	Seizure	Pseudo-seizure
1	Not inducible	Inducible by suggestion and emotional triggers
2	May occur in sleep	Does not occur in sleep
3	Aura present	No aura
4	Impaired consciousness and unresponsive to pain	Consciousness usually preserved but may be fluctuating. Responsive to pain
5	In GTCS- Generalized tonic clonic movements jerky, side with fast small amplitude to slower larger movements occurs. Presentation consistent with respect to other epilepsy syndromes	Nonsynchronous out of phase starting movements (may be mild, jerky, side to side head movements, pelvic thrusting, limping, motionless, unresponsive) Presentation inconsistent with respect to other epilepsy syndromes.
6	Frequent self-injury, tongue bite	Self-protection from any injury
7	Incontinence and tongue bite present	Incontinence and tongue bite not present
8	Post ictal confusion present	Post ictal confusion absent
9	Not always witnessed	Usually witnessed by other people
10	Epileptic changes in EEG in majority with raised serum prolactin	EEG usually normal with normal Serum Prolactin is normal.

differentiating between seizure and pseudo seizure becomes an important parameter.[21]

E. EPILEPSY AND COGNITIVE DISORDERS

Cognitive deficits in epilepsy are common in the setting of newly diagnosed epilepsy, as well as in patients with long-standing seizures.

The most frequent cognitive complaints in adults are–

- feeling slowed down mentally
- memory impairment
- attention problems.

Memory problems are an important symptom of seizures arising from temporal lobe- most common being short term memory. Anti-epileptic medicines have also been known to cause memory problems.[22]

Treatment involves improved seizure control using slower titration rates, lowering dosages, maintaining lower blood levels, and minimizing polypharmacy.[23]

F. INTELLECTUAL DISABILITY AND EPILEPSY

Intellectual disability or mental retardation is the most common psychiatric co-morbidity seen with epilepsy. The complex relation between the two adds up to difficulty in management of symptoms. Both the conditions may be present since birth and go hand in hand for lifetime.

Recurrent episodes of epilepsy and no control over developmental delay adds to the woes of caregivers of these patients. Hence, good control over epileptic symptoms is mandatory for better quality of life.

Intellectual disability, by itself may be associated with myriads of psychiatric symptoms like aggression, psychosis, anxiety and depression to name a few.

Treatment of mental retardation with epilepsy is purely symptomatic. Psychoeducation of the caregivers is the mainstay of the treatment along with compliance to antiepileptic.

G. EPILEPSY SYNDROME- GASTAUT–GESCHWIND SYNDROME:

A group of traits termed the *Gastaut–Geschwind syndrome* occurs in a subset of patients with focal seizures. It is characterized by–

- A sense of the heightened significance of things. These patients are serious, humourless, and overinclusive, and have an intense interest in philosophical, moral, or religious issues.
- Occasionally, epilepsy patients experience multiple religious conversions or experiences.
- In interpersonal encounters, they demonstrate *viscosity*, the tendency to talk repetitively and circumstantially about a restricted range of topics. They can spend a long time getting to the point, give detailed background information with multiple quotations. Viscosity may particularly occur in patients with left-sided or bilateral temporal foci.
- They can write copiously about their thoughts and feelings (hypergraphia).[24]

COMPREHENSIVE OVERVIEW OF PSYCHIATROPIC EFFECT OF ANTIEPILEPTIC MEDICATIONS[14]

Table 58.4

	Negative	**Positive**
Barbiturates	Depression, hyperactivity	Anxiolytic, hypnotic
Carbamazepine—Oxcarbazepine	Irritability	Mood stabilizing, antimanic
Ethosuximide	Behavioral abnormalities, psychosis	–
Felbamate	Depression, anxiety, irritability	–
Gabapentin	Behavioral problems in children	–
Lamotrigine	Insomnia, agitation	Mood stabilizing, antidepressant
Levetiracetam	Irritability, emotional lability	Antimanic?
Phenytoin	Encephalopathy	Antimanic?
Pregabalin	?	Anxiolytic
Tiagabine	Depression (Non-convulsive status epilepticus)	Anti-anxiety?
Topiramate	Depression, psychomotor slowing, psychosis	Mood stabilizing
Valproate	Encephalopathy	Mood stabilizing, antimanic (anxiolytic)
Vigabatrin	Depression, aggression, psychosis	–
Zonisamide	Agitation, depression, psychosis	Antimanic?

BIBLIOGRAPHY

1. Alper K, Schwartz KA, Kolts RL, Khan A. Seizure incidence in psychopharmacological clinical trials: an analysis of Food and Drug Administration (FDA) summary basis of approval reports. Biol Psychiatry. 2007; 62 4: 345- 54
2. Fisher RS, Acevedo C, Arzimanoglou A, et al. A practical clinical definition of epilepsy. Epilepsia 2014; 55:475–82
3. Fisher RS, Boas WV, Blume W, et al. Epileptic seizures and epilepsy: definitions proposed by the International League against Epilepsy (ILAE) and the International Bureau for Epilepsy (IBE). Epilepsia 2005; 46:470–472
4. Fisher, R.S., Cross, J.H., D'Souza, C., French, J.A., Haut, S.R., Higurashi, N., Hirsch, E., Jansen, F.E., Lagae, L., Moshé, S.L. and Peltola, J., 2017. Instruction manual for the ILAE 2017 operational classification of seizure types. Epilepsia, 58(4), pp.531-542
5. Epilepsy auras [Internet]. Epilepsy Society. 2019 [cited 14 December 2019]. Available from: https://www.epilepsysociety.org.uk/epilepsy-auras-0
6. Temporal lobe seizure - Symptoms and causes [Internet]. Mayo Clinic. 2019 [cited 14 December 2019]. Available from: https://www.mayoclinic.org/diseases-conditions/temporal-lobe-seizure/symptoms-causes/syc-20378214
7. Clancy MJ, Clarke MC, Connor DJ, Cannon M, Cotter DR. The prevalence of psychosis in epilepsy; a systematic review and meta-analysis. BMC Psychiatry. 2014; 14:75
8. Kerr M, Mensah S, Besag F, de Toffol B, Ettinger A, Kanemoto K, Kanner A, Kemp S, Krishnamoorthy E, LaFrance WC Jr, Mula M, Schmitz B, Tabertz van Elst L, Troller J, Wilson SJ. (2011) International consensus

clinical practice statements for the treatment of neuropsychiatric conditions associated with epilepsy. Epilepsia 52:2133–2138

9. (Krauss G, Theodore WH. (2010) Treatment strategies in the postictal state. Epilepsy Behav 19:188–190.)
10. Fiest, K. M., Dykeman, J., Patten, S. B., Wiebe, S., Kaplan, G. G., Maxwell, C. J.Jette, N. Depression in epilepsy: a systematic review and meta-analysis. Neurology.2003;80(6): 590–599.
11. Kanner AM. Depression and epilepsy: a bidirectional relation? Epilepsia 2011; 52:21–27
12. Hoppe C, Elger CE. Depression in epilepsy: a critical review from a clinical perspective. Nat Rev Neurol 2011; 7:462–472
13. Grabowska-Grzyb A, Jedrzejczak J, Naganska E, Fiszer U. Risk factors for depression in patients with epilepsy. Epilepsy Behav 2006; 8:411–417
14. Mula, M., & Schmitz, B. (2009). Depression in epilepsy: mechanisms and therapeutic approach. Therapeutic advances in neurological disorders, 2(5), 337–344
15. Barry JJ, Ettinger AB, Friel P, Gilliam FG, Harden CL. Advisory group of the epilepsy foundation as part of its mood disorder: Consensus statement: the evaluation and treatment of people with epilepsy and affective disorders. Epilepsy Behav. 2008;13(1): S1–S29.
16. Barry JJ. Psychiatric uses for anticonvulsants. Merritt-Putnam Lectures. CME monograph. West Hartford, Conn: American Epilepsy Society, 1999:89–105
17. Barry JJ, Lembke A, Huynh N: Affective disorders in epilepsy, in Psychiatric Issues in Epilepsy: A Practical Guide to Diagnosis and Treatment. Edited by Ettinger AB, Kanner AM. Philadelphia, Lippincott Williams & Wilkins, 2001, pp 45–71
18. Jefferson JW, Greist JH, Ackerman DL, et al. Anticonvulsants. In: Lithium encyclopedia for clinical practice. 2nd ed. Washington, DC: American Psychiatric Press, 1987:75–91.
19. Jackson MJ, Turkington D. Depression and anxiety in epilepsy. J Neurol Neurosurg Psychiatry. 2005;76: i45–i47
20. Mula M. Treatment of anxiety disorders in epilepsy: An evidence-based approach. Epilepsia. 2013; 54:13-18.
21. Agrawal N, Govender S. Epilepsy and neuropsychiatric comorbidities. Advances in Psychiatric Treatment. 2011;17(1):44-53.
22. Psychiatric Disorders Associated with Epilepsy: Overview, Psychotic Disorders, Bipolar Affective Disorders [Internet]. Emedicine.medscape.com. 2019 [cited 14 December 2019]. Available from: https://emedicine.medscape.com/article/1186336-overview
23. Dikmen S, Matthews CG. Effect of major motor seizure frequency upon cognitive-intellectual functions in adults. Epilepsia 1977;18(1):21–9,
24. Benson DF. The Geschwind syndrome. Advances in neurology. 1991; 55: 411-21.

59 Neuropsychiatric Aspects of Headache and Migraine

Bindoo S. Jadhav • Navoneela Bardhan

INTRODUCTION

Headache is a common presenting symptom among patients in out-patient as well as emergency basis. It is a major public health burden affecting the most productive years in both men and women. At times, it is chronic with episodic exacerbations. The term "active headache disorder" is used when symptoms of headache are present in the last 12 months. According to the Global Burden of Disease Study 2010 (GBD2010), headache disorders are the third highest cause of disability. The one year and lifetime prevalence have been reported to be as high as 90% and 99% respectively. Majority of the headaches are transient, only 3% of the general population suffer from chronic headache.

The causes of headache are varied ranging from medical & neurological causes to psychiatric disorders. The associated symptomatology depends on the cause of the headache. At times, headache can be the only complaint with no associated systemic involvement. The relationship between headache, psychological factors and psychiatric disorders is well documented and treatment strategies need to focus on this aspect to improve overall prognosis. Considering the impact of headache on people worldwide, "Lifting the Burden: the Global Campaign" to reduce the burden of headache was launched as a collaboration between the World Headache Alliance, the International Headache Society, the European Headache Federation and the World Health Organization.

CLASSIFICATION

The International Headache Society has published the third edition of the International Classification of Headache Disorders (ICHD-3) as the first issue of *Cephalalgia* in 2018. According to this classification, headaches can be broadly classified into 3 categories:

1. **The primary headache disorders:** These are independent disorders not associated with any underlying medical disease or disorder. They are the most common type accounting for almost 90% of all headaches. These include migraine, tension type headache, trigeminal autonomic cephalalgias & other primary headache disorders. The diagnosis is made on the basis of nature of pain, site, duration and severity of headache. A detailed history including aggravating and relieving factors helps in identifying the type of primary headache. The neurological examination and imaging studies usually do not reveal any abnormality.
2. **The secondary headaches:** These are caused by an underlying medical or neurological condition. These headaches are usually sudden in onset and besides headache, the patients present with symptoms of the underlying systemic

illness like disorientation, weakness of limbs, slurred speech, fever, stiffness of neck, rash, seizures, visual complaints or head injury. Detailed neurological and systemic examination reveal abnormalities related to the underlying condition. Laboratory investigations and neuroimaging studies are indicated to confirm the diagnosis. The secondary headaches can be due to head injury or trauma to neck, infections, vascular and non-vascular intracranial disorders, disorders of homeostasis, substance use disorders, or psychiatric disorders like somatoform disorder, depression and anxiety. It is important to distinguish primary from secondary headaches because of its impact on treatment and prognosis.

3. **Neuropathies and facial pains and other headache disorders:** Painful lesions of the cranial nerves can present with headache and facial pain. These include trigeminal neuralgia, glossopharyngeal neuralgia, nervous intermedius neuralgia and occipital neuralgia and other headache disorders. Headache not elsewhere classified and headache unspecified are included under other headache disorders.

ASSESSMENT OF A PATIENT PRESENTING WITH HEADACHE

Every patient who presents with headache should undergo an in depth evaluation, especially when there is presence of red flags. These include new onset headache in patients over 50 years of age, sudden change in nature of headache, increased frequency and intensity of headache, presence of focal neurological signs or papilledema, and headache in patients with systemic illness. A detailed history with special focus on headache features - onset, duration, nature and site of pain, aggravating and relieving factors along with associated symptoms is the first step to help arrive at a diagnosis. It is important to ask about family history, presence of stressors, and any comorbid conditions. This should be followed by an extensive neurological examination so as to be able to distinguish primary from secondary headache disorders. Though not usually indicated in primary headache disorders, laboratory investigations, imaging studies, EEG and lumbar puncture should be done when needed as these may aid in diagnosis. It is imperative to differentiate between primary and secondary headache disorders as the underlying condition in secondary headaches could be life threatening. Early identification helps in formulating an appropriate treatment plan thus improving outcome and functionality.

This chapter will focus mainly on primary headache disorders and its psychiatric aspects.

MIGRAINE

Migraine is a highly disabling primary headache disorder with a one-year worldwide prevalence of 15-18%. The Global Burden of Disease Study found that migraine was the third most prevalent disorder and the third highest cause of disability globally. There is a female preponderance with a ratio of 2:1 to 3:1. Migraine has also been referred to as "sick headache', 'hemicrania' and 'splitting headache'.

The term 'migraine personality' was coined by Wolff in 1963. He described people having migraine as ambitious, successful, perfectionist, rigid, orderly, cautious, emotionally constipated, driven and hence their outbursts take a somatic form. Fromm-Reichmann in 1937 described migraine as a physical expression of unconscious hostility to their beloved ones.

Classification

Migraine is of two major types - migraine with aura and migraine without aura. Migraine with aura is more severe and causes more morbidity than migraine without aura. The typical aura of migraine may exist with headache or without headache. Another subtype of aura is brainstem aura which has been described later. The common variants of migraine are hemiplegic migraine (described later) and retinal migraine. The term chronic migraine is used for migraine attacks occurring for 15 or more days in a month.

Other related conditions are probable migraine without aura, probable migraine with aura. There are episodic syndromes associated with migraine - recurrent gastrointestinal disturbance which includes cyclical vomiting syndrome, abdominal migraine, benign paroxysmal vertigo and benign paroxysmal torticollis.

The complications of migraine are status migrainosus, persistent aura without infarction, migrainous infarction and migraine aura triggered seizure.

Pathophysiology

The most consistent risk factor is a family history of migraine.

Migraine attacks are often triggered by hunger, alcohol, certain types of food, too much or too little sleep, menstruation, environmental factors (bright light, temperature changes, high altitude and certain odors), exhaustion and stress.

These triggers activate the trigeminovascular system and the signals from the vascular nociceptors are transmitted to the bipolar neurons in the trigeminal nerve and then relayed to thalamus and cerebral cortex. Endogenous mediators like vasoactive peptides, neurokinin A, substance P, calcitonin gene related peptide (CGRP), pituitary adenylate cyclase activating peptide and nitric oxide are involved in inflammation of meninges. The brainstem regions including trigeminovascular neurons become sensitised to dural stimuli, which leads to the throbbing nature of a migraine attack.

Clinical Presentation

Classical migraine features are rare before the age of 6 years, headache attacks in children are much shorter than in adults, p ain is less often unilateral and phonophobia is relatively rarely reported.

In adults, a typical migraine attack consists of the following four stages:

1. Premonitory phase
2. Aura phase
3. Headache phase
4. Postdromal phase

1. ***Premonitory phase*** - In this phase, the patient experiences fatigue, muscle tenderness, yawning, mood changes, food cravings, photophobia and phonophobia. These symptoms may precede the headache by upto 3 days and may continue well into the aura phase. Functional neuroimaging (H2O PET) show an increase in hypothalamic blood flow.
2. ***Aura phase*** - The aura of migraine is defined according to the ICHD-3 as *"one or more transient, fully reversible neurological deficits, of which at least one has to have a unilateral localization, that develop over 5*

minutes or more and of which each deficit lasts between 5 and 60 minutes."

The start of an aura is sudden, overwhelming in nature and not congruous to the surroundings and may well continue into the headache phase. The following are the usual symptoms during an aura:

i) Alterations in perception - Most common symptoms of aura are visual (90%) - zoom vision, macropsia (Brobdignagian vision), micropsia, mosaic vision, double vision are typical symptoms. Olfactory and auditory perceptual abnormalities can also be a part of aura.

ii) Neurological symptoms - Tingling and numbness (paraesthesias), apraxia, agnosia, aphasia, motor disturbances have been observed along with disturbances in higher mental functions in some cases.

Cortical spreading depression is associated with the initiation and progression of aura symptoms. It is a wave of depolarisation in the cell membranes of neurons and glial cells that propagates slowly accompanied by ion fluxes that causes suppression of activity as it spreads through the cerebral cortex.

3. ***Headache phase*** - The characteristic headache of migraine is unilateral, beginning as a dull, steady pain progressing to a pulsating or throbbing quality of severe intensity. The associated features of a migraine headache are nausea, vomiting, photophobia, phonophobia, blurring of vision, redness and/or watering from eyes, nasal congestion and occasional diarrhea. The characteristic behavior during this phase is that the patient prefers to stay in a quiet, dark room until the headache subsides.

   Though the headache is mostly unilateral, it may be bilateral too and it may even change sides on different occasions. The usual duration of the headache is 4-72 hours. If the headache phase lasts for more than 72 hours, it is called "status migrainosus".

   The severity and frequency of migraine decrease in the second and third trimester of pregnancy and after menopause.

4. ***Postdrome phase*** - During this phase, the patient is drowsy and experiences tiredness, neck stiffness and difficulties in concentrating.

Migraine with brainstem aura - It is a subtype of migraine with aura including at least two of the following symptoms: speech disturbances, vertigo, tinnitus, hyperacusis, double vision, ataxia and/or decreased level of consciousness.

Hemiplegic migraine - It is a rare subtype which is more severe and accompanied by motor symptoms, e.g., hemiparesis, hemianesthesia, etc. during the attack. Familial hemiplegic migraine is an autosomal dominant subtype. Mutations are found in CACNA1A, ATP1A2 and SCN1A genes, which are involved in encoding ion channel and transport proteins.

Migrainous Neuralgia - This was described by Mollendorf in 1867. Other terms for this condition are histamine headache, sphenopalatine neuralgia, ciliary neuralgia and cluster headache.

Diagnosis

The clinical presentation of a migraine attack is typical and is sufficient for the diagnosis on most occasions. An EEG may be helpful in differentiating an aura from a seizure. If neurological symptoms persist beyond the post-dromal phase, they should be viewed with suspicion and may indicate a disorder of the central nervous system. MIDAS (Migraine Disability Assessment Questionnaire) can be used to assess the impact of migraine on patients' day to day life.

Treatment

I. *Acute (Abortive) Treatment* - The following medications are used to abort a migraine attack:

i) Aspirin (500-1000 mg)
ii) NSAIDs - Acetaminophen (500-1000 mg), ibuprofen (200-400 mg), naproxen (500 mg/day), diclofenac (50 mg/day), mefenamic acid (500mg)
iii) Ergotamines - Dihydroergotamine upto 3 mg/day
iv) Triptans - Sumatriptan (25-200 mg/day), rizatriptan (5-30 mg/day), zolmitriptan (2.5-10 mg/day)
v) Antiemetics - Prochlorperazine, metoclopramide, domperidone.
vi) Intravenous corticosteroids - Dexamethasone (10 mg/day)
vii) Others - Intravenous magnesium, tramadol

In mild to moderate headache, either NSAIDs alone or NSAIDs with antiemetics are recommended. Triptans are a group of selective serotonin receptor agonist which are used during a moderate to severe attack and need to be taken as soon as the headache starts. They provide relief more rapidly as compared to ergotamines. Antiemetics are helpful in reducing nausea and vomiting associated with migraine.

Treatment of status migrainosus may require the use of droperidol, dexamethasone and intravenous valproic acid in addition to the previously described drugs.

During pregnancy, 60-80% of symptoms are alleviated by the third trimester. Sumatriptan is relatively safe during pregnancy while ergotamines are contraindicated.

II. *Prophylactic Treatment* - It is indicated for those who have 6 or more episodes of headache per month. The following drugs are commonly used:

i) Propranolol (40 mg/day)
ii) Antidepressants - Amitriptyline (50-150 mg/day)
iii) Antiepileptics - Valproic acid (500-1800 mg/day), topiramate (25-100 mg/day)
iv) Flunarizine (5-10 mg/day)
v) Others - Magnesium, vitamin B12, naproxen

It takes around 2 months for the prophylactic treatment to show its effectiveness. Treatment should be continued for 3-6 months and tapered off gradually once good migraine control is achieved (less than 1-2 headaches per month).

Propranolol is a beta blocker which has proven to be an effective agent for migraine prophylaxis but is contraindicated in asthma and heart failure. It can be safely used in pregnancy.

Valproic acid is an antiepileptic which suppresses neuronal excitability by increasing the levels of GABA. It has shown to decrease the frequency, severity and duration of the headache. It has teratogenic effect (neural tube defects) and hence preferably avoided during pregnancy.

Topiramate is also effective in reducing the frequency of the headaches.

Antidepressants have an action on norepinephrine and serotonin and thereby also provide relief in migraine. Amitriptyline is most effective among the antidepressants and also helps in treating comorbid anxiety or depression associated with migraine. Other antidepressants that have shown some effect are fluoxetine, fluvoxamine, venlafaxine, mirtazapine. Combined use of triptans and antidepressants should be avoided due to the risk of developing serotonin syndrome.

Non pharmacological approaches are also helpful in acute as well as prophylactic treatment. During an acute attack, patient perceives relief in a dark, quiet room. Various technics like relaxation exercises, biofeedback, and cognitive behavior therapy are also useful in reducing stress which is a major trigger for migraine as well as decreasing the pain sensitivity which is a major mechanism in the development of migraine.

TENSION TYPE HEADACHE

Tension type headache is the most common subtype of primary headache and the lifetime prevalence among the general population ranges from 30-78%. It is more common in females (M:F = 4:5) and in the fourth decade of life. The worldwide prevalence of chronic tension type headache is 1-3% and has a high socio-economic impact. Various terms that are used to describe tension type headache include stress headache, psychogenic headache and muscle contraction headache.

Classification

Tension type headache is classified into - infrequent episodic type, frequent episodic type and chronic type. The differentiation of tension type headache into episodic and chronic types was first described in the International Classification of Headache Disorders. The episodic type was further subdivided into infrequent and frequent types according to the ICHD-II criteria types which differentiates the two groups into having almost no morbidity from those having some morbidity and gives the clinician a guide to when to start prophylactic treatment.

- **Infrequent episodic type** - Episodes occur less than once per month and it has little impact on the functioning and less morbidity. This type may or may not be associated with pericranial tenderness.
- **Frequent episodic type** - In this type, there are 1-14 episodes in a month and requires long term treatment leading to a greater economic burden along with greater disability. This type also may or may not be associated with pericranial tenderness.
- **Chronic type** - It is characterized by more than 15 episodes per month, which may or may not be associated with pericranial tenderness. It is a serious condition with high morbidity and disease burden and poorer quality of life.
- **Probable tension type headache** - This term is used for those headaches when distinguishing a tension type headache from the early phase of migraine becomes difficult or when all clinical features of a tension type headache are not present. Migraine without aura and medication overuse headache need to be ruled out. It may be of episodic as well as chronic type, with the episodic type further subdivided into infrequent and frequent types.

Pathophysiology

Tension type headache was previously thought to be of psychogenic origin but various studies now suggest a strong neurobiological basis. The pathogenesis is multifactorial involving both peripheral and central mechanisms.

- Peripheral mechanisms - The most important factor involved is the myofascial nociception and it plays a role in the episodic type.
- Central mechanisms - These include inadequate pain control and heightened sensitisation and play a role in the development of chronic type.

The factors which make an individual prone to develop tension type headache are - decreased sleep, stressful lifestyle and poor self rated health.

Clinical Presentation

The most significant and consistent finding is the presence of increased pericranial tenderness, typically also present in between the headache episodes but significantly increases during headache and is directly related to the intensity and frequency of the headaches.

The headache is a dull aching, constrictive pain which typically is described as a "band like sensation" by patients. It is not associated with nausea or vomiting but can be associated with irritability and sleep disturbance.

Tension type headache is highly comorbid with anxiety and depression. Stress is a common risk factor for development of tension-type headache as well as depression and anxiety disorders. The presence of these psychiatric comorbidities increases the likelihood of progression to chronic tension-type headache by 2-5 times.

Diagnosis

The diagnosis of tension type headache is mainly clinical and is usually a diagnosis of exclusion. It has to be differentiated from other primary and secondary headache disorders based on the history. Laboratory investigations and neuroimaging studies are usually not warranted in these patients.

Treatment

I. ***Acute (Abortive) Treatment*** - Infrequent episodic type can be managed only by acute therapy but should be restricted to 2-3 times a week for the risk of development of medication-overuse headache that may subsequently result in treatment failure. Pharmacotherapy is the mainstay of acute management.

   Following drugs are used:

   i) Analgesics - Aspirin (500-1000 mg), acetaminophen (500 mg), ibuprofen (200-800 mg), naproxen (200-600 mg) and mefenamic acid. However, gastrointestinal and heamatopoietic side effects may limit its use. In pregnancy, acetaminophen is a safer choice.

   ii) Caffeine (65-200 mg) - It is often used in combination with analgesics. It is effective and fast acting but should be used with caution due to risk of dependence and medication overuse headache.

   iii) Selective COX-2 inhibitors - Rofecoxib and celecoxib

II. ***Prophylactic Therapy*** - Prophylactic therapy should be considered for patients with frequent episodic and chronic tension-type headache where combined pharmacological and non pharmacological modalities are recommended.

- **Pharmacological**

   i) Antidepressants - Antidepressants acting on norepinephrine have proven to be effective prophylactic choices, e.g., tricyclic antidepressants, mirtazapine.

- Tricyclic antidepressants - Amitriptyline (5-75 mg/day), clomipramine (75-150 mg/day), maprotiline (75 mg/day), mianserin (30-60 mg/day)
- NaSSA - Mirtazapine (30 mg/day)

ii) Antiepileptic - Topiramate

iii) Anxiolytics - Alprazolam (0.4 to 1.2 mg/day), etizolam (0.5 to 1 mg/day) provide relief due to their anxiolytic property but continuous use should be avoided due to the risk of dependence.

iv) Muscle relaxants - Tizanidine (3-6 mg/day), eperison (150 mg/day)

- **Non Pharmacological**

A. *Physical therapy* - Massage, exercise, ultrasound and electrical stimulation, improvement of posture, hot and cold packs, and acupuncture may help these patients.

B. *Psychotherapy* - Biofeedback, cognitive behavioral therapy, relaxation training are effective. Biofeedback using electromyography along with relaxation leads to long term relief effectively. Cognitive behavioral therapy targets the relationship between stress and headache.

The comorbid psychiatric disorders also need to be treated.

TRIGEMINAL AUTONOMIC CEPHALGIAS

These are a group of strictly unilateral, short lasting headaches along the distribution of the trigeminal nerve accompanied by ipsilateral autonomic symptoms. The pain is excruciating (one of the most painful conditions) and causes high disability. The conditions included are-

I. Cluster headache

II. Paroxysmal hemicrania

III. SUNCT (*Short lasting unilateral neuralgiform headache attacks with conjunctival injection and tearing)* and SUNA (*Short lasting unilateral neuralgiform headache attacks with cranial autonomic symptoms)*

Pituitary tumors may be an association with trigeminal autonomic neuralgia.

The duration of each attack is highest in cluster headache and lowest in SUNCT while the frequency is highest in SUNCT and lowest in cluster headache.

I. CLUSTER HEADACHE

Cluster headache occurs unilaterally, is excruciatingly painful in nature with cranial autonomic features. It has a characteristic circadian and circannual periodicity. The prevalence of cluster headache ranges from 0.1-0.2%. It is more predominant in females (F:M = 2.5:1) and its usual onset is in the third or fourth decade.

Classification

It is classified into episodic and chronic types depending on the duration of remission.

i) Episodic cluster headache (80-90%) - The patients have recurrent attacks with each episode lasting for more than 1 week, occurring 1-2 times a year with periods of remission lasting more than 4 weeks.

ii) Chronic cluster headache (10-20%) - Here the remission lasts for less than 1 month or the patients do not have a period of remission at all.

Clinical Features

The onset of headache is abrupt, lasting for 45-90 minutes usually and accompanied by cranial autonomic symptoms. The pain is excruciatingly severe, occurring mainly in the orbital and temporal area. The attacks occur in a circadian manner and can be precipitated by exercise, alcohol, nitroglycerine and higher temperatures in the environment. Nausea, vomiting, photophobia and phonophobia as well as aura (similar to migraine), restlessness or even aggressiveness have also been reported.

Treatment

I. *Abortive Treatment*

i) Subcutaneous sumatriptan (6 mg twice daily) is the drug of choice. Sumatriptan and zolmitriptan nasal spray are also used. Subcutaneous sumatriptan does not have the risk of tachyphylaxis or rebound even if required to be used for long term.

ii) 100% oxygen inhaled at 7–12 L/min for 15-30 minutes through a nonrebreathing facial mask is rapidly effective.

iii) Lidocaine (10%) nasal drops or spray deep in the nostril on the painful side provides mild to moderate relief. It is used as an adjunct to others.

iv) Dihydroergotamine nasal spray 1 mg reduces pain intensity

II. *Transitional treatment*

i) Corticosteroids - Oral prednisolone at 1 mg/kg up to a maximum dose of 60 mg daily for 5 days following which tapering the dose by 10 mg every 3 days provides pain relief. The tapering should be achieved by 3 weeks, due to risk of potential adverse effects of corticosteroids. Preventive therapy is also started along with corticosteroids as relapse occurs invariably after stopping prednisolone.

ii) Greater occipital nerve block - A mixture of rapid and long acting betamethasone injected sub-occipitally provides pain relief within a week which is maintained for at least a month in the majority of patients.

iii) IV dihydroergotamine - Complete pain resolution can be achieved by repetitive administration of dihydroergotamine over 3 days. The effect is maintained for over a month in two thirds of patients.

III. *Preventive Treatment*

- **Pharmacotherapy**

i) Verapamil - It is the first line agent used for both episodic and chronic type at doses of 240-960 mg per day. The patients should be carefully monitored for prolongation of PR interval and hence periodic ECG monitoring is recommended to prevent potential heart block.

ii) Second-line agents include: Lithium shows response at doses of 600-1200 mg daily. The response is more robust in chronic than the episodic type. Baseline evaluation of kidney and thyroid function tests should be done prior to starting lithium. Topiramate is also used at doses of 50-200 mg per day.

iii) Methysergide - It is an ideal choice in short cluster bouts, prescribed as a third line agent. Dosage recommended is 1-12 mg per day.

iv) Others - Melatonin and gabapentin are also used at 10 mg/day and upto 900 mg/day respectively.

- **Brain stimulation** - Occipital nerve stimulation and hypothalamic region deep brain stimulation have shown to be effective but are invasive procedures.

II. PAROXYSMAL HEMICRANIA

Paroxysmal hemicrania is a strictly unilateral, excruciating headache that occurs in association with cranial autonomic features. It has a higher frequency and shorter duration than the attacks of cluster headache. It is a rare condition with unknown prevalence and equal gender distribution with onset occurring most commonly in the second or third decade.

Clinical Features

It is a severe, one sided headache which is throbbing, aching or boring in character, located in the ocular, maxillary, temporal and frontal regions and occasionally involving the retro-orbital region, neck or the occiput. The onset and cessation is abrupt, the pain lasts around 10-30 minutes and upto 45 minutes in some cases. Up to 60% of patients experience interictal discomfort or pain. The pain is associated with ipsilateral conjunctival injection, lacrimation, ptosis, eyelid edema, nasal congestion and rhinorrhea. Nausea and phonophobia may be present but vomiting and photophobia are rarely seen. Restlessness and agitation can be seen in 50–80% patients.

Patients usually have more than 5 attacks a day, without nocturnal preponderance (as in cluster headache). The attacks can be precipitated in 10% patients by bending or by rotating the head, by applying external pressure against the C4-5 transverse process or the greater occipital nerve.

Classification

Paroxysmal hemicrania is classified into episodic type (20%) and chronic type (80%) based on the remission period.

- *Episodic type* - There are clear remission periods in between the attacks.
- *Chronic type* - In this type, the remission periods last for less than a month or there is no period of remission within 1 year.

Diagnosis

Paroxysmal hemicrania can be differentiated from other trigeminal autonomic cephalgias with a trial of indomethacin. While both paroxysmal hemicrania and cluster headache respond to indomethacin, they can be differentiated based on the clinical phenotype.

Treatment

The treatment of paroxysmal hemicrania is mainly prophylactic.

Indomethacin is the drug of choice, leading to prompt and complete resolution of headache within 1-2 days at doses of 25-100 mg per day and upto 300 mg per day occasionally. In episodic type, treatment should be continued for a slightly longer duration than the headache bout and tapered subsequently, while in chronic type it is advisable to continue indomethacin long term and gradually tapered once every 6 months. Indomethacin should be prescribed with gastroprotective agents for those requiring long-term treatment.

Other drugs used are cyclooxygenase-2 (COX-2) inhibitors - rofecoxib and celecoxib, which are now sparingly used due to increased risk of myocardial infarction and strokes. Topiramate has also been shown to provide pain relief but not as robust as indomethacin. Greater occipital nerve block has also been tried.

III. SUNCT and SUNA

These are rare primary headache syndromes with strictly unilateral pain associated with both ipsilateral conjunctival injection and lacrimation. SUNCT is considered a subset of SUNA as it may be associated with cranial autonomic symptoms other than conjunctival injection and lacrimation. SUNCT has an onset between 40-70 years with a male to female ratio of 2:1 and is relatively rare with a prevalence of 6.6/100,000.

Clinical Features

It presents as a severe, excruciating, strictly unilateral pain along the ophthalmic branch of the trigeminal nerve in the orbital and periorbital regions. The pain is stabbing, pricking, burning or electric shock like nature, lasting few seconds to minutes. Attacks can be precipitated by touching certain areas along the distribution of the trigeminal nerve, brushing, coughing, talking, shaving and even neck movements. Pain can occur once a day to more than 30 times in an hour, the symptomatic phase lasts few days to months with a completely pain free period in between, though some patients experience a dull ache persistently. Gradually over time, the symptomatic phase increases in frequency and duration. As the illness progresses symptomatic periods increase in frequency and duration.

The pain is associated with cranial autonomic symptoms out of which only conjunctival injection and lacrimation are characteristic of SUNCT. Nausea, vomiting, photophobia and phonophobia are less common.

Diagnosis

SUNCT and SUNA need to be differentiated from trigeminal neuralgia, paroxysmal hemicrania and primary stabbing headache. Secondary causes of SUNCT, e.g., lesions in posterior fossa or pituitary gland should be ruled out, hence MRI brain is an integral part of the diagnostic work up. A trial of indomethacin is helpful in differentiating it from paroxysmal hemicrania.

Treatment

I. *Transitional Treatment*

i) Intravenous lidocaine - It is used short term to avoid breakthrough attacks as well as to abort attacks. It is administered at a dose of 1.3-3.3 mg/kg/hour for about 10 days. It provides a completely pain free period of 6 months and 3 weeks in episodic and chronic SUNCT respectively and 12 weeks in chronic SUNA.

ii) Greater occipital nerve block by injecting lidocaine and steroid sub-occipitally provides pain relief for few weeks to months.

II. *Preventive Treatment* -

i) Antiepileptics - Lamotrigine (25-300 mg/day), topiramate (up to 400 mg/day), gabapentin (800-2700 mg/day) have shown to be effective.

ii) Surgery - As the pathophysiology involves the trigeminal nerve, invasive technics like percutaneous trigeminal ganglion compression, trigeminal ganglion thermocoagulation, retrogasserian glycerol rhizolysis and gamma knife surgery have been tried and has shown to provide complete pain relief, the duration of which lasted around 3 months to 4.5 years.

iii) Neuromodulation - Occipital nerve stimulation and hypothalamic region deep brain stimulation have been tried.

OTHER PRIMARY HEADACHES

These include primary cough headache, primary exercise headache, primary sex headaxhe, primary thunderclap headache, cold stimulus headache, external pressure headache, primary stabbing headache and hypnic headache.

PSYCHIATRIC ASPECTS OF HEADACHE

Various studies have focussed on the relationship between headache and psychiatric disorders. The relationship is complex and all patients with headache should be evaluated for symptoms of psychiatric disorders. Psychiatric disorders are reported to occur at least two to three times more in patients presenting with headache than among the general population. Young adults and female gender are at greater risk for psychiatric comorbidity. In general, most of the studies have shown significantly higher rates of comorbidity between psychiatric conditions and primary headache syndromes. Almost two-thirds of patients with migraine and up to half of the patients with tension type headache have psychiatric comorbidities. Also, psychiatric comorbidities are more likely in patients with greater frequency and intensity of headaches.

Several explanations have been postulated for this co morbidity. A direct causal relationship with the headache resulting in a psychiatric disorder or the psychiatric disorder causing headache is possible. However, literature reviews favour a bidirectional relationship between the two. A common genetic basis could be another potential mechanism considering a higher genetic correlation with psychiatric disorders. Since serotonergic dysfunction, hypothalamic pituitary adrenal axis (HPA) hyperactivity, inflammatory processes, stress, structural and functional changes in different regions of the brain like the anterior cingulate cortex, anterior insula, prefrontal cortex, hippocampus and amygdala, all play a role in the etiopathogenesis of both headaches, especially migraine, and psychiatric disorders, these factors might also combine in a given individual to create a vulnerability to both disorders.

Psychiatry morbidity may manifest in different ways in patients with headache. Headaches that present exclusively during a psychiatric disorder and a causal relationship between the two can be confirmed are coded as 'Headache attributed to psychiatric disorder' i.e. secondary headache syndrome. However, literature on this phenomenon is scarce and uncertainties persist because it is difficult to establish causation. Thus, this category is limited to those few cases in which the headache occurs as a direct consequence of a psychiatric conditions like depression or anxiety. Also, headache which occurs due to substance use, dependence or intoxication and persists for more than 3 months after cessation of substance use is diagnosed as 'Headache attributed to a substance or its withdrawal".

In contrast, if there is no evidence of a causal relationship between the two disorders, but both the headache and psychiatric disorder are present, a dual diagnosis should be made. Stress and negative life events have also been implicated in worsening the course of headaches. Common psychiatric disorders reported in patients with primary headache, especially migraine, include depressive disorders, anxiety disorders, trauma- and stress-related disorders, and somatic symptom and related disorders.

Presence of psychiatric morbidity invariably results in chronicity, poor response to treatment, reduced quality of life and poorer outcome. Hence treatment strategies for headache disorders must include strategies to deal with stress and psychiatric morbidity to improve the overall prognosis in these patients.

Depressive Disorders

Major depressive episodes are characterized by periods of at least two weeks of depressed mood, decreased interest in pleasurable activities, significant loss or gain in weight, increased or decreased sleep, psychomotor agitation or retardation, easy fatiguability or tiredness, feelings of helplessness, hopelessness and worthlessness, inattention or poor concentration and suicidal thoughts, ideas or attempts. Depressive disorders are the most common co morbid psychiatric disorders among patients presenting with headache, especially migraine. Lifetime prevalence of major depression is approximately three times higher in persons with severe headaches compared with controls. The risk of developing depression is more in women. The prevalence estimates of depression in migraine vary considerably and migraineurs are 2-3 times more likely to have comorbid major depressive disorder compared with those not having migraine. Patients having migraine with aura, chronic migraine, medication overuse, and more frequent headaches are more likely to have comorbid major depression. Approximately two thirds of patients with chronic migraine have psychiatric co morbidity. Suicidal behavior is particularly higher in migraine patients with co morbid depression, and 22% to 38% attempt suicide.

Besides migraine, both tension type headache and chronic daily headache are associated with an increase in depression comorbidity. The prevalence is about 13% in episodic TTH while it's almost 30% in chronic TTH, reiterating the impact of chronicity on psychiatric morbidity. Female patients with chronic daily headache tend to have almost two times increase in major depressive disorder. The relationship between headache and depression appears to be bi directional as either disorder can act as a predisposing factor for the other.

Anxiety Disorders

Almost as common as depressive disorders, about 11% of patients with headache develop some anxiety disorder. Migraine patients are two to five times more likely to have a comorbid anxiety disorder compared to the general population. In fact, in patients with migraine, anxiety disorders are more prevalent than depression. Anxiety disorders are more likely to be associated with chronic migraine, medication overuse and comorbid depressive disorders. These disorders probably have a common genetic susceptibility (polymorphism of the serotonin transporter gene) in addition to neurobiological and psychological factors.

Besides migraine, the prevalence of comorbid anxiety is high in patients with tension type headache. The rates of co morbid anxiety vary from 18%-51% in episodic tension type headache with much higher rates reported with chronic TTH.

The various anxiety disorders which have been observed include panic disorder, generalized anxiety disorder (GAD), obsessive compulsive disorder (OCD) and phobic disorder.

Generalized anxiety disorder is characterized by excessive worries for more than six months regarding multiple areas associated with at least three of the following - restlessness, easy fatiguability, disturbed sleep, irritability, muscle tension and concentration problems. The relationship between migraine and GAD is also bidirectional though the prevalence rates vary considerably.

Migraine patients are 12 times more likely to be diagnosed with comorbid panic disorder compared to the general population. Panic disorder comprises of recurrent sudden panic attacks for more than 1 month with at least 4 of the following features - palpitations, tremulousness, shortness of breath, chest discomfort, sweating, nausea, unsteadiness, paraesthesias, hot and cold sensations, fear of dying or going crazy and depersonalization-derealization.

Autonomic symptoms and somatic symptoms are common to both disorders, suggesting shared autonomic dysregulation. Also, panic disorder is more common in chronic migraine patients and migraine with aura.

Other anxiety disorders like OCD and phobic disorder occur with greater frequency in migraine patients, however, not much is known about this relationship.

Bipolar Disorders

Rates of mood disorders tend to be higher in patients with migraine and more so in women. Conversely, the prevalence of migraine is much higher in patients with bipolar disorder with lifetime prevalence being approximately 40%. Bipolar disorders are characterized by episodes of mania or hypomania and depression. Though not much data is available regarding this comorbidity, migraine prevalence is higher in bipolar II disorder (65%) as compared to bipolar I disorder patients. Various studies suggest a shared hereditary hypothesis to explain this association and a positive family history of bipolar disorder has been found to be a risk factor for migraine. Both the illnesses tend to have a more chronic and severe course when comorbid and are more difficult to treat.

Trauma and Stress Related Disorders

Stress is a major trigger for both headache and psychiatric disorders. Higher levels of stress and negative life events are reported in patients with migraine, especially chronic migraine. Acute stress disorder and post traumatic stress disorder (PTSD) develop in response to traumatic life events and a high prevalence (14%-25%) of these disorders has been reported in migraine patients as compared to chronic tension type headache.

In addition, a history of abuse, violence or neglect has been noted in patients with headache disorder. Both physical and psychological abuse may result in increased intensity and frequency of attacks. A childhood history of abuse has been reported in 65% of patients with comorbid migraine and PTSD. Childhood emotional abuse and/or sexual abuse is more common in migraine than tension headache. Physical abuse and sexual abuse have also been reported in 29% and 31% of patients with chronic daily headache respectively. These traumatic events are responsible for some of the comorbidities seen with headache disorders.

Somatic Symptom and Related Disorders

At times, the patients are unable to verbalise their mental symptoms and instead present with physical symptoms, e.g., pain. The diagnosis of "somatic symptom disorder with predominant pain" is made when the patient presents with physical symptoms like headache, associated with health concerns, persistent thoughts about the symptoms and anxiety. These symptoms are not better accounted for by another medical or psychiatric disorder. This group of disorders have also been referred to as 'depressive equivalent'. Headache may also be a prominent feature of illness anxiety disorder or conversion disorder.

Other Psychiatric Comorbidities

Although the actual prevalence of other psychiatric disorders is difficult to determine from available literature, headache disorders may co occur with substance use disorders, personality disorders, sleep disorders and eating disorders. Headache may also be associated with learning and behavioral problems in children but very limited data is available regarding this.

Management of Headache and Comorbid Psychiatric Disorder

Headache disorder when comorbid with a psychiatric disorder, is notoriously difficult to treat.

It is important to target comorbid psychiatric conditions when planning treatment as these are associated with more chronicity, greater financial burden of treatment, significant functional impairment, poorer outcomes and decreased quality of life.

The treatment should be multidisciplinary with various treatment strategies integrated to treat both disorders. A combination of pharmacological and psychological treatments has been found to be beneficial in these patients. The treatment should be tailor made for each patient with the choice of drug for the headache disorder being based on the type of psychiatric comorbidity, potential symbiotic effects, drug-drug interactions and possible adverse effects. A detailed history and evaluation might aid this process. In addition, cognitive behavior therapy, biofeedback, relaxation and stress management technics have documented efficacy in reducing headaches, addressing psychiatric morbidity and improving long term outcomes.

CONCLUSION

Headache disorders are highly prevalent and associated with significant disability. Recent studies have revealed high rates of comorbidity of psychiatric disorders especially depressive and anxiety disorders in patients with primary headache syndromes. The potential mechanisms underlying this association seem to be multi factorial, with biological, psychological and social factors all playing a role. This comorbidity results in more chronic and severe headaches with poor treatment responses along with decreased quality of life. Hence it is essential to evaluate every headache patient for psychiatric morbidity and plan treatment strategies accordingly. Successful long term outcomes require an integrated treatment approach targeting both the disorders.

BIBLIOGRAPHY

1. Classification Subcommittee of the International Headache Society. The International Classification of Headache Disorders. 2nd Edition. Cephalalgia. 2004; 15:1–160.
2. Merikangas KR, Merikangas JR. Neuropsychiatric aspects of headache. In: Sadock BJ, Sadock VA, Ruiz P (eds.). *Kaplan and Sadock's Comprehensive Textbook of Psychiatry: Behavioral Sciences/Clinical Psychiatry.* 11th ed. New York: Wolters Kluwer Health; 2017.
3. Goadsby PJ, Raskin. Headache. In: Kasper DL, Fauci AS, Hauser S, et al (eds.). *Harrison's Principles of Internal Medicine.* 19th ed. New York: Mc Graw-Hill Education; 2015. p. 107-11.
4. Goadsby PJ, Raskin. Migraine and primary headache disorders. In: Kasper DL, Fauci AS, Hauser S, et al (eds.). *Harrison's Principles of Internal Medicine.* 19th ed. New York: Mc Graw-Hill Education; 2015. p. 2586-98.
5. Borsook D, May A, Goadsby PJ, et al. *The Migraine Brain.* Oxford: Oxford University Press; 2012.
6. Young WB, Silberstein SD. *Migraine and other headaches.* New York: AAN Press, American Academy of Neurology. Demos Medical Publishing Inc.; 2004.
7. Sacks O, Sacks OW. *Migraine Revised and Expanded.* 3rd ed. California: University of California Press; 2004.
8. Fernandez-de-las-Penas C, Arendt-Nielsen L, Gerwin RD. *Tension-Type and Cervicogenic Headache Pathophysiology, Diagnosis and Management.* Massachusets: Jones and Bartlett Publishers; 2010.
9. Japanese Neurological Society. *Clinical practice guidelines for chronic headache.* 2013. Available from: https://www.neurology-jp.org/guidelinem/ch/index.html [Accessed 2nd December 2019].

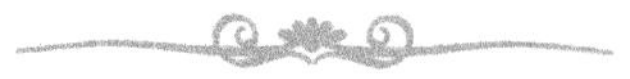

Role of Psychiatric Social Worker in Mental Health

60

Priyanka Anup Bharati

Every branch of medicine has allied health workers such as nursing staff, technicians in various diagnostic work, operation theatre assistant and many others. In the field of mental health too there is requirement of allied health workers who can work along with psychiatrist for better patient care and delivering mental health services at different levels. Clinical Psychologist and Psychiatric Social worker are the integral part of the mental health team.

Psychiatric social worker (PSW) is post graduate in the field of social work with specialization in mental health, either M. Phil or PhD degree. They should have basic skills and knowledge of social work methods and principles, principles of human behavior, interview technics, knowledge of psychiatric assessment, classification of mental and behavior disorders, various diagnostic criteria and treatment modalities used, can write medical case history and mental status examination, principles of individual and group therapy.

These professionals utilize social work principle for the purpose of diagnosis, patient care and treatment in the hospital as well as at the home after the discharge from hospital. They also plan for the rehabilitation of patients in the family and community. They offer counseling, support services and appropriate referrals as per the case.

Psychiatric social worker has following work responsibilities in clinical and non-clinical domains:

1. Intake or Admission in Psychiatric Hospital – PSW can help the patient or relatives at the time of admission process to psychiatric hospital.
2. Case History – PSW should make their own case history by taking appropriate details from patient and relatives.
3. Diagnosis and analysis of patient – after brief history, PSW can formulate their own diagnosis and patient analysis with focus on social needs of the patient.
4. Case Work with Patient – they form adequate rapport with the patient and work on individual counseling, building up insight of the patient, in cases of addiction issues they work on their motivation enhancement.
5. Case Work with Relative – by developing rapport and addressing their concerns related to diagnosis and treatment, PSW can handle relatives own emotional issues too and can work on caregiver burden.
6. Treatment – PSW helps in explaining the treatment plan to patient and family members. They can conduct individual or group counseling sessions for the patient as well as family therapy sessions.
7. Rehabilitation of Patient – This is the core purpose of services from PSW, psychosocial rehabilitation of the patients

suffering from chronic mental illness like schizophrenia, bipolar mood disorder, substance use disorder. Rehabilitation services involve social skills training, encouraging the patients to follow daily routine, keeping them busy in any cognitive task, helping them for vocational work in the home or community settings.

8. Follow- Up or After Care – It is utmost important to focus on post discharge follow up care. PSW do periodic home visits to the patient's home and observe the patient's behavior at home, assess the treatment compliance, addresses issues related to patient care and family members concern, help family members in crisis situations and identification of warning signs of relapse of an illness.

9. Orientation of the Staff – PSW works in collaboration with Psychiatrist and orient the other staff members of hospital for adequate patient care, good communication with patients and their caregivers.

10. Advocating for care and Human Right of Psychiatric Patients – PSW can work in liaison with all other stake holders in mental health care and can advocate for the inclusive care of the mentally ill as well as address their human rights issue.

11. Protecting the vulnerable – PSW during their field visits, can help the wandering or neglected mentally ill persons by working in collaboration with other government agencies, police for providing shelter, food, any other required stuff or hospitalization if required.

    They can also help the wife or other family members of mentally ill person or those having addiction issues by helping them in crisis situation.

12. Working as integral part of team in the management of complex and high-risk cases such as forensic or legal issues such as domestic violence, POCSO, sexual assault victims, cases from family court, prisoners with mental illness, juveniles in conflict with law, LGBT and Gender dysphoria issues.

13. Providing psychosocial treatment and recreational therapies to patients and caregivers by arranging individual or group counseling sessions, Art therapy, Music therapy and other recreational therapies.

14. Promotion of Mental Health – PSW helps in arrangement of various activities such skits, role plays, rallies, lectures for mental health awareness at different public and social platforms such as offices, NGOs, educational institutes, hospital and social organizations.

Also, various workshops for mental health can be arranged for training of volunteers, ASHA workers in the villages, PHCs.

15. Early identification and Providing Referral Services – PSW works for early identification of mental illness, handling the misconceptions towards mental illness and provides adequate referral to mental health care setups.

16. Mental health screening camp – PSW can arrange mental health screening camps at community level, this can help in outreach of mental health services and also could help in stigma reduction. So thus, PSW can work as an administration of community services.

17. Working with other mental health professionals for promotion of positive mental health and preparation of prevention strategies for mental illness and addiction issues.

To summarize, psychiatric social worker has vital role for making mental health care more accessible and available, help improving the capacity and quality of services. Better and inclusive patient care, stigma reduction, preservation of their human rights and maintaining their dignity; this all will help taking the patient and caregivers in to the mainstream of society.

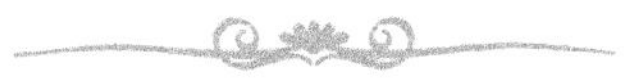

61 Rape - Psychiatric Aspects

Havovi Hyderabadwalla • Avinash De Sousa

In this chapter, we will be discussing sexual assault on adult females and children primarily by adult males. We shall also be throwing light on how health professionals must be equipped to handle these sensitive cases and the way forward for the survivors post the traumatic event and how they can assist them to the best of their ability.

Rape, by the Indian law, CrPC – Criminal Procedure code, is understood to be when a man -

a) Penetrates his penis into the one of the orifices or all - vagina, mouth, urethra or anus of a woman to any extent

b) Makes her to do so with him or any other person or inserts any object or a part of the body, not being the penis, into the above mentioned orifices

c) Makes her to do so with him or any other person or manipulates any part of the body of a woman so as to cause penetration into mentioned orifices or any part of body of such woman

d) Makes her to do so with him or any other person or applies his mouth to one or more orifices mentioned above of a woman or makes her to do so with him or any other person.

The above is generally under the following circumstances -

1) Against the woman's will.
2) Without the woman's consent.
3) With the woman's consent, by obtaining her consent by putting her in fear of death or of hurt or someone concerned to her.
4) With the woman's consent, when the man knows that he is not her husband and that her consent is given because she believes that he is another man to whom she is or believes herself to be lawfully married.
5) With the woman's consent but at the time of giving such consent she is of unsound mind or intoxicated or the administration by the man personally or through another of any stupefying or unwholesome Substance, she is incapable to understand the nature and consequences of which she is consenting to.
6) With or without her consent, when she is under eighteen years of age.
7) When she is inept to communicate.

The labia majora is considered in this context. Consent is understood as an unequivocal voluntary agreement when the woman by words, gestures or any form of verbal or non-verbal communication, communicates willingness to participate in the specific sexual act.

Provided that a woman who does not physically resist to the act of penetration shall not by the reason only of that fact, be regarded as consenting to the sexual activity. Exceptions to the case are medical procedures or interventions shall not constitute rape. Sexual intercourse or sexual acts by a man with his own wife where the wife is not below fifteen years of age.

Marital rape continued to not be considered a crime till the reform in 2013. Article 376B of the 2013 law made forced sexual intercourse by a man with his wife – if she is living separately – a crime, whether under a decree of separation or otherwise, punishable with at least a 2-year prison term.

Forced sex by a man on his wife may also be considered a prosecutable domestic violence under other sections of Indian Penal code, such as Section 498(A) as well as the Protection of Women from Domestic Violence Act 2005. Sexual assault on a child, that is anyone below the age of eighteen, is further outlined and mandatory punishments described in The Protection of Children from Sexual Offences Act 2012.

All sexual acts between the members of the same sex, consensual or forced, was previously a crime under Section 377 of Indian penal code, after the 2013 Criminal Law reform, with punishment the same as that of rape but it was later overturned in a landmark judgment of the Supreme Court on 6 September 2018 which stated all consensual sexual acts between adults who have met the age of consent do not violate Section 377, hence decriminalizing the act of homosexuality in India.

Females are raped and sexually assaulted more often than males. Male rape is often committed by another man, often in prison. Males who are raped are more likely than females to be physically injured, to be unwilling to report the crime, and to have multiple assailants.

SYMPTOMS AND SIGNS

Rape may result in the following physical issues and injuries such extra genitalia injury, Genitalia injury, Sexually transmitted diseases e.g. hepatitis, syphilis, gonorrhea, chlamydial infection, trichomonas', HIV infection at times and/ or pregnancy.

Most physical injuries are relatively minor, but some lacerations of the upper vagina are severe. Additional injuries may result from physical violence during the act of being hit, pushed or shot.

Psychological symptoms of rape are potentially the most prominent. In the short term, most patients experience a combination of fear, bad dreams, sleep issues, anger, humiliation, shame or guilt. Immediately after an assault, a survivor's behavior can range from talkativeness, tenseness, crying, and trembling to shock and disbelief with detachment, dormancy or smiling. The latter responses rarely indicate lack of concern. They reflect avoidance reactions, physical exhaustion, or coping mechanisms that require control of emotion. Anger may be displaced onto hospital staff or family members.

Friends, family members, and officials often react judgmentally, disdainfully, or in another negative way. Such reactions can delay recovery after an assault.

Eventually, most patients recover though long-range effects of rape may include posttraumatic stress disorder (PTSD), particularly among women. PTSD is a trauma-related disorder; symptoms of PTSD include:

- Re-experiencing the trauma (e.g. flashbacks, invasive distressing thoughts or images)
- Avoidance (e.g. of trauma-related situations, thoughts, and feelings)
- Negative effects on cognition and mood (e.g. persistent distorted blame of self or others, inability to experience positive emotions)
- Altered arousal and reactivity (e.g. sleep issues, irritability, focus)

For PTSD to be diagnosed, symptoms must last for more than a month and must not be attributable to the physiological effects of a substance or a medical disorder, and must significantly impair social and occupational functioning. Survivors with PTSD often also have depression and/or other psychological disorders (e.g. substance dependence or abuse).

EVALUATION

Goals of rape evaluation should be to medically assess and treat injuries and prevent STD's and pregnancy. Forensic evidence should be collected cautiously, preserved and sent to forensic laboratories as quick as possible. The integrity and authenticity of the evidence should be maintained at all times. Psychological evaluation would be the need of the hour followed by tremendous psychological support which can be provided by family, friends, neighbors, society, social workers and mental health practitioners.

Patients should be informed not to throw out or change clothing, wash, shower, douche, brush their teeth, clip their fingernails, or use mouthwash as doing so may destroy evidence.

All sexual assault or rape survivors should be referred to a local hospital emergency department. Benefits of a rape evaluation are explained, but patients are free to consent to or decline the evaluation. The police are notified with the patient's consent. Most patients are significantly traumatized, and their care requires sensitivity, empathy and compassion. Patients may feel more comfortable with a doctor of the same sex. A female staff member should accompany all males evaluating a female. Patients are provided privacy and quiet whenever possible.

Medical records may be used in court, therefore forms should be used to record evidences and medical results should be written legibly and in nontechnical language that can be understood by the court.

HISTORY AND EXAMINATION

Before beginning, the examiner must ask for the patient's permission. Because recounting the events often frightens or embarrasses the patient, the examiner must be reassuring, empathetic, and non-judgmental and should not rush the patient. Privacy should be ensured. The examiner prompts specific details such as type of injuries sustained particularly to the mouth, breasts, vagina and rectum or any bleeding from or abrasions on the patient or assailant which would help assess the risk of transmission of HIV and hepatitis. Sensitive topics are touched upon such as the description of the attack e.g. which orifices were penetrated, whether ejaculation occurred or some form of protection was used. An enquiry is made whether the assaulter used any aggression, threats, weapons or violent behavior and whether the survivor is able to recall what the assaulter looked like.

Many rape forms include most or all of these questions posed above. The patient should be told why questions are being asked e.g. information about contraceptive use helps determine risk of pregnancy after rape; information about previous coitus helps determine validity of sperm testing.

The examination should be explained step by step as it proceeds. Results should be reviewed with the patient. When feasible, photographs of possible injuries are taken. The mouth, breasts, genitals, and rectum are examined. Common sites of injury include the labia minora and posterior vagina. Examination using a Wood's lamp may detect semen or foreign debris on the skin. Colposcopy is particularly sensitive for subtle genital injuries. Some colposcopies have cameras attached, making it possible to detect and photograph injuries simultaneously.

TREATMENT

As the treatment plan is aligned for the survivor, psychological support or interventions are planned keeping in mind the physical and mental fitness of the patient. Prophylaxis for STDs and possibly hepatitis B or HIV infection are prescribed from a pharmacological perspective. If required the patient should also be prescribed emergency contraception keeping in time duration that has lapsed post the incident and pregnancy test results.

After the evaluation, the patient is provided with facilities to wash, change clothing, use mouthwash, and urinate or defecate if needed. Most physical injuries are minor and are treated conservatively. If need be vaginal lacerations may require surgical repair.

PREVENTION OF PREGNANCY

Emergency contraception should be offered to all women with a negative pregnancy test. Usually, oral contraceptives are used. If used post seventy-two hours after rape, they are much less likely to be effective. An antiemetic may help if nausea develops. An intrauterine device may be effective if used up to 10 days after rape. If pregnancy results from rape, the patient's attitude toward the pregnancy and abortion should be determined. The option of termination of the pregnancy should be discussed.

UNDERSTANDING IN DEPTH WHAT HEALTH CARE PROFESSIONALS CAN DO FOR SURVIVORS WITH RESPECT TO PSYCHOLOGICAL SUPPORT

Health care providers are responsible to provide first line of support when women disclose the sensitive event and details related. Consultations should be carried out in a private setting ensuring confidentiality. Limits of the confidentiality must be explained to the victim as medical professionals are bound by certain legalities to report information especially in medico legal situations. The victim must be dealt with empathy and sensitivity. A non-judgmental, supportive environment must be created through communication to make the vulnerable victim feel safe. All queries asked by the victim must be addressed with care and reassurance. Medical professionals must tread with caution whilst enquiring about details such as history of the violence. They must listen carefully without pressuring the victim to speak. Knowledge of legal resources and services that may be helpful must be shared. The victim must be encouraged to increase her safety by mobilizing her social support or temporarily moving to a shelter or rehabilitation center. In case a doctor is not present to assist the victim a trained health professional should be assigned to assist the victim in a similar manner as the doctor would. All professionals must understand that it takes a lot of courage for victims to be able to report this gruesome act and recognise the dilemma the survivor maybe facing. Legal rights should be imparted as well so that an informed decision is made by the survivor.

Many repercussions are faced by survivors of sexual violence which are emotional, physical, economic and social in nature. These consequences are not only faced by them but their families as well. Most survivors face tremendous amounts of fear, guilt and shame related to police investigations, the violence and how the society or community may perceive them post the incident. They may fear that most people may doubt them and not believe what they have reported. Many victims may not want to report the incident to the police due to fear of various feelings of fear and threats from perpetrators and the society. It is extremely common for children to not disclose the assault to their family members or guardians. Communication between the Medical professionals and survivors must be transparent. Doctors must prepare all survivors for internal examinations and explain various procedures and stages. Rationales for all procedures must be explained e.g. – USG, X-rays etc. Transparent and clear communication is extremely important between doctors and survivors as the latter faces a sense of grief, loss and powerlessness. Such covert feelings must be recognised and medical procedures must be explained. It allows the survivors to have an understanding of what is happening to them and reasons behind the same. They have a sense of control restored in their system. In case referrals need to be made for different medical assessments confidentiality must be maintained at all times so as to not trigger or embarrass the survivor.

Health professionals must understand that the survivor will present a varied range of emotions. There would either be a fight, flight or frozen response. A relationship of trust must be built to allow the survivor to express themselves and be encouraged to seek crisis counseling. An assessment for suicidal ideation or pathology must be carried out e.g. early signs of depression, psychosis or triggers which could lead to panic attacks or anxiety. Safety plans must be suggested and shared with the survivor. Each survivor copes with sexual violence in a different manner. The healing process depends a lot on family support, friends, community and societal support, job security, financial aid for a fair trial in court etc. it is hard for survivors to express their feelings openly. Medical professionals must educate survivors that they will experience a range of emotions, example – lack of sleep, crying spells, anger, flashbacks triggering nervousness and anxiety and wanting to end one's life post the assault. Such reactions must be explained as being normal post the distressful ordeal. Survivors must be encouraged and try and be as receptive to crisis counseling. Certain myths and false rationales should be dissolved during sessions such as "the victim was asking for it" or "the clothes she wore". A positive and practical delivery and understanding of what has happened would be the need of the hour such as making the survivor understand that she is "not responsible" for the rape. Rebuilding the survivor's self-confidence should be of utmost priority. Survivors should be made to understand that self-blame and feelings of shame about the act should be discarded.

A safety assessment should be carried out and if the same reveal that the survivor maybe unsafe, health professionals must offer substitute measures such as referral to shelter services or temporary admission in the hospital. If the survivor insists on returning home she must be encouraged to mobilize social support e.g. neighbors or friends in case of any recurrence or emergency.

With respect to children, procedures from the POCSO Act, 2012 must be followed. Generally, children (under 18 years of age) are brought to the hospital by parents or guardians. In case the perpetrators are themselves medical professionals must call upon social workers or mental health professionals to discuss a safety plan for the child. A person that the child identifies to trust must be called to the hospital. The police would have to be informed and the social worker would need to inform them about the child's safety and protection. The child may be admitted into a hospital for 24 hours till arrangements for shelter or welfare home is decided.

The role of family, friend and community in helping the survivor cope with the unfortunate event is extremely imperative. Health providers must explain how the survivors well-being is of utmost priority and the importance of their role in helping the survivor readjust to their personal space and environment. Conclusions and allegations made towards with survivor example, "why didn't she resist it" or "she was too open with everyone "make it harder for the survivor to regain her self-esteem and confidence. The journey to recovery becomes a long and arduous one. With respect to child survivors, parents may face a lot of self- blame, guilt, confusion and anger for not paying attention to their child or providing proper care. Health and mental health professionals must help survivors and parents of survivors understand that it is the fault of the perpetrator and not anyone else should be held responsible for the act of sexual violence.

All survivors must be made to understand that with time recovery is possible. Children should be made educated about "Good touch and Bad touch" and how to create boundaries with people and their personal space. In case the child feels unsafe, he/she must come and report any sign of danger to them. Survivors must be encouraged to carry on with their normal routine and life. Mobility must not be restricted and instead survivors must be equipped with safety and trust that they can report any sign of harm to them at any point to the family or individuals who support them. Counseling sessions must be followed up with to continue the healing process as this is a safe space for the survivor to share her inner most feelings, concerns and fears. Conversations about sexual health, STD's and contraception may not always be open discussions amongst family members which can be discussed with counsellors. Caregivers must seek counseling sessions to in case they are dealing with guilt or any concerns to put their minds at ease. Due to fear of recurrence, caregivers may become over protective. Health professionals and mental health professionals must help them create an environment to openly discuss this with the survivor so he/she is informed that she has the choice to make cognizant choices.

BIBLIOGRAPHY

1) The essential handbook of Offender Assessment and Treatment edited by Clive R. Hollin. Wiley publication.
2) The Psychology of Criminal Conduct by Ronald Blackburn, Wiley publication.
3) http://www.indianjpsychiatry.org/article.asp?issn=0019-5545;year=2017;volume=59;issue=1;spage=77;epage=82;aulast=Kamdar
4) https://www.ncbi.nlm.nih.gov/pmc/articles/PMC3777346/
5) http://www.scielo.org.za/scielo.php?script=sci_arttext&pid=S2078-67862015000100004
6) [Internet]. 2022 [cited 23 March 2022]. Available from: http://www.scielo.org.za/scielo.php?script=sci_arttext&pid=S2078-67862015000100004
7) Blackburn R. The psychology of criminal conduct: Theory, research and practice. John Wiley & Sons; 1993.
8) Hollin CR, editor. The essential handbook of offender assessment and treatment.
9) Jiloha RC. Rape: Legal issues in mental health perspective. Indian journal of psychiatry. 2013 Jul;55(3):250.
10) Rao TS, Nagaraj AK. Female sexuality. Indian journal of psychiatry. 2015 Jul;57(Suppl 2):S296.

62 Occupational Therapy in Psychiatry – An Overview

Sushant Sarang

"Man, through the use of his hands, as they are energized by mind and will, can influence the state of his own health."

– Mary Reily,OTR,EdD.

CHAPTER OBJECTIVES

After studying this chapter, the reader will be able to:

1. Discuss the role of occupational therapy in mental health.
2. Identify the different settings in which psychiatry occupational therapist works.
3. Understand the different models/approaches used in Psychiatry occupational therapy.
4. Enlist occupational therapy assessments used in mental health.
5. Recognize the various terminologies/concepts/methods used by occupational therapists in mental health.
6. Understand occupational therapy intervention process.

INTRODUCTION

Shreya failed in all her high school board exam subjects. Shreya lives in a joint family in a Mumbai slum. Her family observed that over the years Shreya had become increasingly defiant and rebellious. She had a lot of angst against her mother who was diagnosed with schizophrenia when Shreya was a child. Shreya also has strained relationship with her alcoholic father who works as a waiter for a living. Shreya attributes her misery to her non caring mother, poor father and a dysfunctional family.

Shreya's mother, Janki, was diagnosed as Schizophrenia when Shreya was three years old. Janki was admitted in the hospital once and later was treated with regular medication on outpatient basis. Though her symptoms were mostly controlled, Schizophrenia affected Janki's daily functioning. Her roles as homemaker, wife, mother, daughter-in-law and neighbor were affected. Due to this, there were constant fights between Janki and her mother-in-law and husband. It affected their family dynamics and thwarted their economic progress. This had a profound effect on Shreya's childhood and she developed her own set of functional problems.

Why did Shreya fail in her exam?

Why did she develop defiance and hatred towards her family members especially her mother?

Did Janki's diagnosis of Schizophrenia affect only her or her entire family?

Did lack of awareness and lack of family centered therapy play a role in the development of the dysfunctional family?

Janki took regular medications. But was it sufficient to maintain her optimal functioning? The above example illustrates the complexities of mental illness. It affects not only the person involved but also his/her family members including the next generation. The recent advances in psychiatric pharmacology has helped control psychiatric symptoms and reduce hospital stay. However, functional deficits developed due to the mental illness, needs a multidisciplinary approach. As part of the mental healthcare team, occupational therapist can play a key role in improving symptoms and helping the person be functionally independent.

WHAT IS OCCUPATIONAL THERAPY?

Man is an active being whose development is influenced by the use of purposeful activity. Occupational therapy (OT) is based on the belief that purposeful activity (occupation), including its interpersonal and environmental components, may be used to prevent and mediate dysfunction, and to elicit maximum adaptation.

OT is a holistic and client-centered health profession concerned with promoting health and well-being through occupation. The primary goal of OT is to enable people to participate in the activities of everyday life. Occupational therapists achieve this goal by working with people and communities to enhance their ability to engage in the occupations they want to, need to, or are expected to do, or by modifying the occupation or the environment to better support their occupational engagement.

occupational therapy is applicable in various musculoskeletal, neurological, cardiorespiratory, developmental and mental health disorders throughout the lifespan.

OCCUPATIONAL THERAPY IN MENTAL HEALTH

Mental recovery is defined as "a journey of healing and transformation enabling a person with a mental health problem to live a meaningful life in a community of his or her choice while striving to reach his or her potential". According to Tina Champagne and Karla Gray, a primary goal of the recovery model is to facilitate resiliency, health, and wellness in the community of the individual's choice, rather than to manage symptoms. The fundamental recovery principles are in full alignment with the philosophy of occupational therapy practice, which is inherently client centered, collaborative, and focused on supporting resiliency, full participation, health promotion, and a wellness lifestyle.

occupational therapy practitioners work collaboratively with people in a manner that helps to foster hope, motivation, and empowerment, as well as system change. Educated in the scientific understanding of neurophysiology, psychosocial development, activity and environmental analysis, and group dynamics, occupational therapy practitioners assume a variety of roles such as direct care therapists, consultants, academic educators, managers and administrators. They may also work in state and national mental health organizations to help assist in local, state and national transformation efforts.

The following are examples of how the knowledge and skill base of occupational therapy is used in the process of assisting individuals in all phases of mental health recovery:

- Teach and support the active use of coping strategies to help manage the effect of symptoms of illness on one's life, including being more organized and able to engage in activities of choice.
- Help to identify and implement healthy habits, rituals, and routines to support a wellness lifestyle.
- Support the identification of personal values, needs and goals to enable informed decision making, such as when considering housing and employment options.

- Support the creation and use of a wellness recovery action plan in group or individual sessions.
- Provide information to increase awareness of community-based resources, such as peer-facilitated groups and other support options.
- Provide information on how to monitor physical health concerns (e.g. diabetes management, smoking cessation), develop strategies to control chronic symptoms, and recognize and respond to acute changes.
- Support the ability to engage in long-term planning (e.g., budget for major purchases, prepare advance medical and mental health directives) that leads to meeting personal recovery goals.

OCCUPATIONAL THERAPY SETTINGS IN MENTAL HEALTH

occupational therapy practitioners provide mental health services in the following settings:

- Acute and long-term care facilities
- Private and public hospitals
- Forensic and juvenile justice centers
- Residential and day programs
- Skilled nursing facilities
- Community-based mental health centers
- Schools
- Military installations
- Employment programs
- Private practice
- Outpatient clinics.

KNOWLEDGE BASE OF OCCUPATIONAL THERAPY IN MENTAL HEALTH

The knowledge base of occupational therapy is drawn from a wide range of disciplines. Occupational therapists use various theories, models and frames of references to guide them in understanding the function-dysfunction and plan evaluation and intervention accordingly. Theories attempt to explain how mental health problems develop and how a therapist may help someone deal with them.

Major Medical And Psychological Theories Used In occupational Therapy Mental Health

1) **Theory of Object relations**:

The theory of object relations is a psychoanalytic theory based on the work of Sigmund Freud and his followers, who believed that mental health and mental illness are determined by our relations with objects in our environment. These objects may be physical (nonhuman) or human. This approach attempts to analyze and change unconscious processes.

occupational therapists who apply object relations theory use symbols in arts, crafts, and everyday activities. As an example, ceramics can provide an opportunity to explore issues of self-control versus control by others. Because wet clay is so similar to feces in color and texture, it can symbolize the anal period, during which the child learns to control the bowels and to cooperate with his or her parents through self-control. People have widely varying reactions to ceramics. Some cannot wait to handle the clay; others shrink back and may try to avoid it altogether.

There are varying ways in which people relate to symbols. A patient's behavior toward an activity may reveal his or her attitudes and feelings about issues that the activity symbolizes. Because people have their own personal histories, they may also have individual or idiosyncratic symbols that are theirs alone.

2) Developmental Theory:

There are several versions of developmental theory. The best known are those of Erikson, Piaget, and Gesell. According to the developmental concepts, human beings mature through a series of stages that occur in a fixed sequence. Specific developmental tasks arise at each stage. The person's experience with these tasks provides a foundation for later development. Problems occur when developmental tasks are not mastered sufficiently well. This causes a lag in development that can interfere with a person's attempts to master other developmental tasks in future stages. A developmental lag can be corrected by exposing the person to a situation that will encourage growth in the deficient area. If the proper conditions are created and the therapist provides corrective guidance, the developmental task can be corrected.

Erikson's and other developmental theories are consistent with many of the basic ideas of occupational therapy. The concept of gradation, of learning through successively more challenging and complex stages, and the focus on solving problems and acquiring skills make developmental theory an appealing choice for working with persons who have poor social relationships and weak skills. Similarly, occupational therapists have long attempted to meet the patient at his or her own level, matching tasks to abilities and interests.

3) Behavioral Theories:

The behavioral theories are derived from the work of Pavlov and Skinner. The central concept of these theories is that all behavior is learned. Behaviors that have pleasurable results tend to be repeated. Actions that have negative or unpleasant consequences tend not to be repeated. According to behavioral theories, each person develops through a process of learning from the results of his or her behavior. If adaptive behaviors are rewarded and maladaptive behaviors punished or ignored, the result should be a mature and responsible human being. Mental disorders, in this theory are defined by abnormal behavior that results because normal or adaptive behavior was not rewarded or did not have pleasurable consequences. In some cases, abnormal behavior occurs because maladaptive behavior was reinforced.

occupational therapists use a variety of technics based on behavioral theory. Sometimes it is called an **action-consequence** approach because the therapist tries to change the person's behavior (action) by changing the consequences of the behavior. The therapist may reward new adaptive behaviors or ignore or not reward the maladaptive behavior (withhold reinforcement). Some therapists use both methods. **Identification of terminal behavior** is the first step in a behavioral treatment program. Terminal behavior is the normal or adaptive behavior that the therapist wants the person to perform. The **baseline** is a known standard or record of how the person behaved before the treatment was started. Next the therapist selects a **reinforcement**. Reinforcement is the consequences of behavior that either encourage or discourage the repetition of the behavior. The therapist then decides how often the reinforcement will be given (**schedule**). Often the terminal behavior seems very far from the way the person is acting now. In such cases, a method called **shaping** is used. Shaping is a method of approaching the terminal behavior gradually, using a series of steps (successive approximations) that lead to the goal. When the terminal behavior involves learning a complicated routine with several steps, the technic of **chaining** can be used. Chaining is a method of teaching a complex activity a step at a time, starting with either the first or the last step. The therapist performs the remaining steps until the person masters the entire sequence. Other strategies that can be used include **systematic desensitization.** This is a technic for reducing fear (desensitizing) by guiding the person to relax, and then gradually increasing exposure to the fear-provoking stimulus.

4) **Cognitive-Behavioral Therapy**:

Cognitive-behavioral treatment is based on the work of psychiatrist Aaron Beck. The many variations of cognitive-behavioral theories share an underlying assumption that human behavior is based on what we think and believe. What we think (cognition) determines how we act (behavior). The theory proposes that people with mental health problems have maladaptive patterns of thinking (cognitions) that lead to unsuccessful behaviors. Cognitive-behavioral therapy helps the person understand and change negative cognitions, and this process brings about a change in behavior. Negative cognitions include **automatic thoughts** that occur without the person recognizing them or challenging their logic. The negative thought triggers negative feelings and maladaptive behaviors.

Cognitive-behavioral approaches link a precipitating event to a person's thoughts about the event and then to the feelings these thoughts evoke.

Events are in themselves neutral; they receive their value from our thoughts about them. When an event occurs, a person has thoughts about it, although these thoughts may occur below the level of conscious awareness. These thoughts are evaluative, attaching an **attribution** or meaning to the event. Thoughts lead to feelings. These feelings stimulate associated behavior.

Cognitive-behavioral treatment focuses on both cognition and behavior and on the relationship between them. Cognitive technics involve challenging and modifying negative automatic thoughts and their underlying assumptions. Behavioral technics focus on identifying behaviors, investigating their consequences, and evaluating their effectiveness.

Cognitive-behavioral therapy has been applied in occupational therapy by Johnston and Taylor and others. Johnston described the teaching of communication skills, assertive training, problem solving, and feeling management in a day treatment setting. These skills were taught in groups and individually. Interventions included role playing; teaching of behaviors; and monitoring of beliefs, assumptions, and self-talk (automatic thoughts).

Taylor's work focused on anger intervention. From a cognitive-behavioral perspective, the link between anger and aggression is learned. Anger intervention teaches nonaggressive management of anger. The major technics used are (a) monitoring physiological arousal, (b) practice in arousal control methods, (c) monitoring escalating self-talk (angry automatic thoughts), (d) promotion of neutral or calming self-talk via humor and diversional activities, (e) identification of anger-arousing stimuli, and (f) learning strategies to avoid these conditions.

In Taylor's approach, the client first

learns to identify and control arousal. Only after arousal has been controlled to some extent are the cognitions behind the arousal addressed. Clients are exposed to activities that induce high and low states of arousal (e.g. physical exercise is generally energizing while listening to soothing music is generally calming). Clients are taught to use both high and low arousal activities for reducing anger. Although Taylor employed crafts and other traditional activities in her approach, she molded them to the goals of cognitive-behavioral therapy. For example, if physical exercise or wedging clay is used, the client is cautioned not to dwell on angry thoughts because these will perpetuate and accelerate angry arousal. The therapist teaches more appropriate self-talk so that the client can learn to use the activity to promote a calm state. Once arousal has been controlled, the client explores the cognitive components of anger and learns to change anger-producing cognitions. The emphasis is on problem solving, stress management, and positive and neutral self-talk.

5) **Client-Centered Therapy:**

One of several humanistic therapies, client-centered therapy was developed by psychologist Carl Rogers. Humanistic therapies are concerned with the individual's view of life and with helping people find satisfaction in whatever way makes most sense for them. Rogers used the word *client* to convey a greater sense of self-determination than does the word *patient,* which suggests a dependent role in a medical relationship.

A central concept of client-centered therapy is that human beings possess the potential for directing their own growth and development. No matter how psychotic or disorganized the behavior may appear, the client is capable of self-understanding and ultimately of changing behavior. Another concept is that people direct their own lives. By being *nondirective* the therapist allows the client to take an individual direction. The therapist does help the client, however, by making the client more aware of feelings and by helping explore the possible consequences of contemplated action. A third and related concept is that mental health problems occur when a person is not aware of feelings and of the available choices. A fourth concept is that a person can become more aware of feelings and choices by experiencing them in a relationship with a therapist who genuinely accepts himself or herself and the client. Therapists must be able to provide **unconditional positive regard**- that is, they must continue to like the client no matter what the client does. The client's relationship with a warm, empathic therapist is the key to the client-centered approach. **Accurate empathy** involves constantly being in the moment so that one can "feel with" the client, sensitively tuning in to the client's feelings and thoughts. Client-centered therapists use several technics that facilitate clients' awareness and expression of feelings. Occupational therapists use some of these technics when interviewing and conversing with clients or patients. These are i) **open invitation to talk** through open questions, ii) **minimal response,** which shows that the therapist is listening to the client and that the client should go on talking. iii) **reflection of feeling**- through this technic, the therapist puts the client's feelings into words and helps him or her experience the emotional content. iv) using **paraphrasing,** the therapist restates in different words what the client has said. v) **witholding judgment** is a technic in which the therapist refrains from giving an opinion about the client's remarks or behaviors.

6) **Neuroscience theories:**

Neuroscience theories are based on the assumption that normal human functioning requires a brain that is anatomically normal, with normal neurophysiology and brain chemicals in the proper proportions. Neuroscientists are finding that some mental disorders are associated with variations from these normal conditions. If mental disorders are caused by brain defects, then intervention should be directed to the brain itself. Treatment of mental disorders, according to the neuroscience model, involves changing the abnormal *somatic* (bodily) conditions through somatic intervention. These interventions include pharmacotherapy, psychosurgery, and electroconvulsive therapy (ECT).

Several occupational therapy treatment approaches have ties to neuroscience theory. One is Lorna Jean King's sensory integration approach to the treatment of schizophrenia. King[41] proposed that games and postural exercises can bring about changes in the sensorimotor functioning of persons with certain types of chronic schizophrenia. She argued that these activities stimulate the part of the central nervous system that processes and organizes sensory information.

A second occupational therapy approach related to neuroscience was developed by Allen[1], who proposed that the problems psychiatric patients have functioning in daily life originate in physical and chemical abnormalities of the brain. She argued that the role of occupational therapy should be to define the person's functional level very precisely and to modify the environment to help the person function as well as possible.

More recently Brown and coworkers building on the work of Dunn and Westman, developed an evaluation of sensory processing for adults and adolescents. These writers offer strategies for modifying the environment and one's behavior to compensate for sensory differences. Two key notions for this approach are **neurological threshold** and **behavioral response**. Neurological threshold is the degree to which the person's nervous system registers sensation from the environment. Behavioral response is the action taken by a person in reaction to sensory information. The sensory processing and modulation approaches now in use also may promote helpful changes in behaviors associated with the autonomic nervous system (excitation vs relaxation).

7) **Psychiatric and Psychosocial Rehabilitation:**

PsyR and psychosocial rehabilitation are common names for what is essentially the same approach. PsyR is an approach documented by William Anthony and others and Farkas and others at the Sargent College of Allied Health Professions, Boston University. It combines principles and concepts from the fields of physical rehabilitation, client-centered therapy, behavioral psychology, and psychosocial rehabilitation. PsyR is *eclectic* (drawing on many sources for technics). As such it is **atheoretical** (without theory), although it uses technics associated with several theories. It is not a **treatment theory** and does not attempt to explain why or how mental disorders occur. Rather, it is a **rehabilitation approach** that focuses on how best to help the person with a mental disorder function optimally in his or her life situation.

PsyR is uncannily similar to occupational therapy in that it is oriented to the present and future, focuses on the development of skills and resources, and uses activities and environmental adaptations as a base for intervention.

PsyR is compatible with the **recovery movement,** a model of behavioral health promoted by the Substance Abuse and Mental Health Services Administration (SAMHSA).

Major occupational Therapy Models Used In Mental Health:

occupational therapists use different theories depending on the area in which they work, the kind of problems they encounter in that setting and their own knowledge, skills and preferences. Participation in occupation is the primary concern of occupational therapy. Hence, any theory useful to occupational therapy practitioners must explain how people's performance of occupations affects their mental health and how their mental health affects their performance of occupations. Occupational therapists have developed specific models that focus on occupation or activity.

1) **Development of Adaptive Skills:**

   The **development of adaptive skills** model was conceived by Anne Cronin Mosey. It is also called recapitulation of ontogenesis and means the stage-by-stage progression of development. The aim of this model is to help the person master, step-by-step, occupation supporting skills not yet acquired. Four basic concepts guide the use of this model:

   1. The therapist must provide an environment that facilitates growth.
   2. The subskills are mastered in order.
   3. Subskills from different areas may be addressed at the same time, provided they are normally acquired at the same chronological age.
   4. The patient's intrinsic motivation or desire for mastery of the subskills must be engaged.

2) **Role Acquisition and Social Skills Training:**

   Role acquisition, a term coined by Mosey, is the learning of the daily life, work and leisure skills that enable one to participate in roles that are social and/or productive. Every person performs many roles like son, daughter, student, parent, worker, employer etc. Having optimum social skills is an important part of performing roles successfully. Social skills training refers to the teaching of interpersonal skills needed to relate to other people effectively in situations as varied as dating and applying for a job.

3) **Sensory Integration:**

   Sensory integration (SI) is a theory and practice model developed by occupational therapist Jean Ayres. Lorna Jean King applied the principles of SI in the treatment of chronic schizophrenia. Sensory Integration is a normal process in the brain that receives and organizes sensory information for use in everyday life. Sensory integration therapy aims to improve symptoms by improving the reception and processing of sensory information within the central nervous system.

4) **Sensory Processing:**

   Sensory processing refers to the coordinated activities of multiple sensory receptors and neurological centers. The sensory processing model may appear similar to the Sensory Integration model, but the focus is different. Whereas SI focuses on the largely unconscious use of all the senses in activity, the model of sensory processing aims to make the person more conscious of how sensation affects activity behavior.

5) Cognitive disabilities:

Developed by occupational therapist Claudia Kay Allen, the theory of cognitive disabilities focuses on the effect of impaired cognition – a frequent symptom of psychiatric disorders – on task performance. Allen states that "just as physical disabilities restrict the physical ability to do a voluntary motion action, a **cognitive disability** restricts the cognitive ability to do a voluntary motor action". Allen maintains that the role of occupational therapy are to (a) identify the cognitive level through evaluation, (b) monitor changes in cognitive level that may result from other treatments such as medications, and (c) adapt the environment to help the person compensate for or accommodate to his or her disability. This may include caregiver instruction and training.

6) Model of Human Occupation (MOHO):

The model of human development, developed by Gary Kielhofner, provides a broad view of human occupation in relation to health. The central organizing principle of the human occupation model is that humans have an innate (inborn) drive to explore and master their environments. This process of exploring, creating, and controlling the environment is termed human occupation. The natural human tendency to engage in activity and the ways in which this tendency can be nourished or thwarted are what the human occupation model seeks to understand and explain.

7) Person-Environment-Occupation Model (PEO):

The PEO model, developed by Mary Law and colleagues, is a person-centered model that focuses on the occupational performance that results from transactions between the person and the environment as the person engages in occupation. The PEO model is concerned with **person-environment fit** or the extent to which the environment is a good match for the person's interests and abilities. The better the fit, the better the occupational performance. The poorer the match, the less satisfactory is the occupational performance. The Canadian occupational Performance Model (COPM) is a PEO evaluation designed for use with the PEO model.

8) Psychoeducation:

Psychoeducation is an educational approach used by many service providers, including occupational therapists, to improve the skills of persons with mental disorders. The psychoeducation model is used by occupational therapists to teach individuals or groups. Padilla elaborates on the many activities of an educator: lecturing; guiding role-playing, discussions, and other in-class activities; one-on -one instruction; social modeling; designing and responding to homework assignments; and creating, administering, and evaluating various outcome measures such as pretests and posttests. In this approach, the goals for intervention focus on specific behavioral objectives or outcomes.

ASSESSMENT

Assessment and outcome measurement are integral parts of the occupational therapy process. An initial assessment is used to evaluate the client's strengths, identify problem areas, set the desired outcomes of intervention and establish a baseline prior to beginning program planning. Ongoing assessment occurs throughout the intervention process, enabling the therapist and client to monitor progress and, if necessary, to gain further specific information, modify intervention or review planned outcomes. Final assessment takes place at the end of the intervention. It is used for measuring whether or not outcome goals have been reached and planning for appropriate follow-up.

occupational therapy assessment includes the client and the client's environment (physical and social environment).

WHAT IS ASSESSED?

- Occupations, routines and habits, abilities
- Strengths and interests, roles
- Volition and motivation
- Aspirations and expectations, areas of dysfunction
- External factors risk.

Some of the Standardized and non-standardized assessments used are given below.

Key Standardized Assessments:

- Adolescent/Adult Sensory Profile, Brown & Dunn,2002
- Allen Cognitive Level Screen (ACLS), Allen, 1985
- Assessment of Motor and Process Skills (AMPS), Pan & Fischer, 1994
- Canadian occupational Performance Measure (COPM), Law et al., 2001
- Kohlman Evaluation of Daily Living Skills (KELS), McGourty,1999
- occupational Performance History and interview (OPHI), Kielhofner et al., 1997
- Binary Individualised Outcome Measure, Spreadbury & Cook, 1995
- Goal Attainment Scaling, Ottenbacher & Cusick,1993.

Non-Standardized Assessments:

- Review of records
- Structured and Unstructured Interviews
- Observation
- Home visits
- Functional analysis
- Checklists, Performance scales and Questionnaires
- Projective technics.

OCCUPATIONAL THERAPY INTERVENTION

Psychiatric illness affects the roles a person played before his/her illness. Roles are patterns of activity associated with social position. A role contributes to the individual's sense of social and personal identity and also influences the way in which occupations are performed.

Occupational therapists help the person fulfil his/her occupational roles to the best of his capacity. The purpose of occupational therapy is to help individuals meet their needs, carry on their life activities, and engage in meaningful occupation.

Rather than merely addressing the symptoms of a presumed underlying pathology. Occupational therapy is concerned with enabling the occupations of day-to-day living. This is done by combining micro- level (client-centred) and macro-level (community-orientated) interventions. In mental health terms this means focusing on promoting individuals' personal skills and resources *and* on addressing the socioeconomic environment; acknowledging how disability, exclusion, and stigmatization operate societally. Examples of micro-level intervention include improving copying skills, social skills, stress management, etc. of the individual. Macro-level intervention includes improving housing, supporting access to education and/or training, and strengthening community networks.

occupational therapy intervention is client-centered i.e. the client and the therapist partner to make goals of intervention. It is highly individualized and varies depending on the context and the setting.

Identifying the symptoms and deciphering the underlying need, antecedent event, or environmental stimulus can help in planning interventions.

The OT process starts with gathering information. An individualized occupational profile of the patient is created. "The occupational profile is a summary of a client's occupational history and experiences, patterns of daily living, interests, values, and needs" (AOTA). The occupational therapist chooses a theory or principle or model (e.g. psychodynamic/development of adaptive skills/cognitive disabilities, etc.) that best explains the client's problems, as a guide in selecting methods of intervention. No one theory is adequate to address every problem, and so it is important to choose the best one for the particular situation.

Assessment is done using standardized and non standardized assessment measures. Short term and long term goals are set collaboratively with the patient and/or with the care giver Goals are documented using the SMART format i.e. specific, measurable, attainable/achievable, relevant/realistic and timely.

The occupational therapist uses therapeutic use of self, environment and activities as tools for intervention. These are prescribed based on clinical reasoning skills and the model/frame of reference the therapist selects for the particular patient in order to understand his function-dysfunction. Also taken into consideration are the patient's presenting symptoms, developmental stage, gender, interest, competency and sociocultural aspect. The immediate outcomes expected may vary depending on the patient, his current state and the therapist.

1) **Therapeutic use of self**

   Although occupational therapists help people with mental illness primarily by occupations and activities, they also help them by the way they relate to them. Being aware of oneself and of the patient and being able to control what one communicates is called **therapeutic use of self.** The therapeutic relationship with the occupational therapist strongly influences the way patients see themselves and their abilities.

2) **Environment**

   Environment is the context in which the interaction with the patient takes place. It includes the presence or absence of other people, the general noise level, the amount of visual stimulation, the quality of the lighting, the arrangement of the furniture, the ventilation and temperature, and the presence of objects. Sometimes, the person needs more stimulation, sometimes less. The occupational therapist modifies the environment in order to make it more or less structured/unstructured.

3) **Activity**

   In occupational therapy, activities are used as the means and as the end. It means that activities are used therapeutically in order to achieve the goal of activities which the person wants to achieve. Activities are potent tools in the armour of an occupational therapist. Activity prescription is as important to the occupational therapist, as is medicine prescription to the psychiatrist.

   Purposeful activities have a much deeper relevance to a person than is visible to a layperson. Activities can be viewed as stepping stones towards achieving self-actualization. Activities may also have a lot of symbolism associated with it. e.g. in the early stages of depression, a fun filled activity of group dance may symbolize pleasure and may increase guilt in the patient. Such an activity can be counterproductive and would be contraindicated in the initial stage.

Activity Selection, Activity Analysis and Activity Grading

Activity Selection - Selection of an appropriate activity is an important part of occupational therapy intervention process. Activities are selected either to provide assessment data or to reach an intervention goal. It is important to have a match or fit between the activity and the client.

Activity Analysis – Activity analysis is 'a process of dissecting an activity into its component parts and task sequence in order to identify its inherent properties and the skills required for its performance, thus allowing the therapist to evaluate its therapeutic potential'.

The occupational therapist analyzes activities to assess the performance components needed to engage in the activity and for judging the relevance of the activity for a particular patient. Activity analysis can vary depending on the theory or practice model used by the therapist. For example, the activity of clay modelling can be analyzed using the theory of object relations and as such would examine the unconscious meanings associated with it. The same activity of clay modelling can be analyzed using the behavioral frame of reference to examine its relevance as a reinforcement.

When a particular theory or practice model is used to plan intervention, the activity must be analyzed from the same perspective.

Activity Grading – The occupational therapist designs a graded activity program in a way that patients begin at a level of their capacity and gradually make a step by step progress towards the goal.

Table 62.1: Selected Occupational Therapy Terminologies/concepts/methods:

Occupational Therapy Terminologies/ concepts/methods	Description
Client-centered practice	Creek (2003) defined client-centered practice as 'a partnership between therapist and client in which the client ... actively participates in negotiating goals for intervention and making decisions [while] the therapist adapts the intervention to meet client needs'.
Activities of Daily Living	The activities of daily living (ADL) is a term used to collectively describe fundamental skills that are required to independently care for oneself such as eating, bathing and mobility. ADL is used as an indicator of a person's functional status. ADL are classified into Basic and Instrumental ADL. **Basic ADLs (BADL)** – are those skills required to manage one's physical needs including personal hygiene or grooming, dressing, toileting, transferring or ambulating and eating. **Instrumental ADL(IADL)** – include more complex activities that are related to the ability to live independently in the community. This includes activities such as managing finances and medications, food preparation, housekeepimg, laundry[5].

(Continued...)

<table>
<tr><th>Occupational Therapy Terminologies/ concepts/methods</th><th>Description</th></tr>
<tr><td>Group therapy</td><td>Group therapy is a planned process for creating changes in individuals by bringing them together for a purpose.

Mosey identified five developmental levels for assisting people in learning group interaction skills: parallel, project,egocentric-cooperative, cooperative, and mature

Cole's Seven Steps addresses facilitation of group therapy: introduction, activity, sharing, processing, generalizing, application, summary.</td></tr>
<tr><td>Projective methods</td><td>Projective methods were developed as a method of assessing emotions, motivations and values, none of which could be measured with existing tools. Projective tests use standard stimuli that allow people to make their own interpretations. The theory behind them is that the person does not know what is expected (i.e. what would constitute a good performance) and therefore performs spontaneously. Occupational therapists generally use projective methods in two ways:

1. Creation of an object by the person, such as a painting; or presentation of a stimulus by the therapist, such as a poem, followed by a period of discussion in which the person is encouraged to express their feelings about the object freely. This is usually done in a group

2. Presentation of a series of standard activities to the person, assessing how they cope with them. Projective methods are an appropriate method of assessment for occupational therapists because they involve doing as well as, or instead of, talking. Most of the projective methods used by occupational therapists involve a phase of creating, which can be structured or unstructured, and a phase of talking about the created object or free-associating about it. The method is used as assessment and as a form of intervention simultaneously, in that therapists help clients to accept projected material as their own and gain insight into how their own perceptions are formed. Examples of projective tests:

- The Azima Battery is a typical projective method developed by an occupational therapist (Azima 1982). This utilizes three tasks: a free pencil drawing, drawings of a person of each gender and a free clay model. These are presented to the client in a standard order and method. The person is given a set period of time to complete each task.

- The Goodman Battery was developed from the Azima Battery and differs from it, in that the tasks given are progressively less structured, thus making it possible to assess cognition and ego functioning under decreasingly structured conditions. It was designed for use with young adults and adults experiencing psychiatric disorders. The four tasks in the battery are: copying a mosaic tile, spontaneous drawing, figure drawing and free clay modelling.</td></tr>
</table>

CASE STUDIES

Case Study 1

43 year old patient named Ravi, was admitted in an acute set up hospital with complaints of abusive, aggressive and assaultive behavior. Patient exhibited auditory hallucinations and persecutory delusion. Ravi was diagnosed as a case of Schizophrenia. Psychiatric treatment in the form of medications and electroconvulsive therapy (ECT) was started. Patient was referred to occupational therapy. The occupational therapist visited the patient in the ward. Information about the patient was gathered from his medical file, patient's wife and patient himself. Occupational history of the patient revealed that Ravi was a commerce graduate and had a history of frequent change of jobs due to his interpersonal problems with co-workers, Currently he stayed in a one room kitchen apartment along with his wife and two children aged 12 and 10 years old. Ravi worked as a clerk in a private firm. Clinical observation of the patient's behavior and functional performance of daily activities was done. An occupational profile was created of Ravi.

Different theoretical models and approaches were used to understand Ravi's function-dysfunction. Assessments and intervention were planned based on the model selected.

Assessments like Comprehensive occupational Therapy Evaluation (COTE), Canadian occupational Performance Measure (COPM), Modified Global Assessment Of Functioning Scale(mGAF) were performed.

Short term and long term goals were documented using the SMART format, in collaboration with Ravi's wife and Ravi. Intervention used the tools of therapeutic use of self, activities (selection, analysis and grading) and environment. Ravi received daily sessions of individual therapy. Later Ravi also attended group therapy sessions. There was gradual improvement in Ravi's symptoms and functioning. Discharge planning was done before his discharge from the acute set up. Post discharge Ravi was asked to follow up in the outpatient section of occupational therapy. Accordingly, Ravi attended OT sessions on OPD basis where the focus was reintegrating him back in society. Ravi received sessions to improve copying skills, interpersonal and social skills and stress management using mindfulness. Family was involved in the therapy and were counseled. Ravi also received prevocational and vocational skills training. Disability evaluation was done for Ravi. Eventually, Ravi started attending work with environmental (mainly social) modifications. He was compliant with the medicines prescribed by the psychiatrist. He visited the outpatient occupational therapy department whenever he felt overwhelmed with the surroundings. Till last count, Ravi did not have a relapse and coped well at home and at work.

Case Study 2

Aarav, aged 5 years was brought by his parents to an occupational therapy clinic. The pediatric OT clinic was specially designed in a large sensory rich area with suspended equipments like various swings, therapy balls, ball pool, toys and activities. The parent's main concern was that Aarav exhibited stereotypical behavior in the form of spinning objects, he lined up his toys, did not adapt to simple changes like not going to the garden. His speech was delayed and he had difficulty using verbal and non verbal communication. Aarav did not socialize and preferred to be in his own world. After the initial parent interview, the occupational therapist conducted Aarav's assessment which involved clinical observation of the child including his play. Standardized and non standardized assessment tools like Sensory profile, Pediatric Evaluation of Disability Inventory (PEDI), Test of Playfulness (ToP) were used.

An occupational profile of Aarav was made. Short term and long term goals were formulated using the SMART format, in collaboration with the parents and Aarav. Aarav's intervention was based on two approaches, namely, Sensory Integration and Behavioral. Aarav received three sessions per week and this continued for several months. Treatment also included sensory diet which is a list of sensory activities which the parent conducts for him at home. Environmental modifications were recommended at school with a few suggestions to the class teacher regarding his behavior modification. Aarav's parents were encouraged to attend regular parent training lectures and workshops, autism awareness programs like Walk for Autism during Autism month of April. They were also advocated about autism support groups, concessions available, etc. Aarav continued to receive occupational therapy for several years, at the end of which he was independent in his daily living and attended a vocational training centre for future pursuits.

Psychiatric Disorders in Pregnancy and related to Menstruation and Menopause

63

Ruksheda Syeda • Rupali Shivalkar

Key Words

Menstruation, PMS, PMDD, Premenstrual Dysphoric Disorder, Pregnancy, Perinatal Psychiatry, Postpartum Depression, Menopause, Anxiety, Psychosis

INTRODUCTION

In the recent years there has been an increased focus on women's health, including particular attention to psychiatric conditions specific to them. Women experience developmental and cyclic changes in hormonal exposures affecting cerebral functions and some aspects of mental health. Some women experience suboptimal central nervous system responses to changes in reproductive hormones during menstruation, pregnancy and menopause, that leads to negative affect and behavior maladaptations (Bloch 2000). Genetic vulnerabilities, life experiences, and cultural and gender expectations, shape subjective resilience. Experiences alter gene expression, contributing to neuro-biological and physiological changes throughout lifespan (Curley 2011).

PSYCHIATRIC MORBIDITY ASSOCIATED WITH MENSTRUATION

The link between mental health and menstruation has long been established. As early as 1827, menstrual mood disorder was one of the legal defences used in cases of filicide (Brockington, 2009). Over past few decades there has been significant research into biological basis and treatment of Premenstrual Syndrome (PMS). It is estimated that nearly 85% women experience transient symptom of discomfort either physical or psychological just prior to or during menstruation. Out of these 20-25% report moderate to severe symptoms classified as Premenstrual syndrome while 5% may fulfil criteria for Premenstrual Dysphoric Disorder (PMDD) (Yonkers and Casper 2019). In India the prevalence of PMDD in different studies range from 3.7% to 12.2% (Andrade 2016). These are most often reported yet under treated conditions in clinical practice.

Premenstrual Syndrome (PMS)

Premenstrual Syndrome (PMS) is broad term that refers to cluster of physical, behavioral and emotional symptoms (**Table 63.1**) occurring in cyclical patterns about 1-2 weeks prior to menstruation and remit in 3-4 days after the onset of menstrual flow (Hartlage et al 2012; Durairaj A & Ramamurthi R 2019).

Premenstrual Dysphoric Disorder

Premenstrual Dysphoric Disorder (PMDD) is a more severe and sometimes disabling form of Premenstrual Syndrome characterized by significant premenstrual mood disturbance along with prominent mood reactivity and irritability. This often results in significant impairment interpersonal, social and occupational functioning requiring intervention (Hantsoo & Epperson 2015).

Table 63.1

Psychological Symptoms	Physical Symptoms	Behavioral Symptoms
Anger	Bloating (usually abdominal)	Fatigue
Anxiety	Appetite disturbance (usually increased)	Forgetfulness
Depression	Breast tenderness	Poor concentration
Irritability	Headaches	
Sense of feeling overwhelmed	Lethargy or fatigue	
Sensitivity to rejection	Muscle aches and/or joint pain	
Social withdrawal	Sleep disturbances (usually hypersomnia)	
	Swelling of extremities	

The prevalence of PMDD among various studies across globe is 3-8%, usually starting in late twenties and worsening over time. Studies from Asia show slightly lower rates 5.3%. However it is considered to be prevalent in all age groups. The major risk factors for PMDD include personal history of a mood or anxiety disorder, family history of premenstrual mood dysregulation, stress, trauma and age in the late 20's to mid-30's (Sharma 1999, Cunningham et al 2011).

PMDD needs to be differentiated from other medical and psychiatric disorders which are likely to present with similar symptom profile. These include Medical illnesses such as chronic fatigue syndrome, fibromyalgia, irritable bowel syndrome and migraine Psychiatric illnesses such as depression or anxiety disorders.

Etiological Theories

Etiological theories of premenstrual dysphoric disorder (PMDD) adapted from psych.theclinics.com
Abnormal response to normal fluctuations of the hypothalamic-pituitary-gonadal axis
Decreased or paradoxic sensitivity of the $GABA_A$ receptor to allopregnanolone
Alterations in serotonin axis response
Altered immune functions, calcium homeostasis, circadian rhythms

Genetic factors
Abnormal responses in brain regions to emotional processing and regulation during luteal phase

Diagnosis

There is no biological tests to diagnose premenstrual syndrome (PMS) or premenstrual dysphoric disorder (PMDD). However it is recommended to screen for medical conditions that may mimic the symptoms. Blood count to rule out anemia or chronic infections, Thyroid function test are usually recommended.

The diagnosis is usually done based on ICD11 or DSM 5 criteria (**Table 63.2**). The symptoms must occur only during the second half (luteal phase) of the menstrual cycle, most often during the five to seven days before the menstrual period, and there must be physical as well as behavioral symptoms.

If the symptoms suggest PMDD, woman may be requested to carefully record her symptoms on a daily basis for two full menstrual cycles

Treatment

Conservative treatments like regular exercise, relaxation technics, and vitamin and mineral supplementation do help in PMS. Among

Table 63.2: DSM-5 criteria (www.endtotext.org)

Timing of symptoms **A**) In the majority of menstrual cycles, at least 5 symptoms must be present in the final week before the onset of menses, start to improve within a few days after the onset of menses, and become minimal or absent in the week post menses
Symptoms **B**) One or more of the following symptoms must be present: 1) Marked affective lability (e.g., mood swings, feeling suddenly sad or tearful, or increased sensitivity to rejection) 2) Marked irritability or anger or increased interpersonal conflicts 3) Markedly depressed mood, feelings of hopelessness, or self-deprecating thoughts 4) Marked anxiety, tension, and/or feelings of being keyed up or on edge **C**) One (or more) of the following symptoms must additionally be present to reach a total of 5 symptoms when combined with symptoms from criterion B above 1) Decreased interest in usual activities 2) Subjective difficulty in concentration 3) Lethargy, easy fatigability, or marked lack of energy 4) Marked change in appetite; overeating or specific food cravings 5) Hypersomnia or insomnia 6) A sense of being overwhelmed or out of control 7) Physical symptoms such as breast tenderness or swelling; joint or muscle pain, a sensation of "bloating" or weight gain
Severity **D)** The symptoms are associated with clinically significant distress or interference with work, school, usual social activities, or relationships with others.
E) Consider Other Psychiatric Disorders The disturbance is not merely an exacerbation of the symptoms of another disorder, such as major depressive disorder, panic disorder, persistent depressive disorder (dysthymia) or a personality disorder (although it may co-occur with any of these disorders).
Confirmation of the disorder **F)** Criterion A should be confirmed by prospective daily ratings during at least 2 symptomatic cycles (although a provisional diagnosis may be made prior to this confirmation)
Exclude other Medical Explanations **G)** The symptoms are not attributable to the physiological effects of a substance (e.g., drug abuse, medication or other treatment) or another medical condition (e.g., hyperthyroidism).

the supplements Vitamin B6 (up 1333rfto 100mg/day), Calcium 1 gm/day Magnesium, L-Tryptophan shows some benefit in mild PMS cases. The rest of the dietary supplements, including evening primrose oil, essential free fatty acids, and ginkgo biloba are recommended but have not been proven to be of any scientific benefits in trials.

In moderate to severe cases medication can be considered. These include –

Antidepressants

Selective serotonin reuptake inhibitors (SSRIs) are a highly effective treatment for the symptoms of PMS and PMDD. SSRI either taken as daily therapy or periodic treatment taken only in luteal phase are proven effective. Fluoxetine, Sertraline, Citalopram, Escitalopram, and Paroxetine all are equally effective. Studies showed that SSRIs reduced the symptoms of PMDD significantly compared with placebo; between 12- 50% of women with PMDD improve with an SSRI. SSRIs reduce emotional symptoms, fatigue, food craving and sleep problems.

SSRIs should be taken for at least two menstrual cycles to measure their benefit. Some women do report difficulty in having orgasm with SSRIs. In such cases lowering dose or using alternative drug from same class may help. Other ADD include Venlafaxine, Clomipramine.

Hormonal Treatment

Among the hormonal treatments oral contraceptive pills are usually recommended. The pill can be taken continuously to avoid having a menstrual period. Taking the pill continuously or minimizing pill free interval prevents the usual cyclical hormone changes that could affect mood. It is thought that mood symptoms are improved with a shorter pill-free interval. Alternatively, Gonadotropin-releasing hormone (GnRH) agonists (e.g., leuprolide acetate or goserelin acetate) can be used. These medications cause the ovaries to temporarily stop making estrogen and progesterone; thus, inducing temporary menopause. This improves the physical symptoms (e.g., bloating) and irritability caused by PMS and PMDD.

Surgical treatment like hysterectomy or salpingo-oophorectomy have also been proposed in severe cases.

PSYCHIATRIC DISORDERS IN PREGNANCY:

With new insights in to maternal and infant mental health and its short and long term impact on women and their offsprings it is recommended that special attention be paid to women's mental health in antenatal, perinatal, and postnatal period. Data suggests that most postpartum psychiatric disorders has its onset in the antenatal and perinatal phases. Perinatal period can be considered the duration before, during and after pregnancy. There is exposure to higher levels of circulating hormones like estrogen, progesterone, androgens, prolactin, allopregnanolone, oxytocin, corticotropin-releasing hormone and others during pregnancy and an abrupt drop in hormones and peptides produced by the placenta after delivery. These changes along with life events and experiences may increase risk of onset of affective, anxiety or psychotic disorders or exacerbate pre existing symptoms.

Depression and Suicide

Depressive illnesses are common during perinatal period and share the same phenomenology of as non-pregnancy depressive disorders.. Antepartum depression has been associated with low maternal weight gain, low birth weight, increased risk of premature births (Payne 2017).

Up to 70% of women experience "baby blues" which is a short lasting condition marked with sadness, irritability, fatigue, crying spells, and anxiety. The symptoms last for a week or two and do not cause interfere with daily activities, resolving without any treatment.

Perinatal depression can occur in 1 in 7 women. Untreated perinatal depression can have disastrous consequences like suicide and in lesser cases infanticide.

Symptoms of depression commonly seen are:

- Feeling sad, hopeless, or overwhelmed
- Crying spells for no apparent reason
- Anxiety
- Mood swings, irritability, anger, restlessness, feelings of guilt

- Change in sleep patterns (oversleeping or insomnia)
- Eating too little, or too much
- Trouble concentrating, forgetfulness, difficulty in making decisions
- Having little or no interest in activities that are usually enjoyable
- Physical aches and pains
- Having trouble bonding with the baby
- Withdrawing from friends and family
- Thinking of harming self or the baby

Risk Factors for Perinatal Depression:

- Genetic vulnerability
- Previous history of affective disorder
- Previous history of perinatal depression
- Low social support
- Low spousal support
- Multiple stressors
- History of abuse
- Family history
- Medical complications during pregnancy or delivery
- Other medical disorders

Diagnosis

An integrative care approach should be adopted by the obstetrician or primary physician where every woman during the perinatal period should be screened for depression. An easy, screening tool, Edinburgh Postnatal Depression Scale (EPDS), which is 10 item self rating scale is used quite commonly.

ICD11 or DSM 5 criteria for Depression (with peripartum onset specifier) is applied to diagnose some with postpartum depression.

Treatment

- Psychoeducation
- Individual Counseling (Cognitive Behavior Therapy CBT, Interpersonal Therapy IPT)
- Couple's Counseling
- Family Counseling

Medications

- Overall use of antidepressants during pregnancy appears to be relatively safe.
- SSRIs are the most commonly and successfully used antidepressants. Sertraline, Fluoxetine, Escitalopram, Fluvoxamine are FDA category C while Paroxetine is category D and hence it is usually not recommended during pregnancy or lactation
- SNRIs like Duloxetine, Mirtazapine, Venlafaxine have limited data but are thought to be effective with a good safety profile
- Others like Bupropion, and tricyclics like Amitriptyline and clomipramine are category C

Anxiety

Anxiety is over looked as a symptom and a disorder in pregnancy and postpartum though it has a prevalence rate of about 13% (Lancet 2014).

OCD

OCD symptoms, especially ruminating thoughts are unusually common in perinatal period, occurring in as high as 35% of women with postpartum depression (Altemus 2013).

Psychosis

There is a marled increase risk of psychosis and mania in the first few weeks postpartum. There is 23-fold increase risk of first episode of affective psychosis in the postpartum period (Sharma 2012). Although some women may experience psychosis only during postpartum.

Treatment

- Antipsychotics, for the most part, appear to be relatively safe and not treating psychosis can be dangerous for the patient.
- Typical APDS
- Haloperidol, Trifluoperazine
- Atypical APDS
- Olanzapine, Aripiprazole, Quetiapine, Risperidone, Paliperidone, Ziprasidone
- Mood stabilizers
- Valproic acid, Divalproex should be avoided
- Lamotrigine is a safer option

PSYCHIATRIC DISORDERS RELATED TO MENOPAUSE

Menopause is permanent cessation of menstruation resulting in loss of ovarian follicular development. Menopausal transition or Perimenopause is defined as period beginning with onset of irregular menstrual cycles interspersed until loss of menstrual period followed by one year period of amenorrhea. This period may vary from 4-7 years and is marked by gradual decline in estrogen and rise in LH and FSH. Postmenopausal period starts after complete cessation of menstrual cycles. In India the average age of menopause is 47.5 years (Dalal & Agarwal 2015; Friedman et al 2018).

WHO define Perimenopause is as the 2–8 years preceding menopause and the 1-year period after final menses, resulting from the loss of follicular activity (WHO,1996) During this period, production of the estrogen and progesterone becomes more irregular, with wide and unpredictable fluctuations in their levels; the levels of follicle-stimulating hormone increase until months after the last menstrual period leading to diminishing fertility and irregularity of menses (Soules at al 2001).

Postmenopausal Symptoms: (Santoro et al 2011; Friedman et al 2018)

Vasomotor symptoms- Hot flushes, headache
Urogenital atrophy – Dry vagina, sexual dysfunction, dyspareunia, dysuria, urinary urgency, stress incontinence
Osteoporotic changes- backache, recurrent fractures with minor trauma, decreased height and mobility
Psychiatric Symptoms- increased mood swings, depression, anxiety
Sleep Disturbances- Insomnia, daytime somnolence, Non-refreshing sleep with frequent awakenings
Memory problems, confusion, concentration difficulties

Depression

Earlier termed as climacteric depression, postmenopausal Depression is reported in nearly 20% women. Perimenopause is considered to be period of heightened risk for clinical as well as subclinical depressive disorders. Young age of menopause, prior depressive episode, surgical menopause, severity of vasomotor symptoms, sleep problems, poor physical health or comorbid chronic medical conditions are some of the common risk factors besides psychosocial stressors. The study of Women's Health across Nations (SWAN) used data from 13 year follow up period found that nearly one third of women who developed depression in this period ultimately had persistent or recurring course (Bromberger & Kravitz 2012; Friedman et al 2018).

Sleep Disorders

Nearly 16-42% women report sleep disturbances associated with perimenopausal period. In post menopause the prevalence could be 35-60%. The sleep problems are often multifactorial in origin and worsen quality of life. Insomnia with somnolence at day time is the commonest problem reported. It is often associated with hot flushes interfering with sleep cycle or associated mood or anxiety symptoms. Increasing rate of sleep apnea in this period has also been one of the factors studied. Anxiety and sleep problems are often identified as contributing factors for psychosocial morbidity among middle aged women (Kravitz & Joffe 2011; Jehan et al 2015).

Anxiety Disorders

Anxiety disorders constitute heterogenous group and often symptoms overlap considerably with mood and stress related disorders. Worsening of existing anxiety disorders, OCD or panic disorder or new onset is commonly noted in peri and postmenopausal period. Irritability, nervousness or tension, fear for no apparent reason, heart pounding are some of the commonest symptoms reported in this period (Bromberger et al 2013; Dalal & Agarwal 2015).

Cognitive Dysfunction

Memory disturbances, concentration difficulties are commonly reported during menopausal transition. Neuropathological changes in brain can cause mild cognitive impairment (MCI) and eventually Dementia. Women are reported to be at higher risk of developing Alzheimer's disease as compared to men. Apart from antioxidants and Cholinesterase Inhibitors, beneficial role of Estrogen replacement in cognitive dysfunction suggest specific association with menopause (Kim & Jung 2015; Friedman et 2018).

Severe Mental Illnesses

Estrogen is considered to be playing neuroprotective role against psychotic and mood disorders. Severe Mental illnesses including schizophrenia and other psychotic disorders may have new onset or exacerbation after 40-50 years of age. Also worsening of preexisting schizophrenia symptoms during menopausal transition suggests estrogen modulatory role. The course of Bipolar disorders during perimenopausal period also associated with greater mood symptom severity, more frequency of depressive episodes and increased risk of rapid cycling. Addition of low dose estrogen and role of selective estrogen receptor modulators as an adjuvant to antipsychotics has been found to be beneficial (Robinson GE 2001; Riecher-Rossler 2009; Dalal & Agarwal 2015, Friedman et al 2018).

Management

In menopause, decreasing estrogen levels correlate with increased mood symptoms, physical symptoms, and psychotic symptoms. Systemic Estrogen therapy is the most effective treatment available for decreasing perimenopausal and postmenopausal symptoms particularly the vasomotor symptoms, sleep disturbances and symptoms associated with urogenital atrophy. Low dose estrogen as 0.3 mg/day orally or 0.025 mg/day as transdermal replacement are often reported to be effective with minimal side effects. Besides estrogen replacement, intermittent low dose progestin treatment is also considered effective option. Hormone replacement have been reported to be associated with increased risk of thromboembolism as well as breast carcinoma and need to be used with caution in at risk individuals. Estrogen is also reported to be effective adjuvant in patients with preexisting or recent onset psychiatric morbidities like Depression, anxiety disorders, OCD as well as SMI like Schizophrenia, Bipolar disorders, cognitive dysfunctions.

Other medications that alter central noradrenergic activity like clonidine as 0.1-0.2 mg/Day orally or 0.1 mg/day Transdermal is also reported effective in alleviating vasomotor symptoms.

Modulation of Serotonin and Norepinephrine using various Anti-depressants is effective in managing neuropsychiatric disorders associated with menopausal transition. SSRIs like Paroxetine, Sertraline; SNRIs like Venlafaxine have shown promising results in randomized controlled trials.

Along with medications biopsychosocial approach is particularly important in menopause. Therapies focusing in life cycle perspective helping women with adjusting to role transition, loss of fertility, changing social and financial status have shown to be highly effective.

CONCLUSION

New data about sex and gender differences in psychiatric disorders in, prevalence, causes, risk factors, clinical presentations, interventions, and treatment outcomes are impacting mental health care for women. The hormonal milieu during puberty, menstruation, pregnancy, lactation (perinatal period), and menopause can be triggers for some women, for onset, recurrence, and increase in psychopathology of conditions like anxiety, affective, and psychotic disorders. PMDD, Perinatal Depression, Affective and Anxiety Disorders in menopause affect a good proportion of women requiring appropriate and timely intervention for better outcomes. The newer research and growing awareness is helping clinicians to implement personalized medicine to women which changes across their life cycle.

BIBLIOGRAPHY

1. Bloch M, Scmidt PJ, Danaceau MA et al. Effects of gonadal steroids in women with a history of postpartum depression. Am J Psychiatry 2000;157:924-30
2. Brockington I. 2009 Obstetric and gynaecological conditions associated with Psychiatric disorder. Gelder MG, Andreasen NC, Lopez-Ibor J, Geddes JR (eds) New Oxford textbook of Psychiatry second edition vol 2,Oxford uni press pp- 1114-1127.
3. Yonkers KA & Casper RF (2019, October 22) Epidemiology and pathogenesis of premenstrual syndrome and premenstrual dysphoric disorder (R. L. Barbieri & W. F. Crowley Jr., Eds.). Retrieved December 04, 2019 from https://www.uptodate.com/contents/epidemiology-and-pathogenesis-of-premenstrual-syndrome-and-premenstrual-dysphoric-disorder?topicRef=7382&source=see_link
4. Durairaj A, Ramamurthi R. (2019) Prevalence, pattern and predictors of premenstrual syndrome (PMS) and premenstrual dysphoric disorder (PMDD) among college girls. The New Indian Journal of OBGYN. 2019; 5(2): 93-8
5. Andrade C (2016) Premenstrual Dysphoric Disorder: General Overview, Treatment strategies and focus on Sertraline for symptom onset dosing, Indian J Psychiatry 2016; 58:329-31.
6. Hantsoo L, Epperson CN. (2015) Premenstrual dysphoric disorder: Epidemiology and treatment. Curr Psychiatry Rep 2015;17:87.
7. Hartlage SA, Freels S, Gotman N, Yonkers K. (2012) Criteria for premenstrual dysphoric disorder: secondary analyses
8. Dalal PK, Agarwal M. Postmenopausal syndrome. Indian J Psychiatry 2015;57:222-32.
9. Sharma I (1999) Premenstrual Dysphoric Disorders. Textbook of Postgraduate Psychiatry second edition; Ed. Vyas JN, Ahuja N; 2011, 376-385
10. American Psychiatric Association Diagnostic and Statistical manual of Mental Disorders IV, Ed. Washington DC: American Psychiatry Press Inc. 1994
11. American Psychiatric Association Diagnostic and Statistical Manual of Mental Disorders (5th Edition). Arlington, VA: American Psychiatric Association. 2013
12. Cunningham J, Yonkers KA, O'Brien S, Eriksson E (2009) Update on research and treatment of Premenstrual dysphoric disorder; Harv Rev Psychiatry. 2009; 17(2): 120–137.
13. World Health Organization. Research on the Menopause in the 1990s (Report of a WHO Scientific Group), WHO Technical Report Series, 886. Geneva: World Health Organization; 1996
14. Soules MR, Sherman S, Parrott E, Rebar R,

Santoro N, Utian W, et al. Executive summary: Stages of Reproductive Aging Workshop (STRAW) Climacteric. 2001;4:267–72. [PubMed]]

15. Friedman SH, Prakash c, Moller-Oslen c (2018, October) Psychiatric considerations in Menopause; Current Psychiatry Vol 17, No 10, 11-17.
16. Santoro N, Taylor ES, Kim Sutton-Tyrrell 2011 Study of Women's Health Across Nation's Recurring Themes, Obstet Gynaecol Clin North Am. Sep;38(3):417-423
17. Bromberger JT, Kravitz HM 2012 Mood and Menopause: Findings from Study of Women's Health Across the Nation (SWAN) over ten years, Obstet Gynaecol Clin North Am. Sep;38(3):609-625
18. Kravitz HM, Joffe H 2011 Sleep during the Perimenopause: A SWAN story. Obstet Gynaecol Clin North Am. Sep;38(3):567-586
19. Jehan S, Masters-Isarilov A, Salifu I, McFarlane SI et al 2015 Sleep Disorders in Postmenopausal Women. J Sleep Disord Ther. Aug;4(5):1000212
20. Bromberger JT, Kravitz HM, Matthews KA et al 2013 Does Risk for Anxiety Increase During the Menopausal Transition? SWAN study. Menopause. May;20(5):488-495
21. Kim SA , Jung H 2015 Prevention of Cognitive Impairment in the Midlife Women. J Menopausal Med.Apr, 21(1): 19-23.
22. Riecher-Rossler A2009 Psychotic Disorders and Menopause: The Untold Story. Soares CN, Warren M (eds) The Menopausal Transition, Interface between Gynaecology and Psychiatry. Key issues in Mental Health, Basel, Karger, vol 175,pp 115-126.
23. The Lancet, Perinatal Mental Health Volume 384, Issue 9956, P1775-1788
24. Altemus M, Neeb C, Davis A, et al. Phenotypic differences between pregnancy-onset and postpartum-onset major depressive disorder. J Clin Psychiatry 2013;73e1485-1491.
25. Sharma V, Pope C. Pregnancy and bipolar disorder: a systemic review. J Clin Psychiatry 2012;73:1447-55.

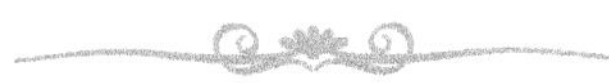

64 Consultation Liaison Psychiatry

Sandeep Grover • Devakshi Dua

INTRODUCTION

Consultation-Liaison Psychiatry (CLP) is a subspecialty of psychiatry which has brought psychiatry very close to the advances in medicine. CLP has brought psychiatry out of mental asylum and has helped in reduction of stigma. The subspecialty of CLP is based on the concept of *"interaction of mind & body"*. CLP as a subspecialty is defined as, *"the area of clinical psychiatry that encompasses clinical, teaching & research activities of psychiatrists and allied mental health professionals in the non-psychiatric divisions of a general hospital"*. *Consultation* refers to the provision of expert opinion about the diagnosis and advice on management regarding a patient's mental state and behavior. *Liaison* refers to linking up of groups for the purpose of effective collaboration, i.e., *mediation between patient and members of the clinical team and between mental health professionals and other health professionals.*

In recent times, the term "psychosomatic medicine" is used interchangeably with CLP. Psychosomatic medicine is understood as *"the interplay of biological and psychosocial factors in the development, course and outcome of all disease(s)"*. Some of the researchers understand, psychosomatic medicine as a non-clinical discipline, whereas, CLP is the practical/clinical arm or the applied form of psychosomatic medicine.

A CL Psychiatrist is a specialist within psychiatry who has specific training and specialized expertise in the diagnosis and treatment of psychiatric disorders in patients with concurrent physical and psychiatric illness. In addition, the CL Psychiatrist has special expertise in treatment modalities that can be carried out in the hospital, outpatient medical-surgical settings or require multidisciplinary collaboration, such as electroconvulsive therapy (ECT) and deep brain stimulation (DBS). In-terms of functioning, CL Psychiatrists are expected to integrate all information available from all the sources to provide optimal health care to patients with various medical and surgical illnesses. A CL Psychiatrist is expected to work in a General Hospital Setting across different specialties, or work at the primary care level to supervise other physicians in providing mental health services.

HISTORY OF CLP/ PSYCHOSOMATIC MEDICINE

History of psychosomatic medicine as a subspecialty is long, dating back to 3rd Century BC. However, in the recent times, history can be traced back to Johann Heinroth (1773-1843), who coined the term "psychosomatic", and the concept of "psychosomatic medicine" was put forth by Felix Deutsch in 1922. The credit of being the first CL psychiatrist is given to Jackson Putnam, who worked in Massachusetts General Hospital (MGH) in the later part of nineteenth century. The clinical aspect of psychosomatic medicine, i.e., CLP, got its recognition in the early part of the 20th century, with the opening of a first ever viable general hospital psychiatric unit (GHPU) at the Albany Hospital in 1902. The founder, JM Mosher, set up the GHPU with the aim of bringing mental health professionals close to other specialists in medicine for the purposes of training and providing psychiatric care. This had a huge impact on the specialty of psychiatry, with the opening up of a large number of GHPUs across the world. CLP flourishes in a GHPU with teaching facility for psychiatry residents.

Lipowski is credited for providing the first formal definition of the subspecialty of CLP. Lipowski in 1967 defined CLP as a sub-specialty of psychiatry that involves providing clinical service, teaching and carrying out research at the borderland of psychiatry and medicine. He described the two inter-related roles of the CL Psychiatrist. According to Lipowski, the term 'consultation' implies giving expert opinion about the diagnosis and advice on management of mental health issues in a patient with medical or surgical illness on the request of the primary physician/surgeon of the patient. The term "liaison" implies linking up of groups of professionals for the purpose of effective collaboration. Over the years, the concept of liaison has been further broadened to involve interpretation and mediation. Accordingly, the mental health professional working as a CL Psychiatrist is expected to mediate between patients, family members and members of the clinical team, and also between mental health and other health professionals.

ROLES AND FUNCTIONS OF A CL PSYCHIATRIST

A good CL Psychiatrist is expected to be a medical expert, a good communicator, a good collaborator, a manager and a supervisor, a health advocate, a professional and a scholar. The functions of a CL Psychiatrist include providing patient care, teaching, supervision, resolving crisis and research (**Box 64.1**). In terms of training, the CL Psychiatrist is expected to improve the knowledge of the psychiatry trainees and trainees in other specialties, and enhance the awareness and knowledge of members of medical and surgical team about mental health issues in patients with various physical illnesses.

Box 64.1: Functions of CL Psychiatrist

- **Patient care:** diagnosis, pharmacological & Non-pharmacological management, assessment of competence
- **Teaching:** Specialists of other specialties, primary care physicians, nurses, other mental and non-mental health professionals
- **Supervision:** Specialists, physicians, primary care health workers
- **Resolving crisis** (interpersonal problems): between patient/family members and other treating team members, between different members of treating team
- **Research**

A CL Psychiatrist is expected to have good knowledge and understanding of medical illnesses and their interaction with mental health and behavioral sciences. A CL Psychiatrist is also expected to have thorough knowledge of psychopharmacology, in terms of pharmacokinetics and pharmacodynamics of various psychotropics, drug-drug interactions with respect to psychotropics and other classes of medications, drug-body interaction, drug-disease interaction and drug-food interaction. CL Psychiatrist is also expected to have good knowledge and skills to carry out psychotherapeutic interaction in patients with different medical conditions. A CL Psychiatrist is also expected to have thorough knowledge about medication-induced psychiatric manifestations, such as steroid induced psychiatric syndromes, chemotherapeutic and immunosuppressant associated psychiatric syndromes and psychiatric manifestations associated with other classes of medications. A CL Psychiatrist is also expected to have good knowledge about medical complications associated with psychotropic medications, such as hyponatremia, gastrointestinal bleeding, Neuroleptic malignant syndrome, falls, osteoporosis, QTc prolongations etc. Details of other expected skills are given in **Box 64.2**.

Box 64.2: Expected Skills in a CL Psychiatrist

History Taking and Examination skills:

- Take a medical-psychiatric history
- Competence in interviewing, examining patients and their family members in inpatient, emergency, outpatient, intensive care unit setting.
- Agitation, catatonia, drug intoxication, drug withdrawal
- Assess neurological dysfunction
- Assess the risk of suicide
- Assess the role of psychological behavioral factors in pain
- Assessing stress
- Role of interpersonal and family issues in clinical manifestation
- Carry out psychological pre & post-transplant assessments

Thorough Medical Knowledge:

- Knowledge of established and evolving biomedical, clinical, epidemiological and social-behavioral sciences, as well as the application of the knowledge to patient care
- Recognize and categorize symptoms in patients with complex medical conditions
- Understand the role of psychological and social variables on physical illness
- Knowledge about psychosocial issues associated with pregnancy, pain, malignancies, chronic physical illnesses, patients undergoing organ transplantation, terminally ill patients etc.
- Knowledge about medication effects and drug–drug interactions
- Models of CL Psychiatry care

Providing Clinical Care to the Medically ill Patients:

- Provide compassionate, appropriate, evidence based, and effective clinical care
- Manage self-harm, drug intoxication, drug withdrawal, pain, delirium, psychotropic related side effects

Interpersonal Communication Skills

- Good interpersonal and communication skills to promote effective transfer of information and collaboration between
  the patients, their families and other specialists
- Is able to work as a member of a multidisciplinary team
- Competency to communicate information about the diagnosis and interventions to other members of the medical team
- Intervene in matters relating to interpersonal conflicts

Diagnostic Skills

- Able to formulate multiaxial diagnoses
- Able to consider all possible differential diagnosis – both medical and psychiatric, for a given clinical presentation

(Continued)

Ethical, Legal & Advocacy skills
- Able to make medicolegal determinations
- Execute ethical decisions in clinically challenging situations
- Advocacy for patients and family members

Intervention skills
- Form a good therapeutic alliance in different clinical settings
- Carry out psychotherapy in medico-surgical setting
- Administer ECT therapy
- Administer drug detoxification protocols
- Prescribe and manage psychopharmacological agents in medico-surgical setting
- Apply systems theory and resolve conflicts
- Competence in management of patients with special needs, various disabilities and chronic physical illnesses
- Breaking bad news

Teaching Skills
- Teach medical postgraduates/undergraduates, as well as of para-professionals and non-professionals

Research
- Able to carry out research in CLP setting
- Able to audit the services from time to time

Models of CLP

Various models of consultation liaison services are described based on the focus of consultation, functions of the CL Psychiatrist and the focus of work of the CL Psychiatrist (**Box 64.3**). Different set-ups follow different models of CLP care, depending on the available resources. In general, it is recommended that psychiatrist should be part of the multidisciplinary team.

Box 64.2: Models of CL Psychiatry

Focus of consultation
- **Patient oriented approach:** assessment of patient, diagnostic interview, assessment of reaction to illness, Assessment of personality
- **Crisis oriented approach**: Rapid assessment of patient's problem and coping styles, Immediate therapeutic intervention to address the problem
- **Consultee-oriented approach**: motive of the consultee and his related difficulties and expectations are the major focus
- **Situation oriented approach:** Focus on interpersonal interactions of all the members of the clinical team involved in the care of the patient for whom consultation had been sought are taken into consideration to understand the patient's behavior and the consultee's concern about it
- **Expanded psychiatric consultation:** Although the central focus is the patient for whom consultation has been sought, the operational group that involves the patient, the clinical staff, other patients, and the patient's family

Functions of CL Psychiatrist
- **Consultation model:** Patient is the focus

(Continued)

- **Liaison model:** Consulting physician as the center of focus, in addition to providing consultation for the patient also involves teaching psychiatric and psychological aspects of patient's problem to the physician and the clinical team
- **Bridge model:** Teaching role of a C-L psychiatrist for the primary care physicians
- **Hybrid model:** Psychiatrist as part of multidisciplinary team
- **Autonomous psychiatric model:** C-L psychiatrist is not affiliated to any department but is hired by primary care services

Focus of work

- **Critical care model:** Psychiatrist involved in patient care and redressal of issues of staff
- **Biological model:** Neuroscience, psychopharmacology and psychological management
- **Milieu model:** Based on interpersonal theory and involves group aspects of patient care, reaction and interaction of staff and understanding of ward environment
- **Integral model:** The integral model is usually agency based and involves providing psychological care as an integral factor of clinical and administrative need

COMMON CLINICAL ENCOUNTERS IN CL PSYCHIATRY

Although all kind of psychiatric disorders can be encountered in CL setting, some of the disorders are seen more commonly. Depending on the treatment setting, specialty and model of care followed, the diagnostic profile of cases varies. Commonly encountered diagnosis in CLP setting include delirium, depression, adjustment disorder, self-harm, substance use disorders (intoxication and withdrawal). In intensive care units as high as 80% of the patients can have delirium. In emergency setting, self-harm and substance use disorders are very common. Besides the diagnosis identified by the nosological systems, a CL Psychiatrist may encounter conditions like demoralization; situations like breaking bad news, evaluating the competence for undergoing certain procedures.

Additionally, the CL Psychiatrists may be involved in evaluating patients prior to organ transplant, in palliative care and in deciding about continuation/discontinuation of psychotropics in patients with mental disorders planned for various surgical procedures.

In emergency setting, besides managing patients coming with self harm, a CL Psychiatrist may be involved in assessment and management of patients presenting with delirium, catatonia, agitation, dissociative disorders, panic disorder, substance intoxication or withdrawal, medication toxicity (e.g., lithium toxicity, anticholinergic syndrome, Neuroleptic malignant syndrome, serotonin syndrome, etc.), acute dystonia and acute akathasia etc.

Contributions of CL Psychiatry in understanding the role of psychological factors in Medicine in General

As a subspecialty, CLP emphasizes the role of psychological and social factors in the development and continuation of symptoms, help seeking, following the treatment advice and overall outcome of various physical illnesses. Some of the most important contributions of CL Psychiatry to medicine are shown in **Box 64.4**. Evidence from CL Psychiatry research suggest that various physical illnesses, especially chronic physical illnesses, such as diabetes mellitus, hypertension, malignancies etc. are influenced by stress. CL Psychiatry research has also demonstrated that psychological and

Box 64.4: Some of the important contributions of CL Psychiatry to practice of Medicine

- Humanism
- Importance of communication skills
- Adhering to medical ethics in difficult situations
- Breaking bad news: policy of "truth telling" in medicine & individualization of information disclosure
- Organ transplant: Pre and postoperative evaluation of the recipient and potential donors
- Pre and post testing counseling for HIV/AIDS
- Mental Health issues as contributory factors in causation of various physical illnesses
- Influence of mental health issues on course and outcome of various medical illnesses
- Psychiatric sequalae of medical disorders
- Discharge related issues- leaving against medical advice, discharge on request
- Physician Burnout: work related stress among doctors
- Identification & appropriate management of delirium → significant reduction in hospital morbidity and health care costs
- Proper identification of causes of delirium → change in designs of ICU and procedural changes in ICU management
- Evolution of concept of Telepsychiatry
- Evolution of *psycho-oncology, transplant psychiatry, psycho-nephrology, cardiac psychiatry*

social factors influence the outcome of various chronic physical illnesses. CL Psychiatry research has also demonstrated that besides use of medications and surgical interventions, outcome of patient is influenced by factors like empathy, communication skills, therapeutic alliance and doctor patient relationship. CL Psychiatry has also brought forward the importance of breaking bad news and how this can influence the outcome of the patient. The role of CL Psychiatrist in organ transplant is of paramount importance in determining the fitness of the donor and the recipient.

CONCLUSION

CL Psychiatry as a subspecialty has led to recognition of psychiatry as a medical specialty. Additionally, it has helped in understanding the role of psychological factors in development of various physical illnesses. It has also helped in understanding how psychological factors influence acceptance and adherence with various medical treatments. It has also shaped the doctor patient encounters by emphasizing the role of empathy, communication skills and therapeutic alliance in medicine.

BIBLIOGRAPHY

1. Alter C, Epstein S. Psychosomatic Medicine. In: Comprehensive Textbook of Psychiatry. 10th ed. Philadelphia: Lippincott Williams & Wilkins; 2017.
2. David AS, Fleminger S, Kopelman MD, Lovestone S, Mellers JDC, Folstein M. A Textbook of Neuropsychiatry. 4th ed. Oxford: Jhn Wiley & Sons; 2009.
3. Grover S. State of consultation-liaison psychiatry in India: Current status and vision for future. Indian Journal of Psychiatry. 2011;53:202.
4. Grover S, Avasthi A. Consultation–liaison psychiatry in India: Where to go from here? Indian J Psychiatry. 2019;61:117–24.

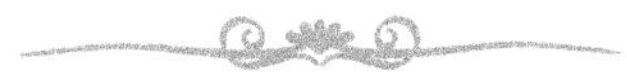

65 Disaster Psychiatry

Fiona Mhapatrao • Aparna Ramakrishnan

"Dread of disaster makes everybody act in the very way that increases the disaster."

–Bertrand Russell

Introduction; Definition of disaster; Classification of disasters – natural/human action associated, magnitude, exposure, duration of impact; *Concept of hazard; Disaster mental health; Phases of disaster response, Individual: normal and abnormal response to disasters; Specific disorders* – grief reaction, acute stress disorder, post traumatic stress disorder, depression, anxiety disorders, substance use, somatic symptoms; *Risk factors for psychological morbidity; Community response.; Etiological factors of psychological morbidity. Phases of intervention, Psychological intervention-* psychological first aid, debriefing, crisis management, cognitive behavior therapy; *Community interventions.; Pharmacotherapy; Resilience; Conclusions, References.*

INTRODUCTION

Disasters are a phenomenon as old as mankind itself. They are a part and parcel of living in a complex unpredictable world. Disasters are often preventable, but they are not a completely inescapable phenomenon. Catastrophic events, ranging from natural disasters like earthquakes and tsunamis to manmade calamities like factory explosions, acts of terrorism can affect large populations resulting in short term and long term physical and psychological consequences. Psychiatrists and other mental health professionals play a vital part in assessing and helping individuals and communities recover from disasters in a healthy manner. Evaluation of and mental health care and psychiatric services provided to the victims of disasters constitutes Disaster Psychiatry.

DEFINITIONS AND CLASSIFICATION

The term **disaster** has multiple and varied definitions. Origins of the word **disaster** are rooted in the astrological concept that unfavourable positioning of stars result in adverse events. The term itself is derived from the Latin "dis" which means against or ill or lack and "astrum" which means stars - loosely translated as evil stars or (Farber 1967) bad luck.[1] Hence many natural disasters are often termed as "acts of God".

The World Health Organization (WHO), in 1992, defined Disaster as: "A severe psychological, ecological and psychosocial disruption, that greatly exceeds the coping capacity of the affected community."

The United Nations Coordinating Committee for Disasters stipulates that a disaster, seen from a sociological point of view, is an event located in time and space, producing conditions under which the continuity of the structures and of the social processes becomes problematic (United Nations Disaster Relief Coordinator Office 1984).[3]

The Disaster Management Act 2005 of India defined disaster as a catastrophe, mishap, calamity or grave occurrence in any area, arising from natural or manmade causes, or by accident or negligence which results in substantial loss of life or human suffering or damage to, and destruction of property, or damage to, or degradation of environment, and is of such a nature or magnitude as to be beyond the coping capacity of the community of the affected area.[4]

From an **ecologica**l point of view, a disaster is an encounter between a hazard (force of harm) and a human population in harm's way.[5]

Oxford dictionary definition of disaster is an unexpected event that kills a lot of people or causes a lot of damage (Oxford Learners thesaurus).[6]

Quarantelli (1985)[7] defined disaster as a "crisis occasion where demands exceed capabilities, " and he offered the following continuum of labels for disasters of varying magnitude relative to community resources (Quarantelli, 2006)[8]:

- Crisis - Capacity exceeds demands – with capacity to spare
- Emergency - Capacity meets or somewhat exceeds demands
- Disaster - Demands exceed capacity
- Catastrophe - Demands overwhelm and may destroy capacity.

Thus, disasters are unpredictable, uncontrollable, overwhelming events characterized by sudden onset, suffering and destruction, and significant losses of life and or property.

CLASSIFICATION OF DISASTERS

DISASTERS can be classified in several ways:

(1) NATURAL DISASTERS

Caused by forces of nature, sometimes referred to as "acts of God", penalty for past deeds).

They can be

a) Hydro meteorological disasters – e.g. floods, landslides

b) Geophysical disasters – e.g. earthquakes, tsunamis

c) Droughts, famines

d) Pandemics

(2) DISASTERS ASSOCIATED WITH HUMAN ACTIONS

Disasters caused or exacerbated by human action.

They can be Non Intentional/Intentional:

a) Non intentional/accidental – e.g. industrial accidents, building/bridge collapses and explosions. These are associated with human errors without malicious intent/intent to harm.

b) Intentional – e.g. war, civil strife, domestic or international terrorism. These are deliberate and willful acts where harm is intended by one human being to other/others.[5,9,10,11]

Complex emergencies - According to the World Health Organization and United Nations, a complex emergency has been defined as a humanitarian crisis in a country, region or society where there is considerable breakdown of authority resulting from internal or external conflict which requires an international response that goes beyond the mandate or capacity of any single agency.[12,13]

Disasters can also be classified according to the

a) **Magnitude** of the catastrophic event:
   1) **LEVEL I** - localized phenomenon, few victims, resources available.
   2) **LEVEL II** - numerous victims, local resources not enough, regional assistance required.
   3) **LEVEL III** - event with cataclysmic impact, local and regional bodies overwhelmed, national or international assistance required.[14]

b) **By exposure:**

   Margins are clear – Fires, explosions

   Destruction occurs in a graded manner – Earthquakes, storms

c) **Pre disaster Warning**

   Brief or absent – Earthquakes, terrorist attacks

   Prolonged – Cyclones, floods

d) **Duration of Impact**

   Brief – Explosions, accidents

   Prolonged – Fires, floods, hurricanes.[15]

The United Nations Development Program used the term **HAZARD** to describe "natural or human-made event that threatens to adversely affect human life, property or activity, to the extent of causing a disaster" which can be of 5 types:

NATURAL: PHYSICAL - Hydrometeorological, Geophysical disasters

NATURAL:BIOTIC, BIOLOGICAL - Pest infestations, epidemics, Pandemics

SOCIO OR PSEUDONATURAL - Human transformation of the natural environment

MANMADE TECHNOLOGICAL - Contamination, explosions

SOCIAL - Conflict including wars, civil strife.[16]

DISASTER MENTAL HEALTH

In the past, the care of disaster victims was limited to rescuing them, attending to their physical injuries, offering shelter, assistance and helping them relocate or resume their previous lives with minimum discomfort. However at present, the intense psychological suffering of the victims is being recognised. The psychosocial burden of the disaster on the individual and the community is being paid heed to. Hence current interventions for disaster management includes medical, psychological and social aspects which are implemented at different stages of the disaster and its aftermath. They attempt to prevent the development of delayed chronic psychological sequelae that would handicap the functioning of the individual or community. Disaster Mental Health has shifted from a curative to a preventive realm.

DISASTER RESPONSE

Immediately after the disaster, there is usually a period of disbelief, denial, fear or confusion and numbness. This is followed by cooperation. The community gets together to help their own. The survivors get actively involved in helping and supporting their fellow victims, in every possible way. This phase usually lasts from a day to weeks depending upon the severity, duration of exposure and availability of the relief sources from various agencies. During this period, family, neighbors and rescue workers are sources of support.

This is followed by a phase wherein external rescue and relief operations commence. Survivors may be relocated to relief camps with free health services, food, shelter and safety. Their plight is given attention and they are reassured by the powers that there will be quick restoration, compensation and rehabilitation. This often gives a sense of relief to the grief stricken survivors and this phase usually lasts for 2-4 weeks. Cleanup and rebuilding process begins. Survivors try to adapt but intrusive recollections of the events may occur resulting in distress.

At the end of this phase, relief materials and resources start weaning and attention to the plight of the survivors starts decreasing. Administration hurdles, bureaucratic delays, discrimination, injustice and corruption may lead to disillusionment. There is disappointment and often resentment when expectations of aid and restoration are not met. Individuals focus on their personal concerns and not that of their fellow victims. This phase can last from a few months to a few years. Mental health professionals play a vital role during this phase of disaster management.[17,18]

Reconstruction phase can take several years as the survivors rebuild their lives and adjust to their new world.

INDIVIDUAL RESPONSE TO DISASTER

NORMAL RESPONSES

In disaster situations, most people will experience transient psychological and behavioral symptoms that represent normal responses to an abnormal event.

In the immediate aftermath of a traumatic event, most people will exhibit symptoms such as difficulty in sleeping, easy irritability, nightmares, restlessness, lack of concentration, anger, disbelief, sadness, anxiety, fear, confusion, increased arousal or numbing, repeated thoughts about the trauma and associated distress.[19] This is often termed as **Sub diagnostic distress** [20] – a normal reaction to abnormal circumstances. Grief reactions will occur. There may also be survivor's guilt, feelings of being overwhelmed, substance use to deal with the stress and death wishes and or suicidal ideations.[18] These are usually a short term phenomenon.

ABNORMAL RESPONSES

In most survivors, the psychological response to trauma is transient and gets resolved with minimum or no significant assistance, in the months following the disaster. However, in some victims there may be chronic psychological sequelae which requires long term management.

The prevalence of psychiatric morbidity in disaster affected population ranges from **8.6 to 57.3** percent which is approximately two to three times higher than the general population.[21] However, mental health disorders occurring in the immediate post disaster period and a few months afterwards are usually self limiting. Several members in the affected community may also show subsyndromal symptoms and unexplained somatic symptoms.[18] Chronic mental health issues, psychological and behavioral changes which persist for months to years after the event, require psychological assistance.

PSYCHIATRIC MORBIDITY IN THE DISASTER AFFECTED

- Abnormal/Complicated Grief/traumatic bereavement.
- Acute stress reactions/disorder.
- Post traumatic stress disorder with or without co-morbidities.
- Post Traumatic Symptoms – Intrusive recollections, trouble concentrating, sleep disturbances, jumpiness.
- Depression, suicidal ideations.
- Adjustment disorders.
- Anxiety disorders – panic disorders, phobic

disorders, hyper vigilance, increased startle response.

- Chronic insomnia, nightmares, night terrors.
- Substance use/abuse/dependence.
- Non specific somatic symptoms - dizziness, headache, body ache.
- Dissociative symptoms
- Relapse of any pre-existing psychiatric disorder.
- Somatoform disorders and somatization.
- Illnesses secondary to physical injury – e.g. Organic mental disorders secondary to head injury, exposure to any toxins, as a response to physical disease.
- Enduring personality change after catastrophic experience/"traumatic neurosis".
- Other behavioral changes – interpersonal conflicts (reduced interaction with family, friends, aggression, violence, family conflict and domestic violence), employment issues (decreased concentration, impaired job performance, absenteesm, quitting), hostility, feelings of frustration and a sense of chaos.
- Survivors are also at risk for developing physical illnesses, particularly hypertension, asthma, chronic pain syndromes and other psychosomatic illnesses.[19,22,23]

RISK FACTORS FOR MENTAL HEALTH ISSUES/PSYCHIATRIC MORBIDITY FOLLOWING DISASTERS

FACTORS RELATED TO **EXPOSURE TO DISASTER**

- **Type** of disaster:

  Studies say natural disasters have the mildest mental health consequences while human errors and technological accidents have moderate consequences on mental health morbidity. Acts of terrorism which are wilful malicious actions of humans against their own species, are associated with most severe mental health sequelae.[11,24]
- **Severity** of disaster – intensity and degree of exposure, number of casualties, injuries and fatalities.

  The greater the size of geographic area involved & magnitude of destruction of life and property, the risk of psychiatric morbidity is higher.

Frequency of Disaster occurrence:

Multiple, simultaneous, serial or cascading events will have more impact than single events.

- Life threatening events, perception of ongoing threat, lack of sense of safety and adequate warning, unpredictability further increases the stress.
- Duration of impact and duration of disruption of vital services, displacement from homes also has a profound impact on the mental health of the disaster affected individuals.

  Knowledge of exposure to toxin – when there is uncertainty of the level of exposure to toxins, the long term effects is also extremely stressful.[25,26]

Other risk factors are:

- **Loss** - Harm or death to spouse/child/ other family members, witnessing/learning of harm to loved ones.
- **Age** - Middle aged individuals – who carry burden of finances and other responsibilities.[15,27]
- **Gender** – women are more prone to PTSD, depression and anxiety disorders.Men are more prone to substance use.[11]
- **Vulnerable population** – children and adolescents, elderly, physically disabled.[28]
- Low educational status

- Belonging to ethnic minority
- Poverty and low socioeconomic status, unemployed or recent job loss
- Substance users
- Poor family and social support, lack of social integration
- Pre existing mental disorders and chronic general medical conditions
- Poor coping skills/capacity
- Continuing difficulties in the aftermath of disasters like delay in getting compensation, reconstruction and difficulty in the rehabilitation of physical injuries.[29,30]
- Individuals working in disaster management operations - rescue workers, paramedics, emergency physicians, hospital employees are also at risk for developing mental health issues due to vicarious exposure to the disaster and observation of its catastrophic aftermath.
- In case of accidents involving human errors, causing death or severe harm to another is a risk factor for the development of psychiatric illness.[5,11,15,18,22,23,31,32]

PROTECTIVE FACTORS

Absence of any past history of psychiatric illness, good social support, healthy coping mechanisms, resilience.[5,15,33]

ABNORMAL GRIEF REACTIONS

Abnormal grief reactions can be delayed, absent, oscillating and exploding grief responses.[18] Excessive yearning for the deceased, difficulty in accepting or denial of death, inability to let go of the loved one and move on in life is seen in abnormal grief. Prolonged grief reaction has been reported in 14–76% of bereaved populations after natural and human caused disasters.[34,35,36,37] Complicated grief interferes in the process of recovery and in the biological, psychological and socio-occupational functioning.

ACUTE STRESS REACTION/DISORDER

It usually occurs within the first two days of traumatic events.[11] It is characterized by dissociative symptoms, a sense of numbing, detachment, or absence of emotional responsiveness, a reduction in awareness of his or her surroundings, depersonalization - derealization, inability to recall important aspects of the trauma, experiencing the traumatic event in the form of recurrent images, thoughts, dreams, flashbacks, distress on exposure to and avoidance of reminders of the traumatic event, anxiety, hyper arousal and significant impairment in socio occupational functioning.[38] These symptoms usually last for less than a month. It is very similar to PTSD but differs in the duration and presence of dissociative symptoms during or after the traumatic event.[18,22,23]

POST TRAUMATIC STRESS DISORDER (PTSD)

PTSD is one of the most important psychological disorder associated with disasters. Post disaster, prevalence of PTSD ranges from 4-60%.[39] When exposed to actual or threatened death or serious injury, or a threat to the physical integrity of self or others (which often happens in disasters), the person often responds with intense fear, helplessness, or horror. The traumatic event is then persistently re-experienced in the form of recurrent, distressing recollections of the event - images, thoughts, dreams, illusions, hallucinations, and flashbacks. There is also intense distress when reminded of the traumatic events and vigorous attempts are made to avoid them. There is a numbing of general responsiveness, trauma related selective amnesia, detachment and a sense of hopelessness. Symptoms of hyperarousal like easy distractibility, insomnia, easy irritability, hypervigilance, exaggerated startle response are also seen. These symptoms last for more than a month. Acute PTSD resolves within 3 months, chronic PTSD lasts for more than 3 months. Delayed onset PTSD shows emergence of symptoms 6 months after the traumatic event.[38] Peritraumatic panic and dissociative symptoms are predictors for subsequent development of PTSD.[40,41] PTSD is often co-morbid with depression, anxiety disorders and substance use.[23] Family history of psychopathology, history of childhood abuse, low IQ, prior exposure to trauma have also found to be risk factors for development of PTSD.[42–46]

DEPRESSION

Depression, adjustment disorder and other mood disorders are common following a disaster.[18,22] Depression is the second most common disorder to emerge in the aftermath of a disaster.[27] Post disaster depression is especially common in individuals who have had a history of major depression in the past.[47,48] It is also seen co-morbid with PTSD, anxiety disorders and substance use which further increases the disability, in the disaster affected population.

ANXIETY DISORDERS

Disaster victims show higher rates of anxiety disorders like panic disorder, phobic disorders as compared to general population. However anxiety disorders are less common than PTSD and Major Depression.[47–49]

SUBSTANCE USE

Several studies have found increased patterns of alcohol, tobacco and use of other drugs following disasters especially in individuals with pre existing substance use.[47–49] Substance abuse is common 6-12 months after the disaster period.[23] However this may often be a form of self medication or an effort to cope with the traumatic events and not necessarily indicate a problem demanding clinical response or intervention.[50,51]

SOMATIZATION

Somatization and medically unexplained physical symptoms are common among disaster survivors.[11,23] Sometimes it may indicate anxiety or depressive disorder and should be managed appropriately.[23]

ENDURING PERSONALITY CHANGE AFTER CATASTROPHIC EXPERIENCE

"Enduring personality change after catastrophic experience" (ICD 10 - F62.0) is characterized by symptoms like a mistrustful attitude toward the world, social withdrawal, feelings of emptiness or of being threatened, and estrangement.[52] There may be associated non-specific symptoms, such as physical, psychological, and sexual asthenia; anxiety, somatic complaints (especially in children).[53]

MENTAL HEALTH OF COMMUNITY

After a disaster the collective behavior of the community may be adaptive or maladaptive. Adaptive collective behavior involves fulfilling one's assigned responsibilities, evacuating the affected area in an orderly fashion, helping others, normal mourning, regaining autonomy, reconstruction and resuming normal professional and social activities. Maladaptive behavior is panic, disorganised flight or freeze reaction, vandalism, violence and aggression, paranoia and hostility, dependency and inability to regain autonomy.[53]

DISASTER AND CHILDREN

Children and adolescents are a biologically and psychologically vulnerable population. Hence effects of disasters on them can be devastating. While they may develop grief reactions, acute stress reaction, PTSD and depression like adult survivours, they also exhibit features of separation anxiety, non specific bodily symptoms, school refusal, deterioration in academic performance, Oppositional Defiant disorder and Conduct disorder. Feelings of guilt and regressive behavior are also common. Their responses are affected by their age, stage of development and the reactions of the significant adults in their lives. Adolescents may engage in risk taking behavior (Pynoos, Nadar 1988, 1992, Norwood et al 2000, Pynoos et al., 2007, Math et Al., 2015).[18,22,54,55,56]

NEUROBIOLOGY OF MENTAL HEALTH MORBIDITY IN DISASTERS

GENETICS

Susceptibility to stress related psychopathology such as PTSD may be associated with genetic factors. There is increased concordance for PTSD in monozygotic twins as compared with dizygotic twins.[57] Studies have shown that children of adults who were Holocaust survivors with PTSD show a greater prevalence of PTSD in response to their own traumatic events.[58] However research regarding specific genes and chromosomes involved are scarce and this remains an interesting area for further research and exploration.

An amplified catecholaminergic response to trauma could be responsible for intense panic, and persons in such a state of fear are likely to misinterpret bodily cues and hence perceive greater danger than which is actually present.

Anticipatory fears, or other predisposing/pre existing cognitive factors might lead to such an exaggerated catecholaminergic response to a calamity.[19]

Sympathetic Nervous System

There is sympathetic hyperactivity in PTSD afflicted individuals during stress (especially stress associated with traumatic reminders). Exposure to trauma related stressors causes exaggerated catecholamine response, increased sympathetic nervous system activation, increased physiological activity (especially heart rate). Prolonged and persistent activation of the sympathetic nervous system may eventually lead to development of PTSD symptoms. Research shows increased 24 hour urinary excretion of epinephrine and Nor Epinephrine and decreased numbers of alpha-2 adrenergic receptors on the surface of platelets, which indicates chronic elevations of epinephrine and nor epinephrine.[19,55]

HPA AXIS

Individuals with low cortisol levels are at risk for development of PTSD. Dexamethasone also shows an exaggerated response in these individuals (during Dexamethasone Suppression test (DST). This is markedly different than findings in major depressive disorders.[59]

Lower circulating cortisol levels may disrupt (or delay) the process of physiological recovery by failing to inhibit the activation of the hypothalamus/pituitary. This failure of inhibition will result in increased corticotropin releasing factor (CRF) which results in higher Adreno Cortico Tropic Hormone (ACTH) response which further stimulates the sympathetic nervous system. Low cortisol leads to longer availability and action of Norepinephrine.[60,61] There is HPA hyper reactivity in PTSD.

Stress sensitization of Sympathetic Nervous system and HPA axis is another contributory factor for PTSD.[59]

Adrenergic activation occurs during periods of arousal associated with trauma. This causes intense panic, fear and distress. Excess of Catecholemine in the presence of low cortisol levels facilitates learning. Hence the intensely distressing traumatic event would be strongly encoded and consolidated in memory. This will result in cognitive distortions which would lead to distressing recollections of the events. When exposed to cues/reminders, the trauma memory and associated distress and fear recur and further make the cognitive distortions and their association with fear stronger.This increases the state of arousal and hinders the recover yprocess.[19,62,63]

Hippocampus and Amygdala are associated with fear and identification of danger. Structural and functional neuroimaging studies in PTSD have shown changes in their volume and/or activation in response to traumatic reminders. Reduced hippocampal volumes, exaggerated blood flow to amygdala and other paralimbic regions, as well as relative decrease in prefrontal cortical regional cerebral blood flow has also been found in studies.[59]

INTERVENTIONS

Intervention during disasters involves four different stages:

(a) **The pre impact phase** - Steps are taken to build "mental immunity"[64] in all members of the vulnerable/at risk community so that they are able to recognise the seriousness and nature of the calamity, organize available resources adequately and perform optimally under adverse circumstances.

(b) **The impact phase** - Evaluation of the impact of the disaster on the individuals and community as a whole is done. Strategies for acute, immediate intervention are planned and executed.

(c) **The phase immediately after** the occurrence of the event - Detailed evaluation of the affected population is done on an individual basis. Strategies are carried out to deal with abnormal responses effectively and prevent development of chronic mental health morbidity.

(d) **The long-term phase** - treatment is provided to survivors who need long-term assistance. Delayed onset or chronic mental health morbidity is treated.[31,65–67]

Mental health professionals play a vital role from pre-disaster phase, well into post disaster period. They have a multidimensional and multifaceted part to play, serving as a bridge between the chaos outside and confusion within the survivors. They serve as a liaison between the various organizations and personnel who are involved in mitigating the suffering of the afflicted. Psychiatrists have to evaluate normal and abnormal reactions to the calamity and decide who are in need of immediate and long term assistance. They have to decide what interventions have to be carried out at an individual and community level and adapt those interventions to the survivors in a pragmatic and fruitful manner to for maximum effectiveness.

DURING PREDISASTER PERIOD

PREPAREDNESS

Mental health professionals are involved in psychoeducation and disbursing practical pre-emptive knowledge to the general public. Psychiatrists conduct various activities to teach community and general population about life skills and about disaster mental health. They also collaborate with various existing agencies like governmental agencies, NGO's and community health workers to form a Disaster Response Network. They also provide disaster response training to the disaster relief personnel especially regarding the ramifications of the disaster on mental health. They train the first responders to identify common mental health issues, make appropriate referrals, first aid skills (both medical and psychological), counseling, stress management and life skill technics. Hence, they work at improving community support systems and resilience.[18] The involvement of psychiatrists in developing disaster response plans in the schools, hospitals and in the community is an ideal way to develop working relationships with local officials and personnel who are the immediate responders to disasters. Training also includes frequent realistic disaster drills to assess preparedness of the community in the face of a calamity.[22]

DURING POST DISASTER PERIOD

IMMEDIATE PHASE

Immediately following disaster, psychiatrists play an important role in disaster relief. They are a part of the multidisciplinary relief team for mitigation of the suffering of the victims. They have to assess the severity of psychological, social impact on the community and organise mental health teams at disaster sites. Needs of the community and resources available and socio cultural aspects of the affected community also have to be evaluated. When necessary a Triage of psychiatric casualties and ‘at risk ’individuals among the survivors has to be done.[53] Medical and psychological first aid and crisis intervention has to be done in this phase. Appraisal and management of any pre-existing mental illness, substance abuse/dependence has to be carried out. Targeted mental health interventions, appropriate referral, promotion of coping and resilience, stress management of the rescue personnel are also necessary at this stage. Disaster outreach activities, adequate dissemination of accurate information to prevent chaos and confusion, collaboration with administrative, funding agencies for support are done.[18,22]

LATER PHASE

At later stages, mental health professionals are involved in treatment of survivors with mental illness and others in need. Psychiatrists continue capacity building activities, train resourceful community members like private physicians/doctors, primary health care workers, school personnel, anganwadi workers and community leaders for adequate and effective management of the psychosocial aftermath of disasters. They also hold community outreach camps to lead the community towards faster recovery.[18,22]

Assessment and intervention should be commenced as early as possible. Initial evaluation and interventions ought to be carried out in the community itself instead of in clinical settings to reduce stigma and resistance to mental heath services.[31] Terms like psychiatric illness/mental illness should be avoided while interacting with the affected community to prevent labeling and stigma associated with mental health issues. This in turn will encourage the afflicted survivors to actively seek recourse for their agony instead of suffering in silence. Socio cultural perspectives, values and belief system of the affected community have to be considered during the disaster management process to facilitate cooperation, prevent severe morbidity and promote early recovery of the afflicted community.[18,32]

Disaster relief workers are also at risk for mental health issues. They are the tertiary victims of disasters and can develop a multitude of stress related issues including compassion fatigue, burnout and vicarious traumatization.[68] Hence adequate evaluation of their physical and psychological health is imperative. Appropriate care and support has to be provided to them also.

PSYCHOLOGICAL INTERVENTIONS

PSYCHOLOGICAL FIRST AID (PFA)

Psychological first aid is one of the initial interventions carried out in disaster survivors. Like physical first aid, its importance cannot be overstated. The main goal of psychological first aid is to relieve immediate distress and to prevent or minimize the development of future psychiatric morbidity.

The main **components** of PFA:

- Getting in touch with survivors in a compassionate, empathetic yet non intrusive manner.
- Providing accurate information about the disaster, about the current disaster response status and resources and services available.
- Protecting survivors from unnecessary exposure to additional trauma or reminders of what they have gone through.
- Immediate physical care and first aid.
- Helping to locate displaced/missing family.
- Encouraging them to talk about their experience for ventilation or processing their experience. However the process is voluntary and they should not be forced to share if they are unwilling.
- Validation/normalization of their reactions when they vent or try to process their experience.
- Psychoeducating survivors on stress and healthy coping which would enable them to feel a sense of better control on their lives.
- Teaching brief relaxation and stress management technics.
- Getting survivors in touch with various support agencies for facilitation of recovery from the calamity.
- Providing practical assistance to vulnerable individuals and identification, monitoring and caring for high risk individuals and those who need more intensive care.
- Focus is on "here and now".[18,31,69]

PSYCHOLOGICAL DEBRIEFING

They are group discussions that occur within 48-72 h after a traumatic event. The survivors are encouraged to talk about the trauma in detail, elaborating not just facts of what they went through but also their thoughts, feelings and emotions during the event. Immediate processing of the catastrophic event is supposed to help the survivor to cognitively restructure the perceived disaster event so that its memory is less traumatic. When these disaster intervention technics are carried out early, there are fewer chances for development of maladaptive coping and behavior patterns. Debriefing and defusing also helps in decreasing sense of isolation, assists emotional release and enhances social support.[18,22,31,64]

CRISIS INTERVENTION AND CRISIS REDUCTION COUNSELING

Crisis reduction counseling is conducted with the individual or the family. The goal is to evaluate the current psychological state, identify mental issues and provide appropriate support.

Crisis intervention helps decrease extreme emotional distress immediately after a disaster. Assessment of the extent of mental health impairment, need for long term assistance is done. Emotional support is provided in a practical manner. Appropriate advice is given on how to maintain emotional equilibrium.[31]

COGNITIVE BEHAVIOR THERAPY (CBT)

Studies have shown that trauma focused CBT

done within 3 months of a traumatic event appears to be effective.[70] CBT is effective in reducing risk of developing subsequent psychopathology.[71,72] Technics used include Stress Inoculation Training (SIT), exposure technics like systematic desensitization, relaxation technics, biofeedback, cognitive restructuring, anger management technics, social skills training.[64,73]

Eye Movement Desensitization and Reprocessing **(EMDR)** is another technic which has been considered for the management of psychological morbidity following disasters. The basis of EMDR is the observation that lateral eye movements help in cognitive processing of trauma. This technic is used to relieve the psychological distress which is associated with the memories of traumatic events.[64,74]

Other interventions include somatic awareness approach (sensory motor psychotherapy)[75] and brief psychoanalytical psychotherapy.[76]

COMMUNITY BASED INTERVENTIONS

Specialized care is required only by a few individuals in the disaster affected population. Hence a significant amount of care is community based, informal and done outside of clinical settings. This helps in reducing the stigma associated with stress related issues and encourages active help seeking behavior. This brings the community together to rebuild their lives in a healthy manner and move forward. Appropriate training of locals and community health workers is an essential component of this process. Simple community-based interventions like group discussions, structuring of daily activities, yoga, meditation, prayers meetings and spiritual activities, family based activities, sports are extremely effective. Displacement of the survivors should be avoided or minimized. Accurate information and facts should be dispensed to them to keep them aware of the going on's and gain their trust. Parents and teachers should be psychoeducated. Children's education should be continued as smoothly as possible. Survivors should be engaged in community based day to day activities. This leads to effective psychosocial rehabilitation which help in management of milder and sub-syndromal symptoms and prevention of serious mental health morbidity. Psychoeducation and working hand in hand with community leaders while helping them cope with their unique stress (due to the leadership roles) also helps in faster recovery of the affected community.[18,22,77]

PHARMACOTHERAPY

While symptomatic treatment is often given to mitigate acute symptoms like anxiety, panic, insomnia, there are no well controlled studies showing that prophylactic use of medicine decreases psychiatric morbidity.[18] Their use may be justified to prevent relapse in pre-existing psychiatric illness, in substance withdrawal and severe depression. But there is paucity of adequate research data for the same. However, if survivors do develop psychiatric morbidity, prompt and appropriate management, in terms of anti-anxiety or antidepressant medications should be administered.

POSITIVE ASPECTS OF DISASTER RESPONSE

Adverse circumstances can also lead to tremendous positive growth. Many survivors consider the traumatic event as a learning experience to prepare them for the vagaries of life. They appreciate the importance of being prepared for adversities, gain a newfound appreciation for life and develop empathy towards others.

RESILIENCE

Resilience is the ability to recover from or adjust to adverse circumstances without significant effort. Factors which characterize resilience are maturity, willingness to consider and be prepared for the unthinkable. Pragmatism and ability to get detached and "let go", ability to accept a situation as it is (What is) instead of lamenting about how they ought to have been (If only) improves resilience.

Resilience also involves an ability to accept lack of control over circumstances and function optimally nonetheless. A resilient individual is flexible and capable of making practical decisions, is independent and self sufficient, optimistic and hopeful towards the future. A supportive, united community with strong selfless leadership, social and family support, minimal displacement or loss of pre existing structure of life and faith are associated with resilience. Resilience is associated with positive outcome in the aftermath of a catastrophe.[15,78–82]

According to a Red Cross report, in the period 1967 to 1991, disaster affected nearly 17, 000, 000 people living in developing countries each year. However in the same period about 700, 000 people in developed countries were impacted by disasters (ratio of 166 to 1).[83] Hence developing countries are a population particularly vulnerable to disasters and their aftermath while developed countries have certain systems in place for timely and adequate disaster response. There is a paucity of the same in most developing countries. This results in enormous losses of life and property in developed nations. Hence the development of a disaster management protocol is of foremost significance. The Indian Psychiatric Society has a taskforce on disaster management to recommend inclusion of mental health care in national strategies for disaster response.[84]

CONCLUSIONS

Disasters are a universal phenomenon in today's world and hence Disaster Psychiatry is of utmost importance. Disaster Psychiatry encompasses a wide range of clinical ventures, from public health preparations to early and long term psychiatric and psychotheraupetic interventions to alleviate stress in child and adult survivors. Psychiatrists have a key role to play in caring for the victims and community after a disaster, building up resilience to bounce back from adversity and move forward towards a better life.

"A great disaster is a symbol to us to remember all the big things of life and forget the small things, of which we have thought too much"

– Jawaharlal Nehru

BIBLIOGRAPHY

1. Farber IJ: Psychological aspects of mass disasters. Journal of the National Medical Association 1967; 59:340–345.
2. World Health Organization. Psychosocial consequences of disasters: Prevention and management. Geneva (Switzerland): World Health Organization; 1992.
3. United Nations Disaster Relief Coordinator Office (1984) Disaster Prevention and Mitigation, Vol. II: Preparedness Aspects. United Nations, New York
4. The. Disaster. Management. act. Available from: http://nidm.gov.in/DM_act2005.pdf 2005
5. Shultz J, Espinel Z, Galea S, Reissman D. Disaster ecology: implications for disaster psychiatry. In: Ursano R, Fullerton C, Wiesaeth L, Raphael B, ed., *Textbook of Disaster Psychiatry*, Cambridge university press; 2007.69-76.

6. Oxford learners thesaurus. Oxford University Press.
7. Quarantelli, E.L. Social support systems: some behavioral patterns in the context of mass evacuation activities. In Disasters and Mental Health: Selected Contemporary Perspectives, ed. Sowder B; 1985.122–136.
8. Quarantelli, E.L. Emergencies, disasters, and catastrophes are different phenomena; 2006. Available at http://www.udel.edu/DRC/preliminary/pp304.pdf
9. Guha-Sapir D, Hargitt D, Hoyois P. Center for Research on the Epidemiology of Disasters. Thirty Years of Natural Disasters: 1974–2003: The Numbers. Louvainla-Neuve: Presses Universitaires de Louvain; 2004.
10. Center for Research on the Epidemiology of Disasters (CRED). EM-DAT Data Base. Brussels: Universite Catholique de Louvain; 2005.
11. North C. Epidemiology of disaster mental health. In: Ursano R, Fullerton C, Wiesaeth L, Raphael B, ed.*Textbook of Disaster Psychiatry*, Cambridge university press; 2007.29-41.
12. United Nations Development Program. Reducing Disaster Risk: A Challenge for Development, 2004. Available at United Nations Development Program, Bureau for Crisis Prevention and Recovery site: www.undp.org/bcpr.
13. World Health Organization. Health action in relation to crises and emergencies. WHO Fifty-Eighth World Health Assembly, Provisional Agenda Item 13.3. Geneva: World Health Organization, 2005.
14. Lopez- Ibor J. What is a Disaster? In: Lopez-Ibor J, Christodoulou G, Maj M, Sartorius N, Okasha A, ed. Disasters and Mental Health. John Wiley and sons Ltd; 2005, 1-9.
15. Mcfarlane A. Psychiatric Morbidity Following Disasters: Epidemiology, Risk and Protective Factors. In: Lopez-Ibor J, Christodoulou G, Maj, Sartorius N, Okasha A, ed. Disasters and Mental Health. John Wiley and sons Ltd; 2005, 37-56.
16. World Health Organization/EHA/EHTP. Emergency Health Training Programe for Africa. Training Modules. Geneva: World Health Organization, 1999.
17. Cohen R, Culp C, Genser S. Human Problems in Major Disasters: A Training Curriculum for Emergency Medical Personnel. US Government Printing Office, Washington, DC, 1987.
18. Math S, Nirmala M, Moirangthem S, Kumar N. Disaster Management: Mental Health Perspective. Indian Journal of Psychological Medicine 2015; 37(3): 261-269.
19. Yehuda R, Bierer L. Re-evaluating the Link between Disasters and Psychopathology. In: Lopez-Ibor J, Christodoulou G, Maj M, Sartorius N, Okasha A, ed. Disasters and Mental Health, John Wiley and sons Ltd; 2005, 65-77.
20. North C.S., Pfefferbaum, B. Research on the mental health effects of terrorism. Journal of the American Medical Association 2002; 288: 633–636.
21. Udomratn P. Mental health and the psychosocial consequences of natural disasters in Asia. Int Rev Psychiatry 2008; 20:441-4.
22. Norwood A, Ursano R, Fullerton C. (2000). Disaster Psychiatry: Principles and Practice. Psychiatric Quarterly, Human Sciences Press, Inc.2000; 71(3):207-224.
23. Ursano R, Fullerton C. Psychological and Psychopathological Consequences of Disasters. In:Lopez-Ibor J, Christodoulou G, Maj M, Sartorius N, Okasha A, ed. Disasters and Mental Health, John Wiley and sons Ltd.2005, 13-30.
24. Baum A, Fleming I. Implications of psychological research on stress and technological accidents. Am Psychol 1993; 48:665-72.
25. Holloway HC, Norwood AE, Fullerton CS, et al. The threat of biological weapons: Prophylaxis and mitigation of psychological and social consequences. Journal of the American Medical Association1997; 278(5):425–427.
26. DiGiovanni J, Cleto. Domestic terrorism with chemical or biological agents: Psychiatric aspects. American Journal of Psychiatry 1999; 156(10):1500–1505.
27. Norris FH, Friedman MJ, Watson PJ, Byrne CM, Diaz E, Kaniasty K. 60, 000 disaster victims speak: Part I. An empirical review of the empirical literature, 1981–2001. Psychiatry: Interpersonal and biological processes 2002; 65(3): 207–239.
28. Suar D, Kar S. Social and behavioral consequences of the Orissa Supercyclone. J

Health Management. 2005; 7:263–75.

29. Burnett K, Ironson G, Benight C, Wynings C, Greenwood D, Carver C, et al. Measurement of perceived disruption during rebuilding following Hurricane Andrew. J Trauma Stress 1997; 10: 673–681.
30. Kwon Y, Maruyama S, Morimoto K. Life events and posttraumatic stress in Hanshin-Awaji earthquake victims. Environ Health Prevent Med, 2001; 6:97–103.
31. Rao TSS. Managing Impact of Natural Disasters: Some Mental Health Issues. Indian Journal of Psychiatry, 2004; 46(4):289-292.
32. Kar N. Indian research on disaster and mental health. Indian J Psychiatry 2010; 52:286-90.
33. Norris F, Kaniasty K. Received and perceived social support in times of stress: a test of the social support deterioration deterrence model. J Person Soc Psychol 1996; 71:498–511.
34. Ghaffari – Nejad A, Ahmadi-Mousavi M, Gandomkar M, Reihani-Kermani H. The prevalence of complicated grief among Bam earthquake survivors in Iran. Archives of Iranian Medicine. 2007; 10:525-528.
35. Johannesson K.B, Lundlin T, Hultman CM, Lindam A, Dyster-Aas J, Arneberg P, Michel P. The effect of traumatic bereavement on tsunami exposed survivors. Journal of Traumatic Stress 2009; 22:497-504.
36. Kristensen P., Wiesaeth L., Heir T. (2009). Psychiatric disorders among disaster bereaved: An interview study of individuals directly or not directly exposed to the 2004 tsunami. Depression and Anxiety 26, 1127-33
37. Kristensen, P, Weisæth L, Heir T. Bereavement and Mental Health after Sudden and Violent Losses: A Review. Psychiatry: Interpersonal and Biological Processes 2012; 75(1), 76–97.
38. American Psychiatric association. Diagnostic and Statistical Manual of Mental Disorders: DSM IV TR.Washington DC: American Psychiatric Association, 2000.
39. Young BH, Ford JD, Ruzek JI, Friedman M, Gusman FD. Disaster mental health services: A guide for clinicians and administrators. National Center for Post-Traumatic Stress Disorder, Palo Alto, California.1998. Available from: http://www. ncptsd.va.gov/publications/disaster/index.html.
40. Galea S, Ahern J, Resnick H, Kilpatrick D, Bucuvalas M, Gold J, et al. Psychological sequelae of the September 11 terrorist attacks. N Engl J Med, 2002; 346: 982–987.
41. Ozer EJ, Best SR, Lipsey TL, Weiss DS. Predictors of posttraumatic stress disorder and symptoms in adults: a meta-analysis. Psychol Bull, 2003; 129: 52-73.
42. Breslau N, Davis GC, Andreski P, Peterson E. Traumatic events and posttraumatic stress disorder in an urban population of young adults. Arch GenPsychiatry 1991; 48: 216–222.
43. Breslau N, Chilcoat HD, Kessler RC, Davis G. Previous exposure to trauma and PTSD effects of subsequent trauma: results from the Detroit Area Survey of Trauma. Am J Psychiatry 1999; 156:902–907.
44. Brewin CR, Andrews B, Valentine JD. Meta-analysis of risk factors for posttraumatic stress disorder in trauma-exposed adults. J Consult Clin Psychol 2000; 68: 748–766.
45. Nishith P, Mechanic MB, Resick PA. Prior interpersonal trauma: the contribution to current PTSD symptoms in female rape victims. J Abnorm Psychol 2000; 109: 20–25.
46. Silva RR, Alpert M, Munoz DM, Singh S, Matzner F, Dummitt S. Stress and vulnerability to posttraumatic stress disorder in children and adolescents. Am J Psychiatry 2000; 157:1229-1235.
47. North CS, Smith EM, Spitznagel EL. Posttraumatic stress disorder in survivors of a mass shooting. American Journal of Psychiatry 1994; 151: 82–88.
48. North CS, Nixon S.J, Shariat S, et al. Psychiatric disorders among survivors of the Oklahoma City bombing. Journal of the American Medical Association 1999; 282: 755-762.
49. David D, Mellman TA, Mendoza LM et al. Psychiatric morbidity following Hurricane Andrew. Journal of Traumatic Stress 1996; 9:607–612.
50. Jacobsen LK, Southwick SM, Kosten TR. Substance use disorders in patients with posttraumatic stress disorder: a review of the literature. American Journal of Psychiatry 2001; 158:1184-1190.

51. Saxon AJ, Davis TM, Sloan KL et al. Trauma, symptoms of posttraumatic stress disorder and associated problems among incarcerated veterans. Am Psychiatric Assoc 2001; 52:959-964.
52. APA 6th edition. World Health Organization. The ICD 10 classification of mental and behavioral disorders: Clinical descriptions and Diagnostic guidelines.Geneva: World Health Organization.1992.
53. Crocq, L, Crocq MA, Chiapello A, Damiani C. Organization of Mental Health Services for Disaster Victims. In: Lopez-Ibor J, Christodoulou G, Maj M, Sartorius N, Okasha A. eds., Disasters and Mental Health. John Wiley and sons Ltd; 2005, 99-120.
54. Pynoos RS, Nader K. Psychological first aid and treatment approach to children exposed to community violence: Research implications. Journal of Traumatic Stress 1988; 4:445–473.
55. Nader K, Pynoos R. School disaster: Planning and initial interventions. Journal of Social Behavior and Personality1992; 8:1-21.
56. Pynoos R, Steinberg A, Brymer M. Children and disasters: public mental health approaches. In: Ursano R, Fullerton C, Wiesaeth L, Raphael B, ed. Textbook of Disaster Psychiatry, Cambridge university press, 2007, 48-65.
57. True WR, Rice J, Eisen SA, Heath AC, Goldberg J, Lyons M.J, et al. A twin study of genetic and environmental contributions to liability for posttraumatic stress disorder. Arch Gen Psychiatry 1993; 50:257–264.
58. Yehuda R, Schmeidler J, Wainberg M, Binder-Brynes K, Duvdevani T. Vulnerability to posttraumatic stress disorder in adult offspring of Holocaust survivors. Am J Psychiatry 1998; 155:1163-1171.
59. Smith R, Katz C, Charney D, Southwick S. Neurobiology of disaster exposure: fear, anxiety, trauma, and resilience. In: Ursano R, Fullerton C, Wiesaeth L, Raphael B, ed., Textbook of Disaster Psychiatry, Cambridge university press, 2007, 97-112.
60. Pacak K., Palkovitz M., Kopin IJ, Goldstein DS. Stress-induced norepinephrine release in the hypothalamic paraventricular nucleus and pituitary-adrenocortical and sympathoadrenal activity: in vivo microdialysis studies. Frontiers in Neuroendocrinology 1995; 16:89-150.
61. Holsboer F. The corticosteroid receptor hypothesis of depression. Neuropsychopharmacology 2001; 23:477-501.
62. Yehuda R. Posttraumatic stress disorder. N Engl J Med, 2002; 346:108-114.
63. Cahill L, Prins B, Weber M, McGaugh JL. Adrenergic activation and memory for emotional events. Nature 1994; 371:702–704.
64. Benyakar M, Collazo C. Psychological Interventions for People Exposed to Disasters. In: Lopez-Ibor J, Christodoulou G, Maj M, Sartorius N, Okasha A ed., Disasters and Mental Health. John Wiley and sons Ltd 2005, 81-94.
65. Solomon Z, Laor N, Weiler D, Muller U, Hadar O, Waysman M, et al. The psychological impact of the Gulf War: a study of acute stress in Israeli evacuees. Arch Gen Psychiatry 1991; 50:320-321.
66. Solomon Z. Immediate and long-term effects of traumatic combat stress among Israeli veterans of the Lebanon War. In Wilson JP, Raphael B Eds., International Handbook of Traumatic Stress Syndromes, Plenum, NewYork, 1993, 321-332.
67. Lebigot F. The advantages of immediate and postimmediate care following psychic trauma. Presented at the 5th World Congress of the International Association for Emergency Psychiatry, Brussels, 15–17 October, 1998.
68. McCann IL, Pearlman LA. Vicarious traumatization. A framework, the psychological effects of working with victims. J Trauma Stress 1990; 3: 131-149.
69. World Health Organization. War Trauma Foundation and World Vision International (2011). Psychological first aid: Guide for field workers. WHO: Geneva. Available from: http://www.searo.who.int/srilanka/documents/psychological_first_aid_guide_for_field_workers.pdf
70. Roberts NP, Kitchiner NJ, Kenardy J, Bisson JI. Systematic review and meta-analysis of multiple-session, early interventions following traumatic events. Am J Psychiatry 2009; 166:293-301.
71. Layne CM, Saltzman WR, Poppleton L, Burlin-

game GM, Pasalic A, Durakovic E, *et al.* Effectiveness of a school-based group psychotherapy program for war-exposed adolescents: A randomized controlled trial. J Am Acad Child Adolesc Psychiatry 2008; 47:1048-62.

72. Duffy M, Gillespie K, Clark DM. Post-traumatic stress disorder in the context of terrorism and other civil conflict in Northern Ireland: Randomised controlled trial. BMJ 2007; 334:1147.
73. Kilpatrick DG, Veronen LJ, Resick PA. Psychological sequelae to rape: assessment and treatment strategies. In Dolays DM, Meredith RL, Ciminero AR, Eds., Behavioral Medicine: Assessment and Treatment Strategies, Plenum Press, New York, 1982, 473-497.
74. Van Etten ML, Taylor S. Comparative efficacy of treatments for posttraumatic stress disorder: a meta-analysis. Clin Psychol Psychother, 1998; 5:126– 145.
75. Ogden P, Minton K. Sensorimotor psychotherapy: one method for processing traumatic memory. Traumatology, 2000, 6.
76. Lindy JD. Focal psychoanalytic psychotherapy of posttraumatic stress disorder. In Wilson JP, Raphael B, Eds., International Handbook of Traumatic Stress Syndromes, Plenum, New York, 1993, 803-810.
77. Math SB, Tandon S, Girimaji SC, Benegal V, Kumar U, Hamza A, *et al.* Psychological impact of the tsunami on children and adolescents from the andaman and nicobar islands. Prim Care Companion. J Clin Psychiatry 2008; 10:31-7.
78. Taylor V. Good news about disaster. Psychol Today, 1977; 11:93–94, 124-126.
79. Ursano RJ. The Vietnam era prisoner of war: precaptivity personality and development of psychiatric illness. Am J Psychiatry 1981; 138:315–318.
80. Ursano RJ. Commentary. Posttraumatic stress disorder: the stressor criterion. J Nerv Ment Dis 1987; 175: 273-275.
81. Quarentelli EL. An assessment of conflicting views on mental health: the consequences of traumatic events. In Figley CR, ed., Trauma and its Wake, Brunner/Mazel, New York.1985, 173-215.
82. Vaillant GE. Mental health. Am J Psychiatry 2003; 160:1373-1384.
83. International Federation of Red Cross and Red Crescent Societies, World Disaster Report, 1993. Nijhoff, Dordrecht.
84. Mohandas E. Roadmap to Indian Psychiatry. Indian J Psychiatry 2009; 51:173-179.

Transcultural Psychiatry 66

Pavitra KS • Shubrata Kalmane

INTRODUCTION

Transcultural Psychiatry is the discipline that deals with the description, definition, assessment and management of psychiatric conditions in relation to the cultural factors in a biopsychosocial context. It helps us in understanding psychopathology and its treatment completely. Though Transcultural Psychiatry deals primarily with cultural issues in psychiatry, the principles from Transcultural Psychiatry can be used to deliver effective patient care in any other medical discipline as well.

The boundaries between what is normal and what is pathological may vary from culture to culture. Whether a behavior is normal or abnormal many a time needs to be decided based on the cultural background of an individual. Likewise, whether the treatment needs to be instituted or not also may depend upon culture.

The awareness of the significance of culture may correct mistaken interpretations of psychopathology. Culture contributes to vulnerability and suffering. It also provides coping strategies and suggests help seeking options. It can affect acceptance or rejection of diagnosis and adherence to treatment. It is important to note that cultural differences between the clinician and patient have implications for the accuracy and acceptance of diagnosis as well as for treatment decisions and clinical outcomes..

BASIC CONCEPTS

Culture - Culture refers to the meanings, values and behavioral norms that are learned and passed on to further generations in the society. It powerfully influences the way we think, feel and behave. It acts as a template to shape and orient future behaviors and perspectives within and between generations. It is important to note that Culture exists in a constant state of change. According to the National Institute of Mental Health's Culture and Diagnosis Group, Culture is the lens through which a person registers experiences that shapes his/her perceptions, understanding and reactions to events.

Disease and illness - In the context of transcultural psychiatry, disease pertains to the constructions of clinical realities of the health care practitioners according to their models. In other words it is the 'Culture of the clinician'. Illness refers to the labeling and experience of behavior of patients and their families.

Validity and reliability - Reliability is the degree of consistency in the observations made by different clinicians Whereas Validity is the accuracy with which these criteria define and differentiate a disease from other diseases. Though reliability may appear more relevant, Validity is a more important construct in transcultural psychiatry. This is because overvaluing a construct, whether it is a diagnostic category, therapeutic technique or questionnaire, when used without testing its validity in different cultures, can create the problem of category fallacy. The concepts of both validity and reliability become more important in Psychiatry since the mainstay of diagnosing a particular disorder is through the mental status examination wherein patient's verbal accounts and non-verbal behaviors need to be assessed.

Emic–Etic- These are the terms used in anthropology to refer to different kinds of data concerning human behavior. Emic refers to the inside view about an issue or a problem. It is the behavior described as seen from the perspective of cultural insiders. This is based on the constructs drawn from their self-understanding. In contrast, etic is the outside view. It explains the behavior from a vantage external to the culture. Hence the constructs here apply equally well to other cultures.

Race and ethnicity - From a biological and socio-cultural points of view, ethnicity is a preferred concept compared to race in cross-cultural research. Ethnicity refers to group of people who share a sense of commonness in identity, ancestry, beliefs, history and traditions.

Idioms of distress - Different cultures can have different ways of expressing feelings of distress. Across cultures there can be different ways to cope up with the life problems . One idiom prevalent almost universally is psychological symptoms expressed through bodily complaints i.e., somatization. This also decides the pathways to care.

HISTORY OF TRANSCULTURAL PSYCHIATRY

The concept of Transcultural Psychiatry is not new. Since a long time, Psychiatrists and Social scientists have been observing how the symptoms of the same illness vary across different cultures. Nineteenth century Psychiatrists believed that insanity is rare among 'primitive' people and more prevalent as civilization evolves. They also believed that mental illnesses could be reaching alarming levels in large European cities.

Almost 100 years ago, Emil Kraepelin, the founder of modern psychiatry, envisioned a new field of comparative psychiatry. He focused on ethnic and cultural aspects of mental health and illness. Study of cultural differences in psychopathology has been done under different names within psychiatry - Transcultural Psychiatry, Cultural psychiatry, Ethno-Psychiatry, Cross-cultural psychiatry. The term Transcultural Psychiatry was introduced by Eric Wittkower of McGill University, Montreal in 1950. Wittkower, Rees and Cameron were interested in the impact of environment on the individual, although in varied contexts. Whitkower's life reflected many of the themes associated with early Transcultural psychiatry.

He was a member of British and German cultures, had emigrated, had seen the distorting effects of environment on personality, and he tried to explain the phenomena by using principles of psychology. The war-time experiences of these social scientists led them to the belief that much of the mental illness which was seen in individuals, was related to the wider sociocultural environment. They proposed that the treatment of these might require a multidisciplinary approach. As a consequence, Psychiatry was seen not only a medical Science but also as a social science. Thus, a new global approach to the world's mental health problems was born.

Esquirol thought that high frequency of mental

illness could be due to disordered life, abuse of alcoholic beverages, consanguineous marriages, social disturbances, revolutions, abrupt changes of habits, customs and values. Maudsley in 1843, published first study on mental illnesses among 'exotic people' based on visits to eastern Mediterranean area.

Winslow, a superintendent of a psychiatric sanatorium in Bengal summarized the ethno psychiatric observations. He observed that the Colonialism was accompanied by the growing interest in special mental illnesses among the native people. The doctors treating these patients noticed contrasts between patients seen in Bengal and those previously seen in Europe. This led to identification of Culture bound syndromes.

Currently there is a growing literature that delineates the impact of sociocultural factors, race and ethnicity on clinical care. But this needs to be implemented in clinical care. The sociocultural differences between patient and clinician are not explored, interpreted ,understood or communicated in a clinician-patient relationship there can be important hurdles in recovery. Patient dissatisfaction, poor adherence to treatment, poor health outcome. Ethnic disparities also need to be looked in to. It also is important to keep in mind the doctors' culture along with the patient's culture . As the culture is dynamic, the field of transcultural psychiatry too is expanding.

THE INTERACTION BETWEEN CULTURE AND HUMAN MIND

It is interesting to see how culture influences psychiatric disorders. There are three important ways in which culture interacts with Psychiatric disorders. They are as follows:

- The expression of psychiatric symptoms is shaped by the Culture.
- The Meanings that are given to symptoms. Are influenced by the Culture.
- The interaction between the patient and the health care system can have a cultural influence.

One must be aware of these possibilities. Clinicians must recognize and respect it during the evaluation and treatment of patients from different ethnic and cultural groups. With respect to the understanding of the aetiology of psychiatric illnesses and conditions the fact that certain ethnic groups relate the origin of mental illnesses to spiritual or religious factors has been well documented in the research so far. In a country like India where the patients with bodily complaints would visit a general practitioner or doctors from other disciplines, this focus becomes even more important. However this does not mean that the treating psychiatrist or doctor should be a member of the culture from which the patient came. It is not always possible or practical. But the treating psychiatrist should make an honest attempt to be knowledgeable about and sensitive about the patient's culture.

There are different ways as to how culture can interact with human psyche to bring about psychiatric symptoms.

Pathogenic Effects

Pathogenic effects refer to the cultural influence on the formation of the disorder. They mean situations in which culture is a direct causative factor in forming or 'generating' psychopathology. Stress from arise from the cultural ideas and beliefs which may lead to psychopathology. Stress can be created by culturally formed anxiety and culturally demanded performance. For example, in India 'Harmful' leaking of semen can produce anxiety, depression and somatic symptoms.

This is known as 'Dhat syndrome'. Similarly, women attending outpatient department of gynaecology with the complaints of white discharge per vagina(female dhat syndrome), with fatigue may have anxiety and depression in the background. In Malaysia, the folk belief that death will result if the penis shrinks into the abdomen is termed 'Koropanic'. So here culture is the direct cause of psychopathology, not of disease per se.

Pathoselective Effects

This is the tendency of people in a society, to select certain culturally influenced reaction patterns while encountering stress. This results in the manifestation of certain psychopathologies. In Japan, it is seen that the cultural influences may lead a family encountering serious stress or a hopeless situation to choose, from among many alternative solutions. One of the them is to commit suicide together, forming the unique psychopathology. Farmer's suicides in the regions of Vidarbha and southern India is also an example of this effect. Thus, Culture has a powerful influence on the choices and decisions people make in reaction to stressful situations. Hence it shapes the nature of the psychopathology that occurs as a result of those choices. But this only applies to minor psychiatric disorders, particularly of culture-related specific syndromes, not to major psychiatric disorders.

Pathoplastic Effect

Pathoplastic effects refer to the ways in which culture contributes to the modelling or 'plastering' of the manifestations of psychopathology. In other words, this involves culture modifying the clinical manifestation. Culture can shape symptom manifestations at the level of the content presented. The content of delusions, auditory hallucinations, obsessions, or phobias may depend on the environmental context which is closely related to culture. For example, in schizophrenia, Paranoid subtype is seen as the most common and over represented in developed countries where as Catatonic and Acute subtypes in developing countries.

Pathoelaborating Effect

This refers to culture elaborating mental conditions into a unique nature. Certain behaviors normal or abnormal may be universal. But some of them may appear exacerbated due to cultural reinforcement in some cultures. This is well demonstrated by the phenomenon of "Trance and possession state" widely seen in the region of South east Asia. It is a culturally sanctioned, way of expressing ego-dystonic impulses and thoughts, reported by various studies.

In western countries and urban areas of developing countries there is increasing concerns with body weight in relation to health. This is due to cultural elaboration through methods of diet control and various tools and ways of physical exercises. In addition to health-related concerns, the culture has shaped a belief that "slim is beautiful" which has further led to "body weight anxiety." This is a common reason of eating disorders in developed countries. This is especially important in adolescent girls. Similar concerns can be seen regarding 'muscles' in young men/adolescent boys.

Pathofacilitative Effects

Culture promoting the frequency of occurrence of the disorder is known as Pathofacilitative effect. The frequent occurrence of certain mental disorders is influenced significantly by the cultural factors. Thedisorder may otherwise exist and may be very well recognized in all cultures, but because of cultural influences, it might become prominent and more prevalent in certain cultures. Thus, 'facilitating' effects make it easier for certain psychopathologies to develop and increase in their frequency. An example can be the liberal attitude towards weapon control. This may result in more weapon-related violence or homicidal behavior. Culturally sanctioned to consume alcohol consumption may lead to an increase the prevalence of problem drinking. Similarly religious sanctioning of Cannabis as a method for transcendence may encourage youth to use cannabis.

Pathoreactive Effects

Culture shaping folk responses to the clinical condition is known as Pathoreactive effect. Many a time how people perceive pathologies and label disorders is shaped by the culture. It also influences how they react to them emotionally. It then guides them in expressing their suffering. One example can be faith healing practices seen in India in cases of major psychiatric disorders. People commonly attribute illness as results of "Black magic". It is also believed in India that marriage will cure patient's mental illness. Their belief is that it will alleviate sexual frustration or problem and there by cure his/her mental illness. But despite these, better prognosis of schizophrenia has been noticed in developing countries like India. The underlying factors of this finding are not yet well understood, but it is speculated that familial, social and cultural factors have pathoreactive effects on Schizophrenia and these may lead to different prognoses in different cultures.

IMPACT OF CULTURE ON DOCTOR-PATIENT RELATIONSHIP

The impact of culture on Doctor-Patient relationship becomes important in different areas;

1. Dependency versus Autonomy
2. Linguistic competence
3. Cognitive style
4. Social support system
5. Material culture
6. Psychological sophistication

Let us now try to look at each component in some detail.

Dependency Versus Autonomy

We notice many differences in seeing patients from different geographical locations as well as urban and rural settings. Unlike in western set ups, in developing countries most patients approach the doctor with the expectation of getting advice and decision regarding the treatment. This is almost like getting guidance from their parents and family elders.

Linguistic Competence

Identification and treatment of mental health disorders requires a full understanding of the culture and language of the person. Clinician needs to master the ability to relate successfully to the person through culture and language. For the treatment to be effective, the barriers in communication need to be looked in to. This requires resources, integrity and sustained effort. Language and thought develop together in to linguistic competence. It is the intrinsic knowledge of language of both the speaker and the listener. Linguistic performance refers to the actual use of language in a given situation.

Mental illness and languages are inter-related. In some disorders like schizophrenia, linguistic competence actually determines the phenomenology of schizophrenia. Language seems to be an essential prerequisite for manifestations of schizophrenic symptomatology as well as the outcome of schizophrenia across cultures. This is well proven through the WHO studies on Schizophrenia.

In Positive Symptom like hallucinations, delusions and other thought phenomena greater linguistic competence leads to increased elaboration of symptoms and hence a better understanding of symptoms. This also can increase the severity of symptoms by elaboration of the delusional content. Positive symptoms have a better prognosis compared to negative symptoms in schizophrenia. Positive correlation has been observed between outcome and linguistic competence. In studies on outcome of Schizophrenia, high linguistic competence was associated with low degree of negative symptoms and increased chances of recovery. High degree of negative symptoms is seen to be associated with low linguistic competence. It is important to note that high degree of negative symptoms are not easily amenable to therapeutic change.

Cognitive Styles

Cognitive styles are the ways in which the mind perceives the environment. It also includes the interpretation and conclusions drawn out of it. Each individual and culture have their unique cognitive style. Two types of cognitive styles are recognized. They are 'analytical' at one extreme and 'synthetic' at the other. In the analytical style of thinking, seen in western autonomous oriented society, the person understands a thing or a phenomenon by breaking it into parts. In synthetic style, one tries to see things or phenomena in the totality. The Indian mind is an example for synthetic cognitive style.

Social Support System

It is a well-known fact that differences across cultures in the social support system has significant impact on course and outcome of various mental illnesses. The traditional and developing societies which have a stronger social support system have shown to have a better prognosis of severe mental illnesses. (WHO 1973, 1979) The expressed emotion (EE) are considered to be an adverse family environment factor It includes the poor quality and abnormal interaction patterns and nature of family relationships among the family, and people with different mental health problems. This has been found to be one of the strong predictors of relapse in schizophrenia.

Material culture

Material Culture means those aspects of the environment that are man-made. This nature of material culture may influence the psychopathology. The subjective environment consists not only of the beliefs, values, norms and myths but also the physical environment which is comprised of structures like roads, bridges, buildings, etc. It is understandable malevolent or evil force which is perceived as spirit of a ghost in a developing society, can be replaced by X-rays and Radio waves in a technologically developed society.

Psychological Sophistication

This is the ability to see conflicts as to be originated in intrapsychic or internal focus. Conflict is perceived as within the mind. It may also be situated between the components of the psychic structure. Here the person recognizes the mind or psyche to be the source of conflict. Psychological sophistication may be related to coping mechanisms and certain types of disorders like dissociative disorders. This helps in the introspection of the self, disorder as a mental attribute to understand and resolve conflicts.

IMPACT OF CULTURE ON MAJOR PSYCHIATRIC DISORDERS

Initial research focussed on Culture bound syndromes, which were considered to be culture specific manifestations of mental illnesses. Later studies have found transcultural differences in incidence, clinical presentation, response to treatment and prognosis in major mental illnesses too. Major Psychiatric disorders consist of Schizophrenia, Bipolar affective disorder, Depressive disorder, Anxiety disorder, Somatoform and dissociative disorders. Here we discuss the impact of culture specifically in relation to these disorders.

Schizophrenia

There have been two Landmark research projects by the Mental Health Division of WHO namely International Pilot Study of Schizophrenia (IPSS) and Study of the Determinants of Outcome of Severe Mental Disorders (DOSMED). These research studies have showed that the syndrome at the beginning defined by Emil Kraepelin and Eugen Bleuler exists in very numerous ethnic and cultural groups. The patho-plastic effects of socio-cultural factors shape the symptom profiles differently in developed and developing countries. Western developed countries have showed a higher frequency of Depressive symptoms, Primary delusions, Thought insertion, Thought broadcasting whereas Non-Western developing countries showed a higher frequency of Visual hallucination and Auditory hallucinations.. The first systematic evaluation of schizophrenia subtypes found that catatonia subtypes are rare in the West, hebephrenic subtypes are common in Japan, and simple subtypes are common in Asia. It is interesting to note that the themes of delusions were related to patients' social background, cultural beliefs, and expectations. Religious delusions were common in Christian societies, whereas these were rarer in Hindu, Muslim, or Buddhist societies. Low rates of religious delusions, grandiose delusions, and delusions of guilt were found in one of the pure Islamic country, Pakistan. However, in contrast to this, religious grandiosity was more frequently seen in African countries.

According to IPSS Study, India had highest percentage with best outcome (66%) and Nigeria had the lowest percentage with worst outcome (10%). Schizophrenic psychoses had a better prognosis in Asian and African than in comparable British patient populations.

The conclusions of DOSMED study were as follows:

- The content of psychotic symptoms, many a time, pointed towards critical problems existing in a particular culture.
- Persecutory delusions and auditory hallucinations are not necessarily indicative of schizophrenia in persons of African cultural background.
- Influence of ethnicity and culture on psychopathology weighs more than geographic proximity, historical relations and racial similarity.
- Even though, the study populations belonged to the same religion, ethnic and cultural differences were reflected in the schizophrenic symptom profiles.

However, studies in Japan, Hong Kong and Singapore demonstrated a more favorable course and outcome than in Europe and North America. These findings are of special interest as they are derived from countries of advanced technological development but from cultures that are still quite different from those of modern Western societies.

It is important to look into specific aspects of modern Western societies that may exert effects conducive to a chronic course and poor final outcome of mental disorders. The crucial difference leading to different outcome is not the difference between societies of high or low technological development. But it is the way these non-western societies have preserved important elements of their traditional culture in the current world. Extreme nuclearization of the family and Covert rejection and social isolation of the mentally ill in spite of public assertions to the contrary may have led to lack of support for mentally ill members. Assumption that a person is insane if beliefs or behavior appear somewhat strange or 'irrational' and Unclear and uncertain role expectation of the youth in Western societies might have added to the poor prognosis in western world.

Acute Transient Psychosis

In developing countries, Acute and transient Psychotic disorders are more common when compared to Schizophrenia. Transient psychotic reactions are of particular interest to comparative cultural psychiatry because they are interwoven with culturally validated beliefs in sorcery and witchcraft. Interestingly these beliefs are seen to exist even after the traditional resources of protection or perceived persecution by magical or supernatural powers are no longer valid as a result of Westernization and urbanization. The individuals experiencing the pressures of rapid social change is steadily increasing because of which many feel unprotected against magical forces in which they still firmly believe. Acute Psychotic episode occurs as a reaction to this emotional trauma and social stress..Instead of rejection and isolation, the surrounding individuals respond to this reaction with sympathy and traditional therapeutic aids. This applies as long as the extended primary social support is still strong in a traditional non-Western society. Once the process of Westernising acculturation becomes irreversible, Transient psychotic reactions evolve into Schizophrenia or Chronic Psychosis.

Affective Disorders-Depression

Culture can heavily influence the way depressive symptoms are expressed.. Depressive illness was assessed in 583 patients at five institutions as part of a WHO collaborative study (Basel, Montreal, Tehran, Nagasaki, and Tokyo). Sadness, anhedonia, a lack of interest and energy, decreased focus, and feelings of worthlessness were also present in the majority of them. In Tehran, guilt feelings and suicide thoughts were the least common. Indian research has discovered that impersonal shame is less common among Indian patients than it is among West Indian patients. Indian belief system supports the concept of Karma-past deeds leading to the present state. Accordingly, instead of attributing the cause of suffering to self-failure as in Western world, the illness was thought over to be the result of one's own 'Karma'. The illness suffering. Physical symptoms are common presenting symptoms in depression.

Bipolar Disorders

Though there is no evidence that individuals belonging to certain ethnic groups present a greater risk of acquiring bipolar disorder, ethno cultural aspects seem to influence the clinical presentation, diagnosis and treatment of the disorder.

Bipolar patients in India have preponderance of mania in contrast to patients in Western countries. They present with delusions of grandeur, persecution and reference, content related to sexual and religious themes more commonly than the patients in the West. The predominant affect seen in in Indians suffering with Mania is one of hostile irritability. There are reports of seasonal occurrence of mania in summer season which is not reported in the west. Recurrent unipolar mania too is a more common condition seen in India and tropical countries.

Anxiety Disorders

Anxiety disorders are highly prevalent mental

health problems seen globally. Ethnic, racial, and cultural factors have a powerful influence in the aetiology of these disorders. This is because of the culturally dependent variations in the beliefs about the underlying physiology of the illness syndromes. the social context and norms a person is exposed to also appear to be important factors.

While evaluating the relationship between culture and anxiety disorders a number of factors need to be considered These factors may relate to ethnopsychology/ethnophysiology or contextual factors. The ideas about bodily systems or symptoms, including psychological signs (e.g., forgetfulness or poor concentration) give rise to ethnophysiology or ethnopsychology factors. Contextual factors relate to the social context and norms that govern the social structure. Contextual and ethnophysiology/ ethnopsychology factors are not independent factors. They are in a complex interactive relationship in different cultures.

Let us take the example of United States of America which is a multi-cultural country. Here, Asian Americans consistently report symptoms of anxiety disorders (social anxiety disorder, generalized anxiety disorder, panic disorder, and post-traumatic stress disorder) less frequently than any of the other racial groups. White Americans consistently describe more symptoms of social anxiety disorder, generalized anxiety disorder and panic disorder more frequently than African Americans, Hispanic Americans, and Asian Americans. These data demonstrate the strong contribution of culture on anxiety disorders.

There are three culturally specific expressions of anxiety disorders which are also listed in the DSM cultural concepts of distress. These include khyâl attacks in the Cambodian population, taijinkyofusho of the Korean and Japanese cultures, and ataques de nervios of the Puerto Rican and Dominican cultures. In the case of TKS, the social norm and setting predominate, whereas in the case of khyâl assaults and ataques de nervios, ethnopsychology/ethnophysiology variables predominate. These disorders demonstrate how culture has a significant impact on anxiety disorders, resulting in distinct manifestations. Although the DSM-5 addresses some of these issues, much more research is needed to fully comprehend when and how culture influences disorders. This has clear consequences not only for the classification of these prevalent illnesses, but also for their treatment.

Dissociative and Somatoform Disorders

The Concept of somatization appears to have its origin in the Cartesian concept of body-mind prevalent in Western societies. Somatoform and dissociative syndromes are heterogeneous. But they are present in all cultures as the most typical sequelae of stress. They are more frequently reported from non-western, developing societies.

Somatic complaints as an expression of personal or social distress is commonly seen in most cultures. Patients tend to develop symptoms that are medically correct and culturally acceptable. Generally, the somatic symptoms tend to be less stigmatizing than psychological symptoms. They are also easier to describe verbally.

Worldwide most common medically unexplained symptoms are Gastrointestinal complaints and abnormal skin sensations. Interestingly, in United States most common medically unexplained somatic symptoms were gynecological complaints, followed by gastrointestinal and cardiovascular symptoms. In Nigeria and India common somatic symptoms are feelings of heat, peppery and crawling sensations, numbness, burning hands and feet,hot, burning sensations in head. It is important to note that these symptoms are extremely rare in Western countries.

Indian studies have observed that most patients with dissociation presented with a "brief dissociative stupor" that coexisted with anxiety and panic symptoms. Multiple Personality Disorder –MPD which is prevalent in North America, is rare or non-existent in other western and non-western countries.

CULTURE AND PERSONALITY

The personality traits play an important role in manifestation and management of mental illness. Cultural influences personality in various ways. When faced with an emotional conflict, a passive-dependent person is more likely to "give up", more prone to break with reality and develop psychotic coping behavior. Later, he is more likely to turn to society for care, develop hysterical and somatoform disorders so as to involve other members of the society in its resolution. This may be different in an autonomous individual. When faced with emotional conflict, he may resist his loss of control, may reject his dependency needs, may try to resolve his conflicts himself from an intrapsychic perspective. He may keep on battling with the anxiety and convert anxiety into development of neurotic-type distress. Thus the Personality configuration may influence the choice of resolution of conflict either individually or culturally. The subsequent elaboration and proliferation of the symptomatology depends upon the various sociocultural factors.

CULTURAL ASPECTS OF INSIGHT

The traditional unidimensional view of insight has been replaced with recent multi-dimensional perspectives. Three dimensions of insight are: – awareness of mental illness, ability to re-label psychotic experience as abnormal, seeking psychiatric treatment. According to Jacob KS, multi-dimensional perspectives of insight employ western concepts of disease and all mental illnesses are considered medical diseases. Alternate explanations pertaining to local and cultural aspects are not considered.

There is a need of cultural standard to assess insight. If a person recognizes a non-visible change in his or her body or mind that affects his or her ability to function socially and socially, and if he or she feels the need for restitution/restoration, we could indeed call this presence of "insight" regardless of the attribution and the pathways of care that the person seeks. Non-delusional explanation for the changes in body or mind is essential for insight. While Diagnosing the non-delusional nature of these changes in body or mind clinician's understanding of the local culture plays an important role. There is a need to use local and cultural standards rather than universal yardsticks to assess insight in people with psychosis.

CULTURAL CONSIDERATION IN CLINICAL PRACTICE

An important classification system in psychiatry, DSM-5 includes an updated version of the cultural formulation outline. It presents an approach to evaluate the cultural issues pertaining to each patient. The instrument used here is the Cultural Formulation Interview. It includes the following components:

1) *Cultural identity of the individual:* Describes the individual's racial, ethnic, or cultural reference groups, linguistic abilities, preferences and patterns of use, identifying difficulties with access to care, social integration and the need for an interpreter. It also includes religious affiliation, socioeconomic background, personal and family places of birth, childhood, migrant status, and sexual orientation.

2) *Cultural conceptualizations of distress:* This term refers to the cultural constructions that influence how a person perceives, understands, and conveys their concerns

to others. Cultural syndromes, distress idioms, and explanatory models or perceived reasons are all possibilities. It is recommended that when assessing coping and help-seeking practises, professionals as well as traditional, alternative, or complementary sources of care be included.

3) *Cultural features of the relationship between the individual and the clinician-* This identifies differences in culture, language and social status between an individual and clinician. These factors may cause difficulties in communication. It may have a strong influence on diagnosis and treatment. Effects of this may include problems in eliciting symptoms, misunderstanding of the cultural and clinical significance of symptoms and behaviors. It may also pose difficulty in establishing and maintaining the rapport.

FUTURE DIRECTIONS AND RESEARCH IN TRANSCULTURAL PSYCHIATRY

Identification of specific fields in general psychiatry that could be the subject of focused research from a cultural perspective forms the future area of research in Transcultural Psychiatry. A number of cultural variables can be considered in conducting cultural psychiatry research like: Language, Religion, Traditions, Beliefs, Ethics, and Gender orientation to name a few.

Five dimensions appear relevant to research in cultural psychiatry. Culture has an impact on each of these. They stand out as relevant indicators at different stages of the clinical evaluation and treatment of mental illnesses and Doctor-patient relationship in all medical disciplines.

1. Culture as a tool for interpretation or explanation of mental illnesses: The ways in which individuals in different cultures see the suffering as well as their causation are explained by these models.
2. Culture as an agent for Pathogenic or Pathoplastic effect: Culture may be a pathogenic agent in the construction of a clinical picture. It may contribute to the production of variety symptoms.
3. Culture as a Diagnostic or Nosological Tool: The DSM-5 cultural formulation is developed as a valuable tool for research as well as for diagnostic purposes.
4. Culture as a Therapeutic or Protective Factor: Culture can be considered as a healing force. A great variety of cultural psychotherapies have emerged. Religion and spirituality as clinical instruments are of great utility in clinical settings. The protective factors against mental illness in each culture are unique to that particular culture and these need to be studied.
5. Culture as a Service or Management Element: – The use of clinicians who belong to the same ethnic group as the patient appears to be at advantage. But the setting in which the clinical encounter occurs deserves more research.

ILLUSTRATING THE IMPORTANCE OF CULTURE IN CLINICAL SETTINGS THROUGH CLINICAL VIGNETTES

CASE ONE

A lady presented with long standing possession symptoms to a psychiatrist. On detailed evaluation the patient had significant depressive symptoms, alcohol dependence in husband and domestic violence. The symptoms served as a relief factor for all these. The family had encouraged the symptomatology because of religious beliefs that 'Devi' possesses the patient on certain days. The patient presented to psychiatry outpatient when the other somatic symptoms, unexplained by any general evaluation, started interfering with the daily routine.

Commentary

While managing this patient, several cultural issues become important in evaluation as well as treatment aspects. It is important for the clinician to understand the cultural model of illness, beliefs associated with possession, substance dependence and domestic violence as being 'normal' parts of rural life. These need to be communicated as possible and important issues to be corrected albeit carefully. Otherwise, the consultation would do more harm than good resulting in increased distress on part of the patient or a possible drop out.

CASE TWO

A middle-aged woman had lost her son aged 23 years in an accident. She presented to a psychiatrist with an intense grief reaction. She had death wishes, fleeting hallucinations of her son's voices, crying repeatedly. The patient was started on Benzodiazepines and Specific serotonin reuptake inhibitors- SSRIs with supportive therapy. She was lost for follow up. She returned to the treating Psychiatrist after three months. She was composed, had come in terms with the loss of her son and had a healthy resolution of grief. She wanted to return the medications which she had not taken. On further clarification, she was staying in a joint family set up with good social support. The religious rituals and frequent visits by her multiple family members had allowed her to ventilate her emotions and aided her in healthy grief resolution.

Commentary

This case is a classical example of how culture can play a protective role in mental health problems. Here the religious beliefs and social rituals allowed the lady to express grief in a healthy way. And hence the problems resolved without pharmacological intervention.

CONCLUSIONS

Psychiatry and people with mental health problems do not exist in isolation but within a larger socio-cultural context that influences their beliefs and behaviors. This context needs to be taken into account both while treating people with mental health problems and when developing healthcare systems. The Clinician needs to have deeper understanding of not only the disease but the cultural underpinnings which play a significant role in the disease process as well as patient's life.

BIBLIOGRAPHY

1. Biju Viswanath and Santosh K. Chaturvedi. Cultural Aspects of Major Mental Disorders: A Critical Review from an Indian Perspective. *Indian Journal of Psychological Medicine* 2012; 34(4)
2. Dinesh Bhugra, *Textbook of Cultural Psychiatry*, 2nd ed. Cambridge: Cambridge University Press; 2016.
3. K. Vijoy Varma. Cultural psychodynamics in health and illness. *Indian J Psychiatry* 1986; 28(1).
4. Rahul Bhattacharya, Dinesh Bhugra. *Clinical topics in cultural psychiatry*, 1 ed. london: The Royal College of Psychiatrists; 2010.
5. Roberto Lewis-Fernández, Neil Krishan Aggarwal et al. *DSM-5® Handbook on the Cultural Formulation Interview*, Washington, DC: American Psychiatric Association Publishing; 2016.
6. Samuel O. Okpaku. *Clinical Methods in Transcultural Psychiatry* . Washington, DC: American Psychiatric Association Publishing; 1998.

Newer Psychiatric Disorders 67

Prerna Khar • Vinyas Nisarga • Swati Shelke

INTRODUCTION

Psychiatry is an ever-evolving branch. The diagnostic and classificatory systems have undergone repeated revisions over the past hundreds of years. The 2 main classificatory systems are the Diagnostic and Statistical Manual of mental disorders (DSM) and the International Classification of diseases (ICD). While these have accommodated most of the disorders, we currently do have an emerging list of disorders, some of which have not yet reached a diagnostic consensus due to socio-cultural differences. Some of them will be discusses in this chapter.

BEHAVIORAL ADDICTIONS

Behavioral addictions refer to those behaviors which are maladaptive, repetitive and associated with reward, loss of control & physical dependence. They are termed so as they share parallels with centrally acting substances (Alcohol, cannabis, stimulants, etc.). The DSM-5 has included Gambling disorder and Binge-eating disorder so far. The other disorders which are currently being explored and will probably make it to the next revision of the DSM are: Internet use disorder (Internet Addiction), Sex addiction, Work addiction, compulsive shopping/buying and exercise addiction.

Behavioral addictions are characterized by the following features:

- *Impaired control* – Craving for the behavior and unsuccessful attempts to quit
- *Socio-occupational impairment* - Narrowing of interests and neglecting other areas of life
- *Risk taking behavior* – Continuing the behavior, despite awareness of its damaging psychological/ physical effect

1) Gambling disorder

It is characterized by persistent and recurrent maladaptive gambling, that causes economic problems and significant disturbance in the personal, social or occupational functioning. There are various types, such as sports betting, office sports pool, sports with bookies, betting on animal fights (cock/ bull/ camel fights etc.), gambling at casinos (slot machines, cards etc.), playing cards, internet games.

Epidemiology

The lifetime prevalence as per Indian literature is 0.4-1.0%. It is more common in men and young adults than in women and older adults.

Clinical Features

Individuals often appear overconfident and free-spending in nature. Often, they may show signs of anxiety, depression and stress. As their gambling increases, they resort to deceit and lies to obtain money and undermine their gambling. In severe cases, they may resort to theft, fraud and other anti-social activities as well. Complications include loss of finances, job, interpersonal issues, estrangement from family members and friends and getting arrested for criminal activities. The various stages of gambling are as follows:

A) The winning phase: Usually ends with a big win, equal to about a year's salary, which encourages the individual to gamble further.

B) The progressive-loss phase: The patients structure their lives around gambling and then move from being excellent gamblers to ones who take considerable risks/borrow money/miss work, and lose jobs.

C) The desperate phase: Gambling large amounts of money and incurring large debts.

D) The hopeless stage: Accepting that losses can never be made up, but the gambling continues because of the associated arousal or excitement.

Diagnostic Criteria

The ICD-10 and DSM 5 diagnostic criteria are summarized in **Table 67.1**.

Comorbidities

Mood disorders- major depression and bipolar disorder, other substance use and addictive disorders (notably, alcohol and stimulant abuse and caffeine and tobacco dependence) and a history of ADHD are commonly associated.

Etiology

Various psychosocial and biological factors have been implicated

a) Psychosocial factors:

- Parental loss due to death/ separation/ divorce, or abandonment before a child is 15 years of age

Table 67.1

Features	DSM-5	ICD-10
Name	Gambling Disorder	Pathologic Gambling
Duration	Symptoms present within a 12-month period	
Symptoms	Minimum 4 of the below: • Needing higher stakes to achieve the same thrill • Becomes irritable when trying to stop • Unsuccessful attempts at reducing • Preoccupation with thoughts about gambling • Gambling in response to distress • Gambling to make up for prior losses • Lying to hide gambling • Losses resulting in socio-occupational and interpersonal functioning • Borrowing/ stealing money from others for gambling	Diagnosis is clinical, characterized by: Pattern that is dominant in the patient's life and resulting in adverse consequences in socio-occupational and interpersonal functioning.
Excludes	Manic episode	Excessive gambling by manic patients and gambling in dissocial personality disorder

- Inappropriate parenting styles -inconsistence/ harsh
- Exposure to, and access to gambling activities during adolescence
- Family emphasis on materialism
- Lack of emphasis on saving/ planning by elders at home

b) Neurobiology: Similar to substance use disorders:
   - Dysregulation of serotonergic pathways
   - Dysfunction of cerebral sites and pathways, which mediate behavioral arousal, inhibition/disinhibition, reward/ reinforcement and psychophysiological stress.

Treatment

a) Pharmacological: Naltrexone and N-Acetyl cysteine (NAC) constitute the first line of treatment. Antidepressants (SSRIs and bupropion) mood stabilizers (lithium and and lamotrigine) and atypical antipsychotics can be used. It is important to treat comorbidities such as mood disorders and anxiety.

b) Psychotherapeutic modalities: These include cognitive behavior therapy (CBT), family therapy, motivational interviewing and enhancement. Support groups such as Gamblers Anonymous (GA) are good when combined with other treatment modalities.

2) Internet use disorder/ Internet Addiction

Excessive internet use has been termed as pathological Internet use, compulsive Internet use, problematic Internet use (PIU), Internet addiction, internet dependency etc. It is characterized by the inability to control one's use of the internet which leads to negative consequences in daily life. As diagnostic criteria have not been defined due to lack of consensus, it is difficult to get an idea of the epidemiology.

Clinical Features

The characteristics of PIU are as follows:

1) Excessive Internet use, often associated with a loss of sense of time or a neglect of basic drives
2) Withdrawal: Feelings of anger, depression and tension when internet is not available
3) Tolerance: Need for better computer equipment, additional software, or more hours of use
4) Adverse consequences: Arguments, lying, poor school or occupational performance, social isolation and fatigue.

Often, the internet is used for gambling, cybersex/ cyber-relational activities or compulsive shopping. These must be kept in mind while assessing the individual.

Comorbidities

Emotional difficulties and poor coping mechanism often manifest as internet use disorder. Depression, anxiety, ADHD are common comorbidities. PIU could lead to loss of physical activity and hence predispose the individual to obesity.

Treatment

a) Psychotherapeutic: Cognitive behavior therapy for internet addiction, Solution-focused Brief Therapy(SFBT), Cognitive Therapy (CT), Reality Therapy (RT) are some of the modalities used. Short-term Treatment for Internet and Computer Game Addiction (STICA) has also been studied across various clinical settings.

b) Pharmacotherapy: Mainly involves using SSRIs (escitalopram) for the underlying depression and anxiety. Stimulants like methylphenidate can be used to treat the underlying ADHD.

3) Binge Eating Disorder

Defined as recurrent binge eating where one eats an abnormally large amount of food over a short time without any inappropriate compensatory behaviors.

Epidemiology

Lifetime prevalence in women is 3.6% and in men is 2.1%. It is most prevalent in females.

Clinical Features and Diagnosis

The DSM5 describes it as recurrent episodes of binge eating with each episode of binge eating characterized by:

- Eating, in a discrete period of time (e.g., within any 2-hour period), large amounts of food than most people would eat during a similar period of time and under similar circumstances.
- A sense of lack of control over eating during the episode (e.g., a feeling that one cannot stop eating or control what or how much one is eating).

The binge eating episodes are associated with eating much more rapidly than normal and until feeling uncomfortably full. They eat large amounts of food when not feeling physically hungry and eat alone because of embarrassment they feel on amount of food they consume. After the episode they feel disgusted with oneself, depressed, or very guilty. The episodes occur on an average, at least once a week for 3 months and experience marked distress regarding binge eating.

It is associated with impulsive personality styles. In ICD-10, the diagnostic name used is Bulimia nervosa, non-purging type.

Severity

Mild : 1-3 binge-eating episodes per week.

Moderate : 4-7 binge-eating episodes per week.

Severe : 8-13 binge-eating episodes per week.

Extreme : 14 or more binge-eating episodes per week.

Differential Diagnosis

- Bulimia Nervosa: In binge-eating disorder patients do not report repetitive compensatory behaviors (vomiting, laxative abuse, or excessive dieting).
- Anorexia nervosa: In binge-eating disorder patients do not exhibit an extreme drive for thinness and are of average weight or are obese.

Comorbidities

- Psychiatric comorbidities: Mood disorders, anxiety disorders and substance use disorders.
- Medical comorbidities: Obesity, metabolic disorders and chronic muscle pain.

Treatment

a) Pharmacotherapy:

  1) Antidepressants: Fluoxetine, fluvoxamine, citalopram, escitalopram, sertraline, duloxetine, and bupropion

  2) Anticonvulsants: Topiramate and zonisamide

3) Stimulants: Lisdexamfetamine

b) Psychotherapy: Cognitive behavior therapy and interpersonal therapy

c) Weight Loss Treatment: Treatment of the associated obesity requires nutritional modification with calorie reduction and an increase in exercise.

4) Sex Addiction

The derivation of early names for sex addiction is from the Greek mythology: satyriasis for male sex addiction after the mythical satyrs who had an uncontrolled sexual behavior and nymphomania for female sex addiction, named after the nymphs who were driven by their desire for others.

Definition

Sex addiction is a behavior involving significant and destructive loss of control of the sexual impulse. It is defined as a non-paraphilic excessive sexual behaviors with features of impulsivity, compulsivity and causing significant personal distress, social or medical comorbidity.

Epidemiology

The estimated prevalence is 3-6%. Male to female ratio is 3-4:1. Cyber sex addiction has almost equal ratio.

Clinical Features, Diagnosis and Course

Sex addiction usually begins in adolescence. The disorder intensifies during 20s to 40s and affects the person's life. The sexual activity is usually kept a secret and they live a double life. There is an exploitative element to the sexual behavior and the person has difficulty in forming intimate relationship. History of chronic affairs, compulsive masturbation, pervasive prostitution use, or habitual online surfing of sex sites is present.

Patients have a tendency to compartmentalize to compartmentalize or dissociate themselves from their behavior. Patients may present for treatment due to an impending divorce from a spouse, threat of loss of a job as they have been caught spending work time sexually interacting on the internet or sexually harassing work colleagues, and confrontations with the legal system. The patient presents the situation as a rare occurrence.

Some of them present with anxiety or depression. The patients may feel their behavior has intensified to a degree that causes them conscious shame and they feel they cannot continue such a way of life and seek treatment.

The course of untreated sex addiction involves hypersexual behavior, interrupted by periods of abstention that involves controlling the addiction, followed by relapses, and further episodes of compulsive sexual activity. They experience a sense of excitement (a high) in sex-seeking behavior even in the absence of an orgasm. The patient invests lot of time in fantasy, preoccupation, preparation and engaging in sexual activity.

After 40 years of age although behavior or acting out diminishes, the fantasies and abnormally heightened preoccupation with sex continues.

DSM-5 has not recognised sex addiction as a disorder whereas, ICD 10 has included the term excessive sexual desire (F52.7). We have summarized the Criteria given by Carnes (1991). below (**Table 67.2**):

Differential Diagnosis

1. Paraphilias: Paraphilic tendencies can also be present in sexual addiction, but they are not the primary symptom whereas deviant sexual preference is the primary complaint in Paraphilias.

Table 67.2

Sexual Addiction Diagnostic Criteria proposed by Carnes (1991)	
A.	**A minimum of three criteria met during a 12-month period:**
1)	Recurrent failure to resist impulses to engage in specific sexual behavior.
2)	Frequent engaging in these behaviors to a greater extent or longer duration than intended.
3)	Persistent desire or unsuccessful efforts to stop, to reduce, or to control behaviors.
4)	Inordinate amount of time spent in obtaining sex, being sexual, or recovering from sexual experiences.
5)	Preoccupation with the behavior or preparatory activities.
6)	Frequently engaging in the behavior when expected to fulfil occupational, academic, domestic, or social obligations.
7)	Continuation of the behavior despite knowledge of having a persistent or recurrent social, financial, psychological, or physical problem that is caused or exacerbated by the behavior.
8)	Need to increase intensity, frequency, number, or risk of behaviors to achieve the desired effect or diminished effect with continued behaviors at the same level of intensity, frequency, number, or risk.
9)	Giving up or limiting social, occupational, or recreational activities.
10)	Distress, anxiety, restlessness, or irritability if unable to engage in the behaviors.
B.	**Has significant personal and social consequences (such as loss of partner, occupation or legal implications)**

2. Affective disorders: Hypersexuality can be present in hypomania, mania and rarely atypical depression which is episodic and accompanied by other symptoms.
3. Substance use disorders: Stimulant, anabolic steroids and other substance abuse can be accompanied by periods of excessive sexual activity.
4. Mental retardation: Lack of inhibition and ability to modulate impulses.
5. Neurological causes: Such as head injury, multiple sclerosis and dementia. Hypersexuality is due to fronto-temporal degeneration or damage leading to lack of inhibition and ability to control.
6. Endocrine: Hyper-testosteronism due to tumor.
7. Drug induced: Testosterone supplementation, GnRH analogues, levodopa and dopamine agonists.
8. Rare genetic disorders: Kleine Levin syndrome.

Comorbidities

Substance use disorders, gambling disorders, mood and anxiety disorders and sexually transmitted disorders.

Investigations

Serology for sexually transmitted infections, toxicology screen and in atypical cases a sex hormone profile may be required (serum FSH, LH, free testosterone and sex hormone binding globulin).

Treatment

a) Pharmacotherapy: Fluoxetine, sertraline and naltrexone.

b) *Psychotherapy:*

- Group therapy: 12 step programs such as Sex Addicts Anonymous (SAA); Sex and Love Addicts Anonymous (SLAA); Sexaholics Anonymous (SA); and Sexual Compulsives Anonymous (SCA).
- Cognitive behavior therapy
- Family therapy
- Marital therapy or couple's therapy.

5) Work addiction

It is characterized by excessive involvement in work leading to a compromise in personal life & social functioning. The overall prevalence across culture & socio-economic classes is estimated to be as high as 10%. This has not yet been classified under ICD-10/ DSM-5, but has been significantly contributed towards burn-out, stress, depression and anxiety. It is also debatable whether to classify it under OCD related disorders or behavioral addictions.

Clinical Features

Such individuals tend to stay busy, have a need to control and are perfectionists. They have difficulty in relationships, relaxing & having fun. It is associated with pre-occupation with work related planning, even while doing recreational activities, and often the individuals have a sense of self-inadequacy.

Etiology

a) Personal factors: Achievement oriented individuals, desire for high self-esteem & perfectionism

b) Environmental factors: Stressful childhood and peer competition

c) Behavioral reinforcement: It is often considered to be a good quality as per societal norms

Treatment

Involves exploring underlying personality traits and using CBT. It is important to look for and treat underlying depression and anxiety, which are common comorbidities.

6) Compulsive buying disorder (CBD)

It is characterized by irrepressible, excessive and uncontrolled buying that continues despite negative consequences.

Clinical Features

CBD is characterized by the following features:

1) Irrepressible Buying: Spending hours shopping and spending each week. The activity is associated with an intense urge to purchase one or multiple items.

2. Uncontrollable Buying: Most individuals have overwhelming and irresistible urges to buy products

3. Negative Consequences of Buying: Failure to change this behavior despite negative consequences across financial and inter-personal functioning.

Epidemiology

Most of the data is from high- income group countries. As per an Indian Council of Medical Research (ICMR) funded survey study, the overall the prevalence in India is 4%. (males -3.2%, females-4.8%)

Etiology

Risk factors include having personality traits of impulsivity and distractibility; and having a preference for materialism.

Comorbidities

Anxiety disorder, mood disorders, substance use disorders and other behavioral addictions should also be screened for.

Treatment

Mainly focuses on treating the underlying co-morbidities. Cognitive behavioral therapy (CBT) focusing on the emotions and feelings associated with the behavior and self-esteem, and financial management has shown results in a few studies.

7) Exercise Addiction

Also known as compulsive exercise, obligatory exercise or exercise abuse. It is more common in individuals related to professional sports. Common comorbidities include eating disorders (anorexia nervosa), substance use disorders and body-dysmorphic disorder. It is often associated with a history of anabolic steroid abuse and repeated overuse injuries. Disruption of social and familial ties is important. It is very difficult to differentiate this at times from individuals who are dedicated in their field and are very competitive and committed in nature. Hence, the diagnostic entity is debatable. Further research is needed to substantiate its existence.

Epidemiology

As per an ICMR funded survey study, the prevalence in India is 5.6%; (7.5% in males & 3.8% in females).

Treatment

Options include CBT and treated existing comorbidities.

DISRUPTIVE MOOD DYSREGULATION DISORDER

Disruptive mood dysregulation disorder (DMDD) is a condition in which children or adolescents experience ongoing irritability, anger, and frequent, intense temper outbursts. Disruptive mood dysregulation disorder (DMDD) was introduced as a new diagnostic

Table 67.3: DSM-5 Diagnostic criteria for DMDD

A. Severe, recurrent temper outbursts (verbal and/or behavioral) that are grossly out of proportion in intensity or duration to the situation/provocation

B. Outbursts are inconsistent with the developmental level

C. Occur three or more times/week

D. Mood between temper outbursts is persistently irritable or angry most of the day, nearly every day, and is observable by others

E. Duration is 12 or more months, without symptom-free interval of three or more consecutive months

F. Symptoms are present in at least two of three settings (home, at school, with peers) and are severe in at least one setting

G. Age at onset, either by history or observation, is before 10 years

H. Diagnosis should not be made for the first time before age 6 years or after 18 years

I. Full symptom criteria for manic/hypomanic episode have never been met for longer than 1 day

J. Behaviors do not occur exclusively during an episode of major depressive disorder and are not better explained by other disorders like dysthymia, autism spectrum disorder, posttraumatic stress disorder, separation anxiety disorder. [Diagnosis cannot coexist with bipolar disorder, intermittent explosive disorder, and Oppositional defiant disorder (ODD)]. Individuals whose symptoms meet the criteria for both DMDD and ODD should only be given the diagnosis of DMDD

K. Symptoms not due to physiological effects of a substance, a medical or neurological condition

entity under the category of depressive disorders in Diagnostic and Statistical Manual of Mental Disorders, Fifth Edition (DSM-5). It was included in DSM-5 primarily to address concerns about the misdiagnosis of chronic irritability with anger outbursts in children as pediatric bipolar disorder, which leads to unnecessary treatment with antipsychotics. ICD 11 does not follow DSM 5 in the introduction of DMDD; a specifier "chronic irritability or anger" is added to the category of oppositional defiant disorder.

Etiology and Risk Factors

- Temperament
- Genetic factors
- Family dysfunction
- Trauma and stressors
- Malnutrition

Epidemiology

The 6 months to 1 year period prevalence is 2-5% of children and adolescents. It is more common in boys.

Assessment

- Assess the duration, frequency and triggers of temper outbursts and also mood between these temper outbursts
- Gather information from the child and parent, as well as from teachers.
- Assess the level of impairment caused by the outbursts, and irritability across home, school, and in other social settings.

Course and Prognosis

DMDD is a chronic disorder. Patients with disruptive mood dysregulation disorder in childhood have a high risk of progressing to major depressive disorder, dysthymic disorder, anxiety disorders and substance use over time. Children with DMDD do not go on to have bipolar disorder in adulthood.

Functional Consequence

Children with DMDD may have trouble in school and experience difficulty maintaining healthy relationships with family or peers.

Differential Diagnosis

- **Bipolar disorder:** children and adolescents with bipolar disorder present with distinct periods of depressed mood and of mania or hypomania.
- **ODD:** Oppositional defiant disorder includes symptoms of annoyance and defiance, which disruptive mood dysregulation disorder does not have.
- **Intermittent explosive disorder (IED):** It does not have persistent disruption of mood between temper outbursts.

Co-morbidities

Attention deficit hyperactivity disorder (ADHD), Anxiety disorders, Depressive disorders.

Treatment

As DMDD is a new diagnosis, data regarding treatment is scarce. Most of the treatment recommendations are extrapolated from related disorders such as severe mood dysregulation, depression, anxiety, ADHD and ODD.

a) Non-Pharmacological treatment:

- Behavior therapy
- *Parent training:* improving parenting skills through parenting programs, psychoeducation providing support to the family
- *School based interventions:* Education and support to teachers

b) Pharmacological treatment:

- It depends on symptomatology and comorbid disorders. If symptomatology resembles unipolar depression and anxiety disorders, then SSRIs are used.
- If the symptomatology is like that of bipolar disorder, then first-line treatments for youth would include atypical antipsychotic agents and mood stabilizers.
- If symptoms of ADHD are significant, specific ADHD treatment can be tried
- Antipsychotics and sodium valproate may be used when there is lack of response to other interventions.

PREMENSTRUAL DYSPHORIC DISORDER (PMDD)

PMDD is a cyclical mood disorder affecting a subset of menstruating women. It is a collection of physical, cognitive, and affective symptoms causing clinically significant distress or interference that occur in the 7 days prior to the onset of menses, after which they become minimal or absent.

Premenstrual Syndrome (PMS): Premenstrual syndrome (PMS) is characterized by psychological and physical symptoms occurring before menses. PMDD is a more severe form of PMS with significant mood symptoms and disability.

Table 67.4

Cognitive & affective	**Behavioral and Physical**
One or more of the following must be present	One or more of the following must be present
1. Markedly depressed mood, feelings of hopelessness, or self-deprecating thoughts **2.** Marked anxiety, tension, feelings of being "keyed up" or "on edge" **3.** Marked affective lability **4.** Persistent and marked anger or irritability or increased interpersonal conflicts	**1.** Hypersomnia or insomnia **2.** Subjective sense of difficulty in concentrating **3.** Lethargy, easy fatigability, or marked lack of energy **4.** Marked change in appetite, overeating, or specific food cravings **5.** A subjective sense of being overwhelmed or out of control **6.** Decreased interest in usual activities (e.g., work, school, friends and hobbies) **7.** Other physical symptoms, such as breast tenderness or swelling, headaches, joint or muscle pain, a sensation of bloating, or weight gain.
At least 5 of the above 11 symptoms should be present during most menstrual cycles in the past year. These symptoms should be confirmed by prospective daily ratings during at least 2 symptomatic cycles.	
These symptoms are severe enough to interfere significantly with social, occupational, sexual or scholastic functioning.	
These symptoms are discretely related to the menstrual cycle and must not merely represent an exacerbation of the symptoms of another disorder, such as major depressive disorder, panic disorder, dysthymic disorder, or a personality disorder (although the symptoms may be superimposed on those of these disorders).	
The symptoms are not attributable to the physiological effects of a substance (e.g., drug abuse, medication or other treatment) or another medical condition (e.g., hyperthyroidism)	

PMDD is listed as a separate entity under Depressive disorders in *Diagnostic and Statistical Manual of Mental Disorders, 5th Edition* (DSM-5) with the criteria for diagnosis as shown in Table 67.4.

Pathophysiology

In women with PMS/PMDD, there is heightened sensitivity to cyclical reproductive hormonal variations. It predisposes them to experience the mood, behavioral, and somatic symptoms even though reproductive hormone release patterns are normal. Normal hormonal fluctuations during menstrual cycle trigger pain, anxiety and depressive symptoms through interaction with serotonin systems.

Risk Factors

- Stress
- Traumatic events and pre-existing anxiety disorders
- Cigarette smoking
- Obesity
- Genetics: polymorphism of the estrogen alpha receptor gene ESR1

Prevalence

In India, the pooled prevalence of PMS and PMDD were 43% and 8% respectively.

Clinical Course and Outcome

Clinical experience suggests that many women have recurrent symptoms until menopause. The longitudinal course of PMS/PMDD is not yet clearly known.

Differential Diagnosis

Bipolar disorder, Major depressive disorder. In these disorders, chronic or intermittent symptoms are not related to menstrual cycle phase.

Treatment

Treatment modalities for PMDD can be divided into 2 categories:

1. **Non-Pharmacological Methods**
   a) Cognitive-behavioral Therapy: These interventions for PMDD include modifying negative cognitions or improving coping strategies.
   b) Exercise: Increases endorphin levels.
   c) Dietary modifications: Increased intake of complex carbohydrates or proteins. Increased consumption of fruits, vegetables, legumes, whole grains, and water is recommended
   d) Stress management: Relaxation/ meditation/ yoga/ breathing technics.
   e) Dietary supplements: Calcium, Magnesium, Vit B6, Vit E
   f) Herbal Products: Chastberry, St. John's wort, evening primrose oil.
2. **Pharmacological Methods**
   a) Psychotropic agents
   - *Serotonin Reuptake Inhibitors (SRIs):* SRIs have been proven to be effective in the treatment of severe mood and somatic symptoms of PMDD. e.g. Clomipramine, SSRIs (Escitalopram, fluoxetine, paroxetine and sertraline), SNRI(Venlafaxine)
   - *Benzodiazepines (BZDs):* Effective only in women with severe anxiety and premenstrual insomnia.

   b) Suppression of Ovulation
   - *Hormonal therapies:* For very severe symptoms, clinicians can use hormonal therapies to provide relief. The aim of hormonal therapy is to inhibit the hypothalamo-gonadal cycle.

- *Oral contraceptive pills (OCPs):* Current evidence suggests that OCs should be considered if symptoms are primarily physical but may not be effective if mood symptoms are more prevalent.
- Transdermal estradiol: High-dose transdermal estradiol 200 μg provided via patch can prevent ovulation and reduce symptoms of PMS/PMDD.
- *Danazol:* This is a synthetic partial androgen agonist/ antagonist and gonadotropin inhibitor that has also shown to be efficacious in treating PMDD by inhibiting ovulation.
- Gonadotropin-releasing hormone agonists

BIBLIOGRAPHY

1. Benegal V. Gambling experiences, problems and policy in India: a historical analysis. Addiction. 2013; 108(12):2062-7
2. American Psychiatric Association. Diagnostic and statistical manual of mental disorders (DSM-5 (R)). 5th ed. Arlington, TX: American Psychiatric Association Publishing; 2013.
3. Ruiz P, Strain EC, Lowinson JH. Lowinson and Ruiz's substance abuse:a comprehensive textbook. Philadelphia: Wolters Kluwer Health/ Lipincott Williams & wilkins,2011
4. Basu D, Dalal PK, Balhara YPS. Clinical practice guidelines on newer and emerging addictive disorders in India: Published by Indian Psychiatric Society, India 2016
5. Carnes PJ : Don't Call It Love. New York, NY: Bantam Books; 1991:181–266.
6. Sharma MK, Anand N, Tadpatrikar A, Thennarasu K, Rao GN, Benegal V, Singh RL, Thomas D, Gupta HK. Work addiction in the community: A trend for India. Indian Journal of Community Medicine. 2021 Apr 1;46(2):338.
7. Spada MM. An overview of problematic Internet use. Addictive Behaviors 2014;39:3-6.
8. Manoj Sharma, Vivek Benegal, Rao T. Behavioral and Technology addiction survey. Bangalore: National Institute of Mental Health and Neurosciences 2013.
9. Adams J, Kirkby R. Exercise Dependence and Overtraining: The Physiological and Psychological Consequences of Excessive Exercise. Sports Medicine, Training and Rehabilitation. 2001;10(3):199-222
10. Black DW. A review of compulsive buying disorder. World Psychiatry. 2007;6(1):14-8.
11. Indian Council for Medical Research. Behavioral addiction in the community: an exploration. Sharma MK, Benegal V, Girish N, Thennarasu K. http://www.icmr.nic.in/final/Behavioral%20addiction%20in%20the%20community .pdf
12. Boland R, Verduin M, Ruiz P. Kaplan & Sadock's Synopsis of Psychiatry. 12th ed. Baltimore, MD: Wolters Kluwer Health; 2021.
13. IACAPAP Textbook of Child and Adolescent Mental Health, ©2015 International Association for Child and Adolescent Psychiatry and Allied Professions. IACAPAP
14. Dutta A, Sharma A. Prevalence of premenstrual syndrome and premenstrual dysphoric disorder in India: A systematic review and meta-analysis. *Health Promot Perspect*. 2021;11(2):161-170.
15. Washington, M., Brown, C., & Ling, F. (2015). Premenstrual syndrome/premenstrual dysphoric disorder. In E. Bieber, J. Sanfilippo, I. Horowitz, & M. Shafi (Eds.), Clinical Gynecology (pp. 27-43). Cambridge: Cambridge University Press.

Mental Health 68

Pragya Lodha • Avinash De Sousa

INTRODUCTION

The long-standing definition of health by the World Health Organization (WHO, 1948) states that health is a state of complete physical, mental and social well-being, and not merely the absence of disease or infirmity. It is often that when we talk about health, we don't address mental health. Mental health, as defined by the World Health Organization (WHO, 2014) is a state of well-being in which every individual realizes his or her own potential, can cope with the normal stresses of life, can work productively and fruitfully, and is able to make a contribution to her or his community. Health is incomplete without mental health. It is crucial to understand that mental health and physical health are interlinked and interdependent on each other. Physical health and mental health affect each other complementarily.

Mental health affects the way we think, feel and act. Our mental health determines how we handle stress, how we maintain our relationships and make choices. Mental health is often called as 'invisible health' because it is not tangible. Mental health is linked to various health conditions. A sound mental health helps cope with other physical health conditions in a better manner. An individual with a sound mental health is able to take care of himself/herself and others in an efficient manner. Mental health is a construct that usually falls on a continuum and is temporal. It changes with situations the person is in, surrounding environment, relationships with people, existing stressors, history of illnesses and various other personal, interpersonal and external factors.

Another term related to mental health is mental illness (also referred to as mental health problems, mental health conditions). Mental illnesses are health conditions involving changes in perception, thinking, emotion or behavior (or a combination of these) which are constituted over a period of time and start affecting the daily functioning of an individual. Mental illnesses are associated with distress and/or problems functioning in social, work or family activities. A mental illness is always a cluster of symptoms presenting together and never one/two symptom(s) standalone. Not all symptoms may be present in every individual. Presentation of mental illnesses differ from patient to patient. The diagnosis of a mental health illness is done with the reference to the Diagnostic Statistical Manual of Mental Disorders- 5 (DSM-5) and/or the International Classification of Disorders-11 (ICD-11) that are the primary references used across the globe. Both, DSM-5 and ICD-11 have diagnostic criterion for mental disorders (cognitive, affective and behavioral disorders) that provide for a sound foundation to a mental health professional to make a diagnosis. Mental illnesses are common (American Psychiatric Association, 2015) and affect the following:

a. **Perception** – People may experience the world with their senses (vision, smell, taste, touch, hearing) in unusual and/or strange ways (e.g., hearing voices, seeing things that others do not see).

b. **Thinking** – Thoughts may occur very quickly/slowly, may be poorly organized, confusing, illogical and/or irrational.

c. **Mood** – All human beings experience a variety of moods (e.g., depression, anxiety, mania) and mood changes. Mental illness can emerge when symptoms cause significant distress over time and impair one's ability to function in daily life.

d. **Behavior** – People suffering from a mental illness may display behavior that may be quite bizarre and confusing for those who do not understand mental illness, such as- psychomotor agitation, psychomotor retardation, tics, compulsions, catatonic stupor and various other behaviors. The behavior may cause disruption of daily functioning for the individual.

MYTHS AND FACTS

The stigma around mental health is prevalent around the globe and more strongly in our country. The stigma to mental health has its roots in the history of the approach towards mental health and mental illnesses in the past. Earlier, people with severe mental illnesses were institutionalized (in hospitals) but unfortunately the treatment given to them there was inhuman. It was only after the deinstitutionalization movement (where it was considered that it was necessary to reinstate people with mental illnesses back to society- rehabilitate them), that patients started receiving dignity care and it is after long years that patients of mental illnesses now have rights for their treatment. Though there have been several strides towards defeating stigmas, they are still prevalent in our societies. Several reasons contribute to the stigma being present, that include- lack of education, limited awareness, belief in witchcraft, wizardry and various superstitious beliefs and media portrayal that leads to a constricted attitude towards approaching mental health services. Some of the most prevalent myths related to mental health are:

Myth #1: Mental illnesses are not real illnesses.

Fact: Mental illnesses are not the regular ups and downs of life. Mental illnesses create distress, don't go away on their own, and are real health problems. When someone is physically injured, they see a doctor. Similarly, mental health problems also require to be seen by a doctor (mental health professional- psychologist/counselor/psychiatrist).

Myth #2: Mental illnesses will never affect me.

Fact: All of us will be affected by mental illnesses. Researchers estimate that as many as one in four Indians will experience a mental illness at some point in their life. You may not experience a mental illness yourself, but it's very likely that a family member, friend or co-worker will experience challenges.

Myth #3: Mental illnesses are just an excuse for poor behavior.

Fact: It's true that some people who experience mental illnesses may act in ways that are unexpected or seem strange to others. We need to remember that the illness, not the person, is behind these behaviors, the reasons for such behaviors are outside the control of the person. People who experience a change in their behavior due to a mental illness may feel extremely embarrassed or ashamed around others. People with a mental illness are like one of us.

Myth #4: Stress causes mental illnesses.
Fact: No one factor can cause mental illnesses. Mental illnesses are complicated conditions that arise from a combination of genetics, biology, environment, and psycho-social factors. Stress may aggravate the mental state or physical state of problem for an individual but is never the sole problem of an illness.

Myth #5: People with mental illnesses are violent and dangerous.
Fact: People who experience a mental illness are no more violent than people without a mental illness. It's also important to note that people who experience mental illnesses are much more likely to be victims of violence than to be violent. Excluding them from the society because they are violent is because of a misunderstanding and stigmatic approach to mental health.

Myth #6: People don't recover from mental illnesses.
Fact: People can and do recover from mental illnesses. Today, there are many different kinds of treatments, services, and support programs available that can help. Effective treatment for mental illnesses is available. Identifying the illness at an earlier stage is way more effective that allows an individual to return to normal in day to day functioning. We must take care to seek help as early as possible.

Myth #7: People who experience mental illnesses are weak, cannot manage and have a characteristic flaw.
Fact: Stress impacts well-being, but this is true for everyone. Many people who experience mental illnesses learn skills like stress management and problem-solving so that they can remain optimally functional. Taking care of yourself and asking for help when you need it are signs of strength, not weakness. Mental illnesses don't determine the character of a person. Mental illnesses, are like other ailments and can be managed.

Myth #8: People who experience mental illnesses cannot go to work or follow a regular lifestyle.
Fact: Mental illnesses do not certify that someone is no longer capable of working. Most people who experience serious mental illnesses want to work but face systemic barriers to finding and keeping meaningful employment. Medical or therapeutic help can allow them to resume work and a manageable lifestyle.

Myth #9: Children cannot have mental illnesses. Those are adult problems.
Fact: Even children can experience mental illnesses. In fact, many

mental illnesses first appear when a person is young. Mental illnesses may look different in children than in adults, but they are a real concern at younger age as well. Unfortunately, many children don't receive the help they need. The onset for most illnesses starts at 14 years of age. It is important to remember that illnesses can occur and be diagnosed as early as 6-8 months of age.

Myth #10: Everyone gets depressed as they grow older. It's just part of the aging process.

Fact: Depression is not a necessary part of aging. Older adults may have a greater risk of depression because they experience so many changes in roles and social networks. If an older adult experiences depression, they need the same support as anyone else.

IDENTIFICATION OF MENTAL ILLNESSES

Mental illnesses can be identified through signs and symptoms. Signs are indicator of illnesses that are visible overtly whereas symptoms are markers that are felt by the individual and may not be seen overtly. There are various ways in which the signs and symptoms of a mental illness may be manifested in an individual- on a physical (or bodily) level, feeling level, thought level, behavioral level and/or imagination level.

Signs and symptoms of an illness tell us that there is some problem or disturbance at a daily functioning level. One must remember that signs and symptoms of any illness may be persistent and seen over a period of several days in order to classify them as a problem. Once

Table 68.1: Signs & symptoms of mental disorder

Physical	Feeling	Thinking	Behavior	Imagining
Tired	Sadness	Excessive worry	Crying	False beliefs
Aches and Pains	Anxiety	Self-blame and criticism	Social withdrawal	Hearing voices
Weight loss	Guilt	Unable to make decisions	Talking to him/ herself	Seeing things not there
Pounding heart	Helplessness	Poor concentration	Aggression	Smelling things not there
Sleep disturbance	Loss of emotion	Thoughts of death & suicide	Poor personal hygiene	Tasting things not there
Stomach ache	Mood swings	Rapid thinking	Avoidance behavior	Feeling things not there
Feeling of short breathe	Hopelessness	Poor judgment	Rapid speaking	
Loss of appetite	Low self esteem		Not making sense to others	
Muscle tension	Excessive fear		Attempting suicide	
Lack of energy	Loss of motivation		Irritability	

signs and symptoms are identified, one must ensure to consult a mental health professional in order to seek the right treatment.

Early intervention is the practice of identifying the signs and symptoms at an earlier time so that the illness does not reach a full-fledged stage where treatment or management of the illness becomes difficult. It is important to identify for early care so that the burden of illness can be reduced. This also helps improve the quality of life of an individual.

Early Intervention → Early Treatment → Better Managed Symptoms → Better Recovery → Lesser Negative Impact → Better Overall Functioning & Well being

MENTAL ILLNESSES

Who does it affect?

Mental illnesses can affect anyone regardless of age, gender, income, social status, race/ethnicity, religion/spirituality, sexual orientation, background or other aspect of cultural identity. While mental illness can occur at any age, three-fourths of all mental illness begins by age 14. It is also important to remember that women and men are prone to some illnesses more than their counterpart because of the biological aspect of the illness and the prevailing socio-cultural factors.

It is equally important to remember that the way an illness is manifested in an individual can vary with minimal differences from person to person. There are several factors that one must consider while understanding the cause and the course of treatment for a mental illness; and it includes:

- Details of patient- age/gender of patient, socio-economic status, where he/she stays
- Onset of illness- when the illness occurred, under what circumstances
- History of patient- birth, childhood, parenting, family, schooling, education, peer relationships, romantic relationships
- History of past illness- previously suffered medical or mental illness
- Details of family members
- Details of his/her personality before and after illness

Etiological Factors

There is never a single cause of any mental illness. There are many factors that are called as 'risk factors' that predispose an individual to mental illnesses. Causation of mental illnesses are understood from the perspective of 2 models-

(i) **bio-psycho-social model** that involves the interplay of biological (genes, neurotransmitters, brain structure), psychological (personality, beliefs, behaviors, life experiences) and social (stress from environment, family and parenting, cultural issues such

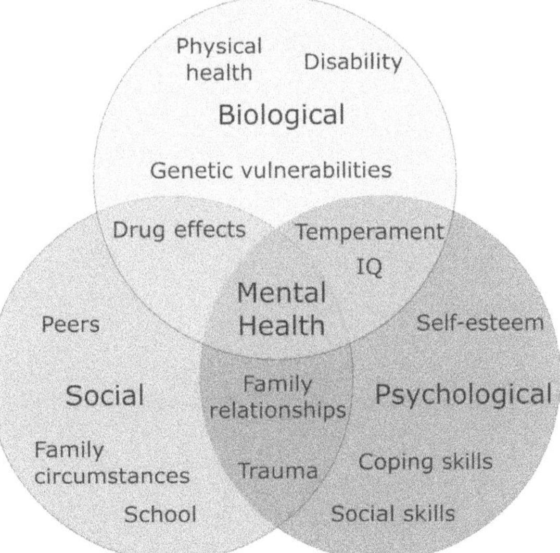

Fig. 68.1

discrimination, racism, etc.) factors in the development and course of the mental illnesses;

(ii) **diathesis stress module** (or vulnerability stress model) which explains the risk factors that an individual bear during birth and the factors in the individual's environment (depending on how healthy versus unhealthy) that are responsible to either increase or decrease the risk of developing a mental illness. Individuals can inherit a genetic predisposition (vulnerability) to mental illness, given a family history of some disorder(s). Given there is a history of illness in the family, environment and life experiences (stress) can trigger the onset/aggravate the mental illness.

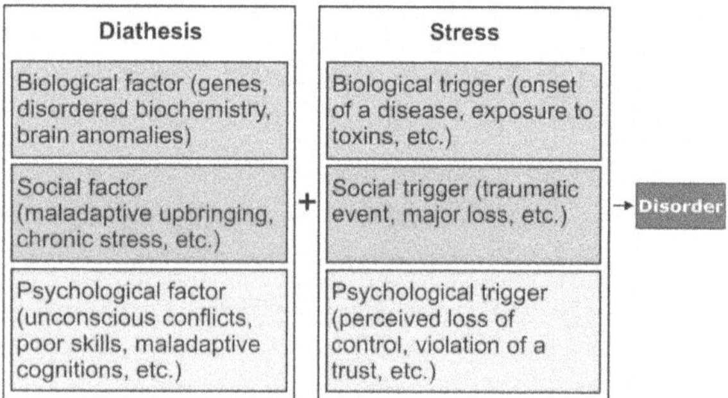

Fig. 68.2

Some of the factors that play a role in the development of a mental illness include the following:

1. **Biological Factors**
   - **Genetics (heredity):** Mental illnesses, many-a-times, run in families, suggesting that people who have a family member with a mental illness may be somewhat more likely to develop one themselves. Mental illness itself occurs from the interaction of multiple genes and other factors - such as stress, abuse, or a traumatic event - which can aggravate, or trigger, an illness in a person who has an inherited susceptibility to it.
   - **Infections:** Certain infections have been linked to brain damage and the development of mental illnesses, or the worsening of its symptoms.
   - **Brain defects or injury:** Defects in or injury to certain areas of the brain, have also been linked to some mental illnesses. These injuries may occur before or during birth or right after birth.
   - **Prenatal damage:** Some evidence suggests that a disruption of early fetal brain development or trauma that occurs at the time of birth - for example, loss of oxygen to the brain, exposure of alcohol to foetus, fetal exposure to substances like lead and mercury - may be factors in the development of certain mental health abnormalities.
   - **Other factors:** Poor nutrition and exposure to toxins, such as lead, may play a role in the development of mental illnesses.
2. **Psychological Factors:**
   - Severe psychological trauma suffered as a child, such as emotional, physical, or sexual abuse
   - An important early loss, such as the loss of a parent due to death or divorce
   - Neglect
   - Feelings of inadequacy, low self-esteem, anxiety, anger or loneliness
   - Poor ability to relate to others
3. **Environmental Factors:**
   - Death or divorce
   - Parenting (authoritarian or neglected)

- A dysfunctional family life
- Bullying and negative behaviors at school
- Changing jobs or schools
- Irrational social or cultural expectations
- Substance abuse by the person or the person's parents

Epidemiology

It is estimated that one in four persons will suffer from a mental illness at some point of time in their lives. Around 450 million people suffer from mental illnesses across the globe. In India, 6.3 million persons suffer from mental illnesses.

Treatment gap in mental health is understood as the difference between how many people need treatment and how many people actually receive the treatment. The treatment gap is huge in India, as less as only 1 out of 10 people receive treatment and more than 75% of people go without receiving any sort of help and treatment for their illness. There are several reasons for the treatment gap, such as-

- Lack of infrastructure
- Lack of professionals
- Lack of quality training
- Lack of access to mental health resources
- Stigma attached to mental health problems
- Ignorance about health care and hygiene
- Superstitious beliefs
- Lack of affordable services

SOME PREVALENT MENTAL ILLNESSES

Some mental health problems are more commonly prevalent than the others, considering epidemiological and etiological factors. At any given time, common mental health disorders can be found in around one in six people in the community, and around half of these have significant symptoms that would warrant intervention from healthcare professionals.

The terms mild, moderate and severe are used to describe different levels of mental health problems, depending on the severity of the illness. Every mental illness is assessed and managed depending on the level of severity that is presented by the patient. A ***mild*** mental health problem is when a person has a lesser number of symptoms that have a limited effect on their daily life and are more manageable. A ***moderate*** mental health problem is when a person has more symptoms that can make their daily life much more difficult than usual and difficulties may be less manageable. A ***severe*** mental health problem is when a person has greater symptoms that can make their daily life extremely difficult. A person may experience different levels at different times.

The cognitive, affective, physiological (somatic) and behavioral symptoms are wide ranging for mental illnesses and differ from one patient to another. The symptomatic presentation also differs with severity and duration of the illness. Factors like personality factors of the patient, available social support, existing environment, genetic make-up, diasthesis stress and several other internal and external contributing factors affect the psychopathogenesis.

Enlisted below are some commonly prevalent mental health disorders:

1. **Depression:** Depression is a common mental disorder and it is estimated as of 2019, that one in three persons is depressed. It is primarily a mood disorder but affects the other areas of functioning as well. Depression involves a low mood

that may persist the entire day or may be present for most of the day; such a mood presentation exists over 6 months. Depression encompasses a wide range of mental health problems, primarily characterized by the following symptoms: sadness of mood/low mood, lack of or excess sleep, lack of or excess appetite, psychomotor agitation/psychomotor retardation, loss of interest in earlier pleasurable activities, helplessness & hopelessness, social withdrawal, crying spells and suicidal ideation.

2. **Generalized Anxiety Disorder (GAD)**: A disorder that has an essential feature of excessive anxiety and worry about day-to-day activities on most days for a period of 6 months. It is an anxiety disorder where the person with GAD finds it difficult to control the anxiety and worry, which is often accompanied by restlessness, being easily fatigued, having difficulty concentrating, irritability, muscle tension and disturbed sleep. Often GAD and depression co-exist. Coexisting mental illnesses are referred to as comorbid conditions. Clinically, 90-95% of patients present with depression and anxiety together. Some clinicians diagnose it as *mixed depression and anxiety disorder*.

3. **Panic Disorder**: panic attack is a sudden, intense feeling of fear or panic that does not have a cause. Panic attacks can be very frightening for the individual and they may peak up to 10 minutes or less. The person experiencing a panic attack may feel that these attacks are life threatening but they are not life threatening. Though experiencing panic attack once or twice may be normal, however, it is a worry when a person may experience panic when there is no real threat or danger. A panic attack becomes a panic disorder when the panic disorders are intermittently present over a period of time. Panic disorder is also a type of anxiety disorder. It is important to discriminate between the different types of anxiety disorders.

4. **Obsessive Compulsive Disorder (OCD)**: OCD is characterized by the presence of either obsessions or compulsions, or both. Commonly, both elements of obsessions and compulsions are present. An obsession is defined as an unwanted intrusive thought, image or urge that repeatedly enters the person's mind. Obsessions are distressing, they are usually regarded by the individual as unreasonable or excessive. Common obsessions in OCD include contamination from dirt, germs, viruses, body fluids and so on, fear of harm (for example, that door locks are not safe), excessive concern with order or symmetry, obsessions with the body or physical symptoms, religious, sacrilegious or blasphemous thoughts, sexual thoughts, an urge to hoard useless or worn out possessions, or thoughts of violence or aggression. Compulsions are repetitive behaviors or mental acts that the person feels driven to perform. A compulsion can either be overt and observable by others, or a covert mental act that cannot be observed. Common compulsions include checking (for example, gas taps), cleaning, washing, repeating acts, mental compulsions (for example, repeating special words or prayers in a set manner), ordering, symmetry or exactness, hoarding/collecting and counting.

5. **Post traumatic Stress Disorder (PTSD):** PTSD often develops in response to one or more traumatic events such as deliberate acts of interpersonal violence, severe accidents, disasters or military action. Primarily, patients with PTSD have an involuntarily re-experience of the

traumatic event in a vivid and distressing way. Symptoms include flashbacks in which the person acts or feels as if the event is recurring; nightmares; and repetitive and distressing intrusive images or other sensory impressions from the event. Reminders of the traumatic event arouse intense distress and/or physiological reactions.

6. **Social Anxiety Disorder (SAD):** SAD is also referred to as social phobia, it is an anxiety disorder where the person experiencing SAD has intense fear in social situations that results in considerable distress and in turn impacts on a person's ability to function effectively in aspects of their daily life. Central to the disorder is a fear of being judged by others and of being embarrassed or humiliated. This leads to the individual avoiding going to social outings or meeting people, resulting in social withdrawal due to anticipated fear. Social anxiety disorder is characterized by a range of physical symptoms including excessive blushing, sweating, trembling, palpitations and nausea.

7. **Specific phobias**: Specific phobias, also a type of anxiety disorder, are unwarranted, extreme and persistent fear of a specific object or situation that is out of proportion to the actual danger or threat that they may pose (sometimes, may not really pose threat). The fear and anxiety occur immediately upon encountering the feared object or situation and tend to lead to avoidance or extreme discomfort. These phobias develop usually due to a negative or aversive reaction of the person towards the object/situation. The person with a specific phobia understands that the fear is excessive and out of proportion to the actual risk.

8. **Schizophrenia:** Schizophrenia is a chronic and severe mental disorder that affects how a person thinks, feels and behaves. People with schizophrenia most usually seem like they have lost touch with reality. Schizophrenia has symptoms that can be classified as positive symptoms- hallucinations, delusions, thought disorders; negative symptoms- flat affect, reduced feelings of pleasure in diurnal activities, difficulty starting activities and difficulty staying motivated; cognitive symptoms- interference in working memory, loss of attention and concentration and difficulty in executive functioning (planning, decision making etc.).

9. **Bipolar Disorder:** Bipolar Disorder is a mood disorder. There is an involvement of clear changes in mood, energy and activity levels. These moods range from periods of extremely "up," elated, and energized behavior (known as manic episodes) to very sad, "down," or hopeless periods (known as depressive episodes). Less severe manic periods are known as hypomanic episodes. People with bipolar disorder experience periods of unusually intense emotion, changes in sleep patterns and activity levels, and unusual behaviors.

10. **Personality Disorders:** personality disorder is a way of thinking, feeling and behaving that deviates from the expectations of the culture, causes distress or problems functioning, and lasts over time. Personality disorders are long-term patterns of behavior and inner experiences that differs significantly from what is expected. The pattern of experience and behavior begins by late adolescence or early adulthood and causes distress or problems in functioning. Without treatment, personality disorders can be long-lasting. Personality disorders affect at least two of these areas: way of thinking about oneself

and others, way of responding emotionally, way of relating to other people and/or way of controlling one's behavior.

11. **Eating Disorders**: Eating disorders involve severe disturbances in people's eating behaviors and related thoughts and emotions. Preoccupation with food, body weight, and shape are also signals of an eating disorder. Common eating disorders include anorexia nervosa, bulimia nervosa, and binge-eating disorder.
12. **Onset of Disorders in Childhood:** There are several disorders that are also seen in children are studied under the specialization of child psychiatry and child psychology. The above-mentioned disorders can also be and are seen in children as well. They are usually then labelled as 'childhood onset' or 'pediatric'. Disorders seen during the onset of childhood include a range of disorders like intellectual developmental disability, attention deficit hyperactivity disorder, learning disability, school refusal, exam anxiety, enuresis, disruptive mood dysregulation disorder, epilepsy, oppositional defiant disorder and others.

TEATMENT OF MENTAL ILLNESSES

Mental illnesses are treatable. It is essential to identify symptoms at an earlier time so that the severity of mental illnesses can be avoided, ensuring faster recovery and better living conditions for the individual. Mental health problems can be treated medically and non-medically. Medically, mental illnesses are treated by a psychiatrist who is a medical doctor trained in psychiatry and only he or she can prescribe medication. Non-medical treatment or therapeutic treatment is given counselors, psychotherapists or clinical psychologists who are trained mental health professionals in talk therapy. They do not prescribe medication.

Other paraprofessionals like social workers in psychiatry, psychiatric nurses and other professionals specialized in specific therapies and alternative treatment, also a play role in providing non-medical management of mental illnesses.

Mental illnesses involve treatment with-

a. **Medication**- various medicines are available for the treatment of mental illnesses. It is important to remember three things about medication for mental illnesses- medicines help in effective management of symptoms; psychiatric medication must not be stopped without the knowledge and approval of the doctor; medications may cause side effects but one must weigh the effectiveness of the medicine when considering for side effects. Psychiatric medication can only be prescribed by a psychiatrist or a general practitioner (with training or background in psychiatry/mental health/psychiatric medication).
b. **Psychotherapy**- several mental illnesses are well managed by the course of psychotherapy which involves a therapeutic relationship between the patient/client and a therapist/counselor. It involves a trained and structured way of conversation along with scientifically approved technics that help in emotion management, behavior management and improving thinking styles. Psychotherapy is done by psychotherapists or psychologists trained in therapy. Therapy sessions may last from 2-12 sessions depending on the needs of the individual.
c. **Combination treatment**- Most mental illnesses are managed by a combination

of medication and psychotherapy, which makes for an effective management of disorders.

d. **Electroconvulsive Therapy (ECT)**: ECT is also one of the frequently used treatment modalities that is administered in the manifestation of several mental illnesses such as OCD, Bipolar Disorder and Schizophrenia. ECT involves the passage of very mild electric currents that initiate a brief seizure. The ECT is administered only with anesthesia and muscle relaxants. Though ECT may have side effects like temporary memory loss. There has been stigma attached with the use of ECT as a treatment from earlier times because it led to severe side effects (as anesthesia and appropriate muscle relaxants were not used); however, in the present times, ECT treatment comes with very few risks. ECT has helped in the recovery of several mental illnesses among people (in Gujarat as well).

e. **Alternative treatments**- Yoga, meditation, relaxation technics, physical exercises and diet/nutritional intake are alternate ways that are accompanied by the first lines of treatment (medication/therapy). These technics help the individual to adjust better with the illness, on a day-to-day basis. These must be undertaken with guidance of the doctor or therapist.

Mental Health First Aid

When a person has an acute physical illness, it can be addressed in the short-term with first aid treatments, such as treatment for snake bite. Mental disorders can also be addressed initially with Mental Health First Aid.

There are many effective ways of responding to people with a mental disorder, and CMHWs have an important role to play in providing assistance and helping the person and his/her family seek appropriate help.

Five basic steps can be taken to help people suffering from a mental disorder:

1. Assess the risk of harm to self or others (and suicide)
2. Listen without judgment
3. Give reassurance and information
4. Encourage the person to get appropriate professional help
5. Encourage self-help treatments

Mental Health First Aid Actions

1. Assess the risk of harm to self or others (and suicide)

People with mental disorders sometimes feel overwhelmed and helpless about their life that the future appears hopeless.

Engage the person in conversation about how they are feeling and let them describe why they are feeling this way.

Ask the person if they are having thoughts of suicide. If they are, find out if they have a plan for suicide. This is not a bad question to ask someone who is mentally unwell. It is important to find out if he/she is having these thoughts in order to refer him/her for help. It is generally a call for help when a person talks about suicide, listen to them, empathize with them.

If you believe the person is at risk of harming him/herself then:

- don't leave the person alone
- listen to the feelings of the person, allow them to talk
- seek immediate help from someone who knows about mental health/disorders

- try to remove the person from access to the means of taking their own life
- avoid the use of alcohol or drugs for the person.

2. **Listen without judgment**

   Listen to what the person describes without being critical or thinking they are weak.

   Don't give advice such as 'just cheer up' or 'pull yourself together.'

   Avoid getting into an argument with the person.

3. **Give reassurance and information**

   Provide hope for the person and their family and talk about a good outcome for that person.

   Tell the person that he/she has an illness that can be treated, and it doesn't mean that he/she is a bad person.

   Let them know that you want to help.

4. **Encourage the person to get appropriate professional help**

   You can encourage the person to consult with a doctor who knows about mental disorders, and who is able to prescribe medication, if necessary. Then you can follow-up by giving ongoing support to the person and their family.

   If the person is very unwell, i.e., you think they are suicidal or psychotic, and he/she is refusing to get any help from a doctor--encourage the family to consult with the doctor so that they can explain the situation and get professional support.

5. **Encourage self-help treatments**

   Suggest actions that the person can perform him/herself that can help relieve the symptoms of mental disorder such as:

   - getting enough sleep
   - eating a healthy diet
   - regular exercise
   - relaxation and breathing exercises e.g. yoga
   - avoiding alcohol, tobacco or nicotine consumption
   - joining support groups for women, men or youth
   - spending time on some hobby each day
   - taking out time for self-time
   - making a schedule and following it

Compliance with Medical Treatment

What must be kept in mind is that it is important to take psychiatric medication. Psychiatric medication may range from 2-5 years and must not be discontinued without the consultation of the doctor. Many a times, people stop taking medication and then relapse into another episode- this further reduces the chance of recovery from the illness and the patient often complaints that the medication is ineffective. It is important to remember that medication must be taken for a prolonged period in order to see the effective change in the condition of the illness.

The myth that psychiatric medication makes an individual dependent on medication also needs to be clarified. Sometimes, taking medication is helpful for the individual to carry out day-to-day activities and must be taken. Another problem reported with psychiatric medication are the side effects. It is important to weigh the risks and benefits of the medication. Modern psychiatric medications have lesser side effects and benefit the patient more. Compliance with medical treatment helps the patient to be receptive of therapy and fastens the rate of recovery from an illness.

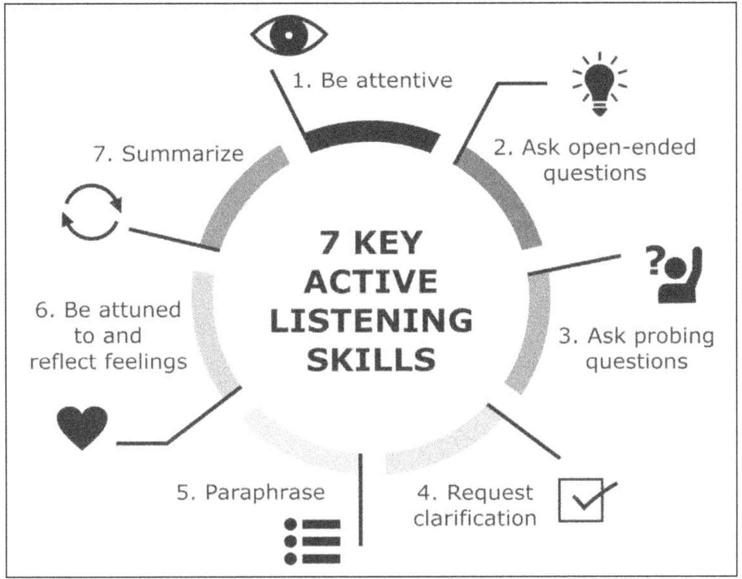

Fig. 68.3

What NOT to do for a person with mental disorder

- Ignore or avoid the person
- Believing the symptoms will just go away
- Thinking that it is part of life and development
- Locking the person away
- Being angry with him/her
- Relying exclusively on practitioners who use magic or faith healing
- Arranging a marriage if they are unmarried
- Giving sleeping tablets or appetite stimulants
- Believing that you can cure the person or that you have all the solutions to their problem
- Believing that time will heal things in the course

Listening is a very important tool when dealing with an individual suffering from a mental health problem. Active Listening can help get most information from the client that can be used effectively in order to help the individual.

Above (**Fig. 68.3**) shows are the tools of active listening that can be incorporated for effective outcomes-

BIBLIOGRAPHY

1. Kaplan BJ. Kaplan and sadock's synopsis of psychiatry. Behavioral sciences/clinical psychiatry. Tijdschrift voor Psychiatrie. 2016;58(1):78-9.
2. Morrison-Valfre M. Foundations of Mental Health Care-E-Book. Elsevier Health Sciences; 2016 Aug 23.
3. Pilgrim D. Key concepts in mental health. SAGE Publications Limited; 2019 Dec 28.
4. Shea SC. Psychiatric Interviewing E-Book: The Art of Understanding: A Practical Guide for Psychiatrists, Psychologists, Counselors, Social Workers, Nurses, and Other Mental Health Professionals, with online video modules. Elsevier Health Sciences; 2016 Sep 19.
5. Thapar A, Pine DS, Scott S, Snowling MJ, Taylor EA, editors. Rutter's child and adolescent psychiatry. John Wiley & Sons; 2017 Dec 26.

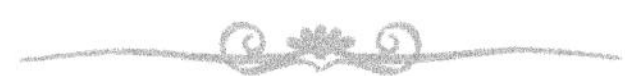

69 Stress – Its Nature and Management

Nahid Dave

DEFINITION

Any threatening situation physical or psychological induces a stress response. Physical expression of this stress is in the form of "flight or fright"[1]. Although in certain psychological situations both flight and fright are not an option, e.g. heavy traffic or unreasonable friend or family member.

Response in such situations depends on nature of the stressor and also on every individual's situational vulnerability. Pre-existing psychological factors play a role in understanding what happens before and after the trauma. In other words, personal context is an essential component in understanding psychological stressors.

Whenever an external event is perceived as debilitating or maladaptive it is perceived as stress. Resilience or the ability to recover from hardships depends to a great extent on childhood relationships and genetic control[2].

EUSTRESS AND DISTRESS

The same stressor can induce eustress and distress in different individuals indicating that stressors are neutral in nature. Individual coping mechanisms and perceptions play an important role.

Eustress is positive stress which motivates us to adapt to the changing environment in a constructive manner instead of anxiety[3].

Distress occurs when the stress exceeds the ability of the body to cope[3].

Classification of Stressors

1. Crisis

   Unforeseen and unpredictable events which are entirely outside the persons control are classified as Crisis stressors[4]. e.g. Natural disasters

2. Major life events

   Life events which bring with them a sense of uncertainty and fear can ultimately lead to stress[4]; e.g. marriage, birth of a child, going to a new college

3. Daily stressors

   Stressors that comprise our everyday life include Minor hassles, routine breakers or lost time[4]; e.g. meeting deadlines, traffic jam.

4. Ambient stressors

   These are chronic yet predictable stressors and are low grade in nature and run in the background[4].

   For pollution, crowding, noise etc.

Psychological conflict of three kinds can contribute to stress:

1. Approach-Approach conflict

   This typically occurs when an individual has to choose between two equally good options i.e whether to see a movie or go for a concert[5].

2. Avoidance- Avoidance conflict

   This typically occurs when an individual has to choose between two equally unattractive options i.e. do the weekly household chores or clean the garage[5].

3. Approach-avoidance conflict

   This typically occurs when an individual is forced to choose something which has its attractive and unattractive traits for i.e. going out to exercise early in the morning[5]. (It has a long term gain as far as health is concerned but has to get up earlier than usual and have an incomplete sleep)

Physiology of Response to Stress[6]

Stress producing trigger

↓

Information to Amygdala (Emotional processing)

↓

Perception of danger

↓

Distress signal to hypothalamus (Command Centre)

↓

Adrenal Glands release epinephrine (Adrenaline)

↓

Sympathetic Nervous System Activation

- Increase heart rate and blood pressure
- Increased rate of breathing + opening of small airways for more oxygen
- Increased blood pumping to heart, muscles and vital organs
- Increased blood to the brain thereby increased alertness and sharpened senses
- Digestion stops

Blood sugar utilization from the temporary storage sites(Epinephrine binds to liver cells and release of glucose)

↓

All the above steps occur within seconds. For e.g.; jumping away from the path of a speeding oncoming car

↓

If stress continues (Chronic Stress)

↓

Hypothalamic-Pituitary-Adrenal Axis

↓

Release of CRH (Corticotropin Releasing Hormone)

↓

Cortisol Release from the Adrenal Glands (Cortisol released until stress lasts) Increases blood sugar, decreases immunity and inflammatory response

↓

Break or Counter stress Parasympathetic system (Rest and Digest response)

Emotional regulation comprises avoiding the threat of stress or to control the level of emotional arousal. Individuals with higher emotional reactivity are more prone to aggression and anxiety.

Psychological Theories of Stress

The usual responses to pain both physical and psychological are 'Blocking' and 'Drowning'

Blocking is when we deny any discomfort caused by the stressor. We try to push through by distracting ourselves or self-medicating with food, alcohol, drugs etc. This response is problematic in itself and doesn't help resolve the primary reason for stress.

Drowning doesn't happen consciously, it typically occurs in situations where we do not have the coping mechanisms to deal with the problem at hand. The person is overwhelmed by the problem and feels hopeless, helpless and in self-doubt.

Quite often one may swing from one to the other without realizing.

Stress may be triggered by a trauma in the present which may make a person relive a past trauma. The ego tries to master it

Psych Endocrinology

The hypothalamus-pituitary-adrenal axis(HPA) plays a vital role in homeostasis and maintaining an adaptive response to challenging stimuli. The response also depends on individual assessment of the stress and coping mechanism.

Corticotropin Releasing Hormone (CRH), Adrenocorticotropic Hormone (ACTH), and cortisol are released in response to physical and mental stress. The HPA axis plays a role in arousal-sleep, memory storage and retrieval, pain.

In Cushing's disease there is an increase in cortisol which may be associated with major depressive disorder, suicidal ideas and psychosis[7].

In Addison's Disease there is adrenal insufficiency which may present clinically as apathy, social withdrawal, decreased sleep and concentration, fatigue[8].

Anti-depressants are known to correct the HPA axis

Psych immunology

Chronic stress increases the susceptibility to common cold, decreased wound healing and decreased response to vaccination. It also increases the mortality and morbidity in HIV, autoimmune diseases, diabetes and cardiovascular diseases. It increases susceptibility to viral infections (e.g., upper respiratory infections, Epstein-Barr virus, herpes simplex virus, cytomegalovirus), may affect HIV progression, and may decrease the ability to fight cancer. Major depressive disorder is shown to decrease immunity and increase the inflammatory response[9].

Locus Ceruleus

Locus Ceruleus acts as a gatekeeper of sympathetic Nervous systems' response to stress. The stress can either be a threatening physiological situation or a cognitive event. Exposure to stressors produces adaptations in its function which ultimately leads to depressive symptoms. Adaptations in locus ceruleus in response to stress may alter individuals' responses to subsequent stress[10].

Consequneces of Stress

Stress and inflammation disrupt the processes of learning, memory, neural plasticity, and neurogenesis.

Stress and Weight Gain

Need for glucose as fuel during stressful situations

↓

Cortisol reduces lean muscle mass

↓

Synthesis of glusoce from protein

↓

Increase in blood sugar

↓

Increase craving for carbohydrates(sugars)

↓

Overeating(unhealthy)

↓

Increased stress after weight gain

Stress and sleep

(Normally) Cortisol level is highest in morning and lowest at night

↓

Chronic stress- cortisol production

↓

Disruption of normal cycle i.e. High levels of cortisol in the night

↓

Insomnia

How Stress Presents Itself[11]

1) Physical symptoms of stress include:

   Fatigue and lethargy

   Aches and pains

   Upset stomach, including diarrhea, constipation, and nausea

   Insomnia

   Frequent infections

   Increased or decreased appetite

2) Cognitive symptoms of stress include:

   Excessive worrying

   Forgetfulness

   Decreased concentration

   Poor judgment

   Seeing only the negative side

3) Emotional symptoms of stress include:

   Easy irritability and provoked on trivial issues

   Feeling overwhelmed, like you are losing control or need to take control

   Low self-esteem, lonely

   Avoiding others

Scales used to Assess Stress

Holmes and Rahe Stress Scale[12]

Perceived Stress Scale

Management of stress

1) Sleep hygiene

The quality of sleep has a direct relationship with alertness during the day and ultimately quality of life and productivity.

Some basic rules of basic sleep hygiene can be followed to reduce the effect of stress on the body

Limit daytime sleep to 30 minutes. Day time naps shouldn't be in the evening or close to dinner time[13].

Stimulants like nicotine, caffeine should be avoided 4-6 hours before bedtime.

A daily routine of aerobic exercise lasting atleast 10 minutes[13].

Dinner should be approximately 3 hours before bedtime. Oily, fatty and spicy food to be avoided in dinner.

Use the bed only for sleeping and sex, all other activities reading, mobile usage talking should be done outside the bed. The purpose is to condition the mind to understand that the bed is associated with sleep induction.

TV, Computer, Mobile or any other gadget usage to be stopped one hour before bedtime.

Have a fixed time of being of the bed each night and a fixed time for waking up each morning.

2) Exercise

It has been studied that even five minutes of aerobic exercise can have anti-anxiety effects. Reduction of stress is same irrespective of the intensity or duration of work out[14].

A theory known as 'time out' is proposed which gives an indicidual a distraction or break from the stressors.

During exercise body releases endorphins, which are opioid neuropeptides (wiki endorphin). They are also known as 'morphine like susbstance which originates from within the body.[15]

After aerobic exercise B endorphin is released from the pituitary, it binds to mu receptors. This binding blocks the neurotransmitter substance P which inhibits the pain signal by the peripheral nerves. The perception of pain diminishes after release of endorphin hence it is known to have analgesic effects.The binding of endorphin to mu receptor also brings about inhibition of GABA neurotransmitter(gamma-aminobutyric acid) which in turn increases the release of Dopamine. Dopamine is the neurotransmitter associated with pleasure

3) **Developing mature Defense Mechanisms**

Defense mechanism is an unconscious psychological mechanism adopted by the body to tide over unacceptable or harmful stressful situations[16].

The psychological process which involves accepting reality even if it is unpleasant falls under mature defense mechanism. Feelings and thoughts are made more conscious and less comfortable. It doesn't occur spontaneously but has to be cultivated.

Altruism

Working constructively in providing service to someone for personal satisfaction.

e.g., "I have been through my own struggles with alcohol, I would like to sponsor another fellow in the AA (Alcohol Anonymous) group struggling with the same".

Anticipation

Having realistic preparation for an anticipated stress in the future.

e.g.; "I have a dental appointment in the evening, it is going to be slightly painful but only for a few minutes and I have been through it once before too."

Sublimation

Unacceptable emotions are thoughts directed towards a positive and constructive activity.

For e.g., "I have a history of diabetes in the family, I will keep a check on my sugar intake and weight at all times".

Suppression

Consciously deciding to push away a disturbing thought to focus on the present. Dealing with the stress at a later time with a more accepting and open mind.

e.g., " I am angry with my brother right now but I shall wait till his friends leave and then talk to him about it"

Humor

Unpleasant thoughts and feelings are expressed in a way which sounds pleasant or amusing to others, while still retaining the innate distress

e.g. "I lost my eye in the accident, now I can dress as a pirate"

4) **Oxytocin**

The hormone oxytocin is associated with stimulating labour and ejection of milk during lactation. The hormone is also stimulated by positive social interaction involving touch and psychological support. It plays a role in decreasing blood pressure and cortisol in the blood, thereby having anxiolytic effect. It is also known to increase pain threshold.[17]

Oxytocin plays a role in maternal bonding with her baby and social affiliation. It has a 'Tend and Befriend' response to stress instead of 'fight and flight'.[18]

5) **Relaxation Technics**

The technic was described by Edmond Jacobson and is based on the premise that mental relaxation is a natural outcome of physical calmness.[19]

Progressive muscular relaxation (PMR) is a simple technic involving tensing and relaxing all the major muscles of the body one after another from foot to the head. It has been researched that relaxing the physical body releases the psychological stress and build resilience.

6) **Mindfulness**

Mindfulness is the practice of being aware of one's body, mind, and feelings in the present moment.[20] Mindfulness skill can be attained with training and meditation only. Mindfulness finds its roots in Buddhist Philosophy, but the practise of mindfulness therapy is entirely secular.

It has been researched that 8 weeks of daily mindful meditation practise for 20 minutes shows neuroplasticity changes in the brain. Mindfulness can be adapted as a way of life, as a means to counter stress and as a form of therapy in psychiatric disorders.

It uses the key concepts of being non-judgmental and having a beginners mind when facing life and situations. Thoughts and feelings are impermanent in nature, yet we obsess over them instead of watching them pass. The skill of observing ones thoughts as they pass and choosing to respond to them instead of reflex reactions.

7) **Psychotherapy**

Psychotherapy explores the meaning of stressors so that earlier traumas can be worked through. It helps individuals adapt to stressors which are not reversible or beyond our control. The focus of therapy remains generating insight and emotional growth.

Rational emotive behavior technics (REBT) and Cognitive behavior technics (CBT) are used most commonly.

8) **Telepsychiatry**

There is a dearth of psychiatrists and mental health facilities in rural settings. Telepsychitary aims at bridging this gap. Outpatients can be provided psychiatric expertise through telephonic or video conferencing.

Red flags

It is important to consider that stress could be a predecessor to psychiatric illnesses. It is important to keep in mind the important signs which may warrant the need to visit a mental health professional. If the symptoms of stress persist more than two weeks and are not mitigated by lifestyle modification and relaxation it is need for concern. Non restorative sleep and persistent low mood could be a warning sign.

BIBLIOGRAPHY

1. McEwen BS. Physiology and neurobiology of stress and adaptation: central role of the brain. Physiological reviews. 2007 Jul;87(3):873-904.
2. Davydov DM, Stewart R, Ritchie K, Chaudieu I. Resilience and mental health. Clinical psychology review. 2010 Jul 1;30(5):479-95.
3. Li CT, Cao J, Li TM. Eustress or distress: An empirical study of perceived stress in everyday college life. InProceedings of the 2016 ACM International Joint Conference on Pervasive and Ubiquitous Computing: Adjunct 2016 Sep 12 (pp. 1209-1217).
4. Pastorino, E. & Doyle-Portillo, S. (2009). What

is Psychology?. 2nd Ed. Belmont, CA: Thompson Higher Education.

5. Aldwin, Carolyn M; Jeong, Yu-Jin; Igarashi, Heidi; Choun, Soyoung; Spiro, Avron (2014). "Do hassles mediate between life events and mortality in older men?". Experimental Gerontology. 59: 74–80. doi:10.1016/j.exger.2014.06.019. PMC 4253863. PMID 24995936.
6. https://www.integrativepro.com/Resources/Integrative-Blog/2016/The-HPA-Axis
7. Starkman MN. The HPA axis and psychopathology: Cushing's syndrome. Psychiatric Annals. 1993 Dec 1;23(12):691-701.
8. Watson S, Mackin P. HPA axis function in mood disorders. Psychiatry. 2006 May 1;5(5):166-70.
9. Goodkin K, Visser AP, editors. Psychoneuroimmunology: stress, mental disorders, and health. American Psychiatric Pub; 2008 Nov 1.
10. Mertz H. Stress and the Gut. UNC School of Medicine. Chapel Hill, NC: www. MED. UNC. EDU/IBS. 2011 Mar.
11. https://www.webmd.com/balance/stress-management/stress-symptoms-effects_of-stress-on-the-body#1
12. Linn MW. Modifiers and Perceived Stress Scale. Journal of consulting and clinical psychology. 1986 Aug;54(4):507.
13. http://healthysleep.med.harvard.edu/healthy/getting/overcoming/tips
14. Weyerer S, Kupfer B. Physical exercise and psychological health. Sports Medicine. 1994 Feb 1;17(2):108-16.
15. Goldstein A, Lowery PJ (September 1975). "Effect of the opiate antagonist naloxone on body temperature in rats". Life Sciences. 17 (6): 927–31. doi:10.1016/0024-3205(75)90445-2. PMID 1195988.
16. Cramer P. The development of defense mechanisms. Journal of personality. 1987 Dec; 55(4):597-614.
17. Uvnas-Moberg K, Petersson M. Oxytocin, a mediator of anti-stress, well-being, social interaction, growth and healing. Z Psychosom Med Psychother. 2005 Jan 1;51(1):57-80.
18. Tori DeAngelis .The two faces of oxytocin. February 2008, Vol 39, No. 2.Print version: page 30.
19. Golombek U. Progressive muscle relaxation (PMR) according to Jacobson in a department of psychiatry and psychotherapy-empirical results. Psychiatrische Praxis. 2001 Nov;28(8):402-4.
20. Baer RA. Mindfulness training as a clinical intervention: A conceptual and empirical review. Clinical psychology: Science and practice. 2003 Jun;10(2):125-43.
21. Hubley S, Lynch SB, Schneck C, Thomas M, Shore J. Review of key telepsychiatry outcomes. World journal of psychiatry. 2016 Jun 22;6(2):269.

Psychology of Learning and Memory 70

Veena Kumar

OUTLINE OF THE CHAPTER

LEARNING:	**MEMORY:**
WHAT IS LEARNING?	WHAT IS MEMORY?
DEFINITIONS OF LEARNING	DEFINITIONS OF MEMORY
NEED TO LEARN AND SIGNIFICANCE OF LEARNING	NEED AND SIGNIFICANCE TO MEMORIZE
THEORIES OF LEARNING	THEORIES OF MEMORY
TYPES OF LEARNING	TYPES OF MEMORY
FACTORS AFFECTING LEARNING	FACTORS AFFECTING MEMORY
ENHANCING LEARNING	ENHANCING MEMORY
TIPS TO LEARN	TIPS TO REMEMBER

OBJECTIVES

1. Mastery of concepts
2. Application of concepts in everyday life: professional and personal
3. Facilitate problem solving
4. Enhancing capabilities to learn and memorize

Learn Unlearn Relearn is what we have been listening and doing in all these years and consciously, unconsciously, knowingly and unknowingly we have been all doing so.

We have been able to learn, unlearn and relearn because of two inseparable and or interconnected phenomena of learning and memory. We learn because there is memory and because there is memory we learn. Thus, learning and memory are two sides of the same coin. Both co-exist to a large extent because of its purpose and meaning to our living except when there is an organic cause for example loss of neurons, reduction in size of the brain, damage and or defective neurons, brain damage, brain abnormalities etc.

It is difficult to separate learning and memory like for example learning ends here and memory begins and or vice versa.

Psychology is defined as the science of human behavior. Behavior refers to covert processes like thoughts, cognitive processes and or physiological responses and overt behavior like action of jumping, walking, talking etc.

Previously Psychology was considered as the study of the soul, mind and because it was unobservable the terms soul mind was substituted as behavior. Initially only observable behavior was considered as it was relatively easy to measure and it was realized that cognitive and or thought processes play a very important role in determining stimuli response and feedback mediated by cognitive factors.

Cognition refers to the processes through which information coming from the senses is "transformed, reduced, elaborated, recovered, and used" (Neisser, 1967). Cognitive processes are mental processes involved in knowing about the world; include short term memory, long term memory, dreaming, decision making, sensation, perception attention etc. Information is sensory data from the environment as well as from within which signals about an activity which is happening.

Cognitive factors
↓
Stimuli → Response → Feedback

For example, a friend of ours generally came 30 mins later than the scheduled time, after a few instances, we are likely to remember this information about this friend and for our next meeting we are either likely to call this friend 30 mins prior and or we are likely to reach 30 mins later. This remembering of information influenced our response and in turn served as a feedback to our future sequence of stimuli and responses.

Educational Psychologists study learners and learning contexts-both within and beyond traditional classrooms and evaluate ways in which factors such as age, gender, culture and physical and social environments influence human learning.

Whereas Developmental Psychologists focus on studying the physical, emotional, social, psychological, cognitive aspects of human learning depending on the age, gender and culture a person belongs to.

WHAT IS LEARNING?

Learning involves knowing information, procedure which helps us in our daily life functioning thus helping us adopt, adapt to our everyday living including adjustment and enhancing our quality of life.

According to International Bureau of Education, Learning is defined as "a process that brings together personal and environmental experiences and influences for acquiring, enriching or modifying one's knowledge, skills, values, attitudes, behavior and worldviews".

Psychologists define learning as the process of acquiring new and relatively enduring information or behaviors (Myers).

Learning is defined as any relatively permanent change in behavior that occurs as a result of practice or experience (Morgan and King), which comprises of three aspects namely learning is a change in behavior for better or worse, change in behavior due to maturation or growth (development) is not learning and the change must be present for a certain amount of time and not due to the influence of drug induced states like alcohol and or alertness, fatigue etc.

In other words any change in behavior which lasts for a relative period of time not because of maturation, drug induced changes are understood as learning, for example, skill based changes like computer knowledge and or literacy, new language, cooking skills, problem solving etc.

WHY DO WE NEED TO LEARN AND SIGNIFICANCE OF LEARNING

Learning comes from the old English leornian

"to get knowledge, be cultivated; to study, read, think about".

Learning enables us to adapt effectively, productively, efficiently to ever changing life situations. T he nature of life is such that as we learn there is change and to adapt to change we learn and so on- a never ending cycle. As we learn we operate on the environment, self which in turn changes the environment, self and thus the need to learn.

Learning, Unlearnig and Relearning helps to modify and build on existing knowledge, procedure and thus there is a change either for better or worse.

Stating very broadly, everything is about learning and memory which includes associative learning, which refers to connecting two events, information which occur together and equally it is true that life and mind can never be fathomed and put into words.

Learning to Solve Problems

Every minute every second every msec there is a change as Universe is constantly changing and so are we.

Learning is highly related to our sensations and perceptions. Sensations are understood as raw sensory data or raw sensory information coming from our sense organs and interpretations of these sensations is perception. Perception is based on personal experiences and association which is highly dependent on the stage, phase of life we are along with gender, age and culture. For example very likely a particular event is interpreted differently last year than the event interpreted at this point of time.

Very often learning moves from being objective to subjective and from being subjective to being objective and hence it is generally stated learning is a lifelong process as we are all still discovering life and its processes.

THEORIES OF LEARNING

We often understand learning as acquired which is true to a large extent, equally true is the role of biology, according to evolutionary psychology is all behaviors (thoughts feelings, actions) are due to the inheritance of genes and chromosomes which determine laying of the basic network essential for learning including flexibility in learning due to neuroplasticity (ability of neurons to form new pathways, network based on practice and usage).

Our nervous system is a network of neurons (though it still remains a mystery of where and how information is coded, encoded and retrieved).Based on the laid neuron network, environment plays a very important role whether a particular behavior will be expressed or not; so it nature and nurture which determines learning and memory rather than nature versus memory.

1. **Behaviorist Perspective-** emphasizes how environment determines what we learn and what we do not learn based on reward and punishments and or reinforcements. If a behavior is learnt the same behavior can be unlearnt too. There are four forms of learning according to behaviorist perspective.

a) Classical Conditioning- Ivan Pavlov a Russian Physiologist explained how behaviors can be acquired through reinforcement. What is rewarding to an organism can bring about certain response and punishment generally refers to inhibition or cessation of responses and both are acquired. Law of association facilitates pairing of two stimuli and the same response is given to a neutral stimulus.

For example:

Dog is presented with food and dog starts salivating

Here food is the unconditioned stimulus and salivation is unconditioned response.

This pairing occurs a few times and then a neutral stimulus bell is presented followed by food and initially dog salivates only at the sight of food. Repeated pairing of bell with food makes the dog salivate at the sound of the bell which is the conditioned stimulus and conditioned response respectively.

Food (UCS) → Salivation (UCR)

Bell + Food (UCS) → Salivation (UCR)

Bell (CS) → Salivation (CR)

Stimulus generalization occurs when the original response to the bell is given to a similar stimulus as it provides reinforcement for example buzzer is presented instead of bell

Food → Salivation

Buzzer + Food → Salivation

Buzzer → Salivation

Generally observed in acquisition of phobias

Stimulus Discrimination occurs when the original response is not given to another stimulus as the organism is not given reinforcement, so the organism learns to differentiate between different stimulus.

For example if Dog is presented with bell and food is given whereas with buzzer no food is given, with time and association the dog learns to salivate at the sound of the bell and not buzzer.

Similarly in real life also we learn to differentiate between stimuli and give different responses accordingly.

Extinction occurs when the stimulus is no longer paired with reinforcements and with time dissociation occurs and the response ceases to exist.

For example if bell is no longer paired with food, initially the dog will salivate because of memory and association and with time only bell is rung and no food is presented then with time dog will stop salivating.

Spontaneous recovery is after a brief interval the response recurs because of reinforcement and it occurs in lesser or fewer trials. For example if food is presented along with bell initially the dog may not salivate and with repeated pairings and in a fewer trials the dog relearns to salivate at the sound of the bell.

b) Operant Conditioning refers to how behavior operates on the environment and depends on the reinforcement received either the behavior is repeated or not repeated.

Law of Effect proposed by Thorndike explains as a behavior is repeated if rewarded and not repeated if not rewarded. e.g. if a study habit leads to scoring better or higher marks we are likely to remain studying in the same habit or pattern than otherwise.

Stimulus generalization, discrimination, extinction and spontaneous recovery occurs based on the reinforcements received after the behavior has occurred.

The primary distinction between classical conditioning and operant conditioning is in reinforcements presented before the behavior occurs and after the behavior has occurred respectively and behavior occurs involuntarily and voluntarily respectively.

Punishment refers to delivery of aversive consequences, which may lead to cessation of behavior.

Positive reinforcement refers to pleasant rewards leading to strengthening of behavior.

Negative reinforcement- removal of unpleasant stimuli to strengthen behavior

Primary reinforcers are generally present since birth and aid survival of the organism e.g. food, water.

Secondary reinforcers- acquire the quality of reinforcement due to association e.g. praise, awards, approval, sanction, acceptance etc.

Schedules of Reinforcement- refers to how reinforcements occur in daily life situations. Interval and ratio occur in combinations. INTERVAL refers to time of reinforcement e.g. every five mins, every two hours.

RATIO refers to number of responses determine reinforcement; e.g. reward given every 4th response, every 12th response etc.

Four forms of schedules of reinforcements are as follows

Fixed interval, Variable ratio, fixed ratio, variable interval

c) Observational learning and or social learning occurs when we acquire behaviors based on seeing how significant or perceiving important people around us behave and or what we see in our environment e.g. parents, siblings, extended family, relatives, teachers, icons, social media etc.

Vicarious learning occurs when we learn to associate the actions of others with their respective reinforcements people receive and hence acquire the behavior indirectly. To a large extent this learning helps as it is not possible to learn everything directly as everything may not happen in the same way as it happens with others.

d) Insight learning- Wolfgang Kohler demonstrated in an experiment on chimpanzee based on previous past experiences, at times we learn some behaviors suddenly without our awareness.

Learning and Memory occurs either implicitly and or explicitly.

2. **Connectivism-** is understood with the help of parallel distributed processing, which is as we are continuously interacting with the outside environment and past experiences combine, we continuously form connections and associations and new learning takes place and/or previous learning is modified.

3. **Cognitive theories-** based on past experiences, how do we evaluate an incoming information explains what is learnt and not learnt. Rational and irrational thoughts, feelings and actions are acquired.

4. **Constructivism-** to understand a new concept and or a phenomena, one uses past experiences to interpret and formulate a relatively new construct, a new understanding which facilitates ones adaptation and functioning in everyday life.

5. **Experiential-** learning by doing or practicing either by modeling or imitation e.g. internship, practicals

6. **Humanistic-** learning is based on the characteristics of learner, learner centric rather than focus on methods and or procedures

7. **Transformative-** combination of new information, life experiences, knowledge of the past and critical reflection we acquire some new information and or skill along with modified information and or skills.
8. **Sociocultural-** which culture we belong to influences what we learn and or not learn. e.g. social skills, occupational skills and or information related to the culture we come from.

   We are all unique individuals and we all learn differently, and distinctly depending on which sensory modality is predominant and often includes relatively "holistic" development.

Piaget enumerates in his theory of learning which includes Accommodation, which refers to modifying or restructuring our previous knowledge so that new information can fit in better and Assimilation occurs when we modify or change new information to fit into our schemes (broad cognitive frameworks for stimuli which includes people, objects, situation); thus keeping the new information and old or previous information bringing about Cognitive Balance.

Factors affecting Learning and Enhancing One's Learning-

1. **Needs and Motivation-** our requirements and goals influence what we learn and unlearn. If we are intrinsically motivated we are likely to learn better and for a longer period of time compared to when we are extrinsically motivated to learn which is likely to be temporary and effective as long as there are external rewards to help us learn.
2. **Learned Helplessness-** Seligman explains as due to repeated failed attempts, we learn that despite any more attempts will not change the outcome we desire,
3. **Schemes-** based on past experiences and association, repeatedly we come to learn that situations, people, objects are the way it is. E.g. four walls, a window, door, fans, furniture is perceived more as a house (as generally this is the experience) rather than a hotel room and or office unless conditioned otherwise.
4. **Law of Association-** two events, two sets of information, two things when they co occur in time space, we tend to perceive it as one. E.g. cat crossing our path and we tripping
5. **Law of effect and reinforcement-** behaviors which are rewarded are likely to be repeated in future and which are not repeated we are not likely to be repeated.
6. **State dependent learning and state congruent learning-** we are likely to learn information and or skill which is consistent with our emotional state known as state congruent learning and state dependent learning is we are likely to retrieve information and or skill consistent with our emotional state.
7. **Contextual cues-** learning and retrieving from same modality and or sensory organs leads to enhanced learning and is likely to be remembered better and recalled better.
8. **Aptitudes and Interests-** information and or skills if it matches our capabilities, liking is likely to be learnt better than otherwise.
9. **Intelligence-** our intelligence determines our learning capabilities as well as capacities. E.g. higher the intelligence higher the ability to learn.
10. **Multimodality-** visualization, imagination is effectively learnt than only verbal mode of learning.

11. **Purpose and meaningfulness of learning**- if the learner perceives meaning and purpose to learn, likelihood of learning will be higher and more durable than otherwise.
12. **Anxiety**- when the learner is in an anxious state less likely to learn compared to when the learner is in a relaxed pleasant state.
13. **Language involved in learning**- when we have a predominant language and being taught in another language may slow one's learning, as we tend to think in the language we are more familiar and comfortable may enhance one's learning.
14. **Prepared and Contraprepared**- through years of evolution certain information skill is easily learnt compared to information, skill which has existed in the last few years.
15. **Avoidance and Escape behavior**- when the consequence is unpleasant, we learn to either not to face it completely (avoidance) and or just manage to avoid (escape) which is maintained by the reduction in anxiety and/or fear.
16. **Habit**- repeated behavior establishes neural pathways consequently creating an automatic behavior
17. **Incidental learning**- when learning takes place without an intention to learn, unintentionally, involuntarily.
18. **Intentional learning**- when learning takes place deliberately, voluntarily and often with the goal of being tested in due time.

Learning Disabilities is a neurological condition which affects the brain's ability to send, receive and process information. A child with a learning disability may have difficulties in reading, writing, speaking, listening, understanding mathematical concepts, and with general comprehension. At times due to neurological deficits, the child is unable to attain developmental milestones and as a result, the child may experience difficulties performing tasks which regular children easily learn. Forms of learning disability are dyscalculia, dysgraphia, dyslexia, non- verbal disabilities, oral/written language disorder and specific reading comprehension deficit and related disorders like attention deficit hyperactivity disorder, dyspraxia, executive functioning etc.

Tips to Learn

We tend to learn better if we are able to understand the learners style, characteristics along with their needs, motives, intelligence, emotional states and there is no one factor that determines what we will learn and not learn along with factors mentioned above.

Breaking a large goal into small manageable goals which will serve as its own reinforcement.

Thus, to summarize Learning is highly influenced by perseverance, will and a realistic understanding of ourselves along with purpose and meaningfulness of the stimuli to be learned.

MEMORY

What is Memory?

Memory means learning to remember which includes recall, recognition, relearning and reconstruction to facilitate future use. Memory is the faculty of the brain by which data or information is encoded, stored, and retrieved when needed, it is the retention of information over time for the purpose of influencing future action.

For learning and memory to occur there are a few steps that need to occur, which includes noticing, attention, encoding, storage and retrieval.

Thus Memory is defined as "is a cognitive system for storing and retrieving information." " Memory is a cognitive system for encoding, storage and retrieval of information."

Memory is generally measured in terms of recall, which is remembering information with minimum and or no cues; e.g. remembering full length essay type answers

Recognition involves retrieval with the help of cues e.g. in multiple choice questions

Relearning involves lesser time to learn an unrehearsed information (already learnt material) for revision at the time of exams and Reconstruction involves filling the gaps in memory by taking a mental walk through the events and or episodes e.g. when reporting in an eye witness testimony.

Very often mind and memory are used synonymously though mind refers to an abstract construct and involves higher order integrative functioning and memory is a part of mind. Often good memory and learning are associated with high intelligence.

Why do we need memory and significance of memory-

1. To help remember, recall and retrieve information in the times to come
2. To fill in gaps for information missing so that there is meaningfulness of the incoming stimuli
3. To facilitate problem solving
4. To use the information in daily living
5. To apply information for effective, productive, efficient use
6. Cost saving in terms of time energy and resources.
7. To prevent learning of the same information, skill every time it is needed.
8. To build up on learning based on memory as every cell has memory

THEORIES OF LEARNING

1. The Information Processing Model/Multi store mode/Modal model- Atkinson and Shiffrin

   Every millisecond our sense organs are constantly bombarded with information and each of the sense organs have their own memory systems. The incoming sensory information, the information is held for very brief period of time maybe 3-5 secs in sensory memory and if paid attention the information gets transferred to a little bigger store called short term memory wherein the information is held for 20-30 secs and if rehearsed either elaborately (rich processing of information), distinctively (novel, unique) and or through maintenance (repeating the information as it is like used in rote learning and rote memory) the information gets transferred to a larger memory store termed as Long term memory; whenever information has to be used, it is remembered either through retrieval cues or recall; the information is brought to short term memory and the information is used. At times information is lost from short term memory especially if there is distraction and or overloading of stimuli.

2. Levels or Depth of Processing model by Craik and Lockhart.

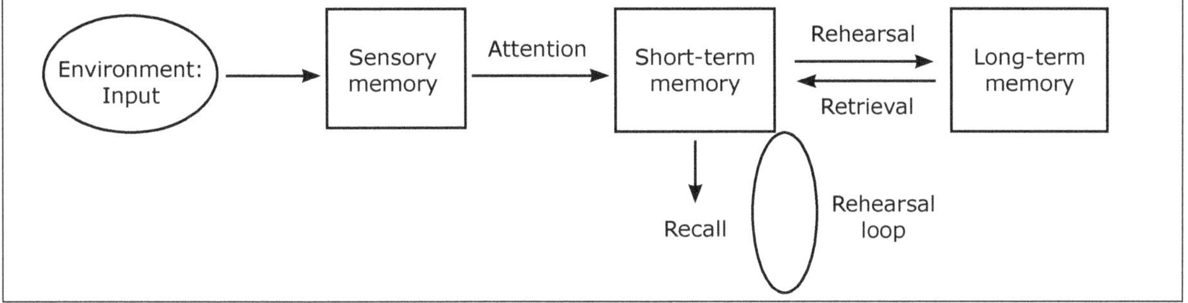

Fig. 70.1

This model explains that any incoming information is processed in one of the three ways namely shallow – processing in terms of physical characteristics of the stimuli

Intermediate/auditory/acoustic- processing in terms of sound which is relatively deeper and deepest being semantic, processing incoming stimuli in terms of its meaning which includes category level processing.

When we process information in terms of its meaning information is retained for a longer period of time followed by acoustic and lowest being for shallow processing; though exceptions are people with photographic memory, acoustic memory and or kinesthetic memory.

3. Self reference effect- the to be learnt material is remembered better when It is applied to oneself
4. Mnemonics- aids to memory, aids and facilitates retrieval e.g. method of loci, peg word, paired associate learning etc.
5. Parallel Distributed Approach by McClelland affirms that information is stored in the form of network and hence a simple retrieval cue can evoke a vast amount of information.

   E.g. tip of the tongue phenomena – information search related to the target word evokes many information related to it including the target word.

FORMS AND TYPES OF MEMORY

a. Sensory memory – all sense organs have a memory store namely visual sensory memory, auditory sensory memory, an olfactory sensory memory, a gustatory sensory memory, and a tactile sensory memory; and a lot of research is done on two sensory storage - Echoic (auditory) and Iconic (eye-conic visual). Sensory memories are modality specific; that is, the visual memory contains visual information; the auditory sensory memory contains auditory information, smell/olfactory sensory memory contains information on smell and so on.

   Sensory memory holds large amounts of information though for a very brief amount of time, very often less than a second.

   Information in sensory memory tends to be relatively processed, meaning that most of it has to do with physical aspects of the stimuli rather than meaningful ones.

b. Short term memory (STM)- holds information for 20-30 secs, George Miller states that the number of items held in STM is 7 ± 2 (seven plus or minus two), Magical number seven and the coding (storage) is acoustic in nature.

c. Long term memory (LTM)- holds large amounts of information for an indefinite amount of time and the information is coded semantically and or in terms of its meaning. Information is highly organized and quite systematic in nature.

d. Episodic memory- information, incidents, experiences related to oneself is stored in this memory.

e. Procedural memory- information related to skills, procedure is stored here.

f. Autobiographical memory- recalling information about one's own lives, story of one's own life.

g. Narrative memory- is a form of episodic and semantic memory which Is characterized by narrative features. E.g. narration of traumatic or an important significant events.

h. Working memory- refers to information in short term memory and we are currently using it to process incoming information and or past, stored information. E.g. visuospatial sketch pad (visual related information in visualization), phonological loop (audition related information)

i. Flashbulb memory- Brown and Kulick (1977) coined this term. Information related to important significant historical events and people find ways to relate to these events with reference to themselves. e.g. In March 2020, when the Janta curfew was announced in India, where we were, with whom we were, what were we doing, what we spoke to our near and dear ones, clothing etc. when recalled is a part of the flashbulb memory.

j. Recovered and false memories- very often memories buried several decades ago are retrieved in few minutes with the help of some retrieval cues and based on information overload, overlap, information consistent and not consistent with schemes at times false memories are created

k. Declarative memory- processes data with reference to names, dates, places, facts, events etc. which are encoded symbolically and are expressed with the help of language; e.g. when we state our graduation year, name of college, which stream/faculty etc.

This memory facilitates fast processing and learning of information.

There is no one specific place and or code in the nervous system for different forms and types of memory as entire nervous system is in the form of a network.. There will be constant interaction, reciprocal influence between various forms of memory depending on the purpose it is being recalled.

Factors Affecting Memory and Enhancing Memory:

1. **Decay theory**- any information which is not used for a considerable period of time is forgotten for e.g. nursery rhymes not rehearsed for a considerable amount of time.

2. **Trace Transformation**- with passage of time the new incoming information does get converted to a more recent information and or skill; e.g. as we receive updates on a certain information, the memory for its original information gets converted and or updated with the more recent information and very often the original message is forgotten. Information in nervous system is stored in the form of a trace.

3. **Proactive and Retroactive interference**- when previously learnt similar information affects RECALL of the current information known as proactive interference or inhibition; e.g. earlier learnt material affecting memory of current learning.

   Retroactive interference refers to when later learnt similar material or information affects recall

   E.g. the later parts of the chapter affects recall of the current information.

   Learning different categories of information is likely to better recall.

4. **Amnesia**- forgetting of information takes place when there is no sufficient rehearsal of information and or due to psychological or organic causes.

   Motivated forgetting refers to forgetting of information which is painful, stressful, threatening to us.

   Anterograde amnesia refers to inability to form new memories that is short term memory is affected, mainly caused by organic factors like brain damage, loss of neurons etc.

   Retrograde amnesia refers to inability to recall old memories which could be psychologically and or organically caused.

   Both forms of amnesia can be caused due to acute reasons namely trauma to brain, infections like meningitis and chronic causes like brain tumors, neurodegenerative diseases like dementia or Alzheimer's, vitamin B1 deficiency –a thiamine can cause Wernicke Korsakoff syndrome.

   Short term amnesia maybe caused due to sedatives, brain injuries affecting hippocampus (plays an important role in memory), encephalitis, surgical removal of certain brain areas.

   Amnesia can also lead to creation of false memories and confabulations, at times to cover up missing information due to confusion and or awareness of ones inability to remember.

   There are a few forms of amnesia which does affect daily life functioning of those suffering from it.

   Global amnesia – combination of retrograde and anterograde amnesia, short term memory and long term memory are collectively lost, thus hampering the person's ability to create new ones e.g. film Ghajini, Amir khan has no memory of the past nor the current times.

   Traumatic Amnesia- generally occurs with brain related injuries in accidents, could be for a short period of time and or for a longer period of time depending on the chronicity and severity of the injury.

   Wernicke-Korsakoff psychosis - chronic and intense use of alcohol subsequently leading to thiamine deficiency causes amnesia.

   Hysterical amnesia- the person forgets his personal identity along with his past identity due to perceived threat, stress present and often the person regains the lost information

   Childhood Amnesia- unable to recollect any information of the persons childhood days, it is progressive and irreversible.

   Post hypnotic amnesia- information related to hypnotic and or trance state is forgotten and often at times creates false memories depending on information shared in the trance or hypnotic state; e.g. in the film Talwar (Arushi Tanwar murder case) the accused were induced to narcotics test and leading questions by the therapist may create false memory.

Prosopamnesia-inability to recognize faces creating insecurity and social distancing in the patient.

5. **Anxiety**- high anxiety is likely to lower memory and a relatively anxious free person is likely to perform better.
6. **Encoding specifity**- when learning and retrieval modality is kept constant then memory is enhanced.
7. **Contextual cues**- the place or situation or context we learn provide rich retrieval cues e.g. a walk or a trip down the memory lane.
8. **Chunking**- holding groups (of related or unrelated) information enhances short term memory.
9. **State/Mood Congruent Memory**- we encode information which is more likely to be consistent with our schemes, mood and or emotional state; e.g. if we are in a happy state likely to store information of a happy kind. (exception is when the stimuli is extremely contrast, novel, distinctive – likely to be stored as an exception and or a subtype)
10. **State/Mood dependent Memory**- we are likely to recollect and or retrieve information which are consistent with our schemes, mood and or emotional state; e.g. when a person is intoxicated recalls information of when he or she was in an intoxicated state (exception is when the stimuli is extremely contrast, novel, distinctive –likely to be recalled as an exception and or a subtype). When a person has been told to learn in a hypnotic state may have no memory when he is not in an hypnotic state and may be able to recollect with accuracy when induced again in an hypnotic state.
11. **Motivated forgetting**- When the information is perceived as stressful, overload, anxiety provoking, threatening, overwhelming, unpleasant and at times we are in a denial we are likely to forget that particular and its related information and very often retrieve when we are relieved of its perceived unpleasantness. E.g. as soon as the perceived exam pressure eases as the exam progresses, we realize we are able to remember all related information easily most often after the bell rings to submit the answer sheet.
12. **Personal Salience/relevance and or self reference effect**- when any information or stimuli is important to us because of past experiences, personal associations and or applicable to us, we are likely to remember and recall information better.
13. **Motives/Needs**- The needs, motives determine what we notice, pay attention, encode, store and retrieve information better; e.g. when we are really wanting to score better marks as we perceive that exam to be important to us, we are likely to learn and retrieve better.
14. **Reinforcement**- When we are rewarded and or punished for a particular information, we are likely to learn and retrieve better.
15. **Emotional Arousal**- when we are in a highly emotionally aroused (pleasant or unpleasant) state, we are unlikely to remember better; e.g. when we are extremely happy or angry or anxious we rarely remember what we said or did in that state.
16. **Serial position effect**- the placement or position of the items in the list at times determines our memory for it. Generally earlier learnt items (primacy effect) are

remembered better as we are likely to be fresh and enough time is there for the information to be transferred to LTM and later learnt items (recency effect) are remembered better as we are motivated to finish learning and the items are more likely to be in STM.

Often it is difficult to remember the middle part of the list as it has items of the previous part and information from the latter part too.

17. **Rehearsal-** When we rehearse the information in a rich elaborative process, we are likely to recollect information better than when it is learnt by rote.

18. **Retrieval cues-** also known as reminders, hints aid memory. Retrieval cues are context based, personal associations, experiences, salience, needs, motives based. Hence we often observe when people are recalling a particular event, different people recall similar details while many recall different details of the same narrated event while some may recall little and or no recall at all.

19. **Attitudes, Interests and Intelligence-** We remember information better which reflects our interests, intelligence of understanding the information as well as our attitudes of wanting to remember or not influences memory.

20. **Difficulty and Ease-** Very often difficult information is forgotten while easy items are remembered better.

21. **Multi-sensorial memory-** When multiple sensory organs are involved in encoding, storage and retrieval, very often memory is enhanced; e.g. learning to cycle when we were in school, till date we remember how to cycle only because multiple sense organs are involved in cycling compared to what we learnt by rote.

22. **Active or Passive learning-** The more we learn actively e.g. in participating, explaining to a few people we are likely to remember better.

23. **Predominance of a sensory organ-** In some people a particular sense organ is sharp and highly effective productive efficient in functioning we are likely to remember information of that particular sensory information e.g. people with photographic memory and or good with auditory sense organs that once they listen they remember the information for a very long period of time.

24. **Brain components-** Hippocampus plays an important part in memory and basal ganglia in emotions; Limbic system plays a critical role in emotions and memory.

25. **Rehearsal-** The more the information is revised, practiced, rehearsed, highly durable will be the memory for it.

26. **Mnemonics-** are aids to memory.

Forgetting Curve- Ebbinghaus states that the decline of memory retention in time if there is no attempt to retain the information.

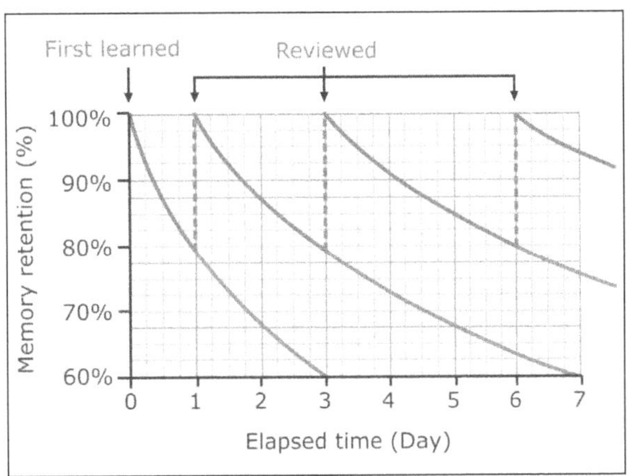

Fig. 70.2

Tips to Remember

a. Time of study- early morning around 4 am helps in better retention

b. Eating appropriately –wholesome nutritious healthy food and lifestyle as what we eat becomes us

c. Appropriate break- Taking break after 45 mins to 60 mins helps to remember better

d. Avoid proactive and retroactive interference so studying information of different content aids memory.

e. Revision- multiple revisions aid recall and every subsequent revision should be of lesser duration which indicates better retention and mastery

f. Adequate sleep rest- produces less load on the brain to process information along with the information learnt.

g. Intention- Make an intention to learn and tell yourself that you are remembering everything you are learning.

h. Pray- Pray and ask your GOD to help you remember better.

i. Style- know your style of learning and memorizing.

j. Distributed learning/practice- avoid learning all at once, space your learning

k. Visualization- Use visual imagery to enhance memory

l. Acronyms- Develop your own retrieval cues as short codes.

Thus to summarize, all these factors in combination with biological and sociocultural factors help us to learn and remember and there will always be an exception to all that has been discussed.

BIBLIOGRAPHY

1. Baron, Branscombe- Social Psychology, fourteenth edition, Pearson Publication. Pages 42-79.
2. Baron A. Robert- Psychology, fifth edition, Pearson Education Asia. Pages 168-243.
3. Galotti M. Kathleen – Cognitive Psychology in and out of the Laboratory- second edition, Brooks/Cole, Wadsworth. An International Thompson Publishing Company. Pages 126-184.
4. Galotti M. Kathleen- Cognitive Psychology in and out of the Laboratory-third edition, Thompson Wadsworth. Pages 130-211.
5. Morgan Clifford and King Richard- Introduction to Psychology-seventh edition, Tata McGraw-Hill Publishing Company Ltd. Pages 140-219
6. Myers David G- Psychology-Tenth edition, MacMillan Publishers India Pvt Ltd. Pages-91-166.
7. Smith, Hoeksema et al. – Introduction to Psychology, 14th edition, Thompson Wadsworth. pages 233-305.
8. Websites on GOOGLE with keywords typed .

Psychology of Motivation 71

Dhruv Parmar • Avinash De Sousa

INTRODUCTION

Motives play a large part in human behavior. Motivation is concerned with why people act and think the way they do. Motivated behavior is *goal-directed*, purposeful behavior. It's difficult to think of any behavior, human or non-human, that isn't motivated in this sense. Motives can range from basic wants, such as hunger and sex, to complicated, long term motives, such as political ambitions, a desire to serve humanity, or a need to master the environment. This suggests that human behavior is driven and pulled towards a goal and such goal-seeking behavior is persistent. This driving or pulling force is *Motivation*.

Motivation refers, in a general sense, to processes involved in the initiation, direction, and energisation of individual behavior (Geen, 1995)

The word 'motive' comes from the Latin for 'move' (*movere*), and this is captured in Miller's (1962)

Definition: *The study of motivation is the study of all those pushes and prods – biological, social and psychological – that defeat our laziness and move us, either eagerly or reluctantly, to action.*

MASLOW'S HIERARCHY OF NEEDS

According to Maslow, we're subject to two quite different sets of motivational states or forces:

1. Those that ensure survival by satisfying basic physical and psychological needs (physiological, safety, love and belongingness, and esteem), and
2. Those that promote the person's self-actualisation – that is, realising one's full potential, 'becoming everything that one is capable of becoming', especially in the intellectual and creative domains.

Behaviors that relate to survival or deficiency needs are engaged in because they satisfy those needs (a means to an end). But those that relate to self-actualisation are engaged in for their own sake, because they are intrinsically satisfying. The hierarchal nature of Maslow's theory highlights that the needs lower down in the hierarchy must be satisfied before we go higher up, higher levels are a later evolutionary development and the higher up we go the more are the needs linked to life experiences and less biological.

THEORIES OF MOTIVATION

Over the years there have been various theories postulated too understand the concept of motivation. These provide a general set of principles to guide our understanding of the urges, wants, needs, desires, strivings, and goals that come under the heading of Motivation.

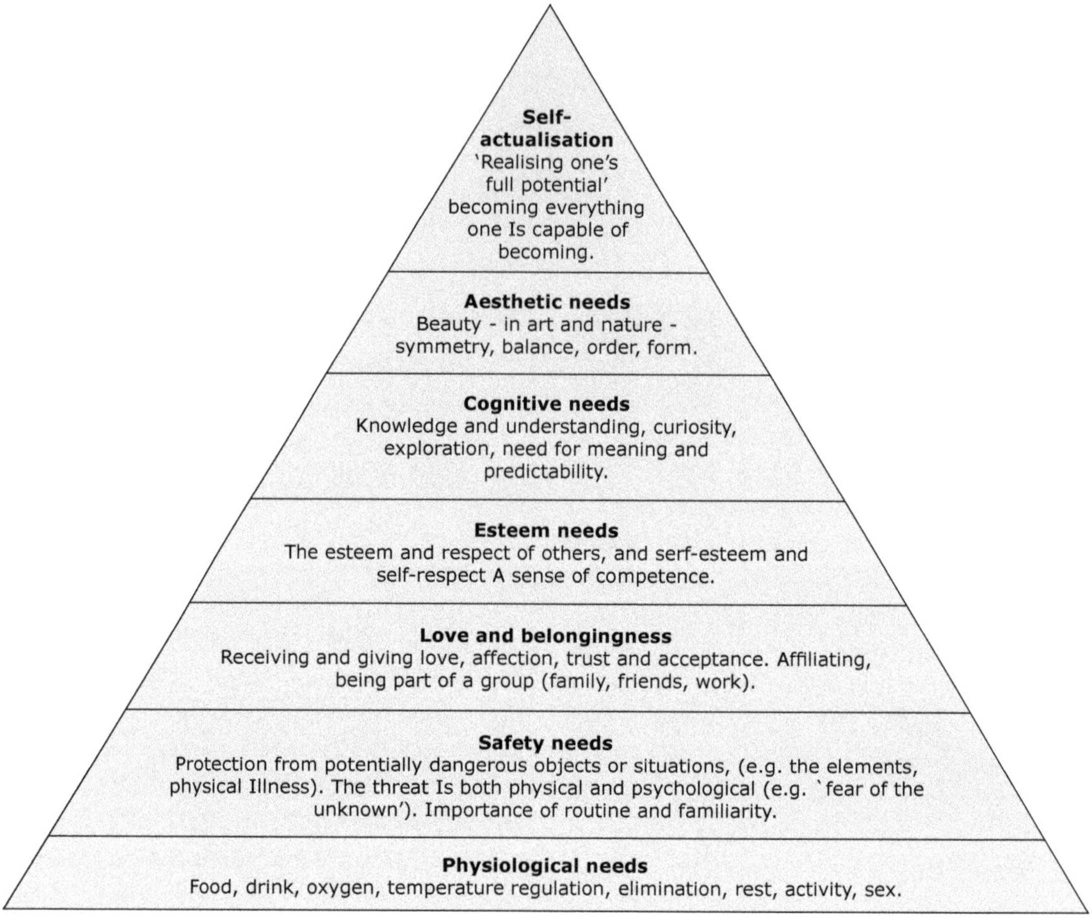

Self-
actualisation
'Realising one's
full potential'
becoming everything
one Is capable of
becoming.
Aesthetic needs
Beauty - in art and nature -
symmetry, balance, order, form.
Cognitive needs
Knowledge and understanding, curiosity,
exploration, need for meaning and
predictability.
Esteem needs
The esteem and respect of others, and serf-esteem and
self-respect A sense of competence.
Love and belongingness
Receiving and giving love, affection, trust and acceptance. Affiliating,
being part of a group (family, friends, work).
Safety needs
Protection from potentially dangerous objects or situations, (e.g. the elements,
physical Illness). The threat Is both physical and psychological (e.g. `fear of the
unknown'). Importance of routine and familiarity.
Physiological needs
Food, drink, oxygen, temperature regulation, elimination, rest, activity, sex.

Fig. 71.1: Maslow's hierarchy of needs.

DRIVE THEORIES

It can be described as the "push" theory of motivation; behavior is pushed towards goals by driving states within the person or animal. When an internal driving state is aroused, the individual is pushed to engage in behavior which will lead to a goal that reduces the intensity of the driving state, which causes satisfaction and pleasure. In the case of human social motives people are said to have learned drives for power, aggression, achievement and other namely social motives. Such learned driving states become enduring characteristics of that particular person and push that person toward appropriate goals

Driving state
(set in motion
by bodily needs
or environmental
stimuli)
Goal Directed
Behavior
Goal
Relief

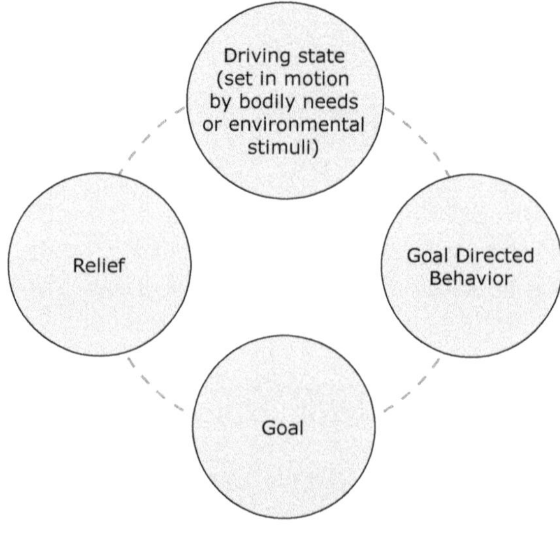

Fig. 71.2: Motivation cycle.

INCENTIVE THEORIES

This applies best to some of the biological motives like hunger, thirst and sex, for example. It says that there is something about the goal itself that motivates behavior. The stimulus characteristics of the goal can sometimes start a train of motivated behavior. Thus, unlike the "push" of the drive theory. Incentive theories are "pull" theories; because of certain characteristics of the goal which pull the behavior towards them. These goal objectives that motivate the behavior are called *incentives*. A major part of this theory is that individuals expect pleasure from the attainment of positive incentives and from avoidance of negative incentives. For example, in a work environment positive incentive such as wages salaries, bonuses, vacations etc.; drives the behavior.

OPPONENT-PROCESS THEORY

It is the *Hedonistic* view of motivation; which says that we are motivated to seek goals which give us good emotional feelings and avoid those resulting in displeasure. The basis of this theory is the observation that many emotional-motivating states are followed by opposing states. For example, feelings of pleasure and happiness follow feelings of fear and dread or vice versa.

As in the figure starting from the baseline it shows the general course followed by emotional states. The peak point of the emotional-motivational state (State A) occurs after the emotion provoking situation is encountered (It can be a pleasant or unpleasant emotional state). Next, the intensity of the state adapts and declines to a steady state. Now the provoking situation terminates and an after reaction occurs in which the emotional motivational state (State B) is the opposite of State A. State B gradually declines until Baseline is again reached. This keeps on repeating.

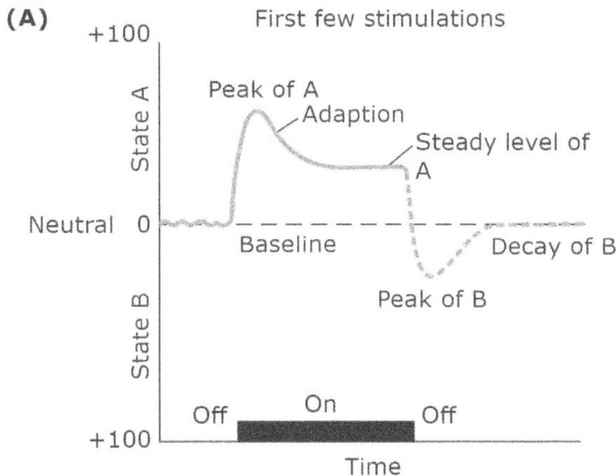

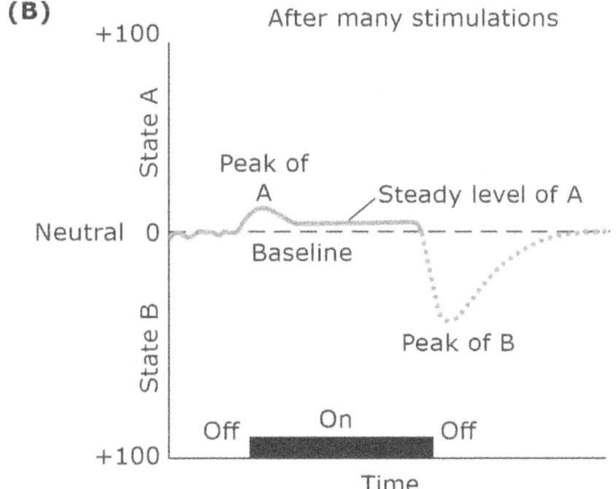

Fig. 71.3: Opponent processes in motivation. The duration of an emotion-provoking situation is shown by the black bars (From Solomon, 1980.)

Now if the same situation has happened many times there is seen a decline in State A and an increase in State B which motivates the person to do the activity again. This explains the basis of some learned motives like addictions and thrill-seeking behavior. Example a heroin addict needs more drug in order to prevent unpleasant consequences of withdrawal and some people acquire the need to seek thrills in order to experience the elation after the danger is over.

OPTIMAL LEVEL THEORIES

These are theories which suggest that there

is a certain optimal or best level of arousal that is pleasurable. Also known as "just right" theories. The individual is motivated to behave in such a way as to maintain the optimal level of arousal. If the arousal is too low, a person will seek situations or stimuli to increase arousal and if the arousal is too high behavior will be directed towards decreasing it. The concept of *homeostasis* is based on this theory. Which is the tendency of the body to maintain its internal physiological processes at optimal levels; departure from such levels can initiate motivated behavior directed towards restoring the state of equilibrium.

BIOLOGICAL MOTIVATION

These are rooted to the physiological state of the body. These motives include hunger, thirst, desire for sex, temperature regulation, sleep, pain avoidance and a need for oxygen.

Biological motives are triggered by departures from balanced physiological conditions of the body. The body always tends to maintain a state of equilibrium called homeostasis. This is crucial for the normal sustenance of life. There are numerous automatic mechanisms that maintain this balance. These automatic mechanisms are supplemented by motivated behavior, for example, fall in body temperature leads to wearing of a sweater, closing the window and so on. When the body lacks substances such as food or water, automatic physiological processes work to conserve the same, but sooner or later these must be obtained from outside. Here the departure from homeostasis creates a drive the pushes a person or animal to seek food and water. Hormones also play a role in arousal of some biological motive states. Sensory stimuli or incentives play a role in arousal of drive states especially in humans. For example, the smell of a savoury dish arouses hunger in a person who isn't biologically hungry.

HUNGER MOTIVATION

Hunger is a primary motive necessary for sustaining life. When the stomach is empty, contractions occur which signal for feelings of hunger. Levels of nutritive substances in blood also are crucial for activating feeling of hunger. Blood sugar levels are important in initiating hunger motivation and feeding. Hypothalamus is critically involved in hunger motivation as it has nerve endings that react to rate of use of glucose. External factors like sight and smell of food also play a major role in motivating hunger. Stomach contains nutrient receptors which provide satiety signals thus motivating the behavior to stop eating.

The lateral hypothalamus is considered to be an excitatory region for hunger motivation, while ventromedial hypothalamus is said to be involved in cessation of eating.

THIRST MOTIVATION

Stimulus factor plays a major role in initiating drinking. A dry mouth or a good tasting beverage is a good stimulation for thirst. Pulled by these incentives we might drink more water than the body needs. Maintaining the level of water in the body is essential for normal functioning of life, body has a set of complicated internal homeostatic processes to regulate the fluid level and drinking behavior. These include the Antidiuretic hormone, cellular dehydration in osmoreceptors in anterior hypothalamus, hypovolemia leading to activation of renin angiotensin mechanism. Drinking stops once the homeostasis is restored.

SEXUAL MOTIVATION

Sexual motives are a complex interplay of biological drive, social and religious beliefs. Sex is not necessary to maintain life of an individual, however it is necessary for the survival of the species. It is not aroused by lack of substances in the body. Sexual motivation is mostly under the influence of sensory information from the environment and incentives. Sex hormones play a major role in the organization of the body and the brain, they influence the secondary sexual characteristics during puberty. The level of sex hormones in the womb and growing baby provide the basis for the gender of the child. A certain level of these hormones must be present for sexual behavior to occur. External stimuli play a major role in activating sexual motivation in higher animals and humans. Hormonally ready humans are sexually aroused based on looks, style, voices, dressing sense and odour. Thus, much of the sexual behavior is based on external stimuli which acts as an incentive. Variability in human sexual behavior is due to people's learning experiences which also plays a role in the social motives.

SOCIAL MOTIVES

Social motives include the complex motive states that are the cause for majority of human actions. These are learned in social groups especially in the family as children when they grow up as it involves other people. These can be said to be general states that lead to particular human behaviors. These persist and one can never be fully satisfied, no sooner is one goal reached than the motive is directed towards another.

Some Major Social Motives

Table 71.1

Motive	Goal and Effects
Abasement	To submit passively to others; to seek and accept injury, blame and criticism
Achievement	To accomplish difficult tasks; to rival and surpass others
Affiliation	To seek and enjoy cooperation with others; to make friends
Aggression	To overcome opposition forcefully; to fight and revenge injury; to belittle, curse or ridicule others
Autonomy	To be free of restraints and obligations; to be independent and free to act according to impulse
Counteraction	To master or makeup for failure by renewed efforts; to overcome weakness and maintain pride and self-respect on a high level
Defense	To defend oneself against attack, criticism, or blame; to justify and vindicate self
Deference	To admire and support a superior person; to yield eagerly to other people
Dominance	To control and influence the behavior of others; to be a leader
Exhibition	To make an impression; to be seen and heard by others; to show off
Harm Avoidance	To avoid pain, physical injury, illness and death
Infavoidance	To avoid humiliation; to refrain from action because of fear of failure
Nurturance	To help and take care of sick or defenceless people; to assist others in trouble
Order	To put things in order; to achieve cleanliness, arrangement and organization
Play	To devote one's free time to sports, games and parties; to laugh and make joke of everything; to be light-hearted and gay
Rejection	To remain aloof and indifferent to an inferior person; to jilt or snub others
Sentience	To seek and enjoy sensuous impressions and sensations; to enjoy the arts genuinely

ACHIEVEMENT MOTIVATION

It was the first social motivation to be studied in detail and research in this continuous till date. People in whom the need for achievement is strong seek to become accomplished and to improve their task performance. These are very task oriented and prefer to work on the tasks that are challenging and in which their performance can be evaluated in some way. Sources of achievement motivation include modelling from parents, peers and other important people and expectation of parents; all as a part of learning experiences of the child.

Characteristics of *n*-achievement (Need for Achievement) People

1. Prefer to work on moderately challenging tasks which promise success
2. Like tasks in which their performance can be compared to that of others and they like a feedback
3. Tend to be persistent in working on tasks they perceive as career related or reflecting personal characteristics.
4. When they are successful, they tend to raise their levels of aspirations in a realistic way to move onto slightly more challenging tasks.
5. Like to work in situations where they have some control over the outcome.
6. Fear of failure as motive inhibits expression of achievement behavior.
7. Competition motivation improves people with low achievement motivation but impairs performance for those in whom achievement motivation is strong.

The need for achievement is related to a society's economic and business growth. Evidence of strong achievement motivation acts as a predictor about economic growth of a society.

POWER MOTIVATION

Social power can be defined as the ability or capacity of a person to produce intended effects (consciously or unconsciously) on the behavior or emotions of another person. Its goals are to influence, control, cajole, persuade, lead, charm others and to enhance one's own reputation in the eyes of other people. People with strong power motivation derive satisfaction from achieving these goals.

Characteristics of *n*-power People

1. Impulsive and aggressive actions.
2. Participation in competitive sports.
3. Joining of organizations and holding office in them.
4. Obtaining and collecting possessions like fancy cars, guns credit cards etc.
5. Association with people not popular with others who can easily be controlled.
6. Choosing occupations that have high impact on others like teaching, diplomacy, business, clergy.
7. Building and disciplining their bodies.
8. Drinking and sexual domination of women (seen in men).

Machiavellianism

People who express their power motivation by manipulating and exploiting others in a deceptive and unscrupulous fashion. It's not the same as power motivation. Machiavels show little warmth in their personal relationships, are weakly guided by conventional morality in their dealings with others, are reality oriented and have little interest in ideologies.

MEASUREMENT OF SOCIAL MOTIVES

To measure social motives psychologists, tend to find themes or common threads which run through samples of action and imagined action.

To find these themes they use

1. Projective Tests
2. Pencil-and-paper questionnaires
3. Observations of actual behavior in certain types of situation to bring out social motives.

Thematic Apperception Test

It is the most common projective technic to assess social motives. In this test, a standard set of pictures depicting various people in various situations is presented, and the person being tested is asked to make up stories describing what is happening in the pictures. Motivational themes are found to run through the stories told about the pictures. These stories and themes can be scored and so different degrees of social motives can be ascertained.

Personality Questionnaire

Several pencil-and-paper tests and inventories have been developed to measure strength of social motives. These consist of questions for people to answer about their typical behavior and preferences in certain situations.

Situational Tests

In this a situation is created in which a person's action will reveal his or her dominant social motives.

BIBLIOGRAPHY

1. Cohen, J. (1970) *Homo Psychologicus*. London:George Allen & Unwin Ltd.
2. Evans, P. (1975) *Motivation*. London: Methuen.
3. Richard Gross Psychology The Science of Mind and Behavior
4. Introduction to Psychology By Cifford T. Morgan, Richard A. King, John R. Weisz, John Schopler

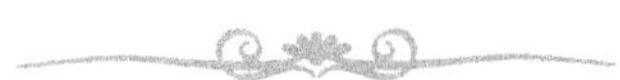

72 Psychology of Emotions

Dhanashree Waghmare • Avinash De Sousa

Guess the emotions felt by the individuals in the Fig. 72.1. Were you able to spot individuals expression? Some common predictions would be happy, sad, thoughtful, shocked etc. As humans, our ancestors developed language as a mode of communication. It is difficult to mark the beginning, but studies show that Languages are linked to each other by shared words or sounds or grammatical constructions.

Imagine a world without words, trying to deliver a message through eyes, expressions, gestures. While language still remains an important tool of survival, before language existed, life on earth survived on emotions. Science suggests that the area of the brain which deals with showing, recognizing and controlling the body's reactions to emotions is called the limbic system. Interestingly limbic system is also responsible for flight and fight response, a skill inbuilt in human body for survival.

In this chapter, we will be understanding a few concepts related to emotions. As future health care facilitators, the sensitivity to emotions

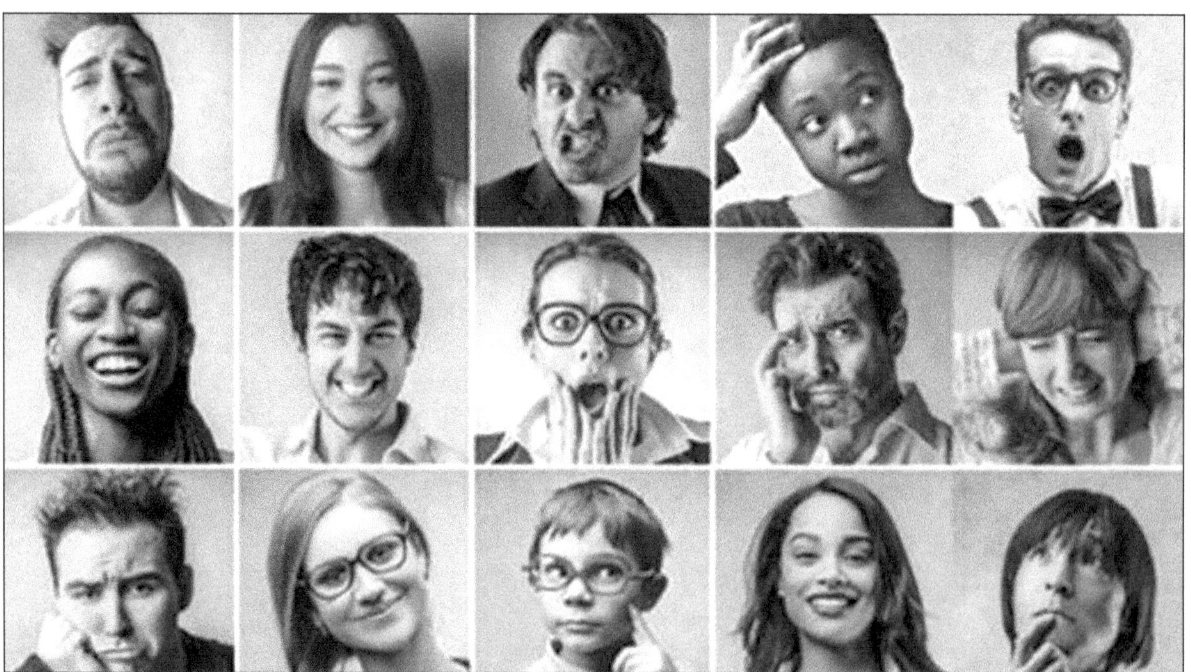

Fig. 72.1

is considered to be one of the key skills. Patients can be difficult, resistant to share. As professionals, pulling out words every time can be hard, observing the signs can aid in your history taking and prognosis.

In Psychology, Emotion can be defined as a response of the whole organism involving physiological arousal, expressive behaviors and conscious experience. They are our body's adaptive response. Perceptions of emotions occurs from various sources. The voice of the individual, screaming could denote fear or excitement, tremor or break in voice could mean sorrow, a loud high pitched sharp voice generally means anger. There are more than 6000 languages in the world, some share dialects, some share foundations, but more or less they differ from one another. There are cultural biases with grammar and semantics. In case of emotions, the problem of biases is relatively low. According to a study done by Izard in 1971, when participants from different cultures were presented with various posed photographs in which actors expressed emotion, it was found that more or less, all the participants identified the primary emotions- anger, disgust, fear, happiness, sadness and surprise irrespective of their origins. Exceptions can exist, for example: one can learn to modify the expressions even for primary emotions. The other is an individual who expresses multiple emotions at once. This blend could be hard to judge. In order to identify the kind of emotion, one must observe the behavior but also know the situation giving rise to the same, making the analysis with rational reasoning.

For instance: It is believed that people who consume too much alcohol are upset. The behavior of drinking could be an issue, but the context of the same makes difference. Drinking at a party gives a different understanding of emotion than just knowing about a person's drinking.

The subject of science focuses on testing and experimenting. It believes in reasoning and factual information. A classic debate in the field of emotions is whether a person feels first and thinks, or thinks first and feels.

Imagine you are sitting inside the examination room. You feel nervous and scared. The invigilator distributes the answer sheets, you mess up the OMR. Your teacher warned you that this error could disrupt your scoring. Invigilator arrives again. Hands you the question paper. And boom! The subject isn't the one you prepared for. What would you do? List the trail of your thoughts? Did you skip your beat first and felt shocked, or were you shocked leading for your heart to skip a beat. Our commonsense understanding of feelings suggests we feel and thereby we respond. But historical theories have a backward interpretation.

According to William James and Carl Lange, for someone to feel emotion, s/he must experience bodily reactions, i.e.; emotions occur as a result of physiological reactions to events. It is said that one doesn't smile because they share teammates' joy, they also share the joy because they are smiling with them. Another theory, popularly known as Cannon-Bard theory of emotion holds a different angle. It suggests that we feel emotions and experience physiological reactions simultaneously. Limitations for the above two theories was concluded by Stanley Schachter and Jerome Singer's two factor theory, emotions have two ingredients: physical arousal and cognitive appraisal. Our physical reactions and our thoughts together create Emotion.

BRAIN AND EMOTION

The modern theories of science have debated over the order of emotion realization for years. Zajonc and Ledouxs' study found that some emotional responses are immediate before any conscious appraisal. The sensory input maybe routed to the cortex via the thalamus for analysis and then transmission to amygdala; or; directly to the amygdala via the thalamus for an instant emotional reaction. Neuroscientist, Oschsner chartered human emotions along two processes-top down (perception driven by cognition) and bottom up (processing sensory information as it is).

According to the definition of Emotion, arousal plays an important role, thereby autonomic nervous system role in arousing and calming. Both Sympathetic and Parasympathetic nervous system contributes in emotional regulation. The Fig. 72.3 will give you a quick view.

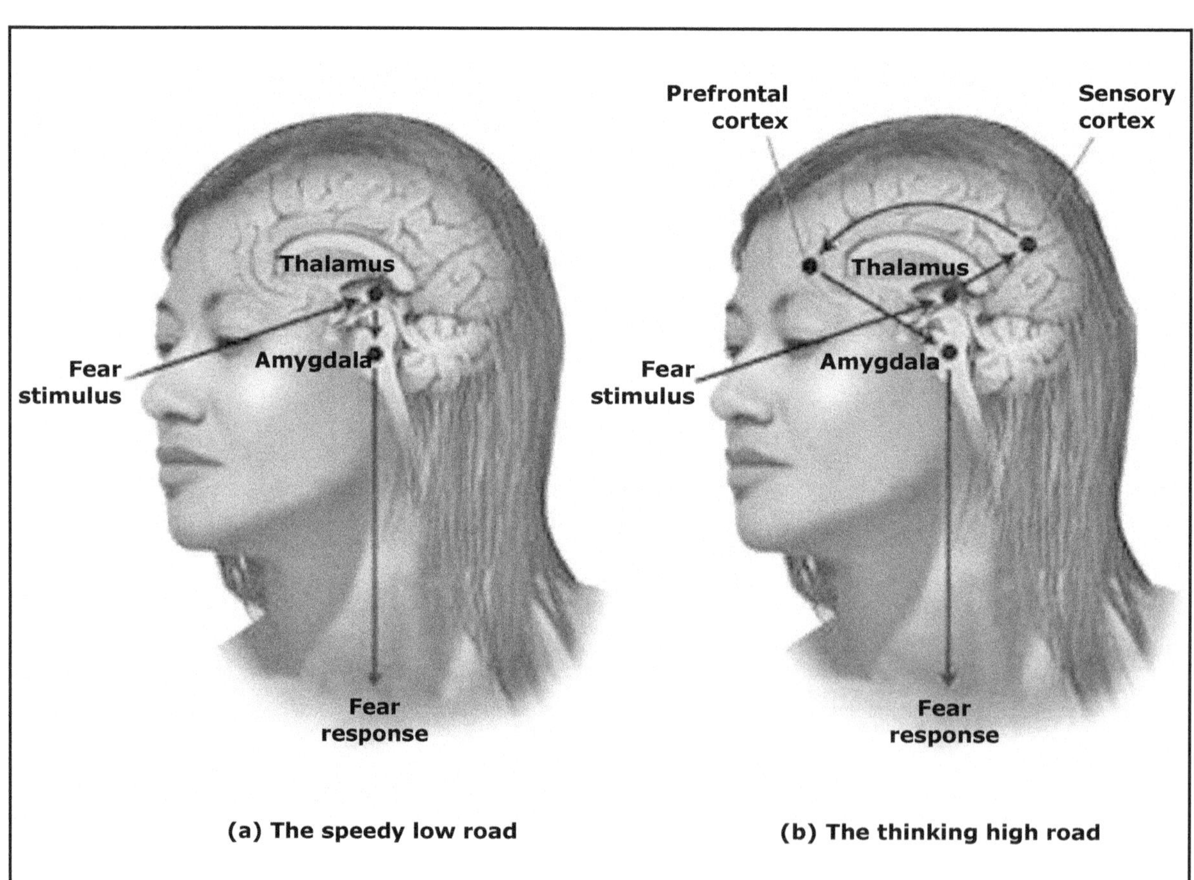

Fig. 72.2: Emotion and the Two-Track Brain.

Arousal can linger. Without being consciously aware of having seen it, we can be influenced by a stimulus flashed too briefly to interpret. A subliminally presented happy face can encourage subjects to drink more than when presented with an angry face (Berridge & Winkeilman, 2003).

Emotions are felt directly through the amygdala (a) or through the cortex (b) for analysis.

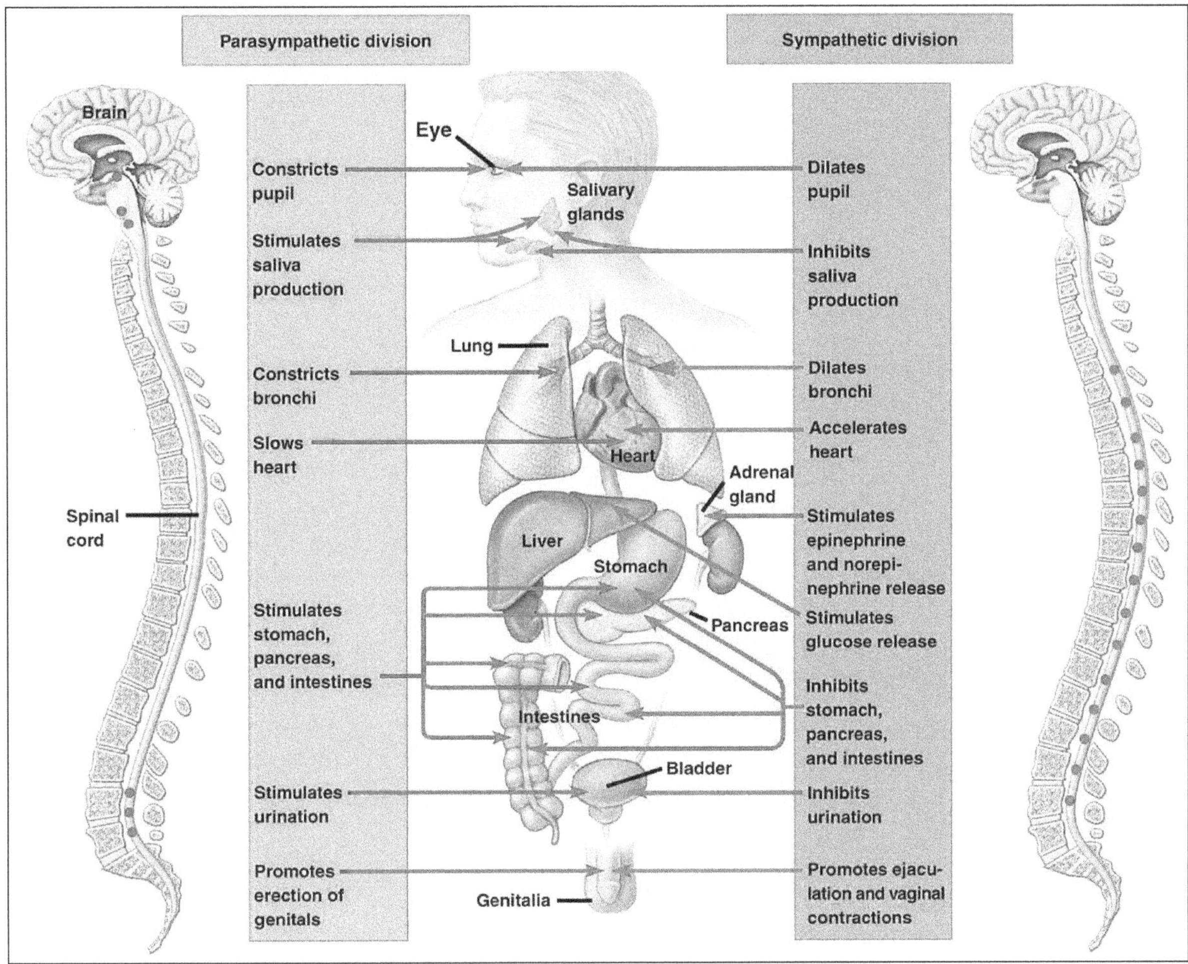

Fig. 72.3: Sympathetic and Parasympathetic nervous system.

Despite all of these diversification, human body works in more complicated patterns. Elated excitement and panicky fear involve similar physiological arousal but the emotion felt is not the same. Research has pointed out some distinctions. Some emotions differ in their brain circuits. The scan studies show that when an individual looks at a fearful face, show more activity in amygdala. Negative emotions like disgust activates the right prefrontal cortex whereas depression prone people with general negative personalities show right frontal activity (Harmon-Jones et.al, 2002) Positive moods trigger left frontal activity.

However established scientific discoveries are, experience can sensitize us to particular emotions. Research suggests individuals who have been abused could recognize angry faces much faster and accurately compared to others.

GENDER DIFFERENCES AND CULTURAL EXPRESSION

Historically women are termed as home-makers and men as bread earners. Thus, qualities like nurturing, caring, understanding and empathetic. On contrary, men are strong willed, powerful, chauvinistic and self-centered.

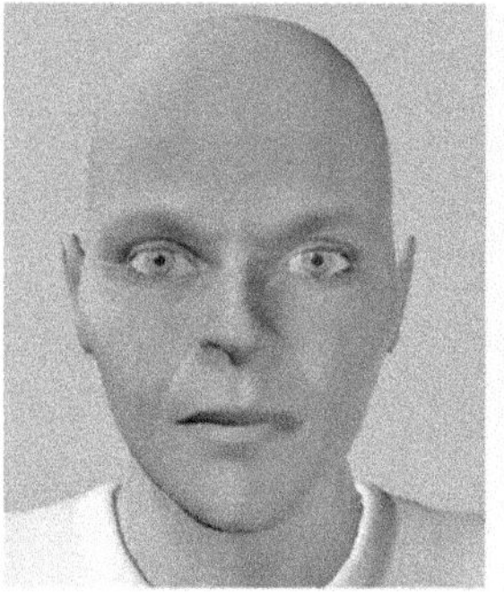
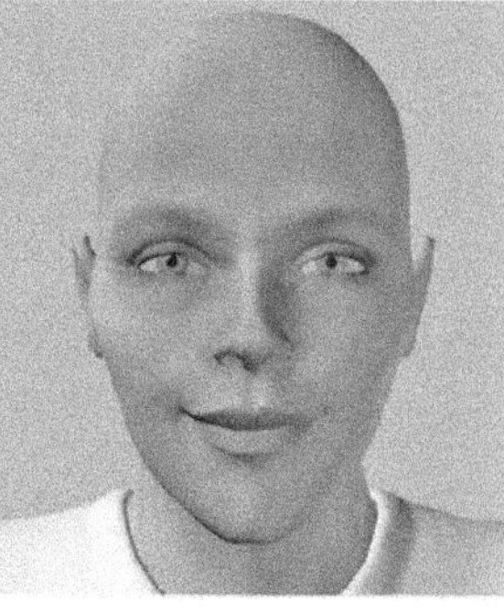

Fig. 72.3: MALE OR FEMALE?
Researchers manipulated a gender neutral face. People were more likely to see it as a male when it wore an angry expression, and as a female when it wore a smile (Becker et al., 2007).

This differentiation brings us to understanding if emotion expression can be different in two sexes.

An experiment was conducted where a gender neutral face was shown to participants. When the expression was of anger, the face was identified of a man whereas when the face wore a smile, the identification changed to that of a female. Judith Halls' study concluded that women surpass men in identifying emotional cues. Their nonverbal sensitivity helps explain their emotional intelligence. Also, unlike men females are more likely to express empathy-to cry and feel distress when observing someone in distress.

Facial expression also convey certain cues that provides an insight into the other's culture. Happy and sad feel happy and sad around the world. Whether one lives in a remote forest or mountains, fast paced music seems happy, and slow paced music depicts sadness. Like most psychological phenomenon, emotion is best understood as a combined study of biological, cognitive and socio-cultural background of the individual.

TESTING EMOTIONAL STATES

There are various ways to test one's emotional state. MRI and FMRIs certainly help in getting an imagery representation of activating areas. On the contrary, due to physiological changes, Polygraph commonly called as lie-detector machine is also used to check an individual's authenticity.

Often used in criminal settings, Polygraph is a machine which records physiological indicators such as blood pressure, pulse, respiration and skin conductivity while a person is asked and answers a series of questions. A baseline condition was recorded and compared to the one when questions were asked. As hypothesized, lying requires arousal and alertness, as the activation occurs, the machine testifies the individuals' response as lie or truth. However, it has been observed that individuals can fake on a polygraph thereby the validity for the same is low. Another tool is called as Emotional Intelligence. A new sub-domain of intelligence given by Salovey and Mayer describing it as a form of social intelligence that involves ability to monitor one's own and other's feelings and emotions, to discriminate among them and to use this information to guide one's thinking and action.

THE FEELINGS CIRCLE

Using intellectual language—words that are not connected to your direct experience—can distance you from your emotions and make it more difficult to know what you are truly feeling. To avoid this, try using simpler, more self-expressive words (emotional language) to explain what you feel. The circle provides some more emotional words you can say in place of intellectual ones.

HERE'S HOW IT WORKS

When a feeling starts to arise, look at the wheel, start with the inner-most wheel and move outward, moving from the core feelings toward any associated feelings that might be coming up for you.

Alternatively if a core emotion is not clear, you can move from the outside in, identifying the associated feeling first and then making your way toward the core emotion. Don't necessarily "hunt" for the right word. Rather, as you look, notice which words resonate with you. **.** *Another way to use the chart is to compare how you're feeling today with how you felt earlier today or even yesterday.*

For example: I'm feeling __________ today, but yesterday I felt __________ and. *Typically you might find that two or even four different emotions apply.* (Refer to Fig. 72.4).

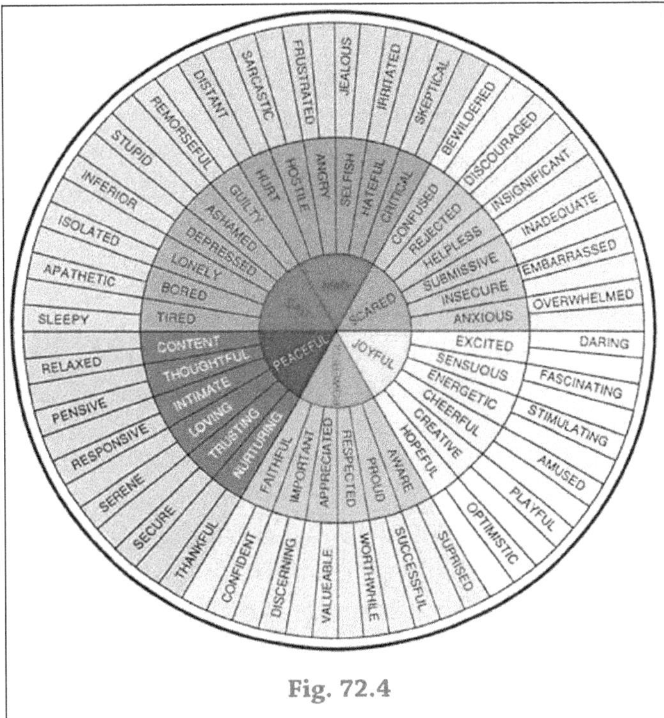

Fig. 72.4

CONCLUSION

Emotions arise from arousal. Both cognitive and biological framework guide the xpression. Experience aids in improving our emotional intelligence.

BIBLIOGRAPHY

1. David G Myers (2013): *Psychology: Motivation and Emotion:* Tenth edition. Macmillan publishers.
2. C. Morgan, R.King et.al. (2017): *Introduction to Psychology: Emotion and Stress.* Indian edition
3. C. Morgan (2011): *A Brief Introduction To Psychology: Arousal, Emotion and Awareness.* Tata McGraw-Hill edition
4. History World: *History of Language:* www.historyworld.net
5. Science Museum: *Which area of the brain controls your emotions:* http://whoami.sciencemuseum.org.uk/
6. November 2019: *The Feelings Wheel- Genius charter for better communication*: www.thechalkboard-mag.com

Psychology of Adolescence 73

Shivani Chande • Avinash De Sousa

Adolescence is the transitional phase between childhood and adulthood. Usually it is viewed as starting just before the teenage years and ending just after them. This period of life evokes excitement, anxiety, glee and despair. It is a time of rapid physical maturation triggered by the onset of puberty. Adolescents are keenly aware of their changing bodies and their cognitive abilities. They crave independence, deal with careening emotions, fluctuating social networks, and the temptation of sex, drugs and alcohol.

PSYCHOLOGICAL EFFECTS OF PUBERTY

One of the main features of adolescence is the onset of puberty. The physical changes that take place during puberty give also rise to various emotional and social changes as well. First, the continuous physical maturation process directly affects the body and brain to alter the adolescent's needs, moods and interests. Then, as they start to look and act differently, an array of social influences further accelerates the emotional and social changes teenagers experience.

As adolescents notice that their bodies are changing, they may experience certain new and unfamiliar social experiences. Reinforced by their initial enjoyable experiences of sexual arousal, and also by their peers and culture, they become involved in forming what can become intense, romantic, and often sexualized relationships with others. Also, as such bodily changes become visible to others around them, adolescents may begin to experience being treated differently by others. For example, an earlier maturing teen may experience an increase in their popularity, while their more slowly maturing peers may experience a decline in popularity. Adolescents may also notice that other people are suddenly paying a great deal more attention to how they look than they used to.

The physical changes accompanying puberty become the source for new emotional experiences. For example, it is common for adolescents to become moodier and more irritable during this period of their lives. This fluctuation in mood is commonly attributed to the sudden and fluctuating hormonal levels. Sex hormones are powerful chemical agents that can affect mood. During puberty, the body adjusts to these fluctuating hormone levels and this fluctuation does create mood swings. However, there are several other physical causes accounting for increased moodiness apart from fluctuating hormones.

Adolescents' fluctuation in mood can be caused by their lack of sleep. There are physical as well as social reasons for why sleep deficits may occur during puberty. First, the body's sleep-wake cycle is dependent upon the "circadian rhythm" which in turn, is influenced by hormones. During puberty, a shift occurs in an adolescent's circadian rhythm that causes them to feel more alert later at night. Unfortunately, they must still wake up early for school and other activities. As a result, they get less than adequate amount of sleep. This takes place just as their educational, extracurricular, and social schedules become more demanding. Teenagers may also develop an irregular sleep pattern, such as wanting to "sleep-in' during the weekends, while simultaneously sleeping less during weeknights. This lack of adequate sleep can increase irritability and decrease concentration ability, and contribute to teens suddenly finding it difficult to complete tasks that were once simple. This new struggle only adds to their frustration and fluctuations in mood.

Studies are accumulating data to support the argument for puberty-associated modifications in brain regions involved in emotion, arousal, response inhibition and the calibration of risks and rewards (Dahl & Spear, 2004). These changes include a rise in the intensity of emotions experienced by adolescents, their sensitivity to emotional influences, and their trouble in regulating emotions in the face of certain conflicting demands (Steinberg, 1989). Studies have shown that puberty has significant effects on emotion processing. There is also evidence that gonadal steroids play a role in the shaping of processes like sexual activity, maternal behavior, social bonding, and social memory (Nelson, Leibenluft, McClure, & Pine, 2005). Sexual hormones play an important role in neural plasticity. For example, neural plasticity in the hypothalamus and the hippocampus is controlled by the ebb and flow of estrogens in females (McEwen, 1994). Both estrogen and androgen influence cognitive abilities like verbal fluency, verbal memory, spatial abilities and motor skills (McEwen & Alves, 1999). There are many areas aside from sexuality that display puberty-specific maturational changes including sensation seeking, mood lability, sleep/arousal regulation (Dahl, 2004), appetite and feeding (Barb, Hausman, & Czaja, 2005), and risk for affective disorders especially among girls (Ge, Kim, Brody, Conger, Simons et al., 2003). Taken together, these findings suggest that puberty is not only a useful milestone for understanding a specific developmental process within the broader group of transformations of adolescence, but also that puberty may trigger rapid changes in the intensity, direction and calibration of multiple emotional and/or motivational domains.

BRAIN AND COGNITIVE DEVELOPMENT

Growth Spurts

There are two major brain growth spurts in the adolescent years. The first one takes place between ages 13 and 15 (Spreen et al., 1995). During this spurt, the cerebral cortex becomes thicker, and the neuronal pathways become more effective. Additionally, more energy is produced and consumed by the brain during this spurt than in the periods that precede and follow it (Fischer & Rose, 1994). Usually, these growth and energy spurts take place in parts of the brain that are responsible for spatial perception and motor functions. Consequently, by the midteens, adolescents' abilities in these areas far surpass those of school-aged children. Neuropsychologists Kurt Fischer and Samuel Rose believe that a qualitatively distinct neural network emerges during the first brain growth spurt that occurs between ages 13 and 15, which enables adolescents to think abstractly and to reflect on their cognitions. (Fischer & Rose, 1994). The 13-to-15 spurt is also linked with profound changes in the prefrontal cortex (PFC) (Gogtay et al., 2004; Kanemura, Aihara, Aoke, Araki, & Nakazawa,

2004). The PFC is responsible for executive processing, a set of information-processing skills which enable us to consciously control and organize our thought processes. Hence, by mid-adolescence, adolescents' executive processing skills far exceed those of middle childhood. studies of patients with damage to the PFC suggest that maturation of this area of the brain contributes to advances in social perception, especially those that involve the interpretation of nonverbal information such as facial expressions (Mah, Arnold, & Grafman, 2005). The next adolescent brain growth spurt initiates around age 17 and continues into early adulthood (van der Molen & Molenaar, 1994). During this spurt, the frontal lobes of the cerebral cortex are seen as focus of development (Davies & Rose, 1999). This part of the brain controls planning and logic. Hence, it is not surprising that older adolescents differ from younger adolescents in terms of how they deal with problems that require such cognitive functions.

Changes in Thinking and Memory

The powerful intellectual tools that emerge during adolescence allow teenagers to make plans and to mentally project themselves into those plans as a way of testing them. According to Piaget, an entirely new form of thought develops between age 12 and age 16. He termed the stage associated with this kind of thought the 'formal operational stage'. Generally, this stage is known as the period during which adolescents learn to reason logically about abstract concepts. Formal operational thinking has a number of key features. One important element of formal operations is systematic problem solving—the capacity to search methodically for the answer to a particular problem. Another facet of this stage is the appearance in the adolescent's repertoire of skills of what is called hypothetico-deductive reasoning, the ability to derive conclusions from hypothetical premises. Psychologist David Elkind hypothesized that another common manifestation of hypothetico-deductive reasoning is a type of thought he termed adolescent egocentrism—the belief that one's thoughts, beliefs, and feelings are unique.

Information processing in adolescents is faster, they use processing resources more efficiently, they understand their own memory processes better, and have more knowledge than do middle school children (Kail, 1990, 1997). Therefore, their working memories operate much more efficiently and they outperform school-aged children even on simple memory tasks as recognizing people's faces (Gathercole, Pickering, Ambridge, & Wearing, 2004; Itier & Taylor, 2004). Furthermore, they are better equipped at using different strategies to help themselves remember things and can more easily remember and understand complex information, such as that given in a textbook. By age 13 or 14, the metacognitive and metamemory skills of adolescents far exceed those of younger school children, and these abilities continue to improve throughout teenage years (and into the adult years) (Weil et al., 2013).

PERSONALITY AND SOCIAL DEVELOPMENT IN ADOLESCENCE

Self-concept and Self-esteem

During Adolescence, self-concept differentiates to include others' view as well as one's own and to include other multiple aspects at the same time. Differentiation of causes confusion as their behavior reflect a complex definition of the self. Teens also differentiate their self-esteem, evaluating certain aspects of themselves differently.

Identity Formation

According to Erik Erikson, adolescents are in an identity-versus-identity-confusion stage, wherein they try to discover their individuality and their identity. They may become confused and exhibit inappropriate or dysfunctional reactions, and they may rely on the advice and information given to them by friends and peers more than on adults. The formation of identity is especially challenging for members of minority groups.

Relationships in Adolescence

During adolescence, teenagers are usually in a quest for autonomy, which often brings tension and conflict to their relationship with their parents.

Peers are essential during adolescence as they provide social comparison and reference groups against which to measure social success. Relationships during adolescence are characterized by the need to belong, and teenagers generally begin to spend time together in groups. Membership in certain cliques or crowds is many a times determined by the degree of similarity with other members of the group. An example of similarity would be substance use. Peer pressure is a complex phenomenon. Adolescents conform to their peers in areas in which they feel their peers have large amounts of knowledge or are experts, and to adults in areas of adult expertise. As adolescents' confidence increase, their conformity to both peers and adults decreases. Not all adolescents commit crimes, however adolescents are seen as disproportionately involved in criminal behaviors.

In adolescence, dating provides intimacy, entertainment as well as prestige. Obtaining psychological intimacy is difficult initially, but becomes easier as adolescents grow and mature, take relationships seriously and gain more confidence.

Sexual orientation develops out of a complex interaction of psychological, genetic and environmental factors. It is seen however that adolescents who are homosexual face a more difficult time that other teens. Society still harbours great ignorance and prejudice against homosexuality, persisting in the idea that people have a choice in their orientation- which they do not have. Gay, lesbian and bisexual teens may be rejected, harassed, victimized, and assaulted by their family and peers. The result is that homosexual adolescents find themselves to be at a greater risk for depression than heterosexual adolescents, and they have lower rates of adjustment.

PSYCHOPATHOLOGY IN ADOLESCENCE

Substance Use Disorder

Adolescence is a time of experimentation, identity formation, exploration, and risk taking. Hence, the incidence of substance abuse in adolescents is higher than that of the general population. Habitual Substance abuse in adolescence is of particular concern to clinicians as it may have adverse long-term effects on adolescents and an intergenerational effect on their future offspring. According to a research carried out by the National Commission for Protection of Child Rights, the most common substance of abuse among children and adolescents are tobacco and alcohol, followed by inhalants and cannabis, least for hard drugs like opium, pharmaceutical opioids, heroin and then substances through injecting into the blood stream. According to results from a prevalence study done in India, 13.1% of people involved with substance abuse are below 20 years of age. Another survey revealed that out of the people seeking treatment for substance abuse, 63.6% were introduced to various drugs and substances at the age of 15 or earlier. There is a distinction between abuse and dependence. Abuse refers to using substances in a way that the individual is harmed, drug dependence refers to situations where there is a compulsive need and pattern of use that may encompass physiological changes that go together with the phenomena of tolerance and withdrawal. Substance abuse is associated with a wide variety of factors which may be defined in terms of the age of onset; the duration of abuse; the range of the substances used; the amount; and the frequency of use. Physiological aspects of substance abuse may be classified into those associated with intoxication; symptoms that follow intoxication; those connected with withdrawal following with the development of dependence; and physiological and medical complications which arise from substance abuse. From an affective level, negative mood states typically follow the euphoria of intoxication, for most types of substances. At a perceptual level, some types of substances, particularly hallucinogens, cause pronounced abnormalities during intoxication and withdrawal. With respect to cognitive processes, common street drugs lead to impairment in concentration, attention, reasoning and judgment during intoxication and withdrawal. Long-term regular drug abuse in many instances leads to impaired cognitive functioning. Substance abuse may have a negative impact on interpersonal functioning leading to family, academic and peer-group-based difficulties. Substance abuse often occurs with other co-morbid psychological issues, including ADHD, conduct disorder, specific learning difficulties, mood disorders, anxiety disorders, schizophrenia and eating disorders like bulimia. The relationship between these co-morbid psychological disorders and substance abuse is complex. Explanations for drug abuse have focused on biological predisposing factors; cognitive behavioral learning processes; intrapsychic deficits; family-systems factors; socio-cultural factors; multiple risk factors; and the change processes involved in recovery and relapse. Studies conducted to test these various theories has led to the identification of biological, psychological and socio-cultural factors which increase vulnerability to substance abuse, may catalyse its onset, or may maintain habitual substance abuse. Because of the complex etiology of substance abuse, a multisystemic approach for assessment and treatment is required. Effective treatment programs for adolescent substance abuse are generally family based and progress through a series of different stages. These include engagement; becoming substance free; facing denial and creating a context for a substance-free lifestyle; reorganization of family; and disengagement. Effective substance abuse prevention programs involve psycho-education, child-focused skills training and parent training, usually conducted within a co-operative, multiagency and multiprofessional, community-wide network.

Mood Disorders and Suicide

Mood disorders adolescents constitute a serious problem because there is a high rate of relapse. While equal numbers of children develop mood problems, during adolescence there is a sharp rise in the prevalence of depression, especially among girls. Prevalence rates may be as high as 8 per cent among teenage girls. The main clinical features involve a low mood; self-defeating behavioral patterns; negative cognitive set; disruption of appetite and sleep; and conflict or social withdrawal from relationships at home and at school. Psychodynamic theories of mood disorders point to the importance of early separation or bereavement, and parenting styles in developing a vulnerability to depression and other mood disorders. According to behavioral theories, a lack of reinforcement or poor self-reinforcement skills are key in the maintenance of depression. Cognitive theories point to the role of negative interpretation of ambiguous events in the development and maintenance of depression. Systems theory highlights the role of problematic family relationships in developing low mood in adolescents. Biological theories highlight the importance, in the etiology of mood disorders, of genetic factors; dysregulation of the neurotransmitter systems in the punishment and reward centers of the nervous system; immune system dysregulation; endocrine dysfunction; disruption of the REM cycle; and in few instances seasonal biological changes. Because of the complexity of mood disorders and the uniqueness of each case, treatment programs should be based on a comprehensive case formulation developed from a thorough multisystemic assessment. Research evidence suggests that with adolescents, multisystemic treatment and intervention based on the principles of family systems therapy, cognitive-behavioral therapy and social learning theory is the preferred treatment. Many adolescents do not respond to anti-depressant medication, and so pharmaceutical intervention should only be considered if psychological therapy is seen to be ineffective.

In India, 33% of the total number of suicides are committed by the youth. When an adolescent present with threats of self-harm or self-injurious behavior, the individual and significant network members should be interviewed. Following this, an exploration of the details of the adolescent's suicidal ideation, suicidal intention and self-injurious behavior should take place. This should be followed by the exploration of the circumstances surrounding the episode that require clarification, and risk factors in the social network. It is important that historical, demographic, health-related risk factors and protective factors are also identified. All these factors should be unified into a formulation, and a plan for reduction of the risk should be studied, developed and implemented.

Eating Disorders

About 1 per cent of adolescent girls have anorexia nervosa and 2–3 per cent are diagnosed with bulimia nervosa. Anorexia nervosa is characterized by self-starvation, while bulimia is characterized by a pattern of dieting, bingeing and purging. Clinical features of eating disorders comprise of a fear of becoming fat, distorted body image, preoccupation and obsessive thoughts of food, a belief that the binge eating behavior is uncontrolled, low self-esteem, low self-efficacy, apprehensions about individuation, perfectionism, self-destructive behavior, depressive affect, lack of interpersonal adjustment, and neuroendocrine abnormalities related to starvation. Important predisposing factors include a genetic predisposition, cultural pressures for thinness, early trauma, perfectionism, low self-esteem, low self-efficacy, and unresolved conflicts about individuation. Stresses related to lifecycle transitions to adolescence or young adulthood may catalyse the onset of eating disorders, and they are maintained by the neurophysiological sequelae of starving oneself, in combination with belief systems characterized by distorted cognitions and rigid and conflict-avoiding patterns of family interaction. The prognosis for less chronic and severe conditions is better, and protective factors include the adolescent's problem-solving and interpersonal skills and the family's and peer group's capacity to support the adolescent with the abnormal eating pattern. For adolescents, the preferred treatment is a highly structured support system family-based treatment programe in which the parents are empowered to refeed the adolescent and later the adolescent is helped to individuate. In extremely severe cases hospitalization for refeeding may be essential, and group therapy may become an important part of a family-based multisystemic intervention programe. Educational prevention programs are required which target adolescents scoring above the cut-off point on a screening test such as the Children's Eating Attitude Test.

Schizophrenia

Schizophrenia is group of disorders which affects around 1 per cent of the population over18 years of age. The onset of schizophrenia takes place in late adolescence or early adulthood. The disorder is marked by positive symptoms such as delusions and hallucination and negative symptoms such as restricted affect, avolition and poverty of speech. During differential diagnosis, it should be differentiated from autism, affective conditions and adolescent precursors of adult personality disorders on the schizophrenia spectrum, such as schizotypal, schizoid and paranoid personality disorder. In the biological domain, genetic factors, dopamine system dysregulation, and neuroanatomical abnormalities associated with pre- and perinatal insults have all been associated with the etiology of schizophrenia. According to the psychological perspective, cognitive deficits, cognitive biases, management of prodromal symptoms, and family-and community-based stresses have all been implicated in the development and maintenance of schizophrenia, and various focal theories have been explored to explain the role of these specific factors. Diathesis-stress theories of schizophrenia have also been constructed, which state that for the symptoms of schizophrenia to occur, an individual with biological vulnerabilities must be exposed to environmental stress. The interaction of the risk factors with the environmental factors leads to the occurrence of the symptoms. Assessment based on multifactorial diathesis-stress models of schizophrenia involve addressing predisposing, precipitating and maintaining factors in the biological, psychological and contextual domains. Intervention programs based on diathesis-stress models involve antipsychotic medication to control the dysregulation of the dopamine system; family intervention to psycho-educate and reduce family-based stress; and individual intervention to enhance personal coping strategies and social skills.

BIBLIOGRAPHY

1. Carr, A. (1999). *The handbook of child and adolescent clinical psychology a contextual approach*. Routledge.
2. Feldman, R. S. (2017). *Development across the life span*. Pearson.
3. Wilmshurst, L. (2017). *Abnormal child and adolescent psychology: A developmental perspective*. Routledge, Taylor & Francis Group.

Parenting - Basics 74

Avinash De Sousa • Sushma Sonavane

Parenting is the process of promoting and supporting the physical, emotional, social, and intellectual development of a child from infancy to adulthood. Parenting refers to the aspects of raising a child aside from the biological relationship. Parenting is usually done by the biological parents of the child in question, although governments and society take a role as well. In many cases, orphaned or abandoned children receive parental care from non-parent blood relations. Others may be adopted, raised in foster care, or placed in an orphanage.

Performing the role of a parent by care-giving, nurturance, and protection of the child by a natural or substitute parent. The parent supports the child by exercising authority and through consistent, empathic, appropriate behavior in response to the child's needs. Parenting differs from child rearing. In child rearing the emphasis is on the act of training or bringing up the children and the interaction between the parent and child, while parenting emphasizes the responsibility and qualities of exemplary behavior of the parent.

PARENTING STYLES

The parenting styles commonly used in psychology today is based on the work of Diana Baumrind, a developmental psychologist at the University of California at Berkeley.

Baumrind's Theory

In the 1960s, Baumrind noticed that pre-schoolers exhibited distinctly different types of behavior. Each type of behavior was highly correlated to a specific kind of parenting. Baumrind's theory is that there is a close relationship between parenting styles and children's behavior, which lead to different outcomes in the children's lives. Based on extensive observation, interviews and analyses, Baumrind initially identified three different parenting styles: authoritative parenting, authoritarian parenting and permissive parenting. Maccoby and Martin (1983) expanded this parenting style model using a two-dimensional framework. They made further distinction by expanding Baumrind's permissive parenting into two different types: permissive parenting (also known as indulgent parenting) and neglectful parenting (also known as uninvolved parenting). These four parenting styles are sometimes called the Baumrind parenting styles or Maccoby and Martin parenting styles.

Parenting styles are categorized based on two dimensions of parenting behavior:

Demandingness refers to the extend parents control their children's behavior or demand their maturity.

Responsiveness refers to the degree parents are accepting and sensitive to their children's emotional and developmental needs.

Diana Baumrind's four Parenting Styles

- Authoritative
- Authoritarian
- Permissive
- Neglectful

Authoritative Parenting

This parenting style is also known as Democratic Parenting Style.

Authoritative parenting is a parenting style characterized by high responsiveness and high demands. Authoritative parents are responsive to the child's emotional needs while having high standards. They set limits and are very consistent in enforcing boundaries.

Authoritative Parents

- Are warm, attuned and nurturing.
- Listen to the children.
- Allow autonomy and encourage independence.
- Reason with children instead of demanding blind obedience.
- Set clear limits on behavior.
- Consistently enforce boundaries.
- Use positive discipline instead of punitive, forceful measures.
- Earn, not demand, children's respect.

Children Raised by Authoritative Parents

- Tend to be happy and content.
- Are independent and self-reliant.
- Develop good social skills.
- Have good emotional regulation and self-control.
- Express warmth and cooperate with peers.
- Explore a new environment without fear.
- Are competent and assertive.
- Achieve higher academic success.
- Engage more in school activities.
- Develop good self-esteem.
- Have better mental health — less depression, anxiety, suicide attempts, delinquency, alcohol and drug use.
- Interact with peers using competent social skills.
- Exhibit less violent tendencies.

Authoritarian Parenting

High demandingness. Low responsiveness. Although authoritarian and authoritative parenting styles have similar names, they have several important differences in parenting beliefs. While both parental styles demand high standards, authoritarian parents demand blind obedience using reasons such as "because I said so ". These parents use stern discipline and often employ punishment to control children's behavior. Authoritarian parents are unresponsive to their children's needs and are generally not nurturing.

Authoritarian Parents

- Authoritarian Parents are Demanding.
- Authoritarian Parents are Cold and Non-Nurturing.
- Authoritarian parents seldom show warmth towards their children, they are often quite cold and harsh.
- Authoritarian parents are controlling.
- Authoritarian Parents Only Allow One-Way Communication.
- Authoritarian Parents Tend to Use Harsh Punishment.
- Authoritarian parents often use fear to control and enforce rules.

Children Raised by Authoritarian Parents

- Are highly compliant and obedient at home and around their parents.
- Tend to be unhappy.
- Are less independent than other children.
- Become hostile and aggressive under pressure.
- Often display aggressive behavior problems outside the home, when the parents are not around.
- Some children appear overly shy or fearful around people.
- Have poor social skills.
- Less likely to feel socially accepted by peers.
- May perform poorly in school[3].
- Develop lower self-esteem[4].
- Are less resilient after failure.
- Have a higher risk for drinking, smoking, substance abuse, or mental health problems like anxiety or suicide attempts. They are also more likely to suffer from depression

Permissive Parenting

Permissive parenting, also known as indulgent parenting, is a parenting style characterized by high responsiveness and low demandingness. Permissive parents are very responsive to the child's emotional needs. But they don't set limits or are very inconsistent in enforcing boundaries.

Permissive Parents

- Responsive to the child's needs
- Rarely say no to the child's demands
- Lenient parents.
- Treat their kids more like peers or friends than children
- Children's freedom over responsibility
- Let children make major decisions alone

Children Raised by Permissive Parents

- Worse academic performance
- More impulsive and aggressive
- More prone to delinquency, substance abuse and alcohol abuse
- Less able to self-regulate
- Worse social skills
- More likely to be overweight

Neglectful Parenting (Uninvolved)

Low demandingness. Low responsiveness. Uninvolved parenting also called neglectful parenting, which obviously carries more negative connotations is a style of parenting where parents don't respond to their child's needs or desires beyond the basics of food, clothing, and shelter. These children receive little guidance, discipline, and nurturing from their parents. And oftentimes kids are left to raise themselves and make decisions big and small on their own. Neglectful parents do not set firm boundaries or high standards.

Neglectful Parents

- Focus on your own problems and desires
- Lack of an emotional attachment
- Lack of interest in child's activities
- No set rules or expectations for behavior
- Too occupied with their own problems
- Are into drugs and other addictions
- Lack of supervision
- Do not express love
- Lack of expectations

Children Raised by Neglectful Parents

- Children feel unloved

- Child becomes directionless
- Difficulty following rules or instructions
- Substance abuse
- Have to take care of themselves
- Heightened emotions
- Hampered brain functioning
- Lack of personality development

Suggestions for Parents

Be a role model for learning: In the early years, parents are their children's first teachers exploring nature, reading together, cooking together, and counting together. When a young child begins formal school, the parent's job is to show him how school can extend the learning you began together at home, and how exciting and meaningful this learning can be. As pre-schoolers grow into school age kids, parents become their children's learning coaches. Through guidance and reminders, parents help their kids organize their time and support their desires to learn new things in and out of school.

Pay attention to what your child loves: One of the most important things a parent can do is notice her child. Is he a talker or is he shy? Find out what interests him and help him explore it. Let your child show you the way he likes to learn,"

Tune into how your child learns: Many children use a combination of modalities to study and learn. Some learn visually through making and seeing pictures, others through tactile experiences, like building block towers and working with clay. Still others are auditory learners who pay most attention to what they hear. And they may not learn the same way their siblings (or you) do. By paying attention to how your child learns, you may be able to pique his interest and explain tough topics by drawing pictures together, creating charts, building models, singing songs and even making up rhymes.

Practice what your child learns at school: Many teachers encourage parents to go over what their young children are learning in a non-pressured way and to practice what they may need extra help with. This doesn't mean drilling them for success, but it may mean going over basic counting skills, multiplication tables or letter recognition, depending on the needs and learning level of your child.

Set aside time to read together: Read aloud regularly, even to older kids. If your child is a reluctant reader, reading aloud will expose her to the structure and vocabulary of good literature and get her interested in reading more. Let kids pick the books they like. Book series are great for reluctant readers. It's okay to read easy, interesting books instead of harder novels.

Connect what your child learns to everyday life: Make learning part of your child's everyday experience, especially when it comes out of your child's natural questions. When you cook together, do measuring math. When you drive in the car, count license plates and talk about the states. When you turn on the blender, explore how it works together. When your child studies the weather, talk about why he felt hot at the beach. Have give-and-take conversations, listening to your child's ideas instead of pouring information into their heads.

Connect what your child learns to the world: Find age-appropriate ways to help your older child connect his school learning to world events. Start by asking questions. For example, ask a second-grader if she knows about a recent event, and what she heard. You might ask a younger child if he's heard about anything in the news, and find out what he knows. This will help your child become a caring learner.

Help your child take charge of his learning: We want to keep children in charge of their learning and become responsible for it. We want them to be responsible for their successes and failures, show them how engaging learning is, and that the motivations for learning should be the child's intrinsic interests, not an external reward.

Don't over-schedule your child: While you may want to supplement school with outside activities, be judicious about how much you let or urge your child to do. Kids need downtime as much as they may need to pursue extra-curricular activities. If a child has homework and organized sports and a music lesson and is part of a youth group in church it can quickly become a joyless race from one thing to another. Therefore, monitor your child to see that he is truly enjoying what he is doing. If he isn't, cut something off the schedule.

Keep TV to a minimum: Watching lots of TV does not give children the chance to develop their own interests and explore on their own, because it controls the agenda. However, unstructured time with books, toys, crafts and friends allows children to learn how to be in charge of their agenda, and to develop their own interests, skills, solutions and expertise.

Learn something new yourself: Learning something new yourself is a great way to model the learning process for your child. Take up a new language or craft, or read about an unfamiliar topic. Show your child what you are learning and how you may be struggling. You'll gain a better understanding of what your child is going through and your child may learn study skills by watching you study. You might even establish a joint study time.

Do Not Shout at Your Child: Instead of shouting at or scolding children, try to calmly reason with them. Give them a time-out if they're being difficult and then sit down and listen to why they were upset in the first place. If it has to do with school, then calmly ask your child to explain the difficulties he/she is facing. Explain to your child why his/her actions are wrong and the larger consequences of those actions.

Give Reasons: If you want your child to do something, then explain to him/her the reasons behind your request. If you want him/her to finish school work before going out to play, then explain the reasons behind it. A great way to explain it would be to say that the second he/she finishes, play time begins. This also works as motivation.

Set Rules: Structure is important for your child's development. However, whatever new rules you do put in place, do make sure to discuss the same with your child. In case you want your child to take up a chore around the house, then have a discussion with him/her about which chore he/she would like to do and to what degree you want that chore to be done. Ask your child to set up a schedule for this new chore. Sticking to this new schedule will boost self-esteem.

Give Your Child Choices: Talk to your child about the different options he/she might have. It can be something small like deciding if he/she wants to go to the park with you the next day. Allowing your child to make choices will boost confidence in making decisions.

Listen: One of the most important aspects of parenting is listening to your child. Even if what your child says seems mundane to you, you must listen, as it might be something important to him/her.

Be a Good Example: Children are known to pick up habits and actions from the people around them. As a parent, your child will be looking up to you for advice on almost everything, particularly in the younger years. Practice healthy habits and your child is bound to pick them up himself/herself.

Role of the Parent in Child Development

All development is interrelated and cannot be defined under water-tight categories. The role of parents in child development is responsive, responsible and never-ending. It governs responses, actions, thinking and decision making of a child in the following areas.

Cognitive Development

When children are growing up, positive parenting improves their cognitive, social and problem-solving skills. Positive parenting also affects their responses and helps them grow up to be better humans. Interaction and stimulation are very important in the early years. It is all about recognizing problems, handling all situations well and picking up the traits of discipline, time management and effective problem-solving through simple routines at home.

Socio-Cultural Development

Children observe spousal interaction and how arguments are settled in the family. It teaches them a variety of good values that are imbibed and crucial to growing up. The child learns how to behave with others, playing to a common goal, team spirit, picking right friends and a lot more.

Physical Development

Reaching age-related milestones is not the only goal. Children learn about being healthy, exercising regularly, being a team player, having the right diet and growing in a conducive environment through the play and learn way. The right guidance from parents can inculcate in children a good regimen of exercise and diet to achieve ideal physical development. Parents should remember that children lead by example.

Mental Development

Parenting styles help the child learn innovatively, accepting failures and overcoming them, understanding discipline, accepting feedback and the award and punishment concept. It governs their response to stimuli, thus moulding their minds.

Spiritual Development

Understanding right from wrong, being empathetic, having the right ethical values, valuing your parents and strengthening goal setting liberates the free spirit in children. Teaching the children to be more accepting and believing in the greater good can help them gain a sense of purpose.

Modern Day Parenting

Concept of Righteousness

The most important axiom in modern-day parenting is that there is no right or wrong way. There is no effective blueprint, as every parent-child relationship is unique and has a distinct quality to it. Admitting your children in a great school or enrolling them in numerous extra-curricular classes does not define parenting. It is about trying to create an emotional bond that transcends material needs, and will remain even if that new phone is not bought or a trip is not planned. Kids are able to perform better when their parents are with them through thick and thin. Children thrive when they have parents who are happy, caring and are keen to enjoy moments together.

Emotional Development

How you are as a parent plays a very important role in shaping the personality of your child as he/she goes into adulthood. A responsible parent is someone who respects the needs and emotions of a child and also encourages the development of the child's self-esteem. In the growing up years, a child's social interaction is the most with his/her parents. Therefore, the style of interaction plays a significant role and leaves an impact on the child during his/her growing up years. However, parenting does not end when a child grows up and enters into adulthood. It is a long-term process and a lifetime commitment that a parent takes up to promote a child's social, emotional, physical and intellectual well-being from infancy to adulthood.

Personal Accountability

Encouraging them to take personal responsibility and ensuring their accountability. For instance, parents should ensure children keep their rooms neat and tidy. Also, children should be motivated to manage small sums of money on their own so they gain financial independence smoothly when they grow up. It is essential that parents should participate enthusiastically in occasions such as festivals etc. and assign specific roles to children, so that the trait of responsibility is inculcated at a young age.

Reward Accomplishments

It is also important to reward children for their accomplishments. Parents need to teach children how to set achievable goals with a reasonable reward. Parents should teach them how to earn their rewards without hurting others and encourage them to pursue some kind of sport that helps them to embrace a competitive spirit.

Parents today are making their job all the more difficult by falling into the trap of comparing between siblings or with other children.

Social Media Battle

Children today are most impressed by likes and followers on social networking sites. Some are even addicted to digital media or pornographic viewing. It is imperative, to communicate to your child. Engage in a healthy conversation whether over a walk in the park or over a game of badminton. Let your kids realize that their parents are keen to listen to them and understand them and they will automatically share things with you. This will enable you to understand their perspective and the reasons behind the choices they make. Parents who are unable to empathize with their child contribute to the development of social anxiety later on in life. Therefore, even if you disagree with your child, use positivity to convince him/her.

Peer Pressure

As the child begins to grow and starts socializing, it is common to find them getting influenced easily. At this juncture, parents need to invest all their experience and maturity to ensure that the child is able to distinguish between right and wrong. This can be achieved by communicating effectively and developing a clear set of family values and beliefs.

CONCLUSION

Parenting is no child's play. It is a continuous learning process that needs a certain level of balance and recognition for the relationship to evolve. Children need time and care to come into their own. Each child is different from the other. With this understanding and by nurturing their talent, encouraging them to take up challenges and fostering in them a sense of individuality, parents can ensure that the child gets the best out of his/her life. Moreover, it ensures that the child gets the best out of the parents

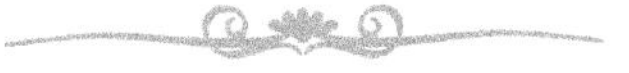

75 Theories of Psychosexual Development

Avinash De Sousa • Sushma Sonavane

The science of psychoanalysis is by no means a simple one. It encompasses a great wealth of knowledge that reveals the total inner nature of human beings. Psychoanalysis in the world of today has taken a back seat due to the advent of various new inventions like the MRI, CT Scan, SPECT and PET Scans. This has resulted in the focus being spread to biological causes for psychiatric disorders rather than psychological ones or those that affect the psyche. There are many issues that are debatable in the world of psychoanalysis. This is so because many of the things mentioned are pure theory and based on speculation. Although these speculations are not mere folly but based on the vast clinical acumen of the distinguished psychologists involved, they have never really been proved on paper. At the same time there is a growing awareness that in the field of psychiatry where biology stops and the mind has to take over. This is where psychology steps in and the study of psychoanalysis plays a vital role. This involves an analysis of the client in totality along with the others who influence his life right from his birth to the present day and this then gives us an idea about the certain obstacles at various levels of development that may have lead to the present state of the patient as of today. Another rather controversial issue in the field of psychoanalysis is whether psychoanalysis is a one person or a two person psychology. When we say one person it merely means that the patient says all that he has to say, without interruptions from the analyst and the analyst maintains a secrecy not stopping the patient nor adding inputs to the patient's story. The two person concept is where both the analyst and the patient are active members in the process and this results in a professional interaction between the two as well as an exchange of views and the personality of the analyst influencing the patient as well as vice versa. Many of the schools of psychology believe that today the science of psychoanalysis is indeed a two person psychology. There is one more major issue at debate being that whether illness occurs in psychiatry due to certain losses or deficiency or whether there are irresistible impulses that are repressed and cause it. It is however agreed worldwide that both have a role to play in the causation of mental illness. While studying the various theories of psychoanalysis and psychological development, one must open one's mind to a large variety of views and thinking and must try to incorporate whatever is possible in the day to day practice of psychiatry. The various theories put forward are by distinguished scholars in their various fields and each being a legend in their own right.

STAGES OF PSYCHOSEXUAL DEVELOPMENT

The birth of the baby results in a change of environment of the baby. The cutting of the umbilical cord results in causing a damming up of energy inside the baby that wants an independent existence. It leaves the dark monotony of the waters of the uterus and comes into the open world. The baby born so has a feeling of being great and independent. This is called as narcissism. But this is not for long as soon it realises that it is helpless in this reckless world. It experiences things that it has never known before. Touch, light, pain and temperature are all new to him. He is not the bundle of the energy that used to float aimlessly in uterus any more. He is a living being that has to survive and face the world on his own. He has to make efforts to survive and even struggle or cry to respire. There is only one person that shall take care of this baby i.e. its mother. The baby soon realises that it depends on its mother for food and its very existence during the first few months of life. It cannot survive if this mother is taken away from him.

THE ORAL PHASE

Here in this phase the baby's main interest is centred round the mouth. The oral phase lasts till the end of the first 18 months. Here the baby experiences pleasure when the breast is brought near the mouth and his hunger needs are satisfied, at the same time experiencing frustration when the breast is absent. The attitude of the mother to her child in this phase is vital for the development of subsequent object relations and growth throughout life. She is the first love object of the infant and is the main provider for his needs and also gives him erotogenic stimuli by allowing him to suck at her nipple. If a warm and affectionate relationship with the mother is set up in the first few months of life, then the stage is set for long lasting affectionate interpersonal relationships throughout life. If the mother is unavailable there are future problems in relationships and the infants grow up with intense feelings of longing to be nurtured and loved. If this stage is not resolved smoothly there are persistent oral traits in the form of thumb sucking, nail biting, oral satisfaction by putting everything in the mouth. This includes traits like a voracious appetite, smoking, drug addiction, alcoholism and tobacco chewing. An oral fixation exists in psychiatric illnesses like Depression, Drug Addiction and Alcoholism.

THE ANAL PHASE

Here the main interests of the baby are located along the anal zone. This period extends from 18-36 months of age. One major difference is that the child here is much passive than he was in the oral phase. Here the mothers make best efforts to teach their babies toilet training with varying resistance. Thus the battle of the chamber pot goes on with hopefully the baby finally giving in but it may be tough if the baby is already fixated at an earlier oral level. The erotization of the anal stage is first in the feeling of evacuating the feces and later in the stimulation of the rectal mucosa caused by retention of feces. There is a strong connection between anal and sadistic drives. The object is the feces and pinching off is the sadism. The child here finds a way to exert power over his parents due to the retaining or excreting the feces. The act of defecation is imbued with a sense of omnipotence and independence and the feces are libidinized with pleasure. The faces are regarded as both 'me' and 'not me'. The child at one point wants to retain the feces and at the same time wants to experience the sensation of pinching off and letting go. Thus he develops a love hate or ambivalent relationship to his parents. The fixation at this stage leads to anal traits like regularity, punctuality, automatic obedience, orderliness, cleanliness, jealousy, lack of trust and a tendency to hoard and miserliness. The psychiatric illnesses that show an anal fixation are sexual perversions, obsessive compulsive disorder, paranoid schizophrenia and homosexuality.

THE URETHRAL STAGE

This is generally viewed as a transition from the anal to the genital pleasure and here a pleasure is derived from the act of urination. Urethral function may be associated with the sadistic urges carried over from the anal stage. Competitiveness and ambition are often viewed as a compensation for the shame associated with loss of urethral control.

THE GENITAL PHASE

This is seen around the age of 3 years. Here the child's interests are around the genital organs. The penis and the clitoris are the main erotogenous zones. There is a greater tolerance to withstand frustration in this phase. There is autoerotism in this phase just like the oral and anal phases but there is also a search for independent love objects that shall determine the later love patterns in life. At the same time it is seen that preferential treatment is meted out to the boys. The boy in this phase realizes that he is strongly attracted to the mother and the girl to her father. The boy wants to possess the mother and hence regards the father as a competitor in this field with him. The converse is true for the girl. The enigma is resolved when the boy identifies with the father and the girl with her mother. If not resolved this goes into adult life with the boy clinging to the mother and the formation of Freud called the Oedipus Complex and the girls cling to their father and form what is called the Electra Complex. The boy here views the father as a rival and may develop murderous attitudes towards the father. This creates a dilemma for the boy as he loves his father too. This produces guilt in the boy and a fear of retaliation from the father who the boy feels may cut off his penis. This results in an anxiety called 'Castration anxiety' and the termination of the Oedipus complex. When the male child has murderous attitude towards the mother who he feels is a rival in the father son relationship, then it is termed as Negative Oedipus Complex. The girl resolves the Electra complex by the awareness of the castrated state. She realizes that she is different from the boys and has lost some part of her. She blames her mother for this loss. The wish to have a baby with her father is then replaced with the wish for a penis. The discovery by the little girl of genital inferiority can lead to a defiant hypermasculinity, neurotic cessation of all sexuality or a normal femininity. The strivings are renounced to maintain the bond with the mother.

THE LATENT PHASE

This starts with 5-6 years and ends at puberty i.e. 12 years. The child recaptures facets of development here and sexual activity is quiescent or latent at this time. Here there is a development of a sense of industry and capacity. The energies are directed in learning various developmental and surviving skills. Contacts with teachers, friends and outside world are broadened here.

THE GENITAL PHASE

This phase begins from around 11-13 years to the onset of adulthood. The physiological maturation of the genital and the hormonal systems occur during this phase. There is an intensifying of drives especially the libidinal ones. There is a regression in personality development where there is opening of conflicts of previous stages of psychosexual development. This stage provides an opportunity for resolution of this conflicts and achieving a mature sexual and adult identity. The main objectives of this stage are a separation from dependence on the parents. Defects in this stage can arise due to a whole spectrum of psychosexual residues that may belong to any earlier stage. A more specific failure may be the identity diffusion. The aim is to achieve a satisfying capacity of self-realization and meaningful participation in areas of work and love more so in the creative and productive spheres.

THE OBJECT RELATIONS THEORY

These theories have some basic fundamental principles that they adhere to. All drives according to them arise in the context of a mother infant relationship and object seeking motivation is equal or even more important than the drive seeking discharge. Conceptualizing object relationship in terms of drive energy does not do justice to the full range of needs and moods associated with relationships. These theories are not interpersonal theories but are one of internal object relationships involving the transformation of interpersonal relationships into interpersonal structures. There is always an association of the object with the self associated with an effect laid down by the child and determined by the child's fantasy. They thus view motivation slightly different from the view of Freud.

These theories involve 2 main defence mechanisms –

1. Introjection.
2. Identification.

There are unconscious conflicts that are perceived as a struggle between different self object-affect units and these strive for center stage of the psyche.

MELANIE KLEIN

Melanie Klein has worked with small children and believed that the fear of annihilation associated with death instinct of Freud was a key factor in the first few months of the infant's life. She said that the ego undergoes a splitting and the derivatives of the death instinct are projected to the mother.

The primary defences used by the child at that stage is projection and introjection. There is a dread of an attack by the mother and this persecutory anxiety is termed by her as the paranoid-schizoid position. He feels that the mother is a good mother when all his needs for care and food are satisfied by her and that she is a tormentor or a persecutor when she fails in this regard. He thus begins to perceive two aspects of the same person and divides them into two different people. Here the good and bad elements of the mother are separated by the child. This occurs in the 1st half of the 1st year. In the 2nd half of the 1st year the child's part object changes. He soon realizes that the mother who was rejecting and loving are in fact two aspects of the same person. He begins to feel that he may have harmed his mother through his hostile tendencies and fears now of losing the love of his mother. This leads to viewing of the mother ambivalently and the child goes into the depressive position.

1st position – concern of external attack.

2nd position – concern of harming the love objects (depressive anxiety).

To deal with guilt there is a reparation to show that love prevails over hate. She says that the Oedipus complex occurs as a means to resolve anxiety and guilt.

There are certain drawbacks of the above theory –

1. The infant in the first year of life has limited sophisticated capacity for abstract and conceptual thinking. The infant's cognition is too rudimentary to develop the fantasies postulated.
2. Klein has emphasized on greed and envy that has clinical utility but the use of

death instinct has fallen out of repute. Klein relies too much on fantasy.

After Melanie Klein there were a group of British psychologists who expanded on her views and theories borrowing little from Freud and many with new formulations of their own. These were called the independent or the middle grouper psychologists. They had some common features in their work –

1. They worked with severely disturbed cases.
2. Focused on pre-oedipal development and dyadic object relations.
3. They were interested more in the theory of deficit.

W.R.D.FAIRBAIRN

His theory had some basic postulates –

1. The mother's failure to provide nurture was more important than a frustration of drives.
2. Infants need love an acceptance and he conceptualized personhood as primary and drives as secondary.
3. Aggression and libido is object seeking rather than pleasure seeking.
4. Fantasy was substitutive.
5. When the mothering figure fails to fulfil the basic needs of the baby the infant splits the ego into various parts. The ego is formed as a whole right from birth.

D.W.WINNICOTT

He believed that the creation of a 'holding environment' by the mother made it possible for the child to develop awareness as a separate person. Mothers play a key role in order to fulfil the infant's needs. Primary attention was paid to the mother infant dyad. Winnicott coined the term 'good enough mothering' for mothers to provide optimal comfort and constancy for infants. He was also responsible for the term 'transitional object' of the infants 'not me' possession that suffices with the mother's scent enabling the child to separate emotionally from the mother through a comfortable maternal object. Transitional phenomena are objects, light, sounds, that are there and art and creativity may derive from here. True self is inherited potential that constitutes the kernel of the child. False self constructed in relation to mother wanted responses develops later. He said that psychopathology developed due to the mother's failures and not due to the integrity conflict.

MICHEAL BALINT

He said that the search for a primary love object underlies all psychological phenomena. He said that people felt that something 'missing' somewhere was the basic fault. He also believed in maternal failure as a cause of all phenomena that followed. He said that libido is always both pleasure as well as object seeking.

When the theories of the British schools reached American shores there were some theories that aimed at encompassing the ego psychology school of the Americans along with object relation schools of the British. These lead to formation of some mixed model theories.

EDITH JACOBSON

He said that the infant's disappointment was viewed not only as a mother's failure but also as a drive determined demand. Good mother child relation carved good images and vice versa. Normal and pathological development are based on self images and object images. The ego and the object images have a reciprocal effect on one another. With ego maturation by the 2nd year the child distinguishes features of a love object and entertains the notion of being like the love object. Ego ideal was a fusion of ideal self images and ideal object images.

OTTO KERNBERG

He postulated that there is a splitting of the ego and separation of the good and bad self configurations. Id is made up of self and object images associated with affects. Goodness and badness precede the drive cathexis. Libido and aggression arise due to the states of love and hate. Infantile development moves from a splitting to an integration of the good and bad images and the result is the formation of ambivalent whole object configurations of the self and others.

The main defence mechanisms used in object relations is splitting and projective identification. The self interacts with objects and the ego interacts with the id and the superego. The self evolves in relational configurations to objects. Identity is the sum of the component array of selves and is a conscious sense of inner solidarity that endures over time. The self is a part of the ego and offers a subjective side to it. The self is viewed as both agency and representational as well. The self is primary and a supraordinate entity implying motivational status. These primitive defence mechanisms are still seen when used by patients of borderline personality disorder.

MARGARET MAHLER

Her findings on her keen observation of infants and their development.

- 1st 2 months – autistic phase of development, where the child is half sleeping and half waking. The stage deals with more on the formation of physiological matters.
- 2-6 months – there is a fusion between the mother and the child called symbiosis or dual unity. This stage starts with the advent of the social smile.
- 6-36 months – this is called the stage of separation individualization and is further subdivided into 4 phases viz.
  1. Differentiation – the mother is seen as a separate person and the child develops attachment to a transitional object. This lasts from the 6th to the 10th month.
  2. Practicing – here the child develops a new found sense of autonomy and there is attainment of locomotor skills. It lasts from the 10th to the 16th months.
  3. Raproachment – there is an obliviousness for the mother and a need for the mother's love. Both the good and bad images of the mother develop here. This stage lasts from the 16th to the 24th months.
  4. Object Constancy and Individuation – there is an integration of the good and the bad self representations and the mother is introjected and a soothing internal presence is felt by the child.

BIBLIOGRAPHY

1. BACAL, H. (1990). Object relations – bridges to self psychology. Columbia University Press. New York.
2. BOWLBY, J. (1965). Child care and the growth of love. Penguin Books. London.
3. FAIRBAIRN, W.R.D. (1952). The study of personality. Routledge & Kegan Paul. London.
4. FREUD, S. The complete psychological works of Sigmund Freud. Hogarth Press. London.
5. FREUD, S. The psychopathology of everyday life. Penguin Books. London.
6. JACOBSON, E. (1964). The self and the object world. International Univeristy Press. New York.
7. KAGAN, J. (1984). The nature of the child. Basic Books. New York.
8. KERNBERG, O.F. (1993). The current status of

psychoanalysis. J.Amer.psychoanl.Assoc. 41: 45-46.

9. KLEIN, M. (1975). Envy, gratitude and other works. Free press. New York.
10. STERN, D.N. (1985). The world of the infant. Basic Books. New York.
11. WINNICOTT, D.W. (1971). Playing and reality. Basic Books. New York.
12. THE PSYCHOANALYTIC STUDY OF THE CHILD – 1982. Butterworth and Hienman.

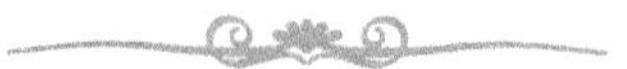

Anger Management 76

Avinash De Sousa • Pragya Lodha

Anger is one of the basic human emotions, as elemental as happiness, sadness, anxiety, or disgust. These emotions are tied to basic survival and were honed over the course of human history. Anger is related to the "fight, flight, or freeze" response. Everyone experiences anger at some point. It becomes problematic, however, when the frequency or severity of anger interferes with relationships, work performance, legal standing or mental health.

Stages of Anger

Each level of anger is different from its predecessor or successor. The triggers and factors associated with various levels of anger provide considerable insight into humans and different emotional states.

Annoyance

Annoyance is the first level of anger and is quite common. People get annoyed at various minute things, such as long lines, traffic jams or hearing someone chew with their mouth open. Generally, annoyance is very mild and tends to subside fairly quickly. Annoyance is the lowest level of anger, and is the easiest to regulate.

Frustration

Frustration is the second level of anger and tends to come along once an annoyance has festered and lasted for too long. A frustrated individual may feel tense or otherwise have a hard time concentrating on certain matters, due to their current negative emotional state. Frustration generally takes longer to subside than annoyance and remaining collected can be much more challenging.

Hostility

After frustration comes hostility which serves as the third stage of anger. Hostility takes place when someone has been consistently subjected to various people or circumstances which displease them or threaten them. In many cases, hostility is the result of pent up anger which hasn't been constructively resolved and is, therefore, seeping out. Screaming, swearing, or even getting physical are signs of hostility which can quickly lead to the fourth stage of anger.

Rage

Rage is the fourth and final stage of anger. By the time someone has reached the point of being enraged, they are verbally confrontational, throwing objects, making threats or even physically lashing out at others. Rage is a dangerous emotional state because it means that someone has lost control of their emotions and is unable to manage their anger. The fourth stage of anger can quickly follow if hostility is allowed to increase and worsen.

Many people have got themselves into trouble because of the words which were said or acts which were committed during fits of rage.

Anger should never reach the point of rage; this is why self-control and dealing with anger before it escalates into its latter stages is critical.

Types of Anger

1. **Aggressive Anger**

   When the person experiences aggressive anger, he tends to get out of control easily and tends to confront the subject of his anger immediately. This is usually another person but could be an object or animal. Defiance, physical harm, and trouble making are the normal ways of behaving for someone expressing aggressive anger.

2. **Chronic Anger**

   Those experiencing chronic anger usually have no definite reason to become angry at all. they just hate themselves & their life, the people next to them, the people around them, the situation they're in, and just the world in general. They seem to just walk around angry all of the time.

3. **Constructive Anger**

   These types of people want to do something with their anger that will be of benefit to others. They work for a cause or promote important changes to right the wrongs that they feel angry about. They want to join a group or some kind of movement to create positive change.

4. **Deliberate Anger**

   This type of anger usually occurs to a person who wants to take control over things, situations or groups. A person who uses this anger wants to have power, however, anger normally subsides if he feels that he can't gain control over things, usually due to opposition by another person.

5. **Judgmental Anger**

   A person with this type of anger expresses his emotion by putting down other people or humiliating others' abilities in front of other people. He would try to show his superiority in these ways.

6. **Overwhelming Anger**

   A person who doesn't like the situation he is in or feels trapped expresses this type of anger. To get out of this uncomfortable situation, he usually finds ways to relieve the pain or stress, usually by hurting himself or other people verbally or physically.

7. **Paranoid Anger**

   Anger of this kind results in hating other people even if they don't do or take away anything from him. They operate out of fear. A person with paranoid anger is generally jealous and intimated by others.

8. **Passive Anger**

   A person who feels this kind of anger doesn't show his anger directly. He doesn't ever confront his anger at all. He often uses other ways to express it in order to always come out looking like the victim. These include using sarcasm or offensive words towards the subject, and treating the subject differently. This is also described as "spitting in someone's soup."

9. **Retaliatory Anger**

   This is the most common type of anger among men. It usually occurs when a person becomes angry because another person is angry with him.

10. **Self-inflicted Anger**

    The consequence of this type of anger is that the person experiencing it tends to hurt himself with a certain thing such as attempting suicide or developing an eating disorder. A person with this type of anger punishes him/herself as they turn the anger inward.

11. Verbal Anger

This anger is expressed merely by words. The person with this type of anger speaks insulting words to the subject of his anger.

12. Volatile Anger

This type of anger is expressed either by physical assault or verbal abuse. But different from other types of anger, this type easily comes and goes. The level of anger also varies from mild to rage. It may explode suddenly or may pass away unnoticed. The magnitude and the duration of this anger depend on how the person handles it.

Physical symptoms of anger

- Clenched jaw or fists
- Muscle tension
- Increase in heart rate
- Increase in respiration
- Increased blood pressure
- Red/flushed face
- Stomach ache
- Shaking
- Dizziness
- Sweating
- Feeling hot in the face or neck
- Heart palpitations or tightening of the chest
- Headaches
- Pressure in the head or sinus cavities
- Fatigue

Causes of Anger

A leading cause of anger is a person's environment. Stress, financial issues, abuse, poor social or familial situations, impoverished childhood, personal discord or health concerns. Disorders such as alcoholism, or Mental disorders such as Bipolar disorder, Borderline personality disorder Post traumatic stress or Schizophrenia may also cause extreme anger. Anger issues may be more prevalent in individuals who were raised by parents with the same disorder. Genetics and your body's ability to deal with certain chemicals and hormones also play a role in how a person would deal with anger.

Effects of Anger

- **Physical health:** Constantly operating at high levels of stress and anger makes you more susceptible to heart disease, diabetes, a weakened immune system, insomnia and high blood pressure.
- **Mental health:** Chronic anger consumes huge amounts of mental energy, and clouds your thinking, making it harder to concentrate or enjoy life. It can also lead to stress, depression and other mental health problems.
- **Career:** Constructive criticism, creative differences, and heated debate can be healthy. But lashing out only alienates your colleagues, supervisors, or clients and erodes their respect.
- **Relationships:** Anger can cause lasting scars in the people you love most and get in the way of friendships and work relationships. Explosive anger makes it hard for others to trust you, speak honestly, or feel comfortable—and is especially damaging to children.

ANGER MANAGEMENT

Anger management is the process of learning to recognize signs that a person is becoming angry, and taking action to calm down and deal with the situation in a productive way. The mental health professional would first take a detailed history of the client, post which he/she would try and find the underlying reasons for the client's anger which the client himself may not be aware off. These feelings would include feelings of detachments, resentment, fear, anguish or sadness. Each individual would also face certain physical symptoms prior to an aggressive bout the therapist help the client to identify the onset of the same.

Methods to Reduce Anger

1. **Think before you speak**

   In the heat of the moment, it's easy to say something you'll later regret. Take a few moments to collect your thoughts before saying anything and allow others involved in the situation to do the same.

2. **Express anger in a calm way**

   Express your frustration in an assertive but nonconfrontational way. State your concerns and needs clearly and directly, without hurting others or trying to control them.

3. **Exercise Regularly**

   Physical activity can help reduce stress that can cause you to become angry. If you feel your anger escalating, go for a brisk walk or run, or spend some time doing other enjoyable physical activities.

4. **Take timeout**

   Timeouts aren't just for kids but adults too. Take short breaks during times of the day that tend to be stressful. A few moments of quiet time help you feel better prepared to handle what's ahead without getting irritated or angry.

5. **Identify possible solutions**

   Instead of focusing on what made you angery, work on resolving the issue at hand. Remind yourself that anger won't fix anything and might only make a situation worse.

6. **Stick with 'I' statements**

   To avoid criticizing or placing blame, which might only increase tension use "I" statements to describe the problem. Be respectful and specific. For example, say, "I'm upset that you left the table without offering to help with the dishes" instead of "You never do any housework."

7. **Don't hold a grudge**

   Forgiveness is a powerful tool. If you allow anger and other negative feelings to crowd out positive feelings, you might find yourself swallowed up by your own bitterness or sense of injustice. But if you can forgive someone who angered you, you might both learn from the situation and strengthen your relationship.

8. **Use humour to release tension**

   Lightening up can help diffuse tension. Use humour to help you face what's making you angry and, possibly, any unrealistic expectations you have for how things should go. Avoid sarcasm, since it can hurt feelings and make things worse.

9. **Practice relaxation skills**

   When your temper flares, put relaxation skills to work. Practice deep-breathing exercises, imagine a relaxing scene, or repeat a calming word or phrase, such as "Take it easy." You might also listen to music, write in a book or do a few yoga poses, whatever it takes to encourage relaxation.

10. **Know when to seek help**

    Learning to control anger is a challenge for everyone at times. Seek help for anger issues if your anger seems out of control or causes you to do things you regret or hurt those around you.

ANGER DISORDER

Anger disorder, more properly known as Intermittent Explosive Disorder (IED) is a psychological condition characterized by sporadic episodes of aggression, violence, and destructive behavior. People who suffer from this disorder are unable to control themselves, exploding with rage in a way which is often out of proportion to the event which triggered the anger. An Anger Disorder is termed when there is pathological aggression, violent or self-destructive behaviors symptomatic of and driven by an underlying and chronically repressed anger or rage. Anger disorders result primarily from the long-term mismanagement of anger, a process in which normal, existential anger grows insidiously over time into resentment, bitterness, hatred and destructive rage. An Anger disorder may also be caused or exacerbated by neurological impairment and substance abuse, both of which can inhibit one's ability to resist aggressive, angry or violent impulses. In certain cases, a doctor may suggest medicines too depending on the needs of the patient. Like other psychological disorders, IED can be treated with help from a psychologist or psychotherapist, but first it needs to be identified as a problem and diagnosed.

77 Parenting – Past, Present and Future

Cicilia Chettiar

FAMILY

Family is the starting point of new life. Across time and cultures, the initiation of new life began with an introduction to the family. A family largely consists of an adult male and adult female who come together physically, financially and temporally. They partner with each other as they go through the various stages of life as decided by the culture they belong to. A family is "a group defined by a sex relationship sufficiently precise and enduring to provide for the procreation and upbringing of children" (MacIver & Page, 1964). This is among one of the earlier definitions of family. The process of parenting is such an essential component of this definition that it appears to be the express reason why two individuals will marry. There are cultural differences in the manner of parenting and the duration of a marriage. Some cultures allow for more than two people to be part of a marriage and the new trend is for both partners in the marriage to belong to the same gender. Family is also when there is a single parent with a child. Across time and cultures, a family has always been meant to include an adult and an offspring. Most often this offspring is biologically connected, in some cases, the offspring may be legally or socially connected.

The highlight of the family is the joint journey undertaken by the adults and the child or children. There are socially relevant milestones along with the developmentally identified ones. In many species besides humans, nurturance of the offspring is the basic function of the parent. This nurturance in humans is part of what is referred to as parenting. Parenting, therefore, is a collection of practices that are meant to allow for the maximum progress of the offspring using a series of tried and tested techniques passed down across time along with the basic instinctual ones. Parenting aims to provide protection and care to the offspring. While in non-humans, parenting is restricted to training in species-specific behaviors; in humans, it encompasses emotional and social training too. The emphasis in parenting could either be biological need satisfaction, emotional fulfillment, or socialization of the child. The aspect that gets maximum importance differs across culture, time and even between parents in the same culture at the same time. Patterns of similarity can however be traced across parents belonging to the same group.

Parenting differences are also due to the changing definition of a family. Once, a family constituted the adult couple, their offspring, their parents and siblings all living together and sharing the responsibilities. Due to societal changes, space constraints and challenges brought by the ever-changing environment, the family kept reducing in size. In the current context, a typical family means an adult and child. It is no longer essential for adults to be in a heterosexual pair. The pair could be of the same gender. Instead of a couple, there could be just one parent figure, male or female; and this could be a choice, not a necessity. Changes in social norms and legal provisions make it easier to do this. There are also vastly deviant family types where the parents could number up to more than two. Both partners could be in polygamous relationships and there could be several children. However, since this is not the norm, nor has it been studied in great detail, this article will only focus on the family type that comprises a heterosexual couple and their children.

INDIAN FAMILIES

Indian culture is representative of Eastern culture. The common yardstick for understanding the nature of a culture is the method provided by Geerst Hofstede (Hofstede, 2011). He identified six measures that aid in understanding any culture and can be used for comparisons between cultures. The first dimension he spoke about was *Power Distance*. This describes how *individuals* in a culture treat people who are not in an equal position as themselves. *Individualism* refers to the amount of interdependence the members of society maintain among themselves. *Masculinity* refers to the value placed on competition and achievement versus the value placed on the quality of life. *Uncertainty Avoidance* reflects how comfortable society is with the concept of the unknown. Those who are uncomfortable with it will attempt to avoid it by establishing beliefs and institutions. *Long-term Orientation* indicates how societies balance the past and the future. Following time-honored traditions and making way for change requires an ability to have a long-term perspective. *Indulgence* is most closely related to the topic of parenting and refers to how children are raised; whether they are restrained or indulged.

If measured according to Hofstede's dimensions, it can be said that India scores about average on Individualism (48), Masculinity (56) and Long-term Orientation (51). It scores high on Power Distance (77) and low on Uncertainty Avoidance (40) and Indulgence (26). A typically Western country like the United States scores low on Power Distance (40) and Long Term Orientation (26). It scores about average on Uncertainty Avoidance (46) and high on Individualism (91), Masculinity (62) and Indulgence (68) (https://geert-hofstede.com/india.html). The low score on indulgence shows that on the whole, Indian parents tend to be more cynical and pessimistic in their parenting style. They also may not put much emphasis on leisure time. Considering these cultural differences, it seems apparent that Indian families would largely differ in their parenting as compared to western practices. Besides, technological change, rural-urban differences, economic position, religious affiliation and ethnic and regional differences all have a part to play in the kind of parenting an Indian child receives. Keeping in mind the fact that the immediate environment will have an impact, Indians living in Western culture may follow a mixed parenting approach.

Ember & Ember (2005) analyzed data from two hundred societies and found an interesting pattern. Those societies that were most violent were most likely to have corporal punishment as an essential part of parenting. The greater the differentiation in power in the society, the more frequent was corporal punishment. It appears that parents wished to teach their children the concept of the hierarchy of power. This is also reflected in our high scores on Power Distance and the increasingly gruesome amounts of violence in our society.

TYPES OF PARENTING

In the earliest stages of research on parenting, the emphasis was on identifying how specific caretaking practices predicted individual differences in the children (Power, 2013). In the 1930s and 1940s, researchers changed their "what" questions to "how" questions. They began to focus on how parents provided their caregiving rather than what their specific caregiving practices were. Based on these researches, parenting came to be understood in terms of the dimensions emphasized. Two dimensions that arose from studying European American parents were parental warmth and control. Three more dimensions arrived at were positive parental involvement, ineffective disciplining and neutral conversations (Power, 2013).

The above dimensions point to some specific characteristics that can be used to study parenting – warmth, control and structure. Each of the three by themselves could be considered multi-dimensional and bring greater detailing to parenting as a concept. Studies later moved from dimensions of parenting to styles of parenting. Currently, research in parenting refers to parenting *styles* and not parenting *dimensions*. The difference between the two is that while dimensions were studied with their correlates, parenting styles acknowledged the multi-dimensionality of parenting and focused on how these dimensions could be classified. Pioneering work in this context was conducted by Diana Baumrind (Baumrind, 1966) and has since been the most frequently used technique to classify parenting. In her later and much-elaborated work (Baumrind, 1967) she explained that parenting can be understood as three different styles: authoritarian, authoritative and permissive. The first two styles can often be confused. Authoritarian is considered quite unhealthy with the emphasis on greater parental control and lower responsiveness. Permissive is the opposite with lesser parental control and a greater expression of acceptance. Authoritative on the other hand was recommended as a balanced style with the parent exhibiting love and care and at the same time ensuring adequate but healthy disciplining of the child. Many pieces of research on parenting followed this system of categorizing the parenting style and used it to understand how it affects the child's well-being and development. Later research by Maccoby and Martin (1983) added another dimension to Baumrind's styles. They focused on the demandingness and responsiveness of the parents in their interactions with their children. This created a fourth style referred to as Uninvolved parenting where the parents were both non-demanding and unresponsive. Although these four types help provide some sort of classification that can help in our understanding of parenting as a concept, it must be remembered that these are not a combination of the demands and the responses of the parents.

Understanding these parenting styles help in the prediction of the well-being of children in terms of their academic performances, social skills, psychological development and overall output as an adult. As mentioned earlier, culture influences the type of parenting that is dominant and this, in turn, creates a particular kind of adult who then parents his or her children in a particular way. This cycle continues and drastic changes have not usually occurred in parenting or the understanding of parenting. One major change, however, was in the use of behavior modification to bring about welcome behavioral changes in children. This was largely due to the theoretical changes that occurred in the understanding of an adult.

Psychodynamic theory was the mainstay when it came to understanding human behavior and it was seemingly difficult to apply to young children. Further, it only helped in predicting adult outcomes based on childhood experiences after prolonged therapeutic efforts. In the case of children, such kind of time investment was neither practical nor possible. Changes in children were required faster and were expected to be sustainable in the long term. Hence when the theoretical world moved towards behaviorism, parenting research also followed suit. The principles of rewards and punishments, positive and negative reinforcement and other behavioral techniques were considered quicker and more practical when dealing with children. Behaviorism as a school quickly gained popularity and it influenced a large part of parenting research. Consequently, parenting practices began to reflect the research output.

Darling and Steinberg (1993) attempted to integrate these theoretical differences and put forth an integrative model that perhaps went back to the research of the early 1920s. They focused on parental behavior which they referred to as parental practices, to see how it impacted the child. Specific child-rearing behaviors are affected by the parenting styles and this is the cause of differences in the child's development. Parenting is best understood from the social learning perspective. The impact of parenting can be observed in the child's socialization skills and is the unit of measurement for the success or failure in parenting. Adolescent outcomes were then considered dependent on the parent's goals and values which affected their parenting habits and styles. It was also important to keep in mind whether the adolescents were willing to be socialized. So a specific parenting style would produce a particular outcome based on the parenting practices followed. Despite this thorough analysis, the process through which a specific parenting style could produce a specific outcome remained a mystery. This impacted future parenting research and the understanding therefore of what parenting is and what it should be.

CHANGING ROLE OF PARENTS

Changes in parenting research have not only reflected the theoretical changes, but they have also reflected the changing perceptions of parents. Parents have been viewed differently at different times by different cultures and sometimes at the same time in the same culture. Parenting has also borrowed from research so that it can be said the perception of a parent has been changing to reflect the changing research findings. This two-way influence has brought much dynamism in parenting in research and reality. Added to this, the cultural changes, technological changes, rapid urbanization, gender role revisions, environmental changes and increasing complexity of modern living have made the role of a current day parent an extremely nebulous one. The basic definition still stays that a couple comes together to give new life and be joint partners in providing and nurturing this life into healthy adulthood. The scientific understanding of parenting as discussed thus far provides a one-sided picture of parenting. The other side includes an understanding of how society and children especially view their parents. The job description of being a parent has changed, some of them pretty drastic, as a result of the greater understanding of the impact of parenting on the adult outcome of human life. The relation between social structure and its treatment of children has been systematically established and can be understood by the evolution of the social structures across the centuries.

Parenting in Hunter-gatherer Societies

Power has defined the direction of relationships, values and social practices in humans and even in animals. In a family, the adult holds more power than the child. In earlier times, parents would be the reigning deities of the home and decide the fate of the offspring. In matters of nutrition, nourishment, education, partner selection and all other events that make up the life of a human being, parents were omniscient. In India, parents are considered next to God and blind obedience to their wishes was the hallmark of an ideal child. When families were part of small communities during the hunting and food gathering era, the life of a child depended entirely on the parent's capability. It was also common for other parents in the group to participate in the rearing of the child. It used to be said that it takes a village to raise a child. Such children were held frequently, nursed, kept outdoors promptly responded to, enjoyed multiple playgroups in early childhood and were all part of the natural childbirth process. The children were breastfed up to the age of five (Hewlett & Lamb, 2005). The amount of freedom given to children was reflected in the amount of reverence paid back to the parent. Such communities emphasized sharing and generosity as the survival of group members depended on the kindness shown to one another. In such an atmosphere children were valued and respected additions to the group and the parents did not feel the need to resort to threats, punishments or "time-outs" to bring about the desired behavior in the child. Children also were initiated into adult life far earlier. The biological clock determined the readiness of the child to step up to the next level of responsibility. Research by Darcia Narvaez and her colleagues (2010) point out the high correlations between such child rearing practices and the development of intelligence, cooperation, conscience, empathy, self-control, aggression and depression in children. Morality is a tree that was planted in infancy and nourished through the early years and the hunter-gatherer societies seemed to have understood this well.

Parenting in Agricultural Societies

Over time, as societies grew more complex and also more settled in agricultural practices, child-rearing habits changed and so did parenting. Agricultural societies saw the rise of patriarchy. It led to increasingly punitive and harsh methods of child-rearing with an emphasis on obedience. Corporal punishment was regularly the means through which obedience was enforced and also led to a devaluation of self. One of the classic anthropological studies (Barry, Child, & Bacon, 1959) carried an interesting hypothesis regarding the state of the economy and its relation to parenting practices. According to the researchers, agricultural societies were largely dependent on following the rules, sticking to a routine and maintaining the practices set forth by the elders. Any amount of creativity or slack in the following of a routine would mean poor crops and hunger for the group for many months to come. In contrast, hunter-gatherer societies relied on the initiative and individualism of the group members to ensure that the group was well-fed for months to come. Agricultural societies and those involved in any form of cattle rearing or routine methods of attempting to control nature have given rise to an interesting possibility. Peter Gray, in his book *Free to Learn: Why Unleashing the Instinct to Play will make our Children Happier* (Gray, 2013) put forth the idea that agriculture brought to our ancestors not just a new way of procuring food but also reintroduced them to nature. Earlier nature was something you worked with and revered so that it would sustain you. Agriculture gave you the feeling that you could make nature work for you if you followed certain rules and you could manipulate it to fulfill your requirements. This put man in a more powerful position. He points out the metaphors common to both raising children and livestock or training them. It also changed the equation in society and made people equate land ownership with power and lack of it with weakness. The relation between the King and his subjects was often equated with that of a father and his children. It was thought that a father can discipline his child to bring him on the right path and that this was a divine right because God also corrected his children when they went astray. The rise of different religions corresponds with the evolution of society. The change from nature worshippers to monotheism was almost a reflection of the increasing need for punitive measures to control the masses.

This societal change affected the way children were treated. The system of educating and training children followed the same process of subjugation and discipline that religions recommended in the following of the divine will. As society found itself increasingly fragmented and differentiated, rules of parenting continued to get harsher. The average human being was taught that he has no power over his destiny and he has to conform and submit to those more powerful than him. At the same time, he was expected to train his next generation to submit in the same manner to his masters. This made harsh parenting common practice and children started losing their voice and their identity in this increasingly adult world ruled by a few powerful people and suffered by the vast majority which often included their parents. It can be said that the snuffing out of the childhood spirit began during this era.

Parenting in Industrial Societies

As parenting grew harsher, societies got more exacting. If you had no wealth, you had no power. Industrialization increased the desire for material goods and the availability of large workforces made it possible to mass-produce goods for consumption. Parents and children worked from dawn to dusk in a feudal system that promoted subservience to authority. Industrialization also brought major reforms in the schooling system more as a means to fulfill the increasing need for skilled workers with technical knowledge. This was the beginning of schooling for jobs. Schools became a means of mass-producing trained workforce that would slog to keep the chimneys of industry smoking and the coffers of industrialists overflowing. This changed parenting goals. Earlier the aim was to produce healthy happy individuals who could work for the well-being of the group. From this point on the aim was to mould children into the best possible version of the required employee. Industrialization gave way to specialization and schools again deferred to industry needs. Parents and children alike started chasing dreams that became more and more individualistic as it became clearer that only a select few would reach the summit of subservient glory. With the understanding of the power of parenting and frequently being given religious sanction, parenting became less about nurturance and more about need fulfillment. Religious and cultural requirements structured the adult life in such a way that every child aimed to grow up, get married, have kids, provide for them till they could grow up and provide for their kids. The method of being the provider was to work in industries and corporations that would periodically reward them. The rat race was nothing but the ploy of clever capitalists to get a workforce that could easily be replaced and hence had everyone clamoring for the few available opportunities. It was the law of demand and supply. Far too many workers and very limited jobs. In this crazy race for economic freedom that was painted by the political and industrial forces, parenting fell to the wayside. The child who was once the central focus of the group, whose well-being was the primary aim of the group now became just another statistic in the population.

Parenting in Post Industrial and Technological Societies

One of the master strokes of industrialization, which also struck the death knell for a healthy child was the introduction of women into the workforce. For centuries women were kept at home to play the role of nurturer for everyone. In the earlier eras, gender equality was better maintained. The role of the woman was as important as the role of the man and there was no need for comparison. Somewhere along the way, women got classified as the weaker sex and the patriarchal system that emerged during the agricultural era slowly washed away the relevance of the woman. She became just another tool that would accomplish certain goals. As the change in technology overlapped with the change in the status of women, more and more women felt the need to prove their worth. This led them to take on the role of a provider along with the role of a nurturer. Somehow, it never occurred to anyone to reverse the roles. Since the woman was considered weaker and since she had to prove herself, it was up to her to take on a new role without giving up the old one.

Women today are quite dominant in the workforce. They head large corporations and they command value that is their due. But this is still a small section of the female population. The large majority are laboring on with their men, trying to fulfill dreams sold by the media, falling prey to the hopes given by ruthless industries and assuming that by doing what the men did for the past few centuries, life will be better. The collateral damage is the child. Raising a child is a time task, with the social, biological, emotional stressors that the child faces, life has become more challenging and complex for the child. Industry continues to question academia on the quality of students turning out and academia continues to rush to pacify industry and fulfill its demands. The problem is that the current education system in India is still producing the students to fulfill the needs of the industrial era while industry has moved on to the next level. It won't be long before the education system catches up and then starts churning out adults that will fit the required industry standards. Parenting has been hijacked. Industry demands a certain type of person with a certain temperament. The various specializations are all about dividing the existing population into various personality types and it is only a certain type that can be considered successful. Parents dutifully rush to fulfill this need.

There are of course challengers to this system. Some refuse to follow the rat race and march out on their own. Surprisingly, the greatest resistance is offered by parents. These individuals who are charting new territory seem to possess the same mindset that children possessed during the hunting-gathering times. They seem to have answered the diktats of their hearts and aligned it with the processing capacity of their brains. Sadly most times, the parents don't seem to follow suit.

CONCLUSION

There is hope. Although parenting has become increasingly challenging and there are an increasing number of adults who refuse to become parents, it has become clear to all that something is not quite right in the system. Parents have started questioning the education and the corporate systems in place. More and more parents are turning to homeschool and experimental schools. Many more are supporting their children's dreams and some even join them as they make personal growth their primary motivation. But we have still a long way to go. Parents may well make it worth their while to look up child-rearing practices in hunter-gatherer societies and see what they can learn from there. There is plenty of technology to assist them in their search.

BIBLIOGRAPHY

1. Albert, I., Trommsdorff, G., & Mishra, R. (2007). Parenting & Adolescent Attachment. (G. Zheng, Ed.) Perspectives and Progress in contemporary cross-cultural psychology, 97-108. Retrieved May 2017, from https://kops.uni-konstanz.de/bitstream/handle/123456789/11271/Parenting_and_adolescent_attachment_in_India_and_Germany_2007_KOPS8373.pdf; sequence=1
2. Barry, H., Child, B., & Bacon, M. (1959). Relation of Child Training to Subsistence Economy. American Anthropology, 51-63. doi:doi/10.1525/aa.1959.61.1.02a00080
3. Baumrind, D. (1966). Effects of Authoritative Parental Control on Child Behavior. Child Development, 37(4), 887-907.
4. Baumrind, D. (1967). Child care practices anteceding three patterns of preschool behavior. Genetic Psychology Monographs, 75(1), 43-88.
5. Coleman, P. K., & Karraker, K. K. (1997). Self-Efficacy and Parenting Quality: Findings and Future Applications. Developmental Review, 18, 47-85. Retrieved May 2017
6. Darling, N., & Steinberg, L. (1993). Parenting Style as Context: An Integratief Model. Psychological Bulletin, 113(3), 487-496.
7. Ember, C. R., & Ember, M. (2005). Explaining Corporal Punishment of Children: A Cross-Cultural Study. American Anthropologist, 107(4), 609–619. https://doi.org/10.1525/aa.2005.107.4.609
8. Espino, J. M. (2012). Two sides of intensive parenting: Present and future dimensions in contemporary relations between parents and children in Spain. Childhood, 22-36. doi:10.1177/0907568212445225
9. Gentina, E., & Singh, P. (2015). How National Culture and Parental Style Affect the Process of Adolescents' Ecological Resocialization. Sustainability, 7, 7581-7603. doi:10.3390/su7067581
10. Givertz, M. (2016). Parenting Styles/Discipline. In C. R. Berger, & M. E. Roloff (Eds.), The International Encyclopedia of Interpersonal Communication. John Wiley & Sons, Inc. doi:10.1002/9781118540190.wbeic0037
11. Gray, P. (2013). Free to Learn: Why Unleashing the Instinct to Play Will Make Our Children Happier More Self-Reliant, and Better Students for Life. New York: Basic Books.
12. Hewlett, B. S., & Lamb, M. E. (2005). Hunter-gatherer Childhoods: Evolutionary, Developmental, and Cultural Perspectives. New Brunswick, New Jersey: Aldine.
13. Hofstede, G. (2011). Dimensionalizing Cultures: The Hofstede Model in Context. International Association of Cross-Cultural Psychology.
14. Hoskins, D. H. (2014). Consequences of Parenting on Adolescent Outcomes. Societies, 4, 506-531. doi:10.3390/soc4030506
15. Kopko, K. (2007). Parenting Styles and Adolescents. Retrieved May 2017, from http://www.human.cornell.edu/pam/outreach/parenting/parents/upload/Parenting-20Styles-20and-20Adolescents.pdf
16. Maccobby, & Martin. (1983). Handbook of Child Psychology.
17. MacIver, R. M., & Page, C. h. (1964). Society: An Introductory Analysis. MacMillan.
18. Mahapatra, S., & Batul, R. (2016, Feb). Psychosocial Consequences of Parenting. IOSR Journal Of Humanities And Social Science, 21(2), 10-17. doi:10.9790/0837-21251017
19. Nixon, E., & Halpenny, A. M. (2010). Children's Perspectives on Parenting Styles and Discipline: A Developmental approach. Dublin: The Stationery Office. Retrieved May 2017
20. Power, T. (2013, August). Parenting Dimensions and Styles: A Brief History and Recommendations for Future Research. Childhood Obesity, 9 (suppl 1), S14-S21. doi: 10.1089/chi.2013.0034
21. Shaffer, A., Kotchick, B. A., Dorsey, S., & Forehand, R. (2001). The Past, Present, And Future Of Behavioral Parent Training:

Interventions For Child And Adolescent Problem Behavior. The Behavior Analyst To day, 91-105. Retrieved May 2017

22. UNICEF (2007). Child poverty in perspective: An overview of child well-being in rich countries, a comprehensive assessment of the lives and well-being of children and adolescents in the economically advanced nations. Report Card 7. Florence, Italy: United Nations Children's Fund Innocenti Research Centre.
23. Van Campen, K. S. (2010). Cultural Differences in Parenting Practices: What Asian American Families Can Teach Us. Frances McClelland Institute for Children. Tucson: Frances McClelland Institute for Children. Retrieved may 2017, from http://McClellandInstitute.arizona.edu
24. https://www.psychologytoday.com/blog/moral-landscapes/201008/the-decline-children-and-the-moral-sense.

Enuresis 78

Sagar Karia • Avinash De Sousa

INTRODUCTION

The term itself is derived from the Greek *enourein*, "to void urine" and has come to imply nocturnal events. Enuresis or Bed Wetting is usually defined as the involuntary passage of urine after the age of three years, and failure to control the urinary bladder during sleep, in the absence of any identifiable physical abnormality. The normal sequence of developing control over bowel and bladder functions is the development of nocturnal fecal continence, diurnal fecal continence, diurnal bladder control, and nocturnal bladder control. A child, generally learns to control his urinary bladder by the age of three years, but in children this inability persists, or gets re-created for certain reasons. The disorder has rightly been considered a psychological one, for the very fact that enuretic children have more psychological problems than non-enuretic ones. The psychological problems generally settle down when psychiatric treatment is instituted, and so does Enuresis. Further, the contributing psychological factors are always multiple that rightly gives this problem the psychological status. Urinary continence is a function of storing urine in the bladder until it is socially appropriate to void. The bladder has thus two main functions i.e. storage and evacuation. Children in the course of their development learn to use the voluntary pelvic musculature to raise the neck of the bladder and thus defer voiding till the time and place are appropriate and at the same time also learn to initiate the process of micturition. The brain structures involved are the cortical centers in the frontal lobe called the paracentral lobule, the pons and the sacral plexus via the cauda equina, pudendal nerves (S2-4) and the hypogastric plexus (T11-L2). It is important to note two facets i.e. an intact neural organization is a must for normal micturition and that normal bladder voiding always occurs more frequently in a day than defecation.

CLASSIFICATION

Enuresis has been divided into -

a) Nocturnal – when it occurs only at night, and this is the common variety of enuresis.

b) Diurnal – when it occurs, while the patient sleeps during the day.

Hallgren (1956) classified Enuresis into –

a) Primary – when the child has never achieved control of the urinary bladder.

b) Secondary or Acquired - when the child after having once obtained control of the urinary bladder, has again lost it.

Martin (1966) also classified enuretics in two groups –

a) Primary- when there was no other problem.

b) Secondary – when there were other causative problems.

Silberstein and Blackman (1956) have described four categories of enuretics –

a) Persistent – when the patient continued to be enuretic into puberty, or even adulthood, with other manifestations of psychopathology.

b) Regressed – when the patient, having acquired control of the urinary bladder, regressed due to emotional conflicts. These patients recovered and repeatedly relapsed using enuresis as primitive resolution of internal conflicts.

c) Ego disturbed – when the patient suffered from serious breaches of ego functioning and psychiatric illness.

d) Organic – when organic disease was the basis for enuresis.

DSM- 5 criteria

A. Repeated voiding of urine into bed or clothes, whether involuntary or intentional.

B. The behavior is clinically significant as manifested by either a frequency of at least twice a week for at least 3 consecutive months or the presence of clinically significant distress or impairment in social, academic (occupational), or other important areas of functioning.

C. Chronological age is at least 5 years (or equivalent developmental level).

D. The behavior is not attributable to the physiological effects of a substance

(e.g., a diuretic, an antipsychotic medication) or another medical condition (e.g., diabetes, spina bifida, a seizure disorder).

Specify whether:

Nocturnal Only: Passage of urine only during night time sleep.

Diurnal Only: Passage of urine only during waking hours.

Nocturnal and Diurnal: A combination of the two subtypes above.

PREVALENCE

Enuresis has been noted in all populations and in all cultures, and in every community, but differences vary from study to study as well as depend on the method of sampling. Studies have reported lower incidence of enuresis among those of Jewish origin and higher incidence among the institutionalized and handicapped children by about 30%. A study conducted at a Child Guidance Clinic in Mumbai, found that out of a total load of 670 children with behavior problems, referred to the clinic over a period of 10 years, 90 of these cases had history of enuresis. Further, enuresis never existed alone, and in 57 of the 63 cases studied in detail, there was evidence of many associated behavior problems.

With increasing age, the likelihood of spontaneous recovery from enuresis decreases like 40% of 2-year-olds with enuresis become dry in the next year and 20% of 3-year-olds become dry before 4 years and only 6% of enuretic 4-year-olds become dry in next year. The chronic nature of the condition is further shown in the study by Rutter and colleagues (1973), in which only 1.5% of 5-year-old bed-wetters became dry during the next 2 years.

ETIOLOGY

The etiology of enuresis is indeed varied as multiple causes contributing to the problem, and enuresis is not the result of a single cause, but the end result of multiple determinant causes.

AGE

The factor of age in the etiology of enuresis can only be considered in certain relative terms for enuresis is known to occur at all ages ranging from 3 - 15 years. The commonest age at the time of referral to a Child Guidance Clinic for treatment of enuresis is between 6 years and puberty, and the age of referral can be considered one of the relative factors referred to above. The frequency of enuresis has also been bracketed with the factor of age. Thus Rutter, Yule and Graham (1973) found that 15% of 7 year old boys wetted less often than once a week, while only 7% wetted more frequently than that.

SEX

Nocturnal enuresis prevalence is equal in boys and girls until the age of 5 years, but by age 11 years, boys outnumber girls (2: 1). Not until the age of 8 years do boys achieve the same levels of night-time continence that are seen in girls by the age of 5 years, probably due to slower physiological maturation in boys. Also the increased incidence of secondary enuresis in boys further affects the sex ratio seen in later childhood. Daytime enuresis occurs more commonly in girls and is associated with higher rates of psychiatric disturbance. Though there is a general impression that enuresis is more common in boys than in girls, it is indeed not true. Perhaps secretiveness and seclusiveness about this complaint in girls, especially in certain communities and in cultures, contributes to the evidence that should be taken with reticence.

GENETIC FACTORS

Hallgren (1956) stressed the role of genetic factors in the causation of enuresis, and found an incidence of 70% in the families of 203 sufferers. The incidence was significantly higher in both siblings of a pair of identical twins, than in both siblings of unidentical twins. The chromosomes that have been identified to date include 13q, 12q, 8, and 22. In some families, an autosomal dominant mode of transmission with penetrance above 90% has been identified. Loeys et al. studied 32 families with extensive histories of nocturnal enuresis, which ranged from two to four generations. Linkage to an area on chromosome 22q11 was noted in nine families, to 13q13-14 in six, and to 12q in four. Evidence of linkage to chromosome 8q could not be established. Deen et al. specifically investigated the aquaporin-2 water channel locus (AQP-2) in six families with a dominant pattern of transmission, as AQP-2 is necessary for concentrating urine and DDAVP enhances AQP2 expression but could not locate mutation in coding sequence.

INTELLIGENCE

High incidences of enuresis were found in children with low I.Q. The question of lower intelligence contributing to the problem is beyond doubt, for with general retardation of milestones seen in the mentally subnormal, chance of urinary bladder control being delayed could be considered the rule. In fact, some authorities would prefer to exclude the mentally subnormal from the realm of enuresis and leave the label only to those who have normal intelligence, considering bed-wetting among the mentally subnormal to be one of 'urinary incontinence'.

IMMATURITY AND DEVELOPMENTAL DYSFUNCTION

General immaturity in various spheres of development, such as speech, behavior etc. and timid and dependent behavior along with emotional immaturity can contribute to enuresis. Studies have shown that primary enuresis was due to improper development of urinary bladder capacity or an infantile urinary bladder. Crosby (1950) was of the opinion that enuresis was due to a specific psychological dysfunction in the act of micturition. He used the term, 'essential' and believed that most enuretics fell into this category.

URINARY TRACT INFECTIONS

The prevalence of enuresis occurred five times more frequently in girls with urinary infections. Therefore before diagnosing enuresis one must always rule out infections of the urogenital tract. There have been recent reports of enterobiasis infection in children with enuresis as the sole presentation.

PHYSICAL DEFECTS, INFECTIONS & INFESTATIONS

Physical defects like spina bifida, meningocele, disorders of the central nervous system, or local defects, like phimosis, hypospadias or epispadias, had been found to be commonly associated with enuresis. Enuresis was also common during severe physical illness, like high fever, and systemic infection. Infestations like thread worms irritating the peri-urethral meatal area, likewise contributed to enuresis. Local growth, in the form of furuncles or small tumors in or around the urinary passages, could contribute to enuresis. Allergy could also be the cause of enuresis according to few.

TOILET TRAINING, FAULTY HABITS & DEPTH OF SLEEP

A child, who was subjected to stringent toilet training, might respond with enuresis during sleep. Faulty toilet training and faulty habits of urination leading to frequency of micturition likewise might contribute to enuresis. An increased fluid intake, and changes in the specific gravity and acidity of urine, often leads to an increased frequency of micturition during the day and enuresis during the night. Chronic tension of the detrusor muscle of the urinary bladder, associated with deep sleep, was the fundamental cause of enuresis. The failure of the parents to enforce toilet training, with emptying of the bladder before going to sleep, contributed in no small manner to enuresis. It has been found that enuresis occurred most often during stage III and IV sleep, and rarely during R.E.M Sleep. However, enuretics were found to wet during all stages of sleep.

E.E.G. ABNORMALITIES

EEG abnormalities have been found in enuretic children. Paroxysmal activity were found at rest in 2.7% of enuretics which increased to 9.1% on photic stimulation, and in 8.7% when drowsy.

CIRCADIAN RHYTHMS IN URINARY OUTPUT

The normal nocturnal fall of urine output to one-third of that during the day, was absent in infants who were enuretic, and excreted urine at a constant rate. Thus immature circadian rhythms and nocturnal polyuria might be the causal factors in enuresis.

STRESS

The stressful life events that received special attention were family break-ups through death or divorce, separation from the mother, birth of a younger sibling, moving home, admission to hospitals, accidents and surgical operations. Enuresis has often been associated with fears of darkness, and accordingly, during the night children are frightened to make the trip to the lavatory as it caused stress, and accordingly tended to be enuretic.

PSYCHIATRIC DISORDERS AND BEHAVIOR PROBLEMS

A frequent combination is that of delinquency, temper tantrums, stubbornness and enuresis. Delinquency and temper tantrums are definite forms of active aggression, while stubbornness and enuresis can be considered forms of passive aggression. Gerrard (1939) found that enuretic children were often distractible at school and sometimes had difficulty in achieving success and showed a tendency for clowning behavior. Stein and Susser (1965) found that enuretic delinquents were more submissive and lacking in dominance and leadership. They had lesser interest in sex and belonged to families who had a larger number of siblings than non-enuretic delinquents.

PARENTS AND GRAND PARENTS

Miller, Walton and Knox (1960) found that insecurity related to parental deprivation and marital instability led to enuresis. Thus, enuresis was found to be associated with nail biting and thumb–sucking that was explained as due to insecurity. Faulty parental attitudes, like rejection, preferential treatment or favoritism often caused hostility and jealousy as a result of sibling rivalry and led to enuresis. Interference by the grandparents (in a joint family more so in India) with the toilet training of their grandchild, with opposition to attitudes and restrictions set by the parents, often contributed to enuresis. Faulty toilet training by the parents themselves was indeed an important causative factor in enuresis. Peculiar notions and false beliefs, like 'weak kidney', held by the parents and grandparents, could lead to perpetuation of problems with no effort to correct it, because of ignorance, indifference or carelessness. These faulty notions and beliefs might also lead to the feeling that enuresis runs in certain families.

SOCIETY AND THE ENVIRONMENT

Enuresis was commoner in the lower socio-economic group, which was associated with adverse environmental conditions. Thus, enuresis occurs more commonly in families, where there are extremes of poverty, repeated disruptions of maternal care, inadequate nutrition and clothing, parental delinquency, large crowded families, alcoholism and drug–taking by the parents and lack of attention to the upbringing of the children.

MULTIFACTORIAL CAUSATION

Though enuresis is a single symptom, the causation is generally multifactorial, and at times, a complex interplay of physical and psychological factors is evident. Psychological factors, nevertheless, hold sway and at times, a number of psychological factors contribute to this single symptom of enuresis. Thus the treatment needs to be multi-pronged, if a cure has to be achieved.

TREATMENT

The treatment of enuresis has not only been multi-pronged, but many non-specific treatments have found application in enuresis from time to time.

These methods consisted of -

1. Mechanical and surgical - It consisted of tying up the prepuce at night or filling the prepuce with collodium during the night, use of a penis clamp, elevation of the foot-end of the bed, catheterization, urinary bladder irrigation, injection of paraffin in to the urinary bladder, distension of the urinary bladder by hydrostatic pressure, lumbar puncture, intra-muscular and epidural injections of large amounts of

physiological saline, urethral dilatation, electrocogaulation of the neck of urinary bladder, pre-sacral neurectomy in persistent cases, tonsillectomy, adenoidectomy, circumcision, electric currents locally, roentgen radiation, ultra-violet radiation, endovesical diathermy, cold baths, hot baths, massage, and a host of other similar therapies, either locally in the surrounding areas, or systemically, depending on the fads and beliefs of the therapist.

2. Drugs - Urotropin, calcium salts, calcium plus iodine, rhus aromatica, bromides, phenobarbital, phenacetin, anti-pyrin, amidopyrin, quinine, camphor, atropine, strychnine, scopolamine; papaverine, transentine, ergotine, ephedrine sulphate, benzedrine sulphate, protein preparations, thyroid, testosterone and pituitary extracts have all been tried from time to time.

DIET THERAPY

A concentrated diet with restriction of fluid, a bland diet with avoidance of seasoned foods, a high water content early in the day and low water content with ample salt late in the day, restriction of fluids in the evening, and so on and so forth, have all been advocated as adjuncts in the therapy of enuresis.

All these methods have put an emphasis on the wetting rather than the wetter, and there has been a total failure to realize the contribution of the wetter to the problem until very recently.

DRUG THERAPY

Drug therapy holds the pride of place. Any patient approaching the medical man for relief and treatment expects a drug to be prescribed and accordingly drug therapy is the most acceptable and suitable to the patients. A number of drugs have been used, as referred to, above, but the degree of success with most drugs was negligible till amphetamines (dexamphetamine and methamphetamine) have been used in doses of 5-10 mgs at bed time or in two or three doses spread over the afternoon and evening hours. It is usual to start with a dose of 2.5 mg and build up the dosage till some degree of control is achieved keeping in mind the requirement of sleep needed by the patient. **Amphetamines** have been used as a remedy for hypersomnia under the belief that keeping the patient in a light state of sleep at night will prevent enuresis. The side- effects of insomnia, loss of weight and appetite, and at times restlessness, have caused Amphetamines to have had their day as the therapeutic agent in enuresis.

With the advent of the **tricyclic antidepressants** and their particular efficacy in enuresis, the final nail in the coffin of amphetamines has been hammered. Among the tricyclic antidepressants, **Imipramine** has been in common use with fair degree of success in a dosage varying from 10-50 mg, at bedtime or spread over the evening hours. The dosage should preferably be tailored to the child's weight or surface area to avoid toxicity. The toxic dose lies between 10-20 mg/kg body weight. Amitriptyline has also been used with similar success. The mode of action of tricyclic antidepressants is far from settled and certain speculations suggest that they possess an antispasmodic action which relaxes and prevents the irritability of the detrusor muscle of the urinary bladder, whose contraction is responsible for enuresis in sleep. Another theory holds that tricyclic antidepressants reduce the depth of sleep. Pharmacological studies have indicated that treatment with imipramine can result in three subtypes of response. There are true responders who have a sustained response, and there are also true nonresponders. There also is a surprisingly large group of transient responders. These children have an initial response to imipramine and then lose it over 2 to 3 weeks.

When the dosage is increased by another 25 mg, they again respond for another 2 to 3 weeks. Eventually, the dosage required to maintain a response becomes prohibitive.

The cure rate with tricyclic antidepressants has been quoted as about 35%–50%. The reason for this low cure rate may lie in the fact that enuresis is a multi-sided problem, as discussed in the etiology, and drug therapy may remedy the local condition like depth of sleep or irritability of urinary bladder, but does not remedy the underlying dynamics. Thus, a relapse often occurs after drug therapy is discontinued, and those cases that remain cured that remain cured perhaps remedy themselves due to coincidental changes of the causative factors.

Desmospressin is an analogue of the naturally occurring anti-diuretic hormone with a longer duration of action and no tendency to produce vasoconstriction. Its dosage is 20-40 ug when given as a nasal spray and 200-400 ug at bedtime as tablets. It is generally safe but needs to be avoided in cardiac patients. Though the side effects are very rare, hyponatremia and hyponatremic seizures have been reported.

Oxybutynin is an anticholinergic drug that increases bladder capacity by an action on the detrusors. Anticholinergic side effects may be troublesome. The advantage lies in the fact that apart from being of value in nocturnal enuresis it has also been used in subjects where there is decreased functional bladder volume secondary to detrusor instability that causes daytime wetting. The dosage is 2.5-5 mg three times a day with the last dose at bedtime.

PSYCHOTHERAPY

Psychotherapy is a must for the patient, his parents and relatives in the management of enuresis. The child is taught through psychotherapy how to accept reality and how to deal with certain situations that cause tension. Both individual and group psychotherapy can be utilized and the psychotherapeutic approach can also be carried out through play therapy, art therapy, group discussion etc. Parents and relatives also need individual and group psychotherapy to get them to understand how their behavior contributes to enuresis, and how exactly they can remedy such behavior. An efficient social worker is indeed a worthy asset in obtaining useful information through interviews at the clinic, home and school visits, which can be used in psychotherapy to bring about a lasting change.

REWARD AND PUNISHMENT

An enuretic child is often helped to remedy his problem through rewards for dry nights. A special chart with day of the week written on one side, and then a gold colored paper star pasted in for each dry night urges the child into a spirit of competition and causes him to sleep lighter and awake and go to lavatory to void his urinary bladder in time, if the need arises during the night. The child tries best, week after week to obtain more and more stars till he has a real 'starry week'. Other forms of rewards consist of extra pocket-money, eatables, toys, clothes, or anything that appeals to the child. Punishment is really of no avail, though at times it is known to work in certain children, but a number of children fail to respond even inspite of the most severe forms of punishment. On the other hand, punishment at times causes the child to be determined to resist all efforts at cure.

DAY TIME TRAINING

Enuresis has been explained as being the result of faulty toilet-training. Over indulgence at this stage of development between 1-3 years of age has the same effect as negligence. Smith (1948) suggested that enuretic children could be treated by training them to postpone going to the toilet during the day, and teaching them to hold the urine, and defer the act of micturition for longer and longer periods. As a result of such forms of therapy, the urinary bladder gets used to the distension and can hold urine easily at night.

SPECIFIC CONDITIONING

Davidson and Douglas (1950) devised a bell and pad apparatus to serve the purpose of conditioning and help the child to wake up whenever his urinary bladder is distended at night. This forms of conditioning works on the principle that the child is first taught to wake up after the active micturition by means of a bell or buzzer. Slowly the child gets conditioned and learns to correlate mounting tension in his urinary bladder with the ringing of the bell. He soon learns to wake up when his bladder is full. The origin of this alarm system is usually credited to Pfaundler (1904). Various theories have been put forward to explain the efficacy of this alarm system which ranged from classical conditioning, avoidance conditioning, punishment training, social training, etc., but the fact that a cure is obtained is indeed important. Sometimes due to the child sleeping in urine and not getting up even with the alarm, this causes stagnation of urine and there have been reports of buzzer ulcers. There are limits to the value of the alarm system that can be removed by a good technic –

1. The treatment is troublesome for both the child and the caretaker. Failure of the treatment is more likely in the course of a disturbed family. The alarm has to be demonstrated before hand and all doubts explained and clarified sensitively.
2. Premature termination of the therapy is quite common. It can be reduced by careful instruction about what to do and arrange regular follow ups. The family must be cautioned that the treatment that they are taking up is a three month commitment and that the treatment may only be gradually successful.
3. The child may fail to wake with the alarm and this can be solved by arrangement of a louder buzzer by the parents.
4. There is a significant relapse rate. 35% children start to wet again. This can be tackled by a repeated course along with overlearning.
5. Butler (1994) cautioned against the use of such alarms when parents are likely to use coercive or punitive responses to them.

REGULATION OF FLUID INTAKE

Restriction of fluid intake especially during the evening hours has often been presented as the means of controlling enuresis. It is not usually appreciated that restriction of fluid intake leads to formation of highly concentrated urine that acts as a stimulus to the urinary bladder receptors and leads to enuresis. On the other hand, intake of plenty of fluids leads to formation of less concentrated urine and helps the urinary bladder to get used to holding more urine.

AWAKENING OF THE CHILD DURING THE NIGHT

Repeated awakening of the child during the night and making him void his urinary bladder in the night to prevent accumulation of urine in the urinary bladder and accordingly to avoid enuresis often has the opposite effect in that the child continues to be enuretic. The reason for this state of affairs is the fact that the urinary bladder does not get a chance to distend, and thus micturition and enuresis occurs even at low thresholds.

HYPNOSIS AND HYPNOTHERAPY

Suggestion and hypnosis have often been advocated as a form of therapy or an adjunct to therapy. This method is indeed only useful in older children with a good attention span.

MANAGEMENT OF DAY TIME WETTING

The management of diurnal enuresis is much the same as nocturnal enuresis. It is important to realize what factors cause it and habit training requires the child to go frequently and regularly

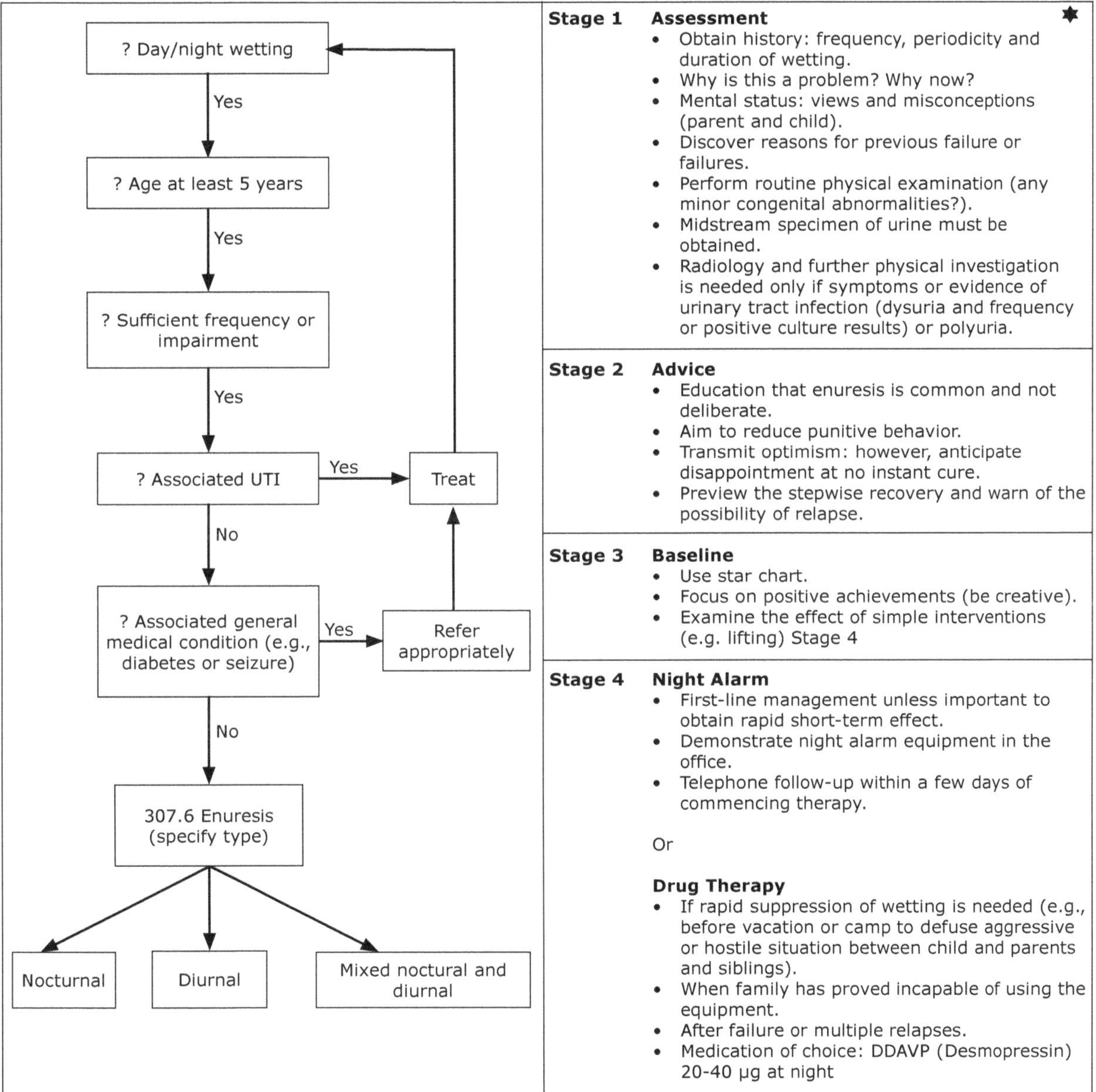

Fig. 78.1

✱Essentials of Psychiatry Jerald Kay and Allan Tasman © 2006 John Wiley & Sons, Ltd. ISBN: 0-470-01854-2

to the toilet at a predetermined time. The use of simple wrist watch alarm for the child to visit the toilet at regular intervals. Bladder training is a method used where there is a regular toileting programe say hourly intervals and gradually increasing the time interval between voiding and subsequent visits. McKenna (1999) has found retention control, sphincter control and biofeedback of little use in enuresis.

Throughout the literature there also are reports of novel treatment approaches such as acupuncture, a prostaglandin synthesis inhibitor, an anticholinergic calcium antagonist and the oral synthetic androgen mesterolone. Although many of these studies are controlled, the use of these approaches in enuresis should still be considered experimental.

CONCLUSION

As mentioned earlier, in a disorder like enuresis, no single treatment module is enough and often a combination of methods may have to be used. It is indeed very important that the therapist must have faith in the method he is using and persist with a method for a sufficient period of time to allow the causative factors to be remedied and the child to appreciate and respond to the changed situation. Perseverance is the watchword without which no cure can be brought and success only comes to those who persevere while treating enuresis.

WEBSITES OF INTEREST

1. The National Enuresis Society Homepage – www.peds.umn.edu
2. Enuresis Resource and Information Centre - www.enuresis.org.uk
3. A public awareness site – www.drynights.com
4. www.stopbedwettingfree.com
5. The Journal of Urology website - www.jurology.com

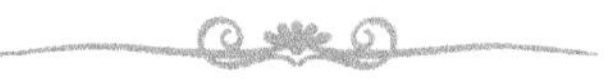

Gaming Disorder 79

Parmod Kumar • Shubham Kamal

WHAT IS GAMING DISORDER? (ICD 11)

Gaming disorder is defined in the 11th Revision of the International Classification of Diseases (ICD-11) as a pattern of gaming behavior ("digital-gaming" or "video-gaming") characterized by impaired control over gaming, increasing priority given to gaming over other activities to the extent that gaming takes precedence over other interests and daily activities, and continuation or escalation of gaming despite the occurrence of negative consequences.

For gaming disorder to be diagnosed, the behavior pattern must be of sufficient severity to result in significant impairment in personal, family, social, educational, occupational or other important areas of functioning and would normally have been evident for at least 12 months.

The proposed symptoms of internet gaming disorder include: **(APA DSM 5)**

- Preoccupation with gaming
- Withdrawal symptoms when gaming is taken away or not possible (sadness, anxiety, irritability)
- Tolerance, the need to spend more time gaming to satisfy the urge
- Inability to reduce playing, unsuccessful attempts to quit gaming
- Giving up other activities, loss of interest in previously enjoyed activities due to gaming
- Continuing to game despite problems
- Deceiving family members or others about the amount of time spent on gaming
- The use of gaming to relieve negative moods, such as guilt or hopelessness
- Risk, having jeopardized or lost a job or relationship due to gaming

Under the proposed criteria, a diagnosis of internet gaming disorder would require experiencing five or more of these symptoms within a year. The condition can include gaming on the internet, or on any electronic device, although most people who develop clinically significant gaming problems play primarily on the internet.

The **IGDS9-SF** was the first brief standardized psychometric tool to assess Internet Gaming Disorder (IGD) according to the nine Internet Gaming Disorder (IGD) criteria as suggested by the American Psychiatric Association in the latest edition of the *Diagnostic and Statistical Manual of Mental Disorders* (DSM-5).

PREVALENCE

'The statistical report on the development of the internet in China' pointed out that China had 486 million people playing internet games by June 2018, accounting for 60.6% of all internet users.[1] A recent systematic review of epidemiological studies on gaming disorder found that the prevalence of gaming disorder was 0.7%–27.5%, and it was mainly among young men.[2] Another group conducted a meta-analysis of 36 studies in China, covering 362 328 internet gamers.[3] The prevalence of online gaming disorder in China was 3.5%–17%. The prevalences of gaming disorder in Europe and the USA were relatively low, for example, the USA was about 0.3%–1.0%,[4] and Germany was 1.16%.[5]

RISK FACTORS

Firstly, the psychological factors associated with IGD need to be understood. IGD can be considered a behavioral addiction[6,7,8,9,10] and has been found to be related to a number of psychological and health problems, including depression, social anxiety, fatigue, loneliness, negative self-esteem, and impulsivity.[11–14] IGD co-occurs with various psychiatric conditions and can lead to a range of negative outcomes. For example, IGD can cause social problems such as lower academic achievement.[15–19] In addition, IGD shares many similarities with other addictions, such as substance use disorder.[20]

Secondly, the Internet gaming characteristics associated with IGD need to be better understood. Research in this area has increased in both quantity and quality. In order to predict, diagnose, and manage IGD, researchers have attempted to identify the causes and negative consequences of excessive gaming as well as risk factors of IGD. Some research, however, has only focused on psychological factors[18,21] or Internet gaming characteristics, such as the level of Internet usage, money spent on gaming, and type of game device.[22] A comprehensive approach based on both psychological factors and Internet gaming characteristics is needed to better understand IGD. Accordingly, the purpose of the present study was to identify risk factors that predict IGD, based on psychological factors and Internet gaming characteristics.

MECHANISMS

Video Game Structure

Some theories focus on the presumed built-in reward systems of video games, such as compulsion loops, to explain their potentially addictive nature.[23] The anticipation of such rewards can create a neurological reaction that releases dopamine into the body, so that once the reward is obtained, the person will remember it as a pleasurable feeling.[24] This has been found to be similar to the neurological reaction of other behavioral addictions such as substance abuse and gambling disorder, although not to the same magnitude and with some differences.[24]

Mark Griffiths has proposed another reason online video games are potentially addictive is because they "can be played all day every day." The fact there is no end to the game can feel rewarding for some, and hence players are further engaged in the game.[25]

Addiction Circuits in the Brain

Long-term internet video game playing affects brain regions responsible for reward, impulse control and sensory-motor coordination.[26] Structural analyses shown modifications in the volume of the ventral striatum, possibly as result of changes in rewards, and video game addicts had faulty inhibitory control and reward mechanisms.[26] Video game playing is associated with dopamine release similar in magnitude to that of drug abuse, and the presentation of gaming pictures activates brain regions similarly to drug pictures for drug addicts.[26] Treatment studies which used fMRI to monitor the brain connectivity changes found a decrease in the activity of the regions associated with cravings.[26] Although there are evidences that video game addiction may be supported by similar neural mechanisms underlying drug abuse, as video game and internet addictions reduce the sensitivity of the dopaminergic reward system, it is still premature to conclude that this addiction is equivalent to substance addictions, as the research is in its early stages.[26] There is evidence of a dual processing model of digital technology addictions characterized by an imbalance between the reactive and the reflective reward systems.[24] Other studies shown increased difficulties in decision making in specific contexts, such as risky situations but not in ambiguous situations, and an increased preference for short-term rewards.[27] Although the number of neuroimaging studies on internet gaming disorder is rising, there are several methodological shortcomings, particularly in the inconsistency of psychometric assessments.[28] Furthermore, the conclusions on reduced inhibition should be moderated, as only one study included a functional control, which then showed no difference in inhibition.[27]

A meta-analytic review of the research concluded the evidence suggests video game addiction arises out of other mental health problems, rather than causing them.[29] Thus it is unclear whether video game addiction should be considered a unique diagnosis.[29]

MANAGEMENT

Treatment of Gaming Disorder

Excessive gaming can damage an individual's daily life and social functioning. Therefore, professional treatment for people with gaming disorder is necessary. Unfortunately, there is currently a lack of recognized treatment measures for gaming disorder.[30] Because the pathogenesis of the gaming disorder is not yet clear, the current intervention measures are basically based on the treatment experience of mental disorders such as substance use disorder. Treatment measures generally include psychobehavioral treatment, drug treatment and comprehensive treatment.[31]

Psychological Therapy

Psychological therapy, including individual and group therapy, is currently the most commonly used method for treating gaming disorder.

Individual Treatment

Among individual treatments, cognitive-behavioral therapy (CBT) is the most commonly used.[32] The main form of the treatment is individual consultation. The typical length of the CBT treatment is several months and generally requires 8–28 treatments, ranging from 1 to 2 hours each time. The treatment content includes: (1) identification of cognitive distortions related to gaming behavior; (2) looking for evidence that can confirm this cognitive distortion; (3) evaluating core beliefs and negative schema; (4) replacement with more adaptive thought patterns; (5) establishing relapse prevention and plan treatment steps; (6) dealing with self-control problems, and so forth. The results show that CBT is effective for people with gaming disorder and can change individuals' cognitions surrounding the game.

Group Therapy

Psychological therapy, also known as team therapy or collective therapy, is conducted in groups or teams. The general framework for these kinds of therapy is 6–10 participants, one to two sessions a week (for 1–2 hours) for at least half a year. Treatment methods include lectures, activities and discussions. Treatment objectives are to reduce the patient's game dependence symptoms, promote the recovery of interpersonal relationships, improve the individual's self-confidence and manage the withdrawal from these games.[33] The American Psychological Association believes that[34] group therapy has certain advantages over individual therapy such as all participants have similar problems and face the same difficulties in life. By sharing game experiences with others, group participants can further recognize their own problems. In addition, group therapy can create a relatively closed and safe environment where sensitive topics about gaming disorder can be openly discussed. Because each person has different ways of dealing with their gaming disorder, group therapy can provide opportunities to learn from others who are dealing with gaming disorder, thereby improving their ability to cope.

Family Therapy

Family therapy provides treatment by using psychological interventions in the family unit. It mainly includes traditional family therapy[35] or marriage and family therapy.[36] Often, a multilevel intervention model of drug abuse is applied,[37] including family counseling and peer support groups. In addition to this, multifamily group therapy[38] has been used to treat gaming disorder.

Multimodal School-Based Group Therapy

It is a group psychotherapy method suitable for the school environment. It involves students, parents and teachers. Each group has 6–10 people. The purpose is to strengthen parent–child communication, promote family harmony, let parents recognize the problems of their children and find out their role in children's gaming behavior as early as possible. Through psychological education, teachers also provide help for treatment.[39]

Pharmacological Treatment

Those who advocate for the use of pharmacological treatment for gaming disorder are usually psychiatrists who believe gaming disorder is a mental disorder.[36] The impulse shown by the person with gaming disorder towards the game has a similar neurobiological mechanism as the impulse of those addicted to substances towards their respective drug.[40] Additionally, those with gaming disorder often have other comorbid mental disorders.[41] This provides the foundation for pharmacological treatment.

Based on the points above, Dell'Osso and colleagues[42] used escitalopram for the treatment of 19 adults with gaming disorder. In the first 10 weeks of drug treatment, the symptoms of game dependence improved in all patients. However, in the following 9 weeks of randomized double-blind controlled trials (half receiving drugs and half receiving placebos), there was no difference in the efficacy of the drug group and the control group. Bipeta and colleagues[43] first treated 38 patients with simple obsessive-compulsive disorder who had gaming disorder or did not have gaming disorder with antianxiety therapy for 3 weeks and then treated with regular antidepressants (selective serotonin reuptake inhibitors or clomipramine) for 1 year. The results found that the patient's compulsive symptoms and game dependence were improved. Han and Renshaw[44] used bupropion for the treatment of 50 patients with severe depression accompanied by excessive online gaming. The results showed that the patient's cravings for games were significantly reduced,[45] the time spent on the internet was shortened and the symptoms of depression were improved. After that,

Han and colleagues[46] used a central nervous stimulant, methylphenidate, to treat 62 children with attention deficit hyperactivity disorder (ADHD) who experienced excessive gaming. It was found that the degree of gaming disorder and the amount of time using the internet decreased significantly, and the symptoms of ADHD were also improved. In addition, there are also studies where the opioid receptor antagonist naltrexone was found to be effective against gaming disorder.[47]

The above limited data suggest that drug therapy (mostly antidepressants) can improve patients' game dependence symptoms, and can significantly shorten the time of internet use and reduce the cravings to play games. However, further research is needed to determine the efficacy, appropriate dose and course of treatment of psychotropic substances in gaming disorder. When the clinician uses drug treatment, he must closely observe the patient's condition and adjust the drug dose in time to prevent adverse reactions.

Combined Therapy

Comprehensive treatment is an intervention that combines CBT with other treatment methods. It includes CBT combined with drug therapy, other forms of psychotherapy or physiotherapy.

CBT Combined Drug Treatment

Kim and colleagues[48] attempted to treat 65 adolescents with depressive disorder with amphetamine combined with CBT and found that it was effective for game dependence symptoms and depression. Santos and colleagues[49] combined antidepressants and antianxiety drugs to treat gaming disorder. In this study, they found that patients' anxiety and gaming dependence symptoms were significantly improved.

CBT Combined Motivation Enhancement Therapy

According to motivation enhancement therapy's (MET) treatment experience with alcohol addiction, Poddar and colleagues[50] first tried this method for gaming disorder. This MET-CBT approach consists of a series of stages[1]: (1) a contemplation stage (i.e., initial sessions of rapport building, a detailed interview and case formulation)[2]; (2) a preparation stage (i.e., sessions delivered in an empathetic atmosphere to emphasize psychoeducation, including managing physiological and emotional arousal through relaxation techniques, and a cost-benefit analysis of game addiction); and[3] (3) a contract stage with the patient, the parents and the therapist (i.e., behavior modification of gaming, reducing time spent online and promoting healthy activities).[19] After treatment, the patient's gaming time was significantly reduced and the learning performance was significantly improved.

CBT Combined Electroacupuncture Therapy

There are people in China who tried to use this method and thought that the combined treatment group in improving game dependence symptoms is better than the individual psychotherapy group. However, the effectiveness and safety of the CBT combined electroacupuncture therapy of gaming disorder need to be verified.[51]

PREVENTION OF GAMING DISORDER

The causes of gaming disorder are complex, involving many biopsychosocial factors, and the treatment is relatively difficult. Therefore, prevention is even more important. The current preventive measures against gaming disorder are as follows:

LIMIT THE USE OF GAMES

In view of the potential addictive nature of computer and games, the long gaming time and the problem of overuse of the internet, limiting usage is a solution.[52] Measures are: (1) prohibition of game access: the government requires game providers to prevent players from accessing their games for a specific period of time during the day; and (2) parental controls: parents control their children's computers through various measures, such as limiting game contents and time.

WARNING MESSAGES

Some gaming companies have released in-game warning information related to the risks of excessive game playing. This information could be similar to the health warning information that appears on tobacco and alcohol packages.[53] Based on the efficiency of cigarette warning labels,[54] it can be assumed that such warning information helps to raise awareness of the harmful consequences of excessive gaming. Király and colleagues suggest that customizing the warnings in games depending on the time gamers spend on gaming.[52] This strategy allows targeting problem behaviors specifically without affecting the non-problematic gamers' enjoyment of a largely healthy pastime activity.[55]

POTENTIAL INTERVENTIONS

In order to reduce the negative consequences of games, the government should promulgate relevant policies requiring all departments to provide appropriate help and treatment for people with gaming disorder.[56] In the case of problematic gaming, the clinician is one of the firsts to identify the potential risks of gaming disorder and provide some help to game players.[52] Since most gaming operators can collect players' data regarding the time spent on gaming, they could contact those gamers who play much more time than the average and offer them contact information for possible referral services.[57] Game companies should also participate in actions to prevent and treat gaming disorder, such as reducing rewards and adding warnings in the game.[58] Game providers should raise game prices and limit minors' premature contact with games. Governments should establish adequate prevention and treatment centres for game dependence, providing preventive education, counseling services and treatment interventions.[59]

MOST ADDICTIVE VIDEO GAMES

- Fortnite
- World of Warcraft
- Minecraft
- Tetris
- Candy Crush Saga
- PUBG
- Call of Duty
- Angry Birds
- League of Legends

BIBLIOGRAPHY

1. China Internet Network Information Center (CNNIC). The 42nd statistical report on the development of China's Internet, 2018.
2. Mihara S, Higuchi S. Cross-sectional and longitudinal epidemiological studies of Internet gaming disorder: a systematic review of the literature. *Psychiatry Clin Neurosci.* 2017;71:425–44.
3. Long J, Liu T, Liu Y, *et al.* Prevalence and correlates of problematic online gaming: a systematic review of the evidence published in Chinese. *Curr Addict Rep.* 2018;5:359–71.
4. Przybylski AK, Weinstein N, Murayama K.

Internet gaming disorder: investigating the clinical relevance of a new phenomenon. *AJP.* 2017;174:230–6
5. Rehbein F, Kliem S, Baier D, *et al.* Prevalence of Internet gaming disorder in German adolescents: diagnostic contribution of the nine DSM-5 criteria in a state-wide representative sample. *Addiction.* 2015;110:842–51.
6. Choi, S.-W.; Kim, H.; Kim, G.-Y.; Jeon, Y.; Park, S.; Lee, J.-Y.; Jung, H.; Sohn, B.; Choi, J.-S.; Kim, D.-J. Similarities and differences among internet gaming disorder, gambling disorder and alcohol use disorder: A focus on impulsivity and compulsivity. J. Behav. Addict. 2014, 3, 246–253.
7. Na, E.; Lee, H.; Choi, I.; Kim, D.J. Comorbidity of internet gaming disorder and alcohol use disorder: A focus on clinical characteristics and gaming patterns. Am. J. Addict. 2017, 26, 326–334.
8. Cho, H.; Kwon, M.; Choi, J.-H.; Lee, S.-K.; Choi, J.S.; Choi, S.-W.; Kim, D.-J. Development of the internet addiction scale based on the internet gaming disorder criteria suggested in DSM-5. Addict. Behav. 2014, 39, 1361–1366. [CrossRef] [PubMed] Int. J. Environ. Res. Public Health. 2018, 15, 40 9 of 11
9. Demetrovics, Z.; Urbán, R.; Nagygyörgy, K.; Farkas, J.; Griffiths, M.D.; Pápay, O.; Kökönyei, G.; Felvinczi, K.; Oláh, A. The development of the problematic online gaming questionnaire (POGQ). PLoS ONE 2012, 7, e36417.
10. Petry, N.M.; O'brien, C.P. Internet gaming disorder and the DSM-5. Addiction. 2013, 108, 1186–1187.
11. Männikkö, N.; Billieux, J.; Kääriäinen, M. Problematic digital gaming behavior and its relation to the psychological, social and physical health of finnish adolescents and young adults. J. Behav. Addict. 2015, 4, 281–288.
12. Brunborg, G.S.; Mentzoni, R.A.; Frøyland, L.R. Is video gaming, or video game addiction, associated with depression, academic achievement, heavy episodic drinking, or conduct problems? J. Behav. Addict. 2014, 3, 27–32.
13. Van Rooij, A.J.; Kuss, D.J.; Griffiths, M.D.; Shorter, G.W.; Schoenmakers, T.M.; Van de Mheen, D. The (co-) occurrence of problematic video gaming, substance use, and psychosocial problems in adolescents. J. Behav. Addict. 2014, 3, 157–165.
14. Park, J.H.; Han, D.H.; Kim, B.-N.; Cheong, J.H.; Lee, Y.-S. Correlations among social anxiety, self-esteem, impulsivity, and game genre in patients with problematic online game playing. Psychiatry Investig. 2016, 13, 297–304.
15. Kardefelt-Winther, D. A conceptual and methodological critique of internet addiction research: Towards a model of compensatory internet use. Comput. Hum. Behav. 2014, 31, 351–354.
16. Lemmens, J.S.; Valkenburg, P.M.; Peter, J. Psychosocial causes and consequences of pathological gaming. Comput. Hum. Behav. 2011, 27, 144–152. [CrossRef]
17. Liu, M.; Peng, W. Cognitive and psychological predictors of the negative outcomes associated with playing mmogs (massively multiplayer online games). Comput. Hum. Behav. 2009, 25, 1306–1311.
18. Caplan, S.E. Relations among loneliness, social anxiety, and problematic internet use. Cyberpsychol. Behav. 2006, 10, 234–242.
19. Kuss, D.J.; Griffiths, M.D. Internet gaming addiction: A systematic review of empirical research. Int. J. Ment. Health Addict. 2012, 10, 278–296.
20. Kardefelt-Winther, D. A critical account of DSM-5 criteria for internet gaming disorder. Addict. Res. Theory. 2015, 23, 93–98.
21. Hyun, G.J.; Han, D.H.; Lee, Y.S.; Kang, K.D.; Yoo, S.K.; Chung, U.-S.; Renshaw, P.F. Risk factors associated with online game addiction: A hierarchical model. Comput. Hum. Behav. 2015, 48, 706–713.
22. Kuss, D.J.; Griffiths, M.D.; Pontes, H.M. DSM-5 diagnosis of internet gaming disorder: Some ways forward in overcoming issues and concerns in the gaming studies field: Response to the commentaries. J. Behav. Addict. 2017, 6, 133–141.
23. King D, Delfabbro P, Griffiths M (1 June 2010). "The Role of Structural Characteristics

in Problem Video Game Playing: A Review". *Cyberpsychology: Journal of Psychosocial Research on Cyberspace* (Review). 4 (1). ISSN 1802-7962.

24. Sussman CJ, Harper JM, Stahl JL, Weigle P (April 2018). "Internet and Video Game Addictions: Diagnosis, Epidemiology, and Neurobiology". *Child and Adolescent Psychiatric Clinics of North America* (Review). 27 (2): 307–326. doi:10.1016/j.chc.2017.11.015. PMID 29502753.
25. Griffiths M (2010). "Online video gaming: what should educational psychologists know?". *Educational Psychology in Practice*. 26 (1): 35–40.
26. Weinstein A, Lejoyeux M (March 2015). "New developments on the neurobiological and pharmaco-genetic mechanisms underlying internet and videogame addiction". *The American Journal on Addictions* (Review). 24 (2): 117–25.
27. Nuyens F, Kuss DJ, Lopez-Fernandez O, Griffiths MD (September 2017). "The experimental analysis of problematic video gaming and cognitive skills: A systematic review". *Journal de Thérapie Comportementale et Cognitive* (Systematic review) (in French). 27 (3): 110–117.
28. Pontes HM, Kuss DJ, Griffiths MD (2017). "Psychometric Assessment of Internet Gaming Disorder in Neuroimaging Studies: A Systematic Review". *Internet Addiction: Neuroscientific Approaches and Therapeutical Implications Including Smartphone Addiction* (Systematic review). Studies in Neuroscience, Psychology and Behavioral Economics. Springer International Publishing: 181–208.
29. Ferguson CJ, Coulson M, Barnett J (December 2011). "A meta-analysis of pathological gaming prevalence and comorbidity with mental health, academic and social problems". *Journal of Psychiatric Research*. 45 (12): 1573–8.
30. Hao W, Zhao M, Li J. *Theory and practice of addiction medicine*. Beijing: People's Medical Publishing House (PMPH), 2016: 238–95
31. Kuss DJ, Lopez-Fernandez O. Internet addiction and problematic internet use: a systematic review of clinical research. *WJP.* 2016;6.
32. Stevens MWR, King DL, Dorstyn D, *et al.* Cognitive-behavioral therapy for Internet gaming disorder: a systematic review and meta-analysis. *Clin Psychol Psychother.* 2018.
33. Fan FM. *Group psychotherapy[M]//Lu L. Shen YuCun's Psychiatry*. 6th edn. Chinese, Beijing: People's Medical Publishing House (PMPH), 2018: 816.
34. American Psychological Association. *Psychotherapy: understanding group therapy*. American Psychological Association, 2015.
35. Tai YP, Kim S, Lee J. Family therapy for an Internet-addicted young adult with interpersonal problems. *J Fam Ther.* 2014;36:394–419
36. Dong GH. *Internet addiction disorder[M]//Lu L. Shen YuCun's Psychiatry*. 6th edn. Chinese: Beijing: People's Medical Publishing House (PMPH), 2018: 691.
37. Shek DT, Tang V M LCY. Evaluation of an Internet addiction treatment program for Chinese adolescents in Hong Kong. *Adolescence.* 2009;44:359–73.
38. Liu Q-X, Fang X-Y, Yan N, *et al.* Multi-family group therapy for adolescent Internet addiction: exploring the underlying mechanisms. *Addictive Behaviors.* 2015;42:1–8.
39. Du Y S JW, Vance A. Longer term effect of randomized, controlled group cognitive behavioral therapy for Internet addiction in adolescent students in Shanghai. *Aust N Z J Psychiatry.* 2010;22:129–34
40. Fauth-Bühler M, Mann K. Neurobiological correlates of Internet gaming disorder: similarities to pathological gambling. *Addictive Behaviors.* 2017;64:349–56.
41. González-Bueso V, Santamaría J, Fernández D, *et al.* Association between Internet gaming disorder or pathological video-game use and comorbid psychopathology: a comprehensive review. *IJERPH.* 2018;15
42. Dell'Osso B, Hadley S, Allen A, *et al.* Escitalopram in the treatment of impulsive-compulsive Internet usage disorder: an open-label trial followed by a double-blind discontinuation phase. *J Clin Psychiatry.* 2008;69:452–6
43. Bipeta R, Yerramilli SS, Karredla AR, *et al.* Diagnostic stability of Internet addiction in obsessive-compulsive disorder: data from a naturalistic one-year treatment study. *Innov Clin*

Neurosci. 2015;12:14–23.

44. Han DH, Renshaw PF. Bupropion in the treatment of problematic online game play in patients with major depressive disorder. *J Psychopharmacol.* 2012;26:689–96.
45. Doug Hyun H, Jun Won H, Renshaw PF. Bupropion sustained release treatment decreases craving for video games and cue-induced brain activity in patients with Internet video game addiction. *Exp Clin Psychopharmacol.* 2010;18.
46. Han DH, Lee YS, Na C, *et al.* The effect of methylphenidate on internet video game play in children with attention-deficit/hyperactivity disorder. *Comprehensive Psychiatry*2009;50:251–6. doi:10.1016/j.comppsych. 2008.08.011
47. Bostwick JM, Bucci JA. Internet sex addiction treated with naltrexone. *Mayo Clinic Proceedings.* 2008;83:226–30.doi:10.1016/S0025-6196(11)60846-X
48. Kim SM, Han DH, Lee YS, *et al.* Combined cognitive behavioral therapy and bupropion for the treatment of problematic on-line game play in adolescents with major depressive disorder. *Computers in Human Behavior.* 2012;28:1954–9. doi:10.1016/j.chb.2012.05.015
49. Santos V, Nardi A, King A. Treatment of Internet addiction in patient with panic disorder and obsessive compulsive disorder: a case report. *CNS Neurol Disord Drug Targets.* 2015;14:341–4. doi:10.2174/1871527314666150225123532
50. Poddar S, Sayeed N, Mitra S. Internet gaming disorder: application of motivational enhancement therapy principles in treatment. *Indian J Psychiatry.* 2015;57
51. Zhu TM, Jin RJ, Zhong XM, *et al.* Effects of electroacupuncture combined with psychologic interference on anxiety state and serum Ne content in the patient of Internet addiction disorder. *Zhongguo Zhen Jiu.* 2008;28.
52. Király O, Griffiths MD, King DL, *et al.* Policy responses to problematic video game use: a systematic review of current measures and future possibilities. *Journal of Behavioral Addictions.* 2018;7:503–17.doi:10.1556/2006.6.2017.050
53. Van Rooij AJ, Meerkerk G-J, Schoenmakers TM, *et al.* Video game addiction and social responsibility. *Addiction Research & Theory.* 2010;18:489–93.doi:10.3109/16066350903168579
54. Azagba S, Sharaf MF. The effect of graphic cigarette warning labels on smoking behavior: evidence from the Canadian experience. *Nicotine & Tobacco Research.* 2013;15:708–17. doi:10.1093/ntr/nts194
55. Billieux J, Schimmenti A, Khazaal Y, *et al.* Are we overpathologizing everyday life? A tenable blueprint for behavioral addiction research. *Journal of Behavioral Addictions.* 2015;4:119–23. doi:10.1556/2006.4.2015.009
56. Policy KDJ. Prevention, and regulation for Internet gaming disorder. *J Behav Addict.* 2018;7:553–5.
57. Auer MM, Griffiths MD. Testing normative and self-appraisal feedback in an online slot-machine pop-up in A real-world setting. *Front. Psychol.* 2015;6.
58. Yousafzai S, Hussain Z, Griffiths M. Social responsibility in online videogaming: what should the videogame industry do?*Addiction Research & Theory.* 2014;22:181–5.doi:10.3109/16066359.2013.812203
59. Dau W, Hoffmann JDG, Banger M. Therapeutic Interventions in the Treatment of Problematic Internet Use—Experiences from Germany[M]// Internet addiction. *Springer, Cham.* 2015:183–217.

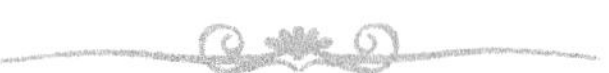

Index

5-hydroxy indole acetic acid 75

A

Aaron Beck 114
Abert Ellis 571
Abnormal grief reactions 677
Abstract 30
Acamprosate 40
Acetylcholine 74
Active Attention 28
Actus rea 539
Acute Stress Reaction 601
Addenbrooke Cognitive Evaluation 431
Adherence 11
Adoption 553
Advance Directive 541
Affect 16
Alcohol 38, 40, 169
Alcoholic Anonymous 186
Alcoholic hallucinosis 182
Aldehyde dehydrogenase 182
Alexithymia 17
Alogia 77, 105
Alprostadil 236
Altruistic 449
Alzheimer's dementia 74
Ambitendency 19
Ambivalence 19, 101
Amnesia 500
Amotivation 105
AMPA 73
Amygdala 71
Anergia 17
Angelman syndrome 310
Anhedonia 77
Anhedonia 17, 105
Annoyance 781
Anomia 390
Anorexia nervosa 39, 216
Anterior cingulate cortex 71, 510
anticonvulsant 42
Anti-social personality Disorder 204
Anxiety 9
Apathy 77, 105
Apomorphine 235
Applied behavioral analysis 304
Apraxia 390
Aripiprazole 474
Aromatherapy 437
Arsenic 394
Artefacts 51
Asenapine 44
Asociality 77
Assertive training 646
Astraphobia 135
Atopic Dermatitis 195
Attention 18
AUDIT: Alcohol Use Disorder Identification Test 179
Aura 609
Authoritarian Parenting 768
Autism spectrum disorder 297
Autobiographical memory 742
Autoimmune 4
Autonomy 536
Autoscopy 27
Autosomal recessive 394
Aversion Therapy 595
Avoidant Personality Disorder 206

Avolition 77
Avolition 105

B

Barbiturates 40
Beck's triad 26
Behavioral addictions 701
Beneficence 536
Benzodiazepines 40
Bereavement 117
Beri-beri 393
Beta-blocker 75
Bhang 170
Binet–Kamat test 278
Binge Eating Disorder 220, 704
Biofeedback 142
Biological 3
Body Dysmorphic Disorder 143, 212
Borderline personality Disorder 203
B-oxidation 89
Bradyphrenia 417
Breath-holding spells 378
Bromocriptine 475
Bulimia Nervosa 39, 218
Bupropion 88

C

Caffeine 624
CAGE 179
Cannabis and synthetic cannabinoids 169
Capacity 9
Capgras' delusion 25
Carbamazepine 38
Carl Jung 61
Carl Rogers 571
Castration anxiety 776
Catalepsy 19, 107
Cataplexy 271
Cerebral Palsy 315
Ceruloplasmin 39
Charas or hashish 170
Checking 144
Child custody 553
Children's Aperception test 279
Child sexual abuse 294, 342
Chlordiazepoxide 40
Chlorpromazine 1
Cholecystokinin 133
Chunking 744
Cingulate gyrus 71
Circadian process 267
Circumstantiality 16
Clang association 16
Classical conditioning 595
Classification 2
Claustrophobia 135
Clonidine 75, 185
Cluster headache 625
Cocaine 169
Cocaine metabolites 40
Cognitive remediation 527
Cognitive retraining 527
Cognitive therapy 110
Coherence 581
Command 27
Communication 33
communication skills 646
Complicated 677
Compulsions 80
Confabulation 18, 390
Confidentiality 11
Conflict 128, 726
Contamination 144
Content 23
Continuous Positive Airway Pressure 273
Coping mechanisms 10
Coprophilia 253
Cortical and Subcortical Dementia 434
Cortical-striatal-thalamic-cortical 145
Cortisol 129
Cotard Syndrome 26
Countertransference 59
Creutzfeldt-Jakob disease 43, 419
Crisis 726
Crisis Intervention 469
Cryptococcal meningitis 389
Culture 4
Cushing's disease 45, 194
Cycloid psychoses 107

Cyclothymia 121
Cynophobia 135
Cytokines 4

D

Dantrolene 475
DAST: Drug Abuse Screening Test 179
D-cycloserine 149
Deep brain stimulation 149, 491
Defense mechanisms 10
Dehydroepiandrosterone 129
Deja entendu 20
Deja vu 20
Delirium 38
Delusional 16
Delusional parasitosis 209
Dementia 42
Dementia Praecox 101
Dependant Personality Disorder 207
Depolarization 505
Depression 17, 79
Dermatitis artefacta 213
Desvenlafaxine 141
Dhat Syndrome 240
Diazepam 40, 141
Digit Span 28
Disruptive mood dysregulation disorder 380, 708
Disulfiram 40, 182
Divorce 798
Donepezil 422
DOPA decarboxylase 89
Dorsolateral prefrontal cortex 71
Down syndrome 308
Doxepine 211
Duloxetine 44, 141
Dyscalculia 325
Dysgraphia 325
Dyslexia 324
Dysthymia 17

E

Eating disorder 39
Ebstein-Barr virus 390
Echolalia 20
Echopraxia 20
Ecstasy 17, 172
Ego dystonic 147
Egoistic and anomic 449
Ego-syntonic 201
Ekbom's Syndrome 26
Ekbom syndrome 210
Elation 17
Electra complex 776
Electroconvulsive therapy 2
Electroencephalography 2
EMDR (Eye Movement Desensitization and Reprocessing) 162
Emile Durkheim 449
Emil Kraeplin 101
Emotionally unstable personality disorder 203
Emotions 9
Empathy 9, 11
Encephalitis 389
Encephalopathies 43
Enuresis 290
Epilepsy 42
Episodic memory 742
Epistemology 581
Erectile dysfunction 231
Eric Berne 571
Erik Erikson 8
Ethics 536
Etomidate 495
Euphoria 17
Eustress 726
Euthymia 17
Exaltation 17
Exhibitionistic Disorder 252
Extinction 596
Extra-campine hallucinations 18
Extrapyramidal symptoms 88
Eye Movement Desensitization and Reprocessing 683

F

Factitious disorder 190, 223
Fading 596
Family therapy 110
Fear 128

Fentanyl 171
Fetishistic Disorder 252
Fibromyalgia 196
Fight 128
Flooding 135, 595
Flumazenil 128, 133
Fluoxetine 1
Flupenthixol 474
Fluphenazine 474
Folie a deux 20, 106, 210
Forensic psychiatry 539
Form 15, 23
Fragile X syndrome 308
Fregoli's delusion 25
Frigidity 239
Frontal lobe 71
Frontotemporal Dementia 414
Frotteuristic Disorder 252
Frustration 781
Functional Neurological Symptom Disorder 189

G

GABA 74
Gabapentin 40
Gambling disorder 701
Gaming 810
Ganja 170
Gastaut-Geschwind syndrome 391
Gateway drugs 175
Gegenhalten 107
Gender Dysphoria 246
Gender identity 244
General Adaptation Syndrome 56
George Engel 55
Geriatric Depression Scale 431
Gerstmann-Sträussler-Scheinker 419
Gestalt Therapy 571
Glossopharyngeal neuralgia 619
Glutamate 74
Glycine 74
Glycopyrrolate 496
Grandiosity 16

H

Habit reversal therapy 152
Hallucination 17
Hallucinogens and Dissociative drugs 169
Haloperidol 44, 474
Hamilton Rating Scale for Depression (Ham-D) 431
Harm minimization 180
Health 7
Hemiplegic migraine 621
Heroin 171
Hindi Mental State Examination 406
Hippocampus 71
Histamine 74
History 1
Histrionic personality Disorder 205
HIV infection 389
Hoarding Disorder 143, 144
Hormones 5
Hostility 781
Human chorionic gonadotropin 45
Human Genome Project 54
Huntington's chorea 435
Hyperpolarization 505
Hypersomnia 271
Hypnogogic 27
Hypnopompic 27
Hypnotherapy 572
Hypocalcemia 39
Hypothalamus 75

I

Illusion 17
Imipramine 475
Immune system 4
Imperative hallucinations 27
Incest 343
Including caffeine 169
Infidelity 25
Insanity 539
Insight 19
Insight oriented psychotherapy 135
Insight oriented therapies 208
Insomnia 268
Intellectual disability 298
Intelligence quotient 8
Intermetamorphosis 26

Intermittent Explosive Disorder 785
Internet gaming 806
Interpersonal therapy 120
Intimacy 62
Investigation 38

J

Jamais entendu 20
Jamais vu 20
Judgment 27
Juveniles 344

K

Kainate receptor 73
Kayser-Fleischer 394
Ketamine 149
Klismaphilia 253

L

La bella indifference 17
Labile 17
Lead 394
Learned Helplessness 738
Leucotomy 508
Lewy Body Dementia 415
Libido 1
Limbic System 71
Lithium 40
Lobotomy 508
Locus ceruleus 75
Long Acting Injectables 474
Long term memory 742
Loosening of associations 15
Lucid interval 540
Lyme disease 389
Lysergic Acid Diethyamide 172
Lysergic acid Diethylamide (LSD) 104

M

Magical Thinking 147
Major life events 726
Malins Intelligence Scale for Indian Children 278
Mammillary bodies 71, 72
Mannerism 107
Marital rape 637
Marriage 551
MAST: Michigan Alcohol Screening Test 179
Masturbation 1
Matchbox sign 210
Mc Naughten's Rule 539
Megaloblastic anemia 393
Melancholia 113
Memantine 149, 422
Memory 28
Menopause 662
Mens rea 539
Mental Health Review Board 504
Mentalization based therapy 142
Mercury 394
Mescaline 104
Methadone 171
Methohexital 495
Methylphenidate 303
Midazolam 498
Migraine 196
Milnacipran 141
Mindfulness meditation 197
Mini Mental State Examination 31, 406
Misidentification 25
Mnemonics 745
Monoamine oxidase 478
Montreal Cognitive Assessment 406
Mood 16
Motivation enhancement therapy 809
Movement disorders 42
Multipurpose workers 531
Munchausen syndrome 190, 224
Music therapy 437
Mutism 19, 107

N

N-acetyl cysteine 152
Naltrexone 304
Narcissistic Personality Disorder 206
Narcolepsy 271
Narcotic Anonymous 186
Narcotic Drugs and Psychotropic Substance Act 544
Narrative memory 742

National Mental Health program 530
Necrophilia 253
Negative reinforcement 596
Negativism 19, 107
Neglect 335
Neglectful Parenting 769
Neologisms 15
Neuroanatomy 70
Neurobehavioral Cognitive Status Examination (NCSE) 32
Neurobiology 2
Neurofibrillary tangles 407, 425
Neuroleptic malignant syndrome 46, 459
Neurosis 15
Neurotics 345
Nicotine 171
Nicotine replacement therapy 185
Nicotine (Tobacco) 169
Nigro-striatal pathway 88
NMDA receptor 73
Nominated representative 541
Non-maleficence 536
Non-rapid eye-movement sleep 263
Non-Suicidal Self-Injury 454
Nucleus accumbens 75, 174
Nymphomania 705

O

Obesity 38
Object relations 777
Obsessions 80
Obstructive sleep apnea 272
Occipital neuralgia 619
Occupational therapy 304, 642
Oedipus Complex 776
Olanzapine 44, 474
Onychophagia 212
Operant Conditioning 593
Ophidiophobia 135
Opiates 40
Opioid 169, 171
Oppositional defiant disorder and Conduct disorder 132, 286
Orbitofrontal cortex 510
Orbitofrontal cortex 71
Orexin 271
Organic 1
Organic disorders 385
Other stimulants 169
Oxidative stress 399

P

Paliperidone 474
Panicogens 133
Papaverine 235
Papez circuit 72
Paraphrase 34
Parasomnias 273
Para suicide 288, 463
Parenting 792
Parkinson's disease 88
Passive Attention 28
Pathoelaborating Effect 692
Pathofacilitative Effects 692
Pathogenic Effects 691
Pathoplastic Effect 692
Pathoreactive effect 692, 693
Pedophilia 344
Pedophilic disorder 252
Peer pressure 773
Pellagra 393
Pentazocine 171
Perception 16
Perimenopause 662
Permissive parenting 769
Pernicious anemia 393
Persecution 25
Perseveration 16
Person-Centered Therapy 571
Phencyclidine 40, 172
Phenylketonuria 311
Phobia 17
Phosphodiesterae type 5 (PDE5) Inhibitors 235
Pick's bodies 414
Pick's disease 435
Pimozide 44
Pimozide 210
Play therapy 132, 292, 594
Polydypsia 38
Polysomnography 38, 42

Poppy plant 171
Porphyria 394
Positive Reinforcement 595
Possession of Thought 23
Post concussional syndrome 386
Posturing 19, 107
Prader–Willi syndrome 310
Pragmatics 580
Prefrontal Cortex 71
Pregabalin 40, 141
Premature ejaculation 236
Premenstrual dysphoric disorder 710
Premenstrual Syndrome 710
Prevalence 15
Priapism 482
Problem solving 646
Procedural memory 742
Progressive multifocal leukoencephalopathy 389
Progressive Muscle Relaxation 142
Prolactin 44
Prolixity 16
Prolonged seizures 498
Promethazine 270
Propofol 495
Protection of children from sexual offences (POCSO) 545
Pseudobulbar palsy 390
Pseudologia Fantastica 224
psilocybin 104
Psychedelics 172
Psychiatric social worker 633
Psychiatry 1
Psychoeducation 57, 560
Psychogenic pruritus 195, 214
Psychological 3
Psychological first aid 682
Psychology 7
Psychoneuroendocrinology 4
Psychopaths 345
Psychosexual 13
Psychosexual development 774
Psychosis 15
Psychosomatic medicine 666
Psychosurgery 508
Psychotics 345
Punishment 596

Q

Quetiapine 44

R

Rage 781
Rape 343
Rapid-eye-movement (REM) sleep 263
Rapport 11, 565
Rational Emotive Behavior Therapy 571
Reboxetine 44
Recall 29
Recent Memory 29
Registration 29
Remedial Education 328
Reminiscence therapy 437
Repetitive Transcranial Magnetic Stimulation (rTMS) 110
Resilience 7, 9, 426
Restless Leg Syndrome 273
Retrograde and anterograde amnesia 500
Reward system 807
Rhinencephalon 71
Riluzole 149
Risperidone 474
Rivastigmine 422
Rorschach Ink Blot Test 279

S

Satyriasis 705
Schizoid Personality Disorder 202
Schizophrenia 42
Schizotypal personality disorder 110, 202
School phobia 475
Sedative Hypnotics 169
Semantics 580
Sensate Focus Therapy 234
Sensory integration 304
Sensory memory 741
Separation anxiety disorder 475
Serotonin syndrome 459
Serotonin transporter (SERT) 74

Sertindole 44
Sex Addiction 705
Sexual Masochism Disorder 252
Sexual Pain Disorders 230
Sexual response 230
Sexual Sadism Disorder 252
Short term memory 741
Sigmund Freud 7, 67
Sildenafil 235
Skin-picking 143, 211
Sleep disorders 42
Sleep Hygiene 270
Social 3
Social Skills Training 526
Sociopaths 345
Sodomy 343
Somatic Symptom Disorder 189
Somnambulism 475
Speech 23
Speech and language therapy 132
Splitting 203
Squeeze technique 238
Standard drink 170
Stereotype 19
Stop-start technique 238
Stream 15, 23
Stress Inoculation Training 683
Stupor 107
Subacute combined degeneration of the cord 393
Subacute sclerosing panencephalitis 53, 390
Succinylcholine 496
Suicide 446
Symmetry 144
Syntax 580
Synthetic cathinones 169
Syphilis 389
Systematic desensitization 135
System Desensitization 595
Sysytemic Lupus Erythematosus 196

T

Tadalafil 235
Tangentiality 16
Tardive Dyskinesias 474
Telepsychiatry 731
Temperament 200
Temper tantrums 377
Temporal lobe 71
Tension type headache 623
Terrorism 676
Testamentary capacity 549
Tetrahydro-cannabinol 40
The Cognitive Capacity Screening Examination (CCSE) 32
The Domestic Violence Act 548
Thematic Apperception Test 753
Theophylline 499
Therapeutic Community 186
Therapeutic drug monitoring 41
Therapeutic index 41
Therapeutic relationship 62
Thiamine 182
Thinking 15
Thiopentone 495
Thioridazine 44
Thought echo 27
Tic disorder 147
Tobacco 38
Token Economy 595
Topiramate 40
Tourette's disorder 149
Toxoplasmosis 389
Transactional Analysis 571
Transcranial Direct Current Stimulation 110
Transcultural Psychiatry 699
Transference 59
Transitional object 778
Transsexualism 245
Transvestic Disorder 252
Traumatic brain injury 385
Trazodone 235
Trichotillomania 143, 212
Trigeminal neuralgia 619
Trypanophobia 135
Tuberculosis 599
Tyrosine 75
Tyrosine hydroxylase 89

U

Urophilia 253
Urticaria 195

V

Vagal Nerve Stimulation 491
Vardenafil 235
Varenicline 185, 489
Vascular Dementia 412
Venlafaxine 44
Ventral tegmental area 75, 174
Verbigeration 107
Verbigeration/word salad 15
Vineland Social Maturity Scale 278
Virtual therapy 135
Volatile Inhalants 169
Voyeuristic Disorder 252

W

Waveforms 52
Waxy flexibility 19, 23
Wernicke's-Korsakoff syndrome 182
Wilson's disease 39, 394
Word Salad 24

Y

Yoga therapy 110
Yohimbine 133, 235

Z

Ziprasidone 44
Zolpidem 270
Zoophilia 253

www.ingramcontent.com/pod-product-compliance
Ingram Content Group UK Ltd.
Pitfield, Milton Keynes, MK11 3LW, UK
UKHW061304190726
13845UKWH00038B/1270